1997-1998

Handbook of

Clinical Drug Data

Eighth Edition

1997-1998
Handbook of
Clinical Drug Data

Eighth Edition

EDITORS

Philip O. Anderson, PharmD, FASHP
Director, Drug Information Service, Department of Pharmacy
University of California Medical Center, San Diego, California
Clinical Professor of Pharmacy
University of California, San Francisco, California
San Diego Program

James E. Knoben, PharmD, MPH
Center for Drug Evaluation and Research
Food and Drug Administration
Rockville, Maryland

ASSOCIATE EDITOR

William G. Troutman, PharmD, FASHP
Regents' Professor of Pharmacy, College of Pharmacy
University of New Mexico, Albuquerque, New Mexico

ASSISTANT EDITOR

Larry Jay Davis, PharmD
Pharmacy Operations Manager
Kaiser Foundation Hospital, San Francisco, California
Associate Clinical Professor of Pharmacy
University of California, San Francisco, California

APPLETON & LANGE
Stamford, CT

Copyright © 1997 by Appleton & Lange
A Simon & Schuster Company
Copyright © 1993 by Drug Intelligence Publications, Inc.
Hamilton, Illinois

We the editors, Philip O. Anderson, PharmD, and James E. Knoben, PharmD, the associate and assistant editors, and the contibutors have written this book in our private capacities. No official support or endorsement by any university, hospital, federal agency, or pharmaceutical company is intended or should be inferred.

98 99 00 01 / 10 9 8 7 6 5 4 3 2

Prentice Hall International (UK) Limited, *London*
Prentice Hall of Australia Pty. Limited, *Sydney*
Prentice Hall Canada, Inc., *Toronto*
Prentice Hall Hispanoamericana, S.A., *Mexico*
Prentice Hall of India Private Limited, *New Delhi*
Prentice Hall of Japan, Inc., *Tokyo*
Simon & Schuster Asia Pte. Ltd., *Singapore*
Editora Prentice Hall do Brasil Ltda., *Rio de Janeiro*
Prentice Hall, *Upper Saddle River, New Jersey*

ISSN 1090–7981

Executive Editor: Cheryl L. Mehalik
Production Editor: Sondra Greenfield
Designer: Mary Skudlarek

PRINTED IN THE UNITED STATES OF AMERICA

Contributors

Brian K. Alldredge, PharmD
Professor of Clinical Pharmacy and Neurology, Departments of Clinical Pharmacy and Neurology, University of California, San Francisco, California

Andrea J. Anderson, PharmD
Section Head, Commercial Liaison, Matrix Services, U.S. Medical Affairs Division, Glaxo Wellcome Inc., Research Triangle Park, North Carolina

Philip O. Anderson, PharmD, FASHP
Director, Drug Information Service, Department of Pharmacy, University of California Medical Center, San Diego, California; Clinical Professor of Pharmacy, University of California, San Francisco, San Diego Program

Lisa W. Ashton, PharmD
Disease Specialist, Integrated Pharmaceutical Services, Foundation Health, Rancho Corona, California; Assistant Clinical Professor, School of Pharmacy, University of California, San Francisco, San Francisco, California, Davis Program

Arasb Ateshkadi, PharmD
Assistant Professor, Department of Pharmacy Practice, College of Pharmacy, University of Utah, Salt Lake City, Utah

Craig R. Ballard, PharmD
Antiviral and Cytokine Program Coordinator, Owen Clinic, University of California Medical Center, San Diego, California; Assistant Clinical Professor of Pharmacy, University of California, San Francisco, San Diego Program

Jerry L. Bauman, PharmD, FACC, FCCP
Professor of Pharmacy Practice, Sections of Cardiovascular Pharmacotherapy and Cardiology, University of Illinois at Chicago, Chicago, Illinois

Rosemary R. Berardi, PharmD, FASHP
Professor of Pharmacy, College of Pharmacy, University of Michigan, Ann Arbor, Michigan; Clinical Pharmacist, Gastroenterology, Department of Pharmacy Services, University of Michigan Health-System, Ann Arbor, Michigan

Lawrence R. Borgsdorf, PharmD, FCSHP
Pharmacist Specialist—Ambulatory Care, Kaiser Permanente Medical Care Program, Bakersfield, California; Adjunct Professor of Clinical Pharmacy, School of Pharmacy, University of the Pacific, Stockton, California

R. Keith Campbell, BPharm, MBA
Associate Dean and Professor of Pharmacy Practice, College of Pharmacy, Washington State University, Pullman, Washington

Larry Jay Davis, PharmD
Pharmacy Operations Manager, Kaiser Foundation Hospital; San Francisco, California; Associate Clinical Professor of Pharmacy, University of California, San Francisco, California

Betty J. Dong, PharmD
Professor of Clinical Pharmacy, Department of Clinical Pharmacy, School of Pharmacy, University of California, San Francisco, California; Clinical Professor of Family and Community Medicine, Division of Family and Community Medicine, School of Medicine, University of California, San Francisco, California

Robert T. Dorr, PhD
Associate Professor of Pharmacology, Director, Pharmacology Research Program, Arizona Cancer Center, University of Arizona, Tucson, Arizona

David G. Dunlop, PharmD
Chief, Pharmacotherapy Services, 81st Medical Group, Keesler AFB, Mississippi

John F. Flaherty, Jr., PharmD, BCPS, FCCP
Associate Professor of Clinical Pharmacy, Department of Clinical Pharmacy, School of Pharmacy, University of California, San Francisco

John G. Gambertoglio, Pharm D
Professor of Pharmacy and Medicine, Department of Clinical Pharmacy, and School of Medicine, University of California at San Francisco, San Francisco, California

Mildred D. Gottwald, PharmD
Neurology Fellow, Department of Clinical Pharmacy, University of California, San Francisco, California

Amy J. Guenette, PharmD, BCPS
Clinical Coordinator, Department of Pharmacy, Wausau Hospital, Wausau, Wisconsin

Philip D. Hansten, PharmD
Professor of Pharmacy, University of Washington, Seattle, Washington

James E. Knoben, PharmD, MPH
Center for Drug Evaluation and Research, Food and Drug Administration, Rockville, Maryland

William E. Murray, PharmD
Pharmacokinetics Service Coordinator, Pharmacy Department, Children's Hospital, San Diego, California; Assistant Clinical Professor of Pharmacy, University of California, San Francisco, San Diego Program

Robert E. Pachorek, PharmD, BCPS
Clinical Pharmacist, Mercy Hospital, San Diego, California; Adjunct Assistant Professor of Pharmacy Practice, University of Southern California, Los Angeles, California; Assistant Clinical Professor of Pharmacy, University of California, San Francisco, San Diego Program

Fred Shatsky, BSPharm, BCNSP
Nutrition Support Pharmacist, Department of Pharmacy, University of California Medical Center, San Diego, California; Assistant Clinical Professor of Pharmacy, University of California, San Francisco, California, San Diego Program

Glen L. Stimmel, PharmD, FCCP
Professor of Clinical Pharmacy and Psychiatry, Schools of Pharmacy and Medicine, University of Southern California, Los Angeles, California

Dianne E. Tobias, PharmD
Corporate Director of Quality Improvement, Regency Health Services, Inc., Tustin, California; Assistant Clinical Professor of Pharmacy, University of California, San Francisco, Irvine Program

William G. Troutman, PharmD, FASHP
Regents' Professor of Pharmacy, College of Pharmacy, University of New Mexico, Albuquerque, New Mexico

John R. White, Jr., PharmD
Associate Professor, Pharmacy Practice, Washington State University, Spokane, Washington; Director, Washington State University/Sacred Heart Medical Center Drug Studies Unit, Spokane, Washington

James M. Wooten, PharmD
Supervisor, Clinical Pharmacy Services, and Clinical Specialist, Department of Pharmacy, Trinity Lutheran Hospital, Kansas City, Missouri; Adjunct Associate Professor, School of Pharmacy, University of Missouri at Kansas City, Kansas City, Missouri

Robin Swett Wooten, PharmD
Clinical Pharmacy Consultant, Department of Pharmacy, Liberty Hospital, Liberty, Missouri

Carolyn R. Zaleon, BSPharm
Ambulatory Care Pharmacist, Department of Pharmacy Services, University of Michigan Health-System, Ann Arbor, Michigan; Clinical Assistant Professor of Pharmacy, College of Pharmacy, University of Michigan, Ann Arbor, Michigan

Contents

Preface

With the publication of the Eighth Edition of the *Handbook of Clinical Drug Data* we embark on a new beginning. For over 20 years, Drug Intelligence Publications has ably served as our publisher. During that time, over 200,000 pharmacists, physicians, and other health professionals have used the *Handbook* as one of their primary clinical drug references.

The 1997–1998 *Handbook of Clinical Drug Data* is now published by Appleton & Lange. Immediately you will see the changes—from the new look of the cover to the reorganization of content between the covers. Consistently rated as one of the most authoritative and well-referenced drug guides available, our goal has been to provide a comprehensive, yet compact source of clinical drug information. With this edition, we have maintained those attributes while adding a more user-friendly approach to locating information. Thus, you will find not only the most up-to-date information on over 1,000 drugs, you will find the information more easily.

Drug Monographs now appear in **Part I.** They have been reorganized as well, so that drugs are now grouped into larger categories that more logically relate similar drugs. Locating drug categories is made easier by a *tabbing guide,* which appears on the back cover of the book. With this new feature, you can tab directly to *drug categories* that have been *alphabetically arranged.* Comprehensive *comparison charts* of the drugs within each class provide the most pertinent information for decision making in a comprehensive *tabular format.* As in previous editions, the alternative way to *search by drug name* is still available by using the *index.* However, you will find that the index format has been revised to make it easier to find drugs by their brand name. The index also includes cross-references to Canadian brand names and British generic names.

The *drug monograph* format has also been *revised* and *expanded.*
- A new heading—*Special Populations*—consolidates dosage information in *Pediatrics, Geriatrics, Renal and Hepatic Disease, Obesity, Pregnancy,* and other pertinent conditions.
- Another new heading—*Drug Interactions*—consolidates information that was previously in the Precautions section or Drug-Drug Interactions chapter.

Clinical Drug Information, now **Part II,** contains the larger chapter groups. Included is specialized, clinically relevant drug information as it relates to specific interactions, disease states, special populations, medical emergencies and nutrition support. Appendices contain useful formulas, nomograms, and reference values.

Bill Troutman and Larry Davis continue to provide valuable editorial support in addition to their authorship duties. Without their assistance and the contributions of our talented and expert clinician-authors, both old and new, this book would not be possible. Cheryl Mehalik, Executive Editor at our new publisher, Appleton & Lange, deserves special recognition for her many efforts in stimulating our thoughts on making the *Handbook* more user-friendly and shepherding it through the production process. We also thank Debra Kent, PharmD, Carol Stoner, PharmD, BCPS, and Lisa Vivero, PharmD, for their help with manuscript preparation at critical junctures.

We welcome readers' comments on the changes in organizations as well as on the book's content. Many improvements in this edition are a direct result of user input. We thank all who have contributed.

Philip O. Anderson
James E. Knoben
October 1996

How to Use This Book

Part I of this book is organized around 10 major drug categories, which have been subdivided into common therapeutic groups. Within these therapeutic groups, drug information is alphabetically presented in three formats: *Monographs, Minimonographs,* and *Comparison Charts.* Monographs and Comparison Charts are *grouped together* to ensure that related drugs are easy to *compare* and *contrast.* Charts are located after the monographs to which they relate. Drug antagonists are grouped together with agonists to help simplify organization and accessibility.

Monographs are used for drugs of major importance and prototype agents.

Minimonographs are used for drugs similar to prototype drugs, those of lesser importance within a therapeutic class, and promising investigational agents.

Comparison Charts are used to present clinically useful information on members of the same pharmacologic class and different drugs with a similar therapeutic use, as well as to present clinically relevant information on certain other topics.

The preferred method to gain access to complete information on a *particular brand* or *generic drug* is to use the index at the end of the book. The index may also direct the user to *other pertinent* information on the drug.

MONOGRAPH FORMAT

CLASS INSTRUCTIONS

This is an optional heading at the beginning of each drug class. It consists of patient instructions that apply to more than one of the drug monographs in this subcategory. If all drugs are not identical in their instructions, only the common information is found here. The Patient Instructions section of each monograph that is affected states, *"See Class Instructions"* as the opening phrase.

GENERIC DRUG NAME   Brand Name(s)

The *nonproprietary (generic)* name is listed on the left, followed by common brand names listed on the right. Brand-name products listed are not necessarily superior or preferable to other brand-name or generic products; *"Various"* indicates the availability of additional brand and/or generic products.

Pharmacology. A description of the chemistry, major mechanisms of action, and human pharmacology of the drug in clinical application.

Administration and Adult Dosage. Route of administration, indications, and usual adult dosage range are given for the most common labeled uses. Dosages correspond to those in the product labeling or in standard reference sources. "Dose" refers to a single administration and "dosage" to a cumulative amount (eg, daily dosage).

Special Populations. Dosages in patient populations other than the typical adult are listed:

Pediatric Dosage (given by age or weight range)

Geriatric Dosage (given by age range)

Other Conditions (renal failure, hepatic disease, obesity, etc.)

Dosage Forms. The most commonly used dosage forms and available strengths are listed, as well as popular combination product dosage forms. Prediluted IV piggyback or large-volume parenteral containers are not listed unless this is the only commercially available product.

Patient Instructions. Key information that should be provided to the patient when prescribing or dispensing. When introductions apply to an entire drug category, see "Class Instructions" at the beginning of that subcategory.

Pharmacokinetics. Data are presented as the mean ± the standard deviation. Occasionally the standard error of the mean (SE) is the only information available on variability, and it is identified as such.

Onset and Duration (time course of the pharmacologic or therapeutic effect)

Serum Levels (therapeutic and toxic plasma concentrations are given)

Fate (The course of the drug in the body is traced. Pharmacokinetic parameters are generally provided as total body weight normalized values. The volume of distribution is either a V_d in a one-compartment system or V_c and $V_{d\beta}$ in a two-compartment system.)

$t_{1/2}$ (terminal half-life is presented)

Adverse Reactions. Reactions known to be dose related are usually given first, then other reactions in decreasing order of frequency. Reaction frequency is classified into three ranges. However, percentages of reactions are provided for reactions that occur more frequently than 1%.

frequent	*(>1/100 patients)*
occasional	*(1/100 to 1/10,000 patients)*
rare	*(<1/10,000 patients)*

Contraindications. Those listed in product labeling are given. "Hypersensitivity" is not listed as a contraindication because it is understood that patients should not be given a drug to which they are allergic or hypersensitive.

Precautions. Warnings for use of the drug in certain disease states and/or patient populations, together with any cross-sensitivity with other drugs. Part II, Chapter 3, "Drug Use in Special Populations." should be consulted for more information particularly regarding pregnancy and breastfeeding.

Drug Interactions. The most important drug interactions are listed. More detailed information on the management or avoidance of the interaction is provided in Part II, Chapter 2, "Drug Interactions and Interferences."

Parameters to Monitor. Important clinical signs and/or laboratory tests to monitor to ensure safe and effective use. The frequency of monitoring may also be given; however, for many drugs the optimal frequency has not been determined.

Notes. Distinguishing characteristics, therapeutic usefulness, or relative efficacy of the drug are presented, as well as unique or noteworthy physicochemical properties, handling, storage, or relative cost.

Part I

DRUG MONOGRAPHS

- ANALGESIC AND ANTIINFLAMMATORY DRUGS
- ANTIMICROBIALS
- ANTINEOPLASTICS, CHEMOPROTECTANTS AND IMMUNOSUPPRESSANTS
- CARDIOVASCULAR DRUGS
- CENTRAL NERVOUS SYSTEM DRUGS
- GASTROINTESTINAL DRUGS
- HEMATOLOGIC DRUGS
- HORMONAL DRUGS
- RENAL AND ELECTROLYTES
- RESPIRATORY DRUGS

Analgesic and Antiinflammatory Drugs

Antimigraine Drugs

DIHYDROERGOTAMINE MESYLATE  D.H.E. 45

Pharmacology. Dihydroergotamine is a semisynthetic ergot alkaloid with α-adrenergic antagonist activity in the peripheral and central nervous systems, smooth muscle, and blood vessels. It is a partial α-adrenergic agonist in veins, inhibits the reuptake of norepinephrine, and is a weak serotonin antagonist. Compared to ergotamine, dihydroergotamine is a weaker vasoconstrictor, is less active as an emetic, and is less oxytocic. In the relief of migraine, it causes vasoconstriction of cranial blood vessels, with a decrease in the amplitude of pulsations.

Administration and Adult Dosage. IM 1 mg initially, then 1 mg q 1 hr prn, to a maximum of 3 mg/day or 6 mg/week. **IV** (for rapid effect) 0.5 mg, may repeat in 1 hr, to a maximum of 2 mg/day or 6 mg/week.

Special Populations. *Pediatric Dosage.* Safety and efficacy not established.

Geriatric Dosage. Same as adult dosage.

Dosage Forms. Inj 1 mg/mL.

Patient Instructions. May cause numbness or tingling in fingers, toes, or face. Notify physician if you are pregnant or have heart disease or high blood pressure. Do not exceed the maximum dosage.

Pharmacokinetics. *Onset and Duration.* Onset under 5 min IV, within 15–30 min after IM; duration 3–4 hr.[1] The pharmacodynamic effect persists even in the absence of measurable serum levels.

Fate. Rapid distribution from the central compartment to the peripheral compartment occurs in about 4 min. $V_{d\beta}$ is 33.2 ± 0.2 L/kg, suggesting distribution into deep tissue compartments; Cl is 1.57 ± 0.17 L/hr/kg. The drug is metabolized to at least 5 metabolites.[1]

$t_{\frac{1}{2}}$ α phase 2.1 ± 1.7 min; ß phase 15 ± 2.8 min.[1]

Adverse Reactions. Nausea, vomiting, diarrhea, and localized edema occur frequently. Occasional numbness and tingling of fingers and toes, muscle pain in the extremities, weakness in legs, pruritus, rash, and infection occur. Rarely precordial distress with pain occurs; pleural and retroperitoneal fibrosis occur rarely and only with prolonged use.

Contraindications. Pregnancy; peripheral vascular disease; coronary artery disease; uncontrolled hypertension; impaired hepatic or renal dysfunction; hypersensitivity to ergot alkaloids.

Precautions. Use caution to avoid overuse by patients with chronic vascular headaches.

Drug Interactions. *See* Ergotamine. Dihydroergotamine may antagonize the anti-anginal effects of nitrates. The risk of bleeding with heparin (eg, wound hematoma, anemia, hematuria) is worsened with coadministration of dihydroergotamine.

Notes. Dihydroergotamine is used when oral agents have failed to abort migraine and for terminating cluster or migraine headache in the emergency room setting. Dihydroergotamine does not cause physical dependence and is associated with a more favorable side effect profile than ergotamine, especially with respect to GI and peripheral vascular effects.[2] Dihydroergotamine has a lower frequency of migraine recurrence than **sumatriptan,** possibly because of the longer half-life of dihydroergotamine.

ERGOTAMINE TARTRATE   Ergomar, Ergostat, Various

Pharmacology. Ergotamine is an ergot alkaloid with α-adrenergic blocking properties in the peripheral and central nervous systems. It is a partial α-adrenergic agonist and antagonist in blood vessels and smooth muscle. It is also a uterine stimulant via its tryptaminergic and α-blocking activity. The mechanism in migraine is thought to be vasoconstriction of cranial blood vessels, with a concomitant decrease in the amplitude of pulsations as well as depression of serotonergic neurons that mediate pain.

Administration and Adult Dosage. **PO for migraine** 2 mg initially, then 1 mg each ½ hr prn, to a maximum of 6 mg/day or 10 mg/week; **PR** 2 mg initially, may repeat in 1 hr prn, to a maximum of 4 mg/attack or 10 mg/week; **SL** 2 mg initially, then 2 mg q 30 min as needed, to a maximum of 6 mg/day or 10 mg/week.[3] Titrate the dosage during several attacks gradually, then administer the minimum effective dosage with subsequent attacks. Patients who routinely require over 2 mg/headache can be given the total effective dosage at the onset of the headache.

Special Populations. *Pediatric Dosage.* Safety and efficacy not established. (Over 12 yr) 1 mg initially, then 1 mg q 30 min prn, to a maximum of 3 mg/attack.

Geriatric Dosage. No specific data are available.

Other Conditions. Decrease dosage by 50% in patients receiving methysergide as prophylaxis.

Dosage Forms. **SL Tab** 2 mg; **Tab** 1 mg with caffeine 100 mg (Cafergot, Ercaf, various); **Supp** 2 mg with caffeine 100 mg (Cafergot, Wigraine).

Patient Instructions. Initiate therapy at the first signs of an attack. Take only as directed and do not exceed recommended dosages. Report tingling or pain in extremities immediately.

Pharmacokinetics. *Onset and Duration.* Onset (oral) 5 hr; (rectal) 1–3 hr.[3]

Serum Levels. 200 ng/L (176 pmol/L) or greater may be therapeutic; a high frequency of adverse reactions has been associated with levels above 1.8 μg/L (1.5 nmol/L).[3]

Fate. Bioavailability 1–2% orally, 5% rectally; relative bioavailability decreases in the following order: PR > PO > SL.[3,4] Peak serum level after 2 mg rectally is 454 ± 407 ng/L (390 ± 350 pmol/L), 50 ± 43 min after the dose. Peak serum level after 2 mg with 100 mg caffeine orally is 21 ± 12 ng/L (18 ± 11 pmol/L), 69 ± 191 min after the dose.[4] V_d is 1.9 ± 0.8 L/kg; Cl is 0.68 ± 0.24 L/hr/kg.[5] The drug is extensively metabolized in the liver, with 90% of metabolites excreted in the bile.

$t_{1/2}$. 1.9 ± 0.3 hr; apparent half-life is 3.4 ± 1.9 hr after rectal administration because of slow absorption.[3,4]

Adverse Reactions. Nausea and vomiting occur frequently. Signs and symptoms of ergotamine intoxication include weakness in legs, coldness and muscle pain in extremities, numbness or tingling of fingers and toes, precordial pain, transient tachycardia or bradycardia, and localized edema; these rarely develop with recommended dosages. Frequent or worsening headaches can occur with frequent, long-term, or excessive dosages. Ergotamine dependence may result in withdrawal symptoms occurring within 24–48 hr following drug discontinuation.[3,6] Rectal or anal ulceration may occur with suppository use.

Contraindications. Pregnancy; peripheral vascular disease; coronary artery disease; hypertension; hepatic or renal impairment; sepsis; severe pruritus.

Precautions. Lactation; avoid excessive dosage or prolonged administration because of the potential for ergotism and gangrene.

Drug Interactions. β-Blockers, dopamine, and epinephrine can cause increased vasoconstriction and increased risk of peripheral ischemia or hypertension. The macrolides (especially erythromycin and troleandomycin) may inhibit the metabolism of ergot alkaloids.

Notes. The stimulant action of preparations containing **caffeine** may keep patients from the beneficial effects of sleep. Caffeine, however, may improve dissolution of the oral formulation. Ergotamine is the most commonly used drug for abortive therapy of migraine and provides relief in 50–90% of patients.[3] **Aspirin** (650 mg) or **naproxen** (750–1250 mg/day) may be effective in aborting migraine headache in mild cases or in patients who cannot take ergotamine. **Sumatriptan** appears to be more effective than ergotamine/caffeine in aborting migraine.[7] For migraine prophylaxis, **propranolol** with an initial dose of 80 mg, to a maximum of 320 mg/day, calcium-channel blocking drugs (**verapamil** or **nimodipine**), and **valproate** have been used successfully.[8]

METHYSERGIDE MALEATE
Sansert

Methysergide is a semisynthetic ergot alkaloid, thought to act centrally as a serotonin agonist and to inhibit blood vessel permeability to humoral factors that affect pain threshold. Unlike other ergots, methysergide does not inhibit reuptake of norepinephrine and has minimal oxytocic, vasoconstrictor, and α-adrenergic blocking effects. Because of its toxicity, methysergide is usually used only after other prophylactic measures fail. Methysergide undergoes extensive liver metabolism to **methylergonovine**, a compound with greater activity and a longer elimination half-life than the parent drug (3.5 hr vs 1 hr). About 56% of an oral dose is eliminated in the urine as unchanged drug and metabolites. Insomnia, postural hypotension, nausea, vomiting, diarrhea, and peripheral ischemia occur frequently. Occasionally heartburn, peripheral edema, rash, or arrhythmias occur. Rarely, mental depression occurs. Long-term (>6 months) therapy may cause retroperitoneal and pleuropulmonary fibrosis, and thickening of cardiac valves. The drug is contraindicated in peripheral vascular, cardiovascular, or pulmonary disease; phlebitis; pregnancy; and impaired liver or kidney function. Precautions and drug interactions are similar to ergotamine. The adult dosage for migraine or cluster headache prophylaxis is 4–8 mg/day with food; a drug-free interval of 3–4 weeks must follow each 6-month course; however, reduce the dosage gradually to avoid rebound headache.[9] Available as 2-mg tablets.

SUMATRIPTAN
Imitrex

Pharmacology. Sumatriptan is a serotonin (5-HT) analogue and a selective agonist at 5-HT_{1D} receptors in cerebral vascular smooth muscle. Receptor activation results in migraine relief by both vasoconstriction of intracranial blood vessels and attenuation of the release of vasoactive peptides responsible for inflammation of sensory nerves.[10–12]

Administration and Adult Dosage. PO for migraine 25–100 mg; a second dose of up to 100 mg may be administered in 2 hr if response is unsatisfactory. If headache returns, additional doses may be given q 2 hr, up to 300 mg in a 24-hr period.[13] **SC for migraine** 6 mg; a second 6-mg injection may be administered 1 hr after the initial dose, but limited to no more than 2 injections within a 24-hr period. Controlled studies have not verified a beneficial effect of a second dose.

Special Populations. *Pediatric Dosage.* Safety and efficacy not established under 18 yr.

Geriatric Dosage. Same as adult dosage.

Dosage Forms. Tab 25, 50 mg; **Inj** 6 mg/0.5 mL.

Patient Instructions. Sumatriptan is used for relief of migraine and not for the prevention of a migraine attack. Do not take this drug if you are pregnant or breastfeeding without consulting with your doctor. Inform your doctor if you have high blood pressure, diabetes, seizures, or heart, liver, or kidney disease. Report pain or tightness in chest, shortness of breath, wheezing, or rash immediately. **Oral.** Do not take more than 300 mg within 24 hours, and allow at least 2 hours after the first tablet. **SC injection.** Do not take more than 2 injections within 24 hours, and allow at least 1 hour between injections. Pain or redness at injection site lasts less than 1 hour.

Pharmacokinetics. *Onset and Duration.* PO 50% of patients respond in 2 hr; peak 1.5 hr. SC 70% of patients respond within 1 hr and 90% within 2 hr;[14] peak 10–15 min.[15]

Fate. Oral bioavailability is 14 ± 3% owing to presystemic metabolism and erratic absorption. Absorption is delayed by about 0.5 hr if taken with food. After a 100-mg oral dose, a peak of 54 ng/mL (0.13 µmol/L) occurs in about 1.5 hr. SC bioavailability is 97 ± 16%; a peak of 74 ng/mL (0.18 µmol/L) occurs in 12 min. Plasma protein binding is 14–21%. V_d is 0.65 ± 0.1 L/kg; Cl is 0.96 ± 0.12 L/hr/kg. Hepatic metabolism is by monoamine oxidase A to an indole acetic acid, followed by glucuronidation and renal elimination. About 40% is found in the feces and 60% excreted renally, 22% unchanged, and 40% as the active indole acetic acid metabolite.[16-18]

$t_{1/2}$. 1.9 ± 0.3 hr.[18]

Adverse Reactions. Frequent side effects include pain and redness at SC injection site, tingling, hot flushes, dizziness, and chest tightness or heaviness. With all routes of administration, occasional weakness, myalgia, burning sensation, tightness in chest, transient hypertension, drowsiness, headache, numbness, neck pain, abdominal discomfort, mouth/jaw discomfort, and sweating occur. Rarely, cardiac arrhythmias, myocardial ischemia, polydipsia, dehydration, dyspnea, skin rashes, dysuria, and dysmenorrhea occur. The drug may accumulate in melanin-rich tissues such as the eye with long-term use.

Contraindications. Ischemic heart disease; Prinzmetal's angina; uncontrolled hypertension; concurrent administration of MAO inhibitors or within 2 weeks of discontinuation; within 24 hr of an ergotamine-containing drug or ergot derivative such as methysergide or dihydroergotamine.

Precautions. Pregnancy. Use with caution in those with impaired hepatic function, seizure disorder, neurologic lesion, or cardiovascular disease, postmenopausal women, or men over 40 yr. Lactation is stated to be a precaution, but recent data indicate that only small amounts appear in milk and risks are minimal.[19]

Drug Interactions. Nonselective MAO inhibitors or MAO-A inhibitors can increase the systemic availability of sumatriptan (especially after oral administration). Theoretically, ergot alkaloids and sumatriptan may cause prolonged vasospastic reactions if used together. *See* Contraindications.

Parameters to Monitor. Renal, hepatic, and cardiovascular status initially and q 6 months.

Notes. Sumatriptan is much more expensive than alternatives. It is effective in the treatment of cluster headache and appears to be more effective than ergotamine/caffeine in aborting migraine.[7]

Nonsteroidal Antiinflammatory Drugs

ACETAMINOPHEN Various

Pharmacology. Acetaminophen is analgesic and antipyretic with weak antiinflammatory action. It has the same potency as aspirin in inhibiting brain prostaglandin synthetase, but very little activity as an inhibitor of cyclooxygenase. Unlike other NSAIDs, it does not inhibit neutrophil activation. These differences may explain its relative lack of antiinflammatory activity. Acetaminophen does not cause the GI erosion and bleeding associated with aspirin and has no effect on platelet function.[20]

Administration and Adult Dosage. **PO for pain or fever** 650–1000 mg q 4–6 hr, to a maximum of 4 g/day. **PR for pain or fever** 650 mg q 4–6 hr, to a maximum of 4 g/day.

Special Populations. *Pediatric Dosage.* **PO for pain or fever** 10–15 mg/kg q 4–6 hr, to a maximum of 5 doses/day; or (up to 3 months) 40 mg/dose, (4–11 months) 80 mg/dose, (12–23 months) 120 mg/dose, (2–3 yr) 160 mg/dose, (4–5 yr) 240 mg/dose, (6–8 yr) 320 mg/dose, (9–10 yr) 400 mg/dose, (11 yr) 480 mg/dose, to a maximum of 5 doses/day. **PR for pain or fever** (3–6 yr) 120 mg q 4–6 hr, to a maximum of 720 mg/day; (6–12 yr) 325 mg q 4–6 hr, to a maximum of 2.6 g/day; (over 12 yr) same as adult dosage.

Geriatric Dosage. Same as adult dosage.

Dosage Forms. **Cap** 500 mg; **Chew Tab** 80 mg; **Tab** 160, 325, 500, 650 mg; **Granules** 80, 325 mg; **Drp** 48, 100 mg/mL; **Elxr** 24, 26, 32, 65 mg/mL; **Syrup** 32 mg/mL; **Supp** 120, 125, 325, 600, 650 mg.

Pharmacokinetics. *Serum Levels.* (Analgesia, antipyresis) 10–20 mg/L (66–132 μmol/L). Serum concentrations over 300 mg/L (2 mmol/L) at 4 hr or 45 mg/L (300 μmol/L) at 12 hr following acute overdosage are associated with severe hepatic damage, whereas toxicity is unlikely if levels are under 120 mg/L (800 μmol/L) at 4 hr or 30 mg/L (200 μmol/L) at 12 hr.[18] *See* Notes.

Fate. Rapidly absorbed from GI tract, with 88 ± 15% bioavailability. Essentially unbound to plasma proteins at therapeutic doses; 20–50% bound in overdose. Extensively metabolized in the liver to inactive conjugates of glucuronic and sulfuric acids (saturable), and to a hepatotoxic intermediate metabolite (first-order) by CYP1A2 and CYP2E1. The intermediate is detoxified by glutathione (saturable). V_d is 0.95 ± 0.12 L/kg; Cl is 0.3 ± 0.084 L/hr/kg, decreased in hepatitis and increased in hyperthyroidism, pregnancy, and obesity; 3% excreted unchanged in urine.[18]

$t_{1/2}$. 2 ± 0.5 hr, decreased in hyperthyroidism and pregnancy, and increased in hepatitis and neonates.[18]

Adverse Reactions. In acute overdose, potentially fatal hepatic necrosis and possible renal tubular necrosis can occur, but clinical and laboratory evidence of hepatotoxicity may be delayed for several days (*see* Serum Levels). Toxic hepatitis has also been associated with long-term ingestion of 5–8 g/day for several weeks or 3–4 g/day for a year. Occasionally, erythematous or urticarial skin reactions occur; methemoglobinemia reported rarely. Analgesic nephropathy has been associated with the consumption of 1–15.3 kg of acetaminophen over periods of 3–23 yr.[21]

Precautions. Use with caution in chronic alcoholics and in patients with G-6-PD deficiency.

Drug Interactions. Chronic alcoholics may be at increased risk for hepatic toxicity.[22] The risk of hepatotoxicity may also be increased by long-term use of other enzyme inducers (eg, barbiturates, carbamazepine, phenytoin, rifampin); acetaminophen's efficacy may also be decreased by these agents.

Notes. For the short-term treatment of osteoarthritis of the knee, acetaminophen 4 g/day has been shown to be comparable to ibuprofen 1.2–2.4 g/day.[23] Management of acute overdosage includes emesis or gastric lavage, if no more than a few hours have elapsed since ingestion. Administration of activated charcoal is not recommended, because it may interfere with the absorption of acetylcysteine, which is used in the treatment of severe acute overdosage. Potentially dangerous acetaminophen levels (*see* Serum Levels) can be managed by the administration of 140 mg/kg acetylcysteine diluted 1:3 in a soft drink or plain water; follow with 70 mg/kg q 4 hr for 17 doses. If administered within 8–16 hr of ingestion, this therapy has been shown to minimize the expected hepatotoxicity, but treatment is still indicated as late as 24 hr after ingestion. The 72-hr oral regimen appears to be as effective as the 20-hr IV regimen, and may be superior when treatment is delayed.[20]

ASPIRIN   Various

Pharmacology. Aspirin is an analgesic, antipyretic, and antiinflammatory agent. Antiinflammatory properties are related to impairment of prostaglandin biosynthesis. Aspirin nonselectively inhibits both cyclooxygenase-1, which is associated with GI and renal effects and inhibition of platelet aggregation, and cyclooxygenase-2, which is associated with the inflammatory response. Unlike other NSAIDs, its antiplatelet effect is irreversible (because of transacetylation of platelet cyclooxygenase) for the life of the platelet (8–11 days). Salicylates without acetyl groups (eg, **sodium salicylate**) have essentially no antiplatelet effect, but retain analgesic, antipyretic, and antiinflammatory activity. Low dosages (1–2 g/day) decrease urate excretion; high dosages (>5 g/day) induce uricosuria.[20,24]

Administration and Adult Dosage. **PO or PR for fever or minor pain** 325–1000 mg q 4 hr, to a maximum of 4 g/day. **PO for arthritis and rheumatic conditions** 3.6–5.4 g/day in divided doses. **PO for acute rheumatic fever** 5–8 g/day in divided doses. **PO for prevention of transient ischemic attacks or stroke** 325–1300 mg/day in divided doses. Although higher dosages (975–1300 mg/day) are associated with slightly higher risk of GI hemorrhage, there is some evidence that they are also more effective.[25] **PO for myocardial infarction risk reduction** (primary prevention in healthy men over 50 yr with cardiovascular risk factors) 160–325 mg/day; (secondary prevention) 160–325 mg/day.[26] **PO for unstable angina** 160–325 mg/day with full dose IV heparin therapy.[26] **PO for prevention of coronary artery bypass graft occlusion** 325 mg/day started 6 hr postoperatively and continued indefinitely.[27] **PO for nonrheumatic atrial fibrillation** (patients who are poor candidates for, or decline, oral anticoagulants only) 325 mg/day; (patients under 65 yr with no stroke risk factors) 325 mg/day, although some experts recommend no antithrombotic therapy in this situation.[28]

Special Populations. *Pediatric Dosage.* **PO for juvenile rheumatoid arthritis** 60–110 mg/kg/day in divided doses. **PO for acute rheumatic fever** 100 mg/kg/day in divided doses initially for 2 weeks, then 75 mg/kg/day in divided doses for 4–6 weeks. PO for Kawasaki disease 80–120 mg/kg/day; decrease to 10 mg/kg/day after fever resolves (*see* Precautions). **PO as an analgesic/antipyretic** 10–15 mg/kg/dose q 4 hr, to a maximum of 60–80 mg/kg/day. Alternatively, **PO** (2–3 yr) 162 mg q 4 hr; (4–5 yr) 243 mg q 4 hr; (6–8 yr) 325 mg q 4 hr; (9–10 yr) 405 mg q 4 hr; (11 yr) 486 mg q 4 hr; (12 yr and over) 650 mg q 4 hr (*see* Precautions).

Geriatric Dosage. Use minimal effective dosages because the elderly are more susceptible to GI bleeding and acute renal insufficiency. **PO for myocardial infarction risk reduction** (healthy men over 50 yr for primary prevention with cardiovascular risk factors) 160–325 mg/day.[26]

Other Conditions. Uremia or reduced albumin levels are likely to produce higher unbound drug levels, which may increase pharmacologic or toxic effects. Dosage reduction may be required in these patients.

Dosage Forms. **Chew Tab** 81 mg; **EC Tab** 81, 165, 325, 500, 650, 975 mg; **SR Tab** 650, 800 mg; **Tab** 81, 325, 500 mg; **Supp** 120, 200, 300, 600 mg.

Patient Instructions. Children and teenagers should not use this medication for chickenpox or flu symptoms before a physician or pharmacist is consulted about Reye's syndrome, a rare but serious illness. Take this drug with food, milk, or a full glass of water to minimize stomach upset; report any symptoms of GI ulceration or bleeding. Do not crush or chew enteric coated or sustained-release preparations.

Pharmacokinetics. *Onset and Duration.* PO onset of analgesia 30 min.[18]

Serum Levels. (Salicylate) 150–300 mg/L (1.1–2.2 mmol/L) for rheumatic diseases, often accompanied by mild toxic symptoms. Tinnitus occurs at 200–400 mg/L (1.5–2.9 mmol/L), hyperventilation at greater than 350 mg/L (2.6 mmol/L), acidosis at greater than 450 mg/L (3.3 mmol/L), and severe or fatal toxicity at levels greater than 900 mg/L (6.6 mmol/L) 6 hr after acute ingestion.[29,30]

Fate. Rapidly absorbed from the GI tract; oral bioavailability of aspirin is 68 ± 3%. A single analgesic/antipyretic dose produces peak salicylate levels of 30–60 mg/L (0.22–0.44 mmol/L). Aspirin is 49% plasma protein bound, decreased in uremia; V_d is 0.15 ± 0.03 L/kg; Cl is 0.56 ± 0.07 L/hr/kg; 1.4% excreted unchanged in the urine. Aspirin is rapidly hydrolyzed to salicylic acid (salicylate), which is also pharmacologically active. Salicylate is metabolized primarily in the liver to four metabolites (salicyluric acid, phenolic and acylglucuronides, and gentisic acid). Salicylate plasma protein binding is dose dependent, 95% at 15 mg/L and 80% at 300 mg/L, and decreased in uremia, hypoalbuminemia, neonates, and pregnancy; V_d is 0.17 ± 0.03 L/kg; Cl is dose dependent, 0.012 L/hr/kg at 134–157 mg/L, and decreased in hepatitis and neonates. From 2 to 30%is excreted unchanged in the urine, depending on dose and urine pH.[18]

$t_{1/2}$. (Aspirin) 0.25 ± 0.03 hr;[18] (salicylate) dose dependent: 2.4 hr with 0.25 g, 5 hr with 1 g, 6.1 hr with 1.3 g, 19 hr with 10–20 g.[31]

Adverse Reactions. Hearing impairment, GI upset, and occult bleeding are frequent, with rare acute hemorrhage from gastric erosion. As with other NSAIDs, aspirin may cause renal dysfunction, particularly in those with preexisting renal disease or CHF.[20] Rare hepatotoxicity occurs, primarily in children with rheumatic fever or rheumatoid arthritis, and adults with SLE or preexisting liver disease;[32,33] the syndrome of asthma, angioedema, and nasal polyps may be provoked in susceptible patients.[34] A single analgesic dose may suppress platelet aggregation and prolong bleeding time for up to 1 week; large dosages may prolong PT.[35]

Precautions. Use with caution in patients with renal disease, gastric ulcer, bleeding tendencies, hypoprothrombinemia, or history of asthma, or during anticoagulant therapy. Because of the association with Reye's syndrome, the use of salicylates in children and teenagers with flulike symptoms or chickenpox is not recommended.[36,37] Those developing bronchospasm to aspirin may develop a similar reaction to other NSAIDs.[34] Sodium salicylate and other nonacetylated salicylates (except diflunisal) are usually well tolerated in these patients.[36,38]

Drug Interactions. Alkalinizing agents (eg, acetazolamide, antacids) can reduce salicylate levels; acetazolamide may also enhance CNS penetration of salicylate. Corticosteroids can reduce serum salicylate levels. Large doses of salicylates can increase oral anticoagulant effect; even small doses can increase risk of bleeding with oral anticoagulants or heparin because of the antiplatelet effect of aspirin. Alcohol and salicylate may cause an enhanced risk of GI blood loss. Salicylates may cause an increased response to sulfonylureas, especially chlorpropamide. Salicylate decreases the uricosuric effect of uricosuric agents. Salicylate, especially in large doses, may decrease renal elimination of methotrexate and displace it from plasma protein binding sites.

Parameters to Monitor. Monitor for occult GI blood loss (periodic hematocrit, stool guaiac) in patients who ingest salicylates regularly. Serum salicylate level determinations are recommended with higher dosage regimens because of the wide variation among patients in serum levels produced. Using tinnitus as an index of maximum salicylate tolerance is *not* recommended.[29]

Notes. Enteric coatings reduce GI bleeding while maintaining reliable absorption.[39]

Pharmacology. Ibuprofen is a nonsteroidal antiinflammatory agent with analgesic and antipyretic properties. It is a nonselective inhibitor of cyclooxygenase-1 and cyclooxygenase-2, and it reversibly alters platelet function and prolongs bleeding time.

Administration and Adult Dosage. **PO for mild to moderate pain** 400 mg q 4–6 hr prn. **PO for primary dysmenorrhea** 400 mg q 4 hr prn. **PO for rheumatoid arthritis and osteoarthritis** 400–800 mg tid or qid, to a maximum of 3.2 g/day.

Special Populations. *Pediatric Dosage.* **PO for fever** (over 12 months) 5–10 mg/kg q 6–8 hr, to a maximum of 40 mg/kg/day. **PO for juvenile arthritis** 30–40 mg/kg/day in 3 or 4 divided doses; 20 mg/kg/day in milder disease.

Geriatric Dosage. Use minimal effective dosages because the elderly are more susceptible to GI bleeding and acute renal insufficiency.

Dosage Forms. **Chew Tab** 50, 100 mg; **Tab** 100, 200, 300, 400, 600, 800 mg; **Drp** 40 mg/mL; **Susp** 20 mg/mL.

Patient Instructions. This drug may be taken with a small amount of food, milk, or antacid to minimize stomach upset. Report any symptoms of GI ulceration or bleeding, skin rash, weight gain, or edema. Dizziness may occur; until the extent of this effect is known, use appropriate caution.

Pharmacokinetics. *Serum Levels.* 10 mg/L (48 µmol/L) for antipyretic effect.[18] Serum concentrations over 200 mg/L (971 µmol/L) 1 hr after acute overdosage may be associated with severe toxicity (apnea, metabolic acidosis, and coma).[40]

Fate. Rapidly absorbed from the GI tract with bioavailability over 80%.[18] Peak serum levels in children of 17–42 mg/L (82–204 µmol/L) following a dose of 5 mg/kg and 25–53 mg/L (121–257 µmol/L) following a dose of 10 mg/kg are achieved in 1.1 ± 0.3 hr.[41] Greater than 99% plasma protein bound; metabolized to at least two inactive metabolites; V_d is 0.15 ± 0.02 L/kg, increased in cystic fibrosis; Cl is 0.045 ± 0.012 L/hr/kg, increased in cystic fibrosis. Less than 1% is excreted unchanged in the urine.[18]

$t_{1/2}$. 2 ± 0.5 hr.[18]

Adverse Reactions. Gastric distress, occult blood loss, diarrhea, vomiting, dizziness, and skin rash occur occasionally; GI ulceration (for all NSAIDs there is a greater risk in the elderly and with higher dosages) and fluid retention have been reported.[42] May occasionally cause renal dysfunction, particularly in those with preexisting renal disease, CHF, or cirrhosis.[43] Rarely, a slight rise in the Ivy bleeding time, elevation of liver enzymes, lymphopenia, agranulocytosis, aplastic anemia, and aseptic meningitis have been reported.[44,45]

Contraindications. Syndrome of nasal polyps; angioedema; bronchospastic reactivity to aspirin or other NSAIDs.

Precautions. Avoid during pregnancy. Use with caution in patients with preexisting renal disease, CHF, or cirrhosis;[43] a history of ulcer disease or bleeding; or risk factors associated with peptic ulcer disease (alcohol and smoking).

Drug Interactions. NSAIDs may inhibit the antihypertensive response to ACE inhibitors, ß-blockers, diuretics, and hydralazine, and also inhibit the natriuretic of diuretics. Possible GI bleeding and the antiplatelet effect of NSAIDs may increase the risk of serious bleeding during anticoagulant therapy. NSAIDs may decrease renal lithium clearance. Some NSAIDs (especially indomethacin and ketoprofen) reduce methotrexate clearance. Indomethacin (and probably other NSAIDs) may reduce renal function when combined with triamterene.

Parameters to Monitor. Monitor for occult blood loss, weight gain, and renal function during long-term use.

Notes. **Misoprostol** is the most effective therapy in preventing NSAID-associated GI ulceration; H_2-receptor antagonists, however, prevent duodenal, but not gastric, ulcerations. The role of **omeprazole** and **sucralfate** for prevention of GI ulceration is not firmly established.[42]

INDOMETHACIN   Indocin, Various

Indomethacin is an indoleacetic acid NSAID that is one of the most potent nonselective inhibitors of cyclooxygenase available. In addition to its antiinflammatory effects, indomethacin has prominent analgesic and antipyretic properties. Indomethacin is approved for treatment of rheumatoid arthritis, ankylosing spondylitis, osteoarthritis, acute gouty arthritis, acute painful shoulder, and pharmacologic closure of persistent patent ductus arteriosus in premature infants. It has also been used to suppress uterine activity and prevent premature labor. Indomethacin is rapidly and well absorbed from the GI tract, with a bioavailability of 98%. Peak serum levels are reached within 2 hr with effective concentrations in the range of 0.3 to 3 mg/L (0.8–8 µmol/L). It is 90% plasma protein bound and has extensive O-demethylation and N-deacylation to inactive metabolites; V_d is 0.29 ± 0.04 L/kg; Cl is 0.084 ± 0.012 L/hr/kg, lower in premature infants, neonates, and the aged; 15 ± 8% is excreted unchanged in the urine. The half-life of the drug is 2.4 ± 0.4 hr, higher in premature infants, neonates, and the aged. A high frequency of adverse effects has been noted, with about 20% of patients unable to tolerate the drug. Frontal lobe headache, drowsiness, dizziness, mental confusion, and GI distress are frequent, especially with dosages greater than 100 mg/day; occasional peripheral neuropathy, occult bleeding, and peptic ulcer occur. Rarely, pancreatitis, corneal opacities, hepatotoxicity, aplastic anemia, agranulocytosis, thrombocytopenia, aggravation of psychiatric disorders, and allergic reactions are reported. The syndrome of asthma, angioedema, and nasal polyps may be provoked in susceptible patients. Precautions, drug interactions, and monitoring are similar to other NSAIDs (*see* Ibuprofen). The oral adult dosage for rheumatoid arthritis, rheumatoid (ankylosing) spondylitis, and osteoarthritis of the hip is 25 mg bid or tid initially. Increase in 25 mg/day increments at weekly intervals until satisfactory response or to a maximum of 150–200 mg/day. Alternatively, up to 100 mg of the daily dosage may be given hs for persistent night or morning stiffness. Oral adult dosage for acute gouty arthritis is 100 mg, followed by 50 mg tid until resolved. The SR capsule 75 mg 1–2 times/day can be substituted for all uses except gouty arthritis, based on the non-SR dosage. Dosage for pharmacologic closure of persistent patent ductus arteriosus in premature infants is 0.2 mg/kg IV, followed by two additional IV doses of 0.1–0.25 mg/kg (depending on age) at 12- to 24-hr intervals. Alternatively, give 0.3 mg/kg as a single dose, or one or more doses of 0.1 mg/kg as a retention enema or via orogastric tube.[18,20,35] Available as 25- and 50-mg capsules; 75-mg SR capsules; 50-mg suppositories; 5 mg/mL suspension; and 1-mg injection.

NAPROXEN	Naprosyn
NAPROXEN SODIUM	Anaprox

Pharmacology. *See* Ibuprofen.

Administration and Adult Dosage. PO for mild to moderate pain, dysmenorrhea, or acute tendinitis or bursitis (naproxen) 500 mg, followed by 250 mg q 6–8 hr, to a maximum of 1250 mg/day; (naproxen sodium) 550 mg, followed by 275 mg q 6–8 hr, to a maximum of 1375 mg/day. **PO for rheumatoid arthritis, osteoarthritis, and ankylosing spondylitis** (naproxen) 250–500 mg bid initially, to a maximum of 1500 mg/day for limited periods; (naproxen sodium) 275–550 mg bid or 275 mg q morning and 550 mg q evening initially, to a maximum of 1650 mg/day for limited periods. If no improvement has occurred after 4 weeks of therapy, consider other drug therapy. **PO for acute gout** (naproxen) 750 mg, followed by 250 mg q 8 hr until resolved; (naproxen sodium) 825 mg, followed by 275 mg q 8 hr until resolved.

Special Populations. *Pediatric Dosage.* **PO for juvenile arthritis** 10 mg/kg/day in 2 divided doses.

Geriatric Dosage. Use minimal effective dosages because the elderly are more susceptible to GI bleeding and acute renal insufficiency.

Dosage Forms. Tab (naproxen) 250, 375, 500 mg; (naproxen sodium) 220, 275, 550 mg; **EC Tab** 375, 500 mg; **SR Tab** (naproxen sodium) 375, 500, 750 mg; **Susp** (naproxen) 25 mg/mL.

Patient Instructions. (*See* Ibuprofen.)

Pharmacokinetics. *Serum Levels.* Though concentrations >50 mg/L (217 μmol/L) are associated with response in rheumatoid arthritis.[18]

Fate. Rapidly absorbed from the GI tract with a bioavailability of about 99%. Greater than 99.7% plasma protein bound, saturable with increasing dosage, increased with uremia, cirrhosis, and in the elderly, and decreased in rheumatoid arthritis and hypoalbuminemia; V_d is 0.16 ± 0.02 L/kg, increased in uremia, cirrhosis, and rheumatoid arthritis. Cl is 0.0078 ± 0.0012 L/hr/kg, increased in rheumatoid arthritis and decreased in uremia; less than 1% is excreted unchanged in urine.[18]

$t_{1/2}$. 14 ± 1 hr, increased in the elderly.[18]

Adverse Reactions. May occasionally cause renal dysfunction, particularly in those with preexisting renal disease, CHF, or cirrhosis.[43] Interstitial nephritis and nephrotic syndrome have been reported.[46,47] (*See* Ibuprofen.)

Contraindications. (*See* Ibuprofen.)

Precautions. (*See* Ibuprofen.)

Drug Interactions. (*See* Ibuprofen.)

Parameters to Monitor. (*See* Ibuprofen.)

Notes. (*See* Ibuprofen and Nonsteroidal Antiinflammatory Drugs Comparison Chart.)

PIROXICAM   Feldene, Various

Piroxicam is an oxicam enolic acid nonsteroidal antiinflammatory drug (non-selective cyclooxygenase inhibitor) chemically and pharmacokinetically distinct from earlier drugs. Piroxicam is effective in patients with rheumatoid arthritis, osteoarthritis, and ankylosing spondylitis. It is 98.5% plasma protein bound. V_d is 0.15 ± 0.03 L/kg; Cl is 0.002 ± 0.0005 L/hr/kg, decreased in cirrhosis. Less than 5% is excreted unchanged in urine. The half-life of the drug is 48 ± 8 hr, which allows a single daily dosage regimen. Adverse effects appear to be similar to other available NSAIDs, although some studies suggest that GI complaints and bleeding may be more frequent. Piroxicam may occasionally cause renal dysfunction, particularly in those with preexisting renal disease, CHF, or cirrhosis. Piroxicam appears to be associated with a high frequency of phototoxic cutaneous eruptions. Precautions, drug interactions, and monitoring are similar to other NSAIDs (*see* Ibuprofen). Dosage is usually 20 mg in single or divided doses. Use with caution and at reduced dosage in the elderly. Available as 10- and 20-mg capsules.[18,20,36,43,48,49]

NONSTEROIDAL ANTIINFLAMMATORY DRUGS COMPARISON CHART

DRUG	DOSAGE FORMS	ADULT DOSAGE	HALF-LIFE (HR)	COMMENTS
ACETIC ACIDS				
Bromfenac DurAct	Cap 25, 50 mg.	PO (pain) 25–50 mg in 1–2 doses.	0.6 ±0.1	Similar to ibuprofen.
Diclofenac Cataflam Voltaren Various	Tab (diclofenac) 25, 50, 75 mg Tab (diclofenac potassium) 50 mg SR Tab (diclofenac sodium) 100 mg.	PO (pain, dysmenorrhea) (Cataflam) 50 mg tid; PO (arthritis) 100– 200 mg/day in 2 doses. PO SR 100 mg once daily. (dosages expressed as diclofenac)	1.1 ±0.2	Increasingly associated with hepatotoxicity. Although it is unclear whether the risk is any greater than with other NSAIDs, careful monitoring of symptoms and liver function tests is recommended.
Etodolac Lodine	Cap 200, 300, 500 mg.	PO (pain) 200–400 mg q 6–8 hr; PO (arthritis) 600–1200 mg/day in 2–3 divided doses.	7.3±4	Recommended for treatment of osteoarthritis; not as effective as other NSAIDs for rheumatoid arthritis.
Indomethacin Indocin Various	Cap 25, 50 mg SR Cap 75 mg Susp 5 mg/mL Supp 50 mg Inj 1 mg.	PO (gouty arthritis) 50 mg tid; PO or PR (arthritis) 50– 200 mg/day in 3 divided doses. SR in 1–2 doses may substitute for equal dosage of non-SR.	2.4±0.4	See monograph. Associated with a high frequency of CNS effects such as drowsiness, dizziness, mental confusion, and frontal lobe headache.

(continued)

NONSTEROIDAL ANTIINFLAMMATORY DRUGS COMPARISON CHART (continued)

DRUG	DOSAGE FORMS	ADULT DOSAGE	HALF-LIFE (HR)	COMMENTS
Ketorolac Toradol	Tab 10 mg Inj 15, 30, 60 mg.	PO (pain, short-term) 10 mg q 4–6 hr prn, to a maximum of 40 mg/day for 5 days (including IM/IV). IM or IV (short-term management of pain) 30 or 60 (IM only) mg once, then 15–30 mg q 6 hr.	4.5	For short-term (up to 5 days) use only. Do not exceed 60 mg/day parenterally in patients 65 yr or over, under 50 kg, or with elevated Cr_s.
Sulindac Clinoril	Tab 150, 200 mg.	PO (arthritis) 300–400 mg/day in 2 divided doses.	15 ± 4 (active sulfide metabolite)	Purported "renal-sparing" effect has been questioned. Because the active sulfide metabolite has a relatively long half-life, renal effects may not be observed for several days.
Tolmetin Tolectin Various	Cap 400 mg Tab 200, 600 mg.	PO (arthritis) 0.6–1.8 g/day in 3–4 divided doses.	4.9 ± 0.3	Higher frequency of anaphylactoid reactions than other NSAIDs.

NONSTEROIDAL ANTIINFLAMMATORY DRUGS COMPARISON CHART (continued)

DRUG	DOSAGE FORMS	ADULT DOSAGE	HALF-LIFE(HR)	COMMENTS
ANTHRANILIC ACIDS (FENAMATES)				
Meclofenamate Meclomen Various	Cap 50, 100 mg.	PO (pain) 50 mg q 4–6 hr; PO (arthritis) 200–400 mg/day in 3–4 divided doses.	3	The fenamates as a group are more toxic than other NSAIDs and associated with headache, dizziness, and hemolytic anemia.
Mefenamic Acid Ponstel	Cap 250 mg.	PO (pain, dysmenorrhea) 250 mg q 6 hr for up to 1 week.	3	Not recommended; *see* Meclofenamate Comments.
NONACIDIC COMPOUNDS				
Nabumetone Relafen	Tab 500, 750 mg Chew Tab 1 g.	PO (arthritis) 1–2 g/day in 1–2 doses.	23 ± 4 (active 6-MNA metabolite)	Some cyclooxygenase-2 selectivity. Reported to have less GI toxicity than other NSAIDs; however, additional well-controlled, double-blind studies are needed.
OXICAMS				
Meloxicam (Investigational)		PO (arthritis) 7.5– 15 mg once daily.	20	Greater cyclooxygenase-2 selectivity than nabumetone. Less mucosal damage than piroxicam.

(continued)

17

NONSTEROIDAL ANTIINFLAMMATORY DRUGS COMPARISON CHART (continued)

DRUG	DOSAGE FORMS	ADULT DOSAGE	HALF-LIFE((HR)	COMMENTS
Piroxicam Feldene Various	Cap 10, 20 mg.	PO (arthritis) 20 mg/day in 1–2 doses.	48±8	Based on postmarketing surveillance data, reported to cause about 12 times more GI adverse effects than ibuprofen. High frequency of phototoxic cutaneous eruptions.
PROPIONIC ACIDS				
Fenoprofen Nalfon	Cap 200, 300 mg Tab 600 mg.	PO (pain) 200 mg q 4–6 hr; PO (arthritis) 1.2–2.4 g/day in 3–4 divided doses.	2.5±0.5	Similar to Ibuprofen.
Flurbiprofen Ansaid	Tab 50, 100 mg.	PO (arthritis) 200–300 mg/day in 2–4 divided doses.	3.8±1.2	Similar to Ibuprofen.
Ibuprofen Motrin Various	Chew Tab 50, 100 mg Tab 100, 200, 300, 400, 600, 800 mg Drp 40 mg/mL Susp 20 mg/mL.	PO (pain, dysmenorrhea) 400 mg q 4–6 hr; PO (arthritis) 1.2–3.2 g/day in 3–4 divided doses.	2±0.5	See monograph.
Ketoprofen Orudis Oruvail Various	Cap 25, 50, 75 mg Tab 12.5 mg SR Cap 100, 150, 200 mg.	PO (pain) 25–50 mg q 6–8 hr; PO (arthritis) 150–300 mg/day in 3 divided doses. PO SR 200 mg/day in 1 dose.	1.8±0.3	Similar to Ibuprofen.

NONSTEROIDAL ANTIINFLAMMATORY DRUGS COMPARISON CHART (continued)

DRUG	DOSAGE FORMS	ADULT DOSAGE	HALF-LIFE((HR)	COMMENTS
Naproxen Aleve Anaprox Naprelan Naprosyn	Tab (naproxen sodium) 220, 275, 550 mg Tab (naproxen) 250, 375, 500 mg EC Tab (naproxen) 375, 500 mg SR Tab (naproxen) 375, 500, 750 mg Susp (naproxen) 25 mg/mL.	PO (pain) 200–250 mg q 8–12 hr; PO (arthritis) 0.5–1.25 g/day in 2 divided doses (doses expressed as naproxen).	14±1	*See* monograph.
Oxaprozin Daypro	Tab 600 mg.	PO (arthritis) 1.2 g/day in 1 dose.	50–60	Similar to other NSAIDs.
SALICYLATES **Aspirin** Various	*See* monograph.	PO (pain) 325–650 mg q 4 hr; PO (arthritis) 3.6–5.4 g/day in 3–4 divided doses.	0.25±0.03 (aspirin) 2–19 (salicylate, dose dependent)	*See* monograph.

(continued)

NONSTEROIDAL ANTIINFLAMMATORY DRUGS COMPARISON CHART (continued)

DRUG	DOSAGE FORMS	ADULT DOSAGE	HALF-LIFE((HR)	COMMENTS
Choline Magnesium Trisalicylate Trilisate	Tab 500, 750 mg, 1 g Liquid 100 mg/mL.	PO (pain, arthritis) 1.5–3 g/day in 1–2 divided doses.*	2–19 (salicylate, dose dependent)	Salicylate is only a weak inhibitor of cyclooxygenase. It therefore has no anti-platelet effect and can usually be administered safely to individuals with aspirin sensitivity. *See also* Aspirin monograph.
Diflunisal Dolobid	Tab 250, 500 mg.	PO (arthritis) 250–500 mg bid.	11±2 (dose dependent)	Not converted to salicylate; similar to other NSAIDs
Magnesium Salicylate Doan's Various	Tab 325, 500, 545 600 mg.	PO (pain, arthritis) 3.6–4.8 g/day in 3–4 divided doses.*	2–19 (salicylate, dose dependent)	*See* Choline Magnesium Trisalicylate comments and Aspirin monograph.
Salsalate Disalcid Various	Cap 500 mg Tab 500, 750 mg.	PO (arthritis) 3 g/day in 2–3 divided doses.*	2–19 (salicylate, dose dependent)	*See* Choline Magnesium Trisalicylate comments and Aspirin monograph.

*Long-term dosage for arthritis should be guided by serum salicylate levels; see Aspirin monograph.
Adapted from references 18, 20, 35, 48–57, and product information.

Opioids

Class Instructions. This drug may cause drowsiness. Until the extent of this effect is known, use caution when driving, operating machinery, or performing other tasks requiring mental alertness. Avoid excessive concurrent use of alcohol and other drugs that cause drowsiness. Prolonged use of this drug may cause constipation, and concurrent use of a stool softening or bulk- forming laxative may be helpful.

CODEINE SALTS
Various

Pharmacology. Codeine is 3-methoxymorphine, a phenanthrene opioid with very low affinity for opioid receptors. Its analgesic activity may be the result of a 10% conversion to morphine. However, its antitussive effect is thought to involve receptors that do bind codeine.[58,59] (*See* Morphine Sulfate.)

Administration and Adult Dosage. PO, SC, IM, or IV for analgesia 15–60 mg q 4–6 hr. **PO or SC for antitussive action** 10–20 mg q 4–6 hr, to a maximum of 120 mg/day.

Special Populations. *Pediatric Dosage.* **PO, SC, or IM for analgesia** (1 yr and older) 0.5 mg/kg q 4–6 hr. **PO for antitussive action** (2–6 yr) 2.5–5 mg q 4–6 hr, to a maximum of 30 mg/day; (7–12 yr) 5–10 mg q 4–6 hr, to a maximum of 60 mg/day; (over 12 yr) same as adult dosage.

Geriatric Dosage. Reduce initial dosage in the elderly.

Other Conditions. Reduce initial dosage in debilitated patients or those with hypoxia or hypercapnia.

Dosage Forms. Tab 15, 30, 60 mg; **Hyp Tab** 15, 30, 60 mg; **Inj** 30, 60 mg/mL. Formulated as phosphate or sulfate salt.

Patient Instructions. (*See* Opioids Class Instructions.)

Pharmacokinetics. *Onset and Duration.* PO, SC onset 15–30 min; IM peak analgesia 0.5–1 hr; duration (all routes) 4–6 hr.[60]

Fate. Well absorbed from GI tract and metabolized in the liver to norcodeine and morphine (10%). A single PO 15-mg dose produces serum levels of 26–33 µg/L (82–104 nmol/L) in 2 hr and 13–22 µg/L (41–69 nmol/L) in 5 hr.[61] The drug is 7% plasma protein bound. Primarily urinary excretion of inactive forms; V_d is 2.6 ± 0.3 L/kg; Cl is 0.66 ± 0.12 L/hr/kg;[18] 3–16% is excreted unchanged in urine.[62]

$t_{1/2}$ 2.9 ± 0.7 hr.[18]

Adverse Reactions. Low toxicity and potential for addiction. Sedation, dizziness, nausea, vomiting, constipation, and respiratory depression occur frequently. Dose-related signs of intoxication include miosis, drowsiness, decreased rate and depth of respiration, bradycardia, and hypotension.

Precautions. (*See* Morphine Sulfate for parenteral codeine precautions.)

Drug Interactions. (*See* Morphine Sulfate.)

FENTANYL	Duragesic, Fentanyl Oralet, Sublimaze, Various

Pharmacology. Fentanyl is a phenylpiperidine opioid agonist with predominant effects on the mu opioid receptor, and is about 80 times more potent as an analgesic than morphine. Other related compounds include **sufentanil** (Sufenta), which is 5–7 times more potent than fentanyl, **alfentanil** (Alfenta), which is less potent than fentanyl but acts more rapidly and has a shorter duration of action, and **remifentanil** (Ultiva) which has 5–10 times the potency of fentanyl and is extremely short acting because of its rapid ester hydrolysis.[58,59] (*See* Morphine Sulfate.)

Administration and Adult Dosage. IV patient-controlled analgesia (PCA) 20–100 μg per activation with 3–10 min lockout period, both titrated to patient response. *See* Patient-Controlled Analgesia Guidelines Chart. **Epidurally for analgesia** 25–150 μg as an intermittent bolus dose or 25–150 μg/hr as a continuous infusion, titrated to patient response.[60] (*See* Intraspinal Narcotic Administration Guidelines Chart.) **Transdermal for analgesia,** calculate the previous 24-hr analgesic requirement and convert this amount to the equal analgesic oral morphine dosage from the Opioid Analgesics Comparison Chart. Use the following table to determine the fentanyl transdermal dosage from the daily equivalent oral morphine dosage:

TRANSDERMAL FENTANYL COMPARISON CHART	
24-HOUR ORAL MORPHINE DOSAGE* (MG/DAY)	FENTANYL TRANSDERMAL DOSAGE (μG/HR)
45–134	25
135–224	50
225–314	75
315–404	100
405–494	125
495–584	150
585–674	175
675–764	200
765–854	225
855–944	250
945–1034	275
1035–1124	300

* Assumes morphine 10 mg IM is equivalent to morphine 60 mg orally; however, because of individual variability, equivalent dosages may vary among patients. *See* Opioid Analgesics comparison chart.

Initiate treatment using the recommended transdermal fentanyl dosage and increase based on response no more frequently than q 3–6 days. Multiple transdermal patches may be used to achieve appropriate dosage (do not cut patches for a partial dosage). To change treatment to another opioid, discontinue the transdermal patch for 12–18 hr and start treatment with the new opioid at about one-half the equianalgesic dosage. **IV for induction and maintenance anesthesia** (loading) 4–20 µg/kg, (maintenance) 2–10 µg/kg/hr, (additional bolus) 25–100 µg.[63] **IM for postoperative (recovery room) pain control** 50–100 µg, q 1–2 hr as needed; **Lozenge for anesthesia premedication or induction of conscious sedation** 5 µg/kg (provides effects similar to 0.75–1.25 µg/kg given IM), to a maximum of 400 µg.

Special Populations. *Pediatric Dosage.* (Under 2 yr) safety and efficacy not established. **IV for induction and maintenance anesthesia** (2–12 yr) 2–3 µg/kg initially, followed by 1–5 µg/kg/hr.[63] Lozenge for anesthesia premedication or induction of conscious sedation (<15 kg) contraindicated; (≥15 kg) 5–15 µg/kg, to a maximum of 400 µg.

Geriatric Dosage. **Lozenge for anesthesia premedication or induction of conscious sedation** (over 65 yr) 2.5–5 µg/kg, to a maximum of 400 µg.

Other Conditions. In patients with head injury, cardiovascular, pulmonary, or hepatic disease, consider a lower dosage of 2.5–5 µg/kg, to a maximum of 400 µg.

Dosage Forms. Inj 50 µg/mL; **SR Patch** 25, 50, 75, 100 µg/hr; **Lozenge** 200, 300, 400 µg.

Patient Instructions. (*See* Opioids Class Instructions.)

Pharmacokinetics. *Onset and Duration.* IM onset 7–15 min; duration 1–2 hr. Epidural onset 5 min; duration 4–6 hr.[60] Transdermal onset 6–8 hr; peak 24–72 hr; duration after a single application 72 hr.[64,65] Greater than 17 hr required for serum levels to fall by one-half after patch removal.

Serum Levels. (Analgesia) 1–3 µg/L (3–9 nmol/L);[64,65] (balanced anesthesia) 6–20 µg/L (18–60 nmol/L).[63]

Fate. Bioavailability is 52% with lozenge and 32% with oral solution. The drug is 84 ± 2% plasma protein bound; it is metabolized rapidly primarily by the liver to norfentanyl and other inactive metabolites; V_d is 4 ± 0.4 L/kg; Cl is 0.78 ± 0.12 L/hr/kg, decreased in the elderly and increased in neonates. Less than 10% excreted unchanged in the urine.[58,64,65]

$t_{½}$. 3.7 ± 0.4 hr, increased in the elderly;[58] 7.1–11 hr during cardiopulmonary bypass surgery.[63]

Adverse Reactions. (*See* Morphine Sulfate.) Unlike other opioids, fentanyl, alfentanil, remifentanil, and sufentanil are not associated with histamine release.[63]

Contraindications. (*See* Morphine Sulfate.) Fentanyl SR patch is contraindicated in acute or postoperative pain, including outpatient surgery; patients under 12 yr or 50 kg; pain that can be managed by conventional analgesics; and doses over 25 µg/hr at the initiation of opioid therapy.

Precautions. (*See* Morphine Sulfate.)

Drug Interactions. (*See* Morphine Sulfate.) The effects of fentanyl may be potentiated by other CNS depressant drugs (eg, barbiturates, general anesthetics, narcotics, and tranquilizers). Carbamazepine may decrease fentanyl's effect during anesthesia for craniotomy.

Parameters to Monitor. Monitor vital signs routinely.

Notes. Pruritus that results from spinal narcotics is thought to be caused in part by histamine release and is probably more common with morphine than fentanyl. Pruritus following spinal opioids can be effectively treated with small doses of IV **naloxone** or IV **nalbuphine,** generally without reversing analgesia.[63]

MEPERIDINE HYDROCHLORIDE   Demerol, Various

Pharmacology. Meperidine is a phenylpiperidine opioid agonist with important antimuscarinic activity and negative inotropic effects on the heart. Its major metabolite, normeperidine, has excitant effects that may precipitate tremors, myoclonus, or seizures. Meperidine's antimuscarinic activity may negate the miosis that occurs with other opioids.[59] (*See* Morphine Sulfate.)

Administration and Adult Dosage. PO, SC, or IM for analgesia 50–150 mg (or very slow IV 50–100 mg, preferably diluted) q 3–4 hr prn. Oral doses are about one-half as effective as a parenteral dose. Reduce dosage when given concomitantly with a phenothiazine or other drugs that potentiate the depressant effects of meperidine. **IM or slow IV for shaking caused by general anesthesia or amphotericin B** 25–50 mg. (*See* Notes.)

Special Populations. *Pediatric Dosage.* PO, SC, or IM for analgesia 1–1.8 mg/kg q 3–4 hr, to a maximum of 100 mg/dose. (*See* Notes.)

Geriatric Dosage. Same as adult dosage.

Dosage Forms. **Syrup** 10 mg/mL; **Tab** 50, 100 mg; **Inj** 10, 25, 50, 75, 100 mg/mL.

Patient Instructions. (*See* Opioids Class Instructions.)

Pharmacokinetics. *Onset and Duration.* PO onset about 15 min; duration 2–3 hr; SC or IM onset about 10 min, peak analgesia 0.5–1 hr, duration 2–3 hr.[18,60]

Serum Levels. From 500 to 700 µg/L (2–2.8 µmol/L) appear to be required for analgesia.[64]

Fate. Well absorbed by parenteral route; hydrolyzed and also metabolized in the liver to normeperidine (an active metabolite), which is also hydrolyzed. Oral bioavailability is about $52 \pm 3\%$, increasing to 80–90% in cirrhosis caused by decreased first-pass metabolism.[18,66] After a single 100-mg IM dose, mean serum levels of 670 µg/L (2.7 µmol/L) and 650 µg/L (2.6 µmol/L) are attained in 1 and 2 hr, respectively.[67,68] $58 \pm 9\%$ plasma protein bound, largely to α_1-acid glycoprotein; decreased in the elderly and in uremia.[18,69] V_d is 4.4 ± 0.9 L/kg, increased in the elderly and premature infants; Cl is 1.02 ± 0.3 L/hr/kg, reduced by 25% in surgical patients and by 50% in cirrhosis, and reduced in acute viral hepatitis.[18] An average of 2% unchanged drug and 1–21% (average 6) normeperidine is excreted in urine.[69]

$t_{1/2}$. (Meperidine) α phase 12 min, ß phase 3.2 hr, increasing to 7 hr in patients with cirrhosis or acute liver disease;[68,70] (normeperidine) 14–21 hr in normals, increasing to 35 hr in renal failure.[71]

Adverse Reactions. (*See* Morphine Sulfate.) Factors that may predispose to normeperidine-induced seizures include dosage >400–600 mg/day, renal failure, history of seizures, long-term administration to cancer patients, or coadministration of agents that increase N-demethylation to normeperidine.[72] Local irritation and induration occur with repeated SC injection.

Contraindications. MAO inhibitors within the past 14 days.

Precautions. (*See* Morphine Sulfate.)

Drug Interactions. *See* Morphine Sulfate. Concurrent use with an MAO inhibitor may cause marked blood pressure alterations, sweating, excitation, and rigidity. Barbiturates, chlorpromazine, and phenytoin may decrease meperidine serum concentrations and increase normeperidine, reducing analgesia and increasing the risk of stimulation and seizures.[73]

Parameters to Monitor. Monitor for signs of respiratory or cardiovascular depression.

Notes. A dose of 75–100 mg of meperidine by the parenteral route is approximately equivalent to 10–15 mg of morphine.[60] All opioids including meperidine and morphine increase biliary tract pressure. Sphincter of Oddi spasm may be less with meperidine than with morphine, but there is little evidence that this has clinical relevance. Unlike other opioids, meperidine is useful in treating the shaking and shivering associated with general anesthesia or amphotericin B administration.[72]

METHADONE HYDROCHLORIDE   Dolophine, Various

Pharmacology. Methadone is a phenylheptamine opioid agonist qualitatively similar to morphine. Analgesic activity of l-methadone is 8–50 times that of the d-isomer. d-Methadone lacks addiction liability, but has antitussive activity. Because methadone is a long-acting narcotic agent, it can be substituted for short-acting narcotic agents for maintenance and detoxification. Methadone abstinence syndrome is similar to morphine; however, onset is slower and duration is longer. (*See also* Morphine Sulfate.)

Administration and Adult Dosage. IM or SC for pain 2.5–10 mg q 3–4 hr. **PO for pain** 5–15 mg q 4–6 hr. **PO for maintenance and detoxification treatment** 5–20 mg initially, followed by supplementary doses of 5–10 mg if withdrawal is not suppressed or signs reappear. After stabilization, 10–40 mg/day in single (for maintenance) or divided (for detoxification) doses is adequate for most patients. Detoxification by dosage reduction of 20% per day is usually well tolerated in hospitalized patients.[74]

Special Populations. *Pediatric Dosage.* Safety and efficacy not established.

Geriatric Dosage. Same as adult dosage.

Dosage Forms. Tab 5, 10 mg; **Dispersible Tab** 40 mg; **Soln** 1, 2, 10 mg/mL; **Inj** 10 mg/mL.

Patient Instructions. (*See* Opioids Class Instructions.)

Pharmacokinetics. *Onset and Duration.* (Analgesia) onset SC or IM 10–20 min, PO 30–60 min; peak IM 0.5–1 hr; duration PO, SC, or IM 4–5 hr after a single dose, may be longer with multiple doses.[64,74]

Serum Levels. Best rehabilitation in methadone maintenance patients has been associated with serum levels above 211 µg/L (682 nmol/L).[75] There is no good correlation between serum levels and analgesia.[76]

Fate. Oral bioavailability is 92 ± 21%; 89% plasma protein bound. V_d is 3.8 ± 0.6 L/kg; Cl is 0.084 ± 0.03 L/hr/kg. Extent of metabolism appears to increase with long-term therapy, resulting in a 15–25% decline in serum levels after 8–10 days. Metabolized to form pyrrolidines and pyrrolines which are excreted in urine and bile. The drug is 24 ± 10% excreted unchanged in the urine, increased by further urine acidification.[18,75,76]

$t_{1/2}$. 35 ± 12 hr.[18]

Adverse Reactions. (*See* Morphine Sulfate.) Methadone administered frequently or for prolonged periods may have cumulative effects.

Precautions. (*See* Morphine Sulfate.)

Drug Interactions. (*See* Morphine Sulfate.) Carbamazepine, phenytoin, rifampin, and other drugs that induce CYP enzymes may decrease methadone serum levels and result in withdrawal symptoms in patient on methadone maintenance programs. Diazepam, erythromycin, fluvoxamine, and possibly other enzyme inhibitors may increase methadone levels and effects.[73]

Parameters to Monitor. Monitor for signs of respiratory or cardiovascular depression. During methadone maintenance, monitor for signs of withdrawal, which include lacrimation, rhinorrhea, diaphoresis, yawning, restlessness, insomnia, dilated pupils, and piloerection.[74]

Notes. For treatment of narcotic addiction in detoxification or maintenance programs, methadone may be dispensed only by approved pharmacies. Maintenance therapy (treatment for longer than 3 weeks) may be undertaken only by approved methadone programs; this does not apply to addicts hospitalized for other medical conditions.

MORPHINE SULFATE	Various

Pharmacology. Morphine and other opioids interact with stereospecific opiate receptors in the CNS and other tissues (*see* Opioid Receptor Specificity Comparison Chart). Analgesia is produced primarily through an alteration in emotional response to pain. The relief of pain is fairly specific, other sensory modalities are essentially unaffected, and mental processes are not impaired (unlike anesthetics), except when given in large doses or to unusually susceptible individuals. The drugs also have antitussive effects, usually at dosages less than those required for analgesia.

Administration and Adult Dosage. **PO for analgesia** 8–20 mg q 4 hr; **SR Tab, 12-hr** (narcotive-naive patients) 30 mg q 8–12 hr initially; (narcotic-tolerant patients) total daily oral morphine dosage equivalent in 2 divided doses q 12 hr; **SR Cap, 24-hr** (narcotic-naive patients) 20 mg q 24 hr initially; (narcotic-tolerant patients) total daily oral morphine dosage equivalent q 24 hr; **SC or IM for analgesia** 5–15 mg q 4 hr (10 mg/70 kg is the optimal initial dose); **PR for analgesia** 10–20 mg q 4 hr. **IV for analgesia** 4–10 mg, dilute and inject slowly over a 4–5-min period. **IV infusion** 1–10 mg/hr;[77] some patients with chronic pain may require a dosage as high as 40–95 mg/hr or more.[78] **IV patient-controlled analgesia (PCA)** 1 mg per activation initially with 5–20 min lockout period, both titrated to patient response.[79,80] Continuous infusion combined with PCA has been shown to be effective in managing chronic cancer pain.[81] **Epidural for analgesia (unpreserved solution)** (intermittent) 5 mg initially, may repeat with 1–2 mg after 1 hr, to a maximum of 10 mg/24 hr; (continuous) 2–4 mg/24 hr initially; additional doses of 1–2 mg may be given if pain is not relieved initially. **Intrathecal for analgesia (unpreserved solution)** usually 1/10 of the epidural dosage.

Special Populations. *Pediatric Dosage.* SC or IM 0.1–0.2 mg/kg/dose, to a maximum of 15 mg; may repeat q 4 hr. **IV** use one-half the IM dosage.

Geriatric Dosage. Reduce initial dosage in elderly patients.

Other Conditions. Reduce initial dosage in debilitated patients.

Dosage Forms. **Soln** 2, 4, 20 mg/mL; **Supp** 5, 10, 20, 30 mg; **Tab** 10, 15, 30 mg; **SR Tab** (8–12 hr) 15, 30, 60, 100, 200 mg; **SR Cap (24 hr)** 20, 50, 100 mg; **Inj** (unpreserved solution) 0.5, 1, 10, 25, 50 mg/mL; (preserved solution) 2, 3, 4, 5, 8, 10, 15, 25, 50 mg/mL.

Patient Instructions. (*See* Opioids Class Instructions.)

Pharmacokinetics. *Onset and Duration.* (Analgesia) onset IM 10–30 min; peak 0.5–1 hr; duration 3–5 hr.[64]

Serum Levels. It is speculated that moderate analgesia requires serum levels of at least 50 µg/L (88 nmol/L).[82]

Fate. Rapid absorption after parenteral administration with rapid disappearance from serum, especially after IV administration. Well absorbed from GI tract, but first-pass conjugation is extensive, reducing oral bioavailability to 24 ± 12%.[18,83] Nebulized morphine by inhalation has a low bioavailability, 5 ± 3%, but a rapid peak at 10 min.[83] After an IM dose of 10 mg, peak morphine levels of about 56 µg/L (98 nmol/L) are reached within 20 min. The drug is 35 ± 2% plasma protein bound, decreased in acute viral hepatitis, cirrhosis, and hypoalbuminemia;[18] V_d is 2.12 L/kg in young normals and 1.16 L/kg in elderly patients; Cl is 2.02 L/hr/kg in young normals and 1.66 L/hr/kg in elderly patients.[77] Inactivated in the liver, primarily by conjugation to morphine-6-glucuronide (active) and morphine-3-glucuronide (inactive).[18,84] Mostly excreted in urine; 14 ± 7% as the active morphine-6-glucuronide and 3.4% (oral) to 9% (parenteral) of a dose is excreted unchanged.[18,84,85]

$t_{1/2}$. 1.9 ± 0.5 hr, increased in neonates and premature infants.[18]

Adverse Reactions. Respiratory and circulatory depression are major adverse effects, the former occurring with therapeutic dosages. Dose-related signs of intoxication include miosis, drowsiness, decreased rate and depth of respiration, bradycardia, and hypotension. Sedation, dizziness, nausea, vomiting, sweating, and constipation occur frequently. Euphoria, dysphoria, dry mouth, biliary tract spasm, postural hypotension, syncope, tachy- or bradycardia, urinary retention, and possible allergic-type reactions are reported occasionally. The majority of allergic-type reactions consist of skin rash and wheal and flare over a vein, which may occur with IV injection; these are caused by direct stimulation of histamine release, are not allergic, and are not a sign of a more serious reactions. True allergy is rare.

Precautions. Use with caution and in reduced dosage when giving concurrently with other CNS depressant drugs. Use with caution in pregnancy; the presence of head injury, other intracranial lesions or preexisting increase in intracranial pressure; patients having an acute asthmatic attack; COPD or cor pulmonale; decreased respiratory reserve; preexisting respiratory depression, hypoxia, or hypercapnia; patients whose ability to maintain blood pressure is already compromised; patients with atrial flutter or other supraventricular tachycardias; patients with prostatic hypertrophy or urethral stricture; elderly or debilitated patients; and in patients with acute abdominal pain, when administration of the drug might obscure the diagnosis or clinical course. Do not administer IV unless a narcotic antagonist and facilities for assisted or controlled respiration are immediately available.

Drug Interactions. Concurrent use of opioids with other CNS depressants (eg, alcohol, antipsychotics, general anesthetics, heterocyclic antidepressants, and sedative-hypnotics) may cause respiratory depression. Cimetidine may increase serum concentration and duration of effect of the opioids.[73]

Parameters to Monitor. Monitor for pain control and signs of respiratory or cardiovascular depression.

NALOXONE HYDROCHLORIDE   Narcan, Various

Pharmacology. Naloxone is an N-allyl derivative of oxymorphone, which is a narcotic antagonist. It competitively binds at opiate receptors. Naloxone is essentially free of narcotic agonist properties and is used to reverse the effects of narcotic agonists and drugs with partial agonist properties.[86]

Administration and Adult Dosage. IV (preferred), IM, or SC for known or suspected narcotic overdose 0.4–2 mg initially, may repeat q 2–3 min. If a total of 10 mg has been given and there is no response, the diagnosis of narcotic overdose should be questioned. If the patient responds, additional doses may be repeated prn with the frequency of repeat doses based on clinical evaluation of the patient. **IV infusion** 2 mg in 500 mL D5W or NS can be used for prolonged therapy; administer at a rate adjusted to patient response. **IV for postoperative narcotic depression** 0.1–0.2 mg initially, may repeat q 2–3 min until desired level of reversal is reached. Subsequent doses may be needed if the effect of the narcotic outlasts the action of naloxone. (*See* Notes.)

Special Populations. *Pediatric Dosage.* **IV for known or suspected narcotic overdose** 0.1 mg/kg, may repeat as needed. **IV for postoperative narcotic depression** 0.005–0.01 mg initially, may repeat q 2–3 min until desired level of reversal is reached. **IV (preferred), IM, or SC for narcotic depression** (neonates) 0.01 mg/kg initially, may repeat q 2–3 min until desired level of reversal is reached.

Geriatric Dosage. Same as adult dosage.

Dosage Forms. Inj 0.02, 0.4 mg/mL.

Pharmacokinetics. *Onset and Duration.* Onset IV within 2–3 min, up to 15 min when given IM or SC; duration variable, but usually 1 hr or less.[87,88]

Fate. 59–67% metabolized by hepatic conjugation and renal elimination of the conjugated compound.[89] V_d is approximately 2–3 L/kg,[18,90] Cl is about 1.3 L/hr/kg.[18]

$t_{1/2}$ 64 ± 12 min in adults;[91] 71 ± 36 min in neonates.[92]

Contraindications. None known.

Precautions. Administration to narcotic-dependent persons (including neonates of dependent mothers) may precipitate acute withdrawal symptoms.

Drug Interactions. None known except for opioid antagonism.

Parameters to Monitor. Respiratory rate, pupil size (may not be useful in mixed drug or narcotic partial agonist overdoses), heart rate, blood pressure, symptoms of acute narcotic withdrawal syndrome.

Notes. Naloxone is effective when administered endotracheally to patients with difficult venous access.[93] It is routinely used in the initial treatment of patients with coma of unknown origin. Its use in clonidine overdose has produced mixed results; use in septic and hemorrhagic shock has been disappointing.[86]

OPIOID PARTIAL AGONISTS

Pharmacology. Opioid partial agonists have analgesic effects with generally lower abuse potential than pure opiate agonists such as morphine. These agents can be classified based on their effects on the opioid receptors: mu, kappa, sigma, and delta (*see* Opioid Receptor Specificity Comparison Chart). Mu receptors are responsible for supraspinal analgesia, morphinelike activity and dependence, and respiratory depression; kappa receptors for supraspinal analgesia, sedation, anesthesia, and respiratory depression; sigma receptors for dysphoria, hallucinations, and confusion; and delta receptors for spinal analgesia and potentiation of mu receptors.[58,60,63,94,95]

Administration, Dosage, and Dosage Forms. (*See* Opioid Analgesics Comparison Chart.)

Patient Instructions. (*See* Opioids Class Instructions.)

Pharmacokinetics. (*See* Opioid Analgesics Comparison Chart.)

Adverse Reactions. Sedation, sweating, dizziness, nausea, vomiting, euphoria, dysphoria (agents with sigma receptor activity), and hallucinations are most frequent. Occasionally, insomnia, anxiety, anorexia, constipation, dry mouth, syncope, visual blurring, flushing, decreased blood pressure, and tachycardia are reported. After parenteral use, diaphoresis, sting on injection, respiratory depression, transient apnea in newborn from use in mother during labor, shock, urinary retention, and alterations in uterine contractions during labor occur rarely. Other rarely reported effects include muscle tremor and toxic epidermal necrolysis. Local skin reactions and ulceration and fibrous myopathy at the injection site have been reported with long-term parenteral use of pentazocine.[58] **Tramadol** adverse reactions include seizures (some after the first dose) with recommended and excessive dosages. Seizure risk is increased in patients taking concomitant medications that may reduce the seizure threshold (eg, heterocyclic antidepressants, selective serotonin reuptake inhibitors, MAO inhibitors, neuroleptics) and with certain medical conditions (eg, epilepsy, head trauma, metabolic disorders, alcohol and drug withdrawal, or CNS infection). In addition, **naloxone** administration for tramadol overdose may increase the risk of seizure. Anaphylactoid reactions have also been observed in tramadol postmarketing surveillance.

Contraindications. (Tramadol) prior allergy to any opiate; acute intoxication with alcohol, hypnotics, centrally acting analgesics, opioids, or psychotropic drugs.

Precautions. (*See* Morphine Sulfate.) Also, use cautiously in patients with myocardial infarction because pentazocine and butorphanol increase cardiac workload. All of these agents may produce dependence and withdrawal symptoms following extended use.[18,94-96]

Drug Interactions. (*See* Morphine Sulfate.) With the possible exception of tramadol, these agents can precipitate acute withdrawal in narcotic-dependent individuals.

Notes. Effects of pentazocine are antagonized by naloxone only (ie, not by nalorphine or levallorphan). Naloxone in the pentazocine tablet is not absorbed orally, but theoretically prevents parenteral abuse of the oral dosage form; however, IV abuse of Talwin Nx plus tripelennamine has been reported.[97]

OPIOID RECEPTOR SPECIFICITY COMPARISON CHART

DRUG	RECEPTOR TYPE		
	MU	*KAPPA*	*SIGMA*
Buprenorphine	Partial agonist-antagonist	Unknown	Minimal activity
Butorphanol	Minimal activity	Agonist	Agonist
Dezocine	Partial agonist-antagonist	Agonist	Minimal agonist activity
Meptazinol* (Investigational)	Partial agonist-antagonist	Minimal activity	Unknown
Morphine	Agonist	Agonist	Agonist
Nalbuphine	Antagonist	Agonist	Agonist
Pentazocine	Antagonist	Agonist	Agonist
Tramadol†	Partial or pure agonist‡	Minimal activity	Unknown

*Also has cholinergic actions that may contribute to analgesia; these effects are antagonized by scopolamine.
†Also blocks norepinephrine and serotonin reuptake.
‡Not a classic agonist-antagonist; has little or no antagonist properties, but appears to have partial mu receptor agonist activity; needs more study.

PATIENT-CONTROLLED ANALGESIA (PCA) GUIDELINES CHART*

DRUG	IV BOLUS DOSE (MG)	LOCKOUT INTERVAL (MINUTES)
Buprenorphine	0.03–0.2	10–20
Fentanyl	0.02–0.1	3–10
Hydromorphone	0.1–0.5	3–15
Meperidine[†]	5–30	5–15
Methadone	0.5–3	10–20
Morphine*	0.5–3	5–20
Nalbuphine	1–5	5–15
Oxymorphone	0.2–0.8	5–15
Pentazocine	5–30	5–15
Sufentanil	0.003–0.015	3–10

*Some clinicians recommend combining PCA with a basal continuous infusion of the narcotic. The hourly dosage is determined by the patient's previous narcotic dose requirements and adjusted q 8–24 hr based on the dose of PCA bolus administered, basal continuous infusion, and pain response. A typical starting hourly basal continuous infusion rate for morphine in a 70-kg adult is 0.5–3 mg/hr.
[†]Use with caution (preferably avoid) for PCA and consider factors that may predispose to seizures which include dosage over 100 mg q 2 hr for longer than 24 hr, renal failure, and history of seizure disorder.
From references 60, 79, 81.

INTRASPINAL NARCOTIC ADMINISTRATION GUIDELINES CHART*

ROUTE AND DRUG	INTRASPINAL BOLUS DOSE (MG)	ONSET (MINUTES)	DURATION (HOURS)
EPIDURAL			
Alfentanil	0.7–2[†]	Rapid	1.5–1.7[‡]
Fentanyl	0.025–0.15	5	2–4
Hydromorphone	1–2	15	10–16
Methadone	1–10	10	6–10
Morphine	1–10	30	6–24
Sufentanil	0.015–0.05	15	4–6
INTRATHECAL (SUBARACHNOID)			
Morphine	0.1–0.5	15	8–24

*Use only preservative-free preparations for intraspinal narcotic administration.
[†]Based on a 70-kg adult body weight (ie, 10–30 µg/kg).
[‡]Very short duration of action; requires epidural infusion to obtain prolonged analgesia. Like fentanyl, prolonged epidural infusions produce high systemic concentrations and appear to have little advantage over IV infusion.
From references 60 and 63.

OPIOID ANALGESICS COMPARISON CHART

DRUG AND SCHEDULE[a]	DOSAGE FORMS	EQUIVALENT IM DOSAGE[b] (MG)	PARENTERAL/ORAL EFFICACY RATIO	DURATION OF ANALGESIA (HOURS)	CARDIAC WORKLOAD	PARTIAL ANTAGONIST ACTIVITY
Buprenorphine (C-V)						
Buprenex	Inj 0.324 mg/mL.	0.3–0.6	—	6–8	↓	yes
Butorphanol (NC)		[0.4–0.8][c]				
Stadol	Inj 1, 2 mg/mL	2	1/16	3–4	↑	yes
Stadol NS	Nasal Spray 10 mg/mL (1 mg/spray).[d]					
Codeine (C-II)	Inj 30, 60 mg/mL	120	1/2–2/3	3–6	↓	no
Various	Hyp Tab 15, 30, 60 mg	[30]				
	Tab 15, 30, 60 mg.					
Dezocine (NC)						
Dalgan	Inj 5, 10, 15 mg/mL.	10–15	—	3–4	0	yes
Fentanyl (C-II)	Inj 50 µg/mL	0.05–0.1	—	1–2	↓	no
Various	SR Patch 25, 50, 75, 100 µg/hr			(patch, 72)		
	Lozenge 200, 300, 400 µg.					
Hydrocodone and Acetaminophen (C-III)	Tab 2.5, 5, 7.5 mg with acetaminophen 500 mg, 7.5 mg with acetamino-phen 750 mg, 10 mg with acetaminophen 650 mg	—	—	4–8	—	no
Vicodin	Cap 5 mg with acetaminophen 500 mg	[5]				
Various	Soln 0.5 mg/mL with acetaminophen 24 mg/mL.					

(continued)

OPIOID ANALGESICS COMPARISON CHART (continued)

DRUG AND SCHEDULE[a]	DOSAGE FORMS	EQUIVALENT IM DOSAGE[b] (MG)	PARENTERAL/ORAL EFFICACY RATIO	DURATION OF ANALGESIA (HOURS)	CARDIAC WORKLOAD	PARTIAL ANTAGONIST ACTIVITY
Hydromorphone (C-II) Dilaudid Various	Inj 1, 2, 3, 4, 10 mg/mL Tab 1, 2, 3, 4, 8 mg/mL Soln 1 mg/mL Supp 3 mg.	1.5 [1]	1/5–1/2	3–5	→	no
Levorphanol (C-II) Levo-Dromoran	Inj 2 mg/mL Tab 2 mg.	2	1/2	4–6	→	no
Meperidine (C-II) Demerol Various	Inj 10, 25, 50, 75, 100 mg/mL Tab 50, 100 mg Syrup 10 mg/mL.	75–100 [50]	1/3–1/2	2–4	→	no
Methadone (C-II) Dolophine Various	Inj 10 mg/mL Tab 5, 10 mg Dispersible Tab 40 mg Soln 1, 2, 10 mg/mL.	10 [3]	1/2	4–6	→	no
Morphine (C-II) Various	Inj 0.5, 1, 2, 3, 4, 5, 8, 10, 15, 25, 50 mg/mL Tab 10, 15, 30 mg Soln 2, 4, 20 mg/mL SR Cap 20, 50, 100 mg SR Tab 15, 30, 60, 100, 200 mg Supp 5, 10, 20, 30 mg.	10 [9]	1/6–1/3	3–5	→	no
Nalbuphine (NC) Nubain Various	Inj 10, 20 mg/mL.	10	1/6	3–6	→	yes

(continued)

OPIOID ANALGESICS COMPARISON CHART (continued)

DRUG AND SCHEDULE[a]	DOSAGE FORMS	EQUIVALENT IM DOSAGE[b] (MG)	PARENTERAL/ORAL EFFICACY RATIO	DURATION OF ANALGESIA (HOURS)	CARDIAC WORKLOAD	PARTIAL ANTAGONIST ACTIVITY
Oxycodone (C-II)	Tab 5 mg	—	1/2	3–4	↓	no
Oxycontin	Soln 1, 20 mg/mL	[5]				
Roxicodone	SR Tab 10, 20, 40 mg.					
Oxymorphone (C-II)	Inj 1, 1.5 mg/mL.	1–1.5	1/6	4–5	↓	no
Numorphan	Supp 5 mg.					
Pentazocine (C-IV)	Inj 30 mg/mL.	30–60	1/3	2–3	↑	yes
Talwin	Tab 50 mg with	[25]				
Talwin Nx	naloxone 0.5 mg.					
Propoxyphene (C-IV)	Cap (HCl) 32, 65 mg	—	—	4–6	—	no
Darvon	Tab (Napsylate) 100 mg	[65 HCl]				
Various	Susp (Napsylate) 10 mg/mL.	[100 Napsylate]				
Sufentanil (C-II)	Inj 50 µg/mL.	0.02	—	2.5–3.5	↓	no
Sufenta						
Tramadol (NC)	Tab 50 mg.	—	3/4	4–6	—	?
Ultram		[25]				

KEY: ↑ = increased, ↓ = decreased, 0 = no change, ? = not well defined, needs more study.
[a]Controlled Substance Schedule designated after each drug (in parentheses); NC = Not Controlled.
[b]Except as noted in c, doses in brackets are oral doses equivalent to about 30 mg of oral codeine; because of individual variability in bioavailability, equivalent doses may differ between patients.
[c]Equivalent sublingual dose.
[d]Recommended dosage is one spray in one nostril, repeated prn in 60–90 min; this cycle may then be repeated q 3–4 hr prn pain.
From references 58, 60, 63–66, 94, 95, 98–101 and product information.

■ REFERENCES

1. Wyss A et al. Pharmacokinetic investigation of oral and IV dihydroergotamine in healthy subjects. *J Clin Pharmacol* 1991;41:597–602.
2. Raskin NH. Repetitive intravenous dihydroergotamine as therapy for intractable migraine. *Neurology* 1986;36:995–7.
3. Perrin VL. Clinical pharmacokinetics of ergotamine in migraine and cluster headache. *Clin Pharmacokinet* 1985;10:334–52.
4. Sanders SM et al. Pharmacokinetics of ergotamine in healthy volunteers following oral and rectal dosing. *Eur J Clin Pharmacol* 1986;30:331-4.
5. Ibraheem JJ et al. Kinetics of ergotamine after intravenous and intramuscular administration to migraine sufferers. *Eur J Clin Pharmacol* 1982;23:235–40.
6. Saper JR. Ergotamine dependency a review. *Headache* 1987;27:435–8.
7. The Multinational Oral Sumatriptan and Cafergot Comparative Study Group. A randomized, double-blind comparison of sumatriptan and Cafergot in the acute treatment of migraine. *Eur Neurol* 1991;31:314–22.
8. Hering R, Kuritzky A. Sodium valproate in the prophylactic treatment of migraine: a double-blind study versus placebo. *Cephalalgia* 1992;12:81–4.
9. Bredberg U et al. Pharmacokinetics of methysergide and its metabolite methylergometrine in man. *Eur J Clin Pharmacol* 1986;30:75–7.
10. Dechant KL, Clissold SP. Sumatriptan. A review of its pharmacodynamic and pharmacokinetic properties, and therapeutic efficacy in the acute treatment of migraine and cluster headache. *Drugs* 1992;43:776–98.
11. Plosker GL, McTavish D. Sumatriptan. A reappraisal of its pharmacology and therapeutic efficacy in the acute treatment of migraine and cluster headache. *Drugs* 1994;47:622–51.
12. Cady RK et al. Treatment of acute migraine with subcutaneous sumatriptan. *JAMA* 1991;265:2831–5.
13. Ferrari et al. Oral sumatriptan: effect of a second dose, and incidence and treatment of headache recurrences. *Cephalalgia* 1994;14:330–8.
14. The Subcutaneous Sumatriptan International Study Group. Treatment of migraine attacks with sumatriptan. *N Engl J Med* 1991;325:316–21.
15. Lacey LF et al. Single dose pharmacokinetics of sumatriptan in healthy volunteers. *Eur J Clin Pharmacol* 1995;47:543–8.
16. Fowler PA et al. The clinical pharmacology, pharmacokinetics and metabolism of sumatriptan. *Eur Neurol* 1991;31:291–4.
17. Dixon CM et al. Disposition of sumatriptan in laboratory animals and humans. *Drug Metab Dispos Biol Fate Chem* 1993;21:761–9.
18. Benet LZ et al. Design and optimization of dosage regimens: pharmacokinetic data. In Hardman JG et al., eds. *Goodman and Gilman's the pharmacological basis of therapeutics,* 9th ed. New York: McGraw-Hill; 1996:1707–92.
19. Wojnarhorton RE et al. Distribution and excretion of sumatriptan in human milk. *Br J Clin Pharmacol* 1996;41:217–21.
20. Insel PA. Analgesic-antipyretic and antiinflammatory agents and drugs employed in the treatment of gout. In Hardman JG et al., eds. *Goodman and Gilman's the pharmacological basis of therapeutics,* 9th ed. New York: McGraw-Hill; 1996: 617–57.
21. Segasothy M et al. Paracetamol: a cause for analgesic nephropathy and end-stage renal disease. *Nephron* 1988;50:50–4.
22. Zimmerman HJ, Maddrey WC. Acetaminophen (paracetamol) hepatotoxicity with regular intake of alcohol: analysis of instances of therapeutic misadventure. *Hepatology* 1995;22:767–73.
23. Bradley JD et al. Comparison of an antiinflammatory dose of ibuprofen, an analgesic dose of ibuprofen, and acetaminophen in the treatment of patients with osteoarthritis of the knee. *N Engl J Med* 1991;325:87–91.
24. Hirsh J et al. Aspirin and other platelet-active drugs. The relationship among dose, effectiveness, and side effects. *Chest* 1995;108:247S–57S.
25. Sherman DG et al. Antithrombotic therapy for cerebrovascular disorders. An update. *Chest* 1995; 108:444S–56S.
26. Cairns JA et al. Antithrombotic agents in coronary artery disease. *Chest* 1995;108:380–400S.
27. Stein PD et al. Antithrombotic therapy in patients with saphenous vein and internal mammary artery bypass grafts. *Chest* 1995;108:424S–30S.
28. Laupacis A et al. Antithrombotic therapy in atrial fibrillation. *Chest* 1995;108:352S–59S.
29. Mongan E et al. Tinnitus as an indication of therapeutic serum salicylate levels. *JAMA* 1973;226:142–5.
30. Done AK. Aspirin-overdosage: incidence, diagnosis, and management. *Pediatrics* 1978;62(suppl):890–7.
31. Levy G. Pharmacokinetics of salicylate elimination in man. *J Pharm Sci* 1965;54:959–67.
32. Levy G, Yaffe SJ. Clinical implications of salicylate-induced liver damage. *Am J Dis Child* 1975;129:1385–6.

33. Jusko WJ, Gretch M. Plasma and tissue protein binding of drugs in pharmacokinetics. *Drug Metab Rev* 1976;5:43–40.

34. Stevenson DD, Mathison DA. Aspirin sensitivity in asthmatics. When may this drug be safe? *Postgrad Med* 1985;78:111–9.

35. Bonica JJ, ed. *The management of pain*, 2nd ed. Philadelphia: Lea & Febiger; 1990.

36. Rahwan GL, Rahwan RG. Aspirin and Reye's syndrome: the change in prescribing habits of health professionals. *Drug Intell Clin Pharm* 1986;20:143–5.

37. Pinsky PF et al. Reye's syndrome and aspirin: evidence for a dose-response effect. *JAMA* 1988;260:657–61.

38. Housholder GT. Intolerance to aspirin and the nonsteroidal anti-inflammatory drugs. *J Oral Maxillofac Surg* 1985;43:333–7.

39. Lanza FL et al. Endoscopic evaluation of the effects of aspirin, buffered aspirin, and enteric-coated aspirin on gastric and duodenal mucosa. *N Engl J Med* 1980;303:136–8.

40. Hall AH et al. Ibuprofen overdose-a prospective study. *West J Med* 1988;148:653–6.

41. Nahata MC et al. Pharmacokinetics of ibuprofen in febrile children. *Eur J Clin Pharmacol* 1991;40:427–8.

42. Hollander D. Gastrointestinal complications of nonsteroidal anti-inflammatory drugs: prophylactic and therapeutic strategies. *Am J Med* 1994;96:274–81.

43. Whelton A et al. Renal effects of ibuprofen, piroxicam, and sulindac in patients with asymptomatic renal failure. *Ann Intern Med* 1990;112:568–76.

44. Stempel DA, Miller JJ. Lymphopenia and hepatotoxicity with ibuprofen. *J Pediatr* 1977;90:657–8.

45. Bernstein RF. Ibuprofen-related meningitis in mixed connective tissue disease. *Ann Intern Med* 1980;92:206–7.

46. Maniglia R et al. Non-steroidal antiinflammatory nephrotoxicity. *Ann Clin Lab Sci* 1988;18:240-52.

47. Brezin JH et al. Reversible renal failure and nephrotic syndrome associated with nonsteroidal anti-inflammatory drugs. *N Engl J Med* 1979;301:1271–3.

48. Halasz CL. Photosensitivity to the nonsteroidal anti-inflammatory drug piroxicam. *Cutis* 1987;39:37–9.

49. Paulus HE. FDA Arthritis Advisory Committee meeting: postmarketing surveillance of nonsteroidal antiinflammatory drugs. *Arthritis Rheum* 1985;28:1168–9.

50. Hart FD, Huskisson EC. Non-steroidal anti-inflammatory drugs. Current status and rational therapeutic use. *Drugs* 1984;27:232–55.

51. Marsh CC et al. A review of selected investigational nonsteroidal antiinflammatory drugs of the 1980s. *Pharmacotherapy* 1986;6:10–25.

52. Litvak KM, McEvoy GK. Ketorolac, an injectable nonnarcotic analgesic. *Clin Pharm* 1990;9:921–35.

53. Brooks PM, Day RO. Nonsteroidal antiinflammatory drugs—differences and similarities. *N Engl J Med* 1991;324:1716–25.

54. Helfgott SM et al. Diclofenac-associated hepatotoxicity. *JAMA* 1990;264:2660–2.

55. Middleton E Jr et al., eds. *Allergy principles and practice*, 3rd ed. St. Louis: CV Mosby; 1988.

56. Quercia RA, Ruderman M. Focus on nabumetone: a new chemically distinct nonsteroidal antiinflammatory agent. *Hosp Formul* 1991;26:25–34.

57. Noble S, Balfour JA. Meloxicam. *Drugs* 1996;51:424–30.

58. Reisine T, Pasternak G. Opioid Analgesics and Antagonists. In, Hardman JG et al., eds. *Goodman and Gilman's the pharmacological basis of therapeutics*, 9th ed. New York: McGraw-Hill; 1996:521-55.

59. Way WL. Opioid analgesics and antagonists. In Katzung BG, ed. *Basic and clinical pharmacology*, 6th ed. Norwalk, CT: Appleton & Lange; 1995:460–75.

60. Bonica JJ, ed. *The management of pain*, 2nd ed. Philadelphia: Lea & Febiger; 1990.

61. Schmerzier E et al. Gas chromatographic determination of codeine in serum and urine. *J Pharm Sci* 1966;55:155–7.

62. Way EL, Adler TK. The pharmacologic implications of the fate of morphine and its surrogates. *Pharmacol Rev* 1968;12:383–446.

63. Bowdle TA et al., eds. *The pharmacologic basis of anesthesiology*, 1st ed. New York: Churchill Livingstone; 1994.

64. Donnelly AJ. Pharmacology of pain management agents. *Anesthesia Today* 1989;1:6–10.

65. Gourlay GK et al. The transdermal administration of fentanyl in the treatment of postoperative pain: pharmacokinetics and pharmacodynamic effects. *Pain* 1989;37:193–202.

66. Edwards DJ et al. Clinical pharmacokinetics of pethidine: 1982. *Clin Pharmacokinet* 1982;7:421–33.

67. Fochtman FW, Winek CL. Therapeutic serum concentrations of meperidine (Demerol). *J Forensic Sci* 1969;14:213–8.

68. Klotz U et al. The effect of cirrhosis on the disposition and elimination of meperidine in man. *Clin Pharmacol Ther* 1974;16:667–75.

69. Julius HC et al. Meperidine binding to isolated alpha$_1$-acid glycoprotein and albumin. *DICP* 1989;23:568–72.

70. McHorse TS et al. Effect of acute viral hepatitis in man on the disposition and elimination of meperidine. *Gastroenterology* 1975;68:775–80.
71. Tang R et al. Meperidine-induced seizures in sickle cell patients. *Hosp Formul* 1980;15:764–72.
72. Clark RF et al. Meperidine: therapeutic use and toxicity. *J Emerg Med* 1995;13:797–802.
73. Quinn DI, Day RO. Drug interactions of clinical importance. An updated guide. *Drug Saf* 1995;12:393–452.
74. Fultz JM, Senay EC. Guidelines for the management of hospitalized narcotic addicts. *Ann Intern Med* 1975;82:815–8.
75. Holmstrand J et al. Methadone maintenance: plasma levels and therapeutic outcome. *Clin Pharmacol Ther* 1978;23:175–80.
76. Berkowitz BA. The relationship of pharmacokinetics to pharmacological activity: morphine, methadone and naloxone. *Clin Pharmacokinet* 1976;1:219–30.
77. Beauclair TR, Stoner CP. Adherence to guidelines for continuous morphine sulfate infusions. *Am J Hosp Pharm* 1986;43:671–6.
78. Holmes AH. Morphine IV infusion for chronic pain. *Drug Intell Clin Pharm* 1978;12:556–7.
79. White P. Use of patient-controlled analgesia for management of acute pain. *JAMA* 1988;259:243–7.
80. Baumann TJ et al. Patient-controlled analgesia in the terminally ill cancer patient. *Drug Intell Clin Pharm* 1986;20:297–301.
81. Kerr IG et al. Continuous narcotic infusion with patient-controlled analgesia for chronic cancer pain in outpatients. *Ann Intern Med* 1988;108:554–7.
82. Berkowitz BA et al. The disposition of morphine in surgical patients. *Clin Pharmacol Ther* 1975;17:629–35.
83. Masood AR, Thomas SHL. Systemic absorption of nebulized morphine compared with oral morphine in healthy subjects. *Br J Clin Pharmacol* 1996;41:250–2.
84. Glare PA, Walsh TD. Clinical pharmacokinetics of morphine. *Ther Drug Monit* 1991;13:1–23.
85. Stanski DR et al. Kinetics of intravenous and intramuscular morphine. *Clin Pharmacol Ther* 1978;24:52–9.
86. Chamberlain JM, Klein BL. A comprehensive review of naloxone for the emergency physician. *Am J Emerg Med* 1994;12:650–60.
87. Longnecker DE et al. Naloxone for antagonism of morphine-induced respiratory depression. *Anesth Analg* 1973;52:447–53.
88. Evans JM et al. Degree and duration of reversal by naloxone of effects of morphine in conscious subjects. *Br Med J* 1974;2:589–91.
89. Fishman J et al. Disposition of naloxone-7,8-^{3}H in normal and narcotic-dependent men. *J Pharmacol Exp Ther* 1973;187:575–80.
90. Vozeh S et al. Pharmacokinetic drug data. *Clin Pharmacokinet* 1988;15:254–82.
91. Ngai SH et al. Pharmacokinetics of naloxone in rats and in man: basis for its potency and short duration of action. *Anesthesiology* 1976;44:398–401.
92. Stile IL et al. The pharmacokinetics of naloxone in the premature newborn. *Dev Pharmacol Ther* 1987;10:454–9.
93. Tandberg D, Abercrombie D. Treatment of heroin overdose with endotracheal naloxone. *Ann Emerg Med* 1982;11:443–5.
94. Schoenle JR, Mullins PM. Dezocine. *P&T* 1990;(Nov):1357–70.
95. Anon. Tramadol-a new oral analgesic. *Med Lett Drugs Ther* 1995;37:59–60.
96. Brogden RN et al. Pentazocine: a review of its pharmacologic properties, therapeutics, efficacy and dependence liability. *Drugs* 1973;5:6–91.
97. Reed DA, Schnoll SH. Abuse of pentazocine-naloxone combination. *JAMA* 1986;256:2562–4.
98. Gourlay GK, Cousins MJ. Strong analgesics in severe pain. *Drugs* 1984;28:79–91.
99. Miller RR. Evaluation of nalbuphine hydrochloride. *Am J Hosp Pharm* 1980;37:942–9.
100. Ameer B, Salter FJ. Drug therapy reviews: evaluation of butorphanol tartrate. *Am J Hosp Pharm* 1979;36:1683–91.
101. Dayer P et al. The pharmacology of tramadol. *Drugs* 1994;47(suppl 1):3–7.

Antimicrobial Drugs

Antibacterial Drugs of Choice

INFECTING ORGANISM	DRUG OF FIRST CHOICE	ALTERNATIVE DRUGS
GRAM-POSITIVE COCCI		
***Enterococcus*[1]**		
Endocarditis or other severe infection	Penicillin G or ampicillin + gentamicin or streptomycin	Vancomycin + gentamicin or streptomycin; teicoplanin[2], quinupristin/dalfopristin[3]
Uncomplicated urinary tract infection	Ampicillin or amoxicillin	Nitrofurantoin; a fluoroquinolone[4]
Staphylococcus aureus* or *epidermidis		
Non-penicillinase-producing	Penicillin G or V[5]	A cephalosporin;[6,7] vancomycin; imipenem; clindamycin; a fluoroquinolone[4]
Penicillinase-producing	A penicillinase-resistant penicillin[8]	A cephalosporin;[6,7] vancomycin; amoxicillin/clavulanic acid; ticarcillin/clavulanic acid; piperacillin/tazobactam; ampicillin/sulbactam; imipenem; clindamycin; a fluoroquinolone[4]
Methicillin-resistant[9]	Vancomycin ± gentamicin ± rifampin	Trimethoprim-sulfamethoxazole; a fluoroquinolone;[4] minocycline[10]
***Streptococcus pyogenes* (group A) and groups C and G[11]**	Penicillin G or V[5]	Clindamycin; erythromycin; a cephalosporin;[6,7] vancomycin; clarithromycin;[12] azithromycin
***Streptococcus*, group B**	Penicillin G or ampicillin	A cephalosporin;[6,7] vancomycin; erythromycin
***Streptococcus*, viridans group[1]**	Penicillin G ± gentamicin	A cephalosporin;[6,7] vancomycin
Streptococcus bovis[1]	Penicillin G	A cephalosporin;[6,7] vancomycin
Streptococcus*, anaerobic or *Peptostreptococcus	Penicillin G	Clindamycin; a cephalosporin;[6,7] vancomycin
***Streptococcus pneumoniae*[13] (pneumococcus)**	Penicillin G or V[5,13]	A cephalosporin;[6,7] erythromycin; vancomycin ± rifampin; trimethoprim-sulfamethoxazole; azithromycin; clarithromycin;[12] clindamycin; chloramphenicol;[14] a tetracycline;[10] quinupristin/dalfopristin
GRAM-NEGATIVE COCCI		
Moraxella* (*Branhamella*) *catarrhalis	Trimethoprim-sulfamethoxazole	Amoxicillin/clavulanic acid; erythromycin; clarithromycin;[12] azithromycin; a tetracycline;[10] cefuroxime;[6] cefotaxime;[6] ceftizoxime;[6] ceftriaxone;[6] cefuroxime axetil;[6] cefixime;[5] a fluoroquinolone[4]

(continued)

INFECTING ORGANISM	DRUG OF FIRST CHOICE	ALTERNATIVE DRUGS
Neisseria gonorrhoeae (gonococcus)	Ceftriaxone[6] or cefixime[6]	Cefotaxime;[6] a fluoroquinolone;[4] spectinomycin; penicillin G
Neisseria meningitidis[15] (meningococcus)	Penicillin G	Cefotaxime;[6] ceftizoxime;[6] ceftriaxone;[6] chloramphenicol;[14] a sulfonamide[16]

GRAM-POSITIVE BACILLI

Bacillus anthracis (anthrax)	Penicillin G	An erythromycin; a tetracycline[10]
Bacillus cereus, subtilis	Vancomycin	Imipenem; clindamycin
Clostridium perfringens[17]	Penicillin G	Clindamycin; metronidazole; imipenem; a tetracycline;[10] chloramphenicol[14]
Clostridium tetani[18]	Penicillin G	A tetracycline[10]
Clostridium difficile[19]	Metronidazole	Vancomycin; bacitracin
Corynebacterium diphtheriae[20]	An erythromycin	Penicillin G
Corynebacterium, JK group	Vancomycin	Penicillin G + gentamicin; erythromycin
Listeria monocytogenes	Ampicillin ± gentamicin	Trimethoprim-sulfamethoxazole

ENTERIC GRAM-NEGATIVE BACILLI
*Bacteroides

Oropharyngeal strains[21, 22]	Penicillin G or clindamycin	Cefoxitin;[6] metronidazole; chloramphenicol;[14] cefotetan;[6] ampicillin/sulbactam
Gastrointestinal strains	Metronidazole	Clindamycin; imipenem; ticarcillin/clavulanic acid; piperacillin/tazobactam; cefoxitin;[6] cefotetan;[6] ampicillin/sulbactam; piperacillin; chloramphenicol;[14] ceftizoxime;[6] cefmetazole[6]
*Campylobacter fetus	Imipenem	Gentamicin
*Campylobacter jejuni	A fluoroquinolone[4] or erythromycin	A tetracycline;[10] gentamicin
*Enterobacter	Imipenem[23]	Cefotaxime,[6,23] ceftizoxime,[6,23] ceftriaxone,[6,23] or ceftazidime;[6,23] gentamicin, tobramycin, or amikacin; trimethoprim-sulfamethoxazole; ticarcillin,[24] mezlocillin,[24] or piperacillin;[24] aztreonam;[23] a fluoroquinolone[4]
*Escherichia coli[25]	Cefotaxime, ceftizoxime, ceftriaxone or ceftazidime[6,23]	Ampicillin ± gentamicin, tobramycin, or amikacin; carbenicillin;[24] ticarcillin,[24] mezlocillin,[24] or piperacillin;[24] gentamicin, tobramycin, or amikacin; amoxicillin/clavulanic acid;[23] ticarcillin/clavulanic acid;[24] piperacillin/tazobactam;[24] ampicillin/sulbactam;[23] trimethoprim-sulfamethoxazole; imipenem;[23] aztreonam;[23] a fluoroquinolone;[4] another cephalosporin.[6,7]

(continued)

INFECTING ORGANISM	DRUG OF FIRST CHOICE	ALTERNATIVE DRUGS
*Helicobacter pylori[26]	Tetracycline HCl[10] + metronidazole + bismuth subsalicylate	Tetracycline HCl + clarithromycin[12] + bismuth subsalicylate; amoxicillin + metronidazole + bismuth subsalicylate
*Klebsiella pneumoniae[25]	Cefotaxime, ceftizoxime, ceftriaxone, or ceftazidime[6,23]	Imipenem;[23] gentamicin, tobramycin, or amikacin; amoxicillin/clavulanic acid;[23] ticarcillin/clavulanic acid;[24] piperacillin/tazobactam;[24] ampicillin/sulbactam;[23] trimethoprim-sulfamethoxazole; aztreonam;[23] a fluoroquinolone;[4] mezlocillin[24] or piperacillin;[24] another cephalosporin[6,7]
*Proteus mirabilis[25]	Ampicillin[27]	A cephalosporin;[6,7,23] ticarcillin,[24] mezlocillin,[24] or piperacillin;[24] gentamicin, tobramycin, or amikacin; trimethoprim-sulfamethoxazole; imipenem;[23] aztreonam;[23] a fluoroquinolone;[4] chloramphenicol[14]
*Proteus, indole-positive (including *Providencia rettgeri,* *Morganella morganii,* and *Proteus vulgaris*)	Cefotaxime, ceftizoxime, ceftriaxone, or ceftazidime[6,23]	Imipenem;[23] gentamicin, tobramycin, or amikacin; carbenicillin,[24] ticarcillin,[24] mezlocillin,[24] or piperacillin;[24] amoxicillin/clavulanic acid;[23] ticarcillin/clavulanic acid;[24] piperacillin/tazobactam;[24] ampicillin/sulbactam;[23] aztreonam;[23] trimethoprim-sulfamethoxazole; a fluoroquinolone[4]
*Providencia stuartii	Cefotaxime, ceftizoxime, ceftriaxone or ceftazidime[6,23]	Imipenem;[23] ticarcillin/clavulanic acid;[24] piperacillin/tazobactam;[24] gentamicin, tobramycin, or amikacin; carbenicillin;[24] ticarcillin,[24] mezlocillin,[24] or piperacillin;[24] aztreonam;[23] trimethoprim-sulfamethoxazole; a fluoroquinolone[4]
*Salmonella typhi[28]	A fluoroquinolone[4] or ceftriaxone[6]	Chloramphenicol;[14] trimethoprim-sulfamethoxazole; ampicillin; amoxicillin
*other Salmonella[29]	Cefotaxime[6] or ceftriaxone[6] or a fluoroquinolone[4]	Ampicillin or amoxicillin; trimethoprim-sulfamethoxazole; chloramphenicol[14]
*Serratia	Cefotaxime, ceftizoxime, ceftriaxone or ceftazidime[6,30]	Gentamicin or amikacin; imipenem;[30] aztreonam;[30] trimethoprim-sulfamethoxazole; carbenicillin,[31] ticarcillin,[31] mezlocillin,[31] or piperacillin;[31] a fluoroquinolone[4]

(continued)

INFECTING ORGANISM	DRUG OF FIRST CHOICE	ALTERNATIVE DRUGS
Shigella	A fluoroquinolone[4]	Trimethoprim-sulfamethoxazole; ampicillin; ceftriaxone[6]
Yersinia enterocolitica	Trimethoprim-sulfamethoxazole	A fluoroquinolone;[4] gentamicin, tobramycin, or amikacin; cefotaxime or ceftizoxime[6]

OTHER GRAM-NEGATIVE BACILLI

Acinetobacter	Imipenem[23]	Amikacin, tobramycin, or gentamicin; ticarcillin,[24] mezlocillin,[24] or piperacillin;[24] ceftazidime;[23] trimethoprim-sulfamethoxazole; a fluoroquinolone;[4] minocycline;[10] doxycycline[10]
Aeromonas	Trimethoprim-sulfamethoxazole	Gentamicin or tobramycin; imipenem; a fluoroquinolone[4]
Bartonella		
Agent of bacillary angiomatosis (Bartonella henselae or quintana)[32]	An erythromycin	Doxycycline[10]
Cat scratch bacillus (Bartonella henselae)[32,33]	Ciprofloxacin[34]	Trimethoprim-sulfamethoxazole; gentamicin; rifampin
Bordetella pertussis (whooping cough)	An erythromycin	Trimethoprim-sulfamethoxazole; ampicillin
Brucella	A tetracycline[10] + streptomycin or gentamicin	A tetracycline[10] + rifampin; chloramphenicol[14] ± streptomycin; trimethoprim-sulfamethoxazole ± gentamicin; rifampin + a tetracycline[10]
Burkholderia cepacia	Trimethoprim-sulfamethoxazole	Ceftazidime;[6] chloramphenicol[14]
Calymmatobacterium granulomatis (granuloma inguinale)	A tetracycline[10]	Streptomycin or gentamicin; trimethoprim-sulfamethoxazole; erythromycin
Eikenella corrodens	Ampicillin	An erythromycin; a tetracycline;[10] amoxicillin/clavulanic acid; ampicillin/sulbactam; ceftriaxone
Francisella tularensis (tularemia)	Streptomycin	Gentamicin; a tetracycline;[10] chloramphenicol[14]
Fusobacterium	Penicillin G	Metronidazole; clindamycin; cefoxitin;[6] chloramphenicol[14]
Gardnerella vaginalis (bacterial vaginosis)	Oral metronidazole[35]	Topical clindamycin or metronidazole; oral clindamycin
Haemophilus ducreyi (chancroid)	Erythromycin or ceftriaxone or azithromycin	A fluoroquinolone[4]
Haemophilus influenzae		
Meningitis, epiglottitis, arthritis and other serious infections	Cefotaxime or ceftriaxone[6]	Cefuroxime[6] (but not for meningitis); chloramphenicol[14]

(continued)

INFECTING ORGANISM	DRUG OF FIRST CHOICE	ALTERNATIVE DRUGS
Upper respiratory infections and bronchitis	Trimethoprim-sulfamethoxazole	Cefuroxime;[6] amoxicillin/clavulanic acid; cefuroxime axetil;[6] cefaclor;[6] cefotaxime;[6] ceftizoxime;[6] ceftriaxone;[6] cefixime;[6] ampicillin or amoxicillin; a tetracycline;[10] clarithromycin;[12] azithromycin; a fluoroquinolone[4]
Legionella species	Erythromycin ± rifampin	Clarithromycin;[12] azithromycin; ciprofloxacin;[34] trimethoprim-sulfamethoxazole
Leptotrichia buccalis	Penicillin G	A tetracycline;[10] clindamycin; erythromycin
Pasteurella multocida	Penicillin G	A tetracycline;[10] a cephalosporin;[6,7] amoxicillin/clavulanic acid; ampicillin/sulbactam
Pseudomonas aeruginosa Urinary tract infection	A fluoroquinolone[4]	Carbenicillin, ticarcillin, piperacillin, or mezlocillin; ceftazidime;[6] imipenem; aztreonam; tobramycin; gentamicin; amikacin
Other infections	Ticarcillin, mezlocillin, or piperacillin + tobramycin, gentamicin, or amikacin[36]	Ceftazidime,[6] imipenem or aztreonam + tobramycin, gentamicin, or amikacin; ciprofloxacin[34]
Pseudomonas mallei (glanders)	Streptomycin + a tetracycline[10]	Streptomycin + chloramphenicol[14]
Pseudomonas pseudomallei (melioidosis)	Ceftazidime[6]	Chloramphenicol[14] + doxycycline[10] + trimethoprim-sulfamethoxazole; amoxicillin/clavulanic acid; imipenem
Spirillum minus (rat bite fever)	Penicillin G	A tetracycline;[10] streptomycin
Stenotrophomonas maltophilia (Pseudomonas maltophilia)	Trimethoprim-sulfamethoxazole	Minocycline;[10] ceftazidime;[6] a fluoroquinolone[4]
Steptobacillus moniliformis (rat bite fever; Haverhill fever)	Penicillin G	A tetracycline;[10] streptomycin
Vibrio cholerae (cholera)[37]	A tetracycline[10]	Trimethoprim-sulfamethoxazole; a fluoroquinolone[4]
Vibrio vulnificus	A tetracycline[10]	Cefotaxime[6]
Yersinia pestis (plague)	Streptomycin	A tetracycline;[10] chloramphenicol;[14] gentamicin

ACID FAST BACILLI

Mycobacterium tuberculosis[38]	Isoniazid + rifampin + pyrazinamide ± ethambutol or streptomycin[14]	Ciprofloxacin or ofloxacin;[34] cycloserine;[14] capreomycin[14] or kanamycin[14] or amikacin;[14] ethionamide;[14] clofazimine;[14] aminosalicylic acid[14]

(continued)

IINFECTING ORGANISM	DRUG OF FIRST CHOICE	ALTERNATIVE DRUGS
Mycobacterium kansasii	Isoniazid + rifampin ± ethambutol or streptomycin[14]	Clarithromycin;[12] ethionamide;[14] cycloserine[14]
Mycobacterium avium complex	Clarithromycin[12] or azithromycin + one or more of the following: ethambutol; rifabutin; ciprofloxacin[34]	Rifampin; clofazimine;[14] amikacin[14]
Prophylaxis	Rifabutin or clarithromycin[12]	Azithromycin
Mycobacterium fortuitum complex	Amikacin + doxycycline[10]	Cefoxitin;[6] rifampin; a sulfonamide
Mycobacterium marinum (balnei)[39]	Minocycline[10]	Trimethoprim-sulfamethoxazole; rifampin; clarithromycin;[12] doxycycline[10]
Mycobacterium leprae (leprosy)	Dapsone + rifampin ± clofazimine	Minocycline;[10] ofloxacin;[34,40] sparfloxacin;[41] clarithromycin[12,42]

ACTINOMYCETES

Actinomyces israelii (actinomycosis)	Penicillin G	A tetracycline;[10] erythromycin; clindamycin
Nocardia	Trimethoprim-sulfamethoxazole	Sulfisoxazole; amikacin;[14] a tetracycline;[10] imipenem; cycloserine[14]

CHLAMYDIAE

Chlamydia psittaci (psittacosis; ornithosis)	A tetracycline[10]	Chloramphenicol[14]
Chlamydia trachomatis (trachoma)	Azithromycin	A tetracycline[10] (topical plus oral); A sulfonamide (topical plus oral)
(inclusion conjunctivitis)	Erythromycin (oral or IV)	A sulfonamide
(pneumonia)	Erythromycin	A sulfonamide
(urethritis, cervicitis)	Doxycycline[10] or azithromycin	Erythromycin; ofloxacin;[34] sulfisoxazole; amoxicillin
(lymphogranuloma venereum)	A tetracycline[10]	Erythromycin
Chlamydia pneumoniae (TWAR strain)	A tetracycline[10]	Erythromycin; clarithromycin;[12] azithromycin

EHRLICHIA

Ehrlichia chaffeensis	A tetracycline[10]	
Agent of human granulocytic ehrlichiosis[43]	A tetracycline[10]	

MYCOPLASMA

Mycoplasma pneumoniae	Erythromycin or a tetracycline[10]	Clarithromycin;[12] azithromycin
Ureaplasma urealyticum	Erythromycin	A tetracycline;[10] clarithromycin[12]

(*continued*)

INFECTING ORGANISM	DRUG OF FIRST CHOICE	ALTERNATIVE DRUGS
RICKETTSIA		
Rocky Mountain spotted fever, endemic typhus (murine), epidemic typhus (louse-borne), scrub typhus, trench fever, Q fever	A tetracycline[10]	Chloramphenicol;[14] a fluoroquinolone[4]
SPIROCHETES		
Borrelia burgdorferi (Lyme disease)[44]	Doxycycline[10] or amoxicillin	Cefuroxime axetil;[6] ceftriaxone;[6] cefotaxime;[6] penicillin G; azithromycin; clarithromycin[12]
Borrelia recurrentis (relapsing fever)	A tetracycline[10]	Penicillin G
Leptospira	Penicillin G	A tetracycline[10]
Treponema pallidum (syphilis)	Penicillin G[5]	A tetracycline;[10] ceftriaxone[6]
Treponema pertenue (yaws)	Penicillin G	A tetracycline[10]

*Resistance may be a problem; susceptibility tests should be performed.

1. Disk sensitivity testing may not provide adequate information; beta-lactamase assays and dilution tests for susceptibility should be used in serious infections.

2. An investigational drug in the US (*Targocid* - Hoechst Marion Roussel).

3. An investigational drug in the US available through Rhone-Poulenc Rorer (610-454-3071).

4. For most infections, ofloxacin or ciprofloxacin. For urinary tract infections, norfloxacin, lomefloxacin, or enoxacin can be used. Ciprofloxacin and ofloxacin are available for intravenous use. None of these agents is recommended for children or pregnant women.

5. Penicillin V is preferred for oral treatment of infections caused by non-penicillinase-producing staphylococci and other gram-positive cocci. For initial therapy of severe infections, penicillin G, administered parenterally, is first choice. For somewhat longer action in less severe infections caused by group A streptococci, pneumococci, or *Treponema pallidum*, procaine penicillin G, an intramuscular formulation, is given once or twice daily. Benzathine penicillin G. a slowly absorbed preparation, is usually given in a single monthly injection for prophylaxis of rheumatic fever, once for treatment of Group A streptococcal pharyngitis and once or more for treatment of syphilis.

6. The cephalosporins have been used as alternatives to penicillins in patients allergic to penicillins, but such patients may also have allergic reactions to cephalosporins.

7. For parenteral treatment of staphylococcal or non-enterococcal streptococcal infections, a "first-generation" cephalosporin such as cephalothin or cefazolin can be used; for staphylococcal endocarditis, some *Medical Letter* consultants prefer cephalothin. For oral therapy, cephalexin or cephradine can be used. The "second-generation" cephalosporins cefamandole, cefprozil, cefuroxime, cefuroxime axetil, cefonicid, cefotetan, cefmetazole, cefoxitin, and loracarbef are more active than the first-generation drugs against Gram-negative bacteria. Cefuroxime and cefamandole are active against ampicillin-resistant strains of *H. influenzae*, but cefamandole has been associated with prothrombin deficiency and occasional bleeding. Cefoxitin, cefotetan, and cefmetazole are active against *B. fragilis*, but cefotetan and cefmetazole have also been associated with prothrombin deficiency. The "third-generation" cephalosporins cefotaxime, cefoperazone, ceftizoxime, ceftriaxone, and ceftazidime have greater activity than the second-generation drugs against enteric Gram-negative bacilli. Ceftazidime has poor activity against many Gram-positive cocci and anaerobes, and ceftizoxime has poor activity against penicillin-resistant *S. pneumoniae* (DW Haas et al, *Clin Infect Dis*, 20:671, 1995. Cefixime and cefpodoxime are oral cephalosporins with more activity than second-generation cephalosporins against facultative Gram-negative bacilli; they have no useful activity against anaerobes or *Pseudomonas aeruginosa*, and cefixime has no useful activity against staphylococci. With the exception of cefoperazone (which, like cefamandole, can cause bleeding) and ceftazidime, the activity of all currently available cephalosporins against *Pseudomonas aeruginosa* is poor or inconsistent.

8. For oral use against penicillinase-producing staphylococci, cloxacillin or dicloxacillin is preferred; for severe infections, a parenteral formulation of nafcillin or oxacillin should be used. Ampicillin, amoxicillin, bacampicillin, carbenicillin, ticarcillin, mezlocillin, and piperacillin are not effective against penicillinase-producing staphylococci. The combinations of clavulanic acid with amoxicillin or ticarcillin, sulbactam with ampicillin, and tazobactam with piperacillin are active against these organisms.

9. Many strains of coagulase-positive staphylococci and coagulase-negative staphylococci are resistant to penicillinase-resistant penicillins; these strains are also resistant to cephalosporins and imipenem.

10. Tetracyclines are generally not recommended for pregnant women or children less than eight years old.

11. For serious soft-tissue infection due to group A streptococci, clindamycin may be more effective than penicillin. Group A streptococci may, however, be resistant to clindamycin; therefore, some *Medical Letter* consultants suggest using both clindamycin and penicillin to treat serious soft-tissue infections. Group A streptococci may also be resistant to erythromycin, azithromycin, and clarithromycin.

12. Not recommended for use in pregnancy.

13. Strains frequently show intermediate or high-level resistance to penicillin. Infections caused by strains with intermediate resistance to penicillin may respond to cefotaxime or ceftriaxone. Cafuroxime or high doses of penicillin may be effective for pneumonia. Highly resistant strains and, before susceptibility is known, all patients with meningitis should be treated with vancomycin with or without rifampin in addition to a cephalosporin. In patients allergic to penicillin, erythromycin, azithromycin or clarithromycin are often useful for respiratory infections, but vancomycin with or without rifampin is recommended for meningitis. Some strains of *S. pneumoniae* are resistant to erythromycin, clindamycin, trimethoprim-sulfamethoxazole, clarithromycin, azithromycin, and chloramphenicol. All strains tested so far are susceptible to quinupristin/dalfopristin.

14. Because of the possibility of serious adverse effects, this drug should be used only for severe infections when less hazardous drugs are ineffective.

15. Rare strains of *N. meningitidis* are resistant or relatively resistant to penicillin. Rifampin is recommended for prophylaxis in close contacts of patients infected by sulfonamide-resistant organisms.

16. Sulfonamide-resistant strains are frequent in the United States; sulfonamides should be used only when susceptibility is established by susceptibility tests.

17. Debridement is primary. Large doses of penicillin G are required. Hyperbaric oxygen therapy may be a useful adjunct to surgical debridement in management of the spreading, necrotic type.

18. For prophylaxis, a tetanus toxoid booster and, for some patients, tetanus immune globulin (human) are required.

19. In order to decrease the emergence of vancomycin-resistant enterococci in hospitals, many *Medical Letter* consultants now recommment use of metronidazole first in treatment of most patients with *C. difficile* colitis, with oral vancomycin used only for seriously ill patients or those who do not respond to metronidazole. Also see *Med Lett*, 31:94, 1989.

20. Antitoxin is primary; antimicrobials are used only to halt further toxin production and to prevent the carrier state.

21. *Bacteroides* species from the oropharynx may be resistant to penicillin; for patients seriously ill with infections that may be caused by these organisms, or when response to penicillin is delayed, clindamycin should be used.

22. When infection is in the central nervous system, metronidazole is generally recommended.

23. In severely ill patients, most *Medical Letter* consultants would add gentamicin, tobramycin, or amikacin.

24. In severely ill patients, most *Medical Letter* consultants would add gentamicin, tobramycin, or amikacin (but see footnote 36).

25. For an acute, uncomplicated urinary tract infection, before the infecting organism is known, the drug of first choice is trimethoprim-sulfamethoxazole.

26. Eradication of *H. pylori* with various antibacterial combinations, usually given concurrently with an H_2-receptor blocker or proton pump inhibitor has led to rapid healing of active peptic ulcers and low recurrence rates (JH Walsh and WL Peterson, *N Engl J Med*, 333:984, 1995).

27. Large doses ($\geq$6 g/day) are usually necessary for systemic infections. In severely ill patients, some *Medical Letter* consultants would add gentamicin, tobramycin, or amikacin.

28. Ampicillin or amoxicillin may be effective in milder cases. Ciprofloxiacin or amoxicillin is the drug of choice for *S. typhi* carriers.

29. Most cases of *Salmonella* gastroenteritis subside spontaneously without antimicrobial therapy.

30. In severely ill patients, most *Medical Letter* consultants would add gentamicin or amikacin.

31. In severely ill patients, most *Medical Letter* consultants would add gentamicin or amikacin (but see footnote 36).
32. KA Adal et al., *N Engl J Med*, 330:1509, 1994.
33. Role of antibiotics is not clear (AM Margileth, *Pediatr Infect Dis J*, 11:474, 1992).
34. Usually not recommended for use in children or pregnant women.
35. Metronidazole is effective for bacterial vaginosis even though it is not usually active against *Gardnerella* in vitro.
36. Neither gentamicin, tobramycin, netilmicin, or amikacin should be mixed in the same bottle with carbenicillin, ticarcillin, mezlocillin, or piperacillin for intravenous administration. When used in high doses or in patients with renal impairment, these penicillins may inactivate the aminoglycosides.
37. Antibiotic therapy is an adjunct to and not a substitute for prompt fluid and electrolyte replacement.
38. For more details, see *Medical Letter*, 37:67, 1995.
39. Most infections are self-limited without drug treatment.
40. B Ji et al., *Antimicrob Agents Chemother*, 38:662, 1994.
41. An investigational drug in the United States.
42. GP Chan et al., *Antimicrob Agents Chemother*, 38:515, 1994.
43. JS Bakken et al., *JAMA*, 272:212, 1994.
44. For treatment of early infection in nonpregnant adults, doxycycline is preferred; for fully developed infection with arthritis or meningitis, ceftriaxone is preferred.

From Anon. The choice of antibacterial drugs. Med Lett Drugs Ther 1996;38:25–34. Reproduced with permission.

Aminoglycosides

AMINOGLYCOSIDES

Pharmacology. Aminoglycosides are aminocyclitol derivatives that have concentration-dependent bactericidal activity against Gram-negative aerobic bacteria via binding to the interface between the 30S and 50S ribosomal subunits; anaerobic bacteria are universally resistant because aminoglycoside transport into cells is oxygen dependent. Dibasic cations (eg, magnesium and calcium) and acidic conditions decrease their in vitro action. Streptomycin and kanamycin have poor activity against some Gram-negative bacteria, especially *Pseudomonas aeruginosa*. Some Gram-positive organisms (eg, streptococci) are relatively resistant to all aminoglycosides; however, in combination with some penicillins or vancomycin, these organisms are often synergistically inhibited or killed. Aminoglycosides have a postantibiotic effect against Gram-negative bacteria, which can be exploited by using less frequent dosage intervals. Resistance is due to transferable plasmid-mediated enzymatic modification or decreased drug uptake.[1,2] (*See* Notes.)

Administration and Adult Dosage. **IM or IV by slow intermittent infusion over 30–60 min,** although 15-min infusions are safe. Newer dosage regimens combine the usual daily dosage into a **single IV infusion administered over 60 min.**[3,4] This method takes advantage of the concentration-related bactericidal effects and post-antibiotic effect of aminoglycosides, and may result in less toxicity.[2–4] **Intrathecal or intraventricular** administration is usually necessary to achieve therapeutic CSF levels. (*See* Aminoglycosides Comparison Chart.)

Special Populations. *Pediatric Dosage.* (*See* Aminoglycosides Comparison Chart.)

Geriatric Dosage. Same as adult dosage, but adjust for age-related reduction in renal function.

Other Conditions. Use of ideal body weight (IBW) for determining the mg/kg dosage appears to be more accurate than dosage based on total body weight (TBW). In morbid obesity, dosage requirement may best be estimated using a dosing weight of IBW + 0.4 (TBW − IBW).[1,2] With conventional dosage methods, serum drug levels should be targeted for high peaks (>6 mg/L with gentamicin and tobramycin) because these may be associated with better outcome in bacteremia, pneumonia, and other systemic infections.[1,2] Critically ill patients with serious infections or in disease states known to markedly alter aminoglycoside pharmacokinetics (eg, cystic fibrosis, burns, or major surgery)[1,2] often have variable distribution and excretion of the drugs. Serum level monitoring is unnecessary in patients with less serious infections without appreciable renal impairment (*see* Aminoglycosides Comparison Chart).

When the drug is administered once daily, very high peak concentrations (>16 mg/L with gentamicin and tobramycin) are achieved; given the lack of association between specific concentrations and therapeutic and/or toxic outcomes, the exact role of serum level monitoring is unclear[3–5] (*see* Aminoglycosides Comparison Chart).

Adjust dosage based on renal function. Individualization is critical because these agents have a low therapeutic index. In renal impairment, the following guidelines may be used to determine initial dosage (modified from reference 6):

1. Select loading dose in mg/kg (lean body weight or dosing weight as above) to provide peak serum levels in the range listed below for the desired aminoglycoside.

AMINOGLYCOSIDE	USUAL LOADING DOSE	EXPECTED PEAK SERUM LEVEL
Tobramycin } Gentamicin } Amikacin }	1.5–2 mg/kg 5–7.5 mg/kg	4–10 mg/L 15–30 mg/L

2. Select maintenance dose (as percentage of chosen loading dose) to continue peak serum levels indicated above, according to desired dosage interval and the patient's corrected Cl_{cr}.

PERCENTAGE OF LOADING DOSE REQUIRED FOR DOSAGE INTERVAL SELECTED				
CL_{CR} (ML/MIN)	HALF-LIFE* (HR)	8 HR	12 HR	24 HR
90	3.1	84%	—	—
80	3.4	80	91%	—
70	3.9	76	88	—
60	4.5	71	84	—
50	5.3	65	79	—
40	6.5	57	72	92%
30	8.4	48	63	86
25	9.9	43	57	81
20	11.9	37	50	75
17	13.6	33	46	70
15	15.1	31	42	67
12	17.9	27	37	61
10[†]	20.4	24	34	56
7[†]	25.9	19	28	47
5[†]	31.5	16	23	41
2[†]	46.8	11	16	30
0[†]	69.3	8	11	21

*Alternatively, 50% of the chosen loading dose may be given at an interval approximately equal to the estimated half-life.

[†]Dosage adjustment for patients with Cl_{cr} under 10 mL/min should be assisted by measured serum levels. Give supplemental doses of 50–75% of the loading dose after each hemodialysis period.

These guidelines are based on population data; serum levels in individual patients may deviate from guideline estimates. No guidelines have been developed for netilmicin or streptomycin.

Dosage Forms. (*See* Aminoglycosides Comparison Chart.)

Patient Instructions. Report any dizziness or sensations of ringing or fullness in the ears.

Pharmacokinetics. *Serum Levels.* (*See* Aminoglycosides Comparison Chart.)

Fate. Absorption after oral or rectal administration is about 0.2–2%; absorption across denuded skin may reach 5%. Irrigation of vascularized areas (eg, peritoneal cavity) results in absorption approximating IM use.[7] IM administration is followed by rapid and complete absorption, with peak serum levels occurring after 0.5–1.5 hr. IV infusions over 0.5–1 hr produce serum levels similar to equal IM doses. Binding of aminoglycosides to plasma proteins is low. These agents distribute rapidly into the extracellular fluid compartment with a V_d of about 0.3 ± 0.08 L/kg, which is increased by fever, edema, ascites, fluid overload, and in neonates.[8] Aminoglycosides accumulate markedly in some tissues, especially the renal cortex, to levels many times those found in the serum,[2,8] particularly with frequent dosage intervals compared with the same dosage given at less frequent intervals.[2,3] Levels in the CSF of patients with meningitis generally do not exceed 25% of serum levels, except in neonates;[2,8] penetration into the eye is inadequate for treatment of intraocular infections. Penetration into lung tissues and sputum is low, and large doses may be necessary to optimally treat pneumonias with relatively insensitive organisms (eg, *Pseudomonas aeruginosa*). Distribution of aminoglycosides into the peritoneal cavity of patients with peritonitis is therapeutically adequate.[7,8] Elimination is via glomerular filtration of unchanged drug;[1,2] Cl is about 80% of Cl_{cr}. After discontinuation, low levels of aminoglycoside can be detected in the urine for several days caused by excretion of drug that had accumulated in deep tissue compartments.[2,8]

$t_{1/2}$. α phase 5–15 min; ß phase (adults) about 2 ± 0.4 hr with normal renal function (1.5–9 hr in neonates under 1 week and 3 hr in older infants); may be more variable in certain groups (eg, obstetric and burn patients) despite normal renal function; 50–70 hr in anuria. A prolonged γ elimination phase is observed when concentrations fall to the lower range of detectability, representing egress from deep tissue compartments and subsequent renal elimination; the half-life of this phase ranges from 60–350 hr (usually 150–200).[2–8] ß phase half-life is most important for use in calculating individualized dosage, but the γ phase may account for the gradual rise of serum levels and apparent increase in half-life with continued therapy, despite stable renal function.[2,8]

Adverse Reactions. Aminoglycoside-induced nephrotoxicity is usually mild and reversible; progression to severe renal disease and dependence upon dialysis is rare. Nephrotoxicity is manifested by elevations in Cr_s, BUN, and aminoglycoside concentrations, and appearance of renal tubular casts, enzymes, and ß₂-microglobulin, and occurs in 5–30% of patients, depending on the criteria used and the population risk factors present.[1,2,9] Duration of therapy, prior aminoglycoside therapy, advanced age, preexisting renal disease, liver disease, volume depletion, and female sex have been identified as risk factors for nephrotoxicity.[1,2] Concomitant use of nephrotoxic drugs also increases the risk of nephrotoxicity. Elevated trough levels are *not* a risk factor, but often a result of nephrotoxicity.[2,10] There is no evidence that there are clinically important differences in nephrotoxicity between gentamicin, tobramycin, netilmicin, and amikacin.[9] Depletion of magnesium and other minerals caused by increased renal excretion occurs. Occasional, but often permanent, vestibular toxicity is reported, usually in association with streptomycin. Subclinical vestibular disturbances can be detected in 40% or more of patients receiving aminoglycosides.[1,2,9] Early cochlear damage can be detected only by sequential audiometric examination, because hearing loss in conversational frequencies is a sign of advanced auditory impairment. Furthermore, early auditory damage is not as apparent in the elderly or others with preexisting high-tone deficits. Risk factors for ototoxicity include duration of therapy, bacteremia, hypovolemia, peak temperature, and liver disease.[1,2] Elevated serum concentrations are apparently not associated with increased ototoxicity risk,[10] nor do there appear to be any clinically important differences between gentamicin, tobramycin, netilmicin, and amikacin.[9] Oral aminoglycosides, primarily neomycin, have been associated with a spruelike malabsorption syndrome.[1,2] Neuromuscular blockade with respiratory failure is rare, except in predisposed patients (*see* Precautions).

Precautions. Pregnancy; preexisting renal impairment; vestibular or cochlear impairment; myasthenia gravis; hypocalcemia; postoperative or other conditions that depress neuromuscular transmission.

Drug Interactions. Concurrent or sequential use of other nephro- or ototoxic agents may increase the risk of aminoglycoside toxicities. Concurrent use of aminoglycosides with neuromuscular blocking agents may potentiate neuromuscular blockade and cause respiratory paralysis.[2] The action of oral anticoagulants may be potentiated by oral neomycin, presumably via reduced absorption or synthesis of vitamin K. Ticarcillin and acylampicillins may degrade aminoglycosides in vitro, resulting in artificially low levels; the extent of degradation is dependent on time, temperature, and ß-lactam concentration.[8,11] Degradation can occur in vivo in patients with renal insufficiency.[12] **Amikacin** is the aminoglycoside least susceptible to ß-lactam inactivation.[8,11]

Parameters to Monitor. Renal function tests before and q 2–3 days during therapy. Audiometry and electronystagmography may be performed in patients able to cooperate. Peak and trough serum aminoglycoside levels are useful for individualizing dosage and assuring the presence of effective serum levels. In neonates or other patients with rapidly changing renal function, obtain serum drug concentrations initially and q 2–3 days until stable. However, with once- or twice-daily dosage and in pediatric patients, trough serum levels may be undetectable and other sampling strategies are necessary.[3–5,13] Routine monitoring may not be cost-effective in patients without underlying disease between 3 and 18 yr of age.[14] (*See also* Special Populations, Other Conditions.)

Notes. Of the available aminoglycosides, gentamicin, tobramycin, netilmicin, and amikacin are the most clinically useful. **Streptomycin** use is largely restricted to the treatment of enterococcal endocarditis (in combination with ampicillin), tuberculosis, brucellosis, plague, and tularemia; however, it is currently available only for compassionate use from the manufacturer. **Amikacin** is often used as part of a combination regimen for treatment of *Mycobacterium avium* complex infection. **Neomycin** is much more toxic than the other aminoglycosides when given parenterally; it is restricted to oral use for gut sterilization and topical use for minor infections. Resistance among Gram-negative organisms, especially *P. aeruginosa*, has virtually eliminated the systemic use of **kanamycin. Tobramycin** is roughly equivalent to gentamicin therapeutically, although it is about 2–4 times more active against *P. aeruginosa* than is gentamicin, is often active against gentamicin-resistant *P. aeruginosa*, and may be preferred because of a superior peak-to-MIC ratio.[15] Resistance of Gram-negative bacilli is lowest with **amikacin;** amikacin use does not appear to result in increased resistance to the drug.[1,2]

AMINOGLYCOSIDES COMPARISON CHART

DRUG	DOSAGE FORMS	ADULT DOSAGE[a]	PEDIATRIC DOSAGE[a]	USUAL THERAPEUTIC SERUM LEVELS (MG/L)[b] Peak[c]	Trough
Amikacin Sulfate Amikin	Inj 50, 250 mg/mL.	IM or IV 15–20 mg/kg/day in 2 equally divided doses; IT 5–20 mg/day.	IM or IV (under 1 week) 15–20 mg/kg/day in 2 equally divided doses q 12 hr; IM or IV (infants over 1 week) 20–25 mg/kg/day in 2–3 equally divided doses q 8–12 hr; IM or IV (children) same as adult mg/kg dosage.	20–35	≤10
Gentamicin Sulfate Garamycin Various	Inj 10, 40 mg/mL IT Inj 2, 10 mg/mL Ophth Oint 3 mg/g Ophth Soln 3 mg/mL Top Crm 1% Top Oint 1%	IM or IV 5–6 mg/kg/day in 3 equally divided doses q 8 hr or in a single dose IV q 24 hr; IM or IV for less serious infections[d] 3–5 mg/kg/day in 3 equally divided doses q 8 hr or in a single dose IV q 24 hr; IT 4–8 mg q 24 hr.	IM or IV (under 1 week) 4–5 mg/kg/day in 2 equally divided doses q 12 hr; IM or IV (infants over 1 week) 6–7.5 mg/kg/day in 3–4 equally divided doses q 6–8 hr; IM or IV (children) 6–7.5 mg/ kg/day (7–10 mg/kg/day in cystic fibrosis) in 3–4 equally divided doses q 6–8 hr; IT 1–2 mg q 24 hr.	6–12	≤2
Netilmicin Sulfate Netromycin	Inj 100 mg/mL.	IM or IV 3[d]–6.5 mg/kg/day in 1–3 equally divided doses q 8–24 hr.	Same as gentamicin.	6–12	≤2

(continued)

AMINOGLYCOSIDES COMPARISON CHART (continued)

DRUG	DOSAGE FORMS	ADULT DOSAGE[a]	PEDIATRIC DOSAGE[a]	USUAL THERAPEUTIC SERUM LEVELS (MG/L)[b] Peak[c]	Trough
Streptomycin Sulfate Various	Inj 400 mg/mL.	IM 15–25 mg/kg/day (usually 1–2 g/day) in 2 equally divided doses q 12 hr; IM for TB 12–15 mg/kg/day to a maximum of 1 g or 22–25 mg/kg to a maximum of 1.5 g 2–3 times/week.	IM (neonates) 20–30 mg/kg/day in 2 equally divided doses q 12 hr; IM (children) 20–40 mg/kg/day in 2 equally divided doses q 12 hr; IM for TB 20–40 mg/kg/day or 25–30 mg/kg 2–3 times/week.	15–30	≤5
Tobramycin Sulfate Nebcin	Inj 10, 40 mg/mL Ophth Oint 3 mg/g Ophth Soln 3 mg/g.	IM or IV 5–6 mg/kg/day in 3 equally divided doses q 8 hr or in a single daily dose IV q 24 hr; IM or IV for less serious infections[d] 3–5 mg/kg/day in 3 equally divided doses q 8 hr or IV q 24 hr; I or IV q 24 hr; T 4–8 mg q 24 hr.	Same as gentamicin.	6–12	≤2

[a]For systemic infections; urinary tract infections (UTIs) are adequately treated with lower dosages.

[b]Based on divided doses given q 8–12 hr; higher peaks and lower (or undetectable) troughs are seen when less frequent dosage intervals are used.

[c]As seen 30 min after a 30-min IV infusion or approximately 1 hr after IM administration of a usual adult dose. Uncomplicated UTIs may be treated with smaller doses that produce much lower serum levels; however, serious infections, such as Gram-negative bacteremia, pneumonia or endocarditis may require doses resulting in serum levels in the higher part of the range. Clinical efficacy appears to increase as the ratio of the peak serum level to the minimum inhibitory concentration (MIC) of the pathogen increases.[15]

[d]These doses conform to those used in published clinical trials, but higher dosages may be necessary in certain patient populations.

Antifungal Drugs

AMPHOTERICIN B	Fungizone
AMPHOTERICIN B LIPID COMPLEX	Abelcet

Pharmacology. Amphotericin B is a polyene antifungal agent that preferentially binds to fungal cytoplasmic membrane sterols (primarily ergosterol), altering their structure and increasing permeability of fungal membranes. Amphotericin B binds somewhat to human cytoplasmic sterols (primarily cholesterol), which accounts for a portion of the drug's toxicity.[16–18] Amphotericin B lipid complex consists of amphotericin B complexed with two phospholipids, dimyristoylphosphatidyl-choline and dimyristoylphosphatidylglycerol, in a 1:1 drug-to-lipid molar ratio. Incorporation of amphotericin B into a lipid complex attempts to attenuate the drug's toxicity. Other liposomal amphotericin B complexes are under development.

Administration and Adult Dosage. **IV** (conventional amphotericin B) 1 mg test dose by slow infusion advocated by some sources; increase in 10–30 mg/day increments at daily intervals to a maximum of 1–1.5 mg/kg/day over 2–6 hr as dictated by severity of infection, clinical response, and tolerance of infusion. More rapid infusions of 1–2 hr duration have been tolerated as well as 4-hr infusions;[19–21] however, use caution in renal failure to avoid hyperkalemia induced by rapid infusion. Increase dosage rapidly to the higher dosages in critically ill patients. During prolonged therapy, the drug may be given every other day.[22] Recommended infusion concentration is 0.1 mg/mL in D5W. Necessary dosages and duration of therapy are not established for many diseases.[17,21,22] A total dose of 10–12 mg/kg of conventional amphotericin B is recommended for an uncomplicated catheter-related bloodstream infection, administered as 0.5–0.8 mg/kg/day over about 2 weeks.[21,23] **Intracavitary for pulmonary aspergilloma** (conventional amphotericin B) 5–50 mg in D5W daily to 3 times/week.[22] **Intrathecally** (conventional amphotericin B) 100–500 µg in 5 mL CSF 2–3 times a week, or 300 µg/day in D5W or D10W infused over 1 hr.[17,22] **Bladder irrigation** (conventional amphotericin B) 50 mg/day in 1 L of sterile water as a continuous irrigation over 24 hr.[22,23] **IV** (amphotericin B lipid complex) initial test dose is not recommended by the manufacturer. Recommended infusion concentration is 1 mg/mL in D5W at a rate of 2.5 mg/kg/hr. If infusion time exceeds 2 hr, the infusion bag needs to be shaken to mix the contents and repeated q 2 hr. An in-line filter can be used but must not have a pore size less than 5 microns. **IV for aspergillosis in patients refractory to or intolerant of conventional amphotericin B** (amphotericin B lipid complex) 5 mg/kg as a single infusion. **PO for oral candidiasis** (oral suspension) 1 mL qid swished and held in the mouth for as long as possible, then swallowed. Continue therapy for 2 weeks, longer if necessary.

Special Populations. *Pediatric Dosage.* **IV** (conventional amphotericin B) same as adult dosage up to 1 mg/kg. **PO for oral candidiasis** (oral suspension) 1 mL qid swished and held in the mouth for as long as possible, then swallowed. Continue therapy for 2 weeks, longer if necessary. **IV** (amphotericin B lipid complex) same as adult dosage, although infusion concentration is 2 mg/mL.

Geriatric Dosage. Same as adult dosage.

Other Conditions. **IV** (conventional amphotericin B) no dosage reduction necessary with impaired renal function, although further impairment may occur as a result of the amphotericin B;[22] however, if Cr_s exceeds 3 mg/dL it is advisable to discontinue the drug or reduce dosage until renal function improves, depending upon the clinical status of the patient. **IV** (amphotericin B lipid complex) for patients with cardiovascular disease, use an infusion concentration of 2 mg/mL. The manufacturer provides no firm guidelines for dosage adjustment in impaired renal function.

Dosage Forms. **Inj** (conventional amphotericin B) 5 mg/mL (when reconstituted); (amphotericin B lipid complex) 5 mg/mL; **Oral Susp** 100 mg/mL; **Top Crm** 30 mg/g; **Top Lot** 30 mg/mL; **Top Oint** 30 mg/g.

Patient Instructions. **Inj** Forewarn patients of expected immediate reactions to infusion, especially with conventional formulation. **Oral Susp** Shake the oral suspension well before use. Swish and hold in the mouth for as long as possible, then swallow. Discontinue if mouth irritation occurs. **Top** This preparation may stain clothing.

Pharmacokinetics. *Serum Levels.* No correlation between serum concentrations and therapeutic or toxic effects for either formulation.

Fate. Poor oral and IM absorption. (Conventional amphotericin B) 370–650 µg/kg/day infused IV over 4–6 hr produces levels of 1.8–3.5 mg/L (1.9–3.8 µmol/L) 1 hr after infusion. Concentrations of 0.5–1.5 mg/L (0.5–1.6 µmol/L) remain 20 hr after infusion is discontinued; serum concentrations are not directly proportional to dose and tend to plateau at doses exceeding 50 mg. V_d is about 4 L/kg. (Amphotericin B lipid complex) 5 mg/kg/day infused IV at 2.5 mg/kg/hr produces peak levels of 1.7 ± 0.8 mg/L and 0.6 ± 0.3 mg/L at the end of dosage interval. V_d is about 131 L/kg. (Both formulations) With usual doses, trough concentrations on alternate day or daily administration schedules are not appreciably different; peaks are generally higher on alternate day schedules. Serum concentrations represent less than 10% of administered dose; the drug is >95% bound to plasma lipoproteins.[17,22] High concentrations of drug are found in many tissues, but much of the drug may be biologically inactive because of tissue binding.[17,22] The drug appears to be stored in the body, very slowly released, metabolized, and slowly excreted by the kidneys. Despite slow elimination, serum concentrations do not increase after repeated administration or in the presence of impaired renal function. When therapy is discontinued, amphotericin B and metabolites continue to appear in the urine for 7–8 weeks.[17,22]

$t_{½}$. (Conventional formulation) ß phase about 24–48 hr; (lipid complex) ß phase about 173 ± 78 hr; (both formulations) γ phase about 15 days, unchanged in renal impairment.[17,22]

Adverse Reactions. (Conventional amphotericin B) frequent during infusion period: fever, chills, headache, anorexia, nausea, vomiting, malaise, and pain at the infusion site. Severity of reactions may be reduced by premedication with an antipyretic, glucocorticoid, and antiemetic. Addition of phosphate buffer and perhaps heparin to solution may reduce phlebitis, but administration through a central line obviates need for buffer or heparin. Rapid infusion (<1 hr) has been carried out safely, but may produce cardiovascular collapse.[22] Prolonged administration times (>6 hr) may produce more reactions.[24,25] IV **meperidine** HCl 25–50 mg rapidly terminates shaking chills in some patients in whom spontaneous disappearance does not occur when the infusion is stopped. **Dantrolene** may also prevent or reduce rigors in patients unresponsive to other measures.[17,22] With repeated administration thrombophlebitis, normocytic, normochromic anemia, impaired renal function with distal tubular acidosis, hyposthenuria, hypokalemia, and hypomagnesemia frequently occur and are generally reversible, although permanent renal impairment may result, especially if total dosage exceeds 4–5 g.[25] Sodium loading in adults using pre- and posthydration with 500 mL of 0.9% sodium chloride solution (or 10 mL/kg 0.9% sodium chloride in children) may prevent or reverse nephrotoxicity.[23,26] Potassium supplementation is usually necessary, and administration of an alkalinizing potassium salt (eg, bicarbonate, gluconate) is often useful in preventing the occurrence of hypokalemic acidosis. Intrathecal administration can produce peripheral nerve pain, paresthesias, nerve palsies, paraplegia, convulsions, and chemical meningitis; bladder irrigations containing amphotericin B have produced no reported toxicity.[24,25] (Amphotericin B lipid complex) frequent during infusion period: fevers, chills, headache, nausea, vomiting, and diarrhea, but reactions appear to be less frequent than with conventional amphotericin B. Premedication is not advocated by the manufacturer, but may be beneficial to some patients if infusion reactions appear. Heparin is not necessary even if infused by peripheral line. Nephrotoxicity appears to be less than with conventional amphotericin B. Other adverse reactions that occur with conventional amphotericin B may also occur with the lipid complex formulation. (Oral amphotericin B) nausea, vomiting, diarrhea, and steatorrhea have been reported. Rarely, urticaria, angioedema, Stevens-Johnson syndrome, and toxic epidermal necrolysis is reported.

Precautions. Impaired renal function. Safety of use during pregnancy not established despite reports of safe use. Avoid rapid infusions in presence of hyperkalemia.

Drug Interactions. Amphotericin B may have additive nephrotoxicity with aminoglycosides, cyclosporine, and possibly other nephrotoxins. Corticosteroids may enhance potassium loss caused by amphotericin B. Amphotericin B-induced potassium loss may contribute to digitalis toxicity;

Parameters to Monitor. Monitor BUN, Cr_s or Cl_{cr} before therapy and at least weekly during therapy; monitor hematocrit, serum (including magnesium), and urine electrolytes periodically. Some sources consider temporary drug discontinuation if renal function becomes severely impaired because of the amphotericin B (Cr_s >3.5 mg/dL or BUN >40 mg/dL). Monitor the total dosage of amphotericin B; toxicity and perhaps efficacy in some infections may be related to total dosage.[24,25]

Notes. Amphotericin B is water insoluble; the conventional commercial product is a colloidal dispersion in bile salts, buffered with sodium phosphate. Store powder in refrigerator; protect from light. Reconstitute with sterile water for injection *without* a bacteriostatic agent; reconstituted drug is stable for 1 week under refrigeration. Do not mix with electrolyte solutions; protection from light unnecessary if infused in less than 24 hr from time of preparation.[22] The drug is probably removed by in-line filters of less than 1 μ pore size, despite contrary claims; therefore, filtration is not recommended. Liposome-encapsulated amphotericin B is less toxic and more efficacious than conventional amphotericin B in some animal models; studies with liposomal amphotericin B (Ambisome) and amphotericin B colloidal dispersion (Amphocil) in humans are promising.[27] Conventional amphotericin B doses have been mixed in 250 mL of Intralipid 20% and suggested as an alternative to liposome-encapsulated amphotericin B. This preparation has been used by some investigators to reduce nephrotoxicity and improve clinical tolerance in some clinical trials;[28-30] however, others have demonstrated that the amphotericin B in Intralipid 20% mixture is unstable and forms particles larger than 10 μ, which could lead to pulmonary capillary occlusion and unpredictable amphotericin B dosage.[31,32] Daily **fluconazole** is superior to amphotericin B given weekly for prevention of recurrence or relapse of cryptococcal meningitis in patients with AIDS.[33]

CLOTRIMAZOLE
Gyne-Lotrimin, Lotrimin, Mycelex

Clotrimazole is an imidazole used for local therapy of fungal infections. The topical formulations are equivalent to other topical antifungals in the treatment of *Candida* spp. or dermatophyte skin infections. For vulvovaginal candidiasis, a 100-mg vaginal tablet is used daily at bedtime for 7 days; alternatively, two 100-mg tablets may be used intravaginally once daily at bedtime for 3 days or a 500-mg vaginal tablet may be used once at bedtime. The vaginal cream is administered as 1 applicatorful (50 mg) at bedtime for 6–14 days. Troches of 10 mg are dissolved in the mouth 5 times a day to treat or prevent oropharyngeal candidiasis. Available as 1% topical cream, lotion, and solution; 1% vaginal cream; 100- and 500-mg vaginal tablets; and 10 mg troches.

FLUCONAZOLE
Diflucan

Pharmacology. Fluconazole is a triazole antifungal agent that is highly water soluble, and is active in vivo against many fungal species (especially *Cryptococcus* spp.). The drug is active against *Candida* spp., *Blastomyces dermatitidis*, *Coccidioides immitis*, and *Histoplasma capsulatum*. Antifungal effects are caused by inhibition of fungal cytochrome P450–dependent enzymes that prevent conversion of lanosterol to ergosterol.[34-36]

Administration and Adult Dosage. PO or IV for oropharyngeal or esophageal candidiasis 200 mg on day 1, then 100 mg/day for 10–14 days. Severe esophageal candidiasis may require 400 mg/day.[34,37] **PO or IV for cryptococcal meningitis**: **acute therapy** 400 mg on day 1, then 200 mg/day for 6–10 weeks; **maintenance therapy in patients with AIDS** 200 mg/day indefinitely. Dosages up to 1 g/day have been used for cryptococcal meningitis. **PO for uncomplicated vaginal candidiasis** 150 mg as a single dose.[36] **PO or IV for coccidioidal meningitis** 400 mg/day indefinitely;[38] dosages up to 800 mg/day have been used. **PO or IV for prophylaxis of candidiasis in bone marrow transplantation** 400 mg/day and continued for 7 days after granulocyte count exceeds 1000/μL. Initiate therapy several days prior to onset of neutropenia.[37]

Special Populations. *Pediatric Dosage.* **PO or IV** limited experience suggests a dosage of 3–6 mg/kg/day.[39]

Geriatric Dosage. (Over 65 yr) although half-life is prolonged, dosage adjustment appears unnecessary.[35]

Other Conditions. Reduce dosage in impaired renal function: for Cl_{cr} of 20–50 mL/min, give the usual dose q 48 hr; Cl_{cr} of 10–19 mL/min, 50–200 mg q 48 hr; Cl_{cr} under 10 mL/min, 50–100 mg q 48 hr. Give a full dose after hemodialysis. Patients on chronic ambulatory peritoneal dialysis may receive 50–200 mg/day.

Dosage Forms. **Tab** 50, 100, 150, 200 mg; **Susp** 10, 40 mg/mL; **Inj** 2 mg/mL.

Patient Instructions. Take with a meal if stomach upset occurs. Report changes in appetite, dark urine, or light stools.

Pharmacokinetics. *Fate.* Rapidly and well absorbed (90%) orally, unaffected by gastric pH. Peak concentrations of 1.8–2.8 mg/L (5.9–9 μmol/L) achieved 2–4 hr after administration of 100–150 mg orally. Plasma protein binding is 11–12%; penetrates well into CSF (over 60% of simultaneous serum levels). V_d is 0.65 ± 0.2 L/kg; Cl is 0.015 ± 0.006 L/hr/kg. About 64–90% of a dose is excreted unchanged in urine.[35]

$t_{1/2}$. 22 ± 4 hr; 37 hr in patients over 65 yr; up to 125 hr in patients with renal impairment.[35]

Adverse Reactions. Occasional nausea, vomiting, diarrhea, abdominal pain, or elevations of liver transaminases occur. Severe hepatitis or exfoliative skin reactions occur rarely.[34,37]

Precautions. Observe patients who develop rash for worsening of the lesions and discontinue the drug if necessary.

Drug Interactions. Rifampin induces the metabolism of fluconazole, and may lead to clinical failure. Fluconazole inhibits metabolism of phenytoin, warfarin, and to a minor extent cyclosporine. Low dosages have been shown to increase the serum levels of tolbutamide, glipizide, glyburide, and possibly other sulfonylureas. This could lead to a greater hypoglycemic effect, and dosage reduction may be necessary.[37]

Parameters to Monitor. Liver function tests weekly initially, then monthly. Monitor renal function tests weekly if abnormal at outset of therapy. (*See* Precautions). Monitor patients with elevated transaminases more carefully for hepatitis.

Notes. Combination therapy with fluconazole and **flucytosine** for treatment of cryptococcal meningitis appears to be superior to single agent therapy;[34] further studies of this combination, as well as fluconazole plus **amphotericin B** are needed. Fluconazole-resistant *Candida albicans* has been clinically demonstrated; increased use of prophylactic fluconazole may increase the likelihood of the emergence of resistant strains such as *Candida krusei.*[37]

FLUCYTOSINE   Ancobon

Pharmacology. Flucytosine (5-FC) is a fluorinated cytosine analogue that appears to be deaminated to the cytotoxic antimetabolite fluorouracil by cytosine deaminase, an enzyme present in fungal but not human cells. It has a narrow spectrum of activity and is used with other antifungals because resistance develops rapidly when used alone in *Candida* and *Cryptococcus* spp. infections.[18]

Administration and Adult Dosage. **PO** 50–150 mg/kg/day in 4 divided doses; the use of higher dosages has been suggested to prevent the emergence of resistance.[16] Duration of therapy must be guided by severity of the infection and response to therapy.

Special Populations. *Pediatric Dosage.* **PO** same as adult dosage in mg/kg.

Geriatric Dosage. Same as adult dosage, but adjust for age-related reduction in renal function.

Other Conditions. Dosage must be reduced in the presence of impaired renal function.[16–18] An approximate dosage reduction can be determined by administering doses at intervals in hours equal to four times the Cr_s in mg/dL. Alternative regimens such as reduced doses at 6-hr intervals have been recommended. In patients on maintenance hemodialysis q 48–72 hr, give 20–50 mg/kg after each dialysis.[16,17] Use normal dosage in liver disease.

Dosage Forms. **Cap** 250, 500 mg.

Patient Instructions. Take the capsules required for a single dose over a 15-min period with food to minimize stomach upset.

Pharmacokinetics. *Serum Levels.* Toxicity most likely over 100 mg/L (780 μmol/L).[16,17] (*See also* Precautions.)

Fate. Rapidly and well absorbed (about 90%), with peak about 1–2 hr after administration of a 500-mg dose to adults averaging 8–12 mg/L (62–93 μmol/L) in patients with normal renal function.[16] Negligible binding to plasma proteins; V_d is 0.7 L/kg.[17] Widely distributed throughout the body, including the CSF and eye. Eliminated almost entirely (average 90%) in the urine by glomerular filtration unchanged, with urine levels many times greater than serum levels. Low serum concentrations of **fluorouracil** have been found in patients taking flucytosine and may be responsible for hematologic toxicity.

$t_{1/2}$. 6 ± 0.6 hr; up to 100 hr or greater with renal impairment.[16,17]

Adverse Reactions. Occasional nausea, vomiting, diarrhea, bone marrow suppression (often dose limiting in HIV-infected patients), and elevated liver function tests (usually asymptomatic and rapidly reversible). Diarrhea occurs occasionally; ulcerating enteritis occurs rarely.[16–18]

Precautions. Pregnancy; severe renal impairment (elimination is highly variable and monitoring of serum levels is recommended, keeping peak concentrations under 100 mg/L);[16,18] impaired hepatic function; hematologic disorders; or history of therapy with myelosuppressive drugs (eg, zidovudine, ganciclovir, cancer chemotherapy) or radiation.

Drug Interactions. Amphotericin B can increase the toxicity of flucytosine by increasing its cellular penetration and impairing its elimination secondary to nephrotoxicity.

Parameters to Monitor. Before, and frequently during therapy, monitor BUN, Cr_s, Cl_{cr}, full hematology and liver function tests. (*See also* Precautions.)

Notes. Flucytosine may be synergistic with **amphotericin B,** depending on the organism involved; the combination is useful in treating cryptococcal meningitis in AIDS and non-AIDS patients,[41] although the superiority of the combination in AIDS patients has not been established. Flucytosine may be additive or synergistic with **fluconazole** for the treatment of cryptococcal meningitis; however, further experience in clinical trials is needed before this combination can be recommended.[34]

GRISEOFULVIN   Fulvicin, Grifulvin V, Grisactin

Griseofulvin is a fungistatic agent that appears to affect mitosis in fungal cells. It is active against dermatophytes and is not useful in the treatment of yeast or other fungal infections. Adverse reactions include occasional nausea and vomiting. Photosensitivity reactions, peripheral neuritis, and leukopenia are rare. The drug may exacerbate acute intermittent porphyria. Oral dosage of the microsize formulation is 0.5–1 g/day in a single or 2–4 divided doses. Ultramicrosize formulation oral dosage is 330–660 mg/day in 1 or 2 divided doses. Pediatric dosage is 11 mg/kg/day of microsize or 7.3 mg/kg/day of ultramicrosize. Therapy usually must be continued for at least 3 weeks; infections of the palms or soles require 4–8 weeks of therapy; nail infections usually require 6–12 months of therapy. Instruct patients to take the drug with meals to enhance absorption, avoid prolonged sun exposure and avoid alcohol.[16,17] Available as microsize formulations in 125, 250 mg capsules, 250- and 500-mg tablets, and 25 mg/mL suspension; ultramicrosize products are 125-, 165-, 250-, and 330-mg tablets.

ITRACONAZOLE   Sporanox

Pharmacology. Itraconazole is a synthetic triazole antifungal agent that is more active than ketoconazole or fluconazole against certain fungi, notably *Aspergillus* spp. It also has activity against *Coccidioides, Cryptococcus, Candida, Histoplasma, Blastomyces,* and *Sporotrichosis* spp. Itraconazole inhibits fungal cytochrome P450–dependent enzymes. This inhibition blocks ergosterol biosynthesis, creating disturbances in membrane function and membrane-bound enzymes, and affecting fungal cell growth and viability.[37,42]

Administration and Adult Dosage. PO for systemic fungal infections 200–600 mg/day, depending on site and severity of infection. Give dosages over 200 mg/day in 2–3 divided doses. **PO for vulvovaginal candidiasis** 200 mg bid for 1 day or 200 mg/day for 7 days. **PO for dermatomycoses** 100 mg/day for 15 days or 200 mg/day for 7 days. **PO for pityriasis versicolor** 200 mg/day for 7 days. **PO for plantar tinea pedis and palmar tinea manum** 100 mg/day for 30 days or 200 mg bid for 7 days. **PO for onychomycosis** 200 once daily for 3 months.[43]

Special Populations. *Pediatric Dosage.* Safety and efficacy not established.

Geriatric Dosage. Same as adult dosage.

Other Conditions. Dosage reduction in patients with hepatic impairment may be necessary, but guidelines are not established. No dosage adjustment is necessary in renal impairment.

Dosage Forms. Cap 100 mg.

Patient Instructions. Take this drug with food to ensure maximal absorption. Do not take with medications that decrease stomach acid (eg, antacids, H_2-blockers, omeprazole). Report symptoms of fatigue, loss of appetite, nausea, vomiting, yellowing of the skin, dark urine, or pale stools.

Pharmacokinetics. *Serum Levels.* Levels under 5 mg/L (7 µmol/L) are associated with treatment failure in *Aspergillus* infections.[44]

Fate. Relative oral bioavailability of the capsules compared to an oral solution is over 70%;[37] the solubility of itraconazole is aided by an acidic environment, and food increases absorption. Peak serum concentration occurs in 4–5 hr; peak concentration is 20 µg/L (28 nmol/L) after a single 100-mg oral dose during fasting, increasing to 180 µg/L (0.26 µmol/L) when taken with food.[42] The drug is over 99% protein bound, primarily to albumin, with only 0.2% available as free drug.[42] It is highly lipid soluble, and concentrations are much higher in tissues than in serum. Itraconazole is metabolized in the liver and exhibits dose-dependent elimination.[37] One metabolite, hydroxyitraconazole, has antifungal activity, and serum concentrations are double those of itraconazole at steady state.

$t_{1/2}$. 24–42 hr; possibly longer with large daily dosages.[37]

Adverse Reactions. Itraconazole is well tolerated with long-term use. Occasional rash, pruritus, nausea, vomiting, abdominal discomfort, headache, dizziness, decreased libido, and hypertension occur. Mild transient elevations of transaminases occur frequently, but hepatotoxicity is rare. There are no apparent adverse effects on testicular or adrenal steroidogenesis.[37,42]

Contraindications. Coadministration with astemizole, cisapride, or terfenadine.

Precautions. Pregnancy; lactation.

Drug Interactions. Itraconazole inhibits CYP3A3/4 and inhibits metabolism of certain drugs such as astemizole, cisapride, cyclosporine, terfenadine, and warfarin (*see* Contraindications). Warfarin dosage reduction may be necessary during concurrent use. Cyclosporine dosage may need to be reduced by 50% with itraconazole dosages over 100 mg/day. Avoid concurrent carbamazepine, phenytoin, or rifampin because they may dramatically reduce the serum itraconazole concentration.[44,45]

Parameters to Monitor. Closely monitor prothrombin time in patients on concurrent warfarin and cyclosporine levels in patients taking these drug. Monitor liver function tests in patients with preexisting hepatic impairment. Serum drug concentrations may be monitored if poor absorption or increased metabolism of itraconazole is suspected.

KETOCONAZOLE   Nizoral

Pharmacology. Ketoconazole is an imidazole antifungal agent that exerts its antifungal effects through inhibition of the synthesis of ergosterol (a fungal cell wall component) by inhibiting fungal cytochrome P450. It is primarily used for mucocutaneous fungal infections, including candidiasis, and in tinea versicolor unresponsive to topical therapy. It is used to treat blastomycosis, histoplasmosis, and paracoccidioidomycosis in immunocompetent patients. It appears to suppress rather than eliminate coccidiomycosis. Because of its poor CSF penetration, keto-conazole is not recommended for fungal infections of the CNS.[18,42] Because of its effects on steroid synthesis (*see* Adverse Reactions) the drug has been used in prostatic cancer and Cushing's syndrome.

Administration and Adult Dosage. **PO** 200–400 mg daily or bid, depending on site and severity of infection. **Top** apply once daily or bid for dermatophytoses, superficial mycoses, or seborrheic dermatitis. **Top for dandruff** apply shampoo twice weekly for 4 weeks.

Special Populations. *Pediatric Dosage.* **PO** (under 2 yr) not established; (over 2 yr) 5–10 mg/kg/day in 1 or 2 divided doses.[23,39] The drug is bioavailable when tablets are crushed and mixed in applesauce or juice.[17] **Top** apply once daily.

Geriatric Dosage. Same as adult dosage.

Other Conditions. Limited data suggest that dosage adjustment is unnecessary in patients with hepatic impairment; however, definitive studies are needed. No adjustment is necessary in renal dysfunction.

Dosage Forms. **Tab** 200 mg; **Cream** 2%; **Shampoo** 1,2%.

Patient Instructions. This drug may be taken with meals if stomach upset occurs, but do not take with medications that decrease stomach acid (eg, antacids, H_2-blockers, omeprazole). Report symptoms of fatigue, loss of appetite, yellowing of the skin, dark urine, or pale stools. Taking this drug with an acidic beverage (eg, a cola drink) can increase the absorption substantially. In patients receiving the drug in 0.1 N HCl to promote absorption, the solution should be sipped through a straw to avoid damaging the teeth.

Pharmacokinetics. *Fate.* Bioavailability is about 75% and is dose dependent. An acidic environment is necessary for dissolution and absorption. Bioavailability appears to be decreased by 20–40% when the drug is administered with food, and is even more markedly reduced if gastric pH is elevated. Poor absorption may occur in AIDS patients because of achlorhydria and other pathologic changes in the GI tract. Peak serum levels of 3.4 ± 0.3 mg/L (6.4 ± 0.6 μmol/L) are attained following a 200-mg dose taken with a meal. The drug is 93–96% plasma protein bound. V_d is estimated to be 0.36 ± 0.1 L/kg with a single dose, increasing to 2.4 ± 1.6 L/kg during long-term therapy; Cl is estimated to be 0.5 ± 0.25 L/hr/kg during long-term therapy. Ketoconazole is extensively metabolized by the liver to inactive metabolites, with only 2–4% of a dose excreted unchanged in urine.[16,17,46,47]

$t_{1/2}$. 8.7 ± 0.2 hr after a single dose, decreasing to 3.3 ± 1 hr during long-term therapy.[17,46]

Adverse Reactions. Generally well tolerated, with the most frequent side effects being nausea, vomiting, pruritus, and abdominal discomfort. Hepatotoxicity, including massive hepatic necrosis, occurs occasionally, but mild elevations of transaminases occur frequently. Gynecomastia occurs, probably caused by ketoconazole-induced suppression of testosterone synthesis.[18] Ketoconazole also blocks cortisol production; however, clinically apparent hypoadrenalism occurs rarely. Irritation, pruritus, and stinging may occur with topical use.

Contraindications. Coadministration with astemizole, cisapride, or terfenadine.

Precautions. Pregnancy; lactation.

Drug Interactions. Ketoconazole inhibits human CYP3A4 and inhibits metabolism of certain drugs such as astemizole, cyclosporine, methylprednisolone, terfenadin and warfarin (*see* Contraindications). Warfarin dosage reduction may be necessary during concurrent use. H_2-receptor antagonists, antacids, and probably omeprazole and lansoprazole may reduce ketoconazole oral absorption.

Parameters to Monitor. Monitor liver function tests before starting therapy and often during therapy. Closely monitor prothrombin time in patients on concurrent warfarin and cyclosporine levels in patients taking this drug.

Notes. Achlorhydric patients may be given the drug with glutamic acid hydrochloride or 0.1 N HCl (using a drinking straw) to increase absorption.[47] An acidic drink (eg, a cola) may also be used to increase ketoconazole absorption by about 65% in achlorhydria.[48]

MICONAZOLE	Monistat IV
MICONAZOLE NITRATE	Monistat, Micatin, Various

Miconazole is an imidazole antifungal agent available in topical preparations and as a solubilized IV preparation in a polyethoxylated castor oil (Cremophor EL). Because of the serious toxicity (eg, cardiorespiratory arrest, hyponatremia) of the parenteral preparation (most likely caused by the vehicle) and data challenging the clinical effectiveness of this agent, restrict parenteral use to treating fungal infections known to be resistant to amphotericin B (eg, *Scadosporium apiospermum*). Phlebitis, pruritus, nausea, vomiting, fever, chills, and rash are frequent side effects of IV miconazole. For vaginal infections, a 7-day course of a 100-mg suppository or 5 g of cream intravaginally once daily at bedtime, or a 3-day course of a 200-mg suppository intravaginally once daily at bedtime can be used. The IV dosage is 1.2–3.6 g/day in 3 divided doses, diluted in at least 200 mL of D5W or NS and infused over 30–60 min.[16,17] Available as 200-mg ampules (10 mg/mL); 2% topical or vaginal cream, spray, or powder; and 100- and 200-mg vaginal suppositories.

NYSTATIN	Mycostatin, Nilstat, Various

Nystatin is a polyene antifungal agent very similar to amphotericin B, but too toxic for parenteral use. Oral absorption is negligible, and there is no absorption through intact skin or mucous membranes. The drug is nontoxic by oral, topical, and vaginal routes; allergic sensitization occurs rarely. For oral candidiasis, the dosage of the suspension is 400,000–600,000 units qid (as a "swish and swallow") in adults, 100,000 units qid for newborn infants, and 200,000–400,000 units qid in older infants and children. Nystatin troches of 200,000–400,000 units 4–5 times/day may also be used. Treatment lasts for at least 48 hr after oral symptoms have cleared and cultures have returned to normal. Immunocompromised patients require a longer duration of therapy (eg, 10–14 days) than patients with normal host defenses. The vaginal tablet has been successfully used orally in place of the oral suspension; its slow dissolution allows prolonged contact time. For GI candidiasis the dosage is 500,000–1,000,000 units tid orally. For vaginal candidiasis the dosage is 100,000 units daily or bid vaginally for 2 weeks.[16] Available as a 100,000 units/mL suspension, 500,000-unit oral tablet, 200,000-unit troche, 100,000-unit vaginal tablet, and 100,000 units/g topical cream, ointment, and powder.

TERBINAFINE   Lamisil

Terbinafine is a synthetic allylamine antifungal agent that exerts its activity by inhibiting fungal ergosterol synthesis through inhibition of squalene epoxidase. Terbinafine is active orally and topically. It has demonstrated activity against dermatophyte infections, but is less active than azole antifungal agents against yeast species. Terbinafine is orally absorbed with approximately 70–80% absorption regardless of the presence of food. Peak concentrations after 250- and 500-mg oral doses are 0.9 and 2 mg/L, respectively, within 2 hr. Terbinafine is highly lipophilic and is widely distributed with a V_d of 13.5 L/kg. Terbinafine is extensively metabolized to inactive metabolites, and its elimination half-life ranges from 11 to 16 hr; however, an additional elimination phase of 200–400 hr may reflect the gradual release of terbinafine from adipose tissue. Frequent adverse reactions during oral therapy are dyspepsia, abdominal pain, diarrhea, skin reactions, malaise, lethargy and taste disturbance. Terbinafine does not appear to affect cytochrome P450 enzymes markedly, but its clearance is increased 100% by rifampin and decreased 33% by cimetidine. Topical therapy is applied once or twice daily for tinea corporis/cruris or cutaneous candidiasis for 1–2 weeks. The oral adult dosage is 250 mg once daily for 6 weeks for onychomycosis of fingernails or 12 weeks for onychomycosis of the toenails. Dosage reduction is necessary in severe hepatic or renal dysfunction.[49] Available as 250-mg tablets and 1% cream.

Antimycobacterial Drugs

CLOFAZIMINE   Lamprene

Clofazimine is a lipophilic rhimophenazine dye approved for treating leprosy and used in atypical *Mycobacterium* infections, discoid lupus erythematosus, and pyoderma gangrenosum. The drug is about 50% bioavailable. A peak serum level of 0.5–2 mg/L (1–4 μmol/L) 2 hr after an oral 100- to 200-mg dose is proposed as evidence of adequate absorption. Clofazimine accumulates in fatty tissues and the reticuloendothelial system, and is eliminated with a half-life of about 70 days. Bodily secretions, skin, conjunctivae, cornea, urine, and feces may turn red to brownish black; an orange-pink skin discoloration is common and may take months to years to disappear after stopping the drug. Dose-related GI pain, nausea, vomiting, and diarrhea may occur because of crystalline deposits in GI tissue. Eosinophilic enteritis and splenic infarction have occurred rarely at dosages greater than 100 mg/day. The usual adult dosage is PO 100 mg/day with food for leprosy, *M. avium* complex infections, and for discoid lupus erythematosus; dosages up to 200 mg/day are used for erythema nodosum leprosum. Dosages of

300–400 mg/day have induced remission of pyoderma gangrenosum, but the manufacturer states that dosages greater than 200 mg/day are not recommended.[50,51] (*See also* Second-Line Antituberculosis Agents Comparison Chart. Available as 50-and 100-mg capsules.)

ETHAMBUTOL   Myambutol

Ethambutol is a tuberculostatic agent that is only active against mycobacteria, including *Mycobacterium avium* complex. It does not directly enhance short course (6–9 months) regimens of isoniazid, rifampin, and pyrazinamide. Ethambutol is recommended to be included as part of a four-drug initial regimen if there is a possibility of drug resistance, and should be continued for 12 months if isoniazid resistance is demonstrated. Ethambutol is also used in combination with clarithromycin to treat disseminated *M. avium-intracellulare* (MAI) infection in patients with AIDS. It is about 80% absorbed from the GI tract with complex disposition characteristics. A peak serum level of 2–6 mg/L (8–25 μmol/L) 2 hr after an oral 15–25 mg/kg dose is proposed as evidence of adequate absorption. Its half-life is 4–6 hr, increasing to 32 hr in severe renal impairment. Approximately 80% is excreted unchanged in urine. Adverse reactions are rare with the recommended dosage of 15–25 mg/kg/day. Optic neuritis (manifested as blurred vision, color blindness, and restricted visual fields) occurs rarely with dosages of 15 mg/kg/day, and is usually reversible with prompt drug discontinuation. Hyperuricemia may occur because of impairment of uric acid excretion. The dosage for tuberculosis is 15–25 mg/kg/day orally as a single dose given in combination with isoniazid and/or rifampin and/or pyrazinamide. Alternatively, 50 mg/kg (to a maximum of 2.5 g) twice weekly may be given in combination with isoniazid and/or rifampin. The dosage for MAI is 15 mg/kg/day orally to a maximum of 1 g/day as a single dose in combination with clarithromycin or azithromycin.[51–55] Available as 100- and 400-mg tablets.

ISONIAZID   Various

Pharmacology. Isoniazid (INH) is a synthetic hydrazine derivative of isonicotinic acid that inhibits the synthesis of mycolic acid, a component of the mycobacterial cell wall; it probably has other actions. Its activity is limited to mycobacteria; it is tuberculostatic or tuberculocidal depending on concentration and reproductive rate of the organism. Resistance is uncommon in preventive therapy, but can develop rapidly if used alone in active tuberculosis. Primary resistance is becoming increasingly common in certain communities, and has occurred in a variety of institutional settings (eg, hospitals, prisons). These settings are characterized by a high prevalence of HIV infection.[51,52,54,56]

Administration and Adult Dosage. **PO for prophylaxis of tuberculosis** 5 mg/kg/day (usually 300 mg) as a single daily dose, to a maximum of 300 mg/day, given as a single agent for 1 yr (*see* Notes).[55,56] **PO for treatment of tuberculosis** same dosage as above combined with rifampin 600 mg/day and pyrazinamide 15–30 mg/kg/day for 8 weeks, followed by 16 weeks of isoniazid and rifampin. Alternatively, give the daily doses of INH, rifampin, ethambutol, and pyrazinamide for 2 weeks, followed by INH 15 mg/kg (to a maximum of 900 mg), rifampin 600 mg, ethambutol 50 mg/kg (to a maximum of 2.5 g), and pyrazinamide 50–70 mg/kg (to a maximum of 4 g) in 2 or 3 divided doses twice weekly for a total of 6 weeks by directly observed therapy (DOT), then continue INH and rifampin twice weekly for 16 weeks by DOT.[53,54] In 3 times a week regimens, Ethambutol dosage is 25–30 mg/kg/day (to a maximum of 2.5g), with isoniazid, rifampin, and pyrazinamide at the same doses as in the twice-weekly regimen, but continued for 6 months by DOT. If pyrazinamide cannot be taken, a 9-month course may be administered in which INH in the above dosage is combined with rifampin 600 mg/day. **IM or IV** (rarely used) same as oral dosage.

Special Populations. *Pediatric Dosage.* **PO for prophylaxis of tuberculosis** 10–15 mg/kg/day as a single dose, to a maximum of 300 mg/day, given as a single agent for a minimum of 6 months.[53] **PO for treatment of pulmonary tuberculosis** same dosage as above, but combine with rifampin 10–20 mg/kg (to a maximum of 600 mg), and pyrazinamide 15–30 mg/kg/day (to a maximum of 2 g) in 2 or 3 divided doses for 8 weeks followed by 16 weeks of isoniazid and rifampin. Alternatively, give the daily doses of INH, rifampin, ethambutol, and pyrazinamide for 2 weeks, followed by INH 20–40 mg/kg (to a maximum of 900 mg), rifampin 10–20 mg/kg (to a maximum of 600 mg), ethambutol 50 mg/kg (to a maximum of 2.5 g), and pyrazinamide 50–70 mg/kg (to a maximum of 4 g) in 2 or 3 divided doses twice weekly for a total of 6 weeks by DOT, then continue INH and rifampin twice weekly for 16 weeks by DOT. In 3 times a week regimens, pyrazinamide dosage is 50–70 mg/kg/day. (to a maximum of 3 g) in 2–3 divided doses. If pyrazinamide cannot be taken, a 9-month course may be administered in which isoniazid in the above dosage is combined with rifampin 10–20 mg/kg (to a maximum of 600 mg).[53,54] **IM or IV** (rarely used) same as oral dosage.

Geriatric Dosage. Same as adult dosage.

Other Conditions. Acetylator phenotype has not been evaluated as a parameter for dosage individualization; however, some sources recommend a dosage of 150–200 mg/day in slow acetylators with renal impairment.[57] In individuals with HIV infection being treated for tuberculosis, treatment regimens are not altered, but should continue for a total of 9 months and at least 6 months beyond culture conversion.

Dosage Forms. **Tab** 50, 100, 300 mg; **Cap** 150 mg with rifampin 300 mg (Rifamate); **Tab** 50 mg with rifampin 120 mg and pyrazinamide 300 mg (Rifater); **Inj** 100 mg/mL.

Patient Instructions. Report any burning, tingling, or numbness in the extremities, unusual malaise, fever, dark urine, or yellowing of the skin or eyes.

Pharmacokinetics. *Serum Levels.* A peak serum level of 3–5 mg/L (22–36 µmol/L) 2 hr postdose is proposed as evidence of adequate absorption.[51]

Fate. Rapid and nearly complete oral absorption with peak serum concentrations of 1–5 mg/L (7–36 µmol/L) 1 hr after a 5 mg/kg dose.[56] Widely distributed in body tissues including the CSF of normal patients and those with meningitis. V_d is 0.67 ± 0.15 L/kg; Cl is 0.22 ± 0.07 L/hr/kg in slow acetylators and 0.44 ± 0.12 L/hr/kg in rapid acetylators.[46] Eliminated primarily by acetylation in the liver to inactive metabolites which are excreted in the urine. Specific pattern of elimination depends on acetylator phenotype of the individual.[57]

$t_{1/2}$. (Rapid acetylators) 1.1 ± 0.1 hr, (slow acetylators) 2.1 ± 1.1 hr. Increased to 4 hr with renal impairment, and 6.7 hr with liver disease.

Adverse Reactions. Pyridoxine-responsive peripheral neuropathy can occur, especially in alcoholics, diabetics, patients with renal failure, malnourished patients, and slow acetylators, and with dosages greater than 5 mg/kg/day.[57] Subclinical hepatitis is frequent (10–20%) and characterized by usually asymptomatic elevation of AST and ALT, which may return to normal despite continued therapy; it may be more frequent with combined INH-rifampin therapy.[58] Clinical hepatitis is rare in those <20 yr, but is strikingly related to age (rising to 2–3% in 50–65-yr-old patients). Rare cases of massive liver atrophy resulting in death usually appear in association with alcoholism or preexisting liver disease; most severe cases occur within the first 6 months.[58] With acute overdosage (usually 6–10 g), INH may produce severe CNS toxicity including coma and seizures as well as hypotension, acidosis, and occasionally death.[57]

Contraindications. Acute or chronic liver disease; previous INH-associated hepatitis.

Precautions. Pregnancy; lactation. Use with caution in daily users of alcohol, elderly patients, and those with a slow acetylator phenotype.

Drug Interactions. Isoniazid may inhibit the metabolism of carbamazepine and phenytoin, increasing the risk of toxicity, particularly of phenytoin in slow acetylators. Mental changes may result from effects of isoniazid and disulfiram on metabolism of adrenergic neurotransmitters; avoid the use of disulfiram in patients who must take isoniazid. Aluminum-containing antacids may interfere with isoniazid absorption. Rifampin may increase the metabolism of isoniazid to hepatotoxic metabolites.

Parameters to Monitor. Question for prodromal signs of hepatitis (eg, fever, malaise) and signs of peripheral neuropathy (eg, burning, tingling, numbness) monthly during therapy. Baseline and monthly AST and ALT are recommended only in high-risk groups (those over 35 yr, daily alcohol users, and those with a history of liver dysfunction),[58] although they are not predictive of clinical hepatitis.

Notes. It is generally recommended that all patients receive INH for prophylaxis of tuberculosis who have had a positive reaction to intermediate strength Purified Protein Derivative (PPD, 5 Tuberculin Units) and who (1) are household contacts of patients with active tuberculosis; (2) converted their PPD to positive within the past 12–24 months; (3) have radiologic evidence of inactive tuberculosis or a history of inadequately treated active tuberculosis; (4) foreign-born persons (and their families) from high-prevalence areas who have entered the United States within the past 2 years; (5) persons with known or suspected HIV infection; (6) persons with medical or iatrogenic conditions that increase the risk of tuberculosis—silicosis, gastrectomy, jejunoileal bypass, weight of 10% or more below ideal, chronic renal failure, diabetes mellitus, corticosteroid or other immunosuppressive therapy, hematopoietic malignancy, other malignancy, and other conditions in which immunosuppression results from the disease or its treatment. Most sources suggest that the use of INH prophylaxis in patients older than 35 yr should be further restricted because of the increased risk of fatal hepatotoxicity, although this is controversial. Limiting the duration of prophylaxis to 6 months appears to be cost-effective compared to 9- or 12-month regimens, and may improve compliance, although HIV-infected patients should receive 12 months of therapy.[56]

To prevent peripheral neuropathy, give **pyridoxine** in a dosage of 50 mg/day to adults receiving large dosages of INH (10 mg/kg/day or more) and those who are predisposed to peripheral neuritis (eg, diabetics, HIV-infected, alcoholics). Pyridoxine IV in a dosage equal to the estimated amount of INH ingested is recommended for acute INH overdose.[59]

Add **ethambutol** or **streptomycin** to the initial treatment regimen until drug susceptibility studies are available, or unless there is little possibility of drug resistance (ie, there is less than 4% primary resistance to isoniazid in the patient's community, and the patient has had no previous treatment with antituberculosis medications, is not from a country with a high prevalence of drug resistance, and has no known exposure to a drug-resistant case).[53,60]

PYRAZINAMIDE Various

Pyrazinamide is a synthetic analogue of niacinamide that is only active against mycobacteria. The mode of action is unknown. The drug is most active at acid pH, and is active against intracellular organisms. Resistance develops rapidly when used alone, but no cross-resistance with isoniazid is observed. The drug is well absorbed from the GI tract with serum levels of 40–50 mg/L (0.3–0.4 mmol/L) achieved about 2 hr after a 1-g dose. A peak serum level of 20–60 mg/L (163–488 μmol/L) 2 hr after an oral 1–2-g dose is proposed as evidence of adequate absorption. The parent compound and several metabolites are excreted in urine. Adverse effects include frequent hyperuricemia, probably caused by prevention of uric acid excretion by one of the metabolites, and occasional dose-dependent hepatotoxicity. As many as 1–5% of patients taking regimens including isoniazid, rifampin, and pyrazinamide may develop laboratory evidence of hepatic damage. Dosage for tuberculosis treatment is found in the isoniazid monograph.[53–56] Available as 500-mg tablets and in combination tablets 300 mg with isoniazid 50 mg and rifampin 120 mg (Rifater).

RIFABUTIN Mycobutin

Rifabutin (formerly ansamycin) is a rifamycin similar to rifampin chemically and in antibacterial spectrum. Rifabutin is more active against mycobacteria than rifampin, including some rifampin-resistant strains of *Mycobacterium tuberculosis* and atypical mycobacteria, and is particularly active against *M. avium intracellulare* (MAI). It is well absorbed orally, but has a low and variable bioavailability of 12–20% because of first-pass metabolism. Rifabutin is widely distributed in the body and is concentrated intracellularly to a greater extent than rifampin. It is 71 ± 2% plasma protein bound and has an estimated V_d of 45 ± 17 L/kg and Cl of 0.69 ± 0.32 L/hr/kg. The drug is hepatically metabolized to a number of compounds, with about 10% excreted unchanged in urine. Its terminal half-life after long-term use is 45 ± 16 hr. It induces its own metabolism as well as the metabolism of some other drugs metabolized via CYP3A4; although the clinical importance of this effect is not clear, it appears to be less than that of rifampin. The most frequent adverse reactions include rash, taste alterations, anorexia, nausea, insomnia, nervous system disorders (facial paralysis, twitching, and peripheral neuritis), leukopenia, and bilirubinemia. Uveitis has occurred with dosages over 300 mg/day. The adult dosage for the prophylaxis of MAI infections in patients with advanced HIV infection is 300 mg/day.[61–64] Available as 150-mg capsules.

RIFAMPIN
Rimactane, Rifadin

Pharmacology. Rifampin is a synthetic rifamycin B derivative that inhibits the action of DNA-dependent RNA polymerase. It is highly active against mycobacteria, most Gram-positive bacteria, and some Gram-negative bacteria, most notably, *Neisseria meningitidis*. It is also used to enhance bactericidal activity of other antistaphylococcal agents in refractory or chronic infections. Antagonism with vancomycin is observed in vitro, but is probably not clinically relevant. Primary resistance is uncommon, but resistance can develop rapidly if used alone.[65]

Administration and Adult Dosage. **PO or IV (rarely used) for treatment of tuberculosis** 600 mg/day as a single daily dose in combination with at least one other antitubercular agent (*see* Isoniazid);[53,54] **PO for prophylaxis of meningococcal meningitis** 600 mg bid for 2 days.[66] **PO for staphylococcal infection** 600 mg/day as a single dose in combination with another antistaphylococcal agent.

Special Populations. *Pediatric Dosage.* **PO for treatment of tuberculosis** (over 5 yr) 10–20 mg/kg/day as a single daily dose, to a maximum of 600 mg/day, in combination with at least one other antitubercular agent.[53,54] **PO for prophylaxis of meningococcal meningitis** (under 1 month) 5 mg/kg bid for 2 days; (1 month–12 yr) 10 mg/kg bid, to a maximum of 600 mg bid, for 2 days.[66]

Geriatric Dosage. Same as adult dosage.

Other Conditions. Accumulation is expected in patients with hepatic dysfunction or biliary obstruction, but dosage guidelines are not available. No dosage adjustment is necessary in patients with impaired renal function.

Dosage Forms. **Cap** 150, 300 mg; **Cap** 300 mg with isoniazid 150 mg (Rifamate); **Tab** 120 mg with isoniazid 50 mg and pyrazinamide 300 mg (Rifater); **Inj** 600 mg.

Patient Instructions. Take this medication with a full glass of water on an empty stomach (1 hour before or 2 hours after meals) for best absorption. It is important to take this medication regularly as directed, because inconsistent use may increase its toxicity. This drug may cause harmless red-orange discoloration of sweat, tears (it may permanently discolor soft contact lenses), saliva, feces, and urine.

Pharmacokinetics. *Serum Levels.* A peak serum level of 8–24 mg/L (10–29 µmol/L) 2 hr after a 600–750 mg oral dose is proposed as evidence of adequate absorption.[51]

Fate. 100% absorbed orally, with a 600-mg dose producing a peak serum concentration of approximately 10 mg/L (12 µmol/L) 1–3 hr after administration. Food delays absorption but does not affect overall bioavailability. First-pass hepatic extraction is substantial but saturated with doses greater than 300–450 mg; thus, larger doses produce disproportionate increases in serum levels. Widely distributed throughout the body; however, useful amounts appear in the CSF only in the presence of inflamed meninges. About 80% plasma protein bound; V_d is 0.97 ± 0.36 L/kg; Cl is 0.21 ± 0.1 L/hr/kg. Eliminated primarily by deacetylation in the liver to a partially active metabolite that is extensively enterohepatically recirculated, producing very high biliary concentrations. About 50–60% of a dose is eventually excreted in the feces. Urinary excretion is variable and appears to increase with the dose. At usual dosages, 12–15% is excreted unchanged in the urine.[64,67]

$t_{1/2}$. 3.5 ± 0.8 hr. Half-life increases with higher doses, but may become shorter over the first few weeks of treatment. It is not changed by renal impairment, but is increased unpredictably by liver disease or biliary obstruction.[64,67]

Adverse Reactions. Adverse reactions are more frequent and severe with intermittent, high-dose administration. GI symptoms are frequent. Acute, reversible renal failure, characterized as tubular damage with interstitial nephritis, sometimes appearing with concomitant hepatic failure has been reported rarely, especially in association with intermittent administration.[56,57] Asymptomatic elevation of liver enzymes occurs frequently, whereas clinical hepatitis is rare, but more common with preexisting liver disease or alcoholism; the effect of INH coadministration on the frequency of hepatitis is unclear.[58] Competition with bile for biliary excretion may produce jaundice, especially with preexisting liver disease. Intermittent therapy is also associated with thrombocytopenia and a flulike syndrome (ie, fever, joint pain, muscle cramps).

Contraindications. Hypersensitivity to any rifamycin derivative.

Precautions. Pregnancy; lactation. Use with caution in daily users of alcohol, those with preexisting liver disease, and those with a history of drug-associated hepatic damage (especially from antituberculars).

Drug Interactions. Rifampin accelerates the metabolism of many drugs such as oral contraceptives, corticosteroids, cyclosporine, digitoxin, HIV protease inhibitors, propranolol, methadone, metoprolol, mexiletine, phenytoin, quinidine, theophylline, tolbutamide, oral verapamil, warfarin, and zidovudine because of potent inducing effects on CYP3A.[68] The dosage of these drugs may need to be increased during concurrent use. Rifampin may increase the metabolism of isoniazid to hepatotoxic metabolites.

Parameters to Monitor. Question for prodromal signs of hepatitis (eg, fever, malaise). Baseline and monthly AST and ALT have been recommended, especially for patients with factors predisposing to hepatotoxicity (eg, alcoholism, preexisting liver disease), although they are not predictive of clinical hepatitis in the absence of symptoms.

Notes. Rifampin is a useful drug for tuberculosis, but should be used only in combination regimens because of rapid emergence of resistant mutants of *Mycobacterium tuberculosis* when it is used alone. The recent emergence of multiple drug resistance among strains of *M. tuberculosis* in patients with AIDS includes high-level rifampin resistance. The routine use of rifampin in methicillin-resistant *Staphylococcus aureus* (MRSA) endocarditis is not recommended except after failure of conventional therapy and possibly with renal, myocardial, splenic, or cerebral abscess. If rifampin is added to vancomycin for treatment of MRSA, add a third drug (eg, gentamicin) to reduce the likelihood of resistance development. In nonendocarditis infections caused by MRSA, do not use rifampin unless there is inadequate response to vancomycin alone.

SECOND-LINE ANTITUBERCULOSIS AGENTS COMPARISON CHART[a]

DRUG	DOSAGE FORMS	ADULT DOSAGE	PEDIATRIC DOSAGE	SERUM LEVELS[b] (MG/L)	HALF-LIFE Normal	HALF-LIFE Renal Impairment	MAJOR ADVERSE EFFECTS
Aminosalicylic Acid Salts Various	Tab 500 mg.	PO 8–12 g/day in 2–4 divided doses (as the acid).	150–300 mg/kg/day in 3–4 divided doses, to a maximum of 12 g/day.	20–60[d] (4 g)	1 hr	—	GI intolerance; hepatitis; lupuslike syndrome. Rarely used.
Capreomycin Sulfate Capastat	Inj 1 g.	Same as streptomycin.	Same as streptomycin.	Same as streptomycin.	2.5 hr	↑	Nephrotoxicity; ototoxicity.
Clofazimine Lamprene	Cap 50, 100 mg.	PO 100–200 mg/day.	Not well established.	0.5–2 (100–200 mg)	70 days	—	Brown-black discoloration of skin and bodily secretions; nausea, vomiting, GI pain because of deposition in GI tissues.
Cycloserine Seromycin	Cap 250 mg.	PO 15–20 mg/kg/day (usually 500 mg) in 2 divided doses, to maximum of 1 g/day.	PO 10–15 mg/kg/day to a maximum of 1 g/day.	20–35 (250–500 mg)	10 hr	↑	CNS (drowsiness, dizziness headache, depression rare seizures and psychosis).
Ethionamide Trecator-SC	Tab 250 mg.	PO 15–20 mg/kg/day (usually 500–750 mg) as a single daily dose, to a maximum of 1 g/day.	PO 15–20 mg/kg/day to a maximum of 1 g/day.	1–5 (250–500 mg)	3 hr	—	GI intolerance; hepatitis; CNS (drowsiness, dizziness headache, depression, rare seizures).

(continued)

SECOND-LINE ANTITUBERCULOSIS AGENTS COMPARISON CHART[a] (continued)

DRUG	DOSAGE FORMS	ADULT DOSAGE	PEDIATRIC DOSAGE	SERUM LEVELS[b] (MG/L)	HALF-LIFE Normal	HALF-LIFE Renal Impairment	MAJOR ADVERSE EFFECTS
Kanamycin Sulfate Kantrex	Inj 37.5, 250, 333 mg/mL.	Same as streptomycin.	Same as streptomycin.	Same as streptomycin.	2–3 hr	80–90 hr	Nephrotoxicity; ototoxicity.
Rifabutin Mycobutin	Cap 150 mg.	PO 300 mg/day as a single dose.	Not well established. (1 yr) 15–25 mg/kg/day; (2–10 yr) 4–19 mg/kg/day; (14–16 yr) 2.8–5.4 mg/kg/day.	—	20–40 hr	—	See monograph.
Streptomycin Sulfate	Inj 400 mg/mL.	IM 12–15 mg/kg/day to a maximum of 1 g, or 22–25 mg/kg to a maximum of 1.5 g 2–3 times/week.	IM 20–40 mg/kg/day to a maximum of 1 g, or 25–30 mg/kg to a maximum of 1.5 g 2–3 times/week.	35–40 (12–15 mg/kg) 65–80 (22–25 mg/kg)	2–3 hr	↑	Vestibular ototoxicity.

[a]Use only in combination with other effective antituberculars.
[b]Peak serum level 1 hr (parenteral) or 2 hr (oral) after the adult dose in parentheses that is evidence of adequate absorption.
[c]Sodium salt contains 73% aminosalicylic acid; increase dosage accordingly. Sodium content is 4.7 mEq/g.
[d]Peak serum level 6 hr after a dose of Paser granules (investigational).
Adapted from references 51–53, 56, and 57.

Antiparasitic Drugs

Class Instructions: Pinworms. Purgation, enemas, or special dietary restrictions are unnecessary with this drug, which may be taken with food or beverages. To avoid reinfestation with pinworms, wash the perianal area thoroughly each morning. Change and wash nightclothes, undergarments, and bedclothes daily. Wash hands and under fingernails thoroughly after bowel movements and before eating. Treat all family members simultaneously and clean bedroom and bathroom floors thoroughly at the end of the course of treatment. In order to demonstrate a cure, no eggs must be found in the anal area at least 5 weeks after the end of treatment.

ALBENDAZOLE
Albenza

Pharmacology. Albendazole is a benzimidazole drug related to mebendazole and has a similar mechanism of action; however, it has a broader range of activity than mebendazole.

Administration and Adult Dosage. **PO for hydatid cyst** 400 mg bid for 28 days, followed by a 2-week drug-free interval; repeat to a total of three cycles. **PO for neurocysticercosis** 400 mg bid for 8–30 days; repeat courses of therapy may be needed.[69]

Special Populations. *Pediatric Dosage.* Safety and efficacy not established. **PO for hydatid cyst** 15 mg/kg/day for 28 days, repeat course of therapy prn. **PO for neurocysticercosis** 15 mg/kg/day in 2–3 divided doses for 8–28 days, repeat course of therapy prn.[69]

Geriatric Dosage. Same as adult dosage.

Dosage Forms. **Tab** 200 mg.

Patient Instructions. Take this drug with a fatty meal to increase absorption and improve effectiveness.

Pharmacokinetics. *Fate.* Absorption is poor, but is enhanced by fat. Oral bioavailability of unchanged albendazole is negligible because of first-pass metabolism to albendazole sulfoxide, the active form of the drug. The sulfoxide has a peak serum level 2–3 hr after a dose. CNS concentrations are 40% of serum levels; concentration in echinococcal cysts is about 25% of serum levels. The absorbed drug is primarily excreted in urine as metabolites.[70]

$t_{\frac{1}{2}}$. (Albendazole sulfoxide) 10–15 hr.[70]

Adverse Reactions. Occasionally diarrhea, abdominal pain, and migration of roundworms through the mouth and nose occurs. Rarely, leukopenia, alopecia, or increased transaminases occur.[69]

Precautions. Pregnancy; liver dysfunction.

Drug Interactions. Concurrent dexamethasone increases serum levels by 50%.[70]

Parameters to Monitor. Monitor hepatic transaminases and WBC count during prolonged therapy.

Notes. Albendazole is also an alternative in ascariasis, capillariasis, cutaneous larva migrans, eosinophilic enterocolitis, giardiasis, hookworm, microsporidiosis (in AIDS), pinworms, strongyloidiasis, trichostrongyloidiasis, and whipworm.[69,71]

MEBENDAZOLE   Vermox, Various

Pharmacology. Mebendazole is active against many intestinal roundworms. It binds to helminth tubulin, and inhibits glucose uptake in the parasite with no effect on blood sugar concentrations in the host.[70]

Administration and Adult Dosage. PO for pinworms 100 mg in a single dose; repeat in 2 weeks. **PO for roundworms, whipworms, and hookworms** 100 mg bid for 3 days.[69]

Special Populations. *Pediatric Dosage.* Safety and efficacy not established under 2 yr. **PO for pinworms, roundworms, whipworms, and hookworms** same as adult dosage.[69]

Geriatric Dosage. Same as adult dosage.

Dosage Forms. Chew Tab 100 mg.

Patient Instructions. (*See* Pinworms Class Instructions.) Chew tablets before swallowing.

Pharmacokinetics. *Fate.* Poorly absorbed orally. Almost all eliminated unchanged in the feces, but up to 10% may be recovered in the urine 48 hr after a dose, primarily as the decarboxylated metabolite.[70]

Adverse Reactions. Occasional abdominal pain and diarrhea in cases of massive infestation and expulsion of worms. Occasionally migration of roundworms through the mouth and nose occurs. Rarely, leukopenia, agranulocytosis, and hypospermia have been reported.[69]

Precautions. Pregnancy.

Drug Interactions. Carbamazepine and hydantoins may reduce mebendazole serum levels.

Parameters to Monitor. When treating whipworm, take a stool sample for egg count 3 weeks after treatment to detect frequent (about 30%) persistent infestation requiring retreatment.[72]

Notes. Mebendazole is the agent of choice for whipworm, producing about a 70% cure rate with a single treatment; the cure rate is 90–100% with roundworms, hookworms, and pinworms. Particularly useful in mixed infestations. It is also used in several other infestations, such as trichinosis, eosinophilic enterocolitis, capillariasis, angiostrongyliasis, and visceral larva migrans.[69,70]

PRAZIQUANTEL   Biltricide

Pharmacology. Praziquantel causes a loss of intracellular calcium, resulting in paralysis and dislodgement of worms from sites of attachment. In higher dosages, it damages the parasite's surface membrane, allowing the host's immune response to destroy the worm.[71,73]

Administration and Adult Dosage. PO for schistosomiasis (*Schistosoma haematobium, S. mansoni*) 40 mg/kg in 2 divided doses the same day, but heavy infestations require 60 mg/kg in 3 divided doses at 4–6 hr intervals;[69,71] (*S. japonicum, S. mekongi*) 60 mg/kg in 3 doses at 4–6 hr intervals. **PO for flukes** (eg, fascioliasis, clonorchiasis, opisthorchiasis) 25 mg/kg tid for 1 day; (paragonimiasis) 25 mg/kg tid for 2 days.[69,71] **PO for tapeworms** (beef, dog, fish, pork) 5–10 mg/kg as a single dose; (dwarf tapeworm) 25 mg/kg as a single dose. **PO for neurocysticercosis** 50 mg/kg/day in 3 doses for 15 days.[69,72] (*See* Notes.)

Special Populations. *Pediatric Dosage.* Safety and efficacy not established under 4 yr. PO same as adult dosage.

Geriatric Dosage. Same as adult dosage.

Dosage Forms. Tab 600 mg.

Patient Instructions. Take with liquid during meals, but do not chew tablets. This drug may cause dizziness or drowsiness. Use caution when driving, operating machinery, or performing other tasks requiring mental alertness.

Pharmacokinetics. *Fate.* The drug is 80% absorbed orally, but undergoes extensive first-pass metabolism. CSF concentrations are 14–20% of serum levels. The drug is metabolized and metabolites are excreted primarily in urine.

$t_{1/2}$. 1.1 ± 0.3 hr.

Adverse Reactions. Side effects are usually mild. Dizziness, headache, and malaise occur frequently after large doses. Occasionally, abdominal discomfort, fever, sweating, and eosinophilia occur. Drowsiness or fatigue may occur because of a structural similarity to benzodiazepines. Pruritus and rash occur rarely.[69] In patients treated for neurocysticercosis, an inflammatory response, presumably caused by dead and dying organisms, occurs that is manifested by headache, seizures, and increased intracranial pressure.

Contraindications. Ocular cysticercosis.

Precautions. Pregnancy; liver disease; avoid breastfeeding for 72 hr after the last dose.

Drug Interactions. Drugs that induce CYP3A3/4 (eg, dexamethasone, carbamazepine, phenobarbital, phenytoin) can increase clearance, decrease bioavailability, and cause treatment failure; drugs that inhibit CYP3A3/4 (eg, cimetidine, ketoconazole, erythromycin) decrease clearance, increase serum levels, and lengthen half-life.[70,71]

Parameters to Monitor. Observe for CNS toxicity when treating neurocysticercosis.

Notes. Concomitant corticosteroid therapy is recommended for patients treated for neurocysticercosis.

PYRANTEL PAMOATE   Antiminth, Various

Pharmacology. Pyrantel is a depolarizing neuromuscular blocker that produces spastic paralysis of the parasite with no similar effects on the host after oral use. It also inhibits acetylcholinesterases.[70]

Administration and Adult Dosage. PO for roundworms and pinworms 11 mg/kg, to a maximum of 1 g in a single dose; **for pinworms** repeat after a 2-week interval. **PO for hookworms and eosinophilic enterocolitis** 11 mg/kg/day, to a maximum of 1 g for 3 days.[69] Doses are expressed as base equivalent.

Special Populations. *Pediatric Dosage.* Safety and efficacy not established under 2 yr. **PO** same as adult dosage.

Geriatric Dosage. Same as adult dosage.

Dosage Forms. Susp 50 mg/mL (strength expressed as base equivalent).

Patient Instructions. (*See* Pinworms Class Instructions.)

Pharmacokinetics. *Fate.* Slight oral absorption. Over 50% is excreted unchanged in feces, and less than 15% of the dose is excreted as parent drug and metabolites in the urine.[70]

Adverse Reactions. Occasional nausea, vomiting, headaches, dizziness, rash, and transient AST elevations.[69,72]

Contraindications. Liver disease.

Precautions. Avoid during pregnancy.

Drug Interactions. Piperazine and pyrantel may be mutually antagonistic in ascariasis.

Notes. Virtually 100% effective for pinworms and roundworms; ineffective for whipworm and *Strongyloides* spp.

THIABENDAZOLE   Mintezol

Pharmacology. Although the exact mechanism is unknown, thiabendazole inhibits the helminth-specific enzyme, fumarate reductase, and may interfere with microtubule assembly and inhibit glucose uptake in the parasite.[70]

Administration and Adult Dosage. PO for strongyloidiasis 25 mg/kg bid for 2 days; continue therapy of disseminated strongyloidiasis for at least 5 days. **PO for cutaneous larva migrans** 25 mg/kg bid for 2–5 days; concomitantly apply thiabendazole oral suspension topically qid directly over the end of the larval tunnel in the skin. **PO for visceral larva migrans** 25 mg/kg bid for 7 days. Do not exceed a dosage of 3 g/day for any indication.[69] (*See* Notes.)

Special Populations. *Pediatric Dosage.* Safety and efficacy under 13.6 kg is not established. **PO** same as adult dosage.

Geriatric Dosage. Same as adult dosage.

Dosage Forms. Susp 100 mg/mL; **Chew Tab** 500 mg.

Pharmacokinetics. *Fate.* Well absorbed after oral administration. Most of the drug is metabolized to inactive glucuronide or sulfate compounds and excreted in urine within 24 hr.

Adverse Reactions. CNS effects such as dizziness, drowsiness, and giddiness occur frequently; nausea and vomiting are also common. Diarrhea, epigastric pain, fever, chills, flushing, and headache occur occasionally, as do allergic manifestations (eg, pruritus, rash, angioedema). Seizures, leukopenia, lymphadenopathy, and liver damage occur rarely.[69]

Precautions. Pregnancy.

Drug Interactions. Thiabendazole may inhibit hepatic metabolism of xanthines (eg, theophylline).

Notes. A systemic corticosteroid may be indicated to reduce inflammation caused by dying larvae when the drug is used to treat visceral larva migrans of the eye.

Antiviral Drugs

ACYCLOVIR	Zovirax
VALACYCLOVIR	Valtrex

Pharmacology. Acyclovir is an acyclic nucleoside analogue of deoxyguanosine that is selectively phosphorylated by the virus-encoded thymidine kinase to its monophosphate form. Cellular enzymes then convert the monophosphate to the active antiviral acyclovir triphosphate, which inhibits viral DNA synthesis by incorporation into viral DNA, resulting in chain termination. Acyclovir has potent activity against herpes simplex virus I and II (HSV), and also herpes zoster virus (varicella-zoster virus [VZV]). Activity against cytomegalovirus, which lacks a specific virus-encoded thymidine kinase, is limited, but resistance can be overcome with high serum concentrations in some patient populations. Acyclovir inhibits Epstein-Barr virus (EBV), but it has not been found clinically useful. Human herpesvirus 6 is resistant.[74–77] Valacyclovir is the L-valyl ester of acyclovir, which undergoes extensive first-pass hydrolysis to yield high serum acyclovir concentrations.

Administration and Adult Dosage. **IV for severe localized HSV infection** (acyclovir) 5 mg/kg q 8 hr for 5 days for nonimmunocompromised patients or 7–10 days for immunocompromised patients; **IV for VZV infection in immunocompromised patients** 10 mg/kg q 8 hr for 7–10 days; **IV for HSV encephalitis** 10 mg/kg q 8 hr for 10–14 days. Dilute to 50–250 mL and infuse over 60 min. Maintain minimum urine output of 500 mL/24 hr for each gram of acyclovir administered. **PO for primary or recurrent genital HSV infection** (acyclovir) 200 mg 5 times/day for 10 days: (valacyclovir, immunocompetent patients) 500 mg bid for 5 days. **PO for prevention of recurrent genital HSV infection** (acyclovir) 400 mg bid or 200 mg 3–5 times/day; **PO for active varicella-zoster (chickenpox) or herpes zoster** (acyclovir) 800 mg q 4 hr 5 times a day for 5 days (chickenpox) or 7–10 days (zoster). **PO for herpes zoster in immunocompetent patients** (valacyclovir) 1 g q 8 hr for 7 days. **Top for initial genital HSV infection and limited non-life-threatening mucocutaneous herpes simplex infections in immunocompromised patients** (acyclovir) 0.5-inch ribbon to cover 4-square-inch affected skin area q 3 hr, 6 times/day for 7 days.

Special Populations. *Pediatric Dosage.* (All dosages apply to acyclovir) **IV for HSV infection** (neonates) 10 mg/kg q 8 hr for 10–14 days;[39,76] (13 months–11 yr) 750 mg/m^2 in 3 divided doses. **IV for varicella-zoster (chickenpox) in immunocompromised children** (13 months–11 yr) 1500 mg/m^2 in 3 divided doses. **IV for HSV encephalitis** (6 months–11 yr) 1500 mg/m^2 in 3 divided doses. **PO for varicella-zoster (chickenpox)** (acyclovir) (over 2 yr and under 40 kg) 20 mg/kg/dose, to a maximum of 800 mg q 6 hr for 5 days; (over 40 kg) same as adult dosage; (valacyclovir) safety and efficacy not established.

Geriatric Dosage. Same as adult dosage, but adjust for age-related reduction in renal function.

Other Conditions. (Acyclovir) In obesity, base dosage on ideal body weight. In renal insufficiency, reduce parenteral and oral dosage as follows: Cl_{cr} 25–50 mL/min, give the usual dose q 12 hr; Cl_{cr} 10–25 mL/min, give the usual dose q 24 hr; Cl_{cr} 0–10 mL/min, give 50% of the usual dose q 24 hr. For patients on hemodialysis, give the usual daily dosage after dialysis. (Valacyclovir) In renal insufficiency, reduce the dosage as follows: Cl_{cr} 30–49 mL/min, 1 g q 12 hr; Cl_{cr} 10–29 mL/min, 1 g q 24 hr; Cl_{cr} <10 mL/min, 500 mg q 24 hr.

Dosage Forms. (Acyclovir) **Cap** 200; **Tab** 400, 800 mg; **Inj** 500 mg, 1 g; **Oint** 5%; **Susp** 40 mg/mL. (Valacyclovir) **Tab** 500 mg.

Patient Instructions. Use a finger cot or latex glove when applying acyclovir ointment to avoid autoinoculation. The ointment may cause transient burning or stinging.

Pharmacokinetics. *Fate.* Oral bioavailability of acyclovir is estimated to be 15–30%; valacyclovir is well absorbed, with a bioavailability of 54%.[78] Valacyclovir is extensively converted to acyclovir after oral administration. After 200–600 mg of acyclovir orally, mean peak steady-state levels are 0.56–1.3 mg/L (2.5–5.9 µmol/L); levels after IV doses of 2.5–15 mg/kg are 5–24 mg/L (23–105 µmol/L). After an oral dose of 1 g of valacyclovir, mean peak steady-state acyclovir level is 5–6 mg/L (22–27 µmol/L).[79] CSF acyclovir concentrations are 25–70% of simultaneous serum level. Decay is biphasic, with a V_{dB} of 0.69 ± 0.19 L/kg; Cl is 0.21 ± 0.03 L/hr/kg with normal renal function;[78] 86–92% is excreted unchanged in urine; the remainder is metabolized to 9-carboxymethoxymethylguanine. Renal clearance is 75–80% of total clearance and is markedly reduced by concomitant probenecid.[80]

$t_{1/2}$. (Acyclovir) α phase 0.34 hr, β phase 2.9 ± 0.8 hr in adult patients, increasing to nearly 20 hr in end-stage renal disease; 5.7 hr on dialysis; about 4 hr in neonates.[80]

Adverse Reactions. (Acyclovir) Nephrotoxicity, thought to be caused by precipitation of acyclovir crystals in the nephron, occurs in about 10% of patients if the drug is given by bolus (<10 min) injection. Phlebitis at injection site occurs frequently with IV infusion because of the high pH (9–11) of the product. Other side effects reported are CNS toxicity (eg, headache, lethargy, tremulousness, delirium, seizures), nausea, vomiting, and skin rash. CNS toxicity occurs primarily in patients with underlying neurologic disease or end-stage renal disease, or with cancer chemotherapy and irradiation to the CNS, and may not be primarily caused by the drug. Topical application to herpes lesions may be painful.[74–76] (Valacyclovir) Adverse reactions appear comparable to acyclovir. Nausea, vomiting, diarrhea, abdominal pain, and headache have been reported frequently with valacyclovir use. Thrombotic thrombocytopenic purpura/hemolytic-uremic syndrome has been reported in patients with advanced HIV disease and in bone marrow and renal transplant patients. This phenomenon has not been reported in immunocompetent patients.[79]

Contraindications. (Valacyclovir) allergy to any component of the drug or to acyclovir.

Precautions. Use with caution in renal impairment, dehydration, and preexisting neurologic disorders. Valacyclovir is not indicated in immunocompromised patients.

Drug Interactions. Zidovudine and acyclovir may result in drowsiness and lethargy. Probenecid may increase oral bioavailability and half-life of acyclovir.

Parameters to Monitor. Monitor renal function and injection site for signs of phlebitis daily. Carefully monitor patients with underlying neurologic diseases for evidence of neurotoxicity (*see* Adverse Reactions).

Notes. Acyclovir-resistant strains of virus that are deficient in thymidine kinase have been isolated from patients after treatment. Although thought to be less virulent than sensitive strains, HSV strains resistant to acyclovir have been described in AIDS patients.[76]

CIDOFOVIR   Vistide

Cidofovir (HPMPC) is a nucleotide analogue with potent in vitro and in vivo activity against cytomegalovirus (CMV) and other herpesviruses. Cidofovir contains a phosphonate group that enables it to bypass initial virus-dependent phosphorylation. Cellular enzymes convert cidofovir to cidofovir diphosphate, the active intracellular metabolite. Peak serum cidofovir concentration averages 26.1 ± 3.2 mg/L after a 5 mg/kg IV infusion with concomitant probenecid and hydration. Cidofovir is not appreciably bound to plasma proteins; V_d averages 0.5 L/kg. Cidofovir is excreted almost entirely unchanged in the urine. The elimination half-life of cidofovir is 3–6 hr when administered with probenecid. Cidofovir diphosphate has a prolonged intracellular half-life, ranging from 17–65 hr, which allows infrequent administration schedules of once weekly to once every other week. Nephrotoxicity is the most frequent adverse reaction, and high-dose probenecid must be used with administration of cidofovir. Probenecid decreases uptake of cidofovir in proximal renal tubular cells, decreasing the risk of nephrotoxicity. Other frequent adverse reactions are proteinuria, elevated Cr_s, nausea, vomiting, fever, asthenia, neutropenia, rash, headache, diarrhea, alopecia, anemia, and abdominal pain. Ocular hypotony and decreased intraocular pressure have been reported occasionally. Nausea, vomiting, fever, rash, and chills are frequent reactions reported with probenecid. It is essential to give the following with cidofovir: PO 2 g of probenecid 3 hr before administration and IV 1 L of NS over 1 hr just prior to administration. If tolerated, give another liter of NS with or after cidofovir administration; finally, give PO 1 g probenecid 2 hr and 8 hr after the end of cidofovir infusion. The IV induction dosage of cidofovir for CMV retinitis is 5 mg/kg infused over 1 hr once weekly for 2 weeks, and the IV maintenance dosage is 5 mg/kg once every other week. Reduce dosage to 3 mg/kg if Cr_s increases by 0.3–0.4 mg/dL above baseline or $\geq$2+ proteinuria occurs.[81–83] Available as a 75 mg/mL injection. Cidofovir is also being investigated as an intravitreal injection for CMV retinitis.

DELAVIRDINE   Rescriptor

Delavirdine is a nonnucleoside reverse transcriptase inhibitor similar to nevirapine and is used in combination with other antiretroviral drugs. It is an inhibitor of CYP3A in vitro. Skin rashes (including Stevens-Johnson syndrome occasionally) occur in about 50% of patients. The dosage is 400 mg PO tid. If rash occurs, the drug is stopped and reinstituted at a dosage of 200 mg tid for one week, then dosage is increased at weekly intervals until the usual dosage is reached. Available as 100 mg dispersible tablets.

DIDANOSINE   Videx

Pharmacology. Didanosine (dideoxyinosine; ddI) is a purine nucleoside that undergoes complex metabolism in vivo to dideoxyadenosine (ddA), which ultimately undergoes metabolism to an active triphosphorylated form (ddATP). Incorporation of ddATP into viral DNA leads to chain termination, and ddATP is a competitive inhibitor of HIV reverse transcriptase, which further contributes to the interference of HIV replication.[84]

Administration and Adult Dosage. PO for HIV infection (60 kg or greater) 200 mg (as 2 tablets) q 12 hr, or 250 mg (as powder) q 12 hr; (under 60 kg) 125 mg (as 2 tablets) q 12 hr, or 167 mg (as powder) q 12 hr. Take each dose as 2 whole (not partial) tablets to provide adequate buffering.

Special Populations. *Pediatric Dosage.* PO for HIV infection (BSA 1.1–1.4 m²) 100 mg (as 2 tablets) q 12 hr, or 125 mg (as pediatric powder) q 12 hr; (BSA 0.8–1 m²) 75 mg (as 2 tablets) q 12 hr, or 94 mg (as pediatric powder) q 12 hr; (BSA 0.5–0.7 m²) 50 mg (as 2 tablets) q 12 hr or 62 mg (as pediatric powder) q 12 hr; (BSA 0.4 m² or less) 25 mg (as 1 tablet) q 12 hr, or 31 mg (as pediatric powder) q 12 hr.[85,86]

Geriatric Dosage. Same as adult dosage, but not studied in this population.

Other Conditions. Consider dosage reduction in patients with renal or hepatic impairment. Some clinicians suggest reduction of didanosine dosage by 75% in patients with severe renal impairment.[87] Didanosine is removed by hemodialysis, but the quantity removed is low and supplemental doses are not recommended.[87]

Dosage Forms. **Chew/Dispersible Tab** 25, 50, 100, 150 mg; **Pwdr for Oral Soln** 100, 167, 250, 375 mg; **Pwdr for Oral Soln (pediatric)** 2, 4 g.

Patient Instructions. Didanosine is not a cure for HIV infection, and opportunistic infections and other complications associated with HIV infection may continue to occur. Didanosine must be taken on an empty stomach 1 hour before or 2 hours after a meal. It is essential that the 2-tablet dose be taken each time to avoid destruction of the drug by stomach acid. For children >1 year use the 2-tablet dose; for those <1 year of age, use the 1-tablet dose. Tablets may be chewed and swallowed, or dissolved in at least 30 mL of water and swallowed immediately. Do *not* swallow the tablets whole. Reconstituted solution may be stored for up to 30 days when refrigerated. Shake solution thoroughly before administering each dose.

Pharmacokinetics. *Fate.* Didanosine is rapidly degraded at acidic pH. Appreciable interpatient variability and dose-dependent characteristics affect didanosine absorption. Oral bioavailability of the buffered powder for oral solution is 33 ± 11%.[88,89] The chewable/dispersible buffered tablets are 20–25% more bioavailable than the buffered powder for solution. The peak serum concentration is 1.1 ± 0.7 mg/L (4.7 ± 2.9 µmol/L) after a 375-mg oral dose of buffered powder for solution. Protein binding is less than 5%. CSF concentration 1 hr after infusion of didanosine averages 21% of the concurrent serum concentration. V_{dB} is 1 ± 0.7 L/kg; Cl is 1 ± 0.08 L/hr/kg.[87] Up to 60% of dose is excreted unchanged in the urine; the remainder is extensively metabolized to ddATP, hypoxanthine, and uric acid.[84,87]

$t_{1/2}$. 1.75 ± 0.99 hr;[87] in vitro intracellular half-life of ddATP is 8–43 hr.[90]

Adverse Reactions. Pancreatitis has occurred at a frequency of 5–9% in clinical trials at or below current recommended dosages and can be fatal. Peripheral neuropathy is frequent and occurs in 16–34% of patients, with 12% requiring dosage reduction. Diarrhea has been reported with the buffered powder for oral solution at a frequency of 34%. In children, pancreatitis and peripheral retinal depigmentation have occurred frequently, although the latter has not been associated with visual impairment.[91] Peripheral neuropathy has not occurred in children.

Precautions. Avoid didanosine tablets in patients with phenylketonuria because these contain phenylalanine. Didanosine has been associated with hyperuricemia; use caution in patients with a history of gout or baseline hyperuricemia; avoid in individuals with a history of pancreatitis.

Drug Interactions. Administration with fluoroquinolones may reduce fluoroquinolone serum levels because of buffers in formulation. Avoid concurrent administration with dapsone, indinavir, itraconazole, ketoconazole, or other medications requiring an acidic environment for absorption because of buffers in didanosine formulation. Both ganciclovir and trimethoprim-sulfamethoxazole appear to increase didanosine's bioavailability, but the clinical importance is unknown. Use with alcohol, high-dose trimethoprim-sulfamethoxazole, or other pancreatitis-associated drugs may increase the risk of pancreatitis.[92,93]

Parameters to Monitor. Obtain serum amylase, lipase, and triglycerides monthly. Symptoms of abdominal pain, nausea, and vomiting may indicate pancreatitis. Symptoms of distal numbness, tingling, or pain in the feet or hands may indicate neuropathy and may necessitate dosage modification. Monitor clinical signs, symptoms, and laboratory markers for progression of HIV-disease to help decide regimen changes in antiretroviral therapy. Baseline CD4 and HIV-1 RNA polymerase chain reaction viral load tests are useful to measure clinical benefit of therapy. Repeat tests after 1 month and q 3–4 months thereafter have been suggested to monitor benefit of antiretroviral therapy.

Notes. At present there are no results from clinical trials regarding the effect of didanosine on the clinical progression of HIV infection, such as frequency of opportunistic infections and improvement of survival. Combination therapy with **zidovudine** has been used by some clinicians to decrease viral resistance and improve clinical benefit. As with other nucleoside reverse transcriptase inhibitors, drug-resistant HIV-1 isolates emerge with long-term didanosine therapy (≥12 months).[86]

| **FAMCICLOVIR** | Famvir |
| **PENCICLOVIR** | Denavir |

Famciclovir is the diacetyl, 6-deoxy ester of the guanosine analogue penciclovir. Famciclovir is absorbed rapidly and converted to penciclovir in the intestinal wall and liver. Viral thymidine kinase converts penciclovir to its monophosphate form. Cellular enzymes then convert the monophosphate to the active antiviral penciclovir triphosphate. The triphosphate inhibits viral DNA synthesis by incorporation into viral DNA, resulting in termination of the chain. Penciclovir has potent activity against herpes simplex virus I and II (HSV) and herpes zoster virus (varicella-zoster). Penciclovir also has some activity against Epstein-Barr virus and cytomegalovirus, but has not demonstrated clinical usefulness against infections with these agents. The absolute bioavailability of penciclovir is 77% after a 500-mg oral dose of famciclovir. Serum peak concentrations achieved were 0.84 ± 0.22 and 3.34 ± 0.58 mg/L 0.75 hr after 125- and 500-mg oral doses of famciclovir, respectively. Penciclovir is less than 20% protein bound, and the V_d is approximately 1 L/kg. Penciclovir is eliminated primarily by renal excretion. The elimination half-life is approximately 2 hr with normal renal function, increasing to over 9 hr in patients with impaired renal function. Frequent adverse reactions include nausea, vomiting, diarrhea, and headache. Pruritus, paresthesias and fatigue occur occasionally. Cimetidine may enhance the bioavailability of famciclovir and its conversion to penciclovir somewhat. For herpes zoster the oral famciclovir dosage is 500 mg q 8 hr for 7 days. In renal insufficiency, reduce the dosage as follows: Cl_{cr} 40–59 mL/min, 500 mg q 12 hr; Cl_{cr} 20–39 mL/min, 500 mg q 24 hr; Cl_{cr} <20 mL/min, insufficient information to recommend a dosage. For recurrent episodes of genital HSV infection the famciclovir dosage is 125 mg bid for 5 days.[93–95] Famciclovir is available as 125-, 250-, and 500-mg tablets. Penciclovir is available as a 10 mg/g cream.

FOSCARNET SODIUM   FOSCAVIR

Pharmacology. Foscarnet sodium (phosphonoformic acid; PFA) is a pyrophosphate analogue. Foscarnet actively inhibits viral DNA polymerases in its parent form and does not require phosphorylation for optimal antiviral activity. It has antiviral activity against herpes simplex virus I and II, human cytomegalovirus (CMV), Epstein-Barr virus, hepatitis B virus, varicella zoster virus, and some retroviruses including the human immunodeficiency virus. Foscarnet sodium inhibits DNA synthesis in CMV and other herpesviruses by inhibiting viral DNA polymerase.[96,97]

Administration and Adult Dosage. IV induction for CMV retinitis in AIDS patients 60 mg/kg q 8 hr or 90 mg/kg q 12 hr for 14–21 days.[98] **IV maintenance for CMV retinitis in AIDS patients** 90–120 mg/kg/day in one dose. **IV for acyclovir-resistant herpes virus infections** 40 mg/kg q 8 hr or 60 mg/kg q 12 hr until clinical resolution.[98] **IV for acyclovir-resistant varicella-zoster infections in immunocompromised patients** 40 mg/kg q 8 hr or 60 mg/kg q 12 hr for 10–21 days or until clinical resolution.[77,99]

Special Populations. *Pediatric Dosage.* Safety and efficacy not established.

Geriatric Dosage. Same as adult dosage, but adjust for age-related reduction in renal function.

Other Conditions. Reduce dosage in renal function impairment (*see* product information).

Dosage Forms. Inj 24 mg/mL.

Patient Instructions. Foscarnet is not a cure for CMV retinitis, and progression of disease may continue during or following treatment. Regular eye examinations are important to monitor for disease progression. Report symptoms of tingling around the mouth or numbness in extremities, which may indicate a need for temporary discontinuation of foscarnet.

Pharmacokinetics. *Fate.* After twice-daily infusion of 90 mg/kg over 2 hr peak serum levels are 98 ± 27 mg/L (577 ± 161 μmol/L) and troughs are 6.4 ± 8.3 mg/L (38 ± 49 μmol/L).[98] Plasma protein binding is 14–17%. CSF concentrations range from 35–103% of simultaneous serum levels. V_{dss} is 0.3–0.7 L/kg; Cl is 0.13 ± 0.05 L/hr/kg. Foscarnet is not metabolized and is 70–90% excreted unchanged in the urine.[98]

$t_{1/2}$. α phase 1.4 ± 0.6 hr, ß phase 6.8 ± 5 hr in patients receiving continuous or intermittent infusions. A terminal half-life of 36–196 hr may represent release of the drug from binding sites in bone.[98]

Adverse Reactions. Abnormal renal function, including decreased Cl_{cr} and acute renal failure, occurs in about one-third of patients. Electrolyte abnormalities including hypocalcemia, hypophosphatemia, hyperphosphatemia, hypokalemia, and hypomagnesemia occur in 6–16% of patients. Seizures have been reported in 10% of patients and may be related to electrolyte abnormalities or underlying disease. Other adverse reactions frequently reported are fever 65%, nausea 47%, anemia 33%, diarrhea 30%, vomiting 26%, headache 26%, and granulocytopenia 17%. Local irritation, inflammation, and pain may occur at the injection site with peripheral administration at a frequency of 1–5%.[98,100,101]

Precautions. Use with extreme caution in patients with renal impairment or nephrotoxic drugs, preexisting cytopenias, preexisting electrolyte abnormalities, or underlying neurologic disorders.

Drug Interactions. Concurrent use of nephrotoxic drugs such as aminoglycosides or radiologic contrast media may increase risk and severity of nephrotoxicity. IV pentamidine may increase the risk of hypocalcemia; avoid this combination, if possible, although inhaled pentamidine does not seem to be a risk factor.[93]

Parameters to Monitor. Monitor Cr_s 2 or 3 times a week during induction therapy and weekly during maintenance therapy. Monitor serum calcium, magnesium, potassium, and phosphorus at the same frequency as Cr_s. Symptoms of perioral tingling, numbness in extremities, or other paresthesias may indicate electrolyte abnormalities and may require more frequent monitoring and a need to obtain ionized calcium levels.

GANCICLOVIR　　　　　　　　　　　　　　　　　Cytovene, Vitrasept

Pharmacology. Ganciclovir (DHPG) is a synthetic acyclic nucleoside analogue of guanine structurally related to acyclovir. The antiviral activity of ganciclovir appears to be a result of its conversion to the triphosphate form, which functions as both an inhibitor of and faulty substrate for viral DNA polymerase. Ganciclovir has antiviral activity both in vitro and in vivo against herpes simplex virus I and II, human cytomegalovirus (CMV), Epstein-Barr virus, and varicella-zoster virus.[74,101]

Administration and Adult Dosage. IV for treatment of CMV retinitis (induction) 5 mg/kg q 12 hr for 14–21 days, then (maintenance) 5 mg/kg once daily for 7 days each week or 6 mg/kg once daily for 5 days each week. Induction treatment may be repeated for patients who experience disease progression. **IV for prevention of CMV disease in transplant recipients** 5 mg/kg q 12 hr for 7–14 days, followed by 5 mg/kg once daily for 7 days each week or 6 mg/kg once daily for 5 days each week. Duration of treatment depends on the duration and degree of immunosuppression. Dilute each IV dose in 100 mL NS or D5W and infuse over 60 min. **PO for CMV retinitis (maintenance after IV induction)** 1 g q 8 hr with food. **PO for prophylaxis of CMV disease** 1 g q 8 hr with food indefinitely.

Special Populations. *Pediatric Dosage.* Safety and efficacy not established. If used, the dosage is the same as adult dosage in mg/kg.[39]

Geriatric Dosage. Same as adult dosage, but adjust for age-related reduction in renal function.

Other Conditions. In renal insufficiency, reduce *parenteral induction* dosage as follows: Cl_{cr} 50–69 mL/min, give 2.5 mg/kg q 12 hr; Cl_{cr} 25–49 mL/min, 2.5 mg/kg q 24 hr; Cl_{cr} under 25 mL/min, give 1.25 mg/kg q 24 hr; for patients on hemodialysis, 1.25 mg/kg 3 times/week. On hemodialysis days, give the dose after hemodialysis because dialysis reduces serum levels by approximately 50%. Reduce *parenteral maintenance* dosage in renal insufficiency as follows: Cl_{cr} 50–69 mL/min, give 2.5 mg/kg q 24 hr; Cl_{cr} 25–49 mL/min, 1.25 mg/kg q 24 hr; Cl_{cr} 10–24 mL/min, 0.625 mg/kg q 24 hr; for patients on hemodialysis, 0.625 mg/kg 3 times a week following hemodialysis. Reduce *oral maintenance* dosage in renal insufficiency as follows: Cl_{cr} 50–69 mL/min, give 1.5 g once daily or 500 mg tid; Cl_{cr} 25–49 mL/min, 1 g/day in 1 or 2 doses; Cl_{cr} 10–24 mL/min, 500 mg/day; Cl_{cr} under 10 mL/min, 500 mg 3 times a week, following hemodialysis.

Dosage Forms. **Cap** 250 mg; **Inj** 500 mg; **Ocular Implant** 4.5 mg (nominal release).

Patient Instructions. Ganciclovir is not a cure for CMV retinitis, and progression of disease may continue during or following treatment. Concurrent use with zidovudine may result in severe reduction in white blood cell count; therefore, report any signs or symptoms of infection, such as fever, chills, or sweats. Take oral ganciclovir with food.

Pharmacokinetics. *Fate.* Ganciclovir is absorbed poorly from the GI tract; oral bioavailability is 6% when taken with food (about 20% greater than when taken on an empty stomach). Average peak serum concentration of 0.34 ± 0.13 mg/L (1.3 ± 0.5 μmol/L) occurs 1–2 hr after a single 1 g oral dose. Mean peak and trough steady-state levels after IV doses of 5 mg/kg q 12 hr in patients with normal renal function are 5.3 ± 2.8 mg/L (21 ± 11 μmol/L) and 1.1 ± 0.4 mg/L (4.3 ± 1.5 μmol/L), respectively. Ganciclovir is 1–2% plasma protein bound; CSF concentration is 24–67% of simultaneous serum level. V_c is 0.26 ± 0.08 L/kg; $V_{dβ}$ is 1.17 ± 0.54 L/kg; Cl is 0.25 ± 0.13 L/hr/kg with normal renal function. The drug is 90–99% excreted unchanged in the urine. Hemodialysis reduces serum levels by 53 ± 12%. Renal excretion occurs principally via glomerular filtration, although limited renal tubular secretion may also occur.[101,102]

$t_{1/2}$. α phase 0.76 ± 0.67 hr; ß phase 3.6 ± 1.4 hr in adult patients, increasing to 11.5 ± 3.9 hr in renal insufficiency.[101,102]

Adverse Reactions. Granulocytopenia (ANC under 1000/μL) occurs in 13–67% of patients and is the most frequent dose-limiting adverse effect.[101] Thrombocytopenia (platelets under 50,000/μL) occurs in 20% of patients. CNS toxicity (headache, lethargy, dizziness, confusion, seizure, coma) has been reported at a frequency of 5–17%. Phlebitis, inflammation, and pain at the site of IV infusion occur frequently because of the high pH of the solution. Anemia, fever, rash, and abnormal liver function tests occur in about 2% of patients.[101,103]

Contraindications. Hypersensitivity to acyclovir or ganciclovir.

Precautions. Use with caution in renal impairment, preexisting cytopenias, or concurrent myelosuppressive drug therapy.

Drug Interactions. Didanosine AUC may be increased when given within 2 hr of ganciclovir. Probenecid may decrease the renal excretion of ganciclovir. Use extreme caution in combination with zidovudine because of additive myelosuppression. Concurrent nephrotoxic drugs (eg, cyclosporine, zidovudine) may increase the nephrotoxicity of ganciclovir. Concurrent cytotoxic drugs may increase the toxicity of ganciclovir. Seizures have been reported with concurrent use of ganciclovir and imipenem-cilastatin.

Parameters to Monitor. Monitor CBC and platelet count twice weekly during induction treatment and at least weekly during maintenance treatment. Monitor renal function at least q 2 weeks. Check injection site for phlebitis and infection daily.

Notes. Ganciclovir-resistant CMV strains have been isolated from patients during treatment.[104] Disease progression caused by these strains has been observed and may require changing therapy to an alternative antiviral (eg, foscarnet).

INDINAVIR   Crixivan

Indinavir is an HIV protease inhibitor with a mechanism of action similar to saquinavir. Indinavir is rapidly absorbed in the fasting state. Administration of indinavir with a meal high in calories, fat, or protein decreases oral absorption by about 75%. The absolute bioavailability has not been determined in humans, but the fasting bioavailability ranges from 14–70% in animals. Indinavir is 60% bound to human plasma proteins. It is primarily metabolized by CYP3A4, and less than 20% is excreted unchanged in the urine; half-life is 1.8 ± 0.4 hr. Frequent adverse reactions include nausea, vomiting, abdominal pain, diarrhea, headache, asthenia, insomnia, taste perversion, transient elevations of hepatic transaminases, asymptomatic hyperbilirubinemia, and nephrolithiasis. Dizziness, somnolence, anorexia, malaise, and dry mouth occur occasionally. Nephrolithiasis occurred in 4% of patients in clinical trials and can be managed with hydration and temporary drug discontinuation. Patients should drink at least 1.5 L/day of liquids to ensure adequate hydration while taking indinavir. Each dose should be taken on an empty stomach with water or other fat-free liquid or with light, fat-free foods (eg, toast, jelly, corn flakes, skim milk, sugar, coffee). Dosage is PO 800 mg q 8 hr. In patients with mild to moderate hepatic insufficiency caused by cirrhosis, the dosage is 600 mg q 8 hr.[105] Available as 200-mg and 400-mg capsules.

LAMIVUDINE   Epivir

Lamivudine (3TC) is a synthetic pyrimidine nucleoside that has activity against HIV-1, HIV-2, and hepatitis B virus. Use of lamivudine alone to treat HIV infection leads to rapid emergence of high-level resistance; therefore, it is used in combination with zidovudine. Resistance to zidovudine is markedly delayed when the drug is used with lamivudine, and the combination has resulted in greater and more sustained elevations in CD4 cell counts than zidovudine monotherapy. Lamivudine is also being studied in combination with other nucleoside analogues, such as stavudine. Lamivudine is metabolized intracellularly to lamivudine triphosphate and acts as a chain terminator of viral DNA. It also acts as a competitive inhibitor of HIV-reverse transcriptase. Oral bioavailability is 82%. V_d is 1.3 L/kg; the serum elimination half-life is 2.5 hr. Excretion is primarily by the renal route, with 68–71% of drug excreted unchanged in urine. The most frequently reported adverse effects have been headache, fatigue, nausea, insomnia, neuropathy, and musculoskeletal pain. When used with zidovudine, lamivudine dosage is 150 mg PO bid with zidovudine 200 mg PO tid.[87,91,106–108] The pediatric dosage is (3 mo–12 yr) 4 mg/kg, to a maximum of 150 mg, PO bid with zidovudine. Available as 150-mg tablets and 10 mg/mL solution.

NEVIRAPINE   Viramune

Nevirapine is a dipyridodiazepinone nonnucleoside HIV-1 reverse transcriptase inhibitor (NNRTI). Nevirapine and other nonnucleoside reverse transcriptase inhibitors are not active against HIV-2 reverse transcriptase. The inhibition by nevirapine is noncompetitive, and the binding site is located near but not directly at the catalytic amino acid residues, which may provide nevirapine activity against HIV-1 mutants that are resistant to nucleoside reverse transcriptase inhibitors. Nevirapine provides added benefit (eg, increased CD4 count, decreased viral load) in combination with zidovudine and didanosine. Oral absorption is not affected by food or antacids; bioavailability is 90%. The median time to peak concentration is 4 hr after a 400-mg dose with average peak concentrations after the first dose of 3.4 ± 1 mg/L. Peak and trough concentrations average 7.2 ± 1.4 mg/L and 4 ± 1.2 mg/L, respectively, after 14 days of therapy. The average elimination half-life is 45 hr in the initial 2-week period and decreases to 25–30 hr thereafter because of metabolic autoinduction mediated by the cytochrome P450 system. Less than 3% of the dose is excreted renally. The most frequent adverse effect is a mild to moderate rash occurring in up to 48% of study patients. Rash may be associated with liver function test elevations and a low frequency of clinical hepatitis. The risk of developing rash is highest within 2 weeks of drug initiation or dosage escalation to 400 mg/day and is reduced by following the recommended dosage escalation schedule. Other occasional adverse reactions include arthralgia, fatigue, fever, myalgia, and somnolence. The adult dosage is PO 200 mg/day for 2 weeks, followed by 200 mg bid. The dosage for children <13 yr is 120 mg/m^2/day for 2 weeks, then bid. Available as 200-mg tablets and 10 mg/mL suspension.[109–112]

RITONAVIR   Norvir

Ritonavir is an HIV protease inhibitor with a mechanism of action similar to saquinavir. Ritonavir is rapidly absorbed, and is increased by approximately 15%

with food. Absolute bioavailability has not been determined in humans, but bioavailability ranges from 30–70% in animals. Ritonavir is 98–99% protein bound, primarily to albumin and α_1-acid glycoprotein. After a 600-mg oral dose taken with food, peak serum concentrations of 11.2 ± 3.6 mg/L occur at 3.3 ± 2.2 hr and the troughs are 3 ± 2.1 mg/L. Serum concentrations may decrease over time because of autoinduction of the CYP3A and CYP2D isoenzymes responsible for metabolism of ritonavir. Frequent adverse reactions include nausea, vomiting, diarrhea, asthenia, anorexia, abdominal pain, taste perversion, perioral paresthesia, peripheral paresthesia, headache, insomnia, and elevated serum triglyceride levels. Occasionally elevations of hepatic transaminases and CPK occur. Ritonavir is a potent inhibitor of several cytochrome P450 enzymes (CYP2C9, 2C19, 2D6, and 3A3/4) and can produce large increases in serum concentrations of highly metabolized drugs. Consult the product information for contraindicated drugs and carefully review patient's medication list for interactions before starting this therapy. For treatment of HIV infection in combination with nucleoside analogues or as monotherapy, ritonavir dosage is PO 600 mg q 12 hr with food. Ritonavir may be better tolerated initially if the dosage is initiated at 300 mg q 12 hr and increased to 600 mg q 12 hr over 1 week. If the 600 mg q 12 hr dosage is not reached after 2 weeks of therapy, discontinue therapy, because the risk of developing viral resistance to ritonavir or cross-resistance to other protease inhibitors is increased with lower dosages.[113,114] Available as 100-mg capsules and 80 mg/mL solution, both of which must be refrigerated.

SAQUINAVIR MESYLATE   Invirase

Pharmacology. Saquinavir inhibits human immunodeficiency viruses (HIV-1 and HIV-2) proteases by binding to the active enzymatic site, preventing cleavage of polyprotein precursors. This cleavage is essential for maturation of infectious virus, and its inhibition results in the formation of immature, noninfectious HIV particles.[115,116]

Administration and Adult Dosage. PO for advanced HIV disease in combination with nucleoside analogues 600 mg q 8 hr.

Special Populations. *Pediatric Dosage.* (Under 16 yr) safety and efficacy not established.

Geriatric Dosage. Not studied, but expected to be the same as adult dosage.

Dosage Forms. Cap 200 mg.

Patient Instructions. This drug must be taken within 2 hours after a full meal to achieve adequate absorption of the drug to inhibit viruses. Do not miss doses or take the drug intermittently, because this may lead to resistance. This medication must be used in combination with another antiviral medication. This drug is not a cure for HIV disease. Opportunistic infections and other complications associated with HIV infection may continue to develop while this medication is taken. This drug may cause sensitivity to the sun, so use protective clothing and sunscreen until the extent of sensitivity is determined.

Pharmacokinetics. *Fate.* Oral absorption of saquinavir is erratic and undergoes extensive first-pass metabolism. Approximately 30% of a 600-mg dose is absorbed when given within 2 hr after food, and absolute bioavailability averages 4%. Saquinavir is 98% plasma protein bound, and concentrations in the CSF are negligible. Saquinavir undergoes rapid metabolism, primarily by CYP3A4. After IV doses of 6, 36, and 72 mg of saquinavir, the systemic clearance was 1.14 L/hr/kg.[117]

$t_{1/2}$. Terminal phase 12 hr; however, the mean residence time is 7 hr.[117]

Adverse Reactions. Abdominal discomfort or pain, diarrhea, anorexia, and nausea are frequent. Occasional reactions include asthenia, rash, elevations of transaminases, and headache. Rare reactions include ataxia, confusion, hemolytic anemia, thrombophlebitis, attempted suicide, seizures, and exacerbation of chronic liver disease.

Contraindications. (*See* Drug Interactions.)

Precautions. Do not use saquinavir as monotherapy because of the greater potential for developing resistance.

Drug Interactions. Do not coadminister saquinavir with rifampin because of decreases in steady-state AUC of saquinavir by 80%. Coadministration with rifabutin reduces saquinavir serum concentrations by 40% and alternatives should be considered. Avoid other drugs that strongly induce CYP3A4, because they may substantially decrease saquinavir serum concentrations. Avoid coadministration with astemizole, cisapride, or terfenadine because of possible prolonged QT intervals and serious cardiovascular adverse events. Concurrent ketoconazole, and possibly other inhibitors of CYP3A4, may increase the bioavailability and half-life of saquinavir. Ingesting grapefruit juice with saquinavir has been suggested to increase the bioavailability of saquinavir by inhibition of CYP3A4. However, the grapefruit juice must be concentrated, taken with every dose of saquinavir, and contain flavinoids to have any benefit. This method is not likely to be palatable to most patients because of gastric irritation.

Parameters to Monitor. Monitor clinical signs, symptoms, and laboratory markers for progression of HIV disease to help decide regimen changes in antiretroviral therapy. Baseline CD4 and HIV-1 RNA polymerase chain reaction viral load tests are useful to measure clinical benefit of therapy. Repeat tests after 1 month and q 3–4 months thereafter have been suggested to monitor benefit of antiretroviral therapy.

Notes. A soft gel capsule dosage form of saquinavir with increased bioavailability is under investigation. Other HIV protease inhibitors include **nelfinavir** (Viracept, Agouron) and VX-478,141W94 (Investigational, Glaxo Wellcome).

STAVUDINE	Zerit

Stavudine (d4T) is a synthetic pyrimidine nucleoside reverse transcriptase inhibitor that is structurally similar to zidovudine and has been shown to inhibit HIV replication in vitro. Stavudine is phosphorylated by cellular enzymes to stavudine triphosphate, which acts both as a competitive inhibitor of HIV reverse transcriptase and as an alternative nucleoside substrate, which leads to premature elongation of viral DNA. It is well absorbed with or without food and oral bioavailability is 82%. Average time to peak concentration is 1 hr with serum concentrations of about 1.2 mg/L after a single 0.67 mg/kg dose. V_d is 0.53 L/kg. Limited data suggest that stavudine distributes into the CSF, with concentrations reaching approximately 40% of serum concentration. Renal clearance is about 40% of total clearance, with the remaining drug metabolized to thymine and eventually to ß-aminoisobutyric acid. The most frequent adverse effect is peripheral neuropathy and occasionally elevated hepatic transaminases.[87,118,119] Dosage is 30 mg q 12 hr for patients under 60 kg and 40 mg q 12 hr for patients >60 kg. Dosage can be reduced to 15 mg q 12 hr for patients <60 kg or 20 mg q 12 hr for patients over 60 kg if at risk for peripheral neuropathy. Reduce dosage also in renal impairment. Available as 15-, 20-, 30-, and 40-mg capsules.

ZALCITABINE   Hivid

Zalcitabine (dideoxycytidine; ddC) is a synthetic pyrimidine nucleoside analogue that inhibits human immunodeficiency virus (HIV) replication in vitro and in vivo. Like that of zidovudine, the mechanism of action of zalcitabine is believed to be through the interaction of ddC-5′-triphosphate with the viral reverse transcriptase. The triphosphate form acts both as a competitive inhibitor of HIV reverse transcriptase and as a chain terminator of viral DNA. Oral bioavailability is 88%. The average elimination half-life is 1.2 hr, and most of the drug appears to be eliminated by renal clearance, with 75% of drug excreted unchanged in urine. Zalcitabine penetrates into the CSF in concentrations of 9–37% of simultaneous serum concentrations. The most frequent adverse effects have been peripheral neuropathy, oral aphthous ulcers, nausea, skin rash, and, less frequently, esophageal ulcers, thrombocytopenia, and elevated serum transaminases. Peripheral neuropathy is the limiting toxicity at a dosage of 0.01 mg/kg q 8 hr or greater.[84,87] The dosage is 0.75 mg PO q 8 hr alone or in combination with zidovudine 200 mg PO q 8 hr for advanced AIDS. Available as 0.375- and 0.75-mg tablets.

ZIDOVUDINE   Retrovir

Pharmacology. Zidovudine (azidothymidine; AZT) is a thymidine analogue that inhibits HIV replication. It is converted to the active monophosphate form by thymidine kinase and ultimately to zidovudine triphosphate by intracellular enzymes. This form exerts its activity at viral DNA polymerase (reverse transcriptase) by competing with other cellular deoxynucleosides and by acting as a chain terminator of DNA synthesis.[84]

Administration and Adult Dosage. The optimal dosage is not established; large interpatient pharmacokinetic variability necessitates individualization of dosage. **PO for HIV infection with CD4 <500 cells/μL** 300–600 mg/day in 3–5 divided doses (usually tid).[84,90] **PO for maternal-fetal HIV transmission (maternal)** 100 mg 5 times daily begun after the 14th week of pregnancy and continued throughout the pregnancy, then **IV during labor** 2 mg/kg over 1 hr, followed by a continuous infusion of 1 mg/kg/hr until delivery (*see also* Pediatric Dosage). **PO for combination therapy with zalcitabine** 200 mg q 8 hr with zalcitabine 0.75 mg q 8 hr. **PO for postexposure prophylaxis** 1–1.5 g/day in 4 or 5 divided doses has been used;[120] however, the effectiveness of this regimen is not confirmed in humans and informed consent should be obtained. **IV for patients unable to take oral medication** 1–2 mg/kg q 4 hr infused over 1 hr, only until oral therapy can be initiated.

Special Populations. *Pediatric Dosage.* **PO for prevention of maternal HIV transmission** 2 mg/kg/dose q 6 hr for first 6 weeks of life, beginning 8–12 hr after birth.[121] **IV for prevention of maternal HIV transmission if unable to receive PO** 1.5 mg/kg/dose q 6 hr until oral therapy can be initiated. **PO for HIV infection** (0–2 weeks) 2 mg/kg/dose q 6 hr; (2–4 weeks) 3 mg/kg/dose q 6 hr; (4 weeks–13 yr) 180 mg/m^2/dose (to a maximum of 200 mg) q 6 hr; (over 13 yr) 100 mg q 4 hr 5 times a day.[86]

Geriatric Dosage. Same as adult dosage, but adjust for age-related reduction in renal function.

Other Conditions. Reduce dosage by 50% in patients with Cl_{cr} under 25 mL/min,[87] and decrease by 75% in cirrhosis.[122]

Dosage Forms. **Cap** 100 mg; **Tab** 300 mg; **Syrup** 10 mg/mL; **Inj** 10 mg/mL.

Patient Instructions. This drug is not a cure for HIV disease. Opportunistic infections and other complications associated with HIV infection may continue to develop. This drug may be taken with food to decrease abdominal discomfort or nausea. It is important to have blood counts followed closely during therapy to monitor for decreases in blood cell counts.

Pharmacokinetics. *Serum Levels.* Not established; intracellular concentrations of zidovudine triphosphate may correlate with therapeutic benefit, but in vivo data are not available.

Fate. Zidovudine undergoes marked presystemic metabolism. Oral bioavailability is 60–70%, possibly reduced with high-fat meals. Peak serum levels are approximately 1.2 mg/L (4.5 µmol/L) after a 250-mg oral dose. Protein binding is less than 25%. CSF concentrations are 24% of serum in children receiving a continuous infusion of drug. V_{dss} is 1.6 ± 0.6 L/kg; Cl is 1.3 ± 0.3 L/hr/kg in adults and 36.4 ± 11.5 L/hr/m^2 in children. Zidovudine (ZDV) is rapidly metabolized to the inactive ether glucuronide (GZDV). GZDV formation is reduced and zidovudine AUC and half-life are increased in patients with cirrhosis. About 60% of an oral dose is excreted as GZDV in urine. GZDV excretion is reduced in patients with renal dysfunction; hemodialysis removes GZDV but not ZDV.[87,122,123]

$t_{1/2}$. (Adults) 1.1 ± 0.2 hr; 2.1 hr in uremia; 2.4 hr in cirrhosis.[87] (Children) 1.5 ± 0.6 hr.

Adverse Reactions. Severe anemia and granulocytopenia occur frequently and may necessitate blood transfusions; epoetin may help alleviate anemia in patients with low serum erythropoietin levels. Other frequent adverse reactions associated with zidovudine in placebo-controlled trials include abdominal discomfort, nausea, vomiting, insomnia, myalgias, and headaches. Adverse reactions that occasionally occur with long-term use (over 12 weeks) include myopathy and nail pigmentation.[84]

Contraindications. Life-threatening allergy to the drug or its components.

Precautions. Pregnancy; lactation. Use with caution in liver disease or hepatomegaly, especially obese women.

Drug Interactions. Several drugs decrease the glucuronidation of zidovudine, including atovaquone, methadone, probenecid, valproic acid, and possibly fluconazole; rifampin increases zidovudine glucuronidation; however, the clinical importance of these interactions is not established.[93] Initial studies showed that prolonged administration of acetaminophen was associated with increased hematologic toxicity from zidovudine, but further study does not support this finding.[124]

Parameters to Monitor. Hemoglobin, hematocrit, MCV, and WBC for hematologic toxicity. Monitor clinical signs, symptoms, and laboratory markers for progression of HIV disease to help decide regimen changes in antiretroviral therapy. Baseline CD4 and HIV-1 RNA polymerase chain reaction viral load tests are useful to measure clinical benefit of therapy. Repeat tests after 1 month and q 3–4 months thereafter have been suggested to monitor benefit of antiretroviral therapy.

Notes. Viral resistance to zidovudine has occurred in vitro with isolates recovered from patients and is associated with prolonged zidovudine use and more advanced disease; correlation between viral resistance in vitro and progression of disease has not been established. Studies with **lamivudine** (3TC) suggest that the combination can delay or prevent HIV-1 viral resistance to zidovudine.

ß-Lactams

AMOXICILLIN
Amoxil, Various

Amoxicillin differs from ampicillin by the presence of a hydroxyl group on the amino side chain. It has activity essentially identical to ampicillin. However, it is completely absorbed, with about 85% bioavailability because of a small first-pass effect. Serum levels are greater than those after equal doses of ampicillin; postabsorptive pharmacokinetics are identical to those of ampicillin. Adverse effects are similar to ampicillin, although diarrhea and rashes are much less frequent with amoxicillin. The usual oral dosage for adults is 250–500 mg q 8 hr, to a maximum of 4.5 g/day. For endocarditis prophylaxis, the dosage is 3 g 1 hr prior to the procedure and 1.5 g 6 hr after the first dose. Oral dosage for children is 20–40 mg/kg/day in 3 equally divided doses q 8 hr. For endocarditis prophylaxis, the dose is 50 mg/kg 1 hr prior to the procedure and 25 mg/kg 6 hr later.[125,126] The drug is available as 250- and 500-mg capsules, 125-and 250-mg chewable tablets, 50 mg/mL drops, and 25 and 50 mg/mL suspension. (*See* ß-Lactams Comparison Chart.)

AMOXICILLIN AND POTASSIUM CLAVULANATE
Augmentin

Clavulanic acid has weak antibacterial activity, but is a potent inhibitor of plasmid-mediated ß-lactamases, including those produced by *Haemiophilus influenzae*, *Moraxella (Branhamella) catarrhalis*, *Staphylococcus aureus*, *Neisseria gonorrhoeae*, and *Bacteroides fragilis*. Thus, when combined with certain other ß-lactam antibiotics, the combination is very active against many bacteria resistant to the ß-lactam alone. Peak serum clavulanate level is 2.6 mg/L 40–60 min following an oral dose of amoxicillin 250 mg/clavulanate 125 mg. Amoxicillin pharmacokinetics are not affected by clavulanic acid. Clavulanic acid half-life is approximately 60 min. Adverse effects of this preparation include those of amoxicillin; however, diarrhea is more frequent with the combination and depends on the dosage of clavulanate. The 875-mg formulation reduces the frequency of diarrhea and allows twice-daily administration. Nausea and diarrhea may occur less frequently when this preparation is administered with food. Adult dosage is one "250" or "500" tablet tid or one "875" tablet bid. Do not substitute combinations of lower dose tablets to make a higher dose, because diarrhea is markedly increased. In children, the dosage is 20–40 mg/kg/day (of the amoxicillin component) in 3 divided doses.[127,128] Available as tablets containing amoxicillin/clavulanic acid: 250 mg amoxicillin/125 mg clavulanic acid, 500 mg amoxicillin/125 mg clavulanic acid, and 875 mg amoxicillin/125 mg clavulanic acid; chewable tablets containing 125 mg amoxicillin/31.25 mg clavulanic acid, and 250 mg amoxicillin/62.5 mg clavulanic acid; and suspension containing 25 mg amoxicillin/6.25 mg clavulanic acid/mL and 50 mg amoxicillin/12.5 mg clavulanic acid/mL. (*See* ß-Lactams Comparison Chart.)

AMPICILLIN Various

Ampicillin has a similar mechanism of action and is comparable in activity to penicillin G against Gram-positive bacteria, but is more active than penicillin G against Gram-negative bacteria. Oral forms are about 50% absorbed in the fasting state; food delays absorption. Plasma protein binding is low, and therapeutic levels are attained in most tissues and fluids including CSF (in the presence of inflammation). About 90% is excreted unchanged in urine. Half-life is 1.2 hr, 2 hr in neonates, increasing to 20 hr in anuric patients. Adverse effects include frequent skin rash (more frequent in patients receiving allopurinol and very frequent in patients with Epstein-Barr virus infection [mononucleosis]). Many of these eruptions are probably not hypersensitivity reactions, but are immunologically mediated. They are generally dose related (higher frequency at higher dosages), macular rather than urticarial, and disappear with continued administration of the drug. Nausea and diarrhea occur frequently with oral therapy. The adult dosage is PO 250–500 mg qid, and the IM or IV dosage is 100–200 mg/kg/day in 4–6 divided doses. In children <20 kg, the IV and oral dosage is 50–100 mg/kg/day in 2–4 divided doses; in those >20 kg, the oral dosage is 100–400 mg/kg/day in 4–6 divided doses and the IV dosage is 400 mg/kg/day in 4–6 divided doses. Give the same dose q 12 hr with a Cl_{cr} <20 mL/min.[125,126] Available as 250- and 500-mg capsules, 125-mg chewable tablets, 100 mg/mL drops, 25, 50, and 100 mg/mL suspension, and 125-, 250-, 500-mg and 1-, 2-, and 10-g injection. (*See* ß-Lactams Comparison Chart.)

AMPICILLIN SODIUM AND SULBACTAM SODIUM Unasyn

Sulbactam is a ß-lactamase inhibitor similar to clavulanic acid. Like clavulanate, it has weak antibacterial activity. Following a 15-min IV infusion of ampicillin 2 g/sulbactam 1 g, peak serum concentrations of ampicillin and sulbactam exceed 94 and 41 mg/L, respectively. Sulbactam half-life is about 1 hr; ampicillin pharmacokinetics are unaltered with concomitant sulbactam administration. Adverse reactions include frequent diarrhea. The adult dosage is IM or IV 1.5–3 g (of the combination) q 6–8 hr. Give these doses q 12 hr with a Cl_{cr} of 15–30 mL/min or q 24 hr with a Cl_{cr} <15 mL/min. The dosage in children is not established.[128,129] Available as injection containing ampicillin/sulbactam 1 g of ampicillin/0.5 g sulbactam and 2 g ampicillin/1 g of sulbactam. (*See* ß-Lactams Comparison Chart.)

ANTISTAPHYLOCOCCAL PENICILLINS

Methicillin, nafcillin, oxacillin, cloxacillin, and dicloxacillin are similar to other penicillins in their mechanism of action. However, these drugs are not hydrolyzed by staphylococcal penicillinases. Therefore, nearly all isolates of *Staphylococcus aureus* and some isolates of coagulase-negative staphylococci are susceptible to these drugs. Methicillin- (actually ß-lactam-) resistant staphylococci have altered penicillin-binding proteins (transpeptidases). Although these drugs are primarily used in staphylococcal infection, they retain good activity against most streptococci, except enterococci. Except for methicillin, these drugs are mostly hepatically eliminated by metabolism and biliary excretion. Interstitial nephritis is frequent with methicillin, but occurs only rarely with the other drugs. Hepatic damage occurs rarely with oxacillin. Nafcillin has a propensity for local irritation at the IV infusion site, and may cause neutropenia more frequently than other antistaphylococcal penicillins. Only cloxacillin and dicloxacillin are adequately absorbed from the GI tract. Oral administration of nafcillin and oxacillin is not recommended because they are poorly absorbed.[125,126,130] (*See* ß-Lactams Comparison Chart.)

AZTREONAM   Azactam

Aztreonam is a monobactam with activity similar to that of third-generation cephalosporins against most Gram-negative aerobic bacteria (including *Pseudomonas aeruginosa*), but inactive against Gram-positive bacteria and anaerobes. Peak serum levels of 164 and 255 mg/L occur after a 30-min IV infusion of 1 and 2 g, respectively. With inflamed meninges, CSF levels are similar to those observed with comparable dosages of third-generation cephalosporins, but experience in treating meningitis is limited. The drug is 60% plasma protein bound and has a V_d of about 0.24 L/kg; 60–70% is excreted in urine unchanged. The half-life is 1.5–2 hr, increasing to 6 hr in renal failure and 3.2 hr in alcoholic cirrhosis. Adverse effects of aztreonam are minimal. Cross-allergenicity between aztreonam and other ß-lactams is low, and aztreonam has been used safely in penicillin- or cephalosporin-allergic patients. The usual adult dosage is IM or IV 500 mg–2 g q 6–12 hr, to a maximum of 8 g/day, depending on severity and site of infection. Reduce maintenance dosage by 50% with a Cl_{cr} of 10–30 mL/min and by 75% with a Cl_{cr} <10 mL/min. One- eighth of the initial dose should be given after hemodialysis. Safety and efficacy are not established in children, but a dosage of 30 mg/kg q 6–8 hr IV has been used successfully in children with serious Gram-negative infections and up to 50 mg/kg q 4–6 hr in *P. aeruginosa* infections.[131–133] Available as injection 500 mg and 1 and 2 g. (*See* ß-Lactams Comparison Chart.)

CEPHALOSPORINS

Pharmacology. Cephalosporin antibiotics have broad spectrum activity against many Gram-positive and Gram-negative pathogens. These agents are generally considered to be bactericidal through binding to various penicillin-binding proteins in bacteria, which results in changes in cell wall structure and function. Members of this class are frequently subdivided into "generations" based on their antimicrobial activity (as well as order of introduction into clinical use).[133–137]

First-generation cephalosporins have activity against Gram-positive bacteria (eg, *Staphylococcus* spp.) as well as a limited, but important, number of species of aerobic Gram-negative bacilli (eg, *Escherichia coli*, *Klebsiella* spp., *Proteus mirabilis*). *Haemophilus influenzae* and most other aerobic Gram-negative bacilli often indigenous to hospitals (eg, *Enterobacter* spp., *Pseudomonas* spp.) are resistant to these drugs. Anaerobic bacteria isolated in the oropharynx are generally susceptible to these agents; however, anaerobes such as *Bacteroides fragilis* are resistant.[133,137]

The second-generation cephalosporins cefamandole, cefonicid, ceforanide, and cefuroxime all differ from first-generation agents in their improved activity against *Haemophilus influenzae* and some strains of *Enterobacter* spp., *Providencia* spp., and *Morganella* spp.[133,137] The oral second-generation cephalosporins cefuroxime axetil, cefprozil, cefonicid, and loracarbef (which is actually a carbacephem) have similar but less potent activity.[138–141] Cefoxitin, cefmetazole, and cefotetan (which are actually cephamycins) have increased activity against anaerobes, including *Bacteroides fragilis*;[133,142,143] the other second-generation cephalosporins have poor activity against this organism.[133]

Third-generation cephalosporins are noteworthy for their marked potency against common Gram-negative organisms (eg, *E. coli*, *K. pneumoniae*) as well as their activity against Gram-negative bacilli resistant to older agents (eg, *Serratia* spp., *P. aeruginosa*).[133,134,136,137] Although grouped together, some agents have better activity against certain organisms (eg, ceftazidime is better against *P. aeruginosa*), and poorer activity against others (eg, cefixime and ceftazidime are poorer against *S. aureus*).[133,134,137]

Fourth-generation cephalosporins have a spectrum similar to the third-generation drugs, plus activity against some Gram-negative strains that are resistant to the third-generation agents, such as *Enterobacter* spp. Their antianaerobic activity is poor.

Resistance to cephalosporins is mediated by ß-lactamase, reduction in outer cell wall membrane permeability, and alteration of the affinity of these agents for penicillin-binding proteins. Resistance among certain ß-lactamase-producing organisms (eg, *Enterobacter* and *Citrobacter* spp.) to third-generation cephalosporins has so increased in recent years that these agents cannot be relied upon to provide effective therapy.[137]

Administration and Adult Dosage. (*See* β-Lactams Comparison Chart.)

Special Populations. *Pediatric Dosage.* (*See* β-Lactams Comparison Chart.)

Geriatric Dosage. Same as adult dosage, but adjust for age-related reduction in renal function.

Other Conditions. Most agents require dosage modification in renal dysfunction; exceptions are ceftriaxone and cefoperazone, which have biliary and renal or primarily biliary elimination, respectively.[136] Dosage reduction of all agents is required in patients with concomitant hepatic and renal dysfunction (*see* β-Lactams Comparison Chart).

Pharmacokinetics. Some of the greatest differences between agents reside in their pharmacokinetic properties.[133,136,137] Of note is the improved CSF penetration of certain newer agents over the first-generation agents.[136,137] Therapeutic CSF concentrations are achieved with cefotaxime, moxalactam, ceftriaxone, and ceftazidime; these agents have proven efficacy in the treatment of meningitis caused by susceptible organisms in adults and children.[133,136,137] Adequate CSF concentrations of ceftizoxime have also been observed, although its use in the treatment of meningitis is less well established.[133] Cefuroxime penetrates adequately into CSF, but is less effective for meningitis than third-generation agents.[133,144] (*See* β-Lactams Comparison Chart.)

Adverse Reactions. Most cephalosporins are generally well tolerated, although a few agents have unique adverse reactions. Hypersensitivity reactions may occur in approximately 10% of patients known to be allergic to penicillin; do not administer these agents to patients with a history of an immediate reaction to penicillin.[145] Nausea and diarrhea occur with all agents; however, diarrhea is more common with ceftriaxone and cefoperazone because of high biliary excretion.[133,136,137] Colitis caused by *Clostridium difficile* has been reported with all the cephalosporins, but may be more common with ceftriaxone and cefoperazone. Nephrotoxicity is rare, particularly when used without other nephrotoxic agents.[137] All agents with an N-methylthiotetrazole (NMTT) moiety in the three position of the cephem nucleus (moxalactam, cefoperazone, cefamandole, cefotetan, and cefmetazole) may produce a disulfiramlike reaction in some patients upon ingestion of alcohol-containing beverages.[133,136,137] In addition, these agents may be associated to varying degrees with bleeding secondary to hypoprothrombinemia, which is corrected or prevented by vitamin K administration.[133,136,137,146] Although controversial, the mechanism of this reaction appears to involve inhibition of enzymatic reactions requiring vitamin K in the activation of prothrombin precursors by NMTT. However, other factors (eg, malnutrition, liver disease) may be more important risk factors for bleeding than the NMTT-containing cephalosporins.[146] Thus, cautious use (and perhaps even avoidance) of agents with the NMTT side chain is recommended in patients with poor oral intake and critical illness. Administration of vitamin K and monitoring of the prothrombin time is indicated with these agents, particularly when therapy is prolonged. Moxalactam has antiplatelet activity, which further increases the risk of bleeding. Positive direct Coombs' tests occur frequently, but hemolysis is rare.[133,137] Ceftriaxone has been associated with biliary pseudolithiasis (sludging), which may be asymptomatic or resemble acute cholecystitis.[147] This adverse effect occurs most often with dosages of 2 g/day or more, especially in patients receiving prolonged therapy or those with impaired gall bladder emptying. The mechanism is caused by ceftriaxone:calcium complex formation, and it is usually reversible upon drug discontinuation.[148] Neonates given ceftriaxone can develop kernicterus caused by displacement of bilirubin from plasma protein binding sites; its use in this population is best avoided. Development of resistance during treatment of infections caused by *Enterobacter* spp., *Serratia* spp., and *P. aeruginosa* has occurred with all these agents.[133,136,137]

Precautions. Penicillin allergy. Use agents with NMTT side chain with caution in patients with underlying bleeding diathesis, poor oral intake, or critical illness.

Use with caution in renal impairment and in those on oral anticoagulants (especially NMTT-containing drugs). Avoid use of ceftriaxone in neonates, particularly premature infants.

Drug Interactions. Avoid concomitant ingestion of alcohol or alcohol-containing products with agents containing the NMTT side chain. Probenecid reduces renal clearance and increases serum levels of most agents, except those that do not undergo renal tubular secretion (eg, ceftazidime, ceftriaxone, moxalactam).

Parameters to Monitor. Monitor prothrombin time 2–3 times a week with agents having an NMTT side chain, particularly when using large dosages; monitor bleeding time with moxalactam and with high dosages of other agents having an NMTT side chain. Obtain antimicrobial susceptibility tests for development of resistance in patients relapsing during therapy. Monitor renal function tests initially and periodically during high-dose regimens or when the drug is used concurrently with nephrotoxic agents. Monitor for diarrhea, particularly with ceftriaxone and cefoperazone; test stool specimen for *C. difficile* toxin if diarrhea persists or is associated with fever or abdominal pain.

CEFAZOLIN SODIUM
Ancef, Kefzol, Various

Cefazolin is a first-generation cephalosporin with activity against most Gram-positive aerobic organisms (eg, streptococci and *Staphylococcus aureus*) and some Gram-negative bacilli (eg, *Escherichia coli*, *Klebsiella* spp., *Proteus mirabilis*). It is 75–85% plasma protein bound, and widely distributed throughout the body with high levels in many tissues and cavities, but subtherapeutic levels in the CSF. Virtually 100% is excreted unchanged in the urine via filtration and secretion, and the half-life is about 1.8 hr, increasing to 30–40 hr in renal impairment. Cefazolin is generally well tolerated. Adult dosage is IM or IV 250 mg–1 g q 6–12 hr (usually 1 g q 8 hr) to a maximum of 6 g/day for treatment, and IM or IV 1 g 30–60 min prior to surgery for prophylaxis, then 500 mg–1 g q 6–8 hr for up to 24 hr postoperatively. Dosage in newborns is IV or IM 20 mg/kg/dose q 8–12 hr and in older children is IM or IV 50–100 mg/kg/day in 3 divided doses given q 8 hr. Decrease dosage in renal impairment, with a dosage of 10–25% of the usual dosage in renal failure.[135,137] (*See* ß-Lactams Comparison Chart.)

CEFEPIME HYDROCHLORIDE
Maxipime

Cefepime is a fourth-generation cephalosporin with a broader spectrum of activity than other cephalosporins. It has similar activity to ceftazidime against Gram-negative bacteria, including *Pseudomonas aeruginosa*, but is also active against some isolates resistant to third-generation cephalosporins (eg, *Enterobacter* spp.). Cefepime has greater potency against Gram-positive organisms (eg, staphylococci) than ceftazidime, and is similar in activity to ceftriaxone. Its anaerobic activity is poor, particularly against *Bacteroides fragilis*. Following a 30-min IV infusion of 1 g, serum concentrations of 79 mg/L are achieved. Cefepime penetrates most tissues and fluids well; CSF concentrations of 3.3–6.7 mg/L were found in patients given 50 mg/kg q 8 hr. About 80% of a dose is eliminated renally by glomerular filtration, and the half-life averages 2.3 hr. Elderly patients have a slightly lower total clearance of cefepime, which parallels Cl_{cr}. The most common adverse reactions are injection site reactions, rash, positive direct Coombs' test without hemolysis, decreased serum phosphorus, increased hepatic enzymes, eosinophilia, and abnormal PT and PTT. Encephalopathy has been reported in patients with renal impairment given full (unadjusted) dosages. Adult dosage is IM or IV 500 mg–2 g q 12 hr; moderate to severe infections are treated with IV 1–2 g q 12 hr. In patients with Cl_{cr} of 30–60 mL/min, the usual dose is given q 24 hr; with a Cl_{cr} of 10–30 mL/min, 50% of the usual dose is given q 24 hr; and with a Cl_{cr} <10 mL/min, 25% of the dose (but no less than 250 mg) is given q 24 hr. Give elderly patients the usual adult dosages, adjusting for age-related renal impairment.[148–150] The safety and efficacy of cefepime have not been established in children <12 yr, and dosage recommendations are not available. (*See* ß-Lactams Comparison Chart.)

CEFOTAXIME SODIUM   Claforan

Cefotaxime is a third-generation cephalosporin with activity against Gram-negative organisms resistant to first- and second-generation cephalosporins (eg, indole-positive *Proteus* spp., *Serratia* spp.). Its desacetyl metabolite (DACM) has good activity and may be synergistic with cefotaxime against certain organisms. The activity of cefotaxime against *Pseudomonas aeruginosa* is inferior to ceftazidime, and against *Staphylococcus aureus* is inferior to cefazolin. Cefotaxime is more active than other cephalosporins (except ceftriaxone) against *Streptococcus pneumoniae* that are intermediately resistant to penicillin G. CSF levels range from 0.3–0.44 mg/L after a 1-g dose, and in higher doses cefotaxime is effective for treatment of meningitis. About 50% of a dose is excreted unchanged in urine and 50% metabolized to DACM. DACM is metabolized to inactive metabolites and excreted unchanged in urine. Cefotaxime is well tolerated, with coagulopathies only rarely reported. Adult dosage is IM or IV 250 mg–2 g q 6–12 hr (usually 1–2 g q 8–12 hr), to a maximum of 12 g/day. Reduce dosage by 50% in patients with a Cl_{cr} <20 mL/min. Dosage in newborns up to 1 week of age is IV 50 mg/kg q 12 hr; from 1–4 weeks IV 50 mg/kg q 8 hr; and in older children IM or IV 50–200 mg/kg/day (200 mg/kg/day for meningitis) given q 6–8 hr.[133,134,136,137,151] (*See* ß-Lactams Comparison Chart.)

CEFOTETAN SODIUM   Cefotan

Cefotetan is a cephamycin, structurally and pharmacologically similar to the cephalosporins, particularly second-generation agents, and it contains an NMTT side chain. It has greater activity against enteric Gram-negative bacteria than first- and second-generation cephalosporins and superior activity against *Bacteroides fragilis* and other anaerobic bacteria (comparable to cefoxitin and cefmetazole). Gram-positive activity is less than cefazolin. It is excreted primarily unchanged in urine, with an elimination half-life of 3.5 hr. Adult dosage is IV or IM 500 mg–2 g 1 q 12–24 hr (usually 1–2 g q 12 hr), to a maximum of 6 g/day for treatment; and IV or IM 1–2 g 30–60 min prior to surgery for prophylaxis, then 1–2 g q 12 hr for up to 24 hr postoperatively. Reconstitute the drug with 0.5% lidocaine for IM administration because IM injection is painful. Reduce dosage by 50% with a Cl_{cr} between 10–30 mL/min, and by 75% in patients with a Cl_{cr} <10 mL/min. The safety and efficacy of cefotetan have not been established in children; the dosage based on clinical studies is IV 40–60 mg/kg/day given in equally divided doses q 12 hr.[133,142,143] *See* β-Lactams Comparison Chart.

CEFTAZIDIME   Ceptaz, Fortaz, Tazicef, Tazidime

Ceftazidime is a third-generation cephalosporin with activity generally similar to cefotaxime, but having superior activity against *Pseudomonas aeruginosa* and inferior Gram-positive (particularly against *Staphylococcus aureus* and penicillin-resistant pneumococci) and anaerobic bacteria. It is less than 30% plasma protein bound and is 80–90% excreted unchanged in urine by filtration, with a half-life of 1.6 hr, increasing to 25–34 hr in renal failure. The drug is generally well tolerated. Conventional formulations of ceftazidime release carbon dioxide during reconstitution; the lysine formulation (eg, Ceptaz) avoids this problem. Adult dosage is IM or IV 500 mg–2 g q 8–12 hr; q 12 hr administration appears to be adequate in the elderly. Reduce dosage by 50% with a Cl_{cr} of 30–50 mL/min; with a Cl_{cr} of 15–30 mL/min, the maximum dosage is 1 g q 24 hr; with a Cl_{cr} <15 mL/min, the dosage is 500 mg q 24–48 hr. Dosage in newborns is IV 30–50 mg/kg q 12 hr; and in older children IM or IV 30–50 mg/kg q 8 hr, to a maximum of 6 g/day (225 mg/kg/day for treatment of meningitis).[133–137,151] (*See* ß-Lactams Comparison Chart.)

CEFUROXIME SODIUM   Kefurox, Zinacef

CEFUROXIME AXETIL   Ceftin

Cefuroxime is a second-generation cephalosporin with greater activity than cefazolin, but less than cefotaxime, against *Haemophilus influenzae*, including β-lactamase-producing strains. The activity of cefuroxime against *Staphylococcus aureus* is slightly less than that of cefazolins. Its activity against anaerobes is poor, similar to the first-generation cephalosporins. In adults, bioavailability appears to be lower with the suspension than the tablets, and food increases the bioavailability of the tablets. Do not interchange the tablets and suspension on a mg/kg basis. After absorption of oral cefuroxime axetil, it is hydrolyzed in the bloodstream to cefuroxime. Cefuroxime's pharmacokinetics are similar to cefazolin's, but CSF concentrations are adequate for treatment of meningitis caused by certain organisms; however, the third-generation agents ceftriaxone and cefotaxime are superior in *H. influenzae* meningitis. Over 95% of the drug is excreted unchanged in the urine and the elimination half-life is 1.2 hr. The drug is well tolerated. Adult dosage is IM or IV 750 mg–1.5 g q 8 hr for treatment; and IV 1.5 g 1 hr prior to surgery for prophylaxis; doses of IM or IV 750 mg may be given q 8 hr for up to 24 hr postoperatively (1.5 g q 12 hr to a total of 6 g for open heart surgery). Reduce parenteral dosage in renal impairment: with a Cl_{cr} of 10–20 mL/min, give the usual dose q 12 hr; with a Cl_{cr} <10 mL/min, give the usual dose q 24 hr. Parenteral dosage in newborns is 10–25 mg/kg q 12 hr; and in older children 50–100 mg/kg/day, to a maximum of 250 mg/kg/day for meningitis in 3–4 divided doses. The oral dosage of cefuroxime axetil is 125–500 mg q 12 hr in adults, and 15–20 mg/kg q 12 hr in children (40 mg/kg/day for otitis media); it may be given in applesauce.[133,137,144,152] (*See* ß-Lactams Comparison Chart.)

EXTENDED-SPECTRUM PENICILLINS

The carboxypenicillins (carbenicillin and ticarcillin) and the acylureidopenicillins (mezlocillin and piperacillin) have the same mechanism of action as other penicillins, but are more active against enteric Gram-negative bacteria and *Pseudomonas aeruginosa*. The carboxypenicillins are not active against *Klebsiella* spp., but the acylureido derivatives do have activity and are generally more potent against susceptible isolates. The acylureidopenicillins also have activity comparable to ampicillin against enterococci. Carbenicillin has the least activity and is available only for oral use in urinary tract infections. The combination of clavulanic acid plus ticarcillin is active against *Klebsiella* spp. as well as ß-lactamase-producing staphylococci, *Haemophilus influenzae*, and *Bacteroides* spp. The combination of tazobactam plus piperacillin is similar to clavulanic acid plus ticarcillin. These two combination products are not appreciably more active against *P. aeruginosa* or *Enterobacter cloacae* than ticarcillin or piperacillin alone. Usual half-life is 1–1.5 hr, which is prolonged in anuria, although acylureido derivatives are partially metabolized and accumulate to a lesser extent. The acylureidopenicillins are also subject to capacity-limited elimination (ie, increasing dosage results in progressive saturation of elimination pathways, resulting in decreased clearance), which allows administration of higher doses at 6- to 8-hr intervals. Adverse effects are similar to other penicillins. Sodium content of the usual daily dosage of parenteral ticarcillin approaches the equivalent of 1 L of NS. The carboxylic acid function in the molecule of the carboxypenicillins produces prolongation in bleeding time with systemic dosages as a result of binding to platelets and preventing aggregation.[125,126,128,153–155] (*See* β-Lactams Comparison Chart.)

IMIPENEM AND CILASTATIN SODIUM   Primaxin

Pharmacology. Imipenem is a carbapenem with an extremely broad spectrum against many aerobic and anaerobic Gram-positive and Gram-negative bacterial pathogens. The commercial preparation contains an equal amount of cilastatin, a renal dehydropeptidase inhibitor that has no antimicrobial activity but prevents imipenem's metabolism by proximal tubular kidney cells, thus increasing urinary imipenem concentrations and possibly decreasing nephrotoxicity.[133,155,156] (*See* Notes.)

Administration and Adult Dosage. IV 1–4 g/day in 3 or 4 divided doses (usually 500 mg q 6–8 hr). For severe, life-threatening infections a dose of 1 g q 6 hr is recommended (not to exceed 60 mg/kg/day).[155] Infuse 250- to 500-mg doses over 20–30 min and 1-g doses over 40–60 min; reduce infusion rate if nausea and/or vomiting develops. **IM** 1–2 g/day in 3 or 4 divided doses.

Special Populations. *Pediatric Dosage.* (Under 12 yr) safety and efficacy not established, but IV 15–25 mg/kg (of imipenem) q 6 hr has been successfully used.[155,157]

Geriatric Dosage. Same as adult dosage, but adjust for age-related reduction in renal function.

Other Conditions. Reduce dosage with renal insufficiency as follows: Cl_{cr} 30–70 mL/min, give 75% of the usual dosage; Cl_{cr} 20–30 mL/min, give 50% of the usual dosage; Cl_{cr} <20 mL/min, give 25% of the usual dosage. Give a supplemental dose following hemodialysis.[155]

Dosage Forms. **Inj (IV)** 250 mg imipenem/250 mg cilastatin, 500 mg imipenem/500 mg cilastatin; **Inj (suspension, IM only)** 500 mg imipenem/500 mg cilastatin, 750 mg imipenem/750 mg cilastatin. (*See* Notes.)

Pharmacokinetics. *Fate.* Peak serum imipenem concentrations are 22 and 52 mg/L after 30-min infusions of 500 mg and 1 g, respectively; levels are <1 mg/L at 6 hr. CSF levels range from 0.5–11 mg/L with inflamed meninges and appear to be adequate to treat meningitis, but experience in treating meningitis is limited and seizures may occur in such patients. Imipenem is 20% plasma protein bound; V_d is 0.26 L/kg. Probenecid increases imipenem serum levels and prolongs its half-life. About 70% of imipenem is excreted unchanged in urine when given with cilastatin, with the remainder excreted as metabolite; cilastatin is excreted 90% unchanged in urine.[155,156]

$t_{1/2}$. (Imipenem) 0.9 ± 0.1 hr; 3–4 hr in renal failure. (Cilastatin) 0.8 ± 0.1 hr; 17 hr in renal failure.[155,156]

Adverse Reactions. Nausea and vomiting occur, sometimes associated with hypotension or diaphoresis, particularly with high doses and rapid infusion.[155,156] Rashes occur occasionally, and cross-allergenicity with penicillins has been documented. Convulsions have occurred, primarily in the elderly, in those with underlying CNS disease, with overdosage in patients with renal failure, or with other predisposing factors.[155,156,158,159]

Precautions. Use with caution in elderly patients, or those with a history of seizures or who are otherwise predisposed. Adjust dosage carefully in renal impairment. Imipenem may cause immediate hypersensitivity reactions in patients with a history of anaphylaxis to penicillin.[159]

Drug Interactions. Concomitant administration with probenecid produces higher and prolonged serum concentrations of imipenem and cilastatin. Imipenem has been shown in vitro to antagonize the activity of other ß-lactams (eg, acylureidopenicillins, most cephalosporins, aztreonam) presumably via ß-lactamase induction; although the clinical relevance is unclear, avoid coadministration.[156] Coadministration of imipenem/cilastatin with ganciclovir has been associated with generalized seizures in a few patients; the mechanism of this interaction is unknown.

Parameters to Monitor. Obtain renal function tests periodically.

Notes. Used alone, emergence of resistance during treatment of *Pseudomonas aeruginosa* infections occurs frequently; however, cross-resistance to other classes (eg, aminoglycosides, cephalosporins) does not occur.[155,156] Addition of an aminoglycoside may prevent development of resistance, but in vitro synergism occurs only infrequently.

Vials may be reconstituted into a suspension using 10 mL of the infusion solution and then further diluted by transferring the suspension into the infusion container; alternatively, the powder in the 120-mL vials can be diluted initially with 100 mL of solution. The initial dilution must be shaken well to ensure suspension/solution. Do not inject the suspension. The resulting solution ranges from colorless to yellow. Reconstituted solutions are stable in dextrose-containing solutions for 4 hr at room temperature and 24 hr under refrigeration, and in normal saline for 10 hr at room temperature and 48 hr under refrigeration. With IM administration use 2 mL of lidocaine 1% injection to reconstitute a 500-mg vial and give the suspension by deep IM injection into a large muscle mass (eg, gluteal muscle).[156]

MEROPENEM   Merrem

Meropenem is a carbapenem with a mechanism of action similar to imipenem. Unlike imipenem, meropenem is not appreciably degraded by renal dehydropeptidase-I, and thus does not require concomitant administration of a dehydropeptidase inhibitor. Meropenem is more active than imipenem against enteric Gram-negative bacilli, the two have equivalent activity against *Pseudomonas aeruginosa* and *Bacteroides fragilis*, and meropenem is slightly less active than imipenem against Gram-positive organisms.[156,160,161] The pharmacokinetics of meropenem are similar to those of imipenem, although meropenem can be given by both infusion and IV bolus.[160,162] After IV infusion of 1 g, peak serum concentration is 55 mg/L; the drug distributes well into most tissues and fluids, including the CSF. Plasma protein binding is low and the V_{dss} is 0.32 ± 0.03 L/kg. Meropenem is primarily eliminated renally by both glomerular filtration and tubular secretion; the elimination half-life is 0.9 ± 0.09 hr. Up to 70% of a dose is recovered unchanged in the urine, with a renal metabolite accounting for the remainder of the dose (up to 30%). Probenecid can increase serum levels and reduce renal clearance of meropenem. The half-life is 6.8–13.7 hr in patients with end-stage renal disease, necessitating dosage reduction. Meropenem is appreciably removed by hemodialysis, and a supplemental dose is required following dialysis. Children have pharmacokinetics similar to adults; increased clearance and reduced half-life occur in cystic fibrotics.[162] Adverse effects are similar to imipenem; the most common include rash, nausea and vomiting, and diarrhea.[156,160] Animal studies suggest that meropenem has a lower epileptogenic potential, which has been supported thus far by a very low frequency of seizures in clinical trials, including studies in patients with meningitis.[160] Use meropenem with caution in patients with hypersensitivity to penicillins.[159] The usual adult dosage is IV 500 mg–1 g q 8 hr; severe or life-threatening infections (eg, meningitis) are treated with IV 2 g q 8 hr; less severe infections can be treated with IM or IV 500 mg–1 g q 8–12 hr. In infants and children 3 months–12 yr, the dosage used in clinical trials is 10–20 mg/kg q 8 hr; in children with meningitis a dosage of 40 mg/kg q 8 hr has been used.[160] Daily dosage in patients with Cl_{cr} of 26–50 mL/min is the normal dose q 12 hr; with Cl_{cr} of 10–25 mL/min the dosage is reduced by 50%; with Cl_{cr} <10 mL/min, give half the dose once daily.[160,162] (*See* β-Lactams Comparison Chart.)

PENICILLIN G SALTS   Various

Pharmacology. Penicillin G has activity against most Gram-positive organisms and some Gram-negative organisms, notably *Neisseria* spp. It acts by interfering with late stages of bacterial cell wall synthesis; resistance is primarily caused by bacterial elaboration of ß-lactamases; some organisms have altered penicillin-binding protein (PBP) targets (eg, enterococci and pneumococci), others have impermeable outer cell wall layers.[125,126]

Administration and Adult Dosage. PO 250–500 mg (400,000–800,000 units) q 6 hr for mild to moderate infections. IV 2–24 million units/day in 4–12 divided doses, depending on infection. **IM not recommended** (very painful); use benzathine or procaine salt form as indicated.

Special Populations. *Pediatric Dosage.* PO (under 12 yr) 25,000–90,000 units/kg/day in 3–6 divided doses; PO (over 12 yr) same as adult dosage. IV **(preferably) or IM** (over 1 month) 100,000–300,000 units/kg/day in 4–6 divided doses.

Geriatric Dosage. Same as adult dosage, but adjust for age-related reduction in renal function.

Other Conditions. With usual oral dosage, no dosage adjustment is required in patients with impaired renal function; however, in treating more severe infections with larger IV dosages, careful adjustment is necessary. In anuric patients, give no more than 3 million units/day.[163]

Dosage Forms. Susp/Syrup (as potassium salt) 40,000 and 80,000 units/mL (reconstituted); Tab (as potassium salt) 200,000, 250,000, 400,000, 500,000, 800,000 units; Inj (as potassium salt) 1, 5, 10, 20 million units; Inj (as sodium salt) 5 million units.

Patient Instructions. Take this (oral) drug with a full glass of water on an empty stomach (1 hour before or 2 hours after meals) for best absorption; refrigerate solution.

Pharmacokinetics. *Fate.* Only 15–30% orally absorbed because of its high susceptibility to gastric acid hydrolysis; peak concentrations of 1.5–2.7 mg/L occur 0.5–1 hr after administration of 500 mg. Widely distributed in body tissues, fluids, and cavities, with biliary levels up to 10 times serum levels; 30–60% plasma protein bound. Penetration into CSF is poor, even with inflamed meninges; however, large parenteral dosages (greater than 20 million units/day) adequately treat meningitis caused by susceptible organisms. From 80–85% of the absorbed dose is excreted unchanged in the urine.[125,126]

$t_{1/2}$. 30–40 min; 7–10 hr in patients with renal failure; 20–30 hr in patients with hepatic and renal failure.[163]

Adverse Reactions. Occasionally nausea or diarrhea occurs after usual oral doses. As with all penicillins, CNS toxicity may occur with massive IV dosages (60–100 million units/day) or excessive dosage in patients with impaired renal function (usually greater than 10–20 million units/day in anuric patients); characterized by confusion, drowsiness, and myoclonus, which may progress to convulsions and result in death. Large dosages of the sodium salt form may result in hypernatremia and fluid overload with pulmonary edema, especially in patients with impaired renal function or CHF. Large dosages of the potassium salt form may result in hyperkalemia, especially in patients with impaired renal function and with rapid infusions. Occasional positive Coombs' reactions with rare hemolytic anemia have been reported after large IV doses. Interstitial nephritis has been rarely reported following large IV dosages. Hypersensitivity reactions (primarily rashes) occur in 1–10% of patients. Most serious hypersensitivity reactions follow injection rather than oral administration.[125,159]

Contraindications. History of anaphylactic, accelerated (eg, hives) or serum sickness reaction to previous penicillin administration. (*See* Notes.)

Precautions. Use caution in patients with a history of penicillin or cephalosporin hypersensitivity reactions, atopic predisposition (eg, asthma), impaired renal function (hence neonates and geriatric patients), impaired cardiac function or preexisting seizure disorder.

Drug Interactions. Physically and/or chemically incompatible with aminoglycosides leading to drug inactivation; never mix them together in the same IV solution or syringe. Probenecid competes with penicillin for renal excretion, resulting in higher and prolonged serum concentrations.[125,126]

Parameters to Monitor. Obtain renal function tests initially when using high dosages. During prolonged high-dose therapy, monitor renal function tests and serum electrolytes periodically.

Notes. A dose of 250 mg equals 400,000 units of penicillin G. Penicillin V potassium is preferred to penicillin G potassium for oral administration because of more complete (60%) and reliable absorption. Skin testing with penicilloyl-polylysine (PPL, Pre-Pen) and minor determinant mixture (MDM) can help determine the likelihood of serious reactions to penicillin in penicillin-allergic individuals.[125,164] Availability of MDM is limited; it is locally available in small amounts only at larger medical centers. Desensitization is recommended in pregnant women with syphilis and may be attempted (rarely) in patients with life-threatening infections that are likely to be responsive only to penicillin, but this is a dangerous procedure and many alternative antibiotics are available.[125] (*See* also β-Lactams Comparison Chart.)

β-LACTAMS COMPARISON CHART

DRUG CLASS AND DRUG	DOSAGE FORMS	ADULT DOSAGE	PEDIATRIC DOSAGE	ADULT DOSAGE IN RENAL IMPAIRMENT[a]	PEAK SERUM LEVELS (MG/L)[b]	PERCENTAGE PROTEIN BOUND	COMMENTS
CARBAPENEMS							
Imipenem and Cilastatin Sodium Primaxin	Inj (IV) 250 plus 250 mg, 500 plus 500 mg; (IM) 500 plus 500 mg, 750 plus 750 mg.	IV 1–4 g/day (1–2/day preferred) in 3 or 4 divided doses; IM 1–2 g/day in 3 or 4 divided doses.	Safety and efficacy not established under 12 yr.	Cl$_{cr}$ 30–70 mL/min: 75% of usual dosage; Cl$_{cr}$ 20–30 mL/min: 50% of usual dosage; Cl$_{cr}$ <20 mL/min: 25% of usual dosage.	22 (IV 500 mg imipenem)	20	Very broad activity against most aerobic and anaerobic bacteria. Frequent nausea and dose-related seizure potential.
Meropenem Merrem	Inj 500 mg, 1 g.	IV 500 mg–1 g q 8–12 hr; 2 g q 8 hr in life-threatening infections.	Safety and efficacy not established. IV (3 mo–12 yr) 10–20 mg/kg q 8 hr; 40 mg/kg q 8 hr in meningitis.	Cl$_{cr}$ 25–50 mL/min: usual dose q 12 hr; Cl$_{cr}$ 10–25 mL/min: 50% of usual dose q 12 hr; Cl$_{cr}$ <10 mL/min: 50% of usual dose q 24 hr.	55	Low	Less active than imipenem against Gm$^+$ and more active against most Gm$^-$ bacteria; equivalent against P. aeruginosa and B. fragilis. Less seizure potential than imipenem.

(continued)

B-LACTAMS COMPARISON CHART (continued)

DRUG CLASS AND DRUG	DOSAGE FORMS	ADULT DOSAGE	PEDIATRIC DOSAGE	ADULT DOSAGE IN RENAL IMPAIRMENT[a]	PEAK SERUM LEVELS (MG/L)[b]	PERCENTAGE PROTEIN BOUND	COMMENTS
CEPHALOSPORINS, FIRST-GENERATION							

Cefadroxil
Duricef
Various
	Cap 500 mg
	Susp 25, 50,
	100 mg/mL
	Tab 1 g.
		PO 500 mg–
		1 g q 12–24
		hr.
			PO 30 mg/kg/day
			in 1 or 2 divided
			doses.
				PO 1 g, then 500
				mg at intervals
				below:
				Cl$_{cr}$ 25–50 mL/min:
				  12 hr;
				Cl$_{cr}$ 10–25 mL/min:
				  24 hr;
				Cl$_{cr}$ <10 mL/min:
				  36 hr.
					12–16	20	Spectrum similar to cefazolin.

Cefazolin Sodium
Ancef
Kefzol
Various
	Inj 250, 500 mg,
	1, 5, 10 g.
		IM or IV 250 mg–
		1 g q 6–12 hr.
			IM or IV (neo-
			nates under 1
			month) 20 mg/kg
			q 8–12 hr;
			(Infants over 1
			month) 50–100
			mg/kg/day in
			3 divided doses.
				Cl$_{cr}$ 10–35 mL/min:
				  50% of usual dose
				  q 12 hr;
				Cl$_{cr}$ <10 mL/min:
				  50% of usual dose
				  q 18–24 hr.
					80–110	75–85	Good Gm$^+$ coverage (including *S. aureus*), plus some Gm$^-$ activity (*E. coli, Klebsiella* spp.). Sodium = 2 mEq/g.

Cephalexin Keflex Keftab	Cap 250, 500 mg Drp 100 mg/mL Susp 25,	PO 250 mg–1 g q 6 hr.	PO 25–50 mg/kg/ day in 4 divided doses.	Cl$_{cr}$ 10–50 mL/min: 50% of usual dosage; Cl$_{cr}$ <10 mL/min:	10–20	6	Oral absorption is almost complete; spectrum similar to cefazolin.

(continued)

β-LACTAMS COMPARISON CHART (continued)

DRUG CLASS AND DRUG	DOSAGE FORMS	ADULT DOSAGE	PEDIATRIC DOSAGE	ADULT DOSAGE IN RENAL IMPAIRMENT[a]	PEAK SERUM LEVELS (MG/L)[b]	PERCENTAGE PROTEIN BOUND	COMMENTS
Various	50 mg/mL Tab 250, 500 mg, 1 g.			25% of usual dosage.			
Cephalothin Sodium Various	Inj 1, 2, 4, 10, 20 g.	IV 500 mg–1 g q 4–6 hr; IM not recommended.	IV (neonates under 7 days) 20 mg/kg q 8–12 hr; (infants over 7 days) 75–125 mg/kg/day in 4–6 divided doses.	Cl$_{cr}$ 10–25 mL/min: 1 g q 6 hr; Cl$_{cr}$ <10 mL/min: 500 mg q 6–8 hr.	15–30	65	Spectrum similar to cefazolin. Painful IM injection. Sodium = 2.8 mEq/g.
Cephapirin Sodium Cefadyl Various	Inj 500 mg–1, 2, 4, 20 g.	IM or IV 500 mg–1 g q 4–6 hr.	Same as cephalothin.	Same as cephalothin.	10–20	45–50	Very similar to cephalothin. Sodium = 2.4 mEq/g.
Cephradine Anspor Velosef Various	Cap 250, 500 mg Susp 25, 50 mg/mL Tab 1 g Inj 250, 500 mg, 1, 2, 4 g.	PO 250 mg–1 g q 6 hr; IM or IV 500 mg–1 g q 4–6 hr.	IM or IV same as cephalothin; PO same as cephalexin.	IM or IV same as cephalothin; PO same as cephalexin.	10–20 (PO) 15–30 (IV)	5–20	Oral form comparable to cephalexin; spectrum similar to cefazolin. Sodium = 6 mEq/g injection.

(continued)

DRUG CLASS AND DRUG	DOSAGE FORMS	ADULT DOSAGE	PEDIATRIC DOSAGE	ADULT DOSAGE IN RENAL IMPAIRMENT[a]	PEAK SERUM LEVELS (MG/L)[b]	PERCENTAGE PROTEIN BOUND	COMMENTS
CEPHALOSPORINS, SECOND-GENERATION							
Cefaclor Ceclor Various	Cap 250, 500 mg Susp 25, 37.5, 50, 75 mg/mL.	PO 250 mg– 1 g q 6–8 hr.	PO 40 mg/kg/day in 3 divided doses.	Cl$_{cr}$ 10–50 mL/min: 50% of usual dosage; Cl$_{cr}$ <10 mL/min: 25% of usual dosage.	10–15	25	Spectrum similar to cefazolin, but includes some ampicillin-resistant *H. influenzae.*
Cefamandole Nafate Mandol	Inj 500 mg, 1, 2, 10 g.	IM or IV 500 mg–1 g q 4–8 hr.	IM or IV 50–150 mg/kg/day in 4–6 divided doses.	Cl$_{cr}$ 10–50 mL/min: 50% of usual dose q 8 hr; Cl$_{cr}$ <10 mL/min: 25% of usual dose q 12 hr.	80–90	56	NMTT side chain. Spectrum similar to cefuroxime. Sodium = 3.3 mEq/g.
Cefonicid Sodium Monocid	Inj 500 mg, 1, 10 g.	IM or IV 500 mg, 2 g/day as a single dose.	Not established.	IM or IV 7.5 mg/kg, then 25–50% of usual dose given: Cl$_{cr}$ 10–50 mL/min: q 24–48 hr; Cl$_{cr}$ <10 mL/min: q 3–5 days	220 (IV bolus)	83–98[c]	Poor activity against *Staphylococcus* spp. Unbound drug levels low and excreted rapidly because of saturable protein binding. Sodium 3.7 mEq/g
Cefotetan Disodium	Inj 1, 2 g.	IM or IV 500 mg–2 g q 12–24 hr.	Not established.	IM or IV give usual dose at intervals below.	140–180 (IV bolus)	78–91[c]	NMTT side chain: spectrum similar to cefoxitin. Sodium = 3.5 mEq/g.

(continued)

107

β-LACTAMS COMPARISON CHART (continued)

DRUG CLASS AND DRUG	DOSAGE FORMS	ADULT DOSAGE	PEDIATRIC DOSAGE	ADULT DOSAGE IN RENAL IMPAIRMENT[a]	PEAK SERUM LEVELS (MG/L)[b]	PERCENTAGE PROTEIN BOUND	COMMENTS
Cefotan				Cl_{cr} 10–30 mL/min: 24 hr; Cl_{cr} <10 mL/min: 48 hr.			
Cefoxitin Sodium Mefoxin	Inj 1, 2, 10 g.	IV 1–2 g q 6–8 hr.	IV 80–160 mg/kg/ day in 4–6 divided doses.	Cl_{cr} 10–50 mL/min: 50% of usual dose q 6–8 hr; Cl_{cr} <10 mL/min: 25% of usual dose q 12 hr.	30–50	75	Gm⁺ activity less than cefazolin, but better Gm⁻ and anaerobic activity. Sodium = 2.3 mEq/g.
Cefprozil Cefzil	Tab 250, 500 mg. Susp 25, 50 mg/mL.	PO 500 mg daily–bid.	PO (6 mo–12 yr) 15 mg/kg q 12 hr.	Cl_{cr} ≤30 mL/min: 50% of usual dose at same interval.	10.5	36	Spectrum similar to cefaclor, but more active against *H. influenzae*.
Cefuroxime Sodium Kefurox Zinacef	Inj 750 mg, 1.5 g.	IM or IV 750 mg–1.5 g q 6–8 hr.	IM or IV (neonates) 10–25 mg/kg q 12 hr; (children) 50–100 mg/kg/day in 3–4 divided doses.	IM or IV: Cl_{cr} 10–20 mL/min: usual dose q 12 hr; Cl_{cr} <10 mL/min: usual dose q 24 hr.	140 (IV bolus)	33	Gm⁺ activity similar to cefazolin, but better Gm⁻ activity, including *H. influenzae*. Sodium = 2.4 mEq/g.
Cefuroxime Axetil Ceftin	Tab 125, 250, 500 mg.	PO 125–500 mg bid.	PO 20–40 mg/kg/ day in 2 divided doses.	—	3.6 (PO)		

(continued)

DRUG CLASS AND DRUG	DOSAGE FORMS	ADULT DOSAGE	PEDIATRIC DOSAGE	ADULT DOSAGE IN RENAL IMPAIRMENT[a]	PEAK SERUM LEVELS (MG/L)[b]	PERCENTAGE PROTEIN BOUND	COMMENTS
Loracarbef Lorabid	Cap 200, 400 mg Susp 20, 40 mg/mL.	PO 200–400 mg q 12 hr.	PO (6 mo–12 yr) 7.5–15 mg q 12 hr.	Cl$_{cr}$ 10–49 mL/min: 50% of usual dosage; Cl$_{cr}$ <10 mL/min: usual dose q 3–5 days	6.8 (PO 200 mg)	25	Carbacephan analogue of cefaclor with similar spectrum. Must be taken on an empty stomach.
CEPHALOSPORINS, THIRD-GENERATION							
Cefixime Suprax	Tab 200, 400 mg Susp 20 mg/mL.	PO 200–400 mg q 12–24 hr. PO for gonorrhea 400 mg once.	PO 8 mg/kg/day in 1 or 2 divided doses.	Cl$_{cr}$ 20–60 mL/min: 75% of usual dosage; Cl$_{cr}$ <20 mL/min: 50% of usual dosage.	4.9	70	More active than cefuroxime or cefaclor against *H. influenzae*, but less Gm$^+$ activity.
Cefoperazone Sodium Cefobid Various	Inj 1, 2 g.	IM or IV 2–8 g/day in 2–4 divided doses.	IM or IV (neonates) 50 mg/kg/dose q 12 hr; (children) 50–75 mg/kg q 8–12 hr.	No change.	125	85–95[c]	Less active than ceftazidime against *P. aeruginosa*. NMTT side chain. Sodium = 1.5 mEq/g.

(continued)

B-LACTAMS COMPARISON CHART (continued)

DRUG CLASS AND DRUG	DOSAGE FORMS	ADULT DOSAGE	PEDIATRIC DOSAGE	ADULT DOSAGE IN RENAL IMPAIRMENT[a]	PEAK SERUM LEVELS (MG/L)[b]	PERCENTAGE PROTEIN BOUND	COMMENTS
Cefotaxime Sodium Claforan	Inj 500 mg, 1, 2, 10 g.	IM or IV 1–2 g q 6–12 hr.	IM or IV (neonates 1 week or under) 50 mg/kg q 12 hr; (neonates 1–4 weeks) 50 mg/kg q 8 hr; (infants over 4 weeks) 50–200 (400 in meningitis) mg/kg/day in 4–6 divided doses.	Cl$_{cr}$ <20 mL/min: 50% of usual dosage.	40	37	Good Gm$^+$ and Gm$^-$ activity except for *P. aeruginosa*; modest antianaerobic activity. Sodium = 2.2 mEq/g.
Desacetyl-cefotaxime					1–65	—	
Cefpodoxime Proxetil Vantin	Tab 100, 200 mg Susp 10, 20 mg/mL.	PO 100–400 mg q 12 hr. PO for gonorrhea 200 mg once.	PO 5 mg/kg q 12 hr.	Cl$_{cr}$ <30 mL/min: usual dose given q 24 hr.	23 (PO 200 mg)	18–30	Spectrum similar to cefixime, but better Gm$^+$ activity.
Ceftazidime Ceptaz Fortaz	Inj 500 mg 1, 2, 6 g.	IM or IV 500 mg–2 g q 8–12 hr.	IM or IV (neonates 1 mo or under) 30–50 mg/kg/dose	Cl$_{cr}$ 30–50 mL/min: 50% of usual dose q 12–24 hr;	80	17	Best activity against *P. aeruginosa*; poor Gm$^+$ activity. Sodium = 2.3 mEq/g.

(continued)

DRUG CLASS AND DRUG	DOSAGE FORMS	ADULT DOSAGE	PEDIATRIC DOSAGE	ADULT DOSAGE IN RENAL IMPAIRMENT[a]	PEAK SERUM LEVELS (MG/L)[b]	PERCENTAGE PROTEIN BOUND	COMMENTS
Tazicef Tazidime			q 12 hr; (infants over 1 month) 30–50 mg/kg/dose q 8 hr.	Cl_cr 15–30 mL/min: 1 g q 24 hr; Cl_cr <15 mL/min: 500 mg q 24–48 hr.			
Ceftibuten Cedax	Cap 400 mg Susp 18, 36 mg/mL.	PO 200–400 mg q 24 hr.	PO 9 mg/kg/day in 1 or 2 divided doses.	Cl_cr 30–49 mL/min: 4.5 mg/kg or 200 mg q 24 hr; Cl_cr 5–29 mL/min: 2.25 mg/kg or 100 mg q 24 hr.	60–77	11 (PO 200 mg)	Spectrum similar to cefixime.
Ceftizoxime Sodium Cefizox	Inj 1, 2 g.	IM or IV 1–2 g q 8–12 hr.	IM or IV (over 6 mo) 50 mg/kg/dose q 6–8 hr.	Cl_cr 10–50 mL/min: 50% of usual dose q 12–24 hr; Cl_cr <10 mL/min: 25–50% of usual dose q 24–48 hr.	75–90	31	Spectrum similar to cefotaxime except slightly more active against anaerobes. Sodium = 2.6 mEq/g.
Ceftriaxone Disodium Rocephin	Inj 250, 500 mg, 1, 2, 10 g.	IM or IV 500 mg–2 g/day as a single dose; IM for gonorrhea 250 mg once.	IM or IV 50–100 (100 in meningitis) mg/kg/day in 2 divided doses.	No change, see Comments.	145	83–96[c]	Spectrum similar to cefotaxime. Reduce dose with concurrent renal and hepatic dysfunction. Sodium = 3.6 mEq/g.

(continued)

111

β-LACTAMS COMPARISON CHART (continued)

DRUG CLASS AND DRUG	DOSAGE FORMS	ADULT DOSAGE	PEDIATRIC DOSAGE	ADULT DOSAGE IN RENAL IMPAIRMENT[a]	PEAK SERUM LEVELS (MG/L)[b]	PERCENTAGE PROTEIN BOUND	COMMENTS
Moxalactam Disodium Moxam	Inj 1, 2, 10 g.	IM or IV 1–2 g q 8–12 hr.	IM or IV (neonates under 1 week) 50 mg/kg q 12 hr; (infants over 1 week) 50 mg/kg q 6–8 hr.	Cl$_{cr}$ 10–50 mL/min: 25–50% of usual dose q 8–12 hr; Cl$_{cr}$ <10 mL/min: avoid.	60–70	50	Best activity against anaerobes. NMTT side chain and antiplatelet effect, with serious bleeding reported. Sodium = 3.8 mEq/g.
CEPHALOSPORINS, FOURTH-GENERATION							
Cefepime Maxipime	Inj 500 mg, 1, 2 g.	IM or IV 500 mg–2 g q 12 hr.	Safety and efficacy not established under 12 yr.	Cl$_{cr}$ 30–60 mL/min: usual dose q 24 hr; Cl$_{cr}$ 10–30 mL/min: 50% of usual dose q 24 hr; Cl$_{cr}$ <10 mL/min: 25% of usual dose q 24 hr.	79	16	Spectrum similar to ceftazidime; more active against Gm+ organisms; also active against resistant Enterobacter spp.
MONOBACTAM							
Aztreonam Azactam	Inj 500 mg, 1, 2 g.	IM or IV 0.5–2 g q 6–12 hr.	Safety and efficacy not established. IV 30 mg/kg q 6–8 hr (50 mg/kg q 4–6 hr in P. aeruginosa) has been used.	Cl$_{cr}$ 10–30 mL/min: 50% of usual dosage; Cl$_{cr}$ <10 mL/min: 25% of usual dosage.	164	60	Spectrum similar to ceftazidime against aerobic Gm− organisms only. No cross-allergenicity in penicillin-allergic patients.

(continued)

DRUG CLASS AND DRUG	DOSAGE FORMS	ADULT DOSAGE	PEDIATRIC DOSAGE	ADULT DOSAGE IN RENAL IMPAIRMENT[a]	PEAK SERUM LEVELS (MG/L)[b]	PERCENTAGE PROTEIN BOUND	COMMENTS
PENICILLIN G AND V							
Penicillin G Potassium Various	Inj 1, 5, 10, 20 million units Tab, Susp *see monograph.*	IV 1–5 million units q 4–6 hr.	IV (neonates) 25,000–75,000 units/kg q 8–12 hr; (children) 100,000–250,000 units/kg/day in 4–6 divided doses.	Cl$_{cr}$ <40 mL/min: dose (in million units/day) = 3.2 + (Cl$_{cr}$ = 7).	1.5–2.7 (IV 500 mg)	60	Gm⁺ (except most *Staph.* strains), some Gm⁻ (*Neisseria* spp.), and anaerobes (except *B. fragilis*). Poor oral absorption. Potassium = 1.7 mEq/million units.
Penicillin G Benzathine Various	Inj 300,000, 600,000, 1.2 million units/mL.	IM for *Strep.* pharyngitis 1.2 million units once. IM for syphilis (early) 2.4 million units once, (late) 2.4 million units/ week for 3 weeks.	IM for *Strep.* pharyngitis (under 27 kg) 300,000–600,000 units once; (over 27 kg) 900,000 units once.	No change.	0.063 (IM 600,000 units)	60	Use limited to syphilis and streptococcal pharyngitis. For IM use only.
Penicillin G Procaine Various	Inj 300,000, 500,000, 600,000 units/mL.	IM 600,000–1.2 million units q 12–24 hr.	IM (neonates) 50,000 units/kg/day in 1–2 divided doses; (over 27 kg) 900,000 units once.	No change.	0.9 (IM 300,000 units)	60	For IM use only.

(continued)

β-LACTAMS COMPARISON CHART (continued)

DRUG CLASS AND DRUG	DOSAGE FORMS	ADULT DOSAGE	PEDIATRIC DOSAGE	ADULT DOSAGE IN RENAL IMPAIRMENT[a]	PEAK SERUM LEVELS (MG/L)[b]	PERCENTAGE PROTEIN BOUND	COMMENTS
Penicillin V Potassium Pen VK Veetids Various	Tab 125, 250, 500 mg Susp 25, 50 mg/mL.	PO 250–500 mg q 6 hr.	PO 15–50 mg/kg/day in 3 or 4 divided doses.	No change.	3–8	78	Spectrum similar to penicillin G. About 60% absorbed; preferred oral form of penicillin.
ANTISTAPHYLOCOCCAL PENICILLINS							
Cloxacillin Sodium Cloxapen Tegopen Various	Cap 250, 500 mg Susp 25 mg/mL.	PO 250–500 mg q 6 hr.	PO (under 20 kg) 100 mg/kg/day in 4 divided doses; (over 20 kg) same as adult dosage.	No change.	7	94	Used primarily for *S. aureus* infections. Suspension may be better tolerated than dicloxacillin.
Dicloxacillin Sodium Dynapen Pathocill Various	Cap 125, 250, 500 mg Susp 12.5 mg/mL.	PO 125–500 mg q 6 hr.	PO 12.5–25 mg/kg/day in 4 divided doses.	No change.	12.4	98	Comparable to cloxacillin.
Methicillin Sodium Staphcillin	Inj 1, 4, 6 g.	IV 100–200 mg/kg/day in 4–6 divided doses.	IV (neonates 14 days and under) 25 mg/kg q 8–12 hr; (neonates 15–30 days) 25 mg/kg q 6 hr; (children) same as adult dosage.	Cl_{cr} <10 mL/min: decrease dosage by 50%.	60	40	Least potent of class; most likely to cause interstitial nephritis. Sodium = 2.9 mEq/g.

(continued)

DRUG CLASS AND DRUG	DOSAGE FORMS	ADULT DOSAGE	PEDIATRIC DOSAGE	ADULT DOSAGE IN RENAL IMPAIRMENT[a]	PEAK SERUM LEVELS (MG/L)[b]	PERCENTAGE PROTEIN BOUND	COMMENTS
Nafcillin **Sodium** Nafcil Unipen	Cap 250 mg Tab 500 mg Inj 500 mg, 1, 2, 10 g.	IV 50–150 mg/kg/day in 4–6 divided doses. PO 50–100 mg/kg/day in 4 divided doses, but not recommended.	IV (neonates under 7 days) 25 mg/kg q 8–12 hr; (neonates over 7 days) 25 mg/kg q 6–8 hr.	No change.	3.4 (PO) 20–40 (IV)	89	Comparable to oxacillin. Reversible neutropenia may be more common with nafcillin. Poorly absorbed orally; cloxacillin or dicloxacillin preferred. IV sodium = 2.9 mEq/g.
Oxacillin **Sodium** Bactocill Prostaphlin	Cap 250, 500 mg Susp 50 mg/mL Inj 250, 500 mg, 1, 2, 4, 10 g.	IV 50–200 mg/kg/day in 4–6 divided doses. PO 250–500 mg q 6 hr, but not recommended.	IV (neonates) same as methicillin; (children) same as adult dosage.	No change.	2.5 (PO) 40 (IV)	92	Poorly absorbed orally; cloxacillin or dicloxacillin preferred. Rare hepatic toxicity. IV sodium 2.9 mEq/g.
AMPICILLIN DERIVATIVES							
Amoxicillin Amoxil Various	Cap 250, 500 mg Chew Tab 125, 250 mg Drp 50 mg/mL Susp 25, 50 mg/mL.	PO 250–500 mg tid, to a maximum of 6 g/day. PO for endocarditis prophylaxis 3 g 1 hr before procedure, then 1.5 g 6 hr later.	PO 20–40 mg/kg/day in 3 divided doses. PO for endocarditis prophylaxis 50 mg/kg 1 hr before procedure, then 25 mg/kg 6 hr later.	No change.	9	20	Spectrum similar to ampicillin, but better bioavailability (85%) and less diarrhea.

(continued)

β-LACTAMS COMPARISON CHART (continued)

DRUG CLASS AND DRUG	DOSAGE FORMS	ADULT DOSAGE	PEDIATRIC DOSAGE	ADULT DOSAGE IN RENAL IMPAIRMENT[a]	PEAK SERUM LEVELS (MG/L)[b]	PERCENTAGE PROTEIN BOUND	COMMENTS
Ampicillin Sodium Various	Cap 250, 500 mg Chew Tab 125 mg Drp 100 mg/mL Susp 25, 50, 100 mg/mL Inj 125, 250, 500 mg, 1, 2, 10 g.	PO 250–500 mg qid. IM or IV 100–200 mg/ kg/day in 4–6 divided doses.	PO (under 20 kg) 50–100 mg/kg/day in 2–4 divided doses; PO or IV (over 20 kg) 100–400 mg/kg/day in 4–6 divided doses.	Cl$_{cr}$ <20 mL/min: same dose q 12 hr.	4 (PO) 58 (IV)	22	About 50% oral bioavailability; GI side effects and rashes are frequent. IV sodium = 3 mEq/g.
Bacampicillin Spectrobid	Tab 400 mg (278 mg ampicillin) Susp 25 mg (17.5 mg ampicillin/ mL.	PO 400–800 mg bid.	PO 25–50 mg/kg/day in 2 divided doses.	No change.	12 (PO 800 mg)	22 (ampicillin)	Inactive ester of ampicillin; essentially equivalent to amoxicillin.
EXTENDED-SPECTRUM PENICILLINS							
Mezlocillin Sodium Mezlin	Inj 1, 2, 3, 4, 20 g.	IV 200–300 mg/kg/day in 3–4 divided doses.	IV (neonates under 7 days) 75 mg/kg q 12 hr; (neonates >7 days) 75 mg/kg q 6–8 hr; (children) same as adult dosage.	Cl$_{cr}$ 10–30 mL/min: 3 g q 8 hr; Cl$_{cr}$ <10 mL/min: 2 g q 8 hr.	263 (IV 4 g)	35	Spectrum similar to ticarcillin, but better enterococcal coverage. Sodium = 1.85 mEq/g.

(continued)

DRUG CLASS AND DRUG	DOSAGE FORMS	ADULT DOSAGE	PEDIATRIC DOSAGE	ADULT DOSAGE IN RENAL IMPAIRMENT[a]	PEAK SERUM LEVELS (MG/L)[b]	PERCENTAGE PROTEIN BOUND	COMMENTS
Piperacillin Sodium Pipracil	Inj 2, 3, 4, 40 g.	IV 200–300 mg/kg/day in 4–6 divided doses.	Not well established. IV (neonates) 100 mg/kg q 12 hr; (children) 200–300 (350–500 in cystic fibrosis) mg/kg/day in 4–6 divided doses.	Cl$_{cr}$ 20–40 mL/min: 4 g q 8 hr; Cl$_{cr}$ <20 mL/min: 4 g q 12 hr.	244 (IV 4 g)	35	Best activity against *P. aeruginosa*. Sodium = 1.85 mEq/g.
Ticarcillin Disodium Ticar	Inj 1, 3, 6, 20, 30 g.	IV 200–300 mg/kg/day in 4–6 divided doses.	IV (neonates ≤7 days and <2 kg) 75 mg/kg q 12 hr; (neonates >7 days and <2 kg or ≤7 days and >2 kg) 75 mg/kg q 8 hr; (neonates >7 days and >2 kg) 100 mg/kg q 8 hr.	Cl$_{cr}$ 30–60 mL/min: 2 g q 4 hr; Cl$_{cr}$ 10–30 mL/min: 2 g q 8 hr; Cl$_{cr}$ <10 mL/min: 2 g q 12 hr.	324 (IV 3 g)	65	Less active than piperacillin against *P. aeruginosa*; no activity against *Klebsiella* spp. More antiplatelet effect than mezlocillin or piperacillin. Sodium = 5.2–6.5 mEq/g.

PENICILLIN AND β-LACTAMASE COMBINATIONS

DRUG CLASS AND DRUG	DOSAGE FORMS	ADULT DOSAGE	PEDIATRIC DOSAGE	ADULT DOSAGE IN RENAL IMPAIRMENT[a]	PEAK SERUM LEVELS (MG/L)[b]	PERCENTAGE PROTEIN BOUND	COMMENTS
Amoxicillin and	Chew Tab 125 mg amoxicil-	PO "250" or "500" tablet tid, or	PO 20–40 mg/kg/day (of amoxicillin)	No change.	9 (PO 500 mg)	20 (amoxicillin)	Active against ampicillin-resistant *S. aureus, B. fragilis,*

(continued)

B-LACTAMS COMPARISON CHART (continued)

DRUG CLASS AND DRUG	DOSAGE FORMS	ADULT DOSAGE	PEDIATRIC DOSAGE	ADULT DOSAGE IN RENAL IMPAIRMENT[a]	PEAK SERUM LEVELS (MG/L)[b]	PERCENTAGE PROTEIN BOUND	COMMENTS
Clavulanic Acid Augmentin	lin plus 31.25 mg clavulanate, 250 mg amoxicillin plus 62.5 mg clavulanate Susp 25 mg amoxicillin plus 6.25 mg clavulanate/mL, 50 mg amoxicillin plus 12.5 mg clavulanate/mL Tab 250 mg amoxicillin plus 125 mg clavulanate, 500 mg amoxicillin plus 125 mg c clavulanate, 875 mg amoxicillin plus 125 mg clavulanate.	"875" tablet bid.	in 3 divided doses.		amoxicillin) 2.6 (PO 125 mg clavulanate)	22 (clavulanate)	and B-lactamase-producing Enterobacteriacae. More diarrhea than with amoxicillin. Do not substitute two "250" tablets for one "500" tablet.
Ampicillin Sodium and Sulbactam Sodium Unasyn	Inj 1 g ampicillin plus 500 mg sulbactam/vial, 2 g ampicillin plus 1 g sulbactam/ vial.	IM or IV 1.5–3 g of the combination q 6–8 hr.	Safety and efficacy not established under 12 yr.	Cl_cr 15–30 mL/min: same dose q 12 hr; Cl_cr 5–14 mL/min: same dose q 24 hr.	58 (IV 1 g ampicillin 30 (IV 500 mg sulbactam	22 (ampicillin) 38 (sulbactam)	Spectrum similar to Augmentin. Sodium = 5 mEq/1.5 g.

(continued)

β-LACTAMS COMPARISON CHART (continued)

DRUG CLASS AND DRUG	DOSAGE FORMS	ADULT DOSAGE	PEDIATRIC DOSAGE	ADULT DOSAGE IN RENAL IMPAIRMENT[a]	PEAK SERUM LEVELS (MG/L)[b]	PERCENTAGE PROTEIN BOUND	COMMENTS
Piperacillin Sodium and Tazobactam Sodium *Zosyn*	Inj 2.25, 3.375, 4.5 g (0.5 g tazobactam per 4 g piperacillin).	IV 3.375 g q 6 hr; 4.5 g q 6 hr for *P. aeruginosa.*	Safety and efficacy not established.	Cl$_{cr}$ 20–40 mL/min: 2.25 g q 6 hr; Cl$_{cr}$ <20 mL/min: 2.25 g q 8 hr.	224 (IV 4 g piperacillin) 34 (IV 0.5 g tazobactam)	20 (piperacillin) 31 (tazobactam)	Similar spectrum to Timentin, but better activity against *P. aeruginosa* and enterococci. Sodium = 2.35 mEq/g of piperacillin.
Ticarcillin Disodium and Clavulanate Potassium *Timentin*	Inj 3.1, 31 g. (100 mg clavulanate per 3 g ticarcillin).	IV 3.1 g q 4–6 hr.	Safety and efficacy not established under 12 yr. IV (>15 mo) 2.07–3.1 g q 6 hr has been used.	Cl$_{cr}$ 30–60 mL/min: 3.1 g q 6 hr; Cl$_{cr}$ 10–30 mL/min: 3.1 g q 8 hr; Cl$_{cr}$ <10 mL/min: 3.1 g q 12 hr.[d]	324 (IV 3 g ticarcillin) 8 (IV 100 mg clavulanate)	65 (ticarcillin) 22 (clavulanate)	Improved activity over ticarcillin against *S. aureus, H. influenzae,* and anaerobes, but not *P. aeruginosa* or *E. cloacae.* Sodium = 4.7 mEq/g of ticarcillin.

[a]Usual *dose* means individual doses given at the specified interval; usual *dosage* means total daily dosage.
[b]Average peak serum concentrations following administration of a 500-mg oral dose or a 1-g IV infusion over 30 min, except as noted.
[c]Concentration dependent.
[d]With dosages recommended in marked renal impairment, clavulanate concentrations may provide ineffective synergism with ticarcillin.[171]
From references 153–155, 165–171, and product information.

Macrolides

AZITHROMYCIN   Zithromax

Pharmacology. Azithromycin is a macrolide with a 15-membered ring (making it an azalide) that is slightly less active than erythromycin against Gram-positive bacteria, but substantially more active against *Moraxella (Branhamella) catarrhalis, Hemophilus* spp., *Legionella* spp., *Neisseria* spp., *Bordetella* spp., *Mycoplasma* spp., and *Chlamydia trachomatis*. The drug also has activity against aerobic Gram-negative bacilli and *Mycobacterium avium*, and is comparable to erythromycin in activity against *Campylobacter* spp. It is the most active macrolide for *Toxoplasma gondii*, including activity against the cyst form.[172-174]

Administration and Adult Dosage. PO for mild to moderate acute bacterial exacerbations of chronic obstructive pulmonary disease, pneumonia, pharyngitis or tonsillitis, and uncomplicated skin and skin structure infections 500 mg as a single dose on the first day followed by 250 mg/day on days 2–5 for a total dosage of 1.5 g. **PO for nongonococcal urethritis and cervicitis caused by** *C. trachomatis* **or for chancroid (***Haemophilus ducreyi***)** 1 g as a single dose.[175] **PO for treatment of** *M. avium* **complex in AIDS patients** 500 mg/day in combination with ethambutol.[176] **PO for prophylaxis of** *M. avium* **complex in AIDS patients** 1.2 g once weekly alone or in combination with rifabutin 300 mg/day.[177]

Special Populations. *Pediatric Dosage.* **PO for otitis media** (6 months and over) 10 mg/kg as a single daily dose on day 1, followed by 5 mg/kg/day as a single dose on days 2–5. **PO for streptococcal pharyngitis/tonsillitis** (2 yr and over) 12 mg/kg/day as a single dose for 5 days.[178-180]

Geriatric Dosage. Same as adult dosage.

Other Conditions. Dosage reduction may be needed in severe hepatic impairment, but guidelines are not available.

Dosage Forms. Cap 250 mg; **Tab** 250, 600 mg; **Susp** 20, 40 mg/mL; **Pwdr for oral soln** 1g.

Patient Instructions. Take the capsules with a full glass of water on an empty stomach (1 hour before or 2 hours after meals) for best absorption. Tablets may be taken without regard to meals. Do not take aluminum- or magnesium-containing antacids with azithromycin.

Pharmacokinetics. *Fate.* Oral bioavailability is 37%. After a 500-mg oral capsule, a peak serum concentration of 0.41 mg/L (0.55 μmol/L) is achieved in 2 hr. Plasma protein binding ranges from 7–50%, primarily to α_1-acid glycoprotein. Azithromycin penetrates both macrophages and polymorphonuclear leukocytes, accounting for intracellular concentrations that are 40-fold extracellular concentrations. Azithromycin is widely distributed throughout the body, and tissue concentrations (including the CNS) range from 10- to 150-fold higher than those in serum. Tissue concentrations peak 48 hr after administration, and high concentrations persist for several days after drug discontinuation. Elimination is polyphasic, reflecting rapid initial distribution into tissues, followed by slow elimination. V_d is 23–31 L/kg; Cl is 38 L/hr in adults. Azithromycin is metabolized in the liver and eliminated largely through biliary excretion; only 6% is excreted unchanged in urine.[173,181,182]

$t_{1/2}$. Terminal phase 11–68+hr.[173,182]

Adverse Reactions. The drug is well tolerated. Frequent adverse effects are mild to moderate diarrhea, nausea, and abdominal pain. Headache and dizziness occur occasionally. Rash, angioedema, hepatomegaly, and cholestatic jaundice are reported rarely.[173]

Contraindications. Hypersensitivity to any macrolide.

Precautions. Use during pregnancy only if clearly needed. Use caution in patients with impaired hepatic function or severely impaired renal function.

Drug Interactions. Azithromycin does not interact with hepatic cytochrome P450 enzymes and, unlike erythromycin and clarithromycin, is not associated with these types of interactions.[183]

Parameters to Monitor. Baseline and periodic liver function tests during prolonged therapy.

Notes. Azithromycin has been used investigationally with success in preventing and treating *M. avium* complex infections in AIDS patients.[176,177]

CLARITHROMYCIN Biaxin

Clarithromycin is a semisynthetic macrolide antibiotic that is slightly more active than erythromycin against Gram-positive bacteria, *Moraxella (Branhamella) catarrhalis*, and *Legionella* spp. It is very active against *Chlamydia* spp., and is superior to other macrolides in its activity against *Mycobacterium avium-intracellulare* (MAI). Clarithromycin is acid-stable and is absorbed well with or without food. Bioavailability is 55%, with peak serum concentrations of about 2 mg/L attained after a 400-mg oral dose. Elimination half-life is about 4.5 hr. The hydroxy metabolite is active and may be synergistic in vitro with the parent drug. The metabolite has a half-life of 4–9 hr. The drug appears to have better gastrointestinal tolerance than erythromycin. Clarithromycin has a lower affinity for CYP3A4 than erythromycin and therefore has fewer clinically important drug interactions; however, its use is contraindicated with astemizole, cisapride and terfenadine. The adult oral dosage for respiratory and skin infections is 250–500 mg bid; for MAI infections, the adult dosage is 500 mg bid. Reduce dosage by 50% with $Cl_{cr} <30$ mL/min. The pediatric oral dosage for community-acquired pneumonia is 15 mg/kg q 12 hr; for other indications the dosage is 7.5 mg/kg bid, to a maximum of 500 mg bid. Clarithromycin is also used in combination with proton pump inhibitors and other drugs in a dosage of 500 mg tid for eradication of *Helicobacter pylori* infections (*see* Gastrointestinal Drugs, Treatment of *Helicobacter pylori* Infection in Peptic Ulcer Disease chart).[173,181,182,184] Available as 250- and 500-mg tablets, and 25 and 50 mg/mL suspensions.

DIRITHROMYCIN Dynabac

Dirithromycin is an oral semisynthetic macrolide antibiotic with antimicrobial activity similar to erythromycin. Dirithromycin is a prodrug that is converted by nonenzymatic hydrolysis to erythromycylamine, which is the microbiologically active moiety. Erythromycylamine binds to the 50S ribosomal subunit, inhibiting protein synthesis of susceptible microorganisms. Bacterial strains resistant to erythromycin are also resistant to dirithromycin. Absorption is slightly enhanced by food, but the absolute bioavailability averages 10%. After a 500-mg oral dose, peak serum concentrations of 0.48 mg/L are reached in 4–5 hr. Protein binding of erythromycylamine ranges from 15 to 30%, and the average V_d is 11.4 L/kg. Erythromycylamine is primarily eliminated in the bile and undergoes little hepatic metabolism. Its elimination half-life averages 42 hr. Frequent adverse reactions are GI, with nausea and abdominal pain most common. Other frequent adverse reactions are headache, diarrhea, and dyspepsia. Neither dirithromycin or erythromycylamine binds to cytochrome P450 isoforms, and clinically important drug interactions have not been reported.[185,186] Dosage for patients over 12 yr is PO 500 mg once daily with food or within 1 hr of having eaten. Do not cut, crush, or chew tablets. Available as 250-mg tablets.

ERYTHROMYCIN AND SALTS   Various

Pharmacology. Erythromycin is a bacteriostatic macrolide antibiotic with a spectrum similar to penicillin G; it is also active against *Mycoplasma pneumoniae* and *Legionella pneumophila*.[187–189] It acts by binding to the 50S ribosomal subunit, inhibiting protein synthesis. Gram-positive organisms develop resistance via R-factor mediated alteration of the binding site. Gram-negative organisms are resistant because of cell wall impermeability.

Administration and Adult Dosage. *See* Erythromycins Comparison Chart. **For gastroparesis** 200 mg IV of the lactobionate salt, 250 mg PO of the ethylsuccinate salt or 500 mg PO of the base 15–120 min before meals and at bedtime appear to be effective.[190]

Special Populations. *Pediatric Dosage.* (*See* Erythromycins Comparison Chart.)

Geriatric Dosage. Same as adult dosage.

Other Conditions. Dosage adjustment is probably unnecessary in renal impairment.[180,187]

Dosage Forms. (*See* Erythromycins Comparison Chart.)

Patient Instructions. Take this drug with a full glass of water on an empty stomach (1 hour before or 2 hours after meals) for best absorption. Refrigerate the suspension.

Pharmacokinetics. *Fate.* Oral absorption varies widely with the salt and dosage form (*see* Erythromycins Comparison Chart), with peak serum concentrations occurring from 30 min (suspension) to 4 hr (coated tablet) after administration. However, enteric-coated erythromycin base tablets, stearate tablets, and estolate capsules produce equivalent erythromycin serum levels when administered to fasting subjects. Food or restricted water intake (ie, 20 mL or less) with a dose dramatically lowers the absorption of the stearate form. The drug is 83 ± 5% plasma protein bound and widely distributed into most tissues, cavities, and body fluids except the brain and CSF (even with meningeal inflammation). V_d is 0.6 ± 0.1 L/kg; Cl is 0.55 ± 0.25 L/hr/kg. Erythromycin is partially metabolized in the liver by CYP3A3/4, and is excreted primarily as unchanged erythromycin with high concentrations in the bile and feces. Only 12–15% of an IV dose is excreted unchanged in urine.[46,187]

$t_{1/2}$. 1.6 ± 0.7 hr; unchanged or slightly prolonged in anuric patients, based on minimal data; prolonged in cirrhosis.[46]

Adverse Reactions. Frequent GI distress. IM form is very painful, despite local anesthetic (butamben) in the product, and may produce sterile abscesses. IV administration frequently produces pain, venous irritation, and phlebitis. Mild elevations of serum hepatic enzymes occur frequently. Transient deafness occurs occasionally with high dosages.[187,191] Rare, but potentially serious, reversible intrahepatic cholestatic jaundice occurs primarily with the estolate and ethylsuccinate forms, usually in adults after 10–14 days of therapy, although it may occur after the first dose if there is a history of previous use. Prodrome includes malaise, nausea, vomiting, fever, and abdominal pain (which may be severe and misdiagnosed as acute surgical abdomen). Symptoms resolve in 1–2 weeks, and serum enzymes return to normal over several months.

Contraindications. Concurrent use with astemizole, cisapride, or terfenadine; IM form in patients with hypersensitivity to local anesthetics of the para-aminobenzoic acid type (eg, procaine); hepatic dysfunction (estolate and ethylsuccinate forms).

Precautions. Pregnancy. Use with caution in patients with liver disease because of possibly impaired excretion.

Drug Interactions. Erythromycin inhibits CYP3A4 and can reduce hepatic metabolism of some drugs, including astemizole, carbamazepine, cisapride, cyclosporine, terfenadine, theophylline, triazolam, warfarin and others.[192] *See* Contraindications.

Parameters to Monitor. Liver function tests in patients who experience prodromal symptoms (*see* Adverse Reactions) while receiving the estolate or ethylsuccinate form; check daily for vein irritation and phlebitis in patients receiving IV forms. Closely monitor the effects of other drugs which interact with erythromycin during concurrent use.

Notes. Avoid injectable forms if at all possible. Erythromycin is more active in an alkaline environment. Unrelated to its antibacterial effect, erythromycin in low doses binds to motilin receptors in the GI tract to stimulate gastric emptying. It is the most prokinetic macrolide and has been used in gastroparesis and in other GI motility disorders.[190,193–196]

ERYTHROMYCINS COMPARISON CHART

DRUG	DOSAGE FORMS	ADULT DOSAGE	PEDIATRIC DOSAGE*	COMMENTS†
Erythromycin *Base* E-Mycin Ery-Tab ERYC Various	EC Tab 250, 333, 500 mg EC Cap Pellets 250 mg.	PO 1 g/day in 2–4 doses, to a maximum of 4 g/day.	PO 30–50 mg/kg/day in 4 doses; may double in severe infection.	Food interferes with absorption of uncoated products; EC products appear to be among the best tolerated erythromycin formulations.
Erythromycin *Estolate* Ilosone Various	Cap 250 mg Susp 25, 50 mg/mL (reconstituted) Tab 500 mg.	PO 250–500 mg q 6 hr, to a maximum of 4 g/day.	PO 30–50 mg/kg/day in 4 doses.	PO well absorbed; unaffected by food and highly resistant to gastric acid hydrolysis; absorbed as propionate ester which predominates in serum (8:1) and may be less active; rare intrahepatic cholestatic jaundice.
Erythromycin *Ethylsuccinate* E.E.S. EryPed Various	Drp 40 mg/mL Susp 40, 80 mg/mL Chew Tab 200 mg Tab (coated) 400 mg.	PO 400 mg q 6 hr, to a maximum of 4 g/day; PO for prevention of endocarditis in patients at risk undergoing dental, oral or upper respiratory tract procedures; and who are allergic to amoxicillin or penicillin 800 mg	PO 30–50 mg/kg/day in 4 doses; may double in severe infection; PO for prevention of endocarditis in children at risk undergoing dental, oral or upper respiratory tract procedures and who are allergic to amoxicillin or peni-	Absorbed better than base; intermediate susceptibility to gastric acid hydrolysis. Absorbed as ester, which predominates in serum (3:1) and may be less active. Rare intrahepatic cholestatic jaundice.

(continued)

ERYTHROMYCINS COMPARISON CHART (continued)

DRUG	DOSAGE FORMS	ADULT DOSAGE	PEDIATRIC DOSAGE*	COMMENTS†
Erythromycin Gluceptate Ilotycin	Inj (IV only) 1 g.	2 hr before procedure, then 400 mg 6 hr later. IV 15–20 mg/kg/day in 4 doses, to a maximum of 4 g/day.	cillin 20 mg/kg 2 hr before procedure, then 10 mg/kg 6 hr later. IV same as adult dosage in 2–4 doses; may double in severe infection.	Painful; phlebitis frequent; avoid use if possible. Infuse over 20–60 minutes.
Erythromycin Lactobionate Erythrocin Various	Inj (IV only) 500 mg, 1 g.	Same as erythromycin gluceptate.	Same as erythromycin gluceptate.	Same as erythromycin gluceptate.
Erythromycin Stearate Erythrocin Various	Tab (film coated) 250, 500 mg.	PO 1 g/day in 2 or 4 doses, to a maximum of 4 g/day. PO for prevention of endocarditis in patients at risk undergoing dental, oral, or upper respiratory tract procedures, and who are allergic to amoxicillin or penicillin 1 g 2 hr before procedure, 500 mg 6 hr later.	PO 30–50 mg/kg/day in 4 doses; may double in severe infections. endocarditis in children at risk undergoing dental, oral, or respiratory tract procedures, and who are allergic to amoxicillin or penicillin same as erythromycin ethylsuccinate.	Absorption about equal to ethylsuccinate, although food interferes markedly with absorption. Hydrolyzed to free base before absorption.

*In newborns, data are available for erythromycin estolate only, suggesting an oral dosage of 40 mg/kg/day in 2–4 divided doses.
†Despite differences in oral absorption, no clinical studies have shown any salt to be clearly superior in any particular therapeutic use.
From references 197–200 and product information.

Quinolones

CIPROFLOXACIN
Cipro

Pharmacology. Ciprofloxacin is a fluoroquinolone that inhibits bacterial DNA-gyrase, an enzyme responsible for the unwinding of DNA for transcription and subsequent supercoiling of DNA for packaging into chromosomal subunits. It is highly active against Enterobacteriaceae, with MICs often less than 0.1 mg/L. It is also active against some strains of *Pseudomonas aeruginosa* and *Staphylococcus* spp., with an MIC$_{90}$ of 0.5–1 mg/L. However, recent reports indicate increasing resistance to this agent in methicillin-resistant *S. aureus*. It has poor activity against streptococci and anaerobes.[201,202]

Administration and Adult Dosage. PO for female acute uncomplicated cystitis 100 mg q 12 hr. **PO for uncomplicated urinary tract infections** 250 mg q 12 hr. **PO for moderate to severe systemic infections** 500–750 mg q 12 hr. **PO for gonorrhea** 500 mg once. **PO for chancroid** 500 mg q 12 hr for 3 days.[175] **IV** 400 mg q 12 hr.

Special Populations. *Pediatric Dosage.* Safety and efficacy not established under 16 yr. Use has been limited because of the potential for arthropathy. Ciprofloxacin has been used in children 6–16 yr old in limited situations to treat serious infections. **IV for *P. aeruginosa* infections in cystic fibrosis** 30 mg/kg/day in 3 divided doses. **PO for *P. aeruginosa* infections in cystic fibrosis** 40 mg/kg/day in two divided doses.[203]

Geriatric Dosage. Reduce dosage for age-related reduction in renal function, although dosage reduction is not necessary with only minor age-related renal function changes.[204]

Other Conditions. Reduce dosage by 50% or double the dosage interval when Cl$_{cr}$ is <30 mL/min; special dosage adjustments in patients with cystic fibrosis are not necessary.[205]

Dosage Forms. *See* Fluoroquinolones Comparison Chart.

Patient Instructions. This drug may be taken with food to minimize stomach upset. Avoid antacid use during treatment; calcium, iron, or zinc supplements may also reduce absorption. Avoid excessive exposure to sunlight during ciprofloxacin treatment. Report any tendon pain or inflammation that occurs during therapy.

Pharmacokinetics. *Serum Levels.* A peak serum level of 4–6 mg/L (12–18 µmol/L) 2 hr after an oral 750- to 1000-mg dose is proposed as evidence of absorption adequate for tuberculosis therapy.[51]

Fate. Approximately 70% absorbed orally; food decreases the rate but not the extent of absorption. Aluminum-, calcium-, or magnesium-containing antacids or sucralfate markedly decrease the extent of absorption. Peak serum concentrations are 3 ± 0.6 mg/L (9 ± 1.8 µmol/L) following a 750-mg oral dose; a 200-mg IV dose infused over 30 min results in a peak concentration of about 3.2 ± 0.6 mg/L. V$_d$ averages 2 L/kg. Renal clearance averages 0.26 L/hr/kg. Less than 30% is plasma protein bound. Ciprofloxacin attains very high concentrations in many body fluids and tissues, most notably urine, prostate, and pulmonary mucosa. CSF concentrations are less than 1 mg/L; experience with the drug in the treatment of meningitis is very limited. From 45–60% of a parenteral dose is recovered unchanged in urine; the remainder is excreted as four metabolites or eliminated in feces.[182,204,205-208]

$t_{1/2}$. 4.2 ± 0.63 hr;[207] 6.9 ± 2.9 hr in severe renal impairment.[208]

Adverse Reactions. GI intolerance (nausea, vomiting, diarrhea, abdominal discomfort) occurs frequently. CNS effects such as headaches and restlessness have occurred in 1–2% of patients. Other CNS effects (eg, dizziness, insomnia, anxiety, irritability, and seizures) have been reported in less than 1% of patients. Skin rashes and photosensitivity occur occasionally. Anaphylaxis occurs rarely.[182]

Contraindications. Hypersensitivity to any quinolone.

Precautions. Pregnancy; lactation.

Drug Interactions. Aluminum-, calcium-, or magnesium-containing antacids markedly reduce oral absorption. Although there is some information that spacing administration by 2 hr or more may minimize these interactions, it is probably best not to use ciprofloxacin in patients taking long-term antacid therapy. Iron supplements and zinc-containing multivitamins may reduce absorption. Theophylline clearance may be reduced in some patients receiving ciprofloxacin. Patients receiving fluoroquinolones and methylxanthines such as theophylline or caffeine may be at increased risk of CNS toxicity (eg, convulsions). Warfarin metabolism may be impaired by ciprofloxacin, although studies with the fluoroquinolone enoxacin indicate that only the metabolism of the less active (R)-warfarin is affected. Use caution when adding ciprofloxacin in a patient taking warfarin. The solubility of ciprofloxacin is reduced at higher pH values; thus, avoid alkalinization of the urine.[206]

Parameters to Monitor. Monitor serum theophylline levels closely in patients receiving theophylline. Monitor prothrombin time and signs of bleeding in patients on warfarin.

OFLOXACIN	Floxin
LEVOFLOXACIN	Levaquin

Ofloxacin is a systemic fluoroquinolone similar to ciprofloxacin, except that ofloxacin has greater bioavailability (over 95%). A peak serum level of 8–12 mg/L (22–33 μmol/L) 2 hr after an oral dose of 600–800 mg is proposed as evidence of absorption adequate for tuberculosis therapy. Ofloxacin is predominantly renally excreted, has a longer elimination half-life, and does not alter hepatic metabolism of methylxanthine compounds (eg, caffeine, theophylline). However, like other fluoroquinolones, cations markedly reduce the absorption of this agent. Use of levofloxacin allows higher dosages of the active form to be given with fewer side effects. Ofloxacin has greater activity against *Chlamydia trachomatis*, *Ureaplasma urealiticum*, *Mycoplasma pneumoniae*, and *Mycobacterium tuberculosis* than ciprofloxacin, but less activity against *Pseudomonas aeruginosa*. The usual IV or PO dosage of ofloxacin for systemic infections is 400 mg bid; urinary tract infections can be treated with a dosage of 200 mg bid. For nongonococcal urethritis, the dosage is 300 mg q 12 hr for 7 days. For levofloxacin, the dosage is 250–500 mg once daily. Reduce dosage of both drugs in patients with renal impairment.[51,182,201,202,209] (*See* Fluoroquinolones Comparison Chart.)

FLUOROQUINOLONES COMPARISON CHART

DRUG	DOSAGE FORMS	ADULT DOSAGE	DOSAGE IN RENAL IMPAIRMENT	PEAK ORAL BIOAVAILABILITY (PERCENT)	SERUM LEVELS (MG/L)*	COMMENTS†
Ciprofloxacin Cipro Cloxan	Tab 100, 250, 500, 750 mg Inj 200, 400 mg Ophth Drp 0.3% (Ciloxan) 2.5, 5 mL.	PO 250–750 mg q 12 hr; PO for gonorrhea 500 mg once; IV 200–400 mg q 12 hr; Ophth 2 drops q 15 min–4 hr.	Cl_{cr} 30–50 mL/min: PO 250–500 mg q 12 hr; IV usual dosage. Cl_{cr} 5–30 mL/min PO 250–500 mg q 18 hr; IV 200–400 mg q 18–24 hr; Dialysis: PO 250–500 mg q 24 hr after dialysis.	60–80	3 ± 0.6 (PO 750 mg) 3.2 ± 0.6 (IV 200 mg)	Most active against *P. aeruginosa*.
Enoxacin Penetrex	Tab 200, 400 mg.	PO 200–400 mg q 12 hr.	Cl_{cr} 5–15 mL/min: usual dose q 24 hr.	83–90	5.5 (PO 400 mg) 8.2 (IV 400 mg)	Most potent inhibitor of theophylline metabolism.
Fleroxacin Megalone (Investigational, Roche)	—	PO or IV 200–400 mg/day in one dose.	Cl_{cr} 15–30 mL/min: 50% of usual dose q 24 hr; Cl_{cr} 5–15 mL/min: 25% of usual dose q 24 hr.	>90	5.6 (PO 400 mg)	Under investigation for single daily dose administration.

(continued)

FLUOROQUINOLONES COMPARISON CHART (continued)

DRUG	DOSAGE FORMS	ADULT DOSAGE	DOSAGE IN RENAL IMPAIRMENT	PEAK ORAL BIOAVAILABILITY (PERCENTAGE)	SERUM LEVELS (MG/L)*	COMMENTS†
Levofloxacin Levaquin	Tab 250, 500 mg Inj 250, 500 mg.	PO, IV 200–500 mg once daily.	Cl$_{cr}$ 20–50 mL/min: 250 mg q 24 hr; Cl$_{cr}$ 10–19 mL/min: 250 mg q 48 hr; Cl$_{cr}$ <20 mL/min: 250 mg q 48 hr.	95–100	1.3 (PO 100 mg)	Active S-(−) isomer of ofloxacin.
Lomefloxacin Maxaquin	Tab 400 mg.	PO 400 mg once daily.	Cl$_{cr}$ <40 mL/min: PO 400 mg once, then 200 mg/day.	95–98	25 (PO 400 mg)	No effect on theophylline metabolism. Long half-life of 8 hr. Relatively weak antibacterial. Phototoxic.
Norfloxacin Noroxin Chibroxin	Tab 400 mg Ophth Drp 0.3% (Chibroxin) 5 mL.	PO 200–400 mg q 12 hr; PO for gonorrhea 800 mg once; Ophth 1 or 2 drops q 2 hr–qid.	Cl$_{cr}$ <30 mL/min: PO 400 mg/day.	35–45 (estimated)	1.4–1.6 (PO 400 mg)	Used in urinary and GI tract infections only because of poor oral bioavailability.
Ofloxacin Floxin Ocuflox	Tab 200, 300, 400 mg Inj 200,	PO or IV 200–400 mg q 12 hr;	Cl$_{cr}$ 10–50 mL/min: usual dose q 24 hr; Cl$_{cr}$ 0 <10 mL/min:	95–100	3.5–5.3 (PO 400 mg)	Most active against *Chlamydia* spp.; little effect on

(continued)

FLUOROQUINOLONES COMPARISON CHART (continued)

DRUG	DOSAGE FORMS	ADULT DOSAGE	DOSAGE IN RENAL IMPAIRMENT	PEAK ORAL BIOAVAILABILITY (PERCENT)	SERUM LEVELS (MG/L)*	COMMENTS†
	400 mg	PO for gonorrhea 400 mg	50% of usual dose q 24 hr			theophylline metabolism.
	Ophth Drp 0.3% (Ocuflox).	400 mg once. Ophth 1 or 2 drops q 2–4 hr for 2 days, then qid up to 5 days.				

*Peak serum concentrations following administration of the dose shown in parentheses.
†All fluoroquinolones are associated with tendon rupture. Discontinue therapy at the first sign of tendon pain or inflammation, and patients should refrain from exercise until the diagnosis of tendinitis can be confidently excluded.[201]
From references 182, 201–211 and product information.

Sulfonamides

TRIMETHOPRIM AND SULFAMETHOXAZOLE

Bactrim,
Septra, Various

Pharmacology. Sulfamethoxazole (SMZ) is a synthetic analogue of para-aminobenzoic acid (PABA) which competitively inhibits the synthesis of dihydropteric acid (an inactive folic acid precursor) from PABA in microorganisms. Trimethoprim (TMP) acts at a later step to inhibit the enzymatic reduction of dihydrofolic acid to tetrahydrofolic acid. The most important determinant of efficacy is usually the level of susceptibility to TMP; resistance to the combination is uncommon, but appears to be increasing worldwide. The combination is active against many bacteria except anaerobes, *Pseudomonas aeruginosa,* and many *Streptococcus faecalis* spp. It is also highly active and effective against the protozoan *Pneumocystis carinii.* TMP/SMZ demonstrates in vitro activity against methicillin-resistant *Staphylococcus aureus* (MRSA), but clinical success has been variable and unpredictable.[212-215]

Administration and Adult Dosage. **PO for UTI** 160 mg of TMP and 800 mg of SMZ q 12 hr for 10–14 days. **PO for prophylaxis of recurrent UTI** 40 mg TMP and 200 of SMZ at bedtime 3 times a week. **PO for shigellosis** 160 mg of TMP and 800 of SMZ q 12 hr for 5 days. **IV for severe Gram-negative infections or shigellosis** 8–10 mg/kg/day of TMP and 40–50 mg/kg/day of SMZ, in 2–4 equally divided doses, q 6–12 hr for 5 days for shigellosis and up to 14 days for severe UTI. **PO or IV for *P. carinii* pneumonia (PCP)** 12.5–20 mg/kg/day of TMP and 62.5–100 mg/kg/day of SMZ, in 2–4 equally divided doses, for up to 21 days. **PO for PCP infection prophylaxis** 160 mg of TMP and 800 mg of SMZ once daily; intermittent dosage (eg, 3 times a week) is also used. In patients with HIV infection, the drug is indicated if there was a previous episode of PCP or CD4 counts are <200/μL.[213] (*See* Notes.)

Special Populations. *Pediatric Dosage.* **PO for UTI or shigellosis** (2 months–12 yr) 8 mg/kg/day of TMP and 40 mg/kg/day of SMZ (Susp 1 mL/kg/day) in 2 equally divided doses; (over 12 yr) same as adult mg/kg dosage. **PO for otitis media** same as UTI. **IV for severe Gram-negative infection or shigellosis** (2 months and over) same as adult mg/kg dosage. **PO or IV for *P. carinii* pneumonia (PCP)** same as adult mg/kg dosage. **PO for *P. carinii* infection prophylaxis** 150 mg/m^2/day of TMP and 750 mg/m^2/day of SMZ, in divided doses, given 3 days a week.[216]

Geriatric Dosage. Reduce dosage for age-related reduction in renal function, although dosage reduction is not necessary with only minor age-related renal function changes. (*See* Precautions.)

Other Conditions. For a Cl_{cr} <30 mL/min, give normal dosage for 1–6 doses; then, with a Cl_{cr} of 15–30 mL/min, follow with 50% of the usual dosage; with a Cl_{cr} <15 mL/min, follow with 25–50% of the usual dosage in 1 or 2 divided doses. Give patients on hemodialysis a normal dose after each dialysis procedure. For systemic infections treated with higher dosages, monitor serum levels.

Dosage Forms. Susp 8 mg/mL of TMP and 40 mg/mL of SMZ; **Tab** 80 mg of TMP and 400 mg of SMZ (single strength), 160 mg of TMP and 800 mg of SMZ (double strength); **Inj** 16 mg/mL of TMP and 80 mg/mL of SMZ.

Patient Instructions. Take this medication with a full 8 fl. oz. glass of water on an empty stomach (1 hour before or 2 hours after meals) for best absorption. Drink several additional glasses of water daily, unless directed otherwise.

Pharmacokinetics. *Serum Levels.* Trimethoprim levels >5 mg/L (>17 μmol/L) and SMZ peak levels of about 100 mg/L (396 μmol/L) may be required in *P. carinii* pneumonia.[213,217]

Fate. TMP and SMZ are 90–100% absorbed orally. In normal adults, peak serum concentrations of 0.9–1.9 mg/L (3.1–6.5 μmol/L) of TMP and 20–50 mg/L (79–198 μmol/L) of SMZ occur about 1–4 hr after 160 mg of TMP and 800 mg of SMZ. An additional 10–20 mg/L of SMZ exists in the serum as inactive metabolites. IV infusion of 160 mg of TMP and 800 mg of SMZ over 1 hr produces peak serum levels of 3.4 mg/L (11.7 μmol/L) of TMP and 46.3 mg/L (183 μmol/L) of SMZ. TMP and SMZ are widely distributed in the body, although TMP is much more widely distributed because of its greater lipophilicity. TMP is 45% plasma protein bound and has a V_d of 1–2 L/kg; SMZ is 60% plasma protein bound and has a V_d of 0.36 L/kg. TMP concentrations in various tissues and fluids (including the prostate, bile, and sputum) are several times greater than concomitant serum concentrations; CSF concentrations in normal adults are approximately 50% of serum concentrations. Nearly all TMP is excreted in the urine within 24–72 hr, 50–75% as unchanged drug. SMZ undergoes extensive liver metabolism, producing N^4-acetylated and N^4-glucuronidated derivatives; 85% is excreted in the urine within 24–72 hr, 10–30% as unchanged drug. The pharmacokinetics of these drugs are essentially unchanged when given in combination. The pH of the urine influences renal excretion of both drugs, but does not markedly alter overall elimination.[213,218]

$t_{1/2}$. 11 ± 2.3 hr for TMP and 8 ± 0.4 hr for SMZ in normal adults.[218] 20–30 hr or more for TMP in severe renal failure; 18–24 hr for SMZ in anuria.[215]

Adverse Reactions. Gastrointestinal irritation including nausea, vomiting, and anorexia occurs frequently, and both the frequency and severity appear to be dose related. Rashes and other hypersensitivity reactions similar to those caused by other sulfonamides occur occasionally. In patients with AIDS, allergic skin reactions, rash (usually diffuse, erythematous or maculopapular, and pruritic) are frequent and may be associated with fever, leukopenia, neutropenia, thrombocytopenia, and increased transaminase levels.[219] Desensitization has been successful, though (*see* Notes). In patients without underlying myelosuppression and treated with conventional dosages, the frequency of megaloblastic anemia and other hematologic disorders is rare, but may be higher in folate-deficient patients. Hepatotoxicity and nephrotoxicity are rare; renal dysfunction may occur in patients with preexisting renal disease, but it is reversible.[215,218] Allergic skin reactions, including toxic epidermal necrolysis, exfoliative dermatitis, Stevens-Johnson syndrome, erythema multiforme, and fixed drug eruptions occur rarely. Other rare adverse effects include cholestatic jaundice, pancreatitis, pseudomembranous colitis, hyperkalemia, myalgia, headache, insomnia, fatigue, ataxia, vertigo, depression, and anaphylaxis.[215]

Contraindications. Pregnancy; infants under 2 months; history of hypersensitivity reaction to sulfonamide derivatives or trimethoprim; megaloblastic anemia caused by folate deficiency. Lactation is stated by manufacturer to be a contraindication, but risk is probably limited to nursing infants under 2 months of age.

Precautions. G-6-PD deficiency; impaired renal or hepatic function. Adverse reactions may be more frequent in the elderly, especially with impaired hepatic or renal function or in those taking thiazide diuretics.

Drug Interactions. The effects of methotrexate, sulfonylureas, and warfarin are increased when used with trimethoprim-sulfamethoxazole. Enhanced bone marrow suppression may occur with the combination of trimethoprim/sulfamethoxazole and mercaptopurine. A decreased effect of cyclosporine and an increased risk of nephrotoxicity may occur. High-dose trimethoprim-sulfamethoxazole with didanosine may increase the risk of pancreatitis. Phenytoin clearance may be decreased with concurrent use.

Parameters to Monitor. Baseline and periodic CBC for patients on long-term or high-dose treatment. Monitor SMZ serum levels in patients treated for PCP if absorption is questionable or response is poor.[213] In patients with AIDS, monitor for hypersensitivity skin reactions (rash and urticaria).

Notes. Protect all dosage forms from light. The efficacy and safety of TMP and SMZ have been demonstrated in numerous infectious conditions (eg, chronic UTI, chronic bronchitis, sepsis, enteric fever, prostatitis, endocarditis, meningitis, and gonorrhea), and the combination is considered an effective alternative to conventional therapy in most cases.[213,218] Efficacy of TMP and SMZ in the treatment of *Pneumocystis carinii* pneumonitis is equivalent to **pentamidine,** which makes the combination the therapy of choice because of its greater safety and lower cost.[217] Oral desensitization or rechallenge with TMP/SMZ has been successful in permitting continued use in patients with AIDS who experience hypersensitivity reactions.[220] Sulfamethoxazole is also available as a single agent (Gantanol **Susp** 100 mg/mL; **Tab** 500 mg).

Tetracyclines

DOXYCYCLINE AND SALTS   Vibramycin

Pharmacology. Tetracyclines are broad-spectrum bacteriostatic compounds that inhibit protein synthesis at the 30S ribosomal subunit. Activity includes Gram-positive, Gram-negative, aerobic, and anaerobic bacteria, as well as spirochetes, mycoplasmas, rickettsiae, chlamydiae, and some protozoa. Many bacteria have developed plasmid-mediated resistance. Most Enterobacteriacae and *Pseudomonas aeruginosa* are resistant. Doxycycline is somewhat more active than other tetracyclines against anaerobes and facultative Gram-negative bacilli.[221,222]

Administration and Adult Dosage. PO 100 mg q 12 hr for 2 doses, then 50–100 mg/day in 1 or 2 doses, depending on the severity of the infection, to a maximum of 200 mg/day. **PO for uncomplicated chlamydial genital infections** 100 mg bid for at least 7 days. **PO for primary and secondary syphilis** 100 mg tid for at least 10 days. **PO for prophylaxis against travelers' diarrhea** 200 mg en route, then 100 mg/day for duration of travel (6 weeks maximum). **PO for malaria prophylaxis in short-term (<4 months) travelers** 100 mg/day beginning 1–2 days before travel to malarious areas, and for 4 weeks after leaving the area. **IV** 200 mg in 1 or 2 divided doses for 1 day, followed by 100–200 mg/day, infused at a concentration of 0.1–1 g/L over 1–4 hr; double maintenance dosage in severe infections. **Intrapleural for pleural effusions** 500 mg in 25–30 mL of NS has been used; most patients require 2–4 infusions for maximum efficacy.[223] **Not for SC or IM use.**

Special Populations. *Pediatric Dosage.* **Not recommended under 8 yr. PO** (>8 yr, <45 kg) 2.2 mg/kg q 12 hr for 2 doses, then 2.2–4.4 mg/kg/day in 1 or 2 divided doses, depending on the severity of the infection; (>45 kg) same as adult dosage. **PO for malaria prophylaxis in short-term (<4 months) travelers** (>8 yr) 2.2 mg/kg/day to a maximum of 100 mg/day beginning 1–2 days before travel to malarious areas, and for 4 weeks after leaving the area. **IV** (<45 kg) 4.4 mg/kg in 1 or 2 divided doses for 1 day followed by 2.2–4.4 mg/kg/day in 1 or 2 divided doses, infused at a concentration of 0.1–1 g/L over 1–4 hr; (>45 kg) same as adult dosage.

Geriatric Dosage. Same as adult dosage.

Other Conditions. No dosage adjustment is necessary in renal impairment.

Dosage Forms. **Cap** (as hyclate) 50, 100 mg; **Tab** (as hyclate) 50, 100 mg; **Susp** (as monohydrate) 5 mg/mL (reconstituted); **Syrup** (as calcium) 10 mg/mL; **Inj** (as hyclate) 100, 200 mg.

Patient Instructions. Take doxycycline by mouth with a full glass of water on an empty stomach, but if stomach upset occurs, the drug may be taken with food or milk, but not antacids or iron products. Avoid prolonged exposure to direct sunlight while taking this drug.

Pharmacokinetics. *Onset and Duration.* Duration of protection against travelers' diarrhea is about 1 week after drug discontinuation.[224]

Fate. About 93% is orally absorbed, producing a peak of 3 mg/L (6.5 μmol/L) 2–4 hr after administration of a 200-mg dose; antacids and iron may markedly impair oral absorption; milk causes about a 30% decrease in bioavailability and food has little effect. Widely distributed in the body, penetrating most cavities including CSF (12–20% of serum levels). The drug is $88 \pm 5\%$ plasma protein bound. V_d is 0.75 ± 0.32 L/kg; Cl is 0.032 ± 0.01 L/hr/kg. About $41 \pm 19\%$ is excreted unchanged in the urine in normal adults; the remainder is eliminated in feces via intestinal and biliary secretion.[46,224,225]

$t_{1/2}$. 16 ± 6 hr in normal adults; slightly prolonged in severe renal impairment.[46,224]

Adverse Reactions. IV administration frequently produces phlebitis. Oral doxycycline causes less alteration of intestinal flora than other tetracyclines, but it may cause nausea and diarrhea with equal frequency. It binds to calcium in teeth and bones, which may cause discoloration of teeth in children, especially during growth; however, doxycycline has a lower potential for this effect than most other tetracyclines. In contrast to other tetracyclines, doxycycline is not very antianabolic and will not further increase azotemia in renal failure. Phototoxic skin reactions occur occasionally.[221,222,224]

Contraindications. Hypersensitivity to any tetracycline.

Precautions. Not recommended in pregnancy or in children ≤8 yr because permanent staining of the child's teeth will occur. Use with caution in severe hepatic dysfunction. The syrup contains sulfites.

Drug Interactions. Antacids containing di- or trivalent cations, bismuth salts, or zinc salts interfere with absorption of oral tetracyclines. Oral iron salts lower doxycycline serum levels, even of IV doxycycline, by interfering with absorption and enterohepatic circulation. Barbiturates, carbamazepine, and phenytoin may enhance doxycycline hepatic metabolism, possibly decreasing its effect. Tetracyclines may interfere with enterohepatic circulation of contraceptive hormones, causing menstrual irregularities and possibly unplanned pregnancies. Combined use of tetracyclines with the bactericidal agents such as penicillins may result in decreased activity in some infections.

Parameters to Monitor. Check for signs of phlebitis daily during IV use.

Notes. Doxycycline is the tetracycline of choice because it is better tolerated than other tetracyclines, although tetracyclines are the drugs of choice for very few infections.[221,222] Each vial contains 480 mg of ascorbic acid per 100 mg of doxycycline hyclate for injection. (*See* Tetracyclines Comparison Chart.)

TETRACYCLINE AND SALTS   Various

Tetracycline has an antimicrobial spectrum of activity similar to doxycycline. Current uses are for treatment of infection caused by *Chlamydia* spp., *Mycoplasma* spp., and *Brucella* spp. It is also used as a treatment for acne and in some regimens against *Helicobacter pylori* (*see* Gastrointestinal Drugs, Treatment of *Helicobacter pylori* Infection in Peptic Ulcer Disease). It is well absorbed from the GI tract. Multivalent cations chelate tetracyclines and inhibit absorption; warn patients to avoid concurrent antacids, dairy products, iron, or sucralfate. The half-life of tetracycline is about 10 hr, increasing to as high as 108 hr in anuria. GI irritation is frequent and may result in esophageal ulceration if the drug is taken at bedtime with insufficient fluid. Disruption of bowel flora occurs frequently and may result in diarrhea, candidiasis, or rarely pseudomembranous colitis. Antianabolic effects produce elevated BUN, hyperphosphatemia, and acidosis in patients with renal failure. Acute fatty infiltration of the liver with pancreatitis occurs rarely with large (over 2 g) IV doses, especially in pregnancy; avoid tetracyclines in pregnancy. Tetracyclines are not recommended for children ≤8 yr because of binding of calcium in teeth and resultant discoloration. Adult dosage is 1–2 g/day in 2–4 divided doses. In children >8 yr, dosage is 25–50 mg/kg/day in 2–4 divided doses. Reduce dosage, or preferably use another drug, in severe renal or hepatic impairment.[46,221,222] (*See* Tetracyclines Comparison Chart.)

TETRACYCLINES COMPARISON CHART

DRUG	DOSAGE FORMS	ADULT DOSAGE	PERCENTAGE ORAL ABSORPTION	HALF-LIFE (HOURS) Normal	HALF-LIFE (HOURS) Anuria	PERCENTAGE EXCRETED UNCHANGED IN URINE	COMMENTS
Demeclocycline **Hydrochloride** Declomycin	Cap 150 mg Tab 150, 300 mg.	PO 600 mg/day in 2–4 divided doses. PO for SIADH 300 mg tid–qid.	66	15	40–60	42	Most phototoxic tetracycline; causes nephrogenic diabetes insipidus rarely.
Doxycycline Calcium **Doxycycline Hyclate** **Doxycycline Monohydrate** Vibramycin Various	Cap 50, 100 mg Tab 50, 100 mg Susp 5 mg/mL Syrup 10 mg/mL Inj 100, 200 mg.	PO 100 mg q 12 hr for 2 doses, then 50–100 mg/day in 1–2 divided doses; IV 200 mg in 1–2 divided doses on day 1, then 100–200 mg/day.	93	16 ± 6	12–22	41	Safest in renal failure because of its lack of accumulation and lack of antianabolic effects. Well tolerated when given IV.
Minocycline **Hydrochloride** Minocin Various	Cap 50, 100 mg Tab 50, 100 mg Susp 10 mg/mL Inj (IV only) 100 mg.	PO or IV 200 mg initially, then 100 mg q 12 hr.	95–100	16 ± 2	11–23	11	Very frequent transient vestibular toxicity.

(continued)

TETRACYCLINES COMPARISON CHART (continued)

DRUG	DOSAGE FORMS	ADULT DOSAGE	PERCENTAGE ORAL ABSORPTION	HALF-LIFE (HOURS) Normal	HALF-LIFE (HOURS) Anuria	PERCENTAGE EXCRETED UNCHANGED IN URINE	COMMENTS
Oxytetracycline Various *Oxytetracycline Hydrochloride* *Oxytetracycline Calcium* Various	Cap 250 mg Inj (IM only, contains 2% lidocaine) 50, 125 mg/mL.	PO 1–2 g/day in 2–4 divided doses; IM 250 mg once daily to 300 mg/day in 2–3 doses.	58	9	47–66	70	Seldom used. IM produces lower serum levels than oral.
Tetracycline Various *Tetracycline Hydrochloride* Various	Cap 100, 250, 500 mg Tab 250, 500 mg Susp 25 mg/mL Top Soln 2.2 mg/mL. Top Oint 3%.	PO 1–2 g/day in 2–4 divided doses. Top (soln) for acne apply in the morning and evening.	77	10.6 ± 5	57–108	60	See monograph.

From references 46, 226 and product information.

Miscellaneous Antimicrobials

ATOVAQUONE
Mepron

Pharmacology. Atovaquone is a highly lipophilic hydroxynaphthoquinone with activity against *Pneumocystis carinii*, *Toxoplasma gondii*, and *Plasmodium* spp. It is a structural analogue of ubiquinone, a small hydrophobic respiratory chain electron carrier molecule found in mitochondria. The mechanism of antipneumocystis activity by atovaquone is unclear, but may be inhibition of the mitochondrial electron transport chain, causing inhibition of pyrimidine synthesis and leading to inhibition of nucleic acid and ATP synthesis.[227,228]

Administration and Adult Dosage. PO for *P. carinii* **pneumonia** 750 mg bid for 21 days.

Special Populations. *Pediatric Dosage.* Safety and efficacy not established.

Geriatric Dosage. (>65 yr) not evaluated, but dosage adjustment appears not to be necessary.

Other Conditions. Dosage alteration is not required with renal or hepatic impairment.

Dosage Forms. Susp 150 mg/mL.

Patient Instructions. It is extremely important to take this medication with food to increase absorption; failure to do so may limit response to therapy. Shake the suspension gently prior to use.

Pharmacokinetics. *Serum Levels.* Steady-state serum levels >14 mg/L (38 µmol/L) are correlated with survival in patients with PCP; serum levels <6 mg/L (16 µmol/L) may be ineffective.[228]

Fate. Atovaquone exhibits slow, irregular absorption, depending on the formulation. A high-fat meal increases absorption of the suspension 2.3-fold compared with the fasting state. A peak concentration of 11.5 mg/L (31 µmol/L) is achieved with a single 750-mg dose of the suspension. Oral administration of 750 mg bid as the suspension produces a steady-state level of 24 mg/L (65 µmol/L). More than 99.9% is protein bound, and the drug does not appear to cross the blood-brain barrier well. It appears to undergo enterohepatic cycling, with greater than 94% excreted over 21 days in the feces, with no metabolite identified, and less than 0.6% renally excreted.[228]

$t_{1/2}$. 67 ± 10 hr.[228]

Adverse Effects. Maculopapular rash occurs frequently, but many patients are able to continue atovaquone therapy, and in most instances, the rash resolves without sequelae. GI disturbances including abdominal pain, nausea, vomiting, and diarrhea occur frequently. Fever, headaches, and insomnia have also been reported frequently. Elevations of hepatic transaminases and hyponatremia occur frequently, but do not require cessation of therapy.

Contraindications. Severe diarrhea or malabsorption syndrome, because preexisting diarrhea is associated with poor outcome, presumably as a result of decreased absorption and serum levels.

Precautions. Lactation. Consider alternative therapy in patients who cannot take the drug with food or with GI disorders that may decrease oral absorption.

Drug Interactions. Rifampin may decrease atovaquone serum levels.

Parameters to Monitor. Baseline and periodic liver function tests for patients on prolonged treatment.

Notes. Atovaquone has been used for prevention of *P. carinii* pneumonia in patients who are unable to tolerate or who have failed other traditional prevention medication; although clinical trials are ongoing, the safety, efficacy, and optimal dosage for this indication are not well established.

CHLORAMPHENICOL AND SALTS

Chloromycetin, Various

Pharmacology. Chloramphenicol is a broad-spectrum bacteriostatic antibiotic isolated from *Streptomyces venezuelae* and is particularly useful against ampicillin-resistant *Haemophilus influenzae*, *Salmonella* spp., rickettsial infections such as Rocky Mountain spotted fever, typhoid fever, and most anaerobic organisms. It inhibits protein synthesis by binding the 50S ribosomal subunit and may be bactericidal against some bacteria including pneumococci, meningococci, and *H. influenzae*. Chloramphenicol has variable activity against vancomycin-resistant enterococcal infection. Resistance occurs because of impermeability of the cell wall or bacterial production of chloramphenicol acetyltransferase, a plasmid-mediated enzyme that acetylates chloramphenicol into a microbiologically inert form.[189,222,229,230]

Administration and Adult Dosage. PO or IV 50–100 mg/kg/day depending on severity, location, and organism in 4 divided doses. **IM not recommended.**

Special Populations. *Pediatric Dosage.* PO or IV (<7 days or 2 kg) 25 mg/kg once daily; (neonates >7 days and 2 kg) 25 mg/kg q 12 hr; (older infants and children) 50–100 mg/kg/day given q 6 hr. These regimens produce unpredictable levels, and serum level monitoring is recommended.[231] **IM not recommended.**

Geriatric Dosage. Same as adult dosage.

Other Conditions. Reduce dosage with impaired liver function as guided by serum levels; no alteration necessary in impaired renal function.[231]

Dosage Forms. **Cap** (as base) 250 mg; **Susp** 30 mg/mL; **Inj** (as sodium succinate) 1 g (100 mg/mL when reconstituted); **Ophth Oint** 10 mg/g; **Ophth Pwdr for Soln** 25 mg/vial; **Ophth Soln** 5 mg/mL; **Otic Soln** 5 mg/mL; **Top Crm** 10 mg/g (expressed as chloramphenicol base).

Patient Instructions. Take this drug with a full glass of water on an empty stomach (1 hour before or 2 hours after meals) for best absorption. May take with food if GI upset occurs. Sore throat, fever, or oral lesions may be an early sign of a severe, but rare, blood disorder and should be reported immediately.

Pharmacokinetics. *Serum Levels.* (*See* Adverse Reactions.)

Fate. Well absorbed orally (75–90%), with peak serum levels averaging 12 mg/L after administration of 1 g to normal adults. The palmitate ester (suspension) must be hydrolyzed before absorption; in newborns, infants, and children, hydrolysis may be inadequate and absorption delayed and unreliable. IV 1 g produces levels of 5–12 mg/L (15–37 µmol/L) 1 hr after administration to normal adults. In infants and young children, hydrolysis of succinate to the active form may be slow and incomplete. IM administration may produce serum levels of active drug that are 50% lower than the equivalent oral dose. The drug attains therapeutic levels in most body cavities, the eye, and CSF; it is 53% plasma protein bound. V_d is 0.94 $\pm$ 0.06 L/kg; Cl is 0.14 $\pm$ 0.01 L/hr/kg; 90% of an oral dose is eliminated by glucuronidation in the liver followed by excretion in the urine; the remainder is excreted in the urine unchanged. The rate of glucuronidation and renal elimination is greatly reduced in neonates; 6.5–80% of succinate may be excreted unhydrolyzed. Urine concentrations may be inadequate to treat UTIs, especially in patients with moderately to severely impaired renal function. A small amount (2–4%) of a dose appears in the bile and feces, mostly as the glucuronide.[46,222]

$t_{1/2}$. 4 $\pm$ 2 hr in healthy adults;[46] extremely prolonged and variable in neonates, infants, and young children. Unpredictable in patients with impaired liver function. Some normal patients and patients with impaired renal function exhibit impaired free drug elimination.

Adverse Reactions. Serum levels >25 mg/L (77 μmol/L) frequently produce reversible bone marrow depression with reticulocytopenia, decreased hemoglobin, increased serum iron and iron-binding globulin saturation, thrombocytopenia, and mild leukopenia.[231] The drug inhibits iron uptake by bone marrow, and anemic patients do not respond to iron or vitamin B_{12} therapy while receiving chloramphenicol. This anemia most often follows parenteral therapy, large dosages, long duration of therapy, or impaired drug elimination. Complete recovery usually occurs within 1–2 weeks after drug discontinuation. Aplastic anemia occurs rarely (1/24,500 to 1/40,000) and may be fatal. It is not dose related and can occur long after a short course of oral or parenteral therapy;[231] its occurrence following ophthalmic use is controversial.[232] Fatal cardiovascular-respiratory collapse (gray syndrome) may develop in neonates given excessive dosages. This syndrome is associated with serum levels of about 50–100 mg/L (155–310 μmol/L).[231] A similar syndrome has been reported in children and adults given large overdoses.

Contraindications. Trivial infections; prophylactic use; uses other than those for which it is indicated.

Precautions. Pregnancy; lactation. Use with caution in patients with liver disease (especially cirrhosis, ascites, and jaundice) or preexisting hematologic disorders, or patients receiving other bone marrow depressants. May cause hemolytic episodes in patients with G-6-PD deficiency; observe dosage recommendations closely in neonates and infants.

Drug Interactions. Chloramphenicol increases serum concentrations of phenytoin, warfarin, and sulfonylurea oral hypoglycemic agents. Both phenytoin and phenobarbital can decrease serum levels of chloramphenicol.

Parameters to Monitor. CBC, with platelet and reticulocyte counts before and frequently during therapy; serum iron and iron-binding globulin saturation may also be useful. Liver and renal function tests before and occasionally during therapy.

CLINDAMYCIN SALTS Cleocin, Various

Pharmacology. Clindamycin is a semisynthetic 7-chloro, 7-deoxylincomycin derivative that is active against most Gram-positive organisms except enterococci and *Clostridium difficile*. Gram-negative aerobes are resistant, but most anaerobes are sensitive. It inhibits bacterial protein synthesis by binding to the 50S ribosomal subunit; it is bactericidal or bacteriostatic depending on the concentration, organism, and inoculum.[233,234]

Administration and Adult Dosage. **PO** 150–450 mg q 6 hr; **PO for prevention of endocarditis in patients at risk undergoing dental, oral, or upper respiratory tract procedures, and who are allergic to penicillin** 300 mg 1 hr before procedure and 150 mg 6 hr later.[199] **IM or IV** 600 mg–2.7 g/day in 2–4 divided doses, to a maximum of 4.8 g/day. Single IM doses >600 mg are not recommended; infuse IV no faster than 30 mg/min. **Top for acne** apply bid. **Vag for bacterial vaginosis** 1 applicatorful hs for 7 days.

Dosage Individualization. *Pediatric Dosage.* **PO** (<10 kg) give no less than 37.5 mg q 8 hr; (>10 kg) 8–25 mg/kg/day in 3 or 4 divided doses; **IM or IV** (<1 month) 15–20 mg/kg/day in 3 or 4 divided doses; the lower dosage may be adequate for premature infants; (>1 month) 15–40 mg/kg/day in 3 or 4 divided doses (not less than 300 mg/day in severe infection, regardless of weight).

Geriatric Dosage. Same as adult dosage.

Other Conditions. Dosage adjustment is unnecessary in renal impairment or cirrhosis, although the effect of acute liver disease is unknown.[225,233,235]

Dosage Forms. **Cap** (as hydrochloride) 75, 150, 300 mg; **Soln** (as palmitate) 15 mg/mL (reconstituted); **Inj** (as phosphate) 150 mg/mL; **Top Soln** (as phosphate) 1%; **Top Gel** (as phosphate) 1%; **Vag Crm** 2%.

Patient Instructions. Report any severe diarrhea or blood in the stools immediately and do *not* take antidiarrheal medication. Do not refrigerate the reconstituted oral solution because it will thicken.

Pharmacokinetics. *Fate.* Absorption is nearly 87% and is the same from the capsule or the solution; food may delay, but not decrease, absorption. The palmitate and phosphate esters are absorbed intact and rapidly hydrolyzed to the active base. Unhydrolyzed phosphate ester usually constitutes less than 20% of the total peak serum level after parenteral clindamycin, but may increase to 40% in patients with impaired renal function. A 500-mg oral dose produces a peak serum level of 5–6 mg/L (12–14 µmol/L) in 1 hr. A 300-mg IM dose produces a peak level of 5–6 mg/L 1–2 hr postinjection. A 600-mg IV dose infused over 30 min produces a peak serum level of 10 mg/L (23 µmol/L). The drug is widely distributed throughout the body except the CSF. It is 94% plasma protein bound; V_d is 1.1 ± 0.3 L/kg; Cl is 0.28 ± 0.08 L/hr/kg. There is hepatic metabolism and excretion of active forms in the bile. From 5–10% of the absorbed dose is recovered as unchanged drug and active metabolites in the urine within 24 hr.[46,225,233–236]

$t_{1/2}$ 2.9 ± 0.7 hr; increased in premature infants;[46] unchanged or slightly increased in severe renal disease; may be increased or unchanged in liver disease.[234]

Adverse Reactions. After oral administration anorexia, nausea, vomiting, cramps, and diarrhea occur frequently.[225,233,235] Oral and, rarely, parenteral clindamycin may cause severe, sometimes fatal, pseudomembranous colitis (PMC), which may be clinically indistinguishable at onset from non-PMC diarrhea.[233] Antibiotic-associated PMC is secondary to overgrowth of toxin-producing *Clostridium difficile*. Symptoms usually appear 2–9 days after initiation of therapy. PMC has been reported after topical administration.[235] PMC is terminated in many patients by discontinuing the antibiotic immediately; however, if diarrhea is severe or does not improve promptly after discontinuation, treat with metronidazole or vancomycin.[233,234] The value of corticosteroids, cholestyramine, and antispasmodics in the management of antibiotic-associated diarrhea and PMC has not been established.[233] Antidiarrheals such as diphenoxylate or loperamide may worsen PMC and should *not* be used.

Precautions. Pregnancy; lactation. Use with caution in neonates under 4 weeks of age, and in patients with liver disease. Discontinue *immediately* if severe diarrhea occurs. Drug accumulation may occur in patients with severe concomitant hepatic and renal dysfunction, but data are lacking.

Drug Interactions. Clindamycin may enhance the action of nondepolarizing neuromuscular blocking agents. Kaolin-pectin mixture delays but does not decrease oral absorption of clindamycin.

Parameters to Monitor. Observe for changes in bowel frequency.

Notes. Oral solution is stable for 2 weeks at room temperature following reconstitution; do not refrigerate.

METRONIDAZOLE	Flagyl, MetroGel, Various

Pharmacology. Metronidazole is a synthetic nitroimidazole active against *Trichomonas vaginalis* (trichomoniasis), *Entamoeba histolytica* (amebiasis), and *Giardia lamblia* (giardiasis); it is bactericidal against nearly all obligate anaerobic bacteria including *Bacteroides fragilis*. It is inactive against aerobic bacteria and requires microbial reduction by a nitroreductase enzyme to form highly reactive intermediates that disrupt bacterial DNA and inhibit nucleic acid synthesis, leading to cell death.[231]

Administration and Adult Dosage. PO or IV for anaerobic infections 15 mg/kg (usually 1 g) initially, followed by 7.5 mg/kg (usually 500 mg) q 8–12 hr, to a maximum of 2 g/day. Infuse each IV dose over 1 hr. **PO for antibiotic-associated colitis** 250 mg qid for 7–10 days.[237] (*See* Notes.) **PO for trichomoniasis** 2 g as a single dose or in 2 doses on the same day, or 500 mg bid for 7 days.[175] **PO for giardiasis** 250 mg tid for 5 days (*see* Notes).[237] **PO for symptomatic intestinal amebiasis** (amebic dysentery) 750 mg tid for 10 days. **PO for extraintestinal amebiasis** 750 mg tid for 10 days;[237] some practitioners include a drug effective against the intestinal cyst form, because occasional failures with metronidazole therapy have been reported. **PO for bacterial vaginosis** 500 mg bid for 7 days, or 2 g as a single dose.[175] **Vag for bacterial vaginosis** 1 applicatorful (5 g) bid for 5 days. **Top for rosacea** apply bid.

Special Populations. *Pediatric Dosage.* IV for anaerobic infections (preterm infants) 15 mg/kg once, followed in 48 hr by 7.5 mg/kg q 12 hr; (term infants) 15 mg/kg once, followed in 24 hr by 7.5 mg/kg q 12 hr; (infants >1 week old and children) same as adult mg/kg dosage. **PO for giardiasis** 15 mg/kg/day in 3 divided doses for 5 days, to a maximum of 750 mg/day. *See* Notes. **PO for amebic dysentery or extraintestinal amebiasis** 35–50 mg/kg/day in 3 divided doses for 10 days, to a maximum of 2.5 g/day.

Geriatric Dosage. (>65 yr) decreased clearance may result in accumulation of the drug. Dosage reduction or changing dosage interval to once or twice daily are reasonable modifications to avoid potential adverse reactions.[238]

Other Conditions. No dosage alteration required with renal impairment. Patients with substantial liver dysfunction metabolize metronidazole slowly, with resultant accumulation of metronidazole and its metabolites in the serum. For such patients, it has been suggested that dosage intervals be increased to 12–24 hr, although specific guidelines are not available.[238]

Dosage Forms. **Tab** 250, 500 mg; **Inj** 500 mg; **Top Gel** 0.75%; **Vag Gel** 0.75%.

Patient Instructions. This drug may be taken with food to minimize stomach upset. It may cause a harmless dark discoloration of the urine and metallic taste in the mouth. Nausea, vomiting, flushing, and faintness may occur if alcohol is taken during therapy with this drug.

Pharmacokinetics. *Serum Levels.* Not used clinically.

Fate. IV 500 mg q 12 hr over 1 hr produces steady-state peak and trough levels of 23.6 mg/L (138 µmol/L) and 6.7 mg/L (39 µmol/L), respectively. IV 500 mg q 8 hr over 1 hr produces steady-state peak and trough levels of 27.4 mg/L (160 µmol/L) and 15.5 mg/L (91 µmol/L), respectively. Well absorbed orally with levels similar to those following IV infusion; 250- and 500-mg doses produce peak concentrations of 4–6 mg/L (23–35 µmol/L) and 10–13 mg/L (58–76 µmol/L), respectively, at 1–2 hr in adults. Bioavailability of vaginal gel is 53–58%. Less than 20% plasma protein bound; wide distribution with therapeutic levels in many tissues, including abscesses, bile, bone, breast milk, CSF, and saliva. V_d is 0.85 ± 0.25 L/kg; Cl is 0.07 ± 0.02 L/hr/kg. Extensively metabolized in the liver by hydroxylation, oxidation and glucuronide formation; 44–80% excreted in the urine in 24 hr, about 6–18% as unchanged drug.

$t_{1/2}$. 6–10 hr in adults; not increased with impaired renal function; prolonged variably with severe hepatic impairment.[46,237,238]

Adverse Effects. Metallic taste in mouth and GI complaints occur frequently with high dosages. Occasional dizziness, vertigo, and paresthesias have been reported with very high dosages. Reversible mild neutropenia reported occasionally.[189,237] Reversible, rare, but severe peripheral neuropathy may occur with high dosages given over prolonged periods. Antibiotic-associated colitis has been reported rarely with oral metronidazole.[237] The IV preparation is occasionally associated with phlebitis at the infusion site. Experimental production of tumors in some rodent species and mutations in bacteria have raised concern regarding potential carcinogenicity; to date, mammalian testing and human epidemiologic research have not detected an appreciable risk, although further data are needed.[237]

Contraindications. First trimester of pregnancy, although there is no direct evidence of teratogenicity in humans or animals.[189]

Precautions. Pregnancy; lactation; active CNS disease or neutropenia.

Drug Interactions. Disulfiramlike reactions are reported with concurrent alcohol use, but are uncommon. Confusion and psychotic episodes have been reported with concurrent disulfiram; avoid this combination, if possible. Metronidazole inhibits CYP3A3/4 and may affect the metabolism of many drugs; the best documented is an enhanced hypoprothrombinemic response to warfarin. Phenytoin metabolism may also be inhibited.

Parameters to Monitor. Before and after the completion of any lengthy or repeated courses of therapy, monitor WBC count. Monitor serum metronidazole levels as well as signs of toxicity in patients with severe liver disease.[238]

Notes. The treatment of *asymptomatic* trichomoniasis is controversial. Signs of endocervical inflammation or erosion on physical examination are considered an indication for treatment. Also, most practitioners treat asymptomatic male consorts, because lack of such treatment may be a cause of treatment failure or recurrent infection of the female partner.[175] Metronidazole has been used in combination regimens to treat *Helicobacter pylori* infected patients with duodenal or gastric ulcers (*see* Treatment of *Helicobacter pylori* in Peptic Ulcer Disease Comparison Chart). Although it is slightly less effective than **vancomycin,** metronidazole is considered by some to be the drug of choice for antibiotic-associated pseudomembranous colitis because of its lower cost[239] and because of the emergence of vancomycin-resistant enterococci because of vancomycin overuse.

NITROFURANTOIN
Macrodantin, Macrobid, Various

Nitrofurantoin is a synthetic nitrofuran that is active against most bacteria that cause UTIs except *Pseudomonas aeruginosa*, *Proteus* spp., many *Enterobacter* spp. and *Klebsiella* spp. The drug is used primarily to prevent recurrent UTIs, but is also effective in the treatment of uncomplicated UTIs. Serum and extraurinary tissue concentrations are subtherapeutic. Nitrofurantoin yields a urine concentration of about 200 mg/L from an average dose. Adverse effects are primarily nausea, vomiting, and diarrhea, and are dose related; use of the macrocrystalline form and administration with food may minimize GI distress. Hypersensitivity reactions, such as rash, occur only rarely. Acute allergic pneumonitis is reversible with discontinuation of therapy. Chronic interstitial pulmonary fibrosis also occurs occasionally with long-term therapy and may be irreversible. Ascending polyneuropathy associated with prolonged high-dose therapy or use of the drug in renal failure is only slowly reversible. Intravascular hemolysis may occur in patients with severe G-6-PD deficiency. Although the drug is mutagenic in mammalian cells, there is no clinical evidence of carcinogenicity or teratogenicity. Adult dosage of macrocrystals is usually PO 50–100 mg qid with meals and hs for treatment, or PO 50–100 mg hs for chronic suppression. Pediatric dosage is PO 5–7 mg/kg/day in 4 divided doses for treatment, or PO 1 mg/kg/day in 1–2 doses for chronic suppression. Adult dosage of Macrobid is 1 capsule bid for 7 days.[240] Available as macrocrystals in 25-, 50-, and 100-mg capsules and 5 mg/mL suspension; and as capsules containing 25 mg as macrocrystals and 75 mg in an SR form (Macrobid).

PENTAMIDINE ISETHIONATE
Pentam 300, NebuPent

Pharmacology. Pentamidine is an aromatic diamidine used in the treatment of trypanosomiasis and *Pneumocystis carinii* pneumonia. Pentamidine inhibits dihydrofolate reductase, interferes with anaerobic glycolysis, inhibits oxidative phosphorylation, and limits nucleic acid and protein synthesis, but the mechanism by which pentamidine kills *P. carinii* is unclear.[241]

Administration and Adult Dosage. IV (preferred) or IM 3–4 mg/kg/day as a single dose for 2–3 weeks; infuse IV over 60 min. **Inhal for** *P. carinii* **pneumonia prophylaxis in high-risk HIV-infected patients** 300 mg q 4 weeks via special nebulizer. *See* Notes.

Special Populations. *Pediatric Dosage.* Same as adult dosage.

Geriatric Dosage. Same as adult dosage.

Other Conditions. Dosage adjustment does not appear necessary in renal impairment.[242]

Dosage Forms. Inj 300 mg; **Inhal** 300 mg.

Pharmacokinetics. *Serum Levels.* Not used clinically.

Fate. Negligible oral absorption. Peak serum levels of 0.5–3 mg/L (1.5–8.8 µmol/L) occur after 4 mg/kg IV infusion. Serum levels are very low after inhalation (<0.1 mg/L). About 70% plasma protein bound; distributed widely in tissues, with highest concentrations found in spleen, liver, kidneys, and adrenal glands. V_c is 3 L/kg; terminal V_d is 190 ± 70 L/kg; Cl is 1.08 ± 0.42 L/hr/kg. There are no data on the effects of liver impairment. Less than 20% of a dose is excreted unchanged in urine.[46,243]

$t_{1/2}$. α phase 1.2 ± 0.6 hr; terminal elimination half-life is up to 29 ± 25 days,[242] suggesting rapid tissue uptake with slow release and subsequent urinary excretion.

Adverse Reactions. With IV administration, nephrotoxicity occurs in up to 25% of patients, hypoglycemia in up to 27%, and hypotension in up to 10% of patients. Fever, rash, leukopenia, and liver damage occur occasionally. Hyperglycemia and insulin-dependent diabetes mellitus have been reported as well as pancreatitis. Pentamidine-induced torsades de pointes has been reported rarely. IM injection frequently produces pain and abscess formation at the injection site. With aerosolized pentamidine, reversible bronchoconstriction and unpleasant taste occur frequently. Severe adverse reactions are less frequent, but reports of pancreatitis, hypoglycemia and cutaneous eruptions have occurred rarely, suggesting some systemic absorption.[241]

Precautions. Use with caution in diabetes mellitus.

Drug Interactions. IV pentamidine may increase the risk of hypocalcemia with foscarnet; avoid this combination, if possible, although inhaled pentamidine does not seem to be a risk factor.

Parameters to Monitor. Obtain serum glucose, Cr_s, BUN, liver function tests, electrolytes, CBC, and platelet count daily. Monitor blood pressure after administration.

Notes. Concomitant therapy with both pentamidine and **trimethoprim-sulfamethoxazole** appears to offer no benefit and may be additively toxic. There is concern about occupational exposure with inhalation therapy. No studies have yet determined the health effects of exposure to pentamidine itself; however, transmission of tuberculosis to health care workers has been attributed partly to the use of aerosolized pentamidine among clinic patients coinfected with HIV and tuberculosis. Health care workers administering aerosolized pentamidine should wear masks and protective eye wear.[241]

QUINUPRISTIN AND DALFOPRISTIN (Investigational, Rhone-Poulenc Rorer) Synercid

Quinupristin and dalfopristin is a combination of two streptogramin antibiotics that are naturally occurring compounds isolated from *Streptomyces pristinaspiralis*. Quinupristin, a derivative of pristinamycin IA, and dalfopristin, a derivative of pristinamycin IIA, are combined in a fixed ratio of 30:70 (w/w). This combination inhibits protein synthesis by sequential binding to the 50S subunit of bacterial ribosomes; its synergistic activity may be caused by binding of dalfopristin, altering conformation of the ribosome such that its affinity for quinupristin is increased. Individually pristinamycin I and pristinamycin II are bacteriostatic, but in combination they are bactericidal against Gram-positive bacteria, including methicillin-resistant *Staphylococcus aureus* (MRSA). Synergy has been reported with vancomycin against MRSA and multiply resistant enterococci. It also has activity against anaerobic organisms, but most Gram-negative organisms such as the Enterobacteriacae, *Acinetobacter* spp. and *Pseudomonas aeruginosa* are resistant. The pharmacokinetics are complex, and half-life appears to average 1.5 hr. Adverse effects reported have been limited to mild to moderate local reactions of itching, pain, and burning at the injection site. Diarrhea and headache have been reported occasionally.[244-246] The dosage used investigationally is IV 7.5 mg/kg q 8 hr infused in D5W over 60 min. It is available from the manufacturer for resistant infections.

TRIMETHOPRIM Proloprim, Various

Trimethoprim is a synthetic folate-antagonist antibacterial (*see* Trimethoprim and Sulfamethoxazole). Trimethoprim is effective in acute UTI. It has a potential advantage over the sulfa-containing combination in patients with allergy or toxicity attributed to sulfonamides; however, the relative potential for trimethoprim alone to permit the development of resistance is unsettled. Used alone, trimethoprim is ineffective against *Pneumocystis carinii*, but in combination with **dapsone** (a sulfone), it is effective in treating mild to moderate *P. carinii* pneumonia (PCP). Occasional adverse effects are mild thrombocytopenia, nausea, fever, and rash; the frequency appears to be dose related. Methemoglobinemia and dose-related hemolysis have occurred in patients with G-6-PD deficiency receiving dapsone with trimethoprim; it is important to check G-6-PD status prior to initiating combination therapy. For uncomplicated acute UTI, the dosage is 200 mg/day in 1 or 2 doses for 10 days. For the treatment of mild to moderate (PaO$_2$ >60 mm Hg) PCP, the dosage is 20 mg/kg/day of TMP in 3 or 4 divided doses with dapsone 100 mg once daily.[218,219] Available as 100- and 200-mg tablets.

TRIMETREXATE Neutrexin

Trimetrexate is a lipophilic analogue of methotrexate that inhibits dihydrofolate reductase, leading to the disruption of purine biosynthesis. It has activity against *Pneumocystis carinii* and *Toxoplasma gondii* and has demonstrated modest efficacy against a number of malignancies. It is approved for the treatment of moderate to severe *P. carinii* pneumonia (PCP) in immunocompromised patients. Trimetrexate has at least two metabolites, both of which inhibit dihydrofolate reductase. It is eliminated primarily by hepatic metabolism; less than one-third is excreted unchanged in urine. The elimination half-life ranges from 4–12 hr in patients with AIDS and PCP, and from 8–26 hr in patients with cancer. The primary toxicity is myelosuppression (neutropenia and thrombocytopenia); myelosuppression is minimized with concurrent administration of **calcium leucovorin.** Anemia, elevated liver function tests, fever, rash, peripheral neuropathy, stomatitis, and nausea or vomiting occur frequently. Hypersensitivity reactions and seizures are reported rarely. The dosage for moderate to severe PCP is 45 mg/m^2/day infused IV over 60–90 min for 21 days. Give IV or PO **calcium leucovorin** 20 mg/m^2 q 6 hr concomitantly and continue it for 3 days after the end of trimetrexate administration.[247,248] Available as 25-mg injection.

VANCOMYCIN HYDROCHLORIDE   Vancocin, Various

Pharmacology. Vancomycin binds irreversibly to the cell wall of in a manner slightly different from ß-lactams. Many Gram-positive cocci and bacilli, including methicillin-resistant *Staphylococcus aureus* and *Clostridium difficile* are inhibited. Most Gram-negative bacteria are resistant, and vancomycin-resistant enterococci have been reported in association with overuse of vancomycin.[215]

Administration and Adult Dosage. IV 20–30 mg/kg/day (usually 2 g/day) in 2–4 divided doses as a dilute infusion over 1–2 hr. **PO for staphylococcal enterocolitis** 2 g/day in 2–4 divided doses. **PO for antibiotic-associated colitis** 125–500 mg q 6 hr for 7–10 days; retreat with a longer course if relapse occurs (*see* Notes). **Not for IM use.**

Dosage Individualization. *Pediatric Dosage.* IV (neonates) 12–15 mg/kg/day; (older infants and children) 40 mg/kg/day in 2–4 divided doses. **PO** 10–50 mg/kg/day in 4 divided doses.

Geriatric Dosage. Same as adult dosage, but adjust for age-related reduction in renal function.

Other Conditions. Adjust dosage carefully in renal impairment; Cl is directly related to Cl_{cr}.[248] Anuric patients on hemodialysis have been given the usual dose q 7–14 days, although one source recommends 8 mg/kg given q 6–24 hr according to renal function.[249] Dosage adjustment is unnecessary in liver disease.

Dosage Forms. **Cap** 125, 250 mg; **Susp** 1, 10 g; **Inj** 500 mg, 1 g.

Patient Instructions. Report pain at infusion site, dizziness, fullness or ringing in ears with IV use; nausea or vomiting with oral use.

Pharmacokinetics. *Serum Levels.* Therapeutic range is not well defined. Ototoxicity has been associated with high serum concentrations, but has also been noted at lower levels.[249,250] Peaks associated with efficacy are between 20–40 mg/L (14–28 µmol/L); troughs >15 mg/L (10 µmol/L) may be excessive.

Fate. Oral absorption is negligible, although appreciable serum levels may be observed in patients with renal dysfunction receiving oral vancomycin for *C. difficile*–induced antibiotic-associated colitis. Fecal concentrations with PO 500 mg q 6 hr reach 3 mg/g. IV 500 mg produces serum levels of 6–10 mg/L (4–7 µmol/L) in 1 hr. Plasma protein binding is 30 ± 10%. The drug is widely distributed, except into the CSF, although some success has been reported in the treatment of meningitis, particularly in children. V_c is 0.1–0.15 L/kg; $V_{d\beta}$ is 0.39 ± 0.06 L/kg; Cl is 0.84 L/hr/kg with normal renal function. In renal impairment, Cl (in mL/min) may be estimated as 0.79 × Cl_{cr} (in mL/min) + 0.22. Metabolism and biliary excretion are negligible; 80–90% is excreted unchanged in the urine within 48 hr.[46,251]

$t_{\frac{1}{2}}$. ß phase 5.6 ± 1.8 hr, 6–10 days with renal impairment. No change with hepatic disease.[46,251]

Adverse Reactions. Chills, fever, nausea, and phlebitis may occur frequently, especially with direct injection of undiluted drug (not recommended). Rapid infusion may cause transient systolic hypotension.[252] The "red man" or "red neck" syndrome of erythema, pruritus, and localized edema is associated with histamine release caused by rapid infusions of doses of 500 mg or greater; it often does not occur or is less severe with subsequent doses.[253] Extravasation causes local tissue necrosis. Ototoxicity (auditory and vestibular) and possibly nephrotoxicity occur, but have not been definitely linked to high serum levels.[250,254] Eosinophilia, neutropenia, and urticarial rashes have been reported frequently. Side effects of vancomycin may not be as prevalent today as in the past, perhaps because of changes in the manufacturing process that eliminated some impurities.[255]

Precautions. Pregnancy. Use with caution in patients with impaired renal function or preexisting hearing loss, or in those receiving other ototoxic or nephrotoxic agents.

Drug Interactions. Administration with an aminoglycoside may increase the risk of nephrotoxicity.[250]

Parameters to Monitor. With IV use, obtain initial renal function tests and repeat twice weekly during therapy. Routine monitoring of serum levels in patients with normal renal function is not recommended because it has questionable value, but is often performed.[254] Check for signs of phlebitis daily.

Notes. An alternative agent for treatment or prophylaxis of staphylococcal or streptococcal infections when a less toxic agent is inappropriate (eg, penicillin or cephalosporin allergy, or resistant organisms) or has not produced an adequate therapeutic response. Use of vancomycin in antibiotic-associated colitis is becoming less desirable because of the emergence of vancomycin-resistant enterococci caused by overuse of vancomycin. Reserve vancomycin for cases refractory to metronidazole.[239]

■ REFERENCES

1. Lortholary O et al. Aminoglycosides. *Med Clin North Am* 1995;79:761–87.
2. Gilbert DN. Aminoglycosides. In Mandell GL et al., eds. *Principles and practice of infectious diseases,* 4th ed. Churchill Livingstone: New York; 1995:279–306
3. Preston SL, Briceland LL. Single daily dosing of aminoglycosides. *Pharmacotherapy* 1995;15:297–306.
4. Nicolau DP et al. Experience with a once-daily aminoglycoside program administered to 2184 patients. *Antimicrob Agents Chemother* 1995;39:650–5.
5. Blaser J et al. Monitoring serum concentrations for once-daily netilmicin dosing regimens. *J Antimicrob Chemother* 1994;33:341–8.
6. Sarubbi FA, Hull JH. Amikacin serum concentrations, predictions of levels and dosage guidelines. *Ann Intern Med* 1978;89:612–8.
7. Walshe JJ et al. Crossover pharmacokinetic analysis comparing intravenous and intraperitoneal administration of tobramycin. *J Infect Dis* 1986;153:796–9.

8. Zaske DE. Aminoglycosides. In Evans WE et al. Applied pharmacokinetics. *Principles of therapeutic drug monitoring,* 3rd ed. Vancouver, WA: Applied Therapeutics;1992: 14-1–14-47.

9. Kahlmeter G, Dahlager JI. Aminoglycoside toxicity—a review of clinical studies published between 1975 and 1982. *J Antimicrob Chemother* 1984;13(suppl A):9–22.

10. McCormack JP, Jewesson PJ. A critical reevaluation of the "therapeutic range" of aminoglycosides. *Clin Infect Dis* 1992;14:320–9.

11. Pickering LK et al. Effect of concentration and time upon inactivation of tobramycin, gentamicin, netilmicin, and amikacin by azlocillin, carbenicillin, mecillinam, mezlocillin, and piperacillin. *J Pharmacol Exp Ther* 1981;217:345–9.

12. Thompson MIB et al. Gentamicin inactivation by piperacillin or carbenicillin in patients with end-stage renal disease. *Antimicrob Agents Chemother* 1982;21:268–73.

13. Erdmay SM et al. An updated comparison of drug dosing methods. Part III. Aminoglycoside antibiotics. *Clin Pharmacokinet* 1991;20:374–88.

14. Massey KL et al. Identification of children in whom routine aminoglycoside serum concentration monitoring is not cost-effective. *J Pediatr* 1986;109:897–901.

15. Moore RD et al. Clinical response to aminoglycoside therapy: importance of the ratio of peak concentration to minimum inhibitory concentration. *J Infect Dis* 1987;155:93–9.

16. Bodey GP. Topical and systemic antifungal agents. *Med Clin North Am* 1988;72:637–60.

17. Benson JM, Nahata MC. Clinical use of systemic antifungal agents. *Clin Pharm* 1988;7:424–38.

18. Terrell CL, Hughes CE. Antifungal agents used for deep-seated mycotic infections. *Mayo Clin Proc* 1992;67:69–91.

19. Oldfield EC et al. Randomized, double-blind trial of 1- vs 4-hr amphotericin B infusion durations. *Antimicrob Agents Chemother* 1990;34:1402–6.

20. Nicholl TA et al. Amphotericin B infusion-related toxicity: comparison of two- and four-hour infusions. *Ann Pharmacother* 1995;29:1081–7.

21. Meyer RD. Current role of therapy with amphotericin B. *Clin Infect Dis* 1992;14(suppl 1):S154–60.

22. Gallis HA et al. Amphotericin B: 30 years of clinical experience. *Rev Infect Dis* 1990;12:308–29.

23. Cross JT et al. Antifungal drugs. *Pediatr Rev* 1995;16:123–29.

24. Clements JS, Peacock JE. Amphotericin B revisited: reassessment of toxicity. *Am J Med* 1990;88(5N): 22N–7.

25. Maddux MS, Barriere SL. A review of complications of amphotericin B therapy: recommendations for prevention and management. *Drug Intell Clin Pharm* 1980;14:177–81.

26. Gardner ML et al. Sodium loading treatment for amphotericin B-induced nephrotoxicity. *DICP* 1990;24:940–6.

27. Lopez-Berestein G et al. Treatment of systemic fungal infections with liposomal amphotericin B. *Arch Intern Med* 1989;149:2533–6.

28. Moreau P et al. Reduced renal toxicity and improved clinical tolerance of amphotericin B mixed with Intralipid compared with conventional amphotericin B in neutropenic patients. *J Antimicrob Chemother* 1992;30: 535–41.

29. Caillot D et al. Efficacy and tolerance of an amphotericin B lipid (Intralipid) emulsion in the treatment of candidaemia in neutropenic patients. *J Antimicrob Chemother* 1993;31:161–9.

30. Caillot D et al. A controlled trial of the tolerance of amphotericin B infused in dextrose or in Intralipid in patients with haematological malignancies. *J Antimicrob Chemother* 1994;33:603–13.

31. Trissel LA. Amphotericin B does not mix with fat emulsion. *Am J Health-Syst Pharm* 1995;52:1463–4.

32. Cleary JD. Amphotericin B formulated in a lipid emulsion. *Ann Pharmacother* 1996;30:409–12.

33. Pasco MT et al. Fluconazole: a new triazole antifungal agent. *DICP* 1990;24:860–7.

34. Powderly WG. Fluconazole. *Infect Med* 1995;12:257, 281–82.

35. Debruyne D, Ryckelynck J-P. Clinical pharmacokinetics of fluconazole. *Clin Pharmacokinet* 1993;24: 10–27.

36. Perry CM et al. Fluconazole. An update of its antimicrobial activity, pharmacokinetic properties, and therapeutic use in vaginal candidiasis. *Drugs* 1995;49:984–1006.

37. Como JA, Dismukes WE. Oral azole drugs as systemic antifungal therapy. *N Engl J Med* 1994;330:263–72.

38. Galgiani JN et al. Fluconazole therapy for coccidioidal meningitis. *Ann Intern Med* 1993;119:28–35.

39. Rhodes KH, Henry NK. Antibiotic therapy for severe infections in infants and children. *Mayo Clin Proc* 1992;67:59–68.

40. Allendoerfer R et al. Combined therapy with fluconazole and flucytosine in murine cryptococcal meningitis. *Antimicrob Agents Chemother* 1991;35:726–9.

41. Bennett JE et al. A comparison of amphotericin B alone and combined with flucytosine in the treatment of cryptococcal meningitis. *N Engl J Med* 1979;301:126–31.

42. Lyman CA, Walsh TJ. Systemically administered antifungal agents. A review of their clinical pharmacology and therapeutic applications. *Drugs* 1992;44:9–35.

43. Haria M et al. Itraconazole. A reappraisal of its pharmacological properties and therapeutic use in the management of superficial fungal infections. *Drugs* 1996;51:585–620.

44. Tucker RM et al. Interaction of azoles with rifampin, phenytoin, and carbamazepine: in vitro and clinical observations. *Clin Infect Dis* 1992;14:165–74.

45. Ducharme MP et al. Itraconazole and hydroxyitraconazole serum concentrations are reduced more than tenfold by phenytoin. *Clin Pharmacol Ther* 1995;58:617–24.

46. Benet LZ et al. Design and optimization of dosage regimens: pharmacokinetic data. In Hardman JG et al., eds. *Goodman and Gilman's the pharmacological basis of therapeutics.* New York: McGraw-Hill; 1996:1707–92.

47. Barriere SL. Pharmacology and pharmacokinetics of traditional antifungal agents. *Pharmacotherapy* 1990;10(suppl):134S–40S.

48. Chin TWF et al. Effects of an acidic beverage (Coca-Cola) on absorption of ketoconazole. *Antimicrob Agents Chemother* 1995;39:1671–5.

49. Balfour JA, Faulds D. Terbinafine: a review of its pharmacodynamic and pharmacokinetic properties, and therapeutic potential in superficial mycoses. *Drugs* 1992;43:259–84.

50. Arbiser JL et al. Clofazimine: a review of its medical uses and mechanisms of action. *J Am Acad Dermatol* 1995;32:241–7.

51. Peloquin CA. Pharmacology of the antimycobacterial drugs. *Med Clin North Am* 1993;77:1253–62.

52. Brausch LM, Bass JB. The treatment of tuberculosis. *Med Clin North Am* 1993;77:1277–90.

53. Treatment of tuberculosis and tuberculosis infection in adults and children. *Clin Infect Dis* 1995;21:9–27.

54. Initial therapy for tuberculosis in the era of multidrug resistance. *MMWR* 1993;42(RR-7):1–8.

55. Heifets LB. Antimycobacterial drugs. *Semin Respir Infect* 1994;9:84–103.

56. van Scoy RE, Wilkowske CJ. Antituberculous agents. *Mayo Clin Proc* 1992;67:179–87.

57. Pratt WB, Fekety R. Drugs that act on mycobacteria. In Pratt WB, Fekety R, eds. *The antimicrobial drugs.* New York: Oxford University Press; 1986:277–316.

58. Alexander MR et al. Isoniazid-associated hepatitis. *Clin Pharm* 1982;1:148–53.

59. Holdiness MR. Neurological manifestations and toxicities of the antituberculous drugs. *Med Toxicol Adv Drug Exp* 1987;2:33–51.

60. O'Brien RJ. Drug-resistant tuberculosis: etiology, management and prevention. *Semin Respir Infect* 1994;9:104–12.

61. Skinner MH et al. Pharmacokinetics of rifabutin. *Antimicrob Agents Chemother* 1989;33:1237–41.

62. Nightingale SD et al. Two controlled trials of rifabutin prophylaxis against *Mycobacterium avium* complex infection in AIDS. *N Engl J Med* 1993;329:828–33.

63. Masur H. Recommendations on prophylaxis and therapy for disseminated *Mycobacterium avium* complex disease in patients infected with the human immunodeficiency virus. Public Health Service Task Force on Prophylaxis and Therapy for *Mycobacterium avium* Complex. *N Engl J Med* 1993;329:898–904.

64. Blaschke TF, Skinner MH. The clinical pharmacokinetics of rifabutin. *Clin Infect Dis* 1996;(suppl 1):S15–22.

65. Thornsberry C et al. Rifampin: spectrum of antibacterial activity. *Rev Infect Dis* 1983;5(suppl 3):S412–7.

66. Beaty HN. Rifampin and minocycline in meningococcal disease. *Rev Infect Dis* 1983;5(suppl 3):S451–8.

67. Acocella G. Pharmacokinetics and metabolism of rifampin in humans. *Rev Infect Dis* 1983;5(suppl 3):S428–32.

68. Venkatesan K. Pharmacokinetic drug interactions with rifampicin. *Clin Pharmacokinet* 1992;22:47–65.

69. Anon. Drugs for parasitic infections. *Med Lett Drugs Ther* 1995;37:99–108.

70. Jernigan JA, Pearson RD. Antiparasitic drugs. In Mandell GL et al., eds. *Principles and practice of infectious diseases,* 4th ed. New York: Churchill Livingstone; 1995:458–92.

71. Liu LX, Weller PF. Antiparasitic drugs. *N Engl J Med* 1996;334:1178–84.

72. Mandell WF, Neu HC. Parasitic infections: therapeutic considerations. *Med Clin North Am* 1988;72:669–90.

73. Tracy JW, Webster LY Jr. Drugs used in the chemotherapy of helminthiasis. In Hardman JG et al., eds. *Goodman and Gilman's the pharmacological basis of therapeutics,* 9th ed. New York: McGraw-Hill; 1996:1009–26.

74. Keating MR. Antiviral agents. *Mayo Clin Proc* 1992;67:160–78.

75. Elion GB. Acyclovir: discovery, mechanism of action, and selectivity. *J Med Virol* 1993;(suppl 1):2–6.

76. Whitley RJ, Gnann JW. Acyclovir: a decade later. *N Engl J Med* 1992;327:782–9.

77. Nikkels AF, Pierard GE. Recognition and treatment of shingles. *Drugs* 1994;48:528–48.

78. Soul-Lawton J et al. Absolute bioavailability and metabolic disposition of valaciclovir, the L-valyl ester of acyclovir, following oral administration to humans. *Antimicrob Agents Chemother* 1995;39:2759–64.

79. Jacobson MA. Valaciclovir (BW256U87): the L-valyl ester of acyclovir. *J Med Virol* 1993;(suppl 1):150–3.

80. Laskin OL. Acyclovir, pharmacology and clinical experience. *Arch Intern Med* 1984;144:1241–6.

81. Cundy KC et al. Clinical pharmacokinetics of cidofovir in human immunodeficiency virus–infected patients. *Antimicrob Agents Chemother* 1995;39:1247–52.

82. Lalezari JP et al. (S)-1-[3-hydroxy-2-(phosphonylmethoxy)propyl]cytosine (cidofovir): results of a phase I/II study of a novel antiviral nucleotide analogue. *J Infect Dis* 1995;171:788–96.

83. Flaherty JF. Current and experimental therapeutic options for cytomegalovirus disease. *Am J Health-Syst Pharm* 1996;53(suppl 2):S4–11.

84. Neuzil KM. Pharmacologic therapy for human immunodeficiency virus infection: a review. *Am J Med Sci* 1994;307:368–73.

85. Working Group on Antiretroviral Therapy: National Pediatric HIV Resource Center. Antiretroviral therapy and medical management of the human immunodeficiency virus–infected child. *Pediatr Infect Dis J* 1993;12:513–22.

86. Johnson VA. Nucleoside reverse transcriptase inhibitors and resistance of human immunodeficiency virus type 1. *J Infect Dis* 1995;171(suppl 2):S140–9.

87. Dudley MN. Clinical pharmacokinetics of nucleoside antiretroviral agents. *J Infect Dis* 1995;171(suppl 2):S99–112.

88. Knupp CA et al. Pharmacokinetics of didanosine in patients with acquired immunodeficiency syndrome or acquired immunodeficiency syndrome–related complex. *Clin Pharmacol Ther* 1991;49:523–35.

89. Hartman NR et al. Pharmacokinetics of 2′,3′-dideoxyinosine in patients with severe human immunodeficiency infection. II. The effects of different oral formulations and the presence of other medications. *Clin Pharmacol Ther* 1991;50:278–85.

90. Stretcher BN. Pharmacokinetic optimisation of antiretroviral therapy in patients with HIV infection. *Clin Pharmacokinet* 1995;29:46–65.

91. van Leeuwen R et al. The safety and pharmacokinetics of a reverse transcriptase inhibitor, 3TC, in patients with HIV infection: a phase I study. *AIDS* 1992;6:1471–5.

92. Moore KHP et al. Pharmacokinetics of lamivudine administered alone and with trimethoprim-sulfamethoxazole. *Clin Pharmacol Ther* 1996;59:550–8.

93. Taburet A-M, Singlas E. Drug interactions with antiviral drugs. *Clin Pharmacokinet* 1996;30:385–401.

94. Pue MA et al. Linear pharmacokinetics of penciclovir following administration of single oral doses of famciclovir 125, 250, 500 and 750 mg to healthy volunteers. *J Antimicrob Chemother* 1994;33:119–27.

95. Perry CM, Wagstaff AJ. Famciclovir: a review of its pharmacological properties and therapeutic efficacy in herpesvirus infections. *Drugs* 1995;50:396–415.

96. Minor JR, Baltz JK. Foscarnet sodium. *DICP* 1991;25:41–7.

97. Jacobson MA et al. Foscarnet treatment of cytomegalovirus retinitis in patients with the acquired immunodeficiency syndrome. *Antimicrob Agents Chemother* 1989;33:736–41.

98. Wagstaff AJ, Bryson HM. Foscarnet. A reappraisal of its antiviral activity, pharmacokinetic properties and therapeutic use in immunocompromised patients with viral infections. *Drugs* 1994;48:199–226.

99. Sasadeusz JJ, Sacks SL. Systemic antivirals in herpesvirus infections. *Dermatol Clin* 1993;11:171–85.

100. Jacobson MA et al. Foscarnet-induced hypocalcemia and effects of foscarnet on calcium metabolism. *J Clin Endocrinol Metab* 1991;72:1130–5.

101. Crumpacker CS. Ganciclovir. *N Engl J Med* 1996;335:721–9.

102. Sommadossi J-P et al. Clinical pharmacokinetics of ganciclovir in patients with normal and impaired renal function. *Rev Infect Dis* 1988;10(suppl 3):S507–14.

103. Morris DJ. Adverse effects and drug interactions of clinical importance with antiviral drugs. *Drug Saf* 1994;10:281–91.

104. Erice A et al. Progressive disease due to ganciclovir-resistant cytomegalovirus in immunocompromised patients. *N Engl J Med* 1989;320:289–93.

105. Moyle G, Gazzard B. Current knowledge and future prospects for the use of HIV protease inhibitors. *Drugs* 1996;51:701–12.

106. Hart GJ et al. Effects of (–)-2′-deoxy-3′-thiacytidine (3TC) 5′-triphosphate on human immunodeficiency virus reverse transcriptase and mammalian DNA polymerases alpha, beta, and gamma. *Antimicrob Agents Chemother* 1992;36:1688–94.

107. Merrill DP et al. Lamivudine or stavudine in two- and three-drug combinations against human immunodeficiency virus type 1 replication in vitro. *J Infect Dis* 1996;173:355–64.

108. Eron JJ et al. Treatment with lamivudine, zidovudine, or both in HIV-positive patients with 200 to 500 CD4+ cells per cubic millimeter. *N Engl J Med* 1995;333:1662–9.

109. Cheeseman S et al. Phase I/II evaluation of nevirapine alone and in combination with zidovudine for infection with human immunodeficiency virus. *J Acquir Immune Defic Syndr Hum Retrovirol* 1995;8:141–51.

110. Havlir D et al. High-dose nevirapine: safety, pharmacokinetics, and antiviral effect in patients with human immunodeficiency virus infection. *J Infect Dis* 1995;171:537–45.

111. Investigational drug brochure: Viramune (nevirapine) expanded access program. Ridgefield, CT: Boehringer Ingelheim, March 1996.

112. D'Aquila RT et al. Nevirapine, zidovudine, and didanosine compared with zidovudine and didanosine in patients with HIV-1 infection. A randomized, double-blind, placebo-controlled trial. *Ann Intern Med* 1996;124:1019–30.

152   ANTIMICROBIAL DRUGS

113. Danner SA et al. A short-term study of the safety, pharmacokinetics, and efficacy of ritonavir, an inhibitor of HIV-1 protease. *N Engl J Med* 1995;333:1528–33.

114. Markowitz M et al. A preliminary study of ritonavir, an inhibitor of HIV-1 protease, to treat HIV-1 infection. *N Engl J Med* 1995;333:1534–9.

115. Kitchen VS et al. Safety and activity of saquinavir in HIV infection. *Lancet* 1995;345:952–5.

116. Vella S. Update on a proteinase inhibitor. *AIDS* 1994;8(suppl 3):S25–9.

117. Investigational drug brochure: Ro 31–8959-saquinavir (Invirase). Third version. Nutley, NJ: Hoffman-LaRoche, April 1995.

118. Sommadossi J-P. Comparison of metabolism and in vitro antiviral activity of stavudine versus other 2′,3′-dideoxynucleoside analogues. *J Infect Dis* 1995;171(suppl 2):S88–92.

119. Murray HW et al. Stavudine in patients with AIDS and AIDS- related complex: AIDS clinical trials group 089. *J Infect Dis* 1995;171(suppl 2):S123–30.

120. Lange JM et al. Failure of zidovudine prophylaxis after accidental exposure to HIV-1. *N Engl J Med* 1990;322:1375–7.

121. Recommendations of the U.S. Public Health Service task force on the use of zidovudine to reduce perinatal transmission of human immunodeficiency virus. *MMWR* 1994;43(RR-11):1–20.

122. Taburet AM et al. Pharmacokinetics of zidovudine in patients with liver cirrhosis. *Clin Pharmacol Ther* 1990;47:731–9.

123. Acosta EP et al. Clinical pharmacokinetics of zidovudine: an update. *Clin Pharmacokinet* 1996;4:251–62.

124. Steffe EM et al. The effect of acetaminophen on zidovudine metabolism in HIV-infected patients. *J Acquir Immune Defic Syndr* 1990;3:691–4.

125. Chambers HF, Neu HC. Penicillins. In Mandell GL et al., eds. *Principles and practice of infectious diseases*, 4th ed. New York: Churchill Livingstone; 1995:233–46.

126. Barza M. Antimicrobial spectrum, pharmacology and therapeutic use of antibiotics. Part 2: Penicillins. *Am J Hosp Pharm* 1977;34:57–67.

127. Weber DJ et al. Amoxicillin and potassium clavulanate: an antibiotic combination. *Pharmacotherapy* 1984;4:122–36.

128. Sutherland R. ß-lactam/ß-lactamase inhibitor combinations: development, antibacterial activity and clinical applications. *Infection* 1995;23:191–200.

129. Noguchi JK, Gill MA. Sulbactam: a ß-lactamase inhibitor. *Clin Pharm* 1988;7:37–51.

130. Neu HC. Antistaphylococcal penicillins. *Med Clin North Am* 1982;66:51–60.

131. Johnson DH, Cunha BA. Aztreonam. *Med Clin North Am* 1995;79:733–43.

132. Brogden RN, Heel RC. Aztreonam. A review of its antibacterial activity, pharmacokinetic properties and therapeutic uses. *Drugs* 1986;31:96–130.

133. Donowitz GR, Mandell GL. Beta-lactam antibiotics (2 parts). *N Engl J Med* 1988;318:419–26, 490–500.

134. Cunha BA. Third-generation cephalosporins: a review. *Clin Ther* 1992;14:616–47.

135. Nightingale CH et al. Pharmacokinetics and clinical use of cephalosporin antibiotics. *J Pharm Sci* 1975;64:1899–927.

136. Barriere SL, Flaherty JF. Third-generation cephalosporins: a critical evaluation. *Clin Pharm* 1984;3:351–73.

137. Karchmer AW. Cephalosporins. In Mandell GL et al., eds. *Principles and practice of infectious diseases*, 4th ed. New York: Churchill Livingstone; 1995:247–64.

138. Rodman DP et al. A critical review of the new oral cephalosporins. *Arch Fam Med* 1994;3:975–80.

139. Fassbender M et al. Pharmacokinetics of new oral cephalosporins, including a new carbacephem. *Clin Infect Dis* 1993;16:646–53.

140. Force RW, Nahata MC. Loracarbef: a new orally administered carbacephem antibiotic. *Ann Pharmacother* 1993;27:321–9.

141. Cooper RDG. The carbacephems: a new beta-lactam antibiotic class. *Am J Med* 1992;92(suppl 6A):2S–6S.

142. DiPiro JT, May JR. Use of cephalosporins with enhanced anti-anaerobic activity for treatment and prevention of anaerobic and mixed infections. *Clin Pharm* 1988;7:285–302.

143. Ward A, Richards DM. Cefotetan. A review of its antibacterial activity, pharmacokinetic properties and therapeutic use. *Drugs* 1985;30:382–426.

144. Schaad UB et al. A comparison of ceftriaxone and cefuroxime for the treatment of bacterial meningitis in children. *N Engl J Med* 1990;322:141–7.

145. Petz LD. Immunologic cross-reactivity between penicillins and cephalosporins: a review. *J Infect Dis* 1978;137(suppl):S74–9.

146. Lipsky JJ. Antibiotic-associated hypoprothrombinemia. *J Antimicrob Chemother* 1988;21:281–300.

147. Schaad UB et al. Reversible ceftriaxone-associated biliary pseudolithiasis in children. *Lancet* 1988;2:1411–3.

148. Shiffman ML et al. Pathogenesis of ceftriaxone-associated biliary sludge. *Gastroenterology* 1990;99:1772–8.

149. Cunha BA, Gill MV. Cefepime. *Med Clin North Am* 1995;79:721–32.

150. Barradell LB, Bryson HM. Cefepime. A review of its antibacterial activity, pharmacokinetic properties and therapeutic use. *Drugs* 1994;47:471–505.

151. Friedland IR, McCracken GH Jr. Management of infections caused by antibiotic-resistant *Streptococcus pneumoniae*. *N Engl J Med* 1994;331:377–82.

152. Smith BR, LeFrock JL. Cefuroxime: antibacterial activity, pharmacology, and clinical efficacy. *Ther Drug Monit* 1983;5:149–60.

153. Drusano GL et al. The acylampicillins: mezlocillin, piperacillin, and azlocillin. *Rev Infect Dis* 1984;6:13–32.

154. Holmes B et al. Piperacillin. A review of its antibacterial activity, pharmacokinetic properties and therapeutic use. *Drugs* 1984;28:375–425.

155. Clissold SP et al. Imipenem/cilastatin. A review of its antibacterial activity, pharmacokinetic properties and therapeutic efficacy. *Drugs* 1987;33:183–241.

156. Norrby SR. Carbapenems. *Med Clin North Am* 1995;79:745–59.

157. Ahonkhai VI et al. Imipenem-cilastatin in pediatric patients: an overview of safety and efficacy in studies conducted in the United States. *Pediatr Infect Dis J* 1989;8:740–7.

158. Calandra GB et al. Review of adverse experiences and tolerability in the first 2,516 patients treated with imipenem/cilastatin. *Am J Med* 1985;78(suppl 6A):73–8.

159. Saxon A. Immediate hypersensitivity reactions to beta-lactam antibiotics. *Ann Intern Med* 1987;107: 204–15.

160. Wiseman LR et al. Meropenem. A review of its antibacterial activity, pharmacokinetic properties and clinical efficacy. *Drugs* 1995;50:73–101.

161. Pryka RD, Haig GM. Meropenem: a new carbapenem antimicrobial. *Ann Pharmacother* 1994;28:1045–54.

162. Mouton JW, van den Anker JN. Meropenem clinical pharmacokinetics. *Clin Pharmacokinet* 1995;28: 275–86.

163. Wright AJ, Wilkowske CJ. The penicillins. *Mayo Clin Proc* 1987;62:806–20.

164. Weiss ME, Adkinson NF Jr. ß-lactam allergy. In Mandell GL et al., eds. *Principles and practice of infectious diseases*, 4th ed. New York: Churchill Livingstone; 1995:272–8.

165. Plaisance KI, Nightingale CH. Pharmacology of cephalosporins. In Queener SF et al., eds. *Beta-lactam antibiotics for clinical use*. New York: Marcel Dekker; 1986:285–347.

166. Dudley MN, Nightingale CH. Effects of protein binding on the pharmacology of cephalosporins. In Neu HC, ed. *New beta-lactam antibiotics: a review from chemistry to clinical efficacy of the new cephalosporins*. Philadelphia: Francis Clarke Wood Institute for the History of Medicine; 1982:227–39.

167. Carver P et al. Comparative pharmacokinetic study of cefotetan and cefoxitin in healthy volunteers. *Infect Surg* 1986;(April suppl):11–4.

168. Wise R. The pharmacokinetics of the oral cephalosporins: a review. *J Antimicrob Chemother* 1990;26(suppl E):13–20.

169. Melikian DM, Flaherty JF. Antimicrobial agents. In Schrier RW, Gambertoglio JG, eds. *Handbook of drug therapy in liver and kidney disease*, 1st ed. Boston: Little, Brown; 1991:14–45.

170. Klepser ME et al. Clinical pharmacokinetics of newer cephalosporins. *Clin Pharmacokinet* 1995;28:361–84.

171. Hardin TC et al. Comparison of ampicillin-sulbactam and ticarcillin-clavulanic acid in patients with chronic renal failure: effects of differential pharmacokinetics on serum bactericidal activity. *Pharmacotherapy* 1994;14:147–52.

172. Bahal N, Nahata MC. The new macrolide antibiotics: azithromycin, clarithromycin, dirithromycin, and roxithromycin. *Ann Pharmacother* 1992;26:46–55.

173. Schlossberg D. Azithromycin and clarithromycin. *Med Clin North Am* 1995;79:803–15.

174. Berry A et al. Azithromycin therapy for disseminated *Mycobacterium avium-intracellulare* in AIDS patients. First National Conference on Human Retroviruses. Washington, DC. 1993. Abstract #292.

175. 1993 Sexually Transmitted Diseases Treatment Guidelines. *MMWR* 1993;42(RR-14):1–102.

176. Centers for Disease Control and Prevention. Recommendations on prophylaxis and therapy for disseminated *Mycobacterium avium* complex for adults and adolescents infected with human immunodeficiency virus. *MMWR* 1993;42(RR-9):14–20.

177. Havlir D et al. Prophylaxis against disseminated *Mycobacterium avium* complex with weekly azithromycin, daily rifabutin, or both. *N Engl J Med* 1996;335:392–8.

178. McLinn S. Double blind and open label studies of azithromycin in the management of acute otitis media in children: a review. *Pediatr Infect Dis J* 1995;14:S62–6.

179. Hopkins SJ, Williams D. Clinical tolerability and safety of azithromycin in children. *Pediatr Infect Dis J* 1995;14:S67–71.

180. Nahata MC. Pharmacokinetics of azithromycin in pediatric patients: comparison with other agents used for treating otitis media and streptococcal pharyngitis. *Pediatr Infect Dis J* 1995;14:S39–44.

181. Piscitelli SC et al. Clarithromycin and azithromycin: new macrolide antibiotics. *Clin Pharm* 1992;11: 137–52.

182. Rodvold KA, Piscitelli SC. New oral macrolide and fluoroquinolone antibiotics: an overview of pharmacokinetics, interactions, and safety. *Clin Infect Dis* 1993;17(suppl 1):S192–9.

183. Dunn CJ, Barradell LB. Azithromycin: a review of its pharmacological properties and use as 3-day therapy in respiratory tract infections. *Drugs* 1996;51:483–505.

184. Markham A, Mctavish D. Clarithromycin and omeprazole as *Helicobacter pylori* eradication therapy in patients with *H. pylori*-associated gastric disorders. *Drugs* 1996;51:161–78.

185. Brogden RN, Peters DH. Dirithromycin. A review of its antimicrobial activity, pharmacokinetic properties and therapeutic efficacy. *Drugs* 1994;48:599–616.

186. Anon. Dirithromycin. *Med Lett Drugs Ther* 1995;37:109–10.

187. Brittain DC. Erythromycin. *Med Clin North Am* 1987;71:1147–54.

188. Washington JA, Wilson WR. Erythromycin: a microbial and clinical perspective after 30 years of clinical use. (2 parts). *Mayo Clin Proc* 1985;60:189–203, 271–8.

189. Smilack JD et al. Tetracyclines, chloramphenicol, erythromycin, clindamycin, and metronidazole. *Mayo Clin Proc* 1991;66:1270–80.

190. Weber FH et al. Erythromycin: a motilin agonist and gastrointestinal prokinetic agent. *Am J Gastroenterol* 1993;88:485–90.

191. Eichenwald HF. Adverse reactions to erythromycin. *Pediatr Infect Dis J* 1986;5:147–50.

192. Amsden GW. Macrolides versus azalides: a drug interaction update. *Ann Pharmacother* 1995;29:906–17.

193. Peeters TL. Erythromycin and other macrolides as prokinetic agents. *Gastroenterology* 1993;105:1886–99.

194. Lartey PA et al. New developments in macrolides: structures and antibacterial and prokinetic activities. *Adv Pharmacol* 1994;28:307–43.

195. Kreek MJ, Culpepper-Morgan JA. Constipation syndromes. In Lewis JH, ed. *A pharmacologic approach to gastrointestinal disorders.* Baltimore: Williams & Wilkins; 1994:179–208.

196. Dive A et al. Effect of erythromycin on gastric motility in mechanically ventilated critically ill patients: a double-blind, randomized, placebo-controlled study. *Crit Care Med* 1995;23:1356–62.

197. Guay DRP. Macrolide antibiotics in paediatric infectious diseases. *Drugs* 1996;51:515–36.

198. Bloomfield G. A comparison of gastrointestinal tolerance to five different forms of erythromycin. *P&T* 1996;(April):209–14.

199. Dajani AS et al. Prevention of bacterial endocarditis. Recommendations by the American Heart Association. *JAMA* 1990;264:2919-22.

200. Ginsburg CM. Pharmacology of erythromycin in infants and children. *Pediatr Infect Dis J* 1986;5:124–9.

201. Just PM. Overview of the fluoroquinolone antibiotics. *Pharmacotherapy* 1993;13:4S–17.

202. Suh B, Lorber B. Quinolones. *Med Clin North Am* 1995;79:869–94.

203. Schaad UB et al. Use of fluoroquinolones in pediatrics: consensus report of an international society of chemotherapy commission. *Pediatr Infect Dis J* 1995;14:1–9.

204. Schentag JJ, Gross TF. Quinolone pharmacokinetics in the elderly. *Am J Med* 1992;92(suppl 4A):33S–7S.

205. Nightingale CH. Pharmacokinetic considerations in quinolone therapy. *Pharmacotherapy* 1993;13:34S–8.

206. Radandt JM et al. Interactions of fluoroquinolones with other drugs mechanisms, variability, clinical significance, and management. *Clin Infect Dis* 1992;14:272-84.

207. Dudley MN et al. Effect of dose on the serum pharmacokinetics of intravenous ciprofloxacin with identification and characterization of extravascular compartments using noncompartmental and compartmental pharmacokinetic models. *Antimicrob Agents Chemother* 1987;31:1782–6.

208. Forrest A et al. Relationships between renal function and disposition of oral ciprofloxacin. *Antimicrob Agents Chemother* 1988;32:1537–40.

209. Davis R, Bryson HM. Levofloxacin. A review of its antibacterial activity, pharmacokinetics and therapeutic efficacy. *Drugs* 1994;47:677–700.

210. Balfour JA et al. Fleroxacin. A review of its pharmacology and therapeutic efficacy in various infections. *Drugs* 1995;49:794–850.

211. Wadworth AN, Goa KL. Lomefloxacin. A review of its antibacterial activity, pharmacokinetic properties and therapeutic use. *Drugs* 1991;42:1018–60.

212. Foltzer MA, Reese RE. Trimethoprim-sulfamethoxazole and other sulfonamides. *Med Clin North Am* 1987;71:1177–94.

213. Cockerill FR, Edson RS. Trimethoprim-sulfamethoxazole. *Mayo Clin Proc* 1991;66:1260–9.

214. Markowitz N et al. Trimethoprim-sulfamethoxazole compared with vancomycin for the treatment of *Staphylococcus aureus* infection. *Ann Intern Med* 1992;117:390–8.

215. Lundstrom TS, Sobel JD. Vancomycin, trimethoprim-sulfamethoxazole, and rifampin. *Infect Dis Clin North Am* 1995;9:747–67.

216. Goodwin SD. *Pneumocystis carinii* pneumonia in human immunodeficiency virus–infected infants and children. *Pharmacotherapy* 1993;13:640–6.

217. Davey RT Jr, Masur H. Recent advances in the diagnosis, treatment, and prevention of *Pneumocystis carinii* pneumonia. *Antimicrob Agents Chemother* 1990;34:499–504.
218. Pratt WB, Fekety R. The antimetabolites. In Pratt WB, Fekety R., eds. *The antimicrobial drugs.* New York: Oxford University Press; 1986:229–51.
219. Masur H. Prevention and treatment of pneumocystis pneumonia. *N Engl J Med* 1992;327:1853–60.
220. Absar N et al. Desensitization to trimethoprim/sulfamethoxazole in HIV-infected patients. *J Allergy Clin Immunol* 1994;93:1001–5.
221. Standiford HC. Tetracyclines and chloramphenicol. In Mandell GL et al. *Principles and practice of infectious diseases,* 4th ed. New York. Churchill Livingstone; 1995:306–17.
222. Kapusnik-Uner JE et al. Antimicrobial agents: tetracyclines, chloramphenicol, erythromycin and miscellaneous antibacterial agents. In Hardman JG et al., eds. *Goodman and Gilman's the pharmacological basis of therapeutics.* New York: McGraw-Hill; 1996:1130–5.
223. Fingar BL. Sclerosing agents used to control malignant pleural effusions. *Hosp Pharm* 1992;27:622–8.
224. Francke EL, Neu HC. Chloramphenicol and tetracyclines. *Med Clin North Am* 1987;71:1155–68.
225. Wilson WR, Cockerill FR. Tetracyclines, chloramphenicol, erythromycin, and clindamycin. *Mayo Clin Proc* 1987;62:906–15.
226. USP-DI, Vol I. Rockville, MD: The United States Pharmacopoeial Convention; 1996.
227. Haile LG, Flaherty JF. Atovaquone: a review. *Ann Pharmacother* 1993;27:1488–94.
228. Spencer CM, Goa KL. Atovaquone. A review of its pharmacological properties and therapeutic efficacy in opportunistic infections. *Drugs* 1995;50:176–96.
229. Norris AH et al. Chloramphenicol for the treatment of vancomycin-resistant enterococcal infections. *Clin Infect Dis* 1995;20:1137–44.
230. Greenfield RA. Symposium on antimicrobial therapy X. Chloramphenicol, clindamycin, and metronidazole. *J Okla State Med Assoc* 1993;86:336–41.
231. Smilack JD et al. Tetracyclines, chloramphenicol, erythromycin, clindamycin and metronidazole. *Mayo Clin Proc* 1991;66:1270–80.
232. Rayner SA, Buckley RJ. Ocular chloramphenicol and aplastic anemia. Is there a link? *Drug Saf* 1996;14:273–6.
233. Pratt WB, Fekety R. Bacteriostatic inhibitors of protein synthesis. In Pratt WB, Fekety R, eds. *The antimicrobial drugs.* New York: Oxford University Press; 1986:184–228.
234. Dhawan VK, Thadepalli H. Clindamycin: a review of 15 years of clinical experience. *Rev Infect Dis* 1982;4:1133–53.
235. Klainer AS. Clindamycin. *Med Clin North Am* 1987;71:1169–76.
236. Van Arsdel PP et al. The value of skin testing for penicillin allergy diagnosis. *West J Med* 1986;144:311–4.
237. Falagas ME, Gorbach SL. Clindamycin and metronidazole. *Med Clin North Am* 1995;79:845–67.
238. Lau AH et al. Clinical pharmacokinetics of metronidazole and other nitroimidazole anti-infectives. *Clin Pharmacokinet* 1992;23:328–64.
239. Wenisch C et al. Comparison of vancomycin, teicoplanin, metronidazole, and fusidic acid for treatment of *Clostridium difficile*-associated diarrhea. *Clin Infect Dis* 1996;22:813–8.
240. Black M et al. Antimicrobial agents: sulfonamides, trimethoprim-sulfamethoxazole, quinolones. In Hardman JG et al., eds. *Goodman and Gilman's the pharmacological basis of therapeutics.* New York: McGraw-Hill; 1996:1069–70.
241. Wispelwey B, Pearson RD. Pentamidine: a review. *Infect Control Hosp Epidemiol* 1991;12:375–82.
242. Conte JE Jr. Pharmacokinetics of intravenous pentamidine in patients with normal renal function or receiving hemodialysis. *J Infect Dis* 1991;163:169–75.
243. Donnelly H et al. Distribution of pentamidine in patients with AIDS. *J Infect Dis* 1988;157:985–9.
244. Chant C, Rybak MJ. Quinupristin/dalfopristin (RP 59500): a new streptogramin antibiotic. *Ann Pharmacother* 1995;29:1022–7.
245. Bryson HM, Spencer CM. Quinupristin-dalfopristin. *Drugs* 1996;52:406–16.
246. Griswold MW et al. Quinupristin-dalfopristin (RP 59500): an injectable streptogramin combination. *Am J Health-syst Pharm* 1996;53:2045–53.
247. Fulton B et al. Trimetrexate. A review of its pharmacodynamic and pharmacokinetic properties and therapeutic potential in the treatment of *Pneumocystis carinii* pneumonia. *Drugs* 1995;49:563–76.
248. Marshall JL, DeLap RJ. Clinical pharmacokinetics and pharmacology of trimetrexate. *Clin Pharmacokinet* 1994;26:190–200.
249. Lake KD, Peterson CD. A simplified method for initiating vancomycin therapy. *Pharmacotherapy* 1985;5:340–4.
250. Rybak MJ et al. Nephrotoxicity of vancomycin, alone and with an aminoglycoside. *J Antimicrob Chemother* 1990;25:679–87.
251. Matzke GR et al. Clinical pharmacokinetics of vancomycin. *Clin Pharmacokinet* 1986;11:257–82.

252. Newfield P, Roizen MF. Hazards of rapid administration of vancomycin. *Ann Intern Med* 1979;91:581.

253. Healy DP et al. Vancomycin-induced histamine release and "red man syndrome": comparison of 1- and 2-hour infusions. *Antimicrob Agents Chemother* 1990;34:550–4.

254. Edwards DJ, Pancorbo S. Routine monitoring of serum vancomycin concentrations: waiting for proof of its value. *Clin Pharm* 1987;6:652–4.

255. Farber BF, Mollering RC. Retrospective study of the toxicity of preparations of vancomycin from 1974–1981. *Antimicrob Agents Chemother* 1983;23:138–41.

Antineoplastics, Chemoprotectants, and Immunosuppressants

Antineoplastics

Antineoplastics. The agents included in this section are those having widespread use in cancer chemotherapy. Agents with therapeutic importance in small patient populations are not included.

Information on the dosage of these drugs has largely been determined empirically, and clinical investigations are continually being performed to find safer and more effective dosage regimens. Thus, dosages in this section should only be considered as guidelines based on the most widely accepted usage at the time of this writing. Because space does not permit detailed discussions of the toxicity, dosage regimens, and other aspects of these drugs, the reader should become familiar with specific agents before initiating treatment.[1] References are provided in this section for more detailed information concerning the proper and safe use of these agents. If specific investigational protocols are available, these may also provide information that is unavailable from other sources, especially with regard to dosage and regimens.

Cancer chemotherapeutic agents as a class are the most toxic drugs in use. Adverse reactions listed represent those most likely to occur with the usual doses and methods of use. Infrequent, but serious reactions are also listed; however, the lists of adverse reactions are not comprehensive. Nausea and vomiting are important side effects of these agents that can be adequately treated by current antiemetics alone or in combination. In order to tailor antiemetic therapy better to the emetic potential of the chemotherapy, a standard rating scale is used in these monographs. Several points to remember are that emetogenicity is dose dependent, combinations of chemotherapeutic agents result in greater emetogenic potential than the drug(s) used alone, and emetogenic potentials are best defined in adults and do not necessarily apply to children. The categories of emetogenicity used are as follows:[2]

CATEGORY	PERCENTAGE OF PATIENTS AFFECTED
High	>90
Moderately high	60–90
Moderate	30–60
Moderately low	10–30
Low	<10

Class Instructions: Antineoplastics. This drug is very potent, and some side effects can be expected to occur with its use. Be sure that you understand the possible dangers as well as the possible benefits of the drug before you begin to take it.

Cytotoxic Agents. Because this drug can decrease your body's ability to fight infections, report any signs of infection such as fever, shaking chills, or sore throat immediately. Also report any unusual bruising or bleeding, shortness of breath, or painful or burning urination. Avoid the use of aspirin-containing products, and avoid alcohol or use it in moderation. Nausea, vomiting, or hair loss may sometimes occur with this drug. The severity of these effects depends on the individual, the dosage, and other drugs that may be given at the same time. This drug may cause temporary or sometimes permanent sterility in men and women. It may also cause birth defects if the father is taking the drug at the time of conception or if the mother is taking it any time during pregnancy. If you are breastfeeding, this drug may appear in the milk and cause problems in your baby; therefore, use an alternate method of feeding your baby.

Alkylating Agents

ALTRETAMINE   Hexalen

Altretamine (formerly hexamethylmelamine) acts primarily as an alkylating agent. It is used in combination chemotherapy of ovarian cancer and is also active in cervical and lung cancers. Oral bioavailability is incomplete and erratic, and may be dose dependent. Altretamine is N-demethylated to pentamethylmelamine by hepatic microsomal enzymes. The serum half-life ranges from 4.7–10.2 hr, with >50% of a dose renally excreted in 24 hr and less than 1% excreted unchanged. Nausea, vomiting, and abdominal cramps may be dose limiting in some patients. Neurotoxic effects are frequent, including agitation, hallucinations, and confusion; these are reversible and amenable to dosage reduction. Anemia, leukopenia, and thrombocytopenia are typically mild. As a single agent, oral dosage is 260 mg/m^2/day in 4 divided doses for as long as 2–5 weeks. Lower dosages are required if altretamine is combined with other myelosuppressive agents.[3–5] It is available as 50-mg capsules. The water-soluble metabolite pentamethylmelamine is now in clinical trials as an injection.

BUSULFAN   Myleran

CHLORAMBUCIL   Leukeran

MELPHALAN   Alkeran

Pharmacology. These drugs are water-soluble compounds that alkylate DNA, forming a variety of covalent cross-links. The drugs are polyfunctional and may form more than one covalent bond to susceptible cell constituents (typically the N^7 position of guanine). They are cell cycle phase nonspecific and chemically stable enough for oral absorption before appreciable alkylator activation occurs.

Administration and Dosage.

	BUSULFAN	CHLORAMBUCIL	MELPHALAN
Administration	PO.	PO.	PO; IV.
Adult Dosage	Up to 8 mg/day (usually 1–3 mg/day).	0.1–0.2 mg/kg/day for 1 day; or 6–12 mg/day maintenance; or 0.4 mg/kg q 2–4 weeks.[6]	PO 7 mg/m² for 4 days; or 2–4 mg/day maintenance for multiple myeloma.[7] IV 16 mg/m² q 2 weeks for for 4 doses, then q 4 weeks.
Pediatric Dosage	CML 0.06–0.12 mg/kg.	Non-Hodgkin's lymphoma, CLL, nephrotic syndrome, rheumatoid arthritis (initial) 0.1–0.2 mg/kg/day.	—
Geriatric Dosage	Same as adult dosage, but adjust for age-related reduction in renal function.		

Special Populations. *Other Conditions.* Elimination is significantly correlated with the GFR. Studies in nephrectomized animals demonstrate markedly increased myelotoxicity with unadjusted melphalan doses. Thus, one group currently recommends a 50% decrease in the melphalan dosage for BUN >30 mg/dL or Cr_s >1.5 mg/dL.[8] Reduce IV melphalan dosage to 75% of normal for WBC counts of 3000–4000/µL or platelet counts of 75,000–100,000/µL, or to 50% for WBC counts of 2000–3000/µL or platelet counts of 50,000–75,000/µL, respectively; do not give it with WBC counts of <2000/µL or platelet counts of <50,000/µL.[9]

Dosage Forms. (Busulfan) **Tab** 2 mg. (Chlorambucil) **Tab** 2 mg. (Melphalan) **Tab** 2 mg; **Inj** 50 mg.

Patient Instructions. *See* Antineoplastics Class Instructions.

Pharmacokinetics. BUSULFAN   CHLORAMBUCIL   MELPHALAN

Fate.

	BUSULFAN	CHLORAMBUCIL	MELPHALAN
Absorption	Reported by manufacturer to be well absorbed orally.	Oral bioavailability is about 87 ± 20% by radiolabeled drug studies;[10,11] reduced by 10–20% if ingested with food.[12]	Oral bioavailability erratic and incomplete, (mean of 56%, range 25–89%); some patients have no levels after standard doses.[13,14]
Distribution	Homogeneous; good ascites penetration; V_d is 0.99 ± 0.23 L/kg;[10] extensively bound to proteins.	V_d is 0.29 ± 0.21 L/kg; 99% plasma protein bound.[10]	V_d is 0.45 ± 0.15 L/kg; 90 ± 5% plasma protein bound.[10]

	BUSULFAN	CHLORAMBUCIL	MELPHALAN
Metabolism	Extensively metabolized, major fraction as methanesulfonic acid. Cl is 0.27 ± 0.05 L/hr/kg.[10]	Rapid metabolism to a number of inactive metabolites. Cl is 0.16 ± 0.04 L/hr/kg.[10]	Not actively metabolized; spontaneous chemical degradation to mono- and dihydroxy products. Cl is 0.31 ± 0.17 L/hr/kg.[10]
Excretion	No unchanged drug found in urine; however, metabolites are renally excreted.	Less than 1% excreted unchanged in urine over 24 hr.	Unchanged drug 24-hr urinary excretion is 10–15% of a dose.
$t_{\frac{1}{2}}$	Rapid initial serum clearance: 90% of dose after 3 min. $t_{\frac{1}{2}\beta}$ is 2.6 ± 0.5 hr.[10]	1.3 ± 0.9 hr (unchanged drug); 2.5 hr (major metabolite, an amino-phenylacetic acid derivative).[9,10]	IV: $t_{\frac{1}{2}\alpha}$ 8 min; $t_{\frac{1}{2}\beta}$ 1.4 ± 0.2 hr.[10,13,14]

Adverse Reactions. Emetic potential is low. Nausea and vomiting are rare with long-term administration, although large single doses can be strongly emetogenic. Dose-limiting toxicity for this group is typically myelosuppression, with nadirs of 14–21 days for leukopenia and thrombocytopenia after pulse dosage regimens; daily administration results in chronic low indices with cumulative effects. Not uncommonly, blood counts continue to drop after drug discontinuation; fatal pancytopenia has been reported. Therefore, hematologic assessments are important with long-term daily regimens. There may be some selectivity for different normal cell lines by these drugs; busulfan, and perhaps chlorambucil, selectively depresses granulocytes, relatively sparing platelets and lymphoid elements. The nadir for melphalan can be prolonged (4–6 weeks); continuous administration frequently leads to severe myelosuppression (especially platelets) that continues after the drug is discontinued. Pulmonary fibrosis can occasionally occur with all these drugs, especially busulfan; symptoms include cough, dyspnea, and fever; histopathologic changes include bilateral fibrosis. A high-dose glucocorticoid may help early evolving pulmonary disease caused by melphalan and chlorambucil, but "busulfan lung" is usually fatal within 6 months of diagnosis.[15–17] Busulfan frequently causes hyperpigmentation (especially of intertriginous areas) and broad suppression of testicular, ovarian, and adrenal function (occasionally leading to Addisonian crisis). Long-term daily administration of these drugs predisposes patients to drug-induced carcinogenesis, often heralded by preleukemic pancytopenia and culminating in acute myelocytic leukemia. Allergic hypersensitivity reported, especially with melphalan. With prolonged use, sterility occurs with all alkylators; women appear more sensitive than men.

Contraindications. Documented hypersensitivity; inadequate marrow reserve.

Precautions. *See* Special Populations for melphalan use in renal impairment.

Drug Interactions. None known.

Parameters to Monitor. WBC and platelet counts at least monthly; reduce dosage at first sign of appreciable myelosuppression (ie, WBC <3000/μL or platelets

<75,000/µL). Conversely, assess patients receiving oral melphalan for evidence of mild to moderate myelotoxicity to ensure that some absorption is occurring.

CARBOPLATIN   Paraplatin

Pharmacology. Carboplatin is a more stable cyclobutane carboxylato derivative of cisplatin that is slowly activated to expose two DNA binding sites on the platinum II coordinate complex. The drug binds to DNA by both inter- and intrastrand crosslinks in a fashion similar to, but more delayed than that with cisplatin.[18] It is more water soluble and commensurately less nephrotoxic than cisplatin. Action is cell cycle phase nonspecific.

Administration and Adult Dosage. **IV for refractory ovarian cancer** 360 mg/m^2 q 4 weeks. Administration by continuous infusion has been reported, but is not commonly used.[19–21]

Special Populations. *Pediatric Dosage.* Although not specifically labeled for pediatric use, carboplatin has been safely administered to children. **IV for recurrent brain tumors** 175 mg/m^2/week for 4 weeks.[22]

Geriatric Dosage. Same as adult dosage, but adjust for age-related reduction in renal function.

Other Conditions. Reduce dosage in patients with reduced renal function, a history of prior myelosuppressive therapy, and/or poor bone marrow reserve. Reduce dosage by about 25% if the prior nadir WBC count is <500/µL or the platelet count is <50,000/µL. When Cl_{cr} is 41–59 mL/min, a dose of 250 mg/m^2 is recommended; for Cl_{cr} of 16–40 mL/min, 200 mg/m^2 is recommended. Two prospectively validated formulas for dosage individualization are available. One formula seeks to achieve different target serum AUC values in untreated or pretreated patients: dose (mg) = AUC × (Cl_{cr} + 25), wherein "desired" AUC ranges are 6–8 mg/mL·min for untreated patients and 4–6 mg/mL·min for previously treated patients.[23] The second does not require Cl_{cr} estimates and uses a complex mathematical formula.[24]

Dosage Forms. Inj 50, 150, 450 mg.

Patient Instructions. *See* Antineoplastics Class Instructions, particularly regarding infection risk.

Pharmacokinetics. *Fate.* About 30% of carboplatin is irreversibly bound to plasma proteins; the half-life of this protein-bound fraction is greater than 5 days.[25] V_d is 16–20 L for carboplatin. Carboplatin is slowly hydrolyzed in vivo to a form with two DNA binding sites; the rate of hydrolysis is much slower than the rate of chloride loss with cisplatin. The free (unbound) fraction of carboplatin and its hydrolyzed species are excreted in urine via both glomerular filtration and tubular secretion. Urinary elimination accounts for over 65% of drug elimination in patients with normal renal function.

$t_{1/2}$. (Unbound) α phase 90 ± 50 min; β phase 180 ± 50 min.[25]

Adverse Reactions. The emetic potential is moderately high to high, but is much less severe than with cisplatin and is easily controlled with antiemetics. Myelosuppression is the primary dose-limiting effect of carboplatin, and thrombocytopenia tends to be more severe than leukopenia; about 25% of previously untreated and 35% of previously treated ovarian cancer patients experience thrombocytopenia. The thrombocytopenic nadir for carboplatin as a single agent is approximately 21 days, and patients with preexisting renal dysfunction or poor bone marrow reserve have an increased risk for severe thrombocytopenia. Anemia of a mild degree can also occur in up to 90% of patients; in some studies over 40% of patients required transfusions and 5% of patients experienced hemorrhage. Diarrhea, abdominal pain, or constipation occur in 6–17% of patients. Nephrotoxicity occurs in 1–22% of patients. Unlike cisplatin, carboplatin does not cause cumulative damage to renal tubules. Transient decreases of 20–30% in some serum electrolytes occur, specifically magnesium, potassium, sodium, and calcium. Hepatic enzyme elevations may occur in one-third of patients, but they are not associated with serious or prolonged liver injury. Peripheral neuropathies occur in less than 10% of patients; however, the risk increases in patients over 65 yr or if large dosages of cisplatin have been administered. CNS symptoms occur in 5% or less of patients, and ototoxicity occurs in 1% of patients. Occasional reactions include allergic hypersensitivity, alopecia, and various cardiovascular events (eg, embolism, cerebrovascular accident, cardiac failure).

Contraindications. The manufacturer lists preexisting renal impairment and myelosuppression as contraindications, but the drug has been given with appropriate dosage modification. *See* Special Populations, Other Conditions.

Precautions. Use with caution in patients with hearing impairment or reduced renal function, or if extensive prior chemotherapy has been administered. Patients with a history of prior cisplatin therapy are at a higher risk for nephrotoxic and neurotoxic sequelae. Vigorous hydration and diuretics are not usually required with carboplatin.

Drug Interactions. Myelotoxicity of carboplatin is additive with other myelotoxic drugs. Concurrent use of other nephrotoxic drugs (such as aminoglycosides) may delay carboplatin elimination and enhance toxicity. Although not well documented, cisplatin interactions may also occur with carboplatin, but at a lesser intensity.

Parameters to Monitor. Measure Cl_{cr} prior to dosage calculation. Monitor platelet and granulocyte counts, and Cr_s during therapy.

CISPLATIN Platinol

Pharmacology. Cisplatin is a planar coordinate dichlorodiammino compound of platinum in the +II valence state. It is aquated in vivo to a positively charged species that can alkylate nucleophilic sites in DNA such as purine and pyrimidine bases. Its action is cell cycle phase nonspecific.

Administration and Adult Dosage. **IV bolus or continuous infusion** (usually with aggressive hydration) single doses of up to 120 mg/m² have been used.[26] **IV in the Einhorn testicular cancer regimen** 20 mg/m²/day for 5 days.[27] *See* Notes.

Special Populations. *Pediatric Dosage.* **IV** 10–20 mg/m²/day for 4–5 days, repeat q 3–4 weeks. **IV** maximum single dose is 100 mg/m² given q 2–3 weeks.[26]

Geriatric Dosage. Same as adult dosage, but adjust for age-related reduction in renal function.

Other Conditions. Reduce dosage in renal impairment; specific dosage reduction guidelines have not been established.

Dosage Forms. Inj 10, 50 mg.

Patient Instructions. *See* Antineoplastics Class Instructions. Be prepared for severe nausea and vomiting following drug administration.

Pharmacokinetics. *Serum Levels.* In vitro cell culture data suggest cytotoxicity at levels of 50 mg/L for 1 hr or 5 mg/L for 8 hr.

Fate. Peak serum levels of free platinum following a 100 mg/m^2 bolus are about 3.4 mg/L when given with mannitol (12.5 g) and 2.7 mg/L without mannitol.[28] Over 90% of platinum is protein bound to RBCs, albumin, and prealbumin. It is freely distributed to most organs including kidneys, liver, skin, and lungs, and has minimal accumulation in CSF only after repeated doses. Cumulative 24-hr urinary excretion of platinum is 20% with mannitol, 40% without.

t$_{1/2}$. Free platinum 48 min (without mannitol); 59 min (with mannitol). Terminal half-life is 58–73 hr, probably reflecting slow release of protein-bound drug.[28,29]

Adverse Reactions. Emetic potential is high. Nausea and vomiting are severe and often prolonged (days), and may be managed with aggressive prophylaxis using a serotonin 5HT$_3$-antagonist, butyrophenone (eg, droperidol), metoclopramide, a high-dose glucocorticoid, or a combination. Primary toxicity is dose-related nephrotoxicity, especially proximal tubular impairment. Ototoxicity and elevated hepatic enzymes occur frequently; total dose-related hypomagnesemia and severe cumulative peripheral neuropathy occur. Slight leukopenia, thrombocytopenia, and frequent anemia also occur. Epoetin alfa is useful in preventing severe anemia caused by cisplatin. Rare toxicities include transient cortical dysfunction (blindness) and hypersensitivity (including anaphylaxis).

Contraindications. Renal insufficiency (Cr$_s$ >1.5–2 mg/dL or Cl$_{cr}$ <60 mL/min); myelosuppression; hearing impairment; previous anaphylaxis. However, some patients with prior anaphylaxis have been successfully retreated with cisplatin and concomitant antihistamine, epinephrine, and glucocorticoid.

Precautions. Use with caution in renal impairment and with other nephrotoxic drugs, especially aminoglycosides.[30] Assure adequate hydration prior to administration. Both furosemide and mannitol are used to decrease platinum nephrotoxicity, although each apparently retards free platinum elimination.

Drug Interactions. Cisplatin may enhance nephrotoxicity and ototoxicity of the aminoglycosides. Use with ifosfamide may increase nephrotoxicity and potassium and magnesium loss, especially in children. Furosemide ototoxicity may be increased by cisplatin. Cisplatin can increase methotrexate serum levels and its toxicity. Cisplatin can decrease absorption and serum levels of valproic acid. Phenytoin serum levels may be decreased following cisplatin-containing combination regimens.

Parameters to Monitor. Assess renal function prior to each dose (eg, serial BUN or Cr$_s$) and serum magnesium levels periodically.

Notes. Reconstitute with sterile water; it may then be mixed in saline-containing solutions. It is stable for 24 hr in mannitol. Do not expose solution to metals (eg, metal drippers or cannulae), because platinum may rapidly plate onto these surfaces. Hydrate the patient with at least 1 L of a saline-containing solution with 20 mEq of KCl and 3 g of $MgSO_4/L$.[31]

CYCLOPHOSPHAMIDE   Cytoxan, Various

Pharmacology. Cyclophosphamide is inactive in vitro and must be enzymatically activated in the liver to yield both active alkylating compounds and toxic metabolites.[32] Cell cycle phase nonspecific.

Administration and Adult Dosage. IV or PO alone or in combination regimens 250–500 mg/m² q 3–4 weeks. **IV (usually) or PO in high-dose intermittent regimens (including bone marrow transplant)** maximum of 40–50 mg/kg given once or over 2–5 days, repeat q 2–4 weeks—these doses are not well tolerated orally. IV doses may be given in any convenient volume of all common IV solutions or by IV push. **Continuous daily administration PO** 1–5 mg/kg/day; during continuous therapy, dosage must be individualized based on patient bone marrow response.

Special Populations. *Pediatric Dosage.* IV, PO for **malignancies** same as adult dosage. **PO for nephrotic syndrome** 2.5–3 mg/kg/day for up to 8 weeks.

Geriatric Dosage. Same as adult dosage.

Other Conditions. No dosage alteration appears necessary in renal impairment, because differences in toxicity between normals and patients with renal failure have not been reported.[33]

Dosage Forms. Tab 25, 50 mg; **Inj** 100, 200, 500 mg, 1, 2 g.

Patient Instructions. *See* Antineoplastics Class Instructions. Drink 2–3 quarts of fluids daily (1–2 quarts in smaller children) and urinate frequently; do *not* take oral doses at bedtime. Report any blood in the urine.

Pharmacokinetics. *Fate.* Oral absorption is 74 ± 22%.[10] Metabolized to active compounds (including the highly toxic nonalkylating aldehyde, acrolein, and the principal alkylator, phosphoramide mustard) primarily by hepatic microsomal mixed-function oxidases. Cyclophosphamide is 13% plasma protein bound; its alkylating metabolites are 50% bound. V_d is 0.78 ± 0.57 L/kg for parent drug; Cl is 0.078 ± 0.03 L/hr/kg.[10] Renal elimination accounts for 6.5 ± 4.3% of unchanged drug and 60% of metabolites,[34] with a mean renal clearance of 0.66 L/hr of unchanged drug.[33] Clearance may be reduced in obese patients. Elimination is linear over a wide range of doses.[32]

$t_{1/2}$. (Serum alkylating activity) 7.5 ± 4 hr, slightly longer in patients on allopurinol or those previously exposed to cyclophosphamide;[10,33,34] unchanged in renal dysfunction.[35]

Adverse Reactions. Emetic potential is moderate to high (>1 g). Nausea, vomiting, and alopecia are frequent and dose dependent. Dose-limiting toxicity is myelosuppression with a WBC nadir of about 10 days; platelets are also suppressed, perhaps to a lesser extent. Transient, reversible blurred vision occurs frequently. The drug is locally nonirritating. Renally eliminated active metabolites occasionally cause sterile hemorrhagic cystitis, which may resolve slowly, often leading to a fibrotic, contracted bladder. Bladder epithelial changes range from minimal to frank neoplasia. An early sign of cystitis is microscopic hematuria, which can lead to hemorrhage. Prophylactic hydration is recommended. To prevent urotoxicity with high-dose regimens, administer **mesna** (*see* Mesna). **Acetylcysteine** (Mucomyst) bladder irrigations may have antidotal activity. Rarely, bladder dysplasia can lead to bladder cancer after very high doses or with concurrent or prior bladder radiation. Cross-allergenicity with other alkylators (eg, mechlorethamine) may occur. Ovarian and testicular function may be permanently lost following high-dose, long-term therapy. Rare reactions include a high-dose fatal cardiomyopathy, "allergic" interstitial pneumonitis, and a transient condition similar to SIADH that is preventable with vigorous isotonic hydration.

Contraindications. Previous life-threatening hypersensitivity to cyclophosphamide; marked leukopenia and thrombocytopenia; hemorrhagic cystitis; severe pulmonary toxicity caused by prior alkylator therapy.

Precautions. Pregnancy. Consider dosage reduction or discontinuation of drug in patients who develop infections.

Drug Interactions. Cyclophosphamide may prolong the action of neuromuscular blocking agents. Allopurinol and cimetidine may enhance cyclophosphamide myelotoxicity.

Parameters to Monitor. Prior to induction therapy, assess the patient for adequate numbers of WBCs ($>3500/\mu L$) and platelets ($>120,000/\mu L$). With long-term use, assess these counts at least monthly. Monitor closely for hematuria, especially if the patient has received a large cumulative dosage.

Notes. Do not dilute with benzyl alcohol–preserved solutions. Diluted solution is stable for 24 hr at room temperature and 6 days under refrigeration. Widely used in both hematologic and solid malignancies, and as an immunosuppressant in a variety of autoimmune disorders.

DACARBAZINE   DTIC-Dome

Dacarbazine is an imidazole analogue of a purine precursor that alkylates DNA via methyldiazonium in a cell cycle phase nonspecific fashion. It is used in malignant melanoma with about a 10–20% objective response rate. The drug is extensively metabolized, some microsomally mediated (50% by N-demethylation); it is 5% plasma protein bound, with 30–45% of a dose excreted unchanged in the urine. The drug has an α half-life of 35 min and a β half-life of about 5 hr; in one patient with renal and hepatic dysfunction, the terminal half-life increased to 7.2 hr. Nausea and vomiting, which are occasionally severe, occur almost invariably; these may decrease in severity with successive courses of therapy. Dose- and duration-dependent sterility, mutagenicity, and teratogenicity have been reported. Pain on injection also occurs. The dose-limiting toxicity is myelosuppression, with a leukopenic nadir at 21–25 days. Occasionally, a flulike syndrome of myalgia, fever, and malaise occurs within 1 week of drug administration. Use dacarbazine with caution in patients with preexisting bone marrow aplasia, and avoid exposure to sunlight because of possible photosensitivity reactions. The drug is light sensitive, therefore minimize exposure to light after reconstitution. The reconstituted solution is clear to pale yellow and is stable for 8 hr after reconstitution at room temperature; pink discoloration denotes drug decomposition. The drug is administered IV as a single dose of up to 850 mg/m^2, repeated in 3–4 weeks. Alternatively, it may be given in a dosage of up to 250 mg/m^2/day for 5 days, repeated in 3–4 weeks. Reduce the dosage in renal and/or hepatic impairment.[36,37] Available as 100-, 200-, and 500-mg injection.

IFOSFAMIDE   Ifex

Pharmacology. Ifosfamide is a structural analogue of the alkylating agent cyclophosphamide (CTX). The rate of hepatic conversion of ifosfamide to the active metabolite 4-hydroxyifosfamide is slightly slower than with CTX, although formation of the bladder toxin acrolein is not reduced. The ultimate metabolite ifosforamide mustard crosslinks DNA to impair cell division. The drug is always given with mesna to prevent urotoxicity. Although labeled for use in refractory testicular cancer, ifosfamide also has useful activity against soft tissue sarcoma, malignant lymphoma, and small cell lung cancer.[38] Ifosfamide is cell cycle phase nonspecific.

Administration and Adult Dosage. IV for refractory testicular cancer 1.2 g/m^2/day over 30 min to 4 hr for 5 days, or 2 g/m^2/day for 3 consecutive days. The recommended concurrent IV mesna dose is 20% of the ifosfamide dose, given 15 min before ifosfamide and again at 4 and 8 hr. It can be directly admixed with ifosfamide. The latter two mesna doses can be given orally at twice the dose (ie, each at 40% of the ifosfamide dose) if patient compliance and a lack of emesis can be assured.[39] **Alternatively, IV by continuous infusion** 5–8 g/m^2 over 24 hr with mesna added at the same concentration as ifosfamide.[40] However, more severe nephrotoxicity may occur with this regimen.[41]

Special Populations. *Pediatric Dosage.* IV for sarcomas (Ewing's and osteosarcoma) 1.2 g/m^2/day over 30 min for 5 days, each with 3 IV mesna doses as above.[42,43]

Geriatric Dosage. Same as adult dosage, but adjust for age-related reduction in renal function.

Other Conditions. Dosage reduction is indicated in patients with reduced renal function, although specific guidelines are not available.

Dosage Forms. Inj 1, 3 g.

Patient Instructions. (*See* Antineoplastics Class Instructions.)

Pharmacokinetics. *Fate.* Ifosfamide, but not its metabolites, penetrates into the CNS; CSF levels are about 38–49% of simultaneous serum levels. Ifosfamide is metabolized to the active alkylating agent ifosforamide mustard by CYP2B6, which converts ifosfamide to 4-hydroxyifosfamide (which may act as the transport form of the molecule). The 4-hydroxy metabolite is then chemically or enzymatically broken down to active and inactive metabolites. Inactive metabolites include 4-carboxyifosfamide and several dechloroethylated species such as thiodiacetic acid. About 60–80% of a dose is excreted in the urine over 72 hr, including up to 50% of unchanged drug. In addition to 4-hydroxyifosfamide, the bladder irritant acrolein is also excreted renally and can accumulate to high concentrations in the urinary bladder.[44,45]

$t_{1/2}$. 6.9 hr.[46]

Adverse Reactions. Emetic potential is moderate; nausea and vomiting can be readily managed with antiemetics. Alopecia occurs in most patients treated with ifosfamide. The major dose-limiting effect of ifosfamide is urotoxicity manifested as hematuria. The frequency of microscopic hematuria with ifosfamide and the chemoprotectant mesna ranges from 5–18% of courses;[38] gross hematuria is less common (<5%) (*see* Mesna). Renal tubular toxicity, manifested by elevations in BUN and Cr_s, occurs in less than 10% of patients. It is more frequent in patients who are poorly hydrated or have preexisting abnormal renal function,[47] those with renal cell cancer,[48] those given high-dose 24-hr continuous ifosfamide infusions,[49] and those receiving concomitant treatment with other nephrotoxins.[47] Myelosuppression primarily involves leukopenia with a 7- to 14-day nadir. This effect is less severe than with cyclophosphamide and rarely affects platelets. However, in combination with other myelosuppressive drugs, additive leukopenia may occur that is not reduced by mesna. Leukopenia has been particularly severe in nephrectomized patients with renal cell cancer.[49] CNS toxicities occur in up to 50% of patients, but risk factors, including dosage, are unclear. The most common effect is a slight sedation or somnolence, which rarely proceeds to coma and death. These signs appear within 2 hr and typically remit 1–3 days after drug administration. Other rare CNS neurotoxicities include cerebellar toxicity (ataxia), urinary incontinence, and seizures.[50] Some of these CNS effects may be caused by the minor metabolite chloracetaldehyde, which is excreted in the urine and accumulates in renal failure.[51] Transient elevation in liver function tests is frequently reported, but is rarely clinically important. Other occasional toxic effects include allergic reactions, diarrhea, peripheral neuropathy, and stomatitis.

Contraindications. Severe preexisting myelosuppression.

Precautions. Because of more severe nephrotoxicity and CNS toxicities, patients with reduced renal function, and particularly nephrectomized renal cell cancer patients, are poor candidates for this agent. Withhold repeat therapy until there is resolution of microscopic hematuria (<10 RBCs per high-power field). An adequate state of hydration is critical to reducing urotoxicity.

Drug Interactions. Use with cisplatin may increase nephrotoxicity and potassium and magnesium loss, especially in children. Nephrotoxicity is also enhanced when ifosfamide is combined with other nephrotoxic drugs.

Parameters to Monitor. Ensure that renal function and peripheral WBC counts are normal prior to administration. During therapy, monitor hematuria daily because dosage reduction or higher mesna dosage may prevent more serious urotoxicity.

Notes. Ifosfamide is compatible with D5W, NS, Ringer's lactate injection, and sterile water. It can also be directly mixed with mesna. Exercise caution to reduce exposure during handling and disposal.

MECHLORETHAMINE HYDROCHLORIDE   Mustargen

Pharmacology. Mechlorethamine (nitrogen mustard; HN_2) is a prototype bischloroethylamine, polyfunctional alkylating agent. In solution, the compound readily ionizes to an active form, which can alkylate at a number of nucleophilic protein sites, principally the N^7 position of guanine in both DNA and RNA. This action is cell cycle phase nonspecific.

Administration and Adult Dosage. **IV for Hodgkin's disease** (in the classical MOPP regimen) 6 mg/m^2 by careful push on days 1 and 8 of a monthly treatment cycle.[52] Irritation, spasm, and sclerosis occur in exposed veins; therefore, it is common to begin venipunctures low on the limb and move up serially, and to administer mechlorethamine last in a combination drug sequence. **IV as a single agent** up to 0.4 mg/kg as a single monthly dose. **Top for mycosis fungoides and psoriasis** 10 mg/60 mL of water, applied to the affected body areas 1 or 2 times a day.[53]

Special Populations. *Pediatric Dosage.* **IV** same as adult dosage.

Geriatric Dosage. Same as adult dosage.

Dosage Forms. **Inj** 10 mg.

Patient Instructions. *See* Antineoplastics Class Instructions.

Pharmacokinetics. *Fate.* Chemical cyclization occurs in vivo to form positively charged carbonium ions, which rapidly react with various cellular components; unchanged drug cannot be detected in the blood within minutes of administration. Less than 0.01% of unchanged drug is recovered in the urine; however, up to 50% of radioactively labeled products may be found in urine within 24 hr.[1]

Adverse Reactions. Emetic potential is high; nausea and vomiting within the first 3 hr are severe and may last over 1 day. The major dose-limiting toxicity is myelosuppression: leukopenic nadir occurs at 6–8 days, thrombocytopenic nadir at 10–16 days. Extravasation causes delayed and protracted (months) ulceration and necrosis; a 1/6 molar sodium **thiosulfate** solution (4 mL of 10% sodium thiosulfate plus 6 mL sterile water) and copious flushing with water may be used as topical antidotes to lessen serious tissue damage. Primary reproductive failure and alopecia are frequent in both males and females. IV or topical use can cause maculopapular rashes and sometimes severe sensitivity reactions (anaphylaxis and occasional cross-reactivity with other alkylating agents).

Contraindications. Prior severe hypersensitivity reactions; preexisting profound myelosuppression; infection.

Precautions. Give patients with lymphomas (especially "bulky" lymphomas) prophylactic allopurinol 2–3 days prior to and throughout therapy to prevent hyperuricemia and urate nephropathy following massive tumor lysis. Make every effort to avoid topical contact with this highly vesicant drug by health personnel.

Drug Interactions. None known.

Parameters to Monitor. Pretreatment and at least monthly assessment of bone marrow function, particularly WBC and platelet counts.

Notes. Mechlorethamine is a powerful vesicant and should be prepared with great caution. Use mask and rubber gloves during preparation and avoid inhalation of dust and vapors, or contact with skin and mucous membranes, especially the eyes. Use the injection within 1 hr of preparation; topical solution and ointment are stable for 1 month under refrigeration.[54] Because of its extreme acute toxicity, use is limited primarily to malignant lymphomas[52] and topically in mycosis fungoides, a cutaneous non-Hodgkin's T-cell lymphoma.[55]

MITOMYCIN   Mutamycin

Mitomycin (mitomycin C) is an antibiotic that contains quinone, urethane, and aziridine groups. It is activated chemically and metabolically to alkylating species; it is cell cycle phase nonspecific, but maximum efficacy is in the G_1 and S phases. Mitomycin is used primarily in GI tract tumors intravenously and in bladder cancer intravesically. Following IV doses of 15 mg/m^2, the peak serum level is about 1 mg/L (3 μmol/L). The drug is eliminated primarily by hepatic clearance, with about 20% hepatic extraction and 10–30% recovery of unchanged drug in the urine. Cl is 0.3–0.4 L/hr/kg. The drug has an α half-life of 5–10 min after IV injection and ß half-life of 46 min. Nausea, vomiting, diarrhea, alopecia, and nephrotoxicity occur frequently. The drug also produces sterility, mutagenicity, and teratogenicity. The dose-limiting toxicities are myelosuppression (with a long leukopenic nadir of 3–4 weeks), thrombocytopenia, and anemia, all of which may be cumulative. Monitor the patient carefully for delayed and prolonged myelosuppression. Severe ulceration may occur if the drug is extravasated (topical **DMSO** may be useful). Interstitial pneumonia, for which a glucocorticoid is helpful, occurs occasionally. Long-term therapy occasionally causes hemolytic-uremic syndrome. Mitomycin is contraindicated in patients with preexisting severe myelosuppression or anemia. As a single agent, mitomycin is given IV in a single dose of 10–15 mg/m^2 and repeated q 6 weeks if hematologic toxicity has resolved. In combination regimens, it is given in doses of 5–10 mg/m^2 repeated in 4–6 weeks. Up to 60 mg/week may be given intravesically in bladder cancer.[56–59] Available as 5-, 20-, and 40-mg injection.

NITROSOUREAS:

CARMUSTINE   BiCNU

LOMUSTINE   CeeNU

Pharmacology. Carmustine (BCNU) and lomustine (CCNU) are highly lipid soluble drugs which are metabolized to active alkylating and carbamoylating moieties. Several key cellular enzymatic steps are inhibited, including those involving DNA polymerase and RNA and protein synthesis. There is typically only partial cross-resistance to classical alkylators. The nitrosoureas are cell cycle phase nonspecific and even have activity on G_0 (resting phase) cells.

Administration and Dosage.

	CARMUSTINE	LOMUSTINE
Administration	IV in 100–200 mL D5W in glass containers only over 15–45 min.	PO only.
Adult Dosage	75–100 mg/m^2/day for 1–2 days or 200 mg/m^2 as a single dose, or 80 mg/m^2/day for 3 days. Repeat at 6- to 8-week intervals.	100–130 mg/m^2 as a single dose, repeat at 6- to 8-week intervals.
Pediatric Dosage	Same as adult dosage.	Same as adult dosage.

	CARMUSTINE	LOMUSTINE
Geriatric Dosage	Reduce dosage by 25–50% and/or increase treatment interval to at least 8 weeks.	Same as adult dosage.
Other Conditions	Treat patients with heavily pretreated bone marrow with 50–75% of the recommended dosage and/or at lengthened treatment intervals (8 weeks minimum).	

Dosage Forms. (Carmustine) **Inj** 100 mg with alcohol diluent. (Lomustine) **Cap** 10, 40, 100 mg—commercial packet contains two of each strength for a total of 300 mg.

Patient Instructions. *See* Antineoplastics Class Instructions. Take lomustine on an empty stomach.

Pharmacokinetics. *Fate.*

	CARMUSTINE	LOMUSTINE
Absorption	—	Complete after 30 min.[60]
Distribution	Both drugs are diffusely distributed with decreasing relative concentrations in spleen, liver, and ovaries; both achieve substantial penetration into CNS with simultaneous CSF levels of >50% of serum for intact carmustine and its metabolites[61] and >30% for intact lomustine and its metabolites;[60] enterohepatic cycling of active metabolites is possible and may explain subsequent peaks in nitrosourea serum levels at 1 and 4 hr.	
Metabolism	Both drugs are rapidly and extensively metabolized (partially by liver microsomal enzymes) to a number of active products which have long serum half-lives compared to the parent compounds.	
Excretion	30% urinary drug recovery as metabolites after 24 hr, 65% after 96 hr.[61]	50% urinary drug recovery as metabolites after 12 hr, 60% after 48 hr; less than 5% fecal excretion.[60]
$t_{1/2}$.	Intact drug 5 min; biologic effect 15–30 min; metabolites, slow decay over 3–4 days.[61]	Intact drug 15 min; cyclohexyl and carbonyl metabolites: α phase 4–5 hr, β phase 30–50 hr; chloroethyl metabolite 72 hr.[60]

Adverse Reactions. Emetic potential is moderately high to high; prophylactic antiemetics are recommended. Major dose-limiting toxicity is delayed and potentially cumulative myelosuppression; nadirs are unusually prolonged, with leukopenia at approximately 35 days and thrombocytopenia at about 30 days. Thus, doses are not repeated more often than q 6 weeks.[62] Carmustine frequently causes severe pain at injection site and venospasm, which may be reduced by slow, dilute infusions. Both drugs may transiently elevate liver enzymes. Pulmonary fibrosis may occur following cumulative dosages over 1 g/m^2; nephrotoxicity consistently occurs following cumulative dosages of 1.5 g/m^2 or more.[63]

Variant carmustine-induced pulmonary fibrosis, highly responsive to early drug discontinuation and a glucocorticoid, has been reported.[64] Other occasional toxicities include CNS effects (eg, confusion, lethargy, ataxia), stomatitis, and alopecia. In animal models, the nitrosoureas are highly carcinogenic and several clinical cases of leukemia after nitrosourea therapy have been reported.

Contraindications. Demonstrated hypersensitivity; marked preexisting myelosuppression.

Precautions. Pregnancy.

Drug Interactions. Experimentally in rats, carmustine, lomustine, and the investigational drug semustine are cleared much more rapidly (with reduced antitumor activity) by pretreatment with phenobarbital, which stimulates microsomal enzymes. Conversely, cimetidine can impair metabolism and increase nitrosourea myelotoxicity. Clinical resistance to carmustine and perhaps other nitrosoureas is reduced by concomitant amphotericin B. Digoxin and phenytoin serum levels may be decreased following carmustine-containing combination regimens.

Notes. Carmustine 3.65% in biodegradable polymer wafers (Gliadel, Rhône-Poulenc Rorer) is used as an adjunct to surgery for recurrent glioblastoma multiforme; eight wafers are implanted intracranially at the time of surgery. Store carmustine under refrigeration; appearance of an oily film in the vial is evidence of decomposition, and such vials should be discarded. Carmustine is incompatible with sodium bicarbonate. Lomustine absorption is rapid; thus, vomiting 45 min or more after ingestion does not require readministration. **Semustine** is an oral investigational methyl derivative of lomustine with no appreciable advantages over presently available agents; it is available from the National Cancer Institute.

PROCARBAZINE HYDROCHLORIDE   Matulane

Procarbazine is an N-methylhydrazine derivative that undergoes autooxidation and microsomal activation to form several alkylating species, including the diazonium ion as well as several oxygen free radicals such as H_2O_2, $\cdot OH$ and $\cdot O_2$ (superoxide). It is cell cycle phase nonspecific and used in brain tumors and Hodgkin's and non-Hodgkin's lymphomas. The drug is rapidly and well absorbed after oral administration; CNS levels are equal to serum after 0.5–1.5 hr. Procarbazine is 70% recovered in the urine, primarily as an acid metabolite, with less than 5% excreted unchanged. Frequent CNS side effects include dizziness, headache, ataxia, nightmares, depression, and hallucinations (in up to 30% of patients). Paresthesias may also occur occasionally. Mild to moderate nausea and vomiting occur in 60–90% of patients, but tolerance usually develops rapidly. Dose- and duration-dependent sterility, mutagenicity, and teratogenicity are reported. The drug predisposes patients to secondary acute nonlymphocytic leukemias. The dose-limiting toxicity is myelosuppression with a pancytopenic nadir at 2–3 weeks. Occasional side effects include a flulike syndrome, allergic pneumonitis, and rash. Procarbazine is contraindicated in patients with *severe* hypersensitivity to the drug or preexisting bone marrow aplasia. Avoid concurrent use with MAO inhibitors, alcohol, heterocyclic antidepressants, sympathomimetics, or tyramine-containing foods. Microsomal enzyme-inducing drugs may augment procarbazine cytotoxicity. Procarbazine potentiates barbiturates, narcotics, and other hepatically metabolized drugs. Periodic evaluations of neurologic status and monthly CBCs may be useful. Procarbazine is given orally in doses of 50–200 mg/m^2/day for 10–25 days, repeated in 3–4 weeks. Calculate the dosage based on ideal body weight and reduce dosage for a BUN over 40 mg/dL, Cr$_s$ over 2 mg/dL, or serum bilirubin over 3 mg/dL.[65] Available as 50-mg capsules.

STREPTOZOCIN   Zanosar

Streptozocin (streptozotocin) is a glucose-containing nitrosourea. It has some selective cytotoxic activity in insulinomas and malignant carcinoid, and is active to a lesser extent in other adenocarcinomas of the GI tract. The drug inhibits DNA synthesis via inhibition of pyrimidine biosynthesis and blockade of key enzymatic reactions in gluconeogenesis pathways. It is cell cycle phase nonspecific. It is highly lipophilic, achieving good CNS penetration. Streptozocin and metabolites have a short distribution phase ($t_{1/2\alpha}$, 6 min) followed by possibly two elimination phases representing active metabolites ($t_{1/2\beta}$, 3.5 hr; $t_{1/2\gamma}$, 40 hr). The drug is rapidly and extensively metabolized (unchanged drug half-life is 35 min), and only 10–20% is excreted unchanged in urine. Frequent acute toxicities include nausea, vomiting, and phlebitis; carefully avoid extravasation. The drug is moderately myelotoxic, but extremely nephrotoxic. Signs of streptozocin nephrotoxicity include various renal tubular defects and proteinuria; adequate hydration may offer some protection. It also selectively destroys pancreatic β cells. The adult dosage as a single agent is IV 1–1.5 g/m^2/week for 6 weeks, followed by a 4-week observation period; in combinations, the dosage is 0.5–1 g/m^2/day for 5 days q 4–6 weeks.[66] Available as 1-g injection.

THIOTEPA

Thiotepa (TESPA, TSPA) is a thiophosphoramide compound that is slowly hydrolyzed to release ethylenimine moieties that alkylate DNA. It is used systemically in the treatment of breast cancer, intracavitarily for bladder or pleural disease and intrathecally for CNS disease. It is also given in high doses with autologous bone marrow transplantation. Thiotepa is slowly metabolized, primarily to TEPA. Total body Cl is 8.5 L/hr/m^2, with 15% recovered in the urine as TEPA in 24 hr. Thiotepa has an α half-life of 7.5 min and a β half-life of 109 min. Mild nausea and vomiting occur frequently. The dose-limiting toxicity is myelosuppression (both granulocytes and platelets). Myelosuppression can occur after intravesicular or intrapleural administration. Anaphylaxis occurs rarely, and mutagenicity, teratogenicity, and sterility have been reported. Thiotepa can be administered IV, IM, or SC in a dosage of 0.5 mg/kg monthly or 6 mg/m^2/day for 4 days. Reduce the dosage by all routes in patients with preexisting bone marrow suppression. The intracavitary dose is 60 mg and the intrathecal dose is 1–10 mg/m^2.[67] Available as a 15-mg injection.

Antimetabolites

CLADRIBINE   Leustatin

Cladribine (2CdA) is the 2-chloro analogue of deoxyadenosine. It is a purine nucleoside that is avidly phosphorylated to toxic metabolites that accumulate intracellularly. Lymphocytes, which lack inactivating deaminase activity, are selectively destroyed by inhibition of both DNA synthesis and repair. Cladribine is highly active in hairy cell leukemia; other responsive tumors include malignant lymphoma and acute and chronic myelogenous leukemias. It is also promising in the treatment of chronic progressive multiple sclerosis. Studies with oral administration indicate a bioavailability of 48%, implying that doubling the IV dose may allow oral administration in hairy cell leukemia. The drug has a V_{dB} of 9.2 ± 5.4 L/kg and biphasic elimination with half-lives of 35 min and 6.7 hr. About 40% of a dose is excreted renally as parent drug and metabolites. Frequent adverse reactions include severe neutropenia with fever and infection (70%), anemia (37%), and thrombocytopenia (12%). A flulike syndrome is also common. Suppression of immune system function because of helper T-lymphocyte depletion can be quite long-lived and presents a risk of systemic opportunistic infections by fungi, bacteria, and/or parasites such as *Pneumocystis carinii*. The IV dosage for hairy cell leukemia is 0.09 mg/kg/day for 7 days by continuous infusion. New dosage regimens are exploring single daily SC injections because of the prolonged intracellular retention of active metabolites.[68–71] Available as a 1 mg/mL 10-mL vial.

CYTARABINE   Cytosar-U

Pharmacology. Cytarabine (cytosine arabinoside, Ara-C) is an arabinose sugar analogue of the natural pyrimidine nucleoside deoxycytidine. Cytarabine is cell cycle S phase specific, with activity markedly enhanced by continuous administration over several days.

Administration and Adult Dosage. **IV for remission induction** 100–150 mg/m^2/day as a continuous infusion for 5–10 days.[72] Experimental therapy has successfully used induction doses of 2–3 g/m^2 q 12 hr as a 2-hr infusion for 4–12 doses in refractory AML.[73] **SC for remission induction** 100 mg/m^2 q 12 hr for 5–10 days. **SC for remission maintenance** 70–100 mg/m^2/day for 5 days in 4 divided doses. **Intrathecal** 70 mg/m^2 (usually 100 mg) 1 or 2 times weekly, diluted with nonpreserved isotonic solutions only (eg, NS, D5W, Ringer's lactate).[74] *See* Notes.

Special Populations. *Pediatric Dosage.* **IV or SC** same as adult dosage. **Intrathecal** ($\geq$3 yr or older) 70 mg/m^2, diluted as above, repeated no more often than q 3–5 days; (2–3 yr) reduce dose by one-sixth; (1–2 yr) reduce dose by one-third; (<1 yr) reduce dose by one-half.

Geriatric Dosage. Same as adult dosage.

Dosage Forms. **Inj** 100, 500 mg, 1, 2 g.

Patient Instructions. *See* Antineoplastics Class Instructions.

Pharmacokinetics. *Serum Levels.* 50–100 mg/L (0.2–0.4 mmol/L) are required for cytotoxic effects.[75]

Fate. Not systemically available following oral absorption. After injection, there is a large interpatient variation in serum levels attained as measured by various assay techniques.[76] Serum levels of 100-400 mg/L (0.4–1.6 mmol/L) are produced by a 60-min continuous infusion of 300 mg/m^2.[77] Serum levels up to 240 mg/L (1 mmol/L) are achieved with high-dose regimens. It is widely distributed and deactivated by cytidine deaminase, primarily in the liver. The CSF to serum ratio is 0.1–0.14:1 with bolus doses and up to 0.4–0.5:1 with continuous infusion. There is slow elimination from the CSF caused by low CNS deaminating activity; however, to attain therapeutic CSF concentrations following standard IV doses, intrathecal administration is required. Tear fluid concentrations are detectable after high-dose therapy. The drug is about 13% plasma protein bound. V_d is 3 ± 1.9 L/kg; Cl is 0.78 ± 0.24 L/hr/kg.[10] The deamination product, uracil arabinoside (ara-U) is inactive and rapidly excreted in the urine; 24 hr after injection, 72% of the dose is recovered in the urine as Ara-U, only $11 \pm 8\%$ as unchanged drug.[10,78] $t_{1/2}$. α phase 1.6–12 min; ß phase 2.6 ± 0.6 hr.[10,77,78] Following intrathecal administration, CNS half-life of 2–11 hr has been reported.[79]

Adverse Reactions. Emetic potential is moderate (<250 mg) to moderately high (250 mg–1 g); prophylactic antiemetics are very effective. The principal side effect is dose-related myelosuppression with a leukopenic nadir of 3–11 days and a thrombocytopenic nadir of 12–14 days; megaloblastosis is typically noted in the recovering bone marrow and in the rare cases in which anemia develops. Ocular toxicity is frequent with high-dose therapy; typically, conjunctival injection and central punctate corneal opacities occur.[80] Concurrent use of glucocorticoid eye drops is recommended with high-dose therapy.[80] Occasionally, mild oral ulceration and a flulike syndrome, manifested by arthralgias, fever, and sometimes rash, occur. Irreversible cerebellar toxicity (ataxia, cognitive dysfunction) is a risk after cumulative doses of 30 g/m² or greater.[81] Hepatic enzyme elevation is rare, even with 3 g/m² doses; one instance of SIADH was reported with this large dose.[73] Intrathecal toxicities are dose related and include transient headache and vomiting.[80] Seizures and paraplegia are rare and involve high-dose, closely spaced treatments.

Precautions. Myelosuppression is *not* a contraindication, because marrow hypoplasia with complete suppression of the leukemic clone is the desired clinical endpoint; however, extensive supportive facilities must be available during therapy, including WBC and platelet transfusion capability.

Drug Interactions. Digoxin bioavailability from tablets may be decreased following cytarabine-containing combination regimens.

Parameters to Monitor. Routine WBC and platelet counts; RBC indices.

Notes. Chemically stable in solution for up to 7 days at room temperature. Do not dilute intrathecal doses with bacteriostatic diluents. Physically incompatible with **fluorouracil;** avoid direct admixture. At neutral pH, the drug can be mixed with sodium **methotrexate** and/or **hydrocortisone** sodium succinate. Patients may be taught sterile technique for self-administration of SC drug for leukemia remission maintenance. The use of small reconstitution volumes (1 mL/100 mg) and rotation of injection sites should be observed. Clinical activity is limited primarily to selected hematologic malignancies (eg, AML, ALL, DHL).

FLOXURIDINE
FUDR, Various

Pharmacology. Floxuridine is the deoxyribose metabolite of fluorouracil. The drug inhibits DNA synthesis by binding to thymidylate synthetase in S phase of cell division.

Administration and Adult Dosage. **Intra-arterially for colon cancer metastases to the liver** 0.1–0.6 mg/kg/day for 1–6 weeks by continuous hepatic artery perfusion.[82] Hospitalize patients for at least the first course of therapy.

Special Populations. *Pediatric Dosage.* Safety and efficacy not established.

Geriatric Dosage. Same as adult dosage.

Other Conditions. Reduce dosage when combined with other myelosuppressive drugs or in patients experiencing severe toxicity (usually mucositis or diarrhea) from previous doses.

Dosage Forms. Inj 500 mg.

Patient Instructions. *See* Antineoplastics Class Instructions.

Pharmacokinetics. *Fate.* Floxuridine has a high degree (69–92%) of hepatic extraction.[83] A large fraction is converted to the active phosphorylated metabolite 5-fluorodeoxyuridylate monophosphate (FdUMP). Ultimately, the drug is almost completely metabolized to inactive compounds, which are eliminated by exhalation (60% of a dose) or by urinary excretion (about 10–30% of a dose).

$t_{1/2}$. <15 min.

Adverse Reactions. Emetic potential with intra-arterial administration is low. Diarrhea and stomatitis occur frequently. Stomatitis can be life-threatening, as can an unusual dermatitis affecting the hands and feet; both toxicities are much more frequent with prolonged infusions. The primary dose-limiting toxicity of floxuridine is myelosuppression, principally leukopenia with some thrombocytopenia. Liver enzyme elevations occur frequently, but they rarely herald serious hepatic complications. Local complications involving the hepatic catheter include thrombosis, leakage, embolism, and infection. Some catheter placements can also result in gastric ulcers or biliary sclerosis if their respective arterioles are inadvertently perfused.[82]

Contraindications. Pregnancy; poor nutrition; preexisting myelosuppression; serious infection.

Precautions. Biliary sclerosis may occur, requiring repositioning or removal of the catheter.

Drug Interactions. None known.

Parameters to Monitor. Monitor WBC count prior to and following each treatment. Observe for diarrhea (fluid and electrolyte status). Monitor for severe hepatic enzyme elevations, which may indicate biliary sclerosis.

Notes. Floxuridine can be administered in NS or D5W and it is compatible with **heparin.**

FLUDARABINE PHOSPHATE   Fludara

Fludarabine is a fluorinated nucleotide analogue of vidarabine. It is rapidly converted to 2-fluoro-ara-A, which is then phosphorylated to 2-fluoro-ara-ATP, which inhibits DNA synthesis. Fludarabine has little cross-resistance with other agents used for chronic lymphocytic leukemia (CLL). The metabolite 2-fluoro-ara-A has a V_d of 98 L/m^2, a Cl of 8.9 L/hr/m^2, and a half-life of about 10 hr. About 23% of a dose is excreted in the urine as unchanged 2-fluoro-ara-A, and clearance is proportional to Cl_{cr}. The most frequent adverse effects are myelosuppression (neutropenia, thrombocytopenia, and anemia), fever and chills, infection, rash, myalgia, nausea, vomiting, and diarrhea. Frequent pulmonary symptoms include pneumonia, cough, and dyspnea. Fludarabine produced severe CNS toxicity (ie, blindness, coma, and death) in 36% of patients treated with a dosage of 4 times the currently recommended dosage. Similar CNS toxicity occurs occasionally (≤0.2% of patients) with recommended dosages. Other CNS effects include weakness, visual disturbances, paresthesias, agitation, confusion, and peripheral neuropathy. Fludarabine is indicated in the treatment of B-cell CLL that has not responded to at least one standard alkylating agent regimen. The dosage of fludarabine for CLL is 25 mg/m^2/day for 5 days given over 30 min in 100–125 mL of D5W or NS. Refrigerate the drug before reconstitution and use within 8 hr after reconstitution. Available as a 50-mg injection.

FLUOROURACIL Various

Pharmacology. Fluorouracil (5-fluorouracil, 5-FU) is a fluorinated antimetabolite of the DNA pyrimidine precursor uracil. It inhibits thymidine formation, thereby blocking DNA synthesis. Some fluorouracil may be incorporated into RNA, inhibiting subsequent protein synthesis. It is cell cycle S phase specific.

Administration and Adult Dosage. Rapid IV 15 mg/kg/week for 4 weeks followed by 20 mg/kg/week until severe toxicity develops. The drug is stopped until resolution is complete, then resumed at 5 mg/kg/week.[84] **IV "loading course"** 12 mg/kg (800 mg maximum) as a single daily dose for 4 days, then 12–15 mg/kg/week is recommended by manufacturer; however, this regimen has been associated with severe, life-threatening bone marrow toxicity.[85] **IV continuous infusion** 1–2 g/day for up to 5 days has been used by special treatment centers; continuous infusion does not consistently increase antitumor efficacy, but does appear to lessen hematologic toxicity.[86] **IV for Dukes' stage C colon cancer following resection in combination with levamisole** 450 mg/m^2/day for 5 days initially, then 450 mg/m^2 once a week beginning in 28 days and continued for 1 yr. *See* Notes. **PO** doses are associated with low bioavailability and short clinical response. **Intra-arterial, intraperitoneal, and intracavitary** administration have also been used, although floxuridine is preferred. **Top for neoplastic keratoses** apply daily for 1–2 weeks as a thin layer with gloved hand or nonmetal applicator. Skin response progresses sequentially through erythema, vesiculation, erosion, ulceration, necrosis, and finally regranulation. Treatment is usually stopped once erosion is evident to allow healing to occur over the next 1–2 months. **Vag for condylomata acuminata** ⅓ applicatorful (1.5 g) of 5% cream once a week hs for 10 weeks.[87]

Special Populations. *Pediatric Dosage.* Generally indicated for adult malignancies, although theoretically, equivalent mg/kg doses could be used in children.

Geriatric Dosage. Same as adult dosage.

Other Conditions. Base dosage on ideal body weight in obesity or if the patient has excessive fluid retention.

Dosage Forms. **Inj** 50 mg/mL; **Top Crm** 1, 5%; **Top Soln** 1, 2, 5%.

Patient Instructions. *See* Antineoplastics Class Instructions. Avoid prolonged exposure to strong sunlight; report any severe sores in the mouth immediately.

Pharmacokinetics. *Fate.* Oral doses are erratically and incompletely absorbed with bioavailability of 28%, worsened by mixing with acidic fruit juices.[87] The drug is 8-12% plasma protein bound. The drug diffuses into effusions and CSF (peak CSF levels of 60–80 nmol/L after a 15 mg/kg IV bolus). V_d is about 25 ± 12 L/kg; Cl is 0.96 ± 0.42 L/hr/kg.[10] Extensively and rapidly metabolized, primarily in the liver, to a variety of inactive metabolites that are renally excreted.

Up to 15% is renally excreted unchanged, 90% within 6 hr of administration. Fluoroacetate and citrate metabolites found in the CSF are believed to mediate rare CNS (cerebellar) toxicities.

$t_{1/2}$. α phase about 8 min; ß phase 11 ± 4 min.[10,88]

Adverse Reactions. Emetic potential is moderately low (<1 g) to moderate (>1 g). Dose-limiting toxicity is myelosuppression (when given by bolus injection) with leukopenic and thrombocytopenic nadirs at 7–14 days. Severe stomatitis 5–8 days after therapy can herald severe impending myelosuppression; this occurs unpredictably with large bolus doses (>12 mg/kg). With continuous infusions, myelosuppression is reduced considerably, but mucositis and diarrhea may be dose limiting. Oral administration increases severity of the frequent mild diarrhea. GI ulceration is occasionally severe. Cutaneous toxicities include mild to moderate alopecia, hyperpigmentation of skin and veins, and rashes that are often worsened by sunlight. Excessive lacrimation is frequent; occasionally tear duct fibrosis develops. Rare toxicities involve CNS dysfunction manifested by ataxia, confusion, visual disturbances, and headache. Cardiotoxicity occurs rarely.

Contraindications. Pregnancy. Preexisting severe myelosuppression (WBCs <2000/μL, platelet count <100,000/μL); poor nutritional state; serious infections.

Precautions. Use with caution in patients with preexisting coronary artery disease.

Drug Interactions. Concurrent allopurinol appears to block one activation pathway, thereby reducing fluorouracil hematologic toxicity. Fluorouracil can inhibit the antipurine effects of methotrexate. The clinical importance of these two interactions is unclear.

Parameters to Monitor. Pretreatment and monthly assessment of bone marrow function, particularly WBC and platelet counts. In the weeks following administration, observe for severe stomatitis, which may herald life-threatening myelosuppression.

Notes. If a precipitate is noted in the ampule, gently warm in a water bath and/or vigorously shake to redissolve. Fluorouracil is physically incompatible with diazepam, doxorubicin, cytarabine, and methotrexate injections. Mild to moderate activity in GI tract tumors and in breast cancer; topical application of cream is often curative in superficial skin cancers. **Leucovorin** has been used with fluorouracil to increase fluorouracil binding to the target enzyme, thymidylate synthetase. **Levamisole** (Ergamisol) is an immunomodulator used to enhance fluorouracil efficacy in Dukes' C colon cancer. It is given orally in a dosage of 50 mg q 8 hr for 3 days, q 14 days for 1 yr.

GEMCITABINE   Gemsar

Pharmacology. Gemcitabine is a difluorinated nucleoside analogue of cytarabine that is phosphorylated by intracellular deoxycytidine kinase to the active di- and triphosphate forms. These antimetabolites inhibit ribonucleotide reductase and reduce the normal pool of deoxycytidine triphosphate, respectively. This leads to an inhibition of DNA synthesis (both replication and repair). Compared to cytarabine, gemcitabine is preferentially phosphorylated and retained intracellularly. It is approved for palliative therapy in pancreatic cancer, and is also active in breast cancer and non–small cell lung cancer.[89–91] *See* Notes.

Administration and Adult Dosage. IV 1 g/m²/week infused over 30 min for 7 consecutive weeks, followed by 1 week rest, then once weekly for 3 weeks with 1 week rest thereafter.

Dosage Forms. Inj 100, 500 mg.

Patient Instructions. *See* Antineoplastics Class Instructions. Take acetaminophen prior to each dose to reduce flulike symptoms.

Pharmacokinetics. *Fate.* A peak serum level of 14.7 mg/L (56 µmol/L) occurs following a 1 g/m² IV dose. The drug is metabolized to active di- and triphosphate forms and also deaminated to inactive difluorodeoxyuridine (dFdU) in liver and blood. Cl is 408 ± 121 L/hr/m² in men, and 31% lower in women. Renal elimination of dFdU is 77% of a dose; 5% of a dose is recovered unchanged in urine.[89]

$t_½$. (Gemcitabine) 8–14 min (dose and infusion duration dependent); (dFdU) 10–14 hr.[89]

Adverse Reactions. Emetic potential is moderately low and is well controlled by antiemetics. Thrombocytopenia is the dose-limiting toxicity; cumulative-dosage anemia is next most common. Neutropenia occurs, but is rarely dose limiting. A transient, acute flulike syndrome consisting of fever, fatigue, chills, headache, and arthralgias occurs in most patients. Fever responds to acetaminophen and usually does not recur. Erythematous pruritic maculopapular rashes on the neck and extremities are frequent, but usually respond to a topical glucocorticoid. Hepatic transaminases may increase in two-thirds of patients, but this is rarely serious. Diarrhea occurs rarely.

Contraindications. Severe preexisting thrombocytopenia.

Precautions. Thrombocytopenia may lead to serious bleeding and anemia, and may require transfusion therapy. Based on a similarity to cytarabine, CNS (cerebellar) toxicities may occur after high cumulative dosages, especially with impaired renal function.

Drug Interactions. None known.

Parameters to Monitor. Monitor platelet count, RBC count, and hemoglobin levels, and serum hepatic transaminase levels monthly.

Notes. Gemcitabine is clinically active in pancreatic cancer, breast cancer, and non–small cell lung cancer, although objective increases in tumor shrinkage and survival are minimal.[89–91] Gemcitabine produces primarily palliative responses such as reduced pain and enhanced quality of life with minimal serious toxicity compared to other cytotoxic agent therapies.

METHOTREXATE   Mexate, Various

Pharmacology. Methotrexate is a folic acid analogue that binds to dihydrofolate reductase, blocking formation of the DNA nucleotide thymidine; purine synthesis is also inhibited. It is most active in S phase.

Administration and Adult Dosage. *Single Agent Therapy.* **IM, IV, or PO for chorio-carcinoma** 15–30 mg/day for 5 days, repeated q 1–2 weeks for 3–5 courses; **IM for mycosis fungoides** 50 mg once weekly or 25 mg twice weekly; **IM, IV, or PO for head and neck cancer** 25–50 mg/m² once weekly (watch for cumulative myelosuppression with continued administration of this regimen). **Intrathecal for meningeal**

leukemia 12 mg/m^2 in a preservative-free, isotonic diluent (eg, Elliott's B solution, patient's own CSF, or D5LR); **IV high-dose therapy** (1–3 g/m^2) with leucovorin rescue should be used only by experts in major research centers; **IM or PO for psoriasis or arthritis** maintenance 5–10 mg initially, then **IM, IV, or PO** 10–25 mg/week, to a maximum of 50 mg/week, depending on clinical response; long-term daily administration results in increased hepatotoxicity compared to weekly oral or parenteral doses. **IM in glucocorticoid-dependent asthma** 7.5 mg, then 15 mg 1 week later, with subsequent weekly doses adjusted to 15–50 mg depending on 24-hr serum levels.[92] **PO for glucocorticoid-dependent asthma** 15 mg/week has been used.[93] **IM for ectopic pregnancy** 50 mg/m^2; some investigators repeat dose in 1 week if ß-hCG levels do not drop.[94,95] **IM for induction of abortion** 50 mg/m^2, followed in 3 or 7 days by misoprostol 800 μg vaginally; exact timing of misoprostol dosage and oral administration of methotrexate are under investigation.[96–98]

Combined Modality Therapy. **For acute lymphocytic leukemia** various schedules are reported for remission-maintenance therapy: **IM or IV** 30 mg/m^2 twice weekly, or 7.5 mg/kg/day for 5 days, or **PO** 2.5 mg/kg/day for 2 weeks; repeat at monthly intervals. **IM, IV, or PO for Burkitt's lymphoma** 0.625–2.5 mg/kg/day for 1–2 weeks, then off drug for 7–10 days; **IM or IV for breast cancer** (combined with cyclophosphamide and fluorouracil) 40 mg/m^2 on days 1 and 8, then repeat monthly.[99]

Special Populations. *Pediatric Dosage.* IM or IV for remission maintenance same as adult dosage for acute lymphoblastic leukemia. **Intrathecally for meningeal cancer** use age-adjusted dosage rather than mg/m^2 dose:[100]

AGE (YR)	IT DOSE (MG)
>3	12
2–3	10
1–2	8
<1	6

Geriatric Dosage. Same as adult dosage, but adjust for age-related reduction in renal function.

Other Conditions. Patients with any "third space" fluid (eg, ascites, pleural effusions) should have fluid removed before drug administration because of drug retention and slow release of drug from these compartments.[101] Reduce dosage in renal impairment as follows:[102]

CREATININE CLEARANCE (ML/MIN)	PERCENTAGE OF DOSAGE RECOMMENDED
>50	60–100 (0–40% reduction)
10–50	30–50 (50–70% reduction)
<10	15 (85% reduction)

Dosage Forms. **Tab** 2.5 mg; **Inj** (as sodium) 2.5, 25 mg/mL (preserved solution); 25 mg/mL (nonpreserved solution); 20, 25, 50, 100, 250 mg, 1 g (nonpreserved powder).

Patient Instructions. *See* Antineoplastics Class Instructions.

Pharmacokinetics. *Serum Levels.* Following high-dose therapy, a threshold for bone marrow and mucosal toxicity is approximately 1 µmol/L 48 hr after administration. To prevent fatal bone marrow toxicity, keep serum levels below 10 µmol/L at 24 hr, 500 nmol/L at 48 hr, and 50 nmol/L at 72 hr.[103]

Fate. PO and IM absorption are rapid, peaking at 1–2 and 0.1–1 hr, respectively. Oral bioavailability is dose related, but averages 30%.[102] Following intrathecal administration, the drug slowly diffuses into the bloodstream. About 34% is plasma protein bound; V_d is 0.55 ± 0.19 L/kg; Cl is 0.126 ± 0.048 L/hr/kg.[10] Over 90% of a dose is excreted in the urine, 90% unchanged after IV administration of high doses. Methotrexate solubility is markedly enhanced in slightly alkaline urine and reduced in acidic urine.

$t_{1/2}$. α phase 0.75 min; β phase 2 hr; γ phase 7.2 ± 2.1 hr.[10,104]

Adverse Reactions. Unless otherwise indicated, these reactions apply to high-dose chemotherapy of malignancies. Emetic potential is moderate. Nearly all reactions are dose and duration related. The primary toxicity is hematologic suppression, principally leukopenia, with the nadir at 7–14 days depending upon the administration schedule (more prolonged with daily administration). Thrombocytopenia and macrocytic anemia, dose-related nephrotoxicity, and ocular irritation occur frequently. Hepatotoxicity occurs frequently. Diarrhea and mucosal ulcerations of the mouth and tongue may occasionally become severe within 1–3 weeks after administration, sometimes heralding severe myelotoxicity. Erythematous rashes have been reported. Leukoencephalopathy occurs rarely with either IV or intrathecal use. Other toxicities following intrathecal use include nausea and vomiting, meningismus, paresthesias, and rarely convulsions. Long-term daily administration in psoriasis has led to hepatocellular damage including fibrotic liver changes and atrophy of the liver; the frequency may be lower with larger intermittent doses. A single low dose for use in medical abortion is generally well tolerated, with none of the severe reactions reported above.

Contraindications. Pregnancy; severe renal or hepatic dysfunction; psoriasis patients with preexisting bone marrow depression.

Precautions. Renal function must be determined prior to administration. Alkalinize the urine prior to high doses to enhance methotrexate solubility.

Drug Interactions. Concomitant vinca alkaloids (vincristine or vinblastine) can impair methotrexate elimination from the CSF and may enhance methotrexate toxicity. Cisplatin, NSAIDs, omeprazole, high-dose penicillins, probenecid, and sulfonamides can increase methotrexate serum levels and toxicity. Salicylate may decrease renal elimination of methotrexate and displace it from plasma protein binding sites. Alcohol may enhance hepatotoxicity of methotrexate. Asparaginase given 1 week prior to or 24 hr after methotrexate appears to reduce methotrexate hematologic toxicities. Cholesterol-binding resins may decrease oral methotrexate absorption. Broad-spectrum antibiotics may decrease methotrexate serum levels and efficacy after oral administration.

Parameters to Monitor. Monitor pretreatment and periodic hepatic, renal, and bone marrow function (including WBCs, platelets, and RBCs). Follow high doses with 24-hr and/or 48-hr serum methotrexate levels and institution of appropriate leucovorin rescue.

Notes. Reconstitute lyophilized forms with NS, D5W, or Elliott's B solution (for intrathecal use). Reconstituted solutions are chemically stable for 7 days at room temperature. Methotrexate is physically incompatible with fluorouracil, prednisolone sodium phosphate, and cytarabine. It is clinically useful in a variety of hematologic and solid tumors as well as nonmalignant hyperplastic conditions such as psoriasis. If overdosage occurs, the antidote is **calcium leucovorin** (citrovorum factor), which can be given IV or IM in methotrexate-equivalent doses up to 75 mg q 6 hr for 4 doses. A delay of greater than 36 hr lessens the chance of rescue.[103]

PENTOSTATIN   Nipent

Pentostatin (formerly 2'deoxycoformycin) is an analogue of a normal purine intermediate involved in the conversion of adenosine to inosine. It is an irreversible inhibitor of the enzyme adenosine deaminase (ADA), which is primarily found in lymphoid cells. Pentostatin-induced inhibition of ADA leads to a buildup of deoxyadenosine and several phosphorylated derivatives that deplete cellular ATP. These metabolic products ultimately inhibit DNA synthesis in lymphatic tumor cells, including chronic lymphocytic leukemia, acute lymphoblastic leukemia, and especially hairy cell leukemia. There are some data to suggest that the cytotoxic effect is cell cycle phase specific for the G_1 phase. Serum levels after doses of 2–10 mg/m^2 average 1.5–4.7 mmol/L. V_d is 20–23 L/m^2; Cl is 3.1 L/hr/kg. The terminal half-life of pentostatin averages 5–10 hr. Up to 90% of a dose is excreted in the urine, and dosage reduction is indicated in patients with reduced renal function. Renal tubular toxicity and myelosuppression are the major dose-limiting toxicities of pentostatin. Renal toxicity manifested by Cr_s elevation is much more frequent at doses over 5 $mg/m^2/day$. Adequate hydration and the avoidance of other nephrotoxins can reduce the frequency and severity of pentostatin-induced nephrotoxicity. Lymphocytopenia is frequent with both B- and T-lymphocytes depressed, possibly explaining the relatively frequent, severe systemic infections with organisms that include Gram-negative bacteria, *Candida albicans*, herpes zoster (varicella), and herpes simplex. Neurologic effects are frequent with pentostatin and include lethargy and fatigue; these rarely progress to coma and are more common and severe with high-dose regimens. Mild to moderate nausea and vomiting also occur frequently, but are easily controlled with standard antiemetic regimens. The usual dosage for hairy cell leukemia refractory to interferon alpha is IV 4 mg/m^2 every other week.[105,106] Available as a 10-mg vial.

PURINE ANALOGUES:

MERCAPTOPURINE   Purinethol
THIOGUANINE

Pharmacology. Mercaptopurine (6-MP), and thioguanine (6-TG) are thiolated purines that act as antimetabolites following metabolic activation to the nucleotide forms (phosphorylated ribose sugar attachment). Subsequently, de novo purine biosynthesis is interrupted at a number of enzymatic sites, including the conversion of inosinic acid to adenine- or xanthine-based ribosides. DNA and RNA synthesis is halted in a cell cycle S phase specific fashion.

Administration and Adult Dosage. (Mercaptopurine) **PO, IV** (investigational) 75–100 mg/m²/day.[107] See Drug Interactions. (Thioguanine) **PO, IV** (investigational) 2–3 mg/kg/day.

Special Populations. *Pediatric Dosage.* Same as adult dosage.

Geriatric Dosage. Same as adult dosage.

Other Conditions. Purine antimetabolite toxicities are not consistently increased in patients with renal failure.[108,109] See Precautions.

Dosage Forms. (Mercaptopurine) **Tab** 50 mg; **Inj** (investigational) 500 mg. (Thioguanine) **Tab** 40 mg; **Inj** (investigational) 75 mg.

Patient Instructions. See Antineoplastics Class Instructions. To maximize absorption, do not take these drugs with meals. Nausea and vomiting are uncommon with usual doses.

Pharmacokinetics. *Fate.* (Mercaptopurine) 12 ± 7% oral bioavailability, increasing to 60% with concurrent allopurinol.[110] The drug is approximately 20–30% plasma protein bound and freely distributed throughout the body including placental transfer; the CSF/serum ratio is 0.19–0.27. Mercaptopurine is metabolized extensively by xanthine oxidase, also methylated to active metabolite and sulfated to inactive thiouric acid. V_d is 0.56 ± 0.38 L/kg; Cl is 0.66 ± 0.24 L/hr/kg; 22% excreted unchanged in urine.[10] (Thioguanine) Oral bioavailability is unknown. The drug is approximately 20–30% plasma protein bound and freely distributed throughout the body, including placental transfer; the CSF/serum ratio is 0.16. Thioguanine is metabolized predominantly to inactive metabolites.

$t_{1/2}$. (Mercaptopurine) 0.9 ± 0.37 hr;[10] (thioguanine) α phase 15 min, ß phase 11 hr.

Adverse Reactions. Emetic potential is low to moderate. The dose-limiting toxicity is myelosuppression (leukopenia and thrombocytopenia). Mild to moderate mucositis occurs with large doses with low daily maintenance doses. Predominantly cholestatic liver toxicities occur frequently with long-term therapy. Marked crystalluria with hematuria has occurred with large IV mercaptopurine doses.[111] A variety of rashes have also been described with these drugs. Long-term immunosuppressive therapy with any of these agents predisposes patients to carcinogenesis; CNS lymphomas and acute myeloid leukemia are the most frequent malignancies.[112]

Contraindications. Pregnancy; preexisting severe bone marrow depression.

Precautions. Investigational use of mercaptopurine for inflammatory bowel disease may predispose to pancreatitis.

Drug Interactions. Patients taking allopurinol *must* receive substantially reduced doses of oral mercaptopurine (25–33% of the normal dose), to avoid life-threatening myelosuppression caused by blocked inactivation. Thioguanine is primarily inactivated by methylation; thus, no dosage reduction is necessary with concomitant allopurinol. Enhanced bone marrow suppression may occur with the combination of trimethoprim/sulfamethoxazole and mercaptopurine.

Parameters to Monitor. WBC and platelet counts and total bilirubin at least monthly.

Notes. There is usually complete cross-resistance between mercaptopurine and thioguanine.

Cytokines

ALDESLEUKIN
Proleukin

Pharmacology. Aldesleukin (interleukin-2; IL-2) is a cytokine produced by activated T-lymphocytes. It binds to T-cell receptors to induce a proliferative response and differentiation into lymphokine activated killer (LAK) cells in the blood and tumor-infiltrating lymphocytes (TIL-cells) in specific tumors. The pharmaceutical product is a nonglycosylated molecule produced by recombinant DNA techniques in *Escherichia coli*.[113,114]

Administration and Adult Dosage. IV for metastatic renal cell carcinoma 600,000 IU/kg over 15 min q 8 hr for 14 doses; repeat after 9 days of rest for a total of 28 doses. **IV infusion** 3–6 million IU/m^2 infused over 6 hr is commonly used.

Special Populations. *Pediatric Dosage.* (<18 yr) safety and efficacy not established.

Geriatric Dosage. Same as adult dosage.

Other Conditions. Interpatient pharmacokinetic differences are not known; however, withholding dose(s) is required if severe cardiovascular collapse, or pulmonary or renal insufficiency, coma, psychosis, or GI toxicity occurs.

Dosage Forms. Inj 22 million IU (1.3 mg protein). *See* Notes.

Pharmacokinetics. *Fate.* Limited human data indicate that the drug undergoes biphasic elimination after IV administration. The kidney is believed to be the major organ of elimination, and the drug undergoes intrarenal metabolism to inactive fragments.[115]

$t_{1/2}$. α phase 14 ± 7.7 min; β phase 80 ± 34 min.[116]

Adverse Reactions. Emetic potential is low. Severe cardiovascular toxicities include fluid retention (over 10% of body weight) and pulmonary interstitial edema. Hypotension requiring treatment has occurred 2–4 hr after treatment with a high-dose bolus or continuous infusions as well as with low-dose SC regimens. Anemia occurs in up to 77% of high-dose bolus IV regimens. Frequently, nausea, vomiting, diarrhea, rash, pruritus, and nasal congestion occur. Abnormal laboratory findings include frequent increased Cr_s, oliguria, eosinophilia, and thrombocytopenia.[113] Increased serum transaminases and bilirubin occur occasionally; hepatic dysfunction occurs rarely. Myocardial ischemia may also occur and fatal MI has been reported. Capillary leak syndrome may occur and requires close monitoring of fluid balance.[113] When combined with adoptive cellular therapy (reinfused LAK cells), immediate fever and chills result; **indomethacin** 50 mg orally or **meperidine** 25–50 mg IM or IV may lessen these.

Precautions. Aldesleukin has produced severe cardiopulmonary toxicity and must be cautiously used in any patient with a history of cardiac insufficiency from any cause. Patients must also be in good general physical condition in order to tolerate the hypotension and pulmonary edema that can complicate high-dose aldesleukin therapy.

Drug Interactions. Glucocorticoids block some aldesleukin actions and are usually reserved for treating severe toxicity.

Parameters to Monitor. Monitor blood pressure, cardiac output, and fluid balance closely.

Notes. Some studies describe IL-2 activity in different units or by weight. Aldesleukin is labeled in IU (18 million IU = 1.1 mg protein), and doses for other IL-2 products should be converted to IU for proper dosage. Aldesleukin is active in metastatic renal cell carcinoma (MRCC) and metastatic malignant melanoma. In MRCC, response rates are 15% (with some complete remissions), lasting a median of 23 months. Response rates are higher in patients with good performance status and especially those with pulmonary metastases as the main site of disease.

INTERFERON ALFA:	
ALFA-2A	Roferon-A
ALFA-2B	Intron A
ALFA-N3	Alferon N

Pharmacology. Alpha interferons are single-chain proteins. The alfa-2 interferons are biosynthetic; alfa-2a has a lysine at position 23, alfa-2b an arginine. Alfa-n3 interferon is a multisubspecies form of natural interferons isolated from human leukocytes. Interferons bind to specific membrane receptors and are then taken up intracellularly to affect diverse cellular functions. These include cell membrane alterations (eg, enhanced antigen expression), cell cycle blockade at the G_1-S portion, enhanced antiviral enzyme synthesis (eg, $2',5'$-oligo-adenylate synthetase with resultant products, which destroy double and single stranded viral RNA), and immunomodulatory activity (eg, increased activity of natural killer [NK] lymphocytes and phagocytic macrophages). General cellular protein synthesis is also decreased, including cytochrome P450 enzymes.[116]

Administration and Adult Dosage. **IM or SC for hairy cell leukemia** (alfa-2a or 2b) 2 million IU/m^2 daily or 3 times a week. **IM or SC for AIDS-related Kaposi's sarcoma** (alfa-2b) slowly increase dose from 5 million IU/day up to 20–36 million IU/day.[117] **Intralesionally for condylomata acuminata** (alfa-2b) 1 million IU/wart 3 times weekly for 3 weeks, to a maximum 5 warts a day (use only the 10 million IU vial); (alfa-n3) 250,000 IU (0.05 mL)/wart twice weekly for up to 8 weeks, to a maximum 0.5 mL/day. **IM or SC for chronic hepatitis B** 5 million IU/day or 10 million IU 3 times a week for 16 weeks.[118] **IM or SC for chronic hepatitis C** 3 million IU 3 times a week for 6 months. **IV and SC for malignant melanoma** (alfa-2b) 20 million IU/m^2 IV 5 times a week for 4 weeks, then 10 million IU/m^2 SC 3 times a week for 48 weeks. **IM or SC for chronic myeloid leukemia** (alfa-2a) 3–6 million IU/day.

Special Populations. *Pediatric Dosage.* (<18 yr) Not recommended.

Geriatric Dosage. Same as adult dosage.

Dosage Forms. (Alfa-2a) **Inj** 3, 6, 10, 36 million IU. (Alfa-2b) **Inj** 3, 5, 10, 18, 25, 50 million IU. (Alfa-n3) **Inj** 5 million IU.

Patient Instructions. (Subcutaneous use) Instruct in proper method of aseptic preparation of vials and syringes, proper technique for SC administration, and proper disposal of syringes and needles. Rotate SC injection sites. Acetaminophen is recommended to reduce frequent flulike symptoms, which usually decrease with continued therapy.

Pharmacokinetics. *Fate.* Alfa-2a and 2b are 100% bioavailable after IM or SC administration, with an absorption half-life of about 6 hr. IM or SC doses of 10 million IU produce peak serum levels of 100–200 IU/mL within 4 hr; the same dose IV produces peak serum levels of 500–600 IU/mL within 15–30 min. Alfa-n3 is not detectable in serum after intralesional administration, although a small amount is probably absorbed. The majority of a dose is thought to be metabolized, with none filtered or secreted by the kidney.[119,120]

$t_{1/2}$. α phase 0.11 hr; β phase (IV or IM) 2 hr, (SC) 3 hr.[119,120]

Adverse Reactions. Emetic potential is negligible. The most frequent reactions include fever to 38–39°C, chills, arthralgias, headache, malaise, and myalgias (flulike syndrome). These reactions are more severe upon initiation of therapy and are ameliorated by acetaminophen or dosage reduction. Anorexia and nausea without vomiting are also frequent. With large doses (generally over 1 million IU), hematologic suppression (eg, mild thrombocytopenia, leukopenia) occurs, as does slight elevation of hepatic enzymes (AST, LDH, alkaline phosphatase), and mild hypertension, occasionally associated with tachycardia. Very high doses (≥30 million IU) are associated with somnolence, dizziness, and confusion. Mild erythema and pruritus at the injection site can also occur. Interferons are not mutagenic nor carcinogenic in standard animal or in vitro models.

Contraindications. Severe hypersensitivity; development of a neutralizing serum antibody (precludes the use of alternate recombinant product, switch to natural interferon alfa-n3, *see* Notes).

Precautions. Pregnancy. Use with caution in patients with cardiovascular disease, seizure disorder, or hepatic or renal impairment. Proper hydration during therapy may help lessen hypotensive reactions. Neutralizing serum antibodies can form after prolonged interferon administration. This has been associated with reduced toxicities and antitumor effects.[121]

Drug Interactions. Interferon may worsen the neutropenia of zidovudine in Kaposi's sarcoma. Interferon may increase theophylline serum levels. Combination with vidarabine may result in increased neurotoxicity.

Notes. A clear dose–response relationship is established for toxicity, but not for antitumor effectiveness (except for Kaposi's sarcoma). Alpha interferons have activity in reducing the symptomatology of hairy cell leukemia; hematologic response rates of 80–90% are possible in this disease. Other cancers responsive to alpha interferon include renal cell cancer (10–30% partial response rate); acute leukemias (15–30% response rate), and the nonblastic phase of CML (40–60% response rate). Although not a labeled use, interferon alfa-n3 can be used systemically and is specifically recommended for antibody-positive patients receiving recombinant products.

DNA Intercalating Drugs

ANTHRACYCLINES:	
DAUNORUBICIN HYDROCHLORIDE	Cerubidine
DOXORUBICIN HYDROCHLORIDE	Adriamycin, Rubex
IDARUBICIN HYDROCHLORIDE	Idamycin

Pharmacology. Daunorubicin (daunomycin), doxorubicin (hydroxydaunomycin) and idarubicin (4-demethoxydaunorubicin) are tetracyclic amino sugar-linked antibiotics that are actively taken up by cells and concentrated in the nucleus; intercalation or fitting between DNA base pairs occurs, which impairs DNA synthesis. Other biochemical lesions produced include quinone moiety-generated production of oxygen and hydroxyl free radicals with lipid peroxidation of cellular membranes. The anthracyclines also interfere with the activity of the G_2-specific enzyme, topoisomerase-II, which leads to the formation of cleavable complexes between enzyme and DNA, resulting in DNA double strand breaks. These agents are primarily cell cycle phase nonspecific, but with slightly greater activity in late S or G_2 phase cells.

Administration and Dosage.

	DAUNORUBICIN	DOXORUBICIN	IDARUBICIN
Administration	IV push, infusion. *These compounds are extremely toxic (potent vesicants) if inadvertently extravasated; very careful IV technique is mandatory.*	IV push, infusion.	IV push, infusion.
Adult Dosage	IV 30–45 mg/m²/day for 1–3 days; generally not repeated more often than q 3 weeks.	IV 60–90 mg/m² for 1 dose or 20–30 mg/m²/day for 3 days; generally not repeated more often than q 3 weeks. Alternatively, 20 mg/m²/week.	IV 12 mg/m²/day for 3 days.[122]
Pediatric Dosage	Same as adult dosage.	Same as adult dosage.	Same as adult dosage.[123]
Cumulative Lifetime Dosage Limits*	550 mg/m², up to 850 mg/m².	550 mg/m². 400 mg/m² with prior chest irradiation or preexisting heart disease.[†]	Unknown.

*Attainment of maximal cumulative dosage generally precludes continued use, despite evidence of continuing drug response; however, some patients may continue to respond without development of cardiomyopathy.[124] Use of dexrazoxane can extend dosage limits in breast cancer (*see* Dexrazoxane).
[†]Low weekly doses or continuous 96-hr infusion[125] appear to be less toxic and may allow attainment of greater cumulative dosages (>550 mg/m²).[126,127]

Special Populations. *Other Conditions.* Cumulative dosages of all agents must be reduced in patients with prior irradiation of the cardiac chest region, preexisting heart disease, or prior large cyclophosphamide dosage. Doxorubicin requires no dosage adjustment for severe renal impairment, whereas with daunorubicin 75% of the dosage is recommended in severe renal impairment. Doxorubicin dosages, however, must be substantially reduced with severe hepatic dysfunction.[128] Idarubicin dosage reductions are indicated for bilirubin of 2.6–5 mg/dL or Cr_s ≥2 mg/dL. For severe mucositis, administration is delayed until mucositis resolves, then dosage is reduced by 25%.

SERUM BILIRUBIN (MG/DL)	PERCENTAGE OF DOSE RECOMMENDED	
	Doxorubicin	*Idarubicin*
≤1.2	100 (no reduction)	—
1.2–3	50	—
>3	25 (75% reduction)	50

Dosage Forms. (Daunorubicin) **Inj** 20 mg. (Doxorubicin) **Inj** 10, 20, 50, 100, 150, 200 mg. (Idarubicin) **Inj** 5, 10 mg.

Patient Instructions. *See* Antineoplastics Class Instructions. Immediately report any change in sensation (eg, stinging) at injection site during infusion (this may be an early sign of infiltration). Red-colored urine does not indicate toxicity.

Pharmacokinetics.

	DAUNORUBICIN	DOXORUBICIN	IDARUBICIN	IDARUBICINOL
Fate.				
Absorption	Extensively degraded to inactive aglycone in GI tract.		About 24% oral bioavailability.[129]	The primary active metabolite of idarubicin.
Distribution	Both drugs enter cells rapidly and concentrate in the nucleus. Tissue concentrations are highest in lung, kidney, small intestine, and liver; trivial amounts found in the CNS. Avid tissue binding is probably responsible for prolonged terminal half-lives and V_d of 500–600 L/m².		Peak serum level of 2 μg/L after a dose of 7–9 mg/m².[130] 94% plasma protein bound; V_d about 1700 L/m².	Peak serum level of 15 μg/L.[130] 94% plasma protein bound; V_d about 1700 L/m².
Metabolism	Both drugs are extensively metabolized, initially to less active alcohol metabolites; further metabolized by liver microsomes to inactive aglycones and demethylated glucuronide and sulfate conjugates.[131]		Both agents are partially metabolized and excreted as glucuronide conjugates. Idarubicin Cl is 60–77 L/hr/m².	
Excretion				
Biliary	20–30% of a dose.	40–60% of a dose.	Primary route of excretion.	Primary route of excretion.

(*continued*)

	DAUNORUBICIN	DOXORUBICIN	IDARUBICIN	IDARUBICINOL
Urinary	14–23% as unchanged drug and metabolites (primarily dauno-rubicinol).	5–10% as metabolites over 5 days.[128]	8% of a dose over 24 hr.	8% of a dose over 24 hr.
$t_{1/2}$.	α 45 min β 18.5 hr (daunorubi-cinol 27 hr).	α 30 min β 3 hr γ 17 hr (metabolites 32 hr).[128]	α 14 min[132] β 19–34 hr.[130,132]	— 65.5 hr.[132]

Adverse Reactions. Emetic potential is moderate to moderately high with all three drugs. Stomatitis, nausea, and vomiting are dose dependent and frequent; prophylactic antiemetics are often helpful. Myelosuppression, affecting both platelets and neutrophils, is the major acute dose-limiting side effect. Typical nadirs range from 9–14 days, with recovery nearly complete within 3 weeks of administration. Hemorrhage occurs in up to 10% of induction courses with idaru-bicin. Excessive lacrimation is reported in about 25% of patients receiving doxo-rubicin. Alopecia usually occurs; during low-dose adjuvant chemotherapy admin-istration, regional scalp hypothermia may decrease hair loss.[133] Severe, protracted ulceration and necrosis can occur with inadvertent perivenous infiltration; par-tially effective local treatments include limb elevation, ice packing, and topical **DMSO** (*see* Notes). Large evolving lesions necessitate early plastic surgery con-sultation. Long-term anthracycline use can lead to severe and often fatal car-diomyopathy (*see* Cumulative Dosage Limits and Notes). Symptoms are nonspe-cific and indicative of advanced CHF such as shortness of breath, edema, and fatigue. The frequency is low (overall 2.2%) when total dosage limits are ob-served and may be lower when monthly doses are given over several days or by continuous 96-hr infusion.[134] Late cardiotoxicity is reported in children receiving total dosages of doxorubicin <500 mg/m².[135] During drug infusion, various non-specific ECG changes may occur; these do not imply an increased risk of car-diotoxicity. Graded endomyocardial biopsy and graded radionuclide angiography have proved most effective for assessment of the emergence of severe cardiomy-opathy. Other reactions include transient erythema and phlebitis during adminis-tration and a radiation-synergy phenomenon involving heightened tissue reac-tions in concurrently or previously irradiated tissues, especially the esophagus (avoid by spacing weeks apart). Urine remains red for 1–2 days after administra-tion.

Contraindications. Preexisting bone marrow suppression (WBCs <3000/μL; platelets <120,000/μL; MI in previous 6 months; history of CHF). Marrow sup-pression is not a contraindication in relapsed leukemia patients.

Precautions. Careful administration technique is mandatory to avoid extravasa-tion and tissue necrosis. Hepatocellular disease or cirrhosis may slow production of alcohol metabolites.

Drug Interactions. A number of drugs may interact with the anthracyclines: vinca alkaloids (cross-resistance), amphotericin B (increased drug uptake), and cyclosporine and streptozocin (reduced drug clearance and increased toxicity).[136] Most of these drug interactions have only been studied in vitro and require clinical confirmation.

Parameters to Monitor. Obtain pretreatment and at least biweekly nadir WBC and platelet counts. Monitor general cardiac status and serial radionuclide scans of the heart in high-risk patients. Add up prior doses to estimate cardiotoxicity dosage limit.

Notes. These drugs are compatible with usual IV solutions but incompatible with heparin, sodium bicarbonate, and fluorouracil. IV push doses are best reconstituted with NS or D5W. These solutions are stable for prolonged periods and can withstand freezing and thawing.[137] Doxorubicin is widely effective in numerous solid tumors, such as ovarian, thyroid, and gastric carcinomas, sarcomas, and cancer of the breast, as well as hematologic malignancies, such as the lymphomas and leukemias. The iron-chelating agent dexrazoxane reduces doxorubicin-induced cardiotoxicity in patients with breast cancer[138] (*see* Dexrazoxane). The activity of idarubicin and daunorubicin is limited primarily to AML. Topical **DMSO** (1.5 mL of a 90% w/v solution q 6 hr for 2 weeks) has been effective at preventing extravasation ulceration in one trial.[139]

DAUNORUBICIN CITRATE, LIPOSOMAL   DaunoXome

Pharmacology. Daunorubicin is encapsulated in the lipid component of this red emulsion formulation, which consists of distearoylphosphatidylcholine and cholesterol in a fixed lipid:daunorubicin ratio of 1:18.6 (in mg/mL). These liposomes are taken up into tumor and reticuloendothelial system cells, which release prolonged but low serum levels of daunorubicin over time.[140] Murine studies suggest selective (enhanced) uptake of liposomal daunorubicin into tumor tissues compared to normal organs.[141] It is used to treat AIDS-related Kaposi's sarcoma.

Administration and Adult Dosage. IV for Kaposi's sarcoma 40 mg/m^2 q 2 weeks.

Special Populations. *Pediatric Dosage.* Safety and efficacy not established.

Geriatric Dosage. Same as adult dosage.

Other Conditions. Based on studies with daunorubicin, reduce dose by 25% for a serum bilirubin of 1.2–3 mg/dL and by 50% for a serum bilirubin or Cr_s >3 mg/dL. Do not administer if absolute granulocyte count is under 750/μL.

Dosage Forms. Inj 50 mg.

Pharmacokinetics. *Fate.* Mean peak serum levels (free plus liposomal) after doses of 20, 40, 60, and 80 mg/m^2 are 8.2, 18.2, 36.2, and 43.6 mg/L, respectively.[140] Compared to equivalent doses of the nonliposomal drug, the free drug levels are 100-fold lower for up to 2.5 days after administration. In adults, V_d is 2.9–4.1 L; Cl ranges from 0.4–0.9 L/hr, about 5% of the Cl of the free drug.[140] Thus, the AUC is increased, Cl is slowed, but peak levels are low with the liposomal formulation.

$t_{1/2}$. 2.8–5.2 hr (total of liposomal plus free drug).

Adverse Reactions. Emetic potential is low to moderate. The most frequent symptoms are mild to moderate fatigue, which occurs in 56% of patients, and low-grade fever in 26% of patients. An acute triad of back pain, flushing, and chest tightness may occur in up to 14% of patients, usually upon initial administration. This liposomal-component reaction subsides with interruption of the infusion and typically does not recur upon restarting at a slower infusion rate. Neutropenia occurs in 17% of patients; mild anemia and thrombocytopenia occur in 7% and 4% of treatment courses, respectively. Diarrhea occurs in 10% of patients; mild liver enzyme elevation occurs in 4% of patients.[140] Cardiac toxicity appears to be less with this formulation than with aqueous daunorubicin.

Contraindications. Previous serious allergy to the drug or any component of the formulation. *See* Anthracyclines, Daunorubicin.

Precautions. Pregnancy; lactation. Do not administer if absolute granulocyte count is under 750/µL.

Drug Interactions. Not well studied with this formulation. *See* Anthracyclines.

Parameters to Monitor. Monitor the number of Kaposi's sarcoma lesions for response or evidence of disease progression (10 or more new lesions or an increase of 25%). Obtain WBC count prior to administration. Monitor left ventricular ejection fraction at cumulative dosages of 320 and 480 mg/m^2, and q 240 mg/m^2 thereafter.

Notes. Mix only in D5W; do not filter.

DOXORUBICIN HYDROCHLORIDE, LIPOSOMAL   Doxil

Pharmacology. Doxorubicin is encapsulated in the aqueous core of small (100-nm) liposomes composed of a phospholipid bilayer with an outer coating of polyethylene glycol (PEG). The small liposome size and PEG coating mask recognition by reticuloendothelial cells, thereby increasing the half-life of the liposomes in vivo. Once the liposomes accumulate in tissues, free doxorubicin is slowly released to exert its antitumor effect. Most toxicities are reduced by the liposomal formulation without compromising efficacy in solid tumors such as Kaposi's sarcoma (*see* Anthracycline Agents).

Administration and Adult Dosage. **IV for AIDS-related Kaposi's sarcoma** 20 mg/m^2 q 3 weeks.

Special Populations. *Pediatric Dosage.* Safety and efficacy not established.

Geriatric Dosage. Same as adult dosage.

Other Conditions. (Liver dysfunction) Reduce dosage 50% for serum bilirubin 1.2–3 mg/dL; reduce dosage by 75% for bilirubin over 3 mg/dL. (Stomatitis) For patients who develop stomatitis, wait 1 week, reevaluate, and readminister at 100% for Grade II severity (painful ulcers, but able to eat), 75% for Grade III severity (painful ulcers and unable to eat), or 50% for Grade IV severity (extensive, disabling stomatitis requiring nutritional support). (Hematologic toxicity) Reduce dose and/or delay administration to allow for ANC and platelet count (PC) to return to at least 1000/µL and 50,000/µL, respectively. Then readminister at 100% of dosage if nadir ANC was 1000–1500/µL and/or PC was 50,000–150,000/µL; 75% of dosage if nadir ANC was 500/µL and/or PC was 25,000–50,000/µL; or 50% of dosage if nadir

ANC was under 500/µL and/or PC was under 25,000/µL, respectively. (Erythrodysesthesia) For Grade I erythrodysesthesia (mild swelling or erythema) present 4 weeks after the dose, administer 75% of standard dosage. For Grade II erythrodysesthesia (erythema or desquamation not precluding physical activity) present 3 weeks after the dose, delay the dose for 1 week; if present 4 weeks after the dose, reduce the next dose by 50%. For Grade III erythrodysesthesia (palmar-plantar [hand/foot] that is severe [diffuse blistering]) 3 weeks after drug administration, hold the next dose for 1 week; if it is still present at 4 weeks, discontinue the drug.

Dosage Forms. Inj 2 mg/mL.

Patient Instructions. *See* Antineoplastics Class Instructions.

Pharmacokinetics. *Fate.* Mean peak serum levels (±SE) after 10 and 20 mg/m^2 doses are 4.1 ± 0.2 and 8.3 ± 0.5 µg/mL, respectively. Most of this level is liposomally encapsulated drug; the assay does not differentiate. Liposomal doxorubicin has a smaller V_d (2.2–4.4 L/m^2) than free doxorubicin; Cl is 0.034–0.108 L/hr/m^2. The AUC for the 10 and 20 mg/m^2 doses are 277 ± 33 (±SE) and 590 ± 59 (±SE) mg·L/hr. A small amount (0.8–2.6 ng/mL) of the doxorubicinol metabolite is found in serum following a dose. Cl of parent drug ranges from 24–35 L/hr/m^2. Tissue concentrations of drug may be 19 times higher in Kaposi's sarcoma lesions than in adjacent normal skin.[142]

$t_{1/2}$. (Liposomal and free drug) α phase 5.2 ± 1.4 hr; ß phase 55 ± 4.8 hr.

Adverse Reactions. Similar to free doxorubicin. Myelosuppression, principally neutropenia, occurs in 49% of patients and sepsis in 5%. Opportunistic infections also occur in AIDS patients, especially those with a high tumor burden, low CD4 count, or preexisting infection. Palmar-plantar erythrodysesthesia is cumulative. It is manifested as painful red soles and palms, which can progress to ulceration and debilitating infection if doses are not reduced and/or delayed. Doxorubicin-induced cumulative dosage cardiomyopathy and inadvertent extravasation necrosis may be lessened, but not entirely eliminated, with the liposomal formulation. Radiation recall soft tissue toxicity has been reported.

Contraindications. *See* Anthracyclines, Doxorubicin.

Precautions. May sensitize soft tissues to radiation damage. To lessen frequency of irreversible cardiomyopathy, observe the cumulative anthracycline dosage limit of 500 mg/m^2. Avoid extravasation, and do not give IM or SC.

Drug Interactions. *See* Anthracyclines.

Parameters to Monitor. Obtain absolute neutrophil count and platelet count, serum bilirubin level, and severity of stomatitis and palmar-plantar erythrodysesthesia prior to administration.

Notes. Do not filter. Overall response rates of 40–60% are reported for patients with AIDS-related Kaposi's sarcoma;[142,143] it may also be effective in other solid tumors in HIV-negative patients.

DACTINOMYCIN   Cosmegen

Dactinomycin (actinomycin D) is a tricyclic, peptide-containing antibiotic that acts as an intercalator of DNA, resulting in decreased mRNA transcription in a phase nonspecific fashion. It is used in the treatment of sarcomas and choriocarcinoma. About 30% of the drug is recovered from the feces and urine after 1 week; there is no CNS penetration, and it is probably concentrated in the bile. The terminal half-life is over 36 hr. Nausea, vomiting, mucositis, diarrhea, and reversible alopecia occur frequently. Dose- and duration-dependent hepatotoxicity and genotoxic effects have been reported. Severe ulceration occurs if the drug is extravasated. The dose-limiting toxicity is myelosuppression with a leukopenic nadir at 7–10 days. Rarely, radiation recall occurs. Reconstitute dactinomycin with preservative-free diluents. It is bound by cellulose filters, so avoid in-line filtration. The adult IV dosage is 2 mg/week or 500 µg/day for up to 5 days, repeated at 3- to 4-week intervals. In children, the IV dosage is 450 µg/m^2/day, to a maximum of 500 µg/day, for up to 5 days; the course is repeated in 3 weeks. Reduce dosage in the presence of hepatobiliary dysfunction.[144,145] Available as a 0.5-mg injection.

MITOXANTRONE   Novantrone

Pharmacology. Mitoxantrone is a substituted salt of a planar anthracene. The drug binds to DNA by intercalation and inhibits topoisomerase II, producing DNA strand breaks; DNA synthesis is impaired in a cell cycle phase nonspecific fashion.[146]

Administration and Adult Dosage. IV for solid tumors 12 mg/m^2 q 4 weeks or 5 mg/m^2/week for 3 weeks. IV for leukemia 10–12 mg/m^2/day for 3 days.

Special Populations. *Pediatric Dosage.* IV for leukemia up to 8 mg/m^2/week for 3 weeks or up to 18 mg/m^2 q 4 weeks.[147]

Geriatric Dosage. Same as adult dosage.

Other Conditions. Reduce doses by approximately 30–50% in patients with abnormal hepatobiliary function and/or appreciable third-space fluid accumulations.[148] Reduced doses are also required in patients with poor bone marrow reserve. No dosage alteration is required with renal function impairment.

Dosage Forms. **Inj** 2 mg/mL.

Patient Instructions. *See* Antineoplastics Class Instructions. This drug may turn urine blue-green for 24 hr after administration because of the dark blue drug color. Discoloration of the whites of the eyes may also occur.

Pharmacokinetics. *Fate.* The drug is over 95% plasma protein bound and exhibits prolonged retention in tissues. Some liver metabolism to glucuronyl and glutathione conjugates occurs. Urinary recovery is less than 8% of a dose; the majority is eliminated in the bile; fecal recovery averages 18% of a dose over 5 days.[148]

$t_{1/2}$. α phase 14 min; β phase 1.1 hr; γ phase 38–43 hr.[148]

Adverse Reactions. Emetic potential is low. Myelosuppression, principally granulocytopenia (nadir at 10–14 days), occurs and is most severe in heavily pretreated or irradiated patients. Mucositis, which is dose limiting, occurs only with weekly regimens. CHF has been reported frequently, most often after prior anthracycline therapy. Cumulative cardiotoxicity limits are not well established, but may approach 125 mg/m^2 with prior anthracyclines and 160 mg/m^2 without.[146] Alopecia and extravasation necrosis are minimal.

Precautions. Reduce the dosage in patients with poor hepatobiliary function. Dosage reduction may also be necessary in patients previously treated with marrow suppressant or cardiotoxic agents.

Drug Interactions. None known.

Parameters to Monitor. Obtain serum bilirubin before each dose. Assess cardiac function in patients with prior anthracycline therapy or severe preexisting cardiovascular disease. Monitor absolute granulocyte levels prior to each dose; nadir counts 7–10 days after the dose are optional.

Notes. Mitoxantrone is not usually a vesicant, although it can rarely cause necrosis and usually tints the tissues a blue color.

PLICAMYCIN   Mithracin

Plicamycin (mithramycin) is a complex, polycyclic, sugar-linked antibiotic that acts by DNA binding in a cell cycle phase nonspecific fashion; it also has a separate calcium-lowering effect. It is used in testicular cancer and to control severe hypercalcemia caused by malignancy. The metabolic fate of the drug is unknown, but the drug penetrates well into the CNS and 40% of radioactivity from a radiolabeled dose appears in the urine. Mild to moderate myelosuppression with a leukopenic nadir at 7–12 days, nausea, and vomiting occur frequently. Dose- and duration-dependent nephrotoxicity (increased Cr_s and proteinuria) and hepatotoxicity (increased LDH and AST) occur frequently. Sterility, mutagenicity, and teratogenicity have been reported. The dose-limiting toxicity is a hemorrhagic tendency characterized by decreased platelet count and responsiveness, and depressed clotting factor synthesis. Rarely, stomatitis, progressive skin thickening, and hyperpigmentation occur. The drug is an irritant, but not a vesicant if extravasated. The drug is contraindicated in patients with preexisting bleeding diatheses, hypocalcemia, or severe renal or hepatic dysfunction. Use cautiously, if at all, with other drugs affecting platelet function (eg, aspirin). The dosage for testicular tumors is 25–30 µg/kg/day for up to 5 days, repeat in 4 weeks if toxicity has resolved. For hypercalcemia, a dose of 25 µg/kg/day is given for 3–4 days. Reduce dosage by 25–50% in moderate to severe renal impairment.[149,150] Available as a 2.5-mg vial. *Note:* dosage is in µg/kg with no single dose over 3 mg.

Hormonal Drugs and Antagonists

AMINOGLUTETHIMIDE   Cytadren

ANASTROZOLE   Arimidex

Pharmacology. Aminoglutethimide and anastrozole inhibit the metabolic conversion of androstenedione to estradiol, which is mediated by aromatase, primarily in peripheral adipose tissues. In postmenopausal women, this deprives hormonally sensitive breast cancers of estrogenic stimulation. Aminoglutethimide is less specific and also blocks the cholesterol-based biosynthesis of all corticosteroid precursors (ie, hydrocortisone, aldosterone) in the adrenal gland and at peripheral sites.[151,152]

Administration and Adult Dosage. (Aminoglutethimide) **PO** 750 mg–1.5 g/day; (Anastrozole) **PO** 1 mg/day.

Dosage Forms. (Aminoglutethimide) **Tab** 250 mg. (Anastrozole) **Tab** 1 mg.

Dosage Modification. *Pediatric Dosage.* (Aminoglutethimide) Safety and efficacy not established, but the following has been used; **PO for adrenal hyperplasia and adrenal tumors** (>2.5 yr) 0.375–1.5 g/day. (Anastrozole) Safety and efficacy not established.

Geriatric Dosage. Same as adult dosage.

Other Conditions. (Anastrozole) No change required in hepatic or renal impairment.

Patient Instructions. (Aminoglutethimide) If severe stress or trauma occurs, increased hydrocortisone dosage may be needed. Marked drowsiness may occur during therapy. Skin rashes are common, especially at the start of therapy.

Pharmacokinetics. *Fate.* (Aminoglutethimide) A 1-g oral dose yields serum levels of 9 µg/mL. Cl averages 5.5 L/hr in adults. About 50% is metabolized in liver to a less active N-acetyl derivative; this and other metabolites are excreted renally.[1,151] (Anastrozole) Extensively metabolized and excreted renally (10% as parent, 60% as metabolites).[152]

$t_{1/2}$. (Aminoglutethimide) α phase 2.5 hr; ß phase 13.3 hr. (Anastrozole) 50 hr.[1,151,152]

Adverse Reactions. (Aminoglutethimide) Lethargy and somnolence (80%); skin rashes (50%); visual blurring, dizziness (15–30%, especially in the elderly); nausea, vomiting, and hypotension (15%); hypothyroidism (5%); hematologic suppression (eg, agranulocytosis, pancytopenia) (<1%). (Anastrozole) Asthenia (16%); nausea (15%); headache (13%); hot flashes (12%); back pain (10%); emesis (9%); dizziness, rash, constipation (<5%).

Contraindications. None known.

Precautions. (Aminoglutethimide) Supplemental **hydrocortisone** 50–100 mg/day and **fludrocortisone** 0.1 mg/day are required during therapy.

Drug Interactions. (Aminoglutethimide) Several drug interactions may occur because of the drug's enhancement of CYP3A metabolism; the effects of dexamethasone, digoxin, medroxyprogesterone, tamoxifen, theophylline, and warfarin may be reduced. Aminoglutethimide also induces its own metabolism, which decreases blood levels and half-lives during long-term therapy.

Parameters to Monitor. (Aminoglutethimide) Monitor thyroid function and blood pressure periodically during therapy.

BICALUTAMIDE	Casodex
FLUTAMIDE	Eulexin

Pharmacology. Bicalutamide and flutamide are nonsteroidal antiandrogens that competitively inhibit binding of testosterone at androgen receptors in the testes and prostate gland, reducing androgen-stimulated cell growth. They are used together with an LHRH analogue (eg, leuprolide or goserelin). Bicalutamide has a longer half-life and fourfold higher affinity than flutamide for the androgen receptor, which allows once-daily administration.[153,154]

Administration and Adult Dosage. **PO for prostate cancer** together with an LHRH analogue (Bicalutamide) 40 mg once daily; (Flutamide) 250 mg q 8 hr.

Special Populations. *Pediatric Dosage.* Safety and efficacy not established.

Geriatric Dosage. Same as adult dosage.

Other Conditions. If prostate-specific antigen (PSA) levels rise together with clinical disease progression, consider discontinuing the antiandrogen temporarily and continuing the LHRH antagonist to reestablish androgen receptor sensitivity. Renal or hepatic impairment does not appear to alter elimination of either drug.

Dosage Forms. (Bicalutamide) **Tab** 50 mg. (Flutamide) **Tab** 125 mg.

Patient Instructions. Take therapy continuously without interruption. Start bicalutamide at the same time as the LHRH agonist. Hot flashes and some feminizing side effects (especially breast enlargement or tenderness) may occur during therapy.

Pharmacokinetics. *Fate.* Both agents are well absorbed orally and absorption is unaffected by food, but absolute bioavailability is unknown. (Bicalutamide) With an oral dose of 50 mg/day, bicalutamide attains a peak serum level of 8.9 mg/L (21 μmol/L) 31 hr after a dose at steady state. Cl of (R)-bicalutamide is 0.32 L/hr. The active (R)-enantiomer of bicalutamide is oxidized to an inactive metabolite, which, like the inactive (S)-enantiomer, is glucuronidated and cleared rapidly by elimination in the urine and feces.[154] (Flutamide) Flutamide attains peak serum levels of 78 μg/L (283 nmol/L) 2–4 hr after a 250-mg dose at steady state, and its metabolite (α-hydroxyflutamide) achieves levels of 0.720–1.68 mg/L. Flutamide and its active metabolite α-hydroxyflutamide are bound to plasma proteins. Both drugs are extensively metabolized. The majority of a flutamide dose is excreted in the urine as 2-amino-5-nitro-4-(trifluoromethyl) phenol (inactive) with little parent and active metabolite (4.2% of a dose) excreted in the bile or feces.[155,156]

$t_{1/2}$. (Bicalutamide) 5.8 days; (Flutamide) 7.8 hr.[154–156]

Adverse Reactions. Both agents are relatively well tolerated. When the drugs are combined with an LHRH agonist, the following side effects occur: hot flashes (50%), general pain (25%), back pain (16%), asthenia (16%), pelvic pain (12%), constipation (15%), diarrhea (10–24%, higher with flutamide, possibly because of lactose intolerance),[157] nausea (11%), nocturia (10%), liver enzyme elevation (6–10%), abdominal pain (8%), and chest pain (5%). Hepatic injury and jaundice occur rarely.

Contraindications. None known.

Precautions. Discontinue these drugs if liver function tests are consistently over twice the upper limits of normal in the absence of hepatic metastases.

Drug Interactions. Dosage adjustment of warfarin, based on INR, may be necessary when bicalutamide is administered because it can displace warfarin from protein binding sites in vitro.

Parameters to Monitor. Monitor prostate specific antigen (PSA) levels q 3 months as an index of disease response. Obtain serum transaminases q 3–4 months to rule out drug-induced hepatic injury.

ESTRAMUSTINE PHOSPHATE   Emcyt

Pharmacology. Estramustine is a conjugate of nor-nitrogen mustard linked by a carbamate bond to the 3 position of the steroidal nucleus of estradiol. Phosphorylation at position 17 adds water solubility. Estramustine was originally thought to act as a hormonally directed alkylating agent, but later studies suggest an alternate effect, impairment of mitotic spindle formation. Dephosphorylated estradiol and estrone metabolites produce typical estrogenic effects.[158]

Administration and Adult Dosage. **PO for prostatic carcinoma** 14 mg/kg/day in 3–4 divided doses.

Special Populations. *Geriatric Dosage.* Same as adult dosage.

Other Conditions. Diabetic and hypertensive patients may require increased doses of insulin or antihypertensives because of estrogenic effects.

Dosage Forms. **Cap** 140 mg.

Patient Instructions. Take this drug on an empty stomach; particularly avoid taking with milk, milk products, or calcium-containing foods or drugs.

Pharmacokinetics. *Fate.* Milk and calcium salts reduce oral bioavailability by forming nonabsorbable calcium complexes. Dephosphorylated during absorption to estradiol and estrone congeners (*see* Estradiol, Estrone).

Adverse Reactions. Emetic potential is low. The major side effects are caused by estrogenic actions. These include very frequent gynecomastia, cardiovascular effects (frequent edema, occasional leg cramps, or thrombophlebitis, and rare pulmonary embolism and infarction), and GI effects (frequent nausea without vomiting, diarrhea, and occasional anorexia). Laboratory abnormalities are minimal; there is no consistent hematologic suppression and only mild increases in AST or LDH in about 30% of patients.[158]

Contraindications. Thrombophlebitis or thromboembolic conditions (except when tumor is the cause).

Precautions. Use with caution in patients with severe underlying cardiovascular diseases. Poorly controlled CHF can also be exacerbated by estrogen-induced fluid retention. Insulin-dependent diabetics and patients on antihypertensive medications may have increased medication requirements for these diseases.

Drug Interactions. Dairy products or calcium salts may reduce estramustine bioavailability.

Parameters to Monitor. Responses in prostate cancer are predominantly subjective, including reduced pain and less urinary retention. Objective responses can be followed with serial acid phosphatase determinations. Attention to cardiovascular or thromboembolic signs and symptoms is important.

Notes. Estramustine phosphate is principally used in the palliative treatment of advanced prostate cancer. Objective partial response rates of 20% are common. The drug can be safely combined with cytotoxic agents.[158]

GONADOTROPIN-RELEASING HORMONE ANALOGUES:	
GOSERELIN ACETATE	Zoladex
LEUPROLIDE ACETATE	Lupron

Pharmacology. Goserelin and leuprolide are synthetic peptide analogues of the natural hypothalamic hormone, gonadotropin-releasing hormone (GnRH). This hormone controls the release of pituitary LH and FSH to stimulate sex hormone production in the testes (testosterone) and ovaries (estradiol, others). Both synthetic agents have d-amino acid and other substitutions to increase stimulatory potency. FSH and LH are initially stimulated, followed by profound inhibition of circulating sex hormones to castration levels. This retards the growth of hormonally dependent organs including the prostate, breast, endometrium, and ovaries.[159,160]

Administration and Adult Dosage. SC for prostatic carcinoma (goserelin) insert 3.6 mg implant into upper abdominal wall q 28 days; (leuprolide aqueous) 1 mg/day. **IM for prostatic carcinoma** (leuprolide depot) 7.5 mg of 1-month formulation q 28–33 days or 22.5 mg of the 3-month formulation q 3 months. **SC for endometriosis** (goserelin) insert 3.6-mg implant into upper abdominal wall q 28 days for 6 months; **IM for endometriosis** (leuprolide depot) 3.75 mg monthly for 6 months.

Special Populations. *Pediatric Dosage.* SC for central precocious puberty (CPP) (leuprolide aqueous) 50 µg/kg/day initially, increasing in 10 µg/kg/day increments until total down-regulation is achieved. **IM for CPP** initial dosage is (≤25 kg) 7.5 mg monthly; (25–37.5 kg) 11.25 mg monthly; (>37.5 kg) 15 mg monthly. Increase in 3.75 mg/month increments until total down-regulation is achieved.

Geriatric Dosage. (Prostatic cancer) Same as adult dosage.

Dosage Forms. (Goserelin) **Implant** 3.6 mg. (Leuprolide) **Inj (aqueous)** 5 mg/mL; **Inj (depot, 1-month formulations)** 3.75, 7.5, 11.25, 15 mg; (**3-month formulation**) 22.5 mg/1.5 mL. (*Note:* do not use a partial dose of the 3-month formulation in place of a 1-month formulation.)

Patient Instructions. Instruct in proper method of aseptic preparation of vials and syringes, proper technique for SC administration, and proper disposal of syringes and needles. (Prostate cancer) Disease symptoms such as bone pain and urinary retention may become worse briefly upon initiation of therapy. (Endometriosis) Do not become pregnant while on this drug; always use a barrier contraceptive. Notify your physician if regular menstruation continues. Because therapy may cause a loss of bone density, calcium supplementation is recommended. (Pediatric CPP) A slight increase in pubertal signs and symptoms may occur initially. Adherence to therapy is critical; symptoms such as menses or breast or testicular development may indicate inadequate therapy.

Pharmacokinetics. *Fate.* Both drugs are inactive orally. The SC, IM, and IV routes provide comparable bioavailability. The metabolism of these compounds has not been described. (Goserelin) Goserelin is slowly absorbed over the first 8 days. Thereafter, absorption is steady for the remaining 28 days with no evidence of dose-to-dose accumulation. Goserelin serum levels of about 2.5 µg/L occur on days 15–16 in males with prostate cancer. (Leuprolide) The absorption profile of leuprolide 3-month formulation is similar to the 7.5-mg 1-month formulation. Leuprolide serum levels after a 7.5-mg depot injection are 20 µg/L at 4 hr and 0.36 µg/L at 4 weeks.

$t_{1/2}$. (Goserelin) 4.2 hr with Cl_{cr} over 70 mL/min; 12.1 hr with Cl_{cr} under 20 mL/min. (Leuprolide) 2.9 hr.

Adverse Reactions. Emetic potential is low; nausea occurs in less than 5% of patients. Prostate cancer symptoms flare initially, causing bone pain or urinary retention. Sexual dysfunction and decreased erections are reported in about 20% of males. Hot flashes may initially occur in up to 80% of patients with endometriosis, who may also experience calcium loss and estrogen deficiency side effects including decreased libido, vaginal discomfort, dizziness, general malaise, emotional lability or depression. Mild injection site reactions are rare, unless the patient is sensitive to benzyl alcohol (leuprolide aqueous only).

Contraindications. Pregnancy, because of an established teratogenic activity in animals. Do not initiate therapy for endometriosis until after negative pregnancy test.

Precautions. Monitor carefully initially in prostate cancer patients. Those with severe metastatic vertebral lesions are subject to spinal cord compression, and those with severe urinary retention may develop renal impairment.

Drug Interactions. None known.

Parameters to Monitor. (Prostate cancer) Monitor serum LH, FSH, estradiol, and testosterone; concentrations should fall to castrate levels with adequate GnRH analogue therapy. Close initial monitoring of disease symptom severity (bone pain, urinary retention) is required. Serum prostate-specific antigen (PSA) levels should fall and remain low in patients who respond. (Endometriosis) Monitor pain and menstrual symptoms.

Notes. In prostate cancer, these drugs are often combined with an androgen receptor antagonist (eg, **bicalutamide**, **flutamide**) to provide complete hormonal blockade.

TAMOXIFEN CITRATE   Nolvadex, Various

Pharmacology. Tamoxifen is a synthetic, nonsteroidal antiestrogen that binds to cytosol or nuclear estrogen receptor (ER) proteins in hormonally sensitive organs including the breast, prostate, uterus, and ovary.[161] The tamoxifen-receptor complex binds to chromatin in the cell nucleus, stopping estrogen-dependent growth-stimulatory mRNA synthesis.

Administration and Adult Dosage. PO for breast cancer usually 20 mg bid in premenopausal patients and 10 mg bid in postmenopausal patients. To rapidly achieve steady-state levels, an initial 2-week course of 40 mg/m^2 bid followed by the standard maintenance dosage has been recommended.[162]

Special Populations. *Geriatric Dosage.* Same as adult dosage.

Dosage Forms. **Tab** 10 mg.

Patient Instructions. In premenopausal patients the chance of becoming pregnant is increased and a barrier contraceptive should be used. You should have regular gynecologic examinations after taking this drug and report any menstrual irregularities, abnormal vaginal discharge or bleeding, or pelvic pain or pressure. Lactation may occur while on tamoxifen.

Pharmacokinetics. *Onset and Duration.* Therapeutic levels are attained in 7 or more days with 10–20 mg/m^2/day, but in 3 hr after the loading dose regimen of 40 mg/m^2 or more bid.[162]

Serum Levels. There does not appear to be a direct relationship between serum levels and response or time to response, but all responders have tamoxifen levels over 180 µg/L (0.48 µmol/L) at the time of remission.

Fate. Well absorbed orally, with a peak of 42 µg/L (0.11 µmol/L; 12 µg/L is N-desmethyl metabolite) achieved 3–4 hr after a 20-mg dose.[163] Initially, the N-desmethyl concentration is only 50% of the tamoxifen level, but after 21 days the metabolite level is higher because of its longer half-life. With low-dose continuous therapy, mean steady-state tamoxifen levels of 260 µg/L (0.7 µmol/L) or more are achieved after 16 weeks. Tamoxifen is slowly but extensively metabolized, mainly to N-desmethyltamoxifen, which is equally antiestrogenic to tamoxifen. Neither is readily conjugated, and both undergo hepatic hydroxylation and conjugation followed by elimination into the bile and feces; levels are measurable for up to 6 weeks after drug discontinuation.[162]

t½. (Tamoxifen) 4 days; (N-desmethyltamoxifen) 9 days.[163] With long-term use, these half-lives increase slightly.[162]

Adverse Reactions. Emetic potential is moderately low. Well tolerated, producing rare minor myelosuppression (usually in heavily pretreated patients). Menopausal symptomatology, including hot flashes, nausea, and rarely vomiting, is produced in one-third of patients. Menstrual difficulties include irregularity, vaginal bleeding, and pruritus vulvae. A serious disease "flare" occurs occasionally during initial therapy involving hypercalcemia and an increase in bone or soft tissue pain;[164] the flare often subsides even with continued therapy and may indicate early tumor response. Retinopathy has occurred, most commonly after very large dosages, but also with usual dosages. The drug appears to produce estrogenlike effects in the bone; thus, skeletal demineralization is not a problem with long-term therapy. An increased risk of secondary uterine cancer has been reported.

Precautions. Pregnancy. Use with caution in patients with preexisting leukopenia and thrombocytopenia.

Drug Interactions. Aminoglutethimide may decrease tamoxifen serum levels. Tamoxifen may attenuate the cytotoxic activities of fluorouracil and doxorubicin.[1]

Notes. The response rate in breast cancer is about 50–70% in ER-positive patients, whereas the rate in ER-negative patients is only about 5–10%.[165] Tamoxifen has also been used in endometrial, stage D prostatic, and renal cell cancers as well as in melanoma.[1] It has also been used investigationally to decrease the size and pain of gynecomastia. **Tormifene citrate** (Fareston) is an antiestrogen very similar chemically and clinically to **tamoxifen**, although it may have less intrinsic estrogenic activity than tamoxifen. It is used in ER-positive or ER-unknown breast cancer. Most tumors exhibit almost complete cross-resistance to the two drugs. The dosage is 60 mg/day orally.

Mitotic Inhibitors

DOCETAXEL   Taxotere

Pharmacology. Docetaxel is a semisynthetic derivative of a taxane extracted from the needles of the yew tree, *Taxus baccata*. It binds to microtubule tubulin sites distinct from paclitaxel with the similar result of enhanced microtubule polymerization, causing clumps to form and halting cell division in metaphase. It is active in refractory breast cancer and in non–small cell lung cancer.[166]

Administration and Adult Dosage. IV for breast cancer 60–100 mg/m^2 infused over 1 hr q 21 days; premedicate with dexamethasone 16 mg/day for 5 days, starting 1 day prior to docetaxel.

Special Populations. *Pediatric Dosage.* Safety and efficacy not established.

Geriatric Dosage. Same as adult dosage.

Other Conditions. Reduce dosage by 25–50% in patients with elevated hepatic enzymes (and probably also with elevated serum bilirubin).

Dosage Forms. Inj 40 mg/mL.

Patient Instructions. Immediately report fever or chills occurring 1–2 weeks after drug administration. This drug may cause swelling of the extremities and tingling sensations.

Pharmacokinetics. *Fate.* Peak serum levels average 3.6 μg/mL following a 1-hr IV infusion of 100 mg/m^2. Over 90% is plasma protein bound. Cl averages 40 L/hr in adults; Cl is reduced by 25% or more in patients with elevated liver function tests (transaminases >1.5 times normal and alkaline phosphatase >2.5 times normal). Most of the drug is metabolized to less active hydroxylated forms and excreted by biliary secretion into the feces; less than 5% is excreted in urine.

t½. α phase 5 min; β phase 38 min; γ phase 12 hr.

Adverse Reactions. Emetic potential is moderate. The dose-limiting toxicity is neutropenia, which is more severe with reduced liver function; the onset of febrile neutropenia can be as soon as 5 days after drug administration. Thrombocytopenia also occurs, but is less severe. Anemia and alopecia also occur, but are not dose limiting. Infusion-associated hypersensitivity symptoms (eg, facial flushing) occur in 50% of patients, whereas dyspnea, chest tightness, and low back pain are rare. A pruritic rash on the forearms, hands, and neck occurs in about 40% of patients. Mucositis and nausea and vomiting occur in about one-third of patients. Peripheral nerve numbness and paresthesia, fluid retention, and edema are cumulative dose-related toxicities. Weight gain initially involves peripheral edema at cumulative dosages over 500 mg/m^2; edema may become prominent after 6 cycles (600 mg/m^2 total dosage) and can proceed to pulmonary edema. Pretreatment with oral dexamethasone (8 mg bid for 5 days, starting 24 hr before docetaxel) retards the development of serious fluid retention.

Contraindications. Severe hypersensitivity to drugs formulated with polysorbate 80; neutropenia <1500/μL; hepatic transaminase levels over 1.5 times the upper limit of normal; hepatic alkaline phosphatase levels over 2.5 times normal; severe preexisting neutropenia, edema, or peripheral neuropathy.

Precautions. Febrile neutropenia is frequent, necessitating careful followup of infectious signs after administration.

Drug Interactions. In vitro, metabolism of docetaxel to its hydroxy metabolites is reduced by inhibitors of CYP3A such as cimetidine, erythromycin, ketoconazole, and troleandomycin. Barbiturates stimulate metabolism of docetaxel.[167] The clinical importance of these findings is not known.

Parameters to Monitor. WBC count, peripheral edema, liver function tests (ALT, APT, alkaline phosphatase) and signs of infection.

ETOPOSIDE	VePesid, Various
ETOPOSIDE PHOSPHATE	Etopophos

Pharmacology. Etoposide (VP-16) is a substituted epipodophyllotoxin derivative from the May apple plant. The major cytotoxic activity is cell cycle phase specific for G_2 and involves the induction of protein-linked DNA strand breaks by inhibiting DNA topoisomerase II enzymes.

Administration and Adult Dosage. IV 200–250 mg/m^2 q 7 weeks, or 70 mg/m^2/day for 5 days. IV of etoposide should be administered over 30–60 min or longer; etoposide phosphate may be administered over 5–210 min. **IV continuous infusion** 125 mg/m^2/day for 5 days.[168] **PO for small cell lung cancer** 2 times the IV dose, rounded to the nearest 50 mg; alternatively, 50 mg/day for 30 days.

Special Populations. *Pediatric Dosage.* Safety and efficacy are not established. However, etoposide has been used in dosages similar to adult body surface area dosages.[169–171]

Geriatric Dosage. Same as adult dosage, but adjust for age-related reduction in renal function.

Other Conditions. With Cl_{cr} ≤20 mL/min give 75% of standard dose; reduced dosage is also required with severe bone marrow compromise. Dosage reduction may also be necessary with altered hepatobiliary function.

Dosage Forms. Inj (Etoposide) 20 mg/mL; (Etoposide phosphate) 100 mg; **Cap** 50 mg.

Patient Instructions. (*See* Antineoplastics Class Instructions.)

Pharmacokinetics. *Fate.* Oral bioavailability is 52 ± 17% with inter- and intrapatient variability. Less than 10% of a dose penetrates into the CNS. V_d is 0.36 ± 0.13 L/kg;[10] Cl is 1.1–1.7 L/hr/m^2 or 0.04 ± 0.014 L/hr/kg.[168,172] Inactive metabolites include the hydroxyacid and cis-lactones. Up to 16% of a dose may be eliminated in bile; 30 ± 5% is eliminated in urine, about 70% of this is unchanged drug.

$t_{1/2}$. 8.1 ± 4.3 hr, increased in uremia.[168,172]

Adverse Reactions. Emetic potential is low. Myelosuppression occurs, with a nadir at 7–10 days (longer with daily regimens), principally affecting the granulocytes, but also affecting platelets, with a nadir at 9–16 days. Myelosuppression may be less frequent with the phosphate form. Mild mucositis and alopecia can occur. Diarrhea is more frequent with oral administration. Hypotension occurs rarely with rapid IV bolus injections. There is one report of radiation recall skin injury in 13 of 23 patients with small cell lung cancer. Long-term administration may result in development of acute leukemia.

Precautions. Pregnancy; decrease dosage in severe renal dysfunction; avoid rapid IV bolus injection.

Drug Interactions. Anaphylaxis and possible synergistic neuropathy with vincristine and/or cardiomyopathy with anthracyclines have been reported. Cyclosporine may increase serum etoposide levels and toxicity. Phenytoin, phenobarbital, and possibly other CYP3A inducers may decrease etoposide serum levels.

Parameters to Monitor. Obtain peripheral granulocyte counts immediately prior to administration on repetitive courses. Nadir counts (1–2 weeks after the dose) are optional.

Notes. Etoposide is indicated in the combination treatment of small cell carcinoma of the lung and refractory nonseminomatous testicular cancer. The drug is also active in lymphomas and in acute leukemias (both lymphoblastic and myeloblastic varieties). Etoposide is not a vesicant. Store capsules under refrigeration. Etoposide and cisplatin are compatible for 24 hr in the same container. Concentrated etoposide solutions (>1 mg/mL) may cause cracking of ABS plastic infusion system components and have short stability times of 2 hr. More dilute solutions in NS or D5W of 0.4–0.6 mg/mL have longer stability times of 8 hr and 48 hr, respectively.

IRINOTECAN   Camptosar

Irinotecan is a water-soluble derivative of camptothecin. It is a prodrug for the despiperidine metabolite SN–38, which is an inhibitor of topoisomerase-1 enzymes. This causes single strand breaks in DNA. Irinotecan is approved for the treatment of patients with advanced colorectal cancer who have failed therapy with fluorouracil. The overall response rate in advanced fluorouracil-refractory colon cancer is about 15%, with a 5.2 month median duration of response. The half-lives of irinotecan and the active SN-38 metabolite are 5.7 and 9.8 hr, respectively, with peak SN-38 levels (2–5% of irinotecan) achieved 1 hr after administration. Renal excretion accounts for less than 10% of a dose as irinotecan and less than 1% as SN-38; hepatic elimination predominates. Diarrhea occurs in 90% of patients and can be severe, requiring aggressive prophylaxis with fluids and multiple doses of loperamide. Leukopenia occurs in one-third of patients, although moderate to severe myelosuppression occurs in only 15 and 11% of patients, respectively. The starting dosage is IV 125 mg/m^2 administered in 500 mL of D5W over 90 min once weekly for 4 consecutive weeks. If no toxicity occurs, subsequent doses are increased by 25–50 mg/m^2; if severe toxicity occurs, dosage is decreased by 25–50 mg/m^2. Available as 20 mg/mL injection.

PACLITAXEL   Taxol

Pharmacology. Paclitaxel is a naturally occurring diterpene taxane obtained from the bark of the pacific yew tree *Taxus brevifolia*. It binds to tubulin proteins to cause abnormal microtubule polymerization and cell cycle arrest in metaphase.[173,174]

Administration and Adult Dosage. IV 135–175 mg/m^2 over 3 or 24 hr q 3 weeks. Doses up to 250 mg/m^2 have been used with hematopoietic colony stimulation factors. Use non-PVC infusion systems.

Special Populations. *Pediatric Dosage.* Safety and efficacy not established.

Geriatric Dosage. Same as adult dosage.

Dosage Forms. **Inj** 6 mg/mL.

Pharmacokinetics. *Fate.* Erratic oral bioavailability precludes oral administration. Cl is 18 L/hr/m^2. It is metabolized to a much less active hydroxylated species by

CYP3A. Eliminated 30–40% by hepatobiliary excretion; only 1–5% excreted in urine.[175]

$t_{1/2}$. α phase 0.2 hr; ß phase 1.9 hr (range 0.5–2.8); γ phase 20.7 hr (range 4–65).[175]

Adverse Reactions. Emetic potential is low. The usual dose-limiting toxicity is neutropenia, with an 8- to 11-day nadir; more severe with prolonged infusion. Dose-limiting toxicity in combination regimens with doxorubicin include neutropenia, inflammation of the cecum (typhlitis), and, with cisplatin, neuropathy. Peripheral neuropathy (eg, numbness, paresthesias) is cumulative, dose related, and more severe with prior vinca alkaloid or concurrent cisplatin therapy. Alopecia can involve all body hair, with an abrupt onset of 2 weeks. Mucositis is dose dependent. Cardiotoxicity, primarily bradycardia, occurs in 10–30% of patients, but rarely requires treatment. Myalgia and arthralgia are common, but usually transient. Hypersensitivity reactions, thought to be caused by Cremophor, may occur within the first few minutes of infusion; symptoms include chest pain, hypotension, bronchospasm, urticaria, and flushing, and can rapidly progress to anaphylaxis. (*See* Precautions.)

Contraindications. Hypersensitivity to Cremophor vehicle; neutropenia (<1500/μL).

Precautions. Recommended premedications include dexamethasone PO 20 mg at 12 and 6 hr before paclitaxel, and diphenhydramine IV 50 mg, plus either cimetidine 300 mg, ranitidine 50 mg, or famotidine 20 mg, 30 min before paclitaxel. Ensure that emergency resuscitation equipment is available at the start of infusion. Use cautiously in patients with heart rhythm disturbances.

Drug Interactions. Ketoconazole may decrease paclitaxel clearance and enhance toxicity. Although their effect is not well studied, use other CYP3A inhibitors with caution. (*See also* Adverse Reactions.)

Parameters to Monitor. Neutrophil count prior to administration.

Notes. Highly effective as a first-line or refractory treatment for ovarian cancer; typically used in platinum-containing regimens; also active in breast cancer, non–small cell lung cancer, lymphoma, and malignant melanoma.[113,174]

TENIPOSIDE	Vumon

Teniposide is a semisynthetic podophyllum derivative that has cell cycle S and G_2 phase specific cytotoxic activities similar to etoposide. Teniposide is over 90% plasma protein bound and is eliminated much more slowly than etoposide. Teniposide half-lives are α phase 45 min, β phase 4 hr, and γ phase 11–30 hr (average 20); 40% of a dose is eliminated in the feces; CSF drug levels are high (27% of serum levels). The dose-limiting side effect of teniposide is myelosuppression, with the leukopenic nadir at 10–14 days. Emetic potential is low; nausea and vomiting are typically mild (more severe after oral etoposide). Hypotension is reported with rapid drug infusions. Rarely severe hypersensitivity reactions (including anaphylaxis), alopecia, and chemical phlebitis during infusion occur. Teniposide is active in adults with lymphomas or acute leukemias and in children with relapsed acute leukemia or neuroblastoma. The dosage in pediatric acute leukemias is IV 165–200 mg/m²/week or 165 mg/m² twice weekly.[172,176,177] Available as 10 mg/mL ampules.

TOPOTECAN	Hycamtin

Topotecan is a topoisomerase I inhibitor that causes single strand breaks in DNA. It is a semisynthetic derivative of camptothecin, which is derived from the bark of the Chinese tree, *Camptotheca acuminata*. Topotecan is approved as a second-line treatment for metastatic ovarian carcinoma after failure of a primary agent and is also being studied in breast and colon cancer. It is rapidly hydrolyzed in plasma. About 70% of the drug is excreted renally as metabolites. The primary dose-limiting side effect of topotecan is neutropenia with a nadir at a mean of 11 days; severe neutropenia occurs in 80% of patients. Severe anemia in 40% of patients and severe thrombocytopenia in 26% have also been reported. Nausea and vomiting occur in most patients; other GI effects include frequent diarrhea, constipation, and abdominal pain. Alopecia occurs in about 60% of patients; fatigue and fever of 101°F or greater are also frequent. Topotecan is contraindicated in pregnancy, breastfeeding, or severe bone marrow depression. The adult dosage is IV 1.5 mg/m^2/day administered over 30 min for 5 days, starting on day 1 of a 21-day course of therapy for a minimum of 4 courses. With a Cl_{cr} between 20–39 mL/min, the dosage is reduced to 0.75 mg/m^2/day; no guidelines exist for Cl_{cr} <20 mL/min. If severe neutropenia occurs, either reduce further doses by 0.25 mg/m^2/day or administer filgrastim with subsequent courses.[1] Available as 4-mg injection.

VINCA ALKALOIDS:	
VINBLASTINE SULFATE	Velban, Various
VINCRISTINE SULFATE	Oncovin, Various
VINORELBINE TARTRATE	Navelbine

Pharmacology. The vinca alkaloids are *Vinca rosea* (periwinkle) plant-derived antimitotic agents; cytotoxic activity is related to specific binding to the microtubule protein tubulin, causing microtubule dissolution. This blocks formation of the mitotic spindle apparatus necessary for cell division. The vincas are lethal to cells at high concentrations and, at lower concentrations, dividing cells are arrested in the metaphase portion of mitosis.

Administration and Dosage.

	VINBLASTINE	VINCRISTINE	VINORELBINE
Administration	IV push, infusion.	IV push.	IV short infusion.
Adult Dosage	IV push 4–12 mg/m^2 as a single agent at monthly intervals; or 1.5–1.7 mg/m^2/day for 5 days as a continuous infusion.[178]	0.4–1.4 mg/m^2/week (2.5 mg typical single dose limit).	30 mg/m^2/week.
Pediatric Dosage	IV push 4–10 mg/m^2 q 1–2 weeks.	1.4–2 mg/m^2/week (2 mg typical single dose limit).	Not used in children.
Geriatric Dosage	Same as adult dosage.	Same as adult dosage.	Same as adult dosage.

Special Populations. *Other Conditions.* Vinblastine and vinorelbine require substantial dosage reduction in heavily pretreated patients (ie, drug or radiation therapy). Reduce vinorelbine dosage by 50% in patients in whom over 75% of the liver is replaced by tumor, or for granulocyte levels on the day of treatment of 1000–1499/μL; do not administer at lower WBC levels.[179] Vinca alkaloids are extensively eliminated in the bile, and the dosages of vinblastine and vincristine must be reduced by approximately 50–75% in the presence of severe hepatobiliary dysfunction. Reduce vinorelbine dosage to 15 mg/m²/week for a serum total bilirubin of 2.1–3 mg/dL, and to 7.5 mg/m²/week for a bilirubin over 3 mg/dL.

Dosage Forms. (Vinblastine) **Inj** 1 mg/mL. (Vincristine) **Inj** 1 mg/mL. (Vinorelbine) **Inj** 10 mg/mL.

Patient Instructions. (*See* Antineoplastics Class Instructions.)

Pharmacokinetics. *Fate.*

Distribution | Pharmacokinetics can be described by a two-compartment open model: an initial short phase with rapid tissue uptake (V_d approximating total body water) and a long terminal phase of greater than 1 day with a large V_d reflecting slow drug release from tissue binding sites—see below. Vincas do not effectively penetrate into the CNS or other fatty tissues and achieve their highest levels in liver, gallbladder, and spleen.

Metabolism | Approximately 50% of renally and fecally excreted products are closely related metabolites. An example is the formation of desacetyl vinblastine (which is more active on a weight basis than vinblastine) following vinblastine administration.

Excretion | The vinca alkaloids appear to be eliminated primarily in the bile and feces, some in the urine.

	VINBLASTINE	VINCRISTINE	VINORELBINE
Pharmacokinetic Parameters.[180–182]			
V_c (L/kg)	0.7	0.33	—
V_d (L/kg)	27.3	8.4	40.1 (V_{dss})
Urine		10% (24 hr)	—
(cumulative)	33% (72 hr)	13% (72 hr)	21% (21 days)
Feces		33% (24 hr)	—
(cumulative)	21% (72 hr)	67% (72 hr)	34–58% (21 days)
$t_{1/2}$.			
$t_{1/2\alpha}$ (min)	<5	<5	<27
$t_{1/2\beta}$ (hr)	0.164	2.3	<1.9
$t_{1/2\gamma}$ (hr)	25	85	40

Adverse Reactions. Emetic potential is low (vincristine) to moderate (vinblastine and vinorelbine). Myelosuppression is the dose-limiting toxicity for vinblastine and vinorelbine, with the leukopenic nadir at 4–10 days; unless patients have been heavily pretreated with drugs or radiation, recovery from leukopenia is rather prompt, sometimes facilitating weekly or semimonthly drug administration. The major toxicity of vincristine is peripheral neuropathy manifested by paresthesias, constipation, jaw pain, decreased deep tendon reflexes, and rarely bladder atony or paralytic ileus; gut neurotoxicity occurs rarely with vinorelbine. All of these neurologic symptoms slowly resolve over a month and necessitate substantial dosage reduction if present at the time of drug administration. Seizures and ocular toxicity presenting as blurred vision or ptosis occur frequently. Mild laxatives or **metoclopramide** may be useful for constipation. The vincas are extremely toxic if inadvertently extravasated; **hyaluronidase** (150 units/mL) may be effective as a local (subcutaneous) antidote. Vinorelbine also causes substantial phlebitis, which may be lessened by a short (6- to 10-min) infusion. Transiently severe pain in tumor masses occurs with vinblastine frequently. Alopecia is frequent with both all agents. Inadvertent intrathecal administration of any vinca alkaloid is fatal.

Contraindications. (Vinblastine) Severe bone marrow compromise from prior therapy; uncontrolled infection. (Vincristine) Severe peripheral nervous system effects from prior doses, particularly paralytic ileus, tingling paresthesias, or decreased deep tendon reflexes; demyelinating form of Charcot-Marie-Tooth Syndrome. (Vinorelbine) Pretreatment granulocyte count <1000/μL.

Precautions. Pregnancy. Use with caution in patients with neurologic deficiencies or hepatic disease.

Drug Interactions. Vinca administration (especially vincristine) has been associated with increased cellular retention of methotrexate (increased even in CNS tissues). Concurrent use of vincristine with zalcitabine may increase neuropathy.

Parameters to Monitor. (Vinblastine and vinorelbine) Obtain pretreatment and at least monthly WBC and hemoglobin/hematocrit assessments; (vincristine) obtain serial peripheral neurologic assessments; (all drugs) assess biliary function prior to drug administration and before making dosage adjustments for impaired hepatobiliary status.

Notes. Protect these drugs from light and store under refrigeration. Place individual vincristine doses in an overwrap (eg, plastic bag) that is labeled, "Do not remove covering until the moment of injection. Fatal if given intrathecally. For intravenous use only." Useful in hematologic neoplasms (primarily vincristine) and in solid tumors, including non–small cell lung cancer in combination with cisplatin (vinorelbine) and refractory breast cancer and Kaposi's sarcoma (vinblastine).[183]

Miscellaneous Antineoplastics

ASPARAGINASE	Elspar
PEGASPARGASE	Oncaspar

Pharmacology. Asparaginase is the levo isomer of a macromolecular protein, isolated from *Escherichia coli* and other bacteria, which hydrolyzes the essential amino acid asparagine in the serum, thus depriving susceptible lymphocyte-derived malignancies of a necessary element for protein synthesis. Pegaspargase is a PEG-modified form of asparaginase that can be given to patients allergic to asparaginase. The drug is cell cycle G phase specific.

Administration and Adult Dosage. IM (preferably) or IV for combination therapy of acute leukemia (asparaginase) 200 IU/kg/day for 28 days,[184] or 1000–6000 IU/m^2/day for 5 days,[185] or 20,000 IU/m^2/week;[186] (pegaspargase) 2500 IU/m^2 q 14 days.

Special Populations. *Pediatric Dosage.* IM (preferably) or IV for combination therapy of acute leukemia (asparaginase) 1000–6000 IU/m^2/day for 5 days,[185,187] up to 20,000 IU/m^2/week; (pegaspargase) 2500 IU/m^2 q 14 days.

Geriatric Dosage. Same as adult dosage.

Dosage Forms. Inj (Asparaginase) 10,000 IU vial. (Pegaspargase) 750 IU/mL.

Patient Instructions. *See* Antineoplastics Class Instructions. Asparaginase often causes allergic reactions, which can be life-threatening. This drug may also alter blood sugar levels and might worsen diabetes mellitus. Report any abdominal pain immediately, because it may be a sign of pancreatitis.

Pharmacokinetics. *Fate.* (Asparaginase) IV and IM produce equivalent serum levels. There is negligible distribution out of the vascular compartment, with minimal urinary and biliary excretion. Clearance is probably immune mediated. Asparaginase remains detectable in serum 13–22 days after administration.[188] (Pegaspargase) Asparaginase is slowly released from pegaspargase and is distributed in the body similarly to native asparaginase.

t$_{1/2}$. (Asparaginase) α phase 4–9 hr; ß phase 1.4–1.8 days.[188] (Pegaspargase) 3.2 ± 1.8 days in patients hypersensitive to asparaginase; 5.7 ± 3.3 days in nonsensitive patients.

Adverse Reactions. Emetic potential is low. Moderate to severe non-dose-related hypersensitivity reactions occur in about 20–35% of patients (IM use may reduce and/or delay allergic complications);[184] a prophylactic antihistamine may sometimes be helpful (*see* Precautions). The drug is usually not myelotoxic. Transient blood sugar lowering followed by a pancreatitis-induced hyperglycemia may occur. Elevated serum cholesterol, severely elevated hepatic enzymes, steatosis, depressed clotting factors (especially profound for fibrinogen), and decreased albumin synthesis occur frequently. Lethargy and somnolence occur and may be more frequent in adults.[189] Fatal hyperthermia has been reported.

Contraindications. Anaphylactic reaction to commercial *E. coli* preparation; severe pancreatitis or history of pancreatitis.

Precautions. Onset of abdominal pain, serum amylase elevation, any changes in mental status, or severe elevation of prothrombin time require drug discontinuation. Some elevations of liver function tests should be anticipated. Anaphylaxis can occur with any dose; ensure that emergency resuscitation equipment is available at the time of each dose. Intradermal scratch tests and desensitization procedures are not reliably predictive or preventive for anaphylaxis.[184,188]

Drug Interactions. None known.

Parameters to Monitor. Monitor serum hepatic enzymes, amylase, glucose, and prothrombin time routinely, and all vital signs during administration.

Notes. Reconstitute with NS or D5W (2-mL maximum for IM use); stable at least 24 hr; do not filter.

BLEOMYCIN SULFATE   Blenoxane

Pharmacology. Bleomycin is a mixture of 13 glycopeptide fractions produced by *Streptomyces verticillus*. Antineoplastic effects include single and double strand DNA scission, producing excision of thymine bases mediated through binding with ferric iron and subsequent production of highly reactive hydroxyl and superoxide radicals. It is cell cycle phase specific, with maximal activity in the G_2 (premitotic) phase.[190]

Administration and Adult Dosage. IM test dose 1–2 units may be useful in malignant lymphoma patients to assess exaggerated hyperpyrexic response. If no reaction occurs in 2–4 hr, give regular dose. **SC, IM, or IV** 10–20 units/m² 1–2 times/week.[190] **IV continuous infusion** 15–20 units/day for 4–5 days.[191] Experimental evidence in animals favors continuous administration to lessen pulmonary toxicity and maximize cell kill. A total lifetime dosage limit of 400 units is recommended to avoid pulmonary fibrosis. **Intracavitary for malignant effusion** 15–240 units (60 units for pleural effusion) in 50–100 mL of NS.[192]

Special Populations. *Pediatric Dosage.* **SC, IM, or IV** 10–20 units/m² 1–2 times a week in combination regimens. **IV continuous infusion** 15–20 units/m²/day for 4–5 days, usually as a single agent.

Geriatric Dosage. Same as adult dosage, but use with caution in patients >70 yr and adjust dosage for age-related reduction in renal function.

Other Conditions. Dosage reduction has been recommended in renal impairment:[193]

SERUM CREATININE (MG/DL)	PERCENTAGE OF DOSE RECOMMENDED
2.5–4	25 (75% reduction)
4–6	20
6–10	5–10 (90–95% reduction)

Dosage Forms. **Inj** 15 units.

Patient Instructions. (*See* Antineoplastics Class Instructions.) Report any coughing, shortness of breath, or wheezing. Skin rashes, shaking chills, or transient high fever may occur following administration. Hyperpigmentation of skin fold areas, scars, pressure areas, or sites of trauma may occur.

Pharmacokinetics. *Fate.* Poorly absorbed topically; roughly one-half of intracavitary-administered drug may be systemically available (use this fraction to calculate lifetime exposure). Following an IV dose of about 15 units/m², serum levels of 10–1000 milliunits/L are obtained.[191] Steady-state levels during continuous infusion of 20 units/day are 50–200 milliunits/L.[194] V_{dB} is 0.27 ± 0.04 L/kg; Cl is 0.066 ± 0.018 L/hr/kg.[10] Tissue inactivation is mediated by specific bleomycin-hydrolase, which is low in skin and lung, the two main toxicity targets of the drug.[191,194] From 50–60% of a dose is recovered in the urine, 68% of this as unchanged drug.[10]

$t_{1/2}$. α phase 24 min; β phase 3.1 $\pm$ 1.7 hr.[10,191,194]

Adverse Reactions. Emetic potential is moderately low. Alopecia and acute fever and generalized erythema with edema, eventually leading to hyperpigmentation and skin thickening, are frequent. The most serious long-term toxicity is pulmonary fibrosis manifested by dry cough, rales, dyspnea, and bilateral infiltrates. Pulmonary function studies show hypoxemia and reduced CO diffusing capacity. Pulmonary toxicity usually does not occur below 150 units/m^2, but the frequency increases to 55% at doses above 283 units/m^2 and 66% at 360 units/m^2;[195] life-threatening pulmonary fibrosis is rare if dosage limits are observed. Prior chest radiotherapy, age >70 yr, and hyperoxic ventilation predispose patients to toxicity. About 1% of high-dose bleomycin-treated patients die from pulmonary fibrosis. Low-dose hypersensitivity pneumonitis, which may be responsive to a glucocorticoid, also occurs.[196]

Precautions. Use with extreme caution in patients with renal or pulmonary disease, in those with lymphoma, and in those >70 yr.

Drug Interactions. Inspired oxygen concentrations >35% may cause acute respiratory failure in bleomycin-treated patients.

Parameters to Monitor. Calculate cumulative dosage before and after each treatment. Monitor temperature initially, especially in lymphoma patients. Assess renal function prior to administering. Pulmonary damage is best monitored with CO diffusing capacity and forced vital capacity; specific serial pulmonary function studies have been suggested prior to and during therapy. Characteristic x-ray findings include changes suggestive of progressive diffuse bilateral fibrosis.

Notes. 1 mg of bleomycin equals 1 unit of activity. Reconstituted solution is stable for 1 month under refrigeration and 2 weeks at room temperature. Incompatible with divalent cations (especially copper), ascorbic acid, and compounds with sulfhydryl groups.

TRETINOIN   Vesanoid

Tretinoin (all-trans-retinoic acid) is a modified form of vitamin A used in the treatment of acute promyelocytic leukemia. It causes immature promyeloblasts to differentiate into mature granulocytes, thereby halting cell division and inducing complete remissions in up to 90% of patients. Resistance rapidly develops during therapy because of accelerated drug catabolism to the 4-oxo metabolite, which is excreted in the urine, increased cellular retinoic acid binding protein (II), and tumors with high levels of a mutated a retinoic acid receptor. Peak serum levels of 294 µg/L occur 1–2 hr after a dose; the serum half-life is 0.8 hr. Adverse reactions include hyperleukocytosis and effects typical of hypervitaminosis A: headache, dry skin and mucosa, cheilitis, bone pain, and hypertriglyceridemia. Tolerance to these effects develops rapidly, and skin creams, lip balms, and eye and nasal drops are helpful. Liver and renal function test elevations occur occasionally. The dosage is 45 mg/m^2/day as a single dose until remission is obtained.[197–199] Available as 10-mg capsules.

Chemoprotectants

AMIFOSTINE Ethyol

Pharmacology. Amifostine is a phosphorothiol compound metabolized by membrane-bound alkaline phosphatase to the reduced thiol actifostine, an active sulfhydryl form capable of binding electrophilic metabolites from DNA-binding anticancer agents or ionizing radiation. It is used prophylactically to block cisplatin-induced nephrotoxicity and neurotoxicity without altering antitumor efficacy in patients with advanced ovarian cancer.[200]

Administration and Adult Dosage. IV to block cisplatin toxicity 910 mg/m² in NS over 15 min, beginning 30 min prior to cisplatin.

Special Populations. *Pediatric Dosage.* Safety and efficacy not established.

Geriatric Dosage. Same as adult dosage, but limited experience exists in patients >70 yr.

Other Conditions. In patients who develop rare symptomatic acute hypocalcemia, reduce dose to 740 mg/m² and extend infusion time. Reduce dosage in patients who developed hypotension (drop of 15–20 mm Hg systolic) with prior courses.

Dosage Forms. Inj 50 mg/mL.

Patient Instructions. The severity of chemotherapy-induced nausea and vomiting may increase with amifostine.

Pharmacokinetics. *Fate.* The mean peak serum level is 100 μmol/L following a 740 mg/m² IV dose. V_{dss} is 6.4 ± 1.5 L; Cl is 2.2 ± 0.4 L/min. Relatively little unchanged drug (1.1% of a dose), actifostine (1.4% of a dose), or disulfide metabolite (4.2% of a dose) is excreted renally.[201]

$t_{1/2}$. α phase 0.88 ± 0.12 min; β phase 8.8 ± 2 min.

Adverse Reactions. Toxic effects are all acute and include transient hypotension, during or immediately following drug infusion, nausea, and vomiting.[202] Prophylactic antiemetics before administration can reduce nausea and vomiting. Stopping the infusion and placing the patient in the Trendelenberg position usually reverses the hypotension. Other less serious but common reactions include sneezing (27%), a flushed sensation (26%), somnolence (10–20%), a sensation of cold hands, or a metallic taste in the mouth (<5% each).

Contraindications. Allergy to aminothiol compounds or mannitol.

Precautions. Do not administer concurrently with or after cisplatin infusion. Use with caution in patients in whom hypotension or nausea might pose a serious risk. There is limited experience in patients with preexisting cardiac or cardiovascular conditions such as CHF, angina pectoris, history of stroke, or TIAs.

Drug Interactions. None known.

Parameters to Monitor. Obtain blood pressure frequently during drug administration and immediately after infusion.

Notes. Amifostine has been safely combined with ionizing radiation, carboplatin, and cyclophosphamide. It is not active as a chemoprotectant for mitomycin. Clinical effects on other anticancer agents are largely unknown.

DEXRAZOXANE

Zinecard

Pharmacology. Dexrazoxane, a cardioprotectant for anthracyclines, is the water-soluble dextro isomer of razoxane. Dexrazoxane's two piperazinedione rings open to form sites that chelate intracellular ferrous ions, blocking the formation of doxorubicin-iron complexes capable of forming membrane-damaging oxygen free radicals. Dexrazoxane can extend doxorubicin cumulative dosage in patients with breast cancer. It does not alter the pharmacokinetics of doxorubicin.[203]

Administration and Adult Dosage. **IV as a cardioprotectant** give in a 10:1 dexrazoxane:doxorubicin mg/m^2 ratio (ie, 500 mg/m^2 dexrazoxane:50 mg/m^2 doxorubicin). Infuse IV over 15 min, beginning not more than 30 min before an IV push of doxorubicin.

Special Populations. *Pediatric Dosage.* Safety and efficacy not established.

Geriatric Dosage. Same as adult dosage.

Dosage Forms. **Inj** 250, 500 mg.

Patient Instructions. (*See* Antineoplastics Class Instructions.)

Pharmacokinetics. *Fate.* The mean peak serum level after a 500 mg/m^2 dose given over 15 min is 36.5 mg/L (136 μmol/L). The drug is not protein bound. V_d is 22 L/m^2 or approximately body water; Cl averages 7.9 L/hr/m^2. About 42% is renally eliminated as parent drug, and mono- and diacid amide metabolites.[204]

$t_{1/2}$. α phase 0.2–0.3 hr; ß phase 2.1–2.5 hr.[204]

Adverse Reactions. Dexrazoxane has little toxicity, but does slightly increase the myelosuppressive and emetogenic toxicities of doxorubicin-containing regimens.

Contraindications. None known.

Precautions. Avoid use with bleomycin. Do not administer *after* doxorubicin.

Drug Interactions. None known.

Parameters to Monitor. WBC counts at nadir (7–11 days) after doxorubicin.

Notes. Dexrazoxane does not reduce the antitumor activity of fluorouracil, doxorubicin, and cyclophosphamide regimens in advanced breast cancer.[203] Effects on other antineoplastics are unknown.

MESNA

Mesnex

Pharmacology. Mesna (2-mercaptoethanesulfonate) is a sulfhydryl compound that minimizes urotoxicity from the alkylating agents cyclophosphamide (CTX) and ifosfamide (IFX) by binding to the irritant metabolite acrolein in the urinary bladder to prevent hemorrhagic cystitis.[35,205]

Administration and Adult Dosage. **IV or PO** (ampule contents dissolved in water or juice) in 3 doses as a percentage of the dose of ifosfamide or cyclophosphamide:

TIME BEFORE OR AFTER CTX OR IFX	PERCENTAGE OF CTX OR IFX DOSE[206]	
	IV Mesna Route	PO Mesna Route
15 min before	20	Not recommended
4 hr after	20	40
8 hr after	20	40

Oral administration is not recommended for patients with poor compliance or those experiencing nausea or vomiting.

Special Populations. *Pediatric Dosage.* Same as adult dosage.[42,207]

Geriatric Dosage. Same as adult dosage.

Dosage Forms. Inj 100 mg/mL.

Patient Instructions. This agent does not have antitumor activity but is essential to reduce or prevent permanent bladder damage from chemotherapy.

Pharmacokinetics. *Fate.* About 48% is orally absorbed.[208] V_d is 0.65 L/kg; Cl is 1.23 L/hr/kg. Mesna is oxidized to the inactive dimer, dimesna, which does not inactivate CTX or IFX metabolites in the serum. About 60% of the dimesna is converted back to mesna in the renal tubule and delivered to the bladder in the active sulfhydryl form. About two-thirds of a dose is excreted in the urine, one-half as mesna and one-half as dimesna.[209]

$t_{1/2}$. (Mesna) 22 min; (dimesna) 1.2 hr.[209]

Adverse Reactions. When administered alone, mesna produces little if any serious toxicity.[209] GI effects (eg, diarrhea, nausea and, rarely, vomiting) of CTX or IFX may be slightly greater when mesna is administered. Other CTX or IFX toxicities such as myelosuppression or alopecia are not altered by mesna. With oral administration, a disagreeable sulfur odor may lessen palatability unless the drug is diluted with cola or juice.

Drug Interactions. Mesna inhibits the antitumor activity of cisplatin and carboplatin, but not other anticancer agents.

Notes. Mesna is compatible with solutions of CTX or IFX and has been administered concurrently as a continuous infusion of both agents at equal doses in the same infusion container.[210] It is stable in D5W or NS for at least 96 hr.

Immunosuppressants

AZATHIOPRINE   Imuran

Pharmacology. Azathioprine is a thiolated purine that acts as an antimetabolite following conversion to mercaptopurine and metabolic activation to the nucleotide form (phosphorylated ribose sugar attachment). Subsequently, de novo purine biosynthesis is interrupted at a number of enzymatic sites, including the conversion of inosinic acid to adenine- or xanthine-based ribosides.

Administration and Adult Dosage. PO or IV for immunosuppression following renal transplantation 3–5 mg/kg/day IV in 1 dose initially, usually starting on the day of transplantation. Change to oral administration as soon as feasible. Maintenance dosage is 1–3 mg/kg/day in 1 dose. **PO for rheumatoid arthritis** 1 mg/kg/day (usually 50–100 mg) in 1–2 divided doses initially; after 6–8 weeks, increase dosage, if necessary and there are no serious toxicities, in 0.5 mg/kg/day increments at 4-week intervals to a maximum of 2.5 mg/kg/day. *Patients taking allopurinol must receive substantially reduced dosages of oral azathioprine (25–33% of the normal dosage) to avoid life-threatening myelosuppression.*

Special Populations. *Pediatric Dosage.* **PO or IV for immunosuppression following renal transplantation** same as adult dosage.

Geriatric Dosage. Same as adult dosage.

Dosage Forms. **Tab** 50 mg; **Inj** 5 mg/mL.

Patient Instructions. This medication may be taken with food to minimize gastrointestinal upset. If nausea, vomiting, diarrhea, skin rash, or joint pains become severe or persistent, contact your physician. Notify your physician if any of the following symptoms occur: unusual bleeding or bruising, fever, sore throat, sores in the mouth, abdominal pain, pale stools, or dark urine. Periodic blood counts are essential while taking this medication.

Pharmacokinetics. *Serum Levels.* Not used clinically.

Fate. Oral bioavailability is $60 \pm 31\%$. In renal transplant patients, azathioprine V_d is 0.81 ± 0.65 L/kg; Cl is 3.4 ± 1.9 L/hr/kg. Azathioprine is rapidly converted to the active metabolite mercaptopurine. Mercaptopurine V_d is 0.56 ± 0.38 L/kg; Cl is 0.66 ± 0.24 L/hr/kg. Less than 2% of azathioprine and $22 \pm 12\%$ of mercaptopurine is excreted unchanged in urine.[10]

$t_{\frac{1}{2}}$. (Azathioprine) 9.6 ± 4.2 min in renal transplant patients; (mercaptopurine) 54 ± 22 min.[10]

Adverse Reactions. The most important toxicities are dose-related bone marrow suppression (leukopenia, thrombocytopenia, macrocytic anemia, or selective erythrocyte aplasia). Serious infections are possible during long-term immunosuppression. GI hypersensitivity (severe nausea and vomiting, diarrhea) along with fever, malaise, myalgia, and liver function test abnormalities occur in up to 10% or more of patients. This usually occurs in the first several weeks and can be minimized by giving the drug in divided doses or after meals. The reaction is reversible upon discontinuation, but can return within hours of a rechallenge with a single dose. Neoplasms can occur during long-term use; lymphoma occurs in more than 0.5% of patients, and other neoplasms occur in over 2.8%. Skin rashes occur in about 2% of patients. Alopecia, fever, arthralgias, and negative nitrogen balance occur occasionally. Hepatotoxicity occurs rarely in rheumatoid arthritis patients and more frequently in transplant patients. Renal failure has occurred in one patient with azathioprine.[211] Restrictive lung disease is also described with azathioprine, which reverses upon drug discontinuation.

Contraindications. Pregnancy in rheumatoid arthritis patients.

Precautions. Pregnancy; lactation.

Drug Interactions. Allopurinol markedly increases the pharmacologic effect and toxicity of azathioprine. Concurrent use of azathioprine and ACE inhibitors may induce severe leukopenia. Methotrexate given with azathioprine may increase serum levels of mercaptopurine. Azathioprine may decrease cyclosporine serum levels. The pharmacologic effects of the nondepolarizing neuromuscular blockers may be decreased by azathioprine. Drugs that affect leukocyte production (eg, trimethoprim/sulfamethoxazole) may cause an exaggerated leukopenia when used concurrently.

Parameters to Monitor. Monitor CBC and platelets weekly for the first month, twice monthly for the next 2 months, then monthly or more frequently if changes in dosage or therapy are made. Obtain serum transaminases, alkaline phosphatase, and bilirubin periodically. Observe for signs of infection regularly.

Notes. Azathioprine has been used investigationally in a number of conditions, including myasthenia gravis, Behcet's syndrome, Crohn's disease, chronic ulcerative colitis, and multiple myeloma.

CYCLOSPORINE   Sandimmune, Neoral

Pharmacology. Cyclosporine is a cyclic polypeptide immunosuppressant that acts by calcium-dependent, reversible inhibition of T-helper-cell production of interleukin-2 (IL-2) and several other cytokines. IL-2 is required for further activation and clonal expansion of T-helper cells and cytotoxic T-cells. Cyclosporine has little effect on B-cells, and lacks clinically important myelosuppressive activity.[212,213]

Administration and Adult Dosage. PO for prophylaxis of organ rejection initial dosage varies depending on the transplanted organ and other immunosuppressive agents included in the protocol; initial dosages (mean ± SD) of Sandimmune or Neoral capsules or oral solutions based on a survey of transplant centers, started 4–12 hr before transplantation or postoperatively and given on a bid schedule, are as follows: **renal transplant** 9 ± 3 mg/kg/day, **liver transplant** 8 ± 4 mg/kg/day, and **heart transplant** 7 ± 3 mg/kg/day. The dosage is subsequently adjusted to achieve a predefined (usually trough) cyclosporine blood concentration and also based on clinical assessments of rejection and tolerability. Neoral maintenance dosages may be lower than Sandimmune because of better Neoral bioavailability. Mix Sandimmune solution with milk, chocolate milk, or orange juice in a glass container and administer immediately after mixing. Rinse the container with the same solution to ensure the total dose is taken. Mix the Neoral solution in orange juice or apple juice (milk may be unpalatable) at room temperature in a glass container and rinse as above. Adjunctive therapy with a glucocorticoid is recommended initially in a tapering dosage schedule. **PO conversion from Sandimmune to Neoral** use the same daily dosage (cautiously in patients receiving a dosage over 10 mg/kg/day) and adjust the dosage to obtain the preconversion whole blood trough concentration using concentration monitoring q 4–7 days. The new cyclosporine blood trough concentration may exceed the target range; titrate the dosage of Neoral individually based on trough concentrations, tolerability, and clinical response. Patients with poor absorption of Sandimmune may have increased absorption of cyclosporine following conversion to Neoral. In this population, monitor the trough concentration at least twice a week (daily if initial dosage exceeds 10 mg/kg/day), until the concentration stabilizes within the desired range. **IV for patients unable to take the medication orally** one-third the oral dosage (or 2–6 mg/kg/day) initially, given as a dilute solution of 50 mg/20–100 mL NS or D5W (diluted just prior to use), and infused over 2–6 hr. Give this dosage once daily until patient can tolerate oral administration (*see* Precautions and Notes).

Special Populations. *Pediatric Dosage.* Safety and efficacy not established, although children as young as 6 months have received the drug with no unusual effects. Infants and children usually require larger weight-adjusted dosages than adults.[214,215]

Geriatric Dosage. Same as adult dosage.

Dosage Forms. **Cap** 25, 100 mg (Neoral, Sandimmune); **Soln** 100 mg/mL (Neoral, Sandimmune); **Inj** 50 mg/mL.

Patient Instructions. Take this medication on a regular schedule in relation to time of day and meals, and do not discontinue its use unless directed. Mixing Sandimmune oral solution (in a glass container only) with milk, chocolate milk, or orange juice improves its palatability. Mix Neoral oral solution in orange or apple juice. Avoid grapefruit and grapefruit juice unless otherwise specified by the prescriber, because they may affect metabolism of cyclosporine. Take either oral solution immediately after mixing. Do *not* refrigerate the oral solution, and use it within 2 months after opening. Take missed doses as soon as possible if remembered within 12 hr; otherwise skip the dose and do not double the next dose. Report fever, sore throat, tiredness, or unusual bleeding or bruising. Do not change the cyclosporine formulation used (between Sandimmue and Neoral) except under clinical supervision, because it may result in the need for a dosage change.

Pharmacokinetics. *Serum Levels.* The serum concentration-response relationship is not well established. It is dependent on assay, biologic fluid, and time posttransplant; and the therapeutic range may be lower when other immunosuppressants are used concurrently. Generally, therapeutic trough levels (HPLC, whole blood) are initially (first 1–3 months) 150–225 µg/L (125–188 nmol/L) after renal transplant, and 225–325 µg/L (188–270 nmol/L) after heart and liver transplant; maintenance levels are 100–175 µg/L (83–145 nmol/L) after renal, heart, and liver transplant. Maintenance levels over 300 µg/L (250 nmol/L) with slowly rising Cr_s suggest nephrotoxicity, and maintenance levels over 400 µg/L (333 nmol/L) are associated with a high probability of toxicity. Levels lower than the ranges above may be associated with increased risk of rejection. [216–222] (*See* Notes.)

Fate. Oral absorption is formulation dependent. Sandimmune has poor and erratic oral bioavailability, averaging about 30% (range 5–90); peak serum concentrations occur 2–6 hr after the dose. Neoral appears less dependent on bile acids for adsorption than Sandimmune and has a bioavailability that varies in different patient populations but is about 25% greater than Sandimmune in stable renal transplant patients; peak serum levels are increased by 70% over Sandimmune and occur earlier. Food may decrease or increase absorption (especially with Sandimmune), which is probably dependent on the dietary composition. Patients with diarrhea, liver dysfunction, or transplantation (bile deficit) and shorter small bowel length (eg, children) may have decreased absorption. In blood, the drug is distributed about 45% in RBCs, 15% in WBCs, and 35% in plasma, where it is highly lipoprotein bound. RBC binding is time, temperature, and hematocrit dependent. Cyclosporine is highly tissue bound with a V_{dss} (HPLC, whole blood) of 4–6 L/kg; Cl (HPLC, whole blood) is 0.3–0.4 L/hr/kg (renal or liver transplants), 0.5–0.6 L/hr/kg (marrow transplants). The drug is extensively metabolized by CYP3A to at least 25 metabolites of unresolved clinical activity, with the majority of cyclosporine and metabolites excreted by the biliary route and less than 1% excreted unchanged in urine. [220,223]

$t_{\frac{1}{2}}$. (HPLC, whole blood, renal transplant) approximately 10.5–15 hr in adults, 7.5 hr in children; prolonged in the elderly and in patients with liver dysfunction. [223]

Adverse Reactions. Nephrotoxicity (usually mild) occurs in about 30% of patients. The more severe nephrotoxicity that occurs early after transplantation is usually responsive to dosage reduction, but persistent elevations in BUN and Cr_s are an indication to discontinue the drug. About 5–15% of transplant recipients fail to show a reduction in a rising Cr_s despite a decrease or discontinuation of cyclosporine therapy. This may be chronic progressive nephrotoxicity, which is characterized by serial deterioration in renal function and morphologic changes in the kidneys (eg, interstitial fibrosis). There appears to be an association between interstitial fibrosis and high cumulative dosage or persistently high circulating trough cyclosporine levels. Hypertension occurs in up to 90% of patients and is occasionally difficult to control; consider calcium-channel blockers as initial therapy for hypertension because they may also help to decrease or prevent nephrotoxicity.[224–226] Cholestasis occurs frequently during the first month of therapy and is usually responsive to dosage reduction. Hirsutism, hyperuricemia and gout,[227] tremors, cramps, convulsions (possibly related to hypomagnesemia),[244] headache, gum hyperplasia, leukopenia, diarrhea, nausea, vomiting, acne, and paresthesias also occur frequently. Occasionally, hyperkalemia, sinusitis, gynecomastia, thrombocytopenia, anemia, and anaphylactic reactions to the drug or to the emulsifying agent in the IV product have been reported. As with other immunosuppressive agents, there is an increased risk of lymphoma/lymphoproliferative disease and infectious complications.

Contraindications. Allergy to cyclosporine or polyoxyethylated castor oil.

Precautions. Pregnancy. Patients with malabsorption may have difficulty achieving therapeutic levels with oral Sandimmune. Use with caution in patients with impaired renal function.

Drug Interactions. Do not use with potassium-sparing diuretics because cyclosporine may cause hyperkalemia. Vaccinations may be less effective during treatment with cyclosporine; avoid the use of live attenuated vaccines. Numerous important drug interactions (eg, with anticonvulsants, antimicrobials, calcium-channel blockers, grapefruit) decrease cyclosporine metabolism and may result in sustained changes in cyclosporine concentrations. These interacting drugs may be given intentionally to lower the dosage (and cost) of cyclosporine.[228–231] Consult a comprehensive drug interaction source before prescribing.

Parameters to Monitor. Continuously observe patients receiving IV cyclosporine for the first 30 min and at frequent intervals thereafter for anaphylaxis; have epinephrine and oxygen readily available. Monitor renal and hepatic function tests repeatedly during therapy. Monitor for hypertension.[224–226] Whole blood drug trough level monitoring has been suggested as follows: q 24–48 hr immediately posttransplant until the patient and levels are stable, then gradually reduce to monthly the first year and q 1–3 months thereafter.[221] More frequent blood or serum level monitoring is required in hepatic transplant patients and in patients with conditions that may affect absorption (eg, diarrhea, bile deficit).[215,221] Monitor whole blood levels more frequently in infants and children.[214,215] (*See* Notes.)

Notes. A glass container may be preferred for IV infusion because of leaching of phthalate from PVC containers.[212] Newer monoclonal assays are more specific for cyclosporine than earlier nonspecific polyclonal assays, which also measured some metabolites.[216] Whole blood trough level ranges with these monoclonal assays are similar to those of the HPLC assay (the standard reference), but all must be used cautiously guided by their approved labeling in conjunction with clinical, laboratory, and histopathologic indices to have prognostic value.[216,219,221] Antirejection drugs, including high-dose **glucocorticoids, antilymphocyte globulin** (Atgam), **muromonab-CD3** (Orthoclone OKT3), and **tacrolimus,** may be useful in management of transplant rejection.[232–234,245] Cyclosporine may be effective in a number of diseases in which immunoregulatory dysfunction may be a factor (eg, acute ocular Behcet's syndrome, endogenous uveitis, psoriasis, atopic dermatitis, rheumatoid arthritis, acute Crohn's disease, nephrotic syndrome, aplastic anemia, and primary biliary cirrhosis).[213]

MYCOPHENOLATE MOFETIL   CellCept

Mycophenolate is an immunosuppressant prodrug that inhibits specific DNA synthesis for T- and B-lymphocytes. Unlike cyclosporine or tacrolimus, it reversibly inhibits inosine monophosphate dehydrogenases, thus interfering with the de novo pathway of purine (guanosine) synthesis. T- and B-lymphocytes are critically dependent on the de novo synthesis of purines whereas other cell types are not. Mycophenolate mofetil is well absorbed in healthy or stable renal transplant patients (bioavailability >90%). Bioavailability in early renal transplant patients (<40 days post) is about 50%. Food does not affect bioavailability, but may decrease peak level by about 40%. Mycophenolate mofetil is rapidly hydrolyzed to active mycophenolic acid (MPA). MPA is highly bound to serum albumin at therapeutic concentrations (99%), and is extensively retained in the plasma. MPA is converted in the liver to the inactive glucuronide metabolite (MPAG). Both MPA and MPAG undergo enterohepatic recycling with MPAG conversion back to active MPA. About 81% of an oral dose of mycophenolate mofetil is excreted in the urine as MPAG. A negligible amount of MPA is excreted in the urine. Cl is 10.6 ± 1.9 L/hr (IV) and and 11.6 ± 2.9 L/hr (PO); the half-life is 16.6 ± 5.8 hr (IV) and 17.9 ± 6.5 hr (PO). In patients with renal insufficiency, increases in serum MPA (50%) and MPAG (three- to sixfold) occur. Diarrhea (31%), nausea, and vomiting occur frequently; however, overall there appears to be very little toxicity to the kidney, liver, or CNS. Lymphoma or lymphoproliferative disease, leukopenia, and tissue-invasive infection with cytomegalovirus occur more frequently than in similar patients receiving azathioprine. GI tract hemorrhage (3%) and severe neutropenia (up to 2%) occur. Monitor the CBC weekly during the first month, followed by twice monthly for the second 2 months, then monthly through the first year. Mycophenolate (in combination with cyclosporine and a glucocorticoid) appears more effective than azathioprine (in the same combination) in preventing acute rejection of transplanted organs. Dosage is 1 g PO bid on an empty stomach, started within 72 hr following renal transplantation, and given concurrently with cyclosporine and a glucocorticoid. 1.5 g bid has been used clinically; however, no efficacy advantage over 1 g bid has been established and the overall safety profile was better at the lower dose. Avoid doses over 1 g bid in severe renal dysfunction (GFR <25 mL/min), outside of the immediate posttransplant period. If neutropenia occurs (ANC <1300/μL), interrupt or reduce the dosage. Available as 250-mg capsules.[222,235–238]

TACROLIMUS   Prograf

Tacrolimus, a macrolide antibiotic with immunosuppressant properties, has a mechanism of action similar to that of cyclosporine, but has no structural similarity. Tacrolimus inhibits T-helper lymphocyte activation after intracellular protein binding and suppression of interleukin-2 (IL-2) and other cytokine production. Tacrolimus is an alternative to cyclosporine for primary transplant immunosuppression and for rescue treatment of grafts failing on cyclosporine. The drug is rapidly absorbed orally, with peak serum levels occurring in 2 hr (range 0.5–6). Oral bioavailability averages 25% (range 4–93) in renal and liver transplant patients; unlike cyclosporine, tacrolimus absorption is not dependent on bile salts. Food reduces the rate and extent (30% decrease) of absorption. Whole blood concentrations are about 15 times (range 4–114) higher then serum levels because of extensive concentration-, temperature-, hematocrit-, and time-dependent binding to RBCs. The drug is 77% bound to plasma proteins. Recommended therapeutic whole blood trough levels (ELISA) at 12 hr postdose are 5–20 µg/L early posttransplant (24-hr trough levels are 33–50% less). Higher levels have been associated with an increased frequency of adverse effects; however, the therapeutic range is not clearly defined. Current immunoassays are nonspecific and crossreact with metabolites. V_{dss} (whole blood) is about 1 L/kg (range 0.5–1.4); Cl (whole blood) averages 0.06 L/hr/kg (range 0.03–0.09). The half-life (whole blood) averages 12 hr (range 4–41). Tacrolimus is primarily metabolized by the liver (mainly by CYP3A4) to at least 15 metabolites (with little or no activity), which are predominately excreted in the bile. Less than 1% of the parent drug is excreted unchanged in the urine. Adverse reactions include frequent nephrotoxicity, hyperkalemia, new onset diabetes mellitus, hypertension (although less than cyclosporine), and alopecia. Anaphylactoid reactions have occurred with the IV product. Routine monitoring of blood pressure, Cr_s, potassium, and glucose is recommended. Whole blood trough level monitoring is recommended and should start on day 2 or 3 of therapy, then 3–7 times weekly for the first 2 weeks, 3 times a week for the following week, then with decreasing frequency as needed. Do not give tacrolimus and cyclosporine concurrently; wait at least 24 hr before switching from one immunosuppressant to the other. Dosage in adult patients unable to take capsules (started 6 hr or later after transplant in combination with a glucocorticoid) is 0.05 mg/kg/day as a continuous IV infusion in non-PVC containers. When oral therapy can be tolerated, start 0.15 mg/kg/day PO in 2 divided doses q 12 hr, starting 8–12 hr after discontinuing the IV drug. Give children 0.1 mg/kg/day by continuous infusion (if unable to take orally), and 0.3 mg/kg/day PO in two divided doses q 12 hr, starting 8–12 hr after discontinuing the IV drug. Adjust dosage in adults and children based on clinical assessment of rejection and tolerability. Give children with hepatic or renal impairment initial dosages at the lower value of the recommended IV and PO dosage range and consider using even lower dosages in adults. Delay therapy up to 48 hr or longer in patients with postoperative oliguria.[222,239–243] Available as 1- and 5-mg capsules, and 5 mg/mL ampules for IV infusion after dilution.

■ REFERENCES

1. Dorr RT, Von Hoff DD, eds. *Cancer chemotherapy handbook*, 2nd ed. Norwalk CT: Appleton & Lange: 1994.

2. Lindley CM et al. Incidence and duration of chemotherapy-induced nausea and vomiting in the outpatient oncology population. *J Clin Oncol* 1989;7:1142–9.

3. Wharton JT et al. Hexamethylmelamine: an evaluation of its role in the treatment of ovarian cancer. *Am J Obstet Gynecol* 1979;133:833–44.

4. Manetta A et al. Hexamethylmelamine as a single second-line agent in ovarian cancer. *Gynecol Oncol* 1990;36:93–6.

5. Ames MM et al. Phase I and clinical pharmacological evaluation of a parenteral hexamethylmelamine formulation. *Cancer Res* 1990;50:206–10.

6. Sawitsky A et al. Comparison of daily versus intermittent chlorambucil and prednisone therapy in the treatment of patients with chronic lymphocytic leukemia. *Blood* 1977;50:1049–59.

7. Alexanian R, Dreicer R. Chemotherapy of multiple myeloma. *Cancer* 1984;53:583–8.

8. Adair CG et al. Renal function in the elimination of oral melphalan in patients with multiple myeloma. *Cancer Chemother Pharmacol* 1986;17:185–8.

9. Hoogstraten B et al. Intermittent melphalan therapy in multiple myeloma. *JAMA* 1969;209:251–3.

10. Benet LZ et al. Design and optimization of dosage regimens: pharmacokinetic data. In Hardman JG et al., eds. *Goodman and Gilman's the pharmacological basis of therapeutics*, 9th ed. New York: McGraw-Hill; 1996:1707–92.

11. McLean A et al. Pharmacokinetics and metabolism of chlorambucil in patients with malignant disease. *Cancer Treat Rev* 1979;6(suppl):33–42.

12. Adair CG et al. Can food affect the bioavailability of chlorambucil in patients with hematological malignancies? *Cancer Chemother Pharmacol* 1986;17:99–102.

13. Alberts DS et al. Oral melphalan kinetics. *Clin Pharmacol Ther* 1979;26:737–45.

14. Alberts DS et al. Kinetics of intravenous melphalan. *Clin Pharmacol Ther* 1979;26:73–80.

15. Taetle R et al. Pulmonary histopathologic changes associated with melphalan therapy. *Cancer* 1978; 42:1239–45.

16. Heard BE, Cooke RA. Busulfan lung. *Thorax* 1968;23:187–93.

17. Lane SD et al. Fatal interstitial pneumonitis following high-dose intermittent chlorambucil therapy for chronic lymphocytic leukemia. *Cancer* 1981;47:32–6.

18. Micetich KC et al. A comparative study of the cytotoxicity and DNA-damaging effects of cis-(diammino) (1,1-cyclobutanedicarboxylato)-platinum(II) and cis- diamminedichloroplatinum(II) on L1210 cells. *Cancer Res* 1985;45:4043–7.

19. Curt GA et al. A phase I and pharmacokinetic study of diamminecyclobutane-dicarboxylatoplatinum (NSC 241240). *Cancer Res* 1983;43:4470–3.

20. Meyers FJ et al. Infusion carboplatin treatment of relapsed and refractory acute leukemia: evidence of efficacy with minimal extramedullary toxicity at intermediate doses. *J Clin Oncol* 1989;7:173–8.

21. Smit E et al. Continuous infusion carboplatin on a 21-day schedule: a phase I and pharmacokinetic study. *J Clin Oncol* 1991;9:100–10.

22. Allen JC et al. Carboplatin and recurrent childhood brain tumors. *J Clin Oncol* 1987;5:459–63.

23. Calvert AH et al. Carboplatin dosage: prospective evaluation of a simple formula based on renal function. *J Clin Oncol* 1989;7:1748–56.

24. Chatelut E et al. Prediction of carboplatin clearance from standard morphological and biological patient characteristics. *J Natl Cancer Inst* 1995;87:573–80.

25. Newell DR et al. Plasma free platinum pharmacokinetics in patients treated with high dose carboplatin. *Eur J Cancer Clin Oncol* 1987;23:1399–405.

26. Calvert AH et al. Early clinical studies with cis-diammine-1,1-cyclobutane dicarboxylate platinum(II). *Cancer Chemother Pharmacol* 1982;9:140–7.

27. Einhorn LH, Donahue J. Cis-diamminedichloroplatinum, vinblastine, and bleomycin combination chemotherapy in disseminated testicular cancer. *Ann Intern Med* 1977;87:293–8.

28. Belt RJ et al. Pharmacokinetics of non-protein-bound platinum species following administration of cis-dichlorodiammineplatinum (II). *Cancer Treat Rep* 1979;63:1515–21.

29. DeConti RC et al. Clinical and pharmacological studies with cis-diamminedichloroplatinum (II). *Cancer Res* 1973;33:1310–5.

30. Gonzalez-Vitale JC et al. Acute renal failure after cis-dichlorodiammineplatinum (II) and gentamicin-cephalothin therapies. *Cancer Treat Rep* 1978;62:693–8.

31. Macaulay VM et al. Prophylaxis against hypomagnesemia induced by cisplatinum combination therapy. *Cancer Chemother Pharmacol* 1982;9:179–81.

32. Brock N et al. Activation of cyclophosphamide in man and animals. *Cancer* 1971;6:1512–29.

33. Grochow LB, Colvin M. Clinical pharmacokinetics of cyclophosphamide. *Clin Pharmacokinet* 1979;4:380–94.

34. Bagley CM et al. Clinical pharmacology of cyclophosphamide. *Cancer Res* 1973;33:226–33.

35. Scheef W et al. Controlled clinical studies with an antidote against the urotoxicity of oxazophosphorines: preliminary results. *Cancer Treat Rep* 1979;63:501–5.

36. Carter SK, Friedman MA. 5-(3,3-dimethyl-l-triazeno)-imidazole-4-carboxamide (DTIC, DIC, NSC-45388)—a new antitumor agent with activity against malignant melanoma. *Eur J Cancer* 1972;8:85–92.

37. Loo TL et al. Mechanism of action and pharmacology studies with DTIC (NSC-45388). *Cancer Treat Rep* 1976;60:149–52.

38. Zalupski M, Baker LH. Ifosfamide. *J Natl Cancer Inst* 1988;80:556–66.

39. Araujo C, Tessler J. Treatment of ifosfamide-induced urothelial toxicity by oral administration of sodium 2-mercaptoethane sulphonate (mesna) to patients with inoperable lung cancer. *Eur J Cancer Clin Oncol* 1983;19:195–201.

40. Stuart-Harris RC et al. High-dose alkylation therapy using ifosfamide infusion with mesna in the treatment of adult advanced soft tissue sarcoma. *Cancer Chemother Pharmacol* 1983;11:69–72.

41. Sangster G et al. Failure of 2-mercaptoethane sulphonate sodium (mesna) to protect against ifosfamide nephrotoxicity. *Eur J Cancer Clin Oncol* 1984;20:435–6.

42. Pratt CB et al. Phase II trial of ifosfamide in children with malignant solid tumors. *Cancer Treat Rep* 1987;71:131–5.

43. Miser JS et al. Ifosfamide with uroprotection and etoposide: an effective regimen in the treatment of recurrent sarcomas and other tumors of children and young adults. *J Clin Oncol* 1987;5:1191–8.

44. Creaven PJ et al. Clinical pharmacology of ifosfamide. *Clin Pharmacol Ther* 1974;16:77–86.

45. Colvin M. The comparative pharmacology of cyclophosphamide and ifosfamide. *Semin Oncol* 1982;9(suppl 1):2–7.

46. Allen LM et al. Studies on the human pharmacokinetics of ifosfamide (NSC-109724). *Cancer Treat Rep* 1976;60:451–8.

47. Wheeler BM et al. Ifosfamide in refractory male germ cell tumors. *J Clin Oncol* 1986;4:28–34.

48. Fossa SK, Talle K. Treatment of metastatic renal cancer with ifosfamide and mesnum with and without irradiation. *Cancer Treat Rep* 1980;64:1103–8.

49. Stuart-Harris RC et al. High dose alkylation therapy using ifosfamide infusion with mesna in the treatment of adult advanced soft tissue sarcoma. *Cancer Chemother Pharmacol* 1983;11:69–72.

50. Meanwell CA et al. Phase II study of ifosfamide in cervical cancer. *Cancer Treat Rep* 1986;70:727–30.

51. Goren MP et al. Dechlorethylation of ifosfamide and neurotoxicity. *Lancet* 1986;2:1219–20.

52. DeVita VT et al. Combination chemotherapy in the treatment of advanced Hodgkin's disease. *Ann Intern Med* 1970;73:881–95.

53. Taylor JR, Halprin KM. Topical use of mechlorethamine in the treatment of psoriasis. *Arch Dermatol* 1972;106:362–4.

54. Taylor JR et al. Mechlorethamine hydrochloride solutions and ointment. *Arch Dermatol* 1980;116:783–5.

55. Van Scott EJ, Kalmanson JD. Complete remissions of mycosis fungoides lymphoma induced by topical nitrogen mustard (HN₂). *Cancer* 1973;32:18–30.

56. Crooke ST, Bradner WT. Mitomycin C: a review. *Cancer Treat Rev* 1976;3:121–39.

57. Buice RG et al. Pharmacokinetics of mitomycin C in non–oat cell carcinoma of the lung. *Cancer Chemother Pharmacol* 1984;13:1–4.

58. Dorr RT et al. Mitomycin C skin toxicity studies in mice. *J Clin Oncol* 1986;4:1399–1404.

59. DeFuria MD et al. Phase I-II study of mitomycin C topical therapy for low-grade, low-stage transitional cell carcinoma of the bladder: an interim report. *Cancer Treat Rep* 1980;64:225–30.

60. Sponzo RW et al. Physiologic disposition of 1-(2- chloroethyl)-3-cyclohexyl-1-nitrosourea (CCNU) and 1-(2-chloroethyl)-3-(4-methyl cyclohexyl)-1-nitrosourea (MeCCNU) in man. *Cancer* 1973;31:1154–9.

61. De Vita VT et al. Clinical trials with 1,3-bis(2-chloroethyl)-1-nitrosourea, NSC-409962. *Cancer Res* 1965;25:1876–81.

62. Oliverio VT. Toxicology and pharmacology of the nitrosoureas. *Cancer Chemother Rep* 1973;4(part 3):13–20.

63. Aronin PA et al. Prediction of BCNU pulmonary toxicity in patients with malignant gliomas. *N Engl J Med* 1980;303:183–8.

64. Durant JR et al. Pulmonary toxicity associated with bischloroethylnitrosourea (BCNU). *Ann Intern Med* 1979;90:191–4.

65. Spivack SD. Procarbazine. *Ann Intern Med* 1974;81:795–800.

66. Schein PS et al. Clinical antitumor activity and toxicity of streptozotocin (NSC-85998). *Cancer* 1974;34:993–1000.

67. Cohen BE et al. Human plasma pharmacokinetics and urinary excretion of thiotepa and its metabolites. *Cancer Treat Rep* 1986;70:859–64.

68. Beutler E. Cladribine (2-chlorodeoxyadenosine). *Lancet* 1992;340:952–6.

69. Saven A et al. Treatment of hairy cell leukemia. *Blood* 1992;79:1111–20.

70. Sipe JC et al. Cladribine in treatment of chronic progressive multiple sclerosis. *Lancet* 1994;344:9–13.
71. Liliemark J et al. On the bioavailability of oral and subcutaneous 2-chloro-2'-deoxyadenosine in humans: alternative routes of administration. *J Clin Oncol* 1992;10:1514–8.
72. Southwest Oncology Group. Cytarabine for acute leukemia in adults. *Arch Intern Med* 1974;133:251–9.
73. Rudnick SA et al. High dose cytosine arabinoside (HDARAC) in refractory acute leukemia. *Cancer* 1979;44:1189–93.
74. Band PR et al. Treatment of central nervous system leukemia with intrathecal cytosine arabinoside. *Cancer* 1973;32:744–58.
75. Wan SH et al. Pharmacokinetics of 1-b-D-arabinofuranosylcytosine in humans. *Cancer Res* 1974;34:392–7.
76. Harris AL et al. Pharmacokinetics of cytosine arabinoside in patients with acute myeloid leukaemia. *Br J Clin Pharmacol* 1979;8:219–27.
77. van Prooijen R et al. Pharmacokinetics of cytosine arabinoside in acute myeloid leukemia. *Clin Pharmacol Ther* 1977;21:744–50.
78. Ho DHW, Frei E. Clinical pharmacology of 1-b-D-arabinofuranosylcytosine. *Clin Pharmacol Ther* 1971;12:944–54.
79. Chabner BA et al. Clinical pharmacology of anticancer drugs. *Semin Oncol* 1977;4:165–91.
80. Ritch PS et al. Ocular toxicity from high-dose cytosine arabinoside. *Cancer* 1983;51:430–2.
81. Lazarus HM et al. Central nervous system toxicity of high-dose systemic cytosine arabinoside. *Cancer* 1981;48:2577–82.
82. Kemeny N et al. Intrahepatic or systemic infusion of fluorodeoxyuridine in patients with liver metastases from colorectal carcinoma. *Ann Intern Med* 1987;107:459–65.
83. Ensminger WD et al. A clinical pharmacological evaluation of hepatic arterial infusions of 5-fluoro-2'-deoxyuridine and 5-fluorouracil. *Cancer Res* 1978;38:3784–92.
84. Jacobs EM et al. Treatment of cancer with weekly 5-fluorouracil; study by the Western Cooperative Cancer Chemotherapy Croup (WCCCG). *Cancer* 1971;27:1302–5.
85. Horton J et al. 5-Fluorouracil in cancer: an improved regimen. *Ann Intern Med* 1970;73:897–900.
86. Seifert P et al. Comparison of continuously infused 5-fluorouracil with bolus injection in treatment of patients with colorectal adenocarcinoma. *Cancer* 1975;36:123–8.
87. Cohen JL et al. Clinical pharmacology of oral and intravenous 5-fluorouracil (NSC-19893). *Cancer Chemother Rep* 1974;58(part 1):723–31.
88. Kirkwood JM et al. Comparison of pharmacokinetics of 5-fluorouracil and 5-fluorouracil with concurrent thymidine infusions in a phase I trial. *Cancer Res* 1980;40:107–13.
89. Abbruzzese JL et al. A phase I clinical, plasma, and cellular pharmacology study of gemcitabine. *J Clin Oncol* 1991;9:491–8.
90. Kaye SB. Gemcitabine: current status of phase I and II trials. *J Clin Oncol* 1994;12:1527–31.
91. Rothenberg ML et al. Gemcitabine: effective palliative therapy for pancreas cancer patients failing 5-FU. *Proc Am Soc Clin Oncol* 1995;14:198.
92. Mullarkey MF et al. Long-term methotrexate treatment in corticosteroid-dependent asthma. *Ann Intern Med* 1990;112:577–81.
93. Hedman J et al. Controlled trial of methotrexate in patients with severe chronic asthma. *Eur J Clin Pharmacol* 1996;49:347–9.
94. Henry MA, Gentry WL. Single injection of methotrexate for treatment of ectopic pregnancies. *Am J Obstet Gynecol* 1994;171:1584–7.
95. Corsan GH et al. Identification of hormonal parameters for successful systemic single-dose methotrexate therapy in ectopic pregnancy. *Hum Reprod* 1995;10:2719–22.
96. Wiebe ER. Abortion induced with methotrexate and misoprostol. *Can Med Assoc J* 1996;154:165–70.
97. Creinin MD. A randomized trial comparing misoprostol three and seven days after methotrexate for early abortion. *Am J Obstet Gynecol* 1995;173:1578–84.
98. Schaff EA. Combined methotrexate and misoprostol for early induced abortion. *Arch Fam Med* 1995;4:774–9.
99. Bonadonna G et al. Combination chemotherapy as an adjuvant treatment in operable breast cancer. *N Engl J Med* 1976;294:405–10.
100. Bleyer WA. Clinical pharmacology of intrathecal methotrexate II. An improved dosage regimen derived from age-related pharmacokinetics. *Cancer Treat Rep* 1977;61:1419–25.
101. Evans WE, Pratt CB. Effect of pleural effusion on high-dose methotrexate kinetics. *Clin Pharmacol Ther* 1978;24:68–72.
102. Campbell MA et al. Methotrexate: bioavailability and pharmacokinetics. *Cancer Treat Rep* 1985;69:833–8. Dosages in the table were derived using the nomogram of Rowland M, Tozer TN. *Clinical pharmacokinetics: concepts and applications.* Philadelphia: Lea & Febiger; 1980:233.
103. Isacoff WH et al. Pharmacokinetics of high-dose methotrexate with citrovorum factor rescue. *Cancer Treat Rep* 1977;61:1665–74.
104. Shen DD, Azarnoff DL. Clinical pharmacokinetics of methotrexate. *Clin Pharmacokinet* 1978;3:1–13.

105. O'Dwyer PJ et al. 2'-deoxycoformycin (pentostatin) for lymphoid malignancies. *Ann Intern Med* 1988;108: 733–43.

106. Malspeis L et al. Clinical pharmacokinetics of 2'-deoxycoformycin. *Cancer Treat Symp* 1984;2:7–15.

107. Wiernik PH, Serpick AA. A randomized clinical trial of daunorubicin and a combination of prednisone, vincristine, 6-mercaptopurine, and methotrexate in adult acute nonlymphocytic leukemia. *Cancer Res* 1967;32:2023–6.

108. Lin S-N et al. Quantitation of plasma azathioprine and 6-mercaptopurine levels in renal transplant patients. *Transplantation* 1980;29:290–4.

109. Bach JF, Dardenne M. The metabolism of azathioprine in renal failure. *Transplantation* 1971;12:253–9.

110. Zimm S et al. Variable bioavailability of oral mercaptopurine. *N Engl J Med* 1983;308:1005–9.

111. Duttera MJ et al. Hematuria and crystalluria after high-dose 6-mercaptopurine administration. *N Engl J Med* 1972;287:292–4.

112. Penn I, Starzl TE. A summary of the status of de novo cancer in transplant recipients. *Transplant Proc* 1972;4:719–32.

113. Rosenberg SA et al. Observations on the systemic administration of autologous lymphokine-activated killer cells and recombinant interleukin-2 to patients with metastatic cancer. *N Engl J Med* 1985;313:1485–92.

114. Winkelhake JL, Gauny SS. Human recombinant interleukin-2 as an experimental therapeutic. *Pharmacol Rev* 1990;42:1–28.

115. Konrad MW et al. Pharmacokinetics of recombinant interleukin-2 in humans. *Cancer Res* 1990;50:2009–17.

116. Goldstein D, Laszlo J. Interferon therapy in cancer: from imaginon to interferon. *Cancer Res* 1986;46:4315–29.

117. Krown SE. The role of interferon in the therapy of epidemic Kaposi's sarcoma. *Semin Oncol* 1987;14:27–33.

118. Perrillo RP et al. A randomized controlled trial of interferon alfa-2b alone and after prednisone withdrawal for the treatment of chronic hepatitis B. *N Engl J Med* 1990;323:295–301.

119. Spiegel RJ. Intron A (interferon alfa-2b): clinical overview. *Cancer Treat Rev* 1985;12(suppl B):5–16.

120. Wills RJ et al. Interferon kinetics and adverse reactions after intravenous, intramuscular, and subcutaneous injection. *Clin Pharmacol Ther* 1984;35:722–7.

121. Quesada JR et al. Antitumor activity of recombinant-derived interferon alpha in metastatic renal cell carcinoma. *J Clin Oncol* 1985;3:1522–8.

122. Berman E et al. Idarubicin in acute leukemia: results of studies at Memorial Sloan-Kettering Cancer Center. *Semin Oncol* 1989;16:30–4.

123. Lambertenghi-Deliliers G et al. Idarubicin plus cytarabine as first-line treatment of acute nonlymphoblastic leukemia. *Semin Oncol* 1989;16:16–20.

124. Blum RH, Carter SK. Adriamycin: a new anticancer drug with significant clinical activity. *Ann Intern Med* 1974;80;249–59.

125. Legha SS et al. Reduction of doxorubicin cardiotoxicity by prolonged continuous intravenous infusion. *Ann Intern Med* 1982;96:133–9.

126. Weiss AJ et al. Studies on adriamycin using a weekly regimen demonstrating its clinical effectiveness and lack of cardiac toxicity. *Cancer Treat Rep* 1976;60:813–22.

127. Von Hoff DD et al. Daunomycin-induced cardiotoxicity in children and adults: a review of 110 cases. *Am J Med* 1977;62:200–8.

128. Benjamin RS et al. Adriamycin chemotherapy—efficacy, safety, and pharmacologic basis of an intermittent single high-dosage schedule. *Cancer* 1974;33:19–27.

129. Smith DB et al. Clinical pharmacology of oral and intravenous 4-demethoxydaunorubicin. *Cancer Chemother Pharmacol* 1987;19:138–42.

130. Robert J et al. Pharmacokinetics of idarubicin after daily intravenous administration in leukemic patients. *Leuk Res* 1987;11:961–4.

131. Huffman DH et al. Daunorubicin metabolism in acute nonlymphocytic leukemia. *Clin Pharmacol Ther* 1972;13:895–905.

132. Lu K et al. Clinical pharmacology of 4-demethoxydaunorubicin (DMDR). *Cancer Chemother Pharmacol* 1986;17:143–8.

133. Dean JC et al. Scalp hypothermia: a comparison of ice packs and the Kold Kap in the prevention of doxorubicin-induced alopecia. *J Clin Oncol* 1983;1(1):33–7.

134. Von Hoff DD et al. Risk factors for doxorubicin-induced congestive heart failure. *Ann Intern Med* 1979;91:710–7.

135. Lipshultz SE et al. Late effects of doxorubicin therapy for acute lymphoblastic leukemia in childhood. *N Engl J Med* 1991;324:808–15.

136. Barlett NL et al. Phase I trial of doxorubicin with cyclosporine as a modulator of multidrug resistance. *J Clin Oncol* 1994;12:835–42.

137. Dorr RT. Anthracycline update: stability and compatibility of adriamycin in solution. *Highlights on Antineoplastic Drugs* 1985;3(2):6–7.

138. Speyer JL et al. Protective effect of the bispiperazinedione ICRF-187 against doxorubicin-induced cardiac toxicity in women with advanced breast cancer. *N Engl J Med* 1988;319:745–52.

139. Olver IN et al. A prospective study of topical dimethylsulfoxide for treating anthracycline extravasation. *J Clin Oncol* 1988;6:1732–5.

140. Gill PS et al. Phase I/II clinical and pharmacokinetic evaluation of liposomal daunorubicin. *J Clin Oncol* 1995;13:996–1003.

141. Forssen EA et al. Selective in vivo localization of daunorubicin small unilamellar vesicles in solid tumors. *Cancer Res* 1992;52:3255–61.

142. Northfelt DW et al. Doxorubicin encapsulated in liposomes containing surface-bound polyethylene glycol: pharmacokinetics, tumor localization, and safety in patients with AIDS-related Kaposi's sarcoma. *J Clin Pharmacol* 1996;36:55–63.

143. Harrison M et al. Liposomal-entrapped doxorubicin: an active agent in AIDS-related Kaposi's sarcoma. *J Clin Oncol* 1995;13:914–20.

144. Frei E. The clinical use of actinomycin. *Cancer Chemother Rep* 1974;58:49–54.

145. Tattersall MHN et al. Pharmacokinetics of actinomycin D in patients with malignant melanoma. *Clin Pharmacol Ther* 1975;17:701–8.

146. Shenkenberg TD, Von Hoff DD. Mitoxantrone: a new anticancer drug with significant clinical activity. *Ann Intern Med* 1986;105:67–81.

147. Vietti TJ et al. Mitoxantrone in children with advanced malignant disease. In Rozencweig M et al., eds. *New anticancer drugs: mitoxantrone and bisantrene.* New York: Raven Press; 1983:93–102.

148. Savaraj N et al. Pharmacology of mitoxantrone in cancer patients. *Cancer Chemother Pharmacol* 1982; 8:113–7.

149. Slayton RE et al. New approach to the treatment of hypercalcemia: the effect of short-term treatment with mithramycin. *Clin Pharmacol Ther* 1971;12:833–7.

150. Kennedy BJ. Metabolic and toxic effects of mithramycin during tumor therapy. *Am J Med* 1970;49:494–503.

151. Asbury RF et al. Treatment of metastatic breast cancer with aminoglutethimide. *Cancer* 1981;47:1954–8.

152. Plourde PV. Arimidex: a potent and selective fourth-generation aromatase inhibitor. *Breast Cancer Res Treat* 1994;30:103–11.

153. Newling DWW et al. The response of advanced prostatic cancer to a new non-steroidal antiandrogen: results of a multicenter open phase II study of Casodex. *Eur Urol* 1990;18:18–21.

154. Cockshott ID et al. The pharmacokinetics of Casodex in prostate cancer patients after single and during multiple dosing. *Eur Urol* 1990;18:10–7.

155. Katchen B, Buxbaum S. Disposition of a new nonsteroid antiandrogen, alpha, alpha, alpha-trifluoro-2-methyl-4'-nitro-m-propionotoluidide (flutamide) in men following a single oral 200 mg dose. *J Clin Endocrinol Metab* 1975;41:373–9.

156. Symchowicz S et al. Single and multiple dose pharmacokinetics of flutamide (Eulexin) in normal geriatric volunteers. *Acta Pharmacol Toxicol (Copenh)* 1986;58:301. Abstract.

157. Yagoda A. Flutamide-induced diarrhea secondary to lactose intolerance. *J Natl Cancer Inst* 1989;81:1839–40. Letter.

158. Hauser AR, Marryman R. Estramustine phosphate sodium. *Drug Intell Clin Pharm* 1984;18:368–74.

159. Ahmann FR et al. Zoladex: a sustained-release, monthly luteinizing hormone-releasing hormone analogue for the treatment of advanced prostate cancer. *J Clin Oncol* 1987;5:912–7.

160. Leuprolide Study Group. Leuprolide versus diethylstilbestrol for metastatic prostate cancer. *N Engl J Med* 1984;311:1281–6.

161. Patterson JS, Battersby LA. Tamoxifen: an overview of recent studies in the field of oncology. *Cancer Treat Rep* 1980;64:775–8.

162. Fabian C et al. Clinical pharmacology of tamoxifen in patients with breast cancer: comparison of traditional and loading dose schedules. *Cancer Treat Rep* 1980;64:765–73.

163. Adam HK et al. Studies on the metabolism and pharmacokinetics of tamoxifen in normal volunteers. *Cancer Treat Rep* 1980;64:761–4.

164. Plotkin D et al. Tamoxifen flare in advanced breast cancer. *JAMA* 1978;240:2644–6.

165. Lippman ME, Allegra JC. Receptors in breast cancer: estrogen receptor and endocrine therapy of breast cancer. *N Engl J Med* 1978;299:930–3.

166. Cortes JE et al. Docetaxel. *J Clin Oncol* 1995;13:2643–55.

167. Royer I. Metabolism of docetaxel by human cytochromes P450: interactions with paclitaxel and other antineoplastic drugs. *Cancer Res* 1996;56:58–65.

168. O'Dwyer PJ et al. Etoposide (VP-16-213): current status of an active anticancer drug. *N Engl J Med* 1985;312:692–700.

169. Rivera GK et al. Epipodophyllotoxins in the treatment of childhood cancer. *Cancer Chemother Pharmacol* 1994;34(suppl):S89–95.

170. Chamberlain MC, Grafe MR. Recurrent chiasmatic-hypothalamic glioma treated with oral etoposide. *J Clin Oncol* 1995;13:2072–6.

171. Snyder DS et al. Fractionated total-body irradiation and high-dose etoposide as a preparatory regimen for bone marrow transplantation for 94 patients with chronic myelogenous leukemia in chronic phase. *Blood* 1994;84:1672–9.

172. Allen LM, Creaven PJ. Comparison of the human pharmacokinetics of VM-26 and VP-16, two antineoplastic epipodophyllotoxin glucopyranoside derivatives. *Eur J Cancer* 1975;11:697–707.

173. Holmes FA et al. Phase II study of taxol in patients with metastatic breast cancer. *Proc Am Soc Clin Oncol* 1991;10:60. Abstract.

174. McGuire WP et al. Taxol: a unique antineoplastic agent with significant activity in advanced ovarian epithelial neoplasms. *Ann Intern Med* 1989;111:273–9.

175. Huizing MT et al. Pharmacokinetics of paclitaxel and metabolites in a randomized comparative study in platinum-pretreated ovarian cancer patients. *J Clin Oncol* 1993;11:2127–35.

176. Rozencweig M et al. VM-26 and VP 16–213: a comparative analysis. *Cancer* 1977;40:334–42.

177. Grem JL et al. Teniposide in the treatment of leukemia: a case study of conflicting priorities in the development of drugs for fatal diseases. *J Clin Oncol* 1988;6:351–79.

178. Yap H-Y et al. Vinblastine given as a continuous 5-day infusion in the treatment of refractory advanced breast cancer. *Cancer Treat Rep* 1980;64:279–83.

179. Robieux I et al. Pharmacokinetics of vinorelbine in patients with liver metastases. *Clin Pharmacol Ther* 1996;59:32–40.

180. Owellen RJ et al. Pharmacokinetics of vindesine and vincristine in humans. *Cancer Res* 1977;37:2603–7.

181. Nelson RL et al. Comparative pharmacokinetics of vindesine, vincristine and vinblastine in patients with cancer. *Cancer Treat Rev* 1980;7(suppl):17–24.

182. Wargin WA, Lucas VS. The clinical pharmacokinetics of vinorelbine (Navelbine). *Semin Oncol* 1994;21(5 suppl 10):21–7.

183. Le Chevalier T et al. Randomized study of vinorelbine and cisplatin versus vindesine and cisplatin versus vinorelbine alone in advanced non-small-cell lung cancer: results of a European multicenter trial including 612 patients. *J Clin Oncol* 1994;12:360–7.

184. Clarkson B et al. Clinical results of treatment with *E. coli* l-asparaginase in adults with leukemia, lymphoma and solid tumors. *Cancer* 1970;25:279–305.

185. Sutow WW et al. Evaluation of dose and schedule of l-asparaginase in multidrug therapy of childhood leukemia. *Med Pediatr Oncol* 1976;2:387–95.

186. Pratt CB et al. Comparison of daily versus weekly l-asparaginase for the treatment of childhood acute leukemia. *J Pediatr* 1970;77:474–83.

187. Nesbit M et al. Evaluation of intramuscular versus intravenous administration of l-asparaginase in childhood leukemia. *Am J Pediatr Hematol Oncol* 1979;1:9–13.

188. Ohnuma T et al. Biochemical and pharmacological studies with asparaginase in man. *Cancer Res* 1970;30:2297–305.

189. Haskell CM et al. L-asparaginase: therapeutic and toxic effects in patients with neoplastic disease. *N Engl J Med* 1969;281:1028–35.

190. Bennett JM, Reich SD. Bleomycin. *Ann Intern Med* 1979;90:945–8.

191. Alberts DS et al. Bleomycin pharmacokinetics in man. *Cancer Chemother Pharmacol* 1978;1:177–81.

192. Paladine W et al. Intracavitary bleomycin in the management of malignant effusions. *Cancer* 1976;38:1903–8.

193. Crooke ST et al. Effects of variations in renal function on the clinical pharmacology of bleomycin administered as an IV bolus. *Cancer Treat Rep* 1977;61:1631–6.

194. Kramer WG et al. The pharmacokinetics of bleomycin in man. *J Clin Pharmacol* 1978;18:346–52.

195. Sostman HD et al. Cytotoxic drug-induced lung disease. *Am J Med* 1977;62:608–15.

196. Yagoda A et al. Bleomycin, an antitumor antibiotic: clinical experience in 274 patients. *Ann Intern Med* 1972;77:861–70.

197. Muindi JRF et al. Clinical pharmacology of oral all-trans retinoic acid in patients with acute promyelocytic leukemia. *Cancer Res* 1992;52:2138–42.

198. Warrell RP et al. Differentiation therapy of acute promyelocytic leukemia with tretinoin (all-trans-retinoic acid). *N Engl J Med* 1991;324:1385–90.

199. Fenaux P et al. Effect of all transretinoic acid in newly diagnosed acute promyelocytic leukemia. Results of a multicenter randomized trial. European APL 91 Group. *Blood* 1993;82:3241–9.

200. Glick J et al. A randomized trial of cyclophosphamide and cisplatin ± amifostine in the treatment of advanced epithelial ovarian cancer. *Proc Am Soc Clin Oncol* 1994;13:432.

201. Shaw LM et al. Pharmacokinetics of WR-2721. *Pharmacol Ther* 1988;39:195–201.

202. Kligerman MM et al. Phase I clinical studies with WR-2721. *Cancer Clin Trials* 1980;3:217–21.

203. Speyer JL et al. ICRF-187 permits longer treatment with doxorubicin in women with breast cancer. *J Clin Oncol* 1992;10:117–27.

204. Hochster H et al. Pharmacokinetics of the cardioprotector ADR-529 (ICRF-187) in escalating doses combined with fixed-dose doxorubicin. *J Natl Cancer Inst* 1992;84:1725–30.

205. Burkert H. Clinical overview of mesna. *Cancer Treat Rev* 1983;10:175–81.

206. Antman KH et al. Phase II trial of ifosfamide with mesna in previously treated metastatic sarcoma. *Cancer Treat Rep* 1985;69:499–504.

207. Pratt CB et al. Phase II trial of ifosfamide in children with malignant solid tumors. *Cancer Treat Rep* 1987;71:131–5.

208. Burkert H et al. Bioavailability of orally administered mesna. *Arzneimittelforschung* 1984;34:1597–600.

209. Pohl J et al. Toxicology, pharmacology and interactions of sodium 2-mercaptoethanesulfonate (mesna). *Curr Chemother* 1981;2:1387–9.

210. Stuart-Harris RC et al. High-dose alkylation therapy using ifosfamide infusion with mesna in the treatment of adults advanced soft-tissue sarcoma. *Cancer Chemother Pharmacol* 1983;11:69–72.

211. Sloth K, Thomsen AC. Acute renal insufficiency during treatment with azathioprine. *Acta Med Scand* 1971;189:145–8.

212. Kahan BD. Cyclosporine. *N Engl J Med* 1989;321:1725–38.

213. Faulds D et al. Cyclosporin. A review of its pharmacodynamic and pharmacokinetic properties, and therapeutic use in immunoregulatory disorders. *Drugs* 1993;45:953–1040.

214. Brodehl J. Consensus statements on the optimal use of cyclosporine in pediatric patients. *Transplant Proc* 1994;26:2759–62.

215. Yee GC. Recent advances in cyclosporine pharmacokinetics. *Pharmacotherapy* 1991;11:130S–4.

216. Kahan BD et al. Consensus document: Hawk's Cay meeting on therapeutic drug monitoring of cyclosporine. *Clin Chem* 1990;36:1510–6.

217. Fahr A. Cyclosporin clinical pharmacokinetics. *Clin Pharmacokinet* 1993;24:472–95.

218. Shaw L et al. Canadian consensus meeting on cyclosporine monitoring: report of the consensus panel. *Clin Chem* 1990;36:1841–6.

219. Woo J. Therapeutic monitoring of cyclosporine. *Ann Clin Lab Sci* 1994;24:60–8.

220. Holt DW et al. Sandimmun Neoral pharmacokinetics: impact of the new oral formulation. *Transplant Proc* 1995;27:1434–7.

221. Oellerich M et al. Lake Louise consensus conference on cyclosporin monitoring on organ transplantation: report of the consensus panel. *Ther Drug Monit* 1995;17:642–54.

222. Tsunoda SM, Aweeka FT. The use of therapeutic drug monitoring to optimise immunosuppressive therapy. *Clin Pharmacokinet* 1996;30:107–40.

223. Yee GC, Salomon DR. Cyclosporine. In Evans WE et al., eds. *Applied pharmacokinetics: principles of therapeutic drug monitoring*, 3rd ed. Vancouver, WA: Applied Therapeutics; 1992:28.1–28.40.

224. Porter GA et al. Cyclosporine-associated hypertension. *Arch Intern Med* 1990;150:280–3.

225. Kahan BD. Optimization of cyclosporine therapy. *Transplant Proc* 1993;25(suppl 3):5–9.

226. First RM et al. Hypertension after renal transplantation. *J Am Soc Nephrol* 1994;4(suppl 1):30–6.

227. Lin H-Y et al. Cyclosporine-induced hyperuricemia and gout. *N Engl J Med* 1989;321:287–92.

228. Yee GC, McGuire TR. Pharmacokinetic drug interactions with cyclosporin (2 parts). *Clin Pharmacokinet* 1990;19:319–32, 400–15.

229. Lake KD. Management of drug interactions with cyclosporine. *Pharmacotherapy* 1991;11(suppl):110S–8.

230. Anon. Grapefruit juice interactions with drugs. *Med Lett Drugs Ther* 1995;37:73–4.

231. Campana C et al. Clinically significant drug interactions with cyclosporin. An update. *Clin Pharmacokinet* 1996;30:141–79.

232. Venkateswara K. Mechanism, pathophysiology, diagnosis, and management of renal transplant rejection. *Med Clin North Am* 1990;74:1039–57.

233. Vogelsang GB et al. Acute graft-versus-host disease: clinical characteristics in the cyclosporine era. *Medicine (Baltimore)* 1988;67;163–74.

234. Rossi SJ et al. Prevention and management of the adverse effects associated with immunosuppressive therapy. *Drug Saf* 1993;9:104–31.

235. Anon. Mycophenolate mofetil—a new immunosuppressant for organ transplantation. *Med Lett Drugs Ther* 1995;37:84–6.

236. Shaw LM et al. Mycophenolate mofetil: a report of the consensus panel. *Ther Drug Monit* 1995;17:690–9.

237. Sollinger HW et al. Mycophenolate mofetil for the prevention of acute rejection in primary cadaveric renal allograft recipients. *Transplantation* 1995;60:225–32.

238. Friman S, Bäckman L. A new microemulsion formulation of cyclosporin. Pharmacokinetic and clinical features. *Clin Pharmacokinet* 1996;30:181–93.

239. Anon. Tacrolimus (FK506) for organ transplants. *Med Lett Drugs Ther* 1994;36:82–3.

240. Jusko WJ et al. Consensus document: therapeutic monitoring of tacrolimus (FK506). *Ther Drug Monit* 1995;17:606–14.

241. Hooks MA. Tacrolimus, a new immunosuppressant—a review of the literature. *Ann Pharmacother* 1994;28:501–11.

242. Venkataramanan R et al. Clinical pharmacokinetics of tacrolimus. *Clin Pharmacokinet* 1995;26:404–30.

243. Peters DH et al. Tacrolimus. A review of its pharmacology, and therapeutic potential in hepatic and renal transplantation. *Drugs* 1993;46:746–94.

244. Hauben M. Cyclosporine neurotoxicity. *Pharmacotherapy* 1996;16:576–83.

245. Shoker AS. Immunopharmacologic therapy in renal transplantation. *Pharmacotherapy* 1996;16:562–75.

Cardiovascular Drugs ℞

Antiarrhythmic Drugs

ADENOSINE
Adenocard

Adenosine is a purinergic agonist, acting on the purine P_1 and P_2 receptors (although P_1 receptors are more sensitive to adenosine). Pharmacologic effects include coronary and peripheral vasodilation, negative inotropic actions, and depression of sinus node and AV nodal conduction. It is used most frequently for supraventricular tachycardia caused by reentry (ie, AV nodal reentry or AV reentry associated with an extranodal pathway). In these instances, restoration of sinus rhythm occurs in 85–95% of patients. The drug may also be helpful in diagnosing wide-QRS tachycardias believed to be supraventricular in origin. Adenosine is rapidly metabolized in blood to inactive adenosine monophosphate and inosine; elimination half-life is about 1–10 seconds. Frequent, but short-lived, subjective complaints include chest discomfort, dyspnea, flushing, and headache. Postconversion arrhythmias are also frequent, but transient, and include ventricular ectopy, sinus bradycardia, AV block, atrial fibrillation, and rapid reinitiation of supraventricular tachycardia. Adenosine is contraindicated in patients with preexisting sinus node dysfunction or second- or third-degree heart block without a functioning pacemaker, because of the risk of prolonged sinus arrest or AV block. Also use adenosine with caution in asthmatics because it may precipitate bronchospasm, and in patients with atrial fibrillation with an accessory AV pathway because it may accelerate ventricular response. **Dipyridamole,** which blocks the cellular uptake of adenosine, enhances the pharmacologic effect; **theophylline,** a purine antagonist, inhibits the therapeutic actions of adenosine. For supraventricular tachycardia, administer adenosine over 1–2 sec through an IV line with minimal dead space, followed by a saline flush; the initial dose is 6 mg (3 mg if administered through a central line); if this is ineffective, 12 mg can be given 2 min later and repeated again if necessary. An average effective dose of 1 mg has been reported in patients receiving concurrent dipyridamole.[1-4] Pediatric dosage is 50 µg/kg IV, increased in 50 µg/kg increments q 2 min prn, to a maximum of 250 µg/kg. Available as 3 mg/mL injection.

AMIODARONE HYDROCHLORIDE
Cordarone

Pharmacology. Amiodarone is a type III antiarrhythmic that prolongs the effective refractory period of atrial and ventricular tissue by blocking potassium conductance. It decreases sinus rate and slows conduction through the AV node by β-adrenergic blockade. Amiodarone also blocks sodium and calcium channels. The antiarrhythmic actions may be caused by interruption of reentrant substrate or abolition of premature beats that trigger reentry.

Administration and Adult Dosage. PO loading dosage 800–1600 mg/day in divided doses for 1–2 weeks. Maintenance dosage 100–600 mg/day (usually 300–400 mg/day for recurrent ventricular tachycardia and 100–200 mg/day for supraventricular tachycardias such as atrial fibrillation). Some suggest a 600–800 mg/day priming dosage for 1–2 months after the initial loading period and prior to maintenance therapy.[5] **IV for treatment or prevention of refractory ventricular tachycardia or fibrillation** 150 mg over 10 min, then 360 mg over the next 6 hr, followed by 540 mg over the next 18 hr. Initiate amiodarone only during hospitalization for the first several days of the loading phase.

Special Populations. *Pediatric Dosage.* Safety and efficacy not established. **PO** 10–15 mg/kg/day for 10 days, then 5 mg/kg/day maintenance therapy has been used.[6]

Geriatric Dosage. Same as adult dosage.

Dosage Forms. **Tab** 200 mg; **Inj** 50 mg/mL.

Patient Instructions. Report any shortness of breath, tiredness, abdominal discomfort, or visual abnormalities. Avoid intense sunlight; use sunscreen. Divided daily dosage during loading or maintenance dosage phases may reduce gastrointestinal upset.

Pharmacokinetics. *Onset and Duration.* Onset is variable, from several days to a month; full effect may not occur for several months.[7]

Serum Levels. 1–2.5 mg/L (1.6–4 μmol/L) is proposed, although the therapeutic range is not well established.[8] Peak serum concentrations occur in 3–7 hr. Desethylamiodarone accumulates to serum levels similar to or greater than the parent drug.

Fate. Oral absorption is erratic and incomplete; bioavailability is 46 ± 22%. The drug is 99.9% plasma protein bound;[7,9] V_d is 66 ± 44 L/kg; Cl is 0.11 ± 0.024 L/hr/kg.[7,9,10] Amiodarone is primarily hepatically eliminated with at least one active metabolite, desethylamiodarone. No unchanged amiodarone or desethylamiodarone is found in urine.[7]

$t_{1/2}$. α phase 4–12 hr; ß phase varies with duration of therapy and study sampling. Reported variously as 25 ± 12 days and 53 ± 23 days.[7,9,10] Similar for desethylamiodarone.[7,10]

Adverse Reactions. Corneal microdeposits occur in virtually all patients and are not reason for stopping treatment; however, visual disturbances are reported in about 5%.[10] Neurologic effects occur frequently and include tremor, ataxia, paresthesias, and nightmares, which may be more common during the loading phase.[10] Anorexia, nausea, vomiting, and/or constipation occur frequently. Transient elevations in hepatic enzymes occur in over 50% of patients, but clinical hepatitis occurs only occasionally.[11] Photosensitivity occurs frequently, and a blue-gray skin pigmentation (sometimes irreversible) develops in 2–4% of patients.[10] Hypothyroidism (low-T_3 syndrome) or hyperthyroidism may occur frequently.[12] Proximal muscle weakness and myopathy have been reported occasionally. Symptomatic pulmonary fibrosis has been reported in 1–6% of patients; it is probably not immunologic in etiology and seems to occur more often in patients with underlying lung disease.[10,13] Pulmonary symptoms usually improve upon drug discontinuation, but up to 10% of cases result in death.[10,13] Aggravation of ventricular tachycardia and drug-induced torsades de pointes may occur.[10,14] Severe sinus bradycardia (requiring a pacemaker) or AV block has been reported occasionally.

Contraindications. Sick sinus syndrome or second- or third-degree heart block in the absence of a ventricular pacemaker; patients in whom bradycardia has caused syncope; long-QT syndrome.

Precautions. Electrophysiologic studies may not predict the long-term efficacy of amiodarone.[15]

Drug Interactions. Amiodarone increases cyclosporine, digoxin, flecainide, phenytoin, procainamide, and quinidine serum levels, and potentiates warfarin's anticoagulant effects; the initial dosage of warfarin should be reduced by one-third to one-half.

Parameters to Monitor. Monitor ECG daily during loading phase for heart rate, PR, QRS, and QT duration. Baseline and periodic thyroid function tests and liver enzymes (especially if symptoms present). Obtain baseline pulmonary function tests; repeat chest x-ray and clinical examination q 3–6 months.[10,13]

Notes. After the results of CAST,[16] many clinicians use type III antiarrhythmics (eg, amiodarone, sotalol) as first-line therapy in both supraventricular and ventricular arrhythmias.

BRETYLIUM TOSYLATE   Bretylol, Various

Pharmacology. Bretylium is a type III antiarrhythmic with actions thought to be caused by an initial catecholamine release and subsequent catecholamine depletion and/or direct effect independent of the adrenergic nervous system. Direct actions may be mediated by blockade of potassium channels. Bretylium causes an initial increase in blood pressure, heart rate, and myocardial contractility (catecholamine release) followed by hypotension (neuronal blockade). Its greatest usefulness is in severe ventricular tachyarrhythmias resistant to other antiarrhythmics. Bretylium can be effective for ventricular fibrillation, but is usually ineffective against ventricular tachycardia.

Administration and Adult Dosage. **IV loading dose** 5 mg/kg push with additional dose of 10 mg/kg if no response. **Maintenance dosage** can be given as IM or IV (over 8 min or more) 5–10 mg/kg q 6 hr, or as an IV infusion of 1–2 mg/min.

Special Populations. *Pediatric Dosage.* Not well established, although the following has been suggested: **IV loading dosage for ventricular fibrillation** 5 mg/kg, followed by 10 mg/kg at 15- to 30-min intervals, to a maximum total dosage of 30 mg/kg, then **IV maintenance dosage** 5–10 mg/kg q 6 hr.

Geriatric Dosage. Same as adult dosage.

Other Conditions. In renal impairment, lower dosages may be required.[17] A nomogram for dosage in renal insufficiency has been described.[18]

Dosage Forms. **Inj** 50 mg/mL.

Pharmacokinetics. *Onset and Duration.* IV onset usually 5–10 min, but may be delayed to 20–60 min; myocardial levels increase gradually over 6–12 hr.[17,19] Duration is usually 6–12 hr after a single dose. Because of persistent myocardial levels, duration after multiple doses may be much longer.[19]

Fate. 23 ± 9% is orally absorbed.[9,17] The drug is not bound to plasma proteins.[17,20] V_d is 5.9 ± 0.8 L/kg;[21] Cl is 0.61 ± 0.11 L/hr/kg.[9] After IV administration, bretylium is primarily cleared renally, with 77 ± 15% excreted in the urine unchanged.[21] Disposition is probably route and concentration dependent.[17,22]

$t_{1/2}$. α phase about 25 min; ß phase 8.9 ± 1.8 hr,[17,21] mean of 33.4 hr in renal insufficiency.[18]

Adverse Reactions. Hypotension (usually orthostatic) via adrenergic blockade occurs in up to 50% of patients. The drop in mean arterial pressure is usually not more than 20 mm Hg; however, sometimes it can be severe, necessitating drug discontinuation. Nausea and vomiting occur frequently after rapid IV administration.

Contraindications. Suspected digitalis-induced ventricular tachycardia (may increase the rate of ventricular tachycardia or the likelihood of ventricular fibrillation).

Precautions. Use with caution if hypotension exists prior to administration. Keep patient supine until tolerance to hypotension develops. Prolonged effects may occur, and dosage reduction in patients with impaired renal function may be required.

Drug Interactions. The pressor effects of catecholamines are enhanced by bretylium.

Parameters to Monitor. Close monitoring of blood pressure and constant ECG monitoring is required.

DIGITOXIN
Crystodigin, Various

Digitoxin is a digitalis glycoside with a mechanism of action similar to digoxin. It is about 15% absorbed from the stomach and 70% from the small bowel; 14% of the absorbed drug is enterohepatically recycled. IV onset is 25–120 min, and peak is in 4–12 hr, somewhat slower after oral administration. Therapeutic serum levels are 15–30 µg/L (20–40 nmol/L); toxicity occurs over 35 µg/L (46 nmol/L), although considerable overlap exists between toxic and therapeutic ranges. Because 97 ± 0.5% is plasma protein bound, the V_d is less than that of digoxin, about 0.54 ± 0.14 L/kg; Cl is 0.0033 ± 0.0011 L/hr/kg. Digitoxin is eliminated primarily by hepatic metabolism; 32 ± 15% is excreted in urine as unchanged drug. About 8% of daily losses of digitoxin are caused by metabolic conversion to digoxin; however, even in severe renal dysfunction, clinically important accumulation of digoxin does not occur. The drug's α-phase half-life is 1–2 hr and β-phase half-life is 6.7 ± 1.7 days. Adverse reactions, precautions, contraindications, and patient monitoring are similar to digoxin. β-Blockers may worsen CHF or digitalis-induced bradycardia. Potassium loss caused by amphotericin B or diuretics may contribute to digitoxin toxicity. Cholesterol-binding resins may bind digitoxin in the gut. Quinidine may increase digitoxin levels. Rifampin may increase digitoxin metabolism. Spironolactone may decrease digitoxin renal elimination. The adult oral loading dosage is 0.8–1.4 mg in divided doses over 12–24 hr at intervals of 6–8 hr. Alternatively, give a 10–15 µg/kg loading dosage in divided doses. The daily maintenance dosage is 10% of the total digitalizing dosage. In children, use the following digitalizing dosages: (premature and full-term newborn) 22 µg/kg; (2 weeks–1 yr) 45 µg/kg (1–2 yr) 40 µg/kg; (>2 yr) 30 µg/kg. Give the loading

dosage in divided doses over 12–24 hr at intervals of 6–8 hr. The daily maintenance dosage is 10% of the total digitalizing dosage. Unlike digoxin, maintenance
dosage changes are not needed in patients with impaired renal function.[9,23–26]
Available as 0.1-mg tablets.

DIGOXIN
Lanoxin, Various

Pharmacology. Digitalis glycosides exert positive inotropic effects through improvement of availability of calcium to myocardial contractile elements, thereby increasing cardiac output in CHF. Antiarrhythmic actions of digitalis glycosides are
primarily caused by an increase in AV nodal refractory period via increased vagal
tone, sympathetic withdrawal, and direct mechanisms. Additionally, digitalis exerts
a moderate direct vasoconstrictor action on arterial and venous smooth muscle.

Administration and Adult Dosage. **IV loading dosage** 10–15 µg/kg in divided
doses over 12–24 hr at intervals of 6–8 hr.[27] **PO loading dosage** adjust dosage for
percent oral absorption (*see* Fate). Usually, 0.5 mg is given initially, then 0.25 mg
q 6 hr until desired effect or total digitalizing dosage is achieved. **Maintenance
dosage** = (total body stores) $\times$ (% lost/day), where total body stores is the original
calculated loading dosage and % lost/day is 14 + ($Cl_{cr}/5$). Usual maintenance
dosage ranges from 0.125–0.5 mg/day.[27] A dosage nomogram has also been described.[28] **IM not recommended.**

Special Populations. *Pediatric Dosage.* Base all dosages on ideal body weight.
Total digitalizing dosage (TDD) PO (premature newborn) 20–30 µg/kg; (full-
term newborn) 25–35 µg/kg; (1–24 months) 35–60 µg/kg; (2–5 yr) 30–40 µg/kg;
(5–10 yr) 20–35 µg/kg; (>10 yr) 10–15 µg/kg. Give ½ TDD initially, then ¼
TDD q 8–18 hr twice. **PO maintenance dosage** (premature newborn) 5–7.5
µg/kg/day; (full-term newborn) 6–10 µg/kg/day; (1–24 months) 10–15 µg/kg/day;
(2–5 yr) 7.5–10 µg/kg/day; (5–10 yr) 5–10 µg/kg/day; (>10 yr) 2.5–5 µg/kg/day.
In children <10 yr, give in 2 divided doses per day. **IV** (all ages) 75% of PO
dosage.

Geriatric Dosage. Maintenance dosage may be lower because of age-related decrease in renal function.[29,30]

Other Conditions. Decrease loading and maintenance dosage in renal impairment.
Base dosage on ideal body weight in obese individuals.

Dosage Forms. **Cap** 0.05, 0.1, 0.2 mg; **Elxr** 50 µg/mL; **Tab** 0.0625, 0.125,
0.1875, 0.25, 0.375, 0.5 mg; **Inj** 0.1, 0.25 mg/mL.

Patient Instructions. Report feelings of tiredness, appetite loss, nausea, abdominal discomfort or visual disturbances such as hazy vision, light sensitivity, spots,
halos, or red-green blindness.

Pharmacokinetics. *Onset and Duration.* IV onset 14–30 min; peak 1.5–5 hr;[25]
somewhat slower after oral administration.

Serum Levels. Therapeutic 0.5–2 µg/L (0.6–2.5 nmol/L); toxic, greater than 3 µg/L
(3.8 nmol/L). Considerable overlap exists between therapeutic and toxic ranges.[31]
Signs or symptoms of digitalis toxicity may be evident below 3 µg/L, especially if
other risk factors are present.[31] Obtain blood samples for digoxin levels at least 4

hr after an IV dose and 6–8 hr after an oral dose to allow central and tissue compartment equilibration. Digoxin concentrations (digitalislike immunoreactive substance) have been detected in patients with renal failure, neonates, pregnant women, and those with severe liver disease not receiving digitalis glycosides.[32]

Fate. Oral absorption is 70 ± 13% from tablets; 85% from elixir; 95% from capsules.[9,33] Enterohepatic recycling of digoxin may be as high as 30%.[34] Protein binding to albumin is 25 ± 5%; V_d is 7–8 L/kg; Cl is 0.16 ± 0.036 L/hr/kg; both are dependent on renal function.[33] The drug is excreted 60 ± 11% unchanged in the urine in patients with normal renal function.[33] Active metabolites include digitoxigenin, bisdigitoxoside, digoxigenin monodigitoxoside, and dihydrodigoxin.[33]

$t_{1/2}$. α phase 0.5–1 hr; ß phase 39 ± 13 hr;[9,33] ß phase 3.5–4.5 days in anephric patients.[27]

Adverse Reactions. Arrhythmias, listed by decreasing prevalence, are premature ventricular beats, second- and third-degree heart block, AV junctional tachycardia, atrial tachycardia with block, ventricular tachycardia, and SA nodal block.[35] Visual disturbances are serum level related and occur in up to 25% of patients with digoxin intoxication. They include blurred vision, yellow or green tinting, flickering lights or halos, or red-green color blindness. GI symptoms occur frequently and include abdominal discomfort, anorexia, nausea, and vomiting. CNS side effects occur frequently, yet are nonspecific, such as weakness, lethargy, disorientation, agitation, and nervousness. Hallucinations and psychosis have been reported. Rare reactions include gynecomastia, hypersensitivity, and thrombocytopenia.

Contraindications. Hypertrophic obstructive cardiomyopathy; suspected digitalis intoxication; second- or third-degree heart block in the absence of mechanical pacing; atrial fibrillation with accessory AV pathway; ventricular fibrillation.

Precautions. Electrolyte abnormalities predisposing to digitalis toxicity include hypokalemia, hypomagnesemia, and hypercalcemia. Hypothyroidism may reduce digoxin requirements because of lower V_d and clearance.[33] Direct current cardioversion carries little risk in the absence of digitalis toxicity.[36] Use with caution in patients with pulmonary disease, because hypoxia may sensitize the myocardium to arrhythmias and increase the risk of toxicity.[37] Serious bradyarrhythmias may occur with sick sinus syndrome, but controversy exists concerning the clinical importance of its effects on the SA node. Digitalis glycosides may increase infarct size in the nonfailing heart.

Drug Interactions. ß-Blockers may worsen CHF or digitalis-induced bradycardia. Potassium loss caused by amphotericin B or diuretics may contribute to digoxin toxicity. Spironolactone may decrease digoxin renal elimination. Amiodarone, bepridil, diltiazem, nitrendipine, quinidine, and verapamil increase digoxin levels. Oral antacids, kaolin-pectin, oral neomycin, and sulfasalazine may impair digoxin absorption. Penicillamine may decrease serum digoxin levels.

Parameters to Monitor. Digitalis glycoside serum levels need only be obtained when compliance, effectiveness, or systemic availability is questioned or toxicity is suspected (*see* Serum Levels).[38,39] Monitor heart rate, ECG for digitalis-induced arrhythmias, subjective complaints of toxicity, renal function; serum electrolytes (especially potassium) should be monitored frequently initially, then q 1–2 months when stabilized.

Notes. Treatment of severe or life-threatening digitalis (digoxin or **digitoxin**) toxicity should include IV digoxin **immune Fab** (Digibind). About 40 mg (one vial) of digoxin-specific Fab fragments bind 0.6 mg of the glycoside. Exact dosage can be calculated based upon estimated total body stores.

DISOPYRAMIDE PHOSPHATE   Norpace, Various

Pharmacology. Disopyramide has qualitatively the same electrophysiologic actions as procainamide and quinidine and is effective for both ventricular and (unlabeled) supraventricular tachycardia. It causes an increase in systemic vascular resistance through vasoconstriction; additionally, it may exert a profound negative inotropic effect[40] and has marked anticholinergic properties systemically and on the heart. Disopyramide's isomers have stereospecific pharmacologic actions.[41]

Administration and Adult Dosage. **PO loading dosage** 300–400 mg. **PO maintenance dosage** 400–800 mg/day, to a maximum of 1.6 g/day. Give daily dosage in 4 equally divided doses q 6 hr with non-SR cap, or in 2 equally divided doses q 12 hr with SR cap. Initiate disopyramide during hospitalization.

Special Populations. *Pediatric Dosage.* **PO** (<1 yr) 10–30 mg/kg/day, (1–4 yr) 10–20 mg/kg/day, (4–12 yr) 10–15 mg/kg/day, (12–18 yr) 6–15 mg/kg/day. Daily dosage is divided into 4 equal doses q 6 hr (*see* Notes).

Geriatric Dosage. Decreased dosage is probably necessary because elderly may not tolerate anticholinergic side effects.

Other Conditions. In patients who weigh less than 50 kg, or with hepatic disease or moderate renal insufficiency (Cl_{cr} over 40 mL/min), load with 150–200 mg, then give 400 mg/day in 2 or 4 divided doses, depending on the dosage form used. Initial daily dosage in patients with hepatic disease is about 4.4 mg/kg/day.[42,43] In patients with severe renal insufficiency, give maintenance dosages as follows (non-SR cap):

CREATININE CLEARANCE	DAILY MAINTENANCE DOSAGE
30–40 mL/min	300 mg
15–30 mL/min	200 mg
<15 mL/min	100 mg

Dosage Forms. **Cap** 100, 150 mg; **SR Cap** 100, 150 mg. (*See* Notes.)

Patient Instructions. Report any symptoms such as difficulty in urination, constipation, blurred vision, or dry mouth. Report shortness of breath, weight gain, or edema also. Do not crush or chew SR capsules. SR capsule core may appear in the stool, but this does not mean there was a lack of absorption.

Pharmacokinetics. *Onset and Duration.* PO onset is within 1 hr. Duration varies with individual differences in drug disposition, but is usually 6–12 hr.

Serum Levels. Usual range is 2–5 mg/L, (6–15 µmol/L),[43,44] with toxicity more likely over 4 mg/L. Therapeutic range of unbound drug is 0.5–2 mg/L (1.5–6 µmol/L).[42] Monitoring unbound concentrations eliminates variability caused by concentration-dependent disposition.[43,45]

Fate. Oral absorption is rapid; systemic availability is 83 ± 11%.[43,44] Unbound drug in serum varies from 19–46% over a serum concentration range of 2–8 mg/L and is also age dependent.[46] V_d (unbound) is 1.4–1.7 L/kg in normal subjects;[9,43] Cl (unbound) is about 0.25 L/hr/kg;[43] Cl is stereospecific.[47] The major metabolite is a mono-N-dealkylated form that has weak antiarrhythmic but potent anticholinergic activity; 55 ± 6% is excreted unchanged in the urine.[9]

$t_{1/2}$. α phase 2–4 min (IV);[47] ß phase is concentration dependent, usually 6 ± 1 hr;[9] 11–17 hr in renal impairment, depending on severity.[46]

Adverse Reactions. Nausea or anorexia occur frequently. Dry mouth, urinary retention, blurred vision, and constipation are dose-related anticholinergic effects that may occur in up to 70% of patients, and result in drug discontinuation in about 20%.[48] Through its vagolytic action, disopyramide may cause sinus tachycardia. Severe bradycardia, AV nodal block, or asystole may also occur, especially in patients with SA or AV nodal disease. Exacerbation of CHF is most prevalent (20–40%) in patients with left ventricular systolic dysfunction.[40] Torsades de pointes, similar to quinidine syncope, has been reported.[49] Rarely, rash, hepatic cholestasis, psychosis, or peripheral neuropathy occur. Hypoglycemia has also been reported.

Contraindications. History of disopyramide-induced heart block or serious ventricular arrhythmias; second- or third-degree heart block in the absence of a ventricular pacemaker; long-QT syndrome; cardiogenic shock or severe CHF.

Precautions. In atrial fibrillation or flutter, give digitalis or drugs that slow AV nodal conduction prior to disopyramide. Use very cautiously, if at all, in patients with CHF, because of negative inotropic and vasoconstrictive actions.[40] The drug may worsen sick sinus syndrome or aggravate underlying ventricular arrhythmias. If possible, use other antiarrhythmics in patients with prostatic hypertrophy or preexisting urinary retention. Disopyramide may exacerbate glaucoma or myasthenia gravis.

Drug Interactions. Erythromycin inhibits disopyramide metabolism. Phenytoin may decrease disopyramide serum levels and increase its anticholinergic effects. Rifampin, barbiturates, and other enzyme inducers may decrease disopyramide serum levels. Concurrent use of disopyramide and quinidine may increase disopyramide serum levels or decrease quinidine serum levels.

Parameters to Monitor. Because of concentration-dependent protein binding, total drug levels unreliably reflect active drug concentration, and monitoring unbound drug concentrations is preferable. Monitor serum levels and symptoms or signs of toxicity closely in patients with altered states of drug disposition such as renal dysfunction. When initiating therapy, observe ECG daily for 3–4 days for QT, QRS, or PR prolongation. Obtain frequent vital signs initially for evidence of adverse hemodynamic effects (eg, CHF), and less frequently when a maintenance dosage is attained. Question the patient about anticholinergic manifestations, such as urinary and visual abnormalities.

Notes. A 1–10 mg/mL suspension, prepared from capsules, in cherry syrup is stable for 1 month under refrigeration in an amber bottle.

FLECAINIDE ACETATE   Tambocor

Pharmacology. Flecainide is a type Ic antiarrhythmic that predominantly slows conduction velocity with minimal effect on refractoriness (*see* Electrophysiologic Actions of Antiarrhythmics Comparison Chart). Compared to type Ia or Ib antiarrhythmics, it binds to and dissociates from the sodium channel very slowly. It can decrease cardiac output by a negative inotropic action.

Administration and Adult Dosage. PO 50 mg q 12 hr initially, then increase in 50-mg increments q 12 hr q 4–7 days until desired response. Usual maintenance dosage is 100 mg PO q 12 hr, to a maximum of 300 mg/day. Initiate flecainide during hospitalization.

Special Populations. *Pediatric Dosage.* Safety and efficacy not established. **PO** 100–200 mg/m^2/day (average 140 mg/m^2/day) in 2 divided doses has been used.[50]

Geriatric Dosage. Same as adult dosage.

Other Conditions. Lower maintenance dosage requirements are expected in patients with CHF, liver disease, or renal insufficiency. Start these patients with 50–100 mg q 12–24 hr and cautiously increase dosage as required with the aid of serum levels.[43,51]

Dosage Forms. **Tab** 50, 100, 150 mg.

Patient Instructions. Report any symptoms of dizziness, extra or rapid heart beats, or visual disturbances. Report symptoms of worsening shortness of breath or exercise intolerance.

Pharmacokinetics. *Onset and Duration.* Onset 1–6 hr (average 3); duration 12–30 hr.[51]

Serum Levels. (Therapeutic trough) 0.2–1 mg/L (0.5–2.5 μmol/L).[51,52]

Fate. Oral bioavailability is 70 ± 11%.[9,52] From 37–55% is plasma protein bound, but the percentage may be higher (61%) post-MI because of increases in α_1-acid glycoprotein.[51] V_d is 8–10 L/kg;[51] Cl is reported as 0.34 ± 0.1 L/hr/kg,[9] and 0.61 ± 0.23 L/hr/kg;[43,51] Cl decreases in CHF, renal failure, and liver disease. Flecainide is about 60% stereoselectively metabolized by the liver through the CYP2D6 isozyme[53] and about 30% excreted unchanged in urine.

$t_{1/2}$. α phase 3–8 min; ß phase 14±5 hr. ß phase is 20±4 hr with ventricular ectopy; 37.8 ± 39.7 hr in patients with severe renal dysfunction.[54]

Adverse Reactions. Neurologic side effects, which include dizziness and visual abnormalities, occur frequently. Exacerbation of CHF in patients with underlying left ventricular dysfunction occurs frequently. Nausea, dyspnea, and headache may also occur frequently. Flecainide has proarrhythmic effects, which may result in new sustained ventricular tachycardia or aggravation of underlying ventricular arrhythmias. These reactions occur more frequently in patients with left ventricular dysfunction, coronary disease, or ventricular arrhythmias.[16,55] Risk may be sustained over time and not limited to the several days after initiation of therapy. Flecainide-induced ventricular tachycardia may be unresponsive to cardioversion or pacing, but may respond to lidocaine therapy or sodium bicarbonate. Aggravation of underlying conduction disturbances may also occur.

Contraindications. Second- or third-degree AV block or bifasicular block in the absence of a ventricular pacemaker; severe CHF; history of type Ic–induced arrhythmia.

Precautions. Use with caution in patients with sick sinus syndrome and in combination with other negative inotropic drugs, such as calcium blockers or β-blockers, or following recent therapy with a type Ia antiarrhythmic. Flecainide may increase pacemaker capture threshold.[56] (*See* Notes.)

Drug Interactions. Amiodarone, flecainide, and cimetidine may increase flecainide serum concentrations; flecainide slightly elevates serum digoxin levels.

Parameters to Monitor. Frequent or continuous (preferred) ECG when therapy initiated, then periodically on an ambulatory basis. Obtain a baseline evaluation of left ventricular function prior to starting flecainide. Obtain periodic trough serum levels (particularly in those with renal or liver disease and CHF) once an individual's effective level is determined. Observe closely for neurologic toxicities and CHF symptoms when initiating therapy.

Notes. Because the results of CAST show an increase in mortality in patients with asymptomatic ventricular arrhythmias post-MI given flecainide,[16] it should be reserved for individuals with life-threatening ventricular arrhythmias such as sustained ventricular tachycardia refractory to other drugs.

IBUTILIDE FUMARATE   Corvert

Ibutilide is a class III antiarrhythmic that selectively prolongs atrial and ventricular repolarization by increasing sodium influx (the window current). It may also block potassium channels. It is indicated for the acute termination of atrial fibrillation or atrial flutter of recent onset. In these arrhythmias, sinus rhythm is restored in about 50% of patients. Ibutilide has a large V_d of 11 ± 4 L/kg and is approximately 40% bound to plasma proteins. It is entirely metabolized by the liver. Although many metabolites have been identified, only a hydroxylated form has shown activity. Less than 10% is excreted unchanged in urine. Elimination half-life is about 6 hr (range 2–12). The major side effect is drug-induced proarrhythmia; torsades de pointes (sustained or nonsustained) occurs in 4–5% of patients. Risk factors are hypokalemia and underlying left ventricular dysfunction. Monitor QT interval closely, and do not give ibutilide with other drugs known to delay repolarization or prolong QT interval (eg, terfenadine, astemizole). Heart block and heart failure have occurred rarely. Patients with atrial fibrillation of more than 2 days' duration must be anticoagulated with warfarin for 3 weeks prior to the administration of ibutilide. Normalize serum magnesium and potassium concentrations prior to the administration of ibutilide. The IV dose in patients weighing ≥60 kg is 1 mg over 10 min; in those weighing <60 kg, the dose is 0.01 mg/kg. If the tachycardia is not terminated 10 min after the end of the initial infusion, the dose may be repeated.[57,58] Available as 0.1 mg/mL injection.

LIDOCAINE HYDROCHLORIDE   Xylocaine, Various

Pharmacology. Lidocaine's electrophysiologic actions differ in healthy and diseased cardiac tissues (*see* Electrophysiologic Actions of Antiarrhythmics

Comparison Chart). Most of its antiarrhythmic activity is caused by frequency-dependent blockade of the fast sodium channel in Purkinje fibers. In comparison to other antiarrhythmics, lidocaine binds to and dissociates from the sodium channel very quickly. It is used in the acute treatment of ventricular arrhythmias associated with MI or digitalis intoxication. Effectiveness in the treatment of supraventricular arrhythmia is limited.

Administration and Adult Dosage. **IV loading dose for ventricular tachycardia or fibrillation** 100 mg (1–1.5 mg/kg) over 1 min; if ineffective, may repeat with 50–100 mg q 5–10 min, to a maximum of 300 mg.[59] **IV maintenance** 2–4 mg/min infusion.[59] **IV for neuropathic pain** 5 mg/kg/hr for 60–90 min has been used.[60] (*See* Notes.)

Special Populations. *Pediatric Dosage.* **IV (or intratracheal) loading dose** 1 mg/kg, may repeat q 10–15 min, to a maximum of 5 mg/kg. **IV maintenance dosage** 20–50 μg/kg/min infusion.

Geriatric Dosage. Same as adult dosage. Elderly may be at increased risk of toxicity because of decreased clearance.

Other Conditions. In CHF, use one-half of IV loading dose. In liver disease or CHF, initial maintenance infusion is 1 mg/min, to a maximum of 2–3 mg/min.[59] In MI without CHF, maintenance infusion rate may need to be decreased by 30–50% in 24 hr;[59] however, empiric dosage alterations in MI are not recommended because of increases in α_1-acid glycoprotein and lidocaine binding.[61]

Dosage Forms. Inj 10, 20, 40, 100, 200 mg/mL. Also available premixed in D5W in concentrations of 2, 4, 8 mg/mL.

Patient Instructions. Report side effects such as drowsiness, perioral numbness or tingling, dizziness, and nausea during maintenance infusion.

Pharmacokinetics. *Onset and Duration.* IV onset is immediate; duration after initial IV bolus is 10–20 min. IM onset is 10 min; duration is 3 hr.[62]

Serum Levels. Therapeutic (total) 1.5–6 mg/L (7–28 μmol/L);[44] (unbound) 0.5–1.5 mg/L (2–7 μmol/L).[61] Toxic reactions are more likely at total concentrations >5 mg/L (22 μmol/L).[59] See Adverse Reactions.

Fate. The drug is well absorbed orally; however, a large hepatic first-pass effect limits systemic availability to 35 ± 11%.[63] IM absorption half-life is 12–28 min.[59] The drug is 70 ± 5% plasma protein bound;[59] V_d is 1.3 ± 0.4 L/kg in normals, 0.9 ± 0.2 L/kg in CHF.[64] Cl is 0.55 ± 0.14 L/hr/kg, decreased in CHF, liver disease, and during long-term infusion.[59,64,65] Lidocaine is primarily metabolized in the liver, with 2 ± 1% excreted unchanged in the urine.[64] The major metabolites, monoethylglycinexylidide (MEGX) and glycinexylidide (GX), both have neurotoxic[66] and antiarrhythmic[67] actions. Accumulation of these metabolites in renal impairment or during prolonged infusions may contribute to lidocaine toxicity.

$t_{\frac{1}{2}}$. α phase about 8 min;[62,64] β-phase 98 ± 24 min.[59,64] The β phase in CHF or liver disease may be prolonged to 4.5 ± 2.4 hr and 6.6 ± 1.1 hr, respectively.[59,64] Elimination half-life of total lidocaine increases to an average of 3.2 ± 0.5 hr, 24 hr after MI without CHF; and up to 10.2 ± 2 hr after MI with CHF.[68] In MI, the rise in total lidocaine half-life is greater than that of unbound lidocaine.[69]

Adverse Reactions. Serum level–related neurologic side effects including dizziness, nausea, drowsiness, speech disturbances, perioral numbness, muscle twitching, confusion, vertigo, and tinnitus are frequent at total serum levels over 5 mg/L. Serious toxicities including psychosis, seizures, and respiratory depression occur at serum levels over 9 mg/L.[59] Sinus arrest or severe bradycardia is associated with sinus node disease, toxic drug levels, or concomitant therapy with other antiarrhythmics. Complete AV block may occur, especially in patients with preexisting bifasicular bundle branch block, AV nodal block, or inferior wall MI.[70,71]

Contraindications. History of hypersensitivity to any amide-type local anesthetic (rare); second- or third-degree heart block unless the site of block can be localized to the AV node itself[70] or ventricular pacemaker is functional; severe sinus node dysfunction; Stokes-Adams syndrome; atrial fibrillation in association with Wolff-Parkinson-White syndrome.

Precautions. Lidocaine administered to prevent ventricular fibrillation in acute myocardial infarction is no longer recommended.[71] Toxicity during bronchoscopy because of tracheal lidocaine absorption has been reported.

Drug Interactions. Propranolol decreases lidocaine clearance, so close monitoring is necessary with concomitant administration of these drugs. Cimetidine may decrease lidocaine clearance, but empiric dosage reduction with concomitant cimetidine is not recommended.[72] Phenytoin may decrease lidocaine serum levels and also increase myocardial depression.

Parameters to Monitor. Monitor serum levels and signs or symptoms of toxicity closely in patients with altered drug disposition such as CHF, hepatic disease, acute MI, or prolonged IV infusion (>24 hr). Monitoring unbound levels is preferable post-MI. Minor subjective and objective toxicities are extremely important because they are often subtle and may forecast more serious toxicities (eg, psychosis or seizures). Continuously observe ECG for therapeutic and/or toxic actions. Monitor vital signs such as blood pressure, heart rate, and respiration frequently.

Notes. IV lidocaine has been used to treat pain of peripheral origin such as neuropathies and burns.[60,73] Oral mexiletine has been used for ongoing treatment if lidocaine is successful (*see* Mexiletine).

MEXILETINE HYDROCHLORIDE   Mexitil, Various

Pharmacology. Mexiletine has electrophysiologic actions similar to lidocaine and tocainide. Depression of conduction is accentuated in ischemic/hypoxic tissue. It also has a slight negative inotropic action. It is used in the treatment of ventricular arrhythmias; effectiveness in supraventricular tachycardias is limited.

Administration and Adult Dosage. PO loading dose 400 mg once, followed by maintenance dosage in 8 hr; **PO maintenance dosage** 200–300 mg q 8 hr, to a maximum of 400 mg q 8 hr. **PO for neuropathic pain** 450 mg/day;[74] dosages as high as 10 mg/kg/day have been used to treat the thalmic pain syndrome.[75] (*See* Notes.) Initiate mexiletine during hospitalization.

Special Populations. *Pediatric Dosage.* Safety and efficacy not established.

Geriatric Dosage. Same as adult dosage.

Other Conditions. Reduce maintenance dosage by 30–50% in patients with hepatic disease or severe CHF.[43,76] Dosage may also need to be decreased with $Cl_{cr} < 10$ mL/min.[77]

Dosage Forms. Cap 150, 200, 250 mg.

Patient Instructions. Report numbness, drowsiness, dizziness, or tingling. Nausea or loss of appetite may occur and may be reduced by taking the drug with food. Report any abnormal bruising.

Pharmacokinetics. *Onset and Duration.* PO onset 1–4 hr (average 2); duration 8–16 hr.

Serum Levels. 0.5–2 mg/L (3–11 μmol/L), although not well correlated with therapeutic or toxic effects.[78]

Fate. Oral bioavailability is 87 ± 13%, and, unlike lidocaine, mexiletine undergoes less than 10% first-pass hepatic elimination.[78,79] Absorption can be incomplete in MI patients receiving narcotic analgesics.[78,79] The drug is 63 ± 3% plasma protein bound;[9] V_d is large and variably reported as 6.6 ± 0.9 L/kg and 10.8 ± 7.2 L/kg.[78,79] Cl is variable, ranging from 0.4–0.6 L/hr/kg,[43] decreasing in both CHF and liver disease.[79] Mexiletine is predominantly metabolized in the liver, where it undergoes polymorphic metabolism, primarily via the CYP2D6 isozyme;[80] 10–20% is excreted unchanged in urine, depending on urinary pH.[78,79]

$t_{1/2}$. α phase 3–12 min; β phase 9.2 ± 2.1 hr,[81] 18.5 hr in poor metabolizers.[80] β phase 15.7 ± 4.9 hr in severe renal dysfunction,[77] 15 ± 0.6 hr in CHF with or without MI,[82,83] and may be prolonged in cirrhosis.

Adverse Reactions. Neurologic toxicities are frequent and include tremor, ataxia, drowsiness, confusion, paresthesias, and occasionally psychosis or seizures. Minor CNS side effects may occur in up to 40% of patients.[84] Nausea, vomiting, and anorexia are frequent. Mexiletine may aggravate underlying ventricular arrhythmias or conduction disturbances. Thrombocytopenia has been reported rarely.[84] Mexiletine is an ether analogue of lidocaine, so cross-sensitivity between mexiletine and tocainide or lidocaine is not expected.[85]

Contraindications. Second- or third-degree AV block in the absence of a ventricular pacemaker; cardiogenic shock.

Precautions. Worsening of sick sinus syndrome may occur. Mexiletine can increase pacemaker capture threshold and alter the effectiveness of internal defibrillators.[56]

Drug Interactions. Mexiletine increases theophylline concentrations by 30–50% by decreasing theophylline metabolism.[86] Phenytoin and rifampin may increase mexiletine metabolism. Quinidine and theophylline occasionally increase serum mexiletine levels.

Parameters to Monitor. ECG for 3–5 days when therapy is initiated, then q 3–6 months on an ambulatory basis. Obtain periodic serum levels once an individual's effective level is determined. Observe closely for neurologic toxicities when initiating therapy.

Notes. The efficacy of mexiletine for ventricular tachycardia can be increased by the addition of a type Ia antiarrhythmic, such as quinidine.[87] Mexiletine has been used to treat neuropathic pain such as diabetic neuropathy and for thalmic pain syndrome.[74,75]

MORICIZINE HYDROCHLORIDE   Ethmozine

Pharmacology. Moricizine is a phenothiazine-like type I (probably Ic)[88] antiarrhythmic that (in normal tissue) slows conduction velocity by blocking sodium channels in a frequency-dependent manner. Its effects appear to be accentuated by ischemia.

Administration Adult Dosage. PO 200 q 8 hr initially, then increase daily dosage q 3 days by 150 mg until desired effect or toxicity occurs, to a usual maintenance dosage of 200–300 mg q 8 hr. Initiate moricizine during hospitalization.

Special Populations. *Pediatric Dosage.* Safety and efficacy not established. **PO** 200–600 mg/m^2/day has been used.[89]

Geriatric Dosage. Same as adult dosage.

Other Conditions. Not well studied; patients with hepatic disease may require a lower dosage.

Dosage Forms. Tab 200, 250, 300 mg.

Patient Instructions. Report any dizziness, rapid heartbeat, or gastrointestinal upset.

Pharmacokinetics. *Onset and Duration.* Onset is variable, from 2–20 hr after multiple doses; duration is 12–36 hr after long-term use.[90]

Serum Levels. Correlation between serum levels and therapeutic effect is not well established, but 0.2–3.6 mg/L (0.5–8.4 μmol/L) has been suggested.[91]

Fate. Moricizine is well absorbed after oral administration, but the large hepatic first-pass metabolism limits bioavailability to 34–38%. About 81–90% is bound to plasma proteins.[92] V_d is 5.9 ± 3.2 and 11.6 ± 6.7 L/kg after 1 and 13 days of therapy, respectively.[93] Cl is 3.8 ± 1.8 to 4.7 ± 2.3 L/hr/kg, depending on length of therapy.[94] Moricizine undergoes extensive hepatic metabolism and appears to induce its own metabolism. Over 40 metabolites appear in small quantities systemically;[94] At least two, including moricizine sulfoxide, are active and probably account for some of the drug's antiarrhythmic activity and for its long duration of action. Less than 1% appears in the urine unchanged.[93,94]

$t_{1/2}$. α phase 4–20 min; β phase 1.6 ± 0.2 hr.[93,94]

Adverse Reactions. Frequent noncardiac side effects include nausea, anorexia, and dizziness. Dizziness may be lessened by administering more frequent, smaller doses. Moricizine has proarrhythmic actions, which result in new or worsened ventricular tachycardia in 2–5% of patients. Exacerbation of CHF occurs occasionally. Worsening of underlying conduction disturbances such as AV block, ventricular conduction defects, or sick sinus syndrome may occur. Drug fever has been reported.[95]

Contraindications. Second- or third-degree AV block or bifasicular block in the absence of a ventricular pacemaker; cardiogenic shock; hypersensitivity to phenothiazines.

Precautions. Use with caution in patients with sick sinus syndrome. Because of the final results of CAST II,[96] moricizine is indicated only for life-threatening ventricular arrhythmias such as sustained ventricular tachycardia, where there is a clear benefit to therapy.

Drug Interactions. Cimetidine may increase moricizine serum levels. Moricizine decreases theophylline levels.

Parameters to Monitor. Daily ECG for the first 2–4 days when therapy is initiated, then q 3–6 months on an ambulatory basis, observing for PR and QRS lengthening. Observe for GI side effects and dizziness.

Notes. Limited data exist on the use of moricizine in supraventricular tachycardias.

PROCAINAMIDE HYDROCHLORIDE   Procanbid, Procan SR, Pronestyl, Various

Pharmacology. Procainamide is a class Ia antiarrhythmic that alters conduction in normal and ischemic tissues by sodium-channel blockade in a fashion similar to quinidine. It may decrease systemic blood pressure by causing peripheral ganglionic blockade;[97] it also has weak anticholinergic action and a slight negative inotropic action. The active metabolite N-acetylprocainamide (NAPA) has primarily type III antiarrhythmic activity, predominantly delaying repolarization by blocking potassium conductance.

Administration and Adult Dosage. **PO loading dose** (Cap, Tab) 1 g over 2 hr in 2 divided doses. **PO maintenance dosage** (Cap, Tab) 1–6 g/day in 4–6 divided doses, to a maximum of 9 g/day;[98] (SR Tab) may be given q 6–8 hr (Procan-SR, Pronestyl-SR) or q 12 hr (Procanbid), to a maximum of 50 mg/kg/day. **IV loading dose** 1–1.5 g at 20–50 mg/min;[97] alternatively, 15–20 mg/kg. **IV maintenance dosage** 1.5–5 mg/min (20–80 µg/kg/min) infusion.[97] **Intermittent IV or IM** 1–6 g/day in 4–6 divided doses, to a maximum of 9 g/day. Initiate procainamide during hospitalization.

Special Populations. *Pediatric Dosage.* Safety and efficacy not established. **PO** 15–50 mg/kg/day in 4–8 divided doses, to a maximum of 4 g/day; **IV loading dose** 3–6 mg/kg over 5 min (up to 100 mg/dose), may repeat q 5–10 min, to a maximum of 15 mg/kg. **IV maintenance dosage** 20–80 µg/kg/min infusion, to a maximum of 2 g/day. **IM maintenance dosage** 20–30 mg/kg/day in 4–6 divided doses, to a maximum of 4 g/day.[99]

Geriatric Dosage. Generally the same as adult dosage, although lower dosages may be required because of age-related decrease in renal function.

Other Conditions. Reduce maintenance dosage in liver disease. In renal insufficiency, procainamide and its active metabolite accumulate, necessitating a lower maintenance dosage.[43] Recent data imply no need for decreasing loading and maintenance dosages in CHF and MI.[100]

Dosage Forms. **Cap, Tab** 250, 375, 500 mg; **SR Tab** (6-hr; Procan-SR, Pronestyl-SR, various) 250, 500, 750, 1000 mg; (12-hr; Procanbid) 500, 1000 mg; **Inj** 100, 500 mg/mL.

Patient Instructions. Report any symptoms such as nausea, vomiting, fever, sore throat, joint pain, rash, chest or abdominal pain, and shortness of breath. Do not chew, split, or crush SR tablets. The SR tablet shell may appear in the stool, but this does not mean there was a lack of absorption.

Pharmacokinetics. *Onset and Duration.* IV onset is immediate; PO and IM onset within 1 hr; SR Tab preparations are somewhat slower. Duration is usually 3–6 hr.

Serum Levels. Therapeutic range is 4–10 mg/L (17–43 µmol/L);[44] toxicity is more likely at serum levels over 12 mg/L (51 µmol/L).[101] In some arrhythmias (eg, recurrent ventricular tachycardia), levels of 20 mg/L (85 µmol/L) or greater may be required for prevention of arrhythmias, with average effective levels of 13 mg/L.[98] Effective serum levels of NAPA are 15–25 mg/L (53–88 µmol/L), with overlap between the toxic and therapeutic ranges.[102]

Fate. Oral bioavailability is $83 \pm 16\%$;[9] about $16 \pm 5\%$ is bound to plasma proteins; V_d is 1.9 ± 0.3 L/kg.[9] The drug is $67 \pm 8\%$ excreted in the urine as unchanged drug; the remainder is metabolized, mostly to active NAPA by the liver, with smaller amounts excreted as para-aminobenzoic acid. Cl is highly variable depending upon acetylator status and renal function. The total quantity of NAPA produced depends on liver function and acetylator phenotype.[9,103]

$t_{1/2}$. (Procainamide) α phase about 6 min; β phase in normals 3 ± 0.6 hr; 5.3–20.7 hr in renal dysfunction, with anephric patients averaging 12.5 ± 1.4 hr. (NAPA) 7 ± 1 hr, 41.5 ± 7.8 hr in renal failure.[9,102,103]

Adverse Reactions. About 50–80% of patients develop a positive antinuclear antibody (ANA), with 30–50% developing SLE symptoms; genetically slow acetylators more rapidly develop positive ANA and SLE symptoms.[104] Common SLE symptoms or signs are rash, arthralgias, fever, pericarditis, and pleuritis. Although drug cessation usually reverses these symptoms in about 2 weeks, some patients have prolonged manifestations and for others the SLE syndrome may be initially life-threatening.[104] Hypotension may occur frequently after rapid IV administration. Severe bradycardia, AV nodal block, or asystole have been reported. Procainamide can aggravate underlying ventricular arrhythmias and cause torsades de pointes.[105] GI symptoms occur frequently and include nausea and vomiting; drug fever and dermatologic reactions may occur occasionally.[105] Agranulocytosis is reported occasionally and is potentially fatal. Whether or not the SR product carries a higher risk of neutropenia than the fast-release preparation is controversial.[106] Hepatitis has been reported rarely.

Contraindications. SLE (including drug-induced); second- or third- degree heart block in the absence of a ventricular pacemaker; long-QT syndrome; severe sinus node dysfunction or torsades de pointes caused by other type Ia antiarrhythmics.

Precautions. In atrial fibrillation or flutter, procainamide may paradoxically increase ventricular rate; administer digoxin or other drugs that slow AV nodal conduction prior to procainamide. Procainamide may worsen symptoms of sick sinus syndrome; it may also exacerbate myasthenia gravis.

Drug Interactions. Amiodarone, trimethoprim, cimetidine, and, to a lesser extent, ranitidine may increase procainamide levels; alcohol may decrease levels.

Parameters to Monitor. Monitor serum levels and symptoms or signs of toxicity in patients with suspected altered drug disposition such as hepatic disease or renal dysfunction. Monitor ECG continuously (with IV) or daily initially (with PO) for QRS, QT, or PR prolongation; monitor oral therapy less frequently once maintenance dosage is established. Monitor blood pressure frequently when therapy is initiated (especially with IV), and less frequently once a maintenance dosage is established. Periodically monitor WBC counts and signs of infection for the development of drug-induced agranulocytosis. Observe closely for symptoms of drug-induced SLE.

PROPAFENONE HYDROCHLORIDE   Rhythmol

Pharmacology. Propafenone is a sodium-channel blocker that predominantly slows atrial and ventricular conduction velocity without appreciably prolonging repolarization. It is therefore classified as a type Ic antiarrhythmic, similar to flecainide. Propafenone is administered as a racemate; the enantiomers and the 5-hydroxy metabolite are all equipotent sodium channel blockers. Propafenone, particularly the (S)-enantiomer, and its active 5-hydroxy metabolite also have variable, nonselective β-blocking actions.[107]

Administration and Adult Dosage. PO 150 mg q 8 hr initially, increasing q 3–4 days to desired effect or toxicity. **PO maintenance** 150–200 mg q 8 hr, to a maximum of 1.2 g/day.[108] Initiate propafenone during hospitalization.

Special Populations. *Pediatric Dosage.* Safety and efficacy not established. **PO** 10–20 mg/kg/day in 2–3 divided doses has been used.[109]

Geriatric Dosage. Same as adult dosage. Lower initial dosages have been suggested.[110]

Other Conditions. Bioavailability and half-life are increased in patients with hepatic disease and dosage reduction of 50% has been suggested,[111] but this has been questioned.[108] Lower initial dosages have been suggested for patients with renal dysfunction.[108]

Dosage Forms. **Tab** 150, 225, 300 mg.

Patient Instructions. Report any symptoms of dizziness, rapid heartbeat, blurred vision, or shortness of breath.

Pharmacokinetics. *Onset and Duration.* Onset 2–4 hr; peak 2–6 hr; duration 4–22 hr.[108,110]

Serum Levels. No established therapeutic range. Levels of parent compound and metabolite are highly variable, depending on genetically determined variations in hepatic metabolism. Mean minimal effective concentration was 0.2 mg/L (6 μmol/L) in one study.[112] Side effects are more frequent when trough propafenone level exceeds 0.9 mg/L (26 μmol/L).[113]

Fate. Completely absorbed after oral administration, but large hepatic first-pass metabolism limits bioavailability to $12.1 \pm 11\%$. First-pass elimination appears saturable, so bioavailability is highly variable and increases with larger oral doses and long-term therapy.[108,110,113] About 85–95% is bound to plasma proteins, primarily α_1-acid glycoprotein.[108] V_d is 3.6 ± 2.6 L/kg.[114] The parent drug undergoes polymorphic hepatic metabolism via the CYP2D6 isozyme. Extensive metabolizers (EMs, about 90% of patients) form clinically important quantities of the active metabolite 5-hydroxypropafenone; poor metabolizers (PMs, about 10% of patients) form little of this compound.[110,113] Another active metabolite, N-desethylpropafenone, is not subject to genetic polymorphism.[108,113] Cl is 0.96 ± 1.08 L/hr/kg in EMs and 0.23 ± 0.042 L/hr/kg in PMs.[115] Cl is also stereospecific. $t_{1/2}$. α phase 5 min; β phase (EMs) 5.5 ± 2 hr; (PMs) 17 ± 8 hr.[113]

Adverse Reactions. Frequent noncardiac side effects include metallic or bitter taste in 15–20% of patients, and nausea and CNS toxicity such as dizziness and headache in 10–15% of patients.[114] Because of the ß-blocking activity of propafenone, worsening of asthma or obstructive lung disease may occur.[107,114] Propafenone has proarrhythmic actions (sometimes life-threatening), which may result in new or worsened ventricular tachycardia. This may occur in 5–15% of patients, particularly in those with poor left ventricular function caused by structural heart disease or with underlying ventricular tachycardia. Worsening of existing CHF or underlying conduction disturbances, such as AV block or sick sinus syndrome, may occur. Cholestatic jaundice occurs rarely.[116]

Contraindications. Second- or third-degree AV block or bifasicular block in the absence of a ventricular pacemaker; history of type Ic induced arrhythmia; bronchospastic disorders; uncontrolled CHF; cardiogenic shock; marked hypotension; sick sinus syndrome; bradycardia; electrolyte imbalance.

Precautions. Propafenone may increase pacemaker capture threshold and affect the efficacy of internal defibrillators.[56] Because of the results of CAST (although not studied in this trial), propafenone is indicated only for arrhythmias where there is a clear benefit to therapy.

Drug Interactions. Propafenone inhibits hepatic enzymes and reportedly increases the serum concentrations of digoxin, theophylline, warfarin, and β-blockers.[110]

Parameters to Monitor. Daily or continuous (preferred) ECG for 3–4 days initially, then q 3–6 months on an ambulatory basis. Observe closely for CNS symptoms such as dizziness.

Notes. Although not a labeled indication, propafenone can be effective for some supraventricular arrhythmias.

QUINIDINE SULFATE	Various
QUINIDINE GLUCONATE	Duraquin, Quinaglute, Quinora, Various

Pharmacology. Quinidine is a class Ia antiarrhythmic that slows conduction velocity, prolongs effective refractory period, and decreases automaticity of normal and diseased fibers (*see* Electrophysiologic Actions of Antiarrhythmics Comparison Chart). The cellular mechanism appears to be frequency-dependent blockade of the fast sodium channel. Quinidine also blocks potassium conductance, particularly at low concentrations. AV nodal conduction may be increased reflexly through vasodilation, attributed to peripheral α-adrenergic blockade or vagolytic action. Slight negative inotropic action may be clinically important in patients with severe CHF.

Other Conditions. Reduce frequency of administration in patients with renal insufficiency as follows: Cl_{cr} 30–60 mL/min, q 24 hr; Cl_{cr} 10–30 mL/min, q 36–48 hr.[125] Use with caution, if at all, in patients with Cl_{cr} <10 mL/min.

Dosage Forms. Tab 80, 160, 240 mg.

Patient Instructions. Report any symptoms of fainting, dizziness, shortness of breath, or fatigue.

Pharmacokinetics. ***Onset and Duration.*** PO onset 1–3 hr; duration 12–18 hr.

Serum Levels. 1–3 mg/L (3.7–11 μmol/L), although not well correlated with therapeutic effect. Concentrations required to achieve delay in repolarization may be greater than for β-blockade.[124]

Fate. Bioavailability is 90–100% with negligible first-pass metabolism.[125] AUC is decreased 20% by food.[125] The drug is not bound to plasma proteins. V_d is 1.2–2.4 L/kg; Cl is 0.13 ± 0.04 L/hr/kg;[125–127] 80–90% is excreted unchanged in urine.[125] The disposition of the d-isomer is similar to that of the racemate.[126,127]

$t_{1/2}$. α phase 3–5 min; β phase variously reported as 7.5 ± 0.8 to 17.5 ± 9.7 hr.[127,128] Half-life is highly dependent on renal function: 22.7 ± 6.4 hr for Cl_{cr} 30–80 mL/hr; 64 ± 27 hr for Cl_{cr} 10–30 mL/hr; and 98 ± 57 hr for Cl_{cr} <10 mL/min.[128]

Adverse Reactions. Fatigue, dyspnea, and bradycardia occur frequently, probably caused by the β-blocking actions of sotalol.[129] Exacerbation of CHF (1.7%) and asthma may also occur (*see* Propranolol). Sotalol induces arrhythmias, usually torsades de pointes, in 4.6% of patients.[129] Risk factors for torsades de pointes are hypokalemia, hypomagnesemia, concurrent diuretic usage, and high sotalol dosages.[130]

Contraindications. Asthma; symptomatic sinus tachycardia; second- and third-degree AV block in the absence of a ventricular pacemaker; long-QT syndrome; uncontrolled CHF.

Precautions. Use with caution in sinus node dysfunction. Because of its β-blocking actions, use sotalol with caution in patients with diabetes, depressed left ventricular function, obstructive pulmonary disease, or peripheral vascular disease. Do not abruptly discontinue the drug in patients with coronary artery disease. Use with caution with electrolyte disorders, other drugs that prolong QT interval, or preexisting QT prolongation. Escalate dosage only after perceived steady state (2–3 days).[131]

Drug Interactions. Because of its β-blocking actions, observe β-blocker interaction precautions (*see* Propranolol).

Parameters to Monitor. Baseline and daily ECG for first 2–5 days when therapy is initiated or dosage adjusted, then q 3–6 months on ambulatory basis. QT prolongation to over 550 msec is an indication to discontinue sotalol because of the risk of torsades de pointes.

Notes. After the results of CAST,[16] many clinicians use type III antiarrhythmics (eg, amiodarone, sotalol) as first-line therapy in both supraventricular and ventricular arrhythmias. Most antiarrhythmics currently under investigation are similar to sotalol in structure and electrophysiologic actions.[58]

TOCAINIDE
Tonocard

Pharmacology. Tocainide has electrophysiologic actions similar to lidocaine and mexiletine. Depression of conduction is accentuated in ischemic/hypoxic tissue. Antiarrhythmic actions are somewhat stereospecific. It also has a slight negative inotropic action. It is used in the treatment of ventricular arrhythmias, but it has limited effectiveness in supraventricular tachycardias. There may be a concordance of response (and nonresponse) between tocainide and lidocaine.[132]

Administration and Adult Dosage. PO 400 mg q 8 hr initially; usual maintenance dosage is 1.2–1.8 g/day, to a maximum of 2.4 g/day in 2–3 divided doses. **PO during lidocaine to tocainide conversion** 600 mg q 6 hr for 3 doses, then 600 mg q 12 hr; discontinue lidocaine infusion at the time of the second oral dose of tocainide.[133] Initiate tocainide during hospitalization.

Special Populations. *Pediatric Dosage.* Safety and efficacy not established.

Geriatric Dosage. Same as adult dosage.

Other Conditions. Reduce initial maintenance dosage by 50% in severe liver disease, by 25% in patients with Cl_{cr} of 10–30 mL/min, and by 50% in patients with Cl_{cr} <10 mL/min.[134] Dosages may have to be slightly reduced in CHF, but more data are needed.[135]

Dosage Forms. Tab 400, 600 mg.

Patient Instructions. Report any symptoms of numbness, drowsiness, dizziness, or tingling. Nausea or loss of appetite may occur and may be reduced by taking the drug with food. Report sore throat, mouth sores, fever, or abnormal bruising.

Pharmacokinetics. *Onset and Duration.* PO onset 1–2 hr (delayed by food); duration 12–24 hr.

Serum Levels. 3–10 mg/L (16–52 μmol/L), although not well correlated with therapeutic or toxic effects.[44,136]

Fate. Oral bioavailability is 89 ± 5% with negligible first-pass metabolism.[134-136] The drug is 10 ± 15% plasma protein bound.[9,137] V_d is 3 ± 0.2 L/kg, slightly lower in CHF;[134,135] Cl is 0.16 ± 0.03 L/hr/kg;[9] 38 ± 7% of the drug is excreted unchanged in urine, and 50–60% is hepatically eliminated.[134,136] Renal clearance is dependent on urine pH; hepatic metabolism is stereospecific, with the (S)-enantiomer eliminated more quickly.[138]

$t_{1/2}$. α phase 5–10 min;[137] β phase 13.5 ± 2.3 hr, 14–19 hr with ventricular arrhythmia or CHF,[136] 22 ± 3.1 hr in severe renal insufficiency.[139]

Adverse Reactions. Neurologic toxicities, which include dizziness, tremor, ataxia, drowsiness, confusion, and paresthesias, are frequent (30–50%); psychosis and seizures occur occasionally. The neurologic toxicities of lidocaine and tocainide may be additive.[140] Nausea, vomiting, and anorexia occur frequently. Tocainide may exacerbate underlying ventricular arrhythmias or conduction disturbances. Agranulocytosis and other forms of bone marrow depression have been reported in about 0.18% of patients.[136] Pulmonary fibrosis or interstitial pneumonitis occurs in 0.03–0.11% of patients.[133] Rash and fever occur occasionally, with cross-sensitivity between lidocaine and tocainide possible.[85]

Contraindications. Second- or third-degree AV block in the absence of a ventricular pacemaker.

Precautions. Worsening of sick sinus syndrome may occur. May worsen CHF.

Drug Interactions. Cimetidine may decrease tocainide serum levels; rifampin may decrease levels.

Parameters to Monitor. Monitor ECG daily for 2–4 days when therapy is initiated, then q 3–6 months on an ambulatory basis. Obtain periodic serum levels once an individual's effective level is determined. Observe closely for neurologic toxicities when initiating therapy. Monitor WBC counts frequently, particularly during the first 3 months of therapy.[136] Obtain baseline chest x-ray; repeat if pulmonary symptoms arise.

Notes. Because of reports of bone marrow toxicity, pulmonary fibrosis, and hypersensitivity reactions, the indications for tocainide are restricted to patients with life-threatening ventricular arrhythmias.

ELECTROPHYSIOLOGIC ACTIONS OF ANTIARRHYTHMICS COMPARISON CHART

CLASS AND DRUG[a,b]	CONDUCTION VELOCITY	REFRACTORY PERIOD	AUTOMATICITY	AV NODAL CONDUCTION
Ia (Intermediate Sodium-Channel Blockers)				
Disopyramide	↓↓	↑↑	↓↓	↓
Procainamide	↓↓	↑↑	↓↓	↑/↓
Quinidine	↓	↑↑	↓↓	↑/↓
Ib (Fast On-Off Sodium-Channel Blockers)				
Lidocaine				
Normal Tissue	0	→	→	0
Ischemic Tissue	↓↓	←	↓↓	0
Mexiletine	0	→	→	0
Phenytoin				
Normal Tissue	0	→	→	←
Ischemic Tissue	↓↓	←	↓↓	←
Tocainide	0	→	→	0

(continued)

ELECTROPHYSIOLOGIC ACTIONS OF ANTIARRHYTHMICS COMPARISON CHART (continued)

CLASS AND DRUG[a,b]	CONDUCTION VELOCITY	REFRACTORY PERIOD	AUTOMATICITY	AV NODAL CONDUCTION
Ic (Slow On-Off Sodium-Channel Blockers)				
Flecainide	↓↓	0	↓	0
Moricizine[c]	↓↓↓	↓/0	↓	0
Propafenone[e]	↓↓↓	0	↓	0
II (β-Blockers)				
Propranolol[d]	→ →	↓ (acute) ↑ (chronic)	→ →	↓↑ ↓↑
III (Potassium-Channel Blockers)				
Amiodarone[e-g]	0/↓	↑↑	0	→
Bretylium	0	↑↑	↑/0	↑/0
Ibutilide	0	↑↑	0	0
Sotalol[e,f]	0	↑	0	→

(continued)

ELECTROPHYSIOLOGIC ACTIONS OF ANTIARRHYTHMICS COMPARISON CHART (continued)

CLASS AND DRUG[a,b]	CONDUCTION VELOCITY	REFRACTORY PERIOD	AUTOMATICITY	AV NODAL CONDUCTION
IV (Calcium-Channel Blockers)				
Diltiazem	0	0	0	↓
Verapamil	0	0	0	↓↓

↑ = increase, ↓ = decrease, 0 = minimal or no effect, ↑/↓ = variable.

[a]Classification system from references 141 and 142.

[b]Type I antiarrhythmics are subdivided into Ia, Ib, and Ic based upon their actions on repolarization in normal ventricular tissue and their binding characteristics to the sodium channel: type Ia prolongs repolarization; type Ib shortens repolarization; type Ic, no change in repolarization.

[c]Classification of moricizine is controversial; it also has type Ia characteristics.

[d]When caused by sympathetic stimulation.

[e]Amiodarone, propafenone, and sotalol also have type II or β-adrenergic blocking activity.

[f]Most investigational antiarrhythmics are potassium-channel blockers, many of which are analogues of sotalol (*see* reference 58).

[g]Amiodarone also has type Ib sodium-channel blocking activity.

Antihypertensive Drugs

Class Instructions: Antihypertensives. This medication can control hypertension, but it will not cure the disease. Long-term treatment is necessary to control hypertension and prevent damage to several body systems. Do not start or stop taking medications or change the dosage without medical supervision, and avoid running out of medications. Some prescription and nonprescription medications may interact with medications for hypertension; make sure that your physician and pharmacist know the names of any other medications that you are taking.

α_1-ADRENERGIC ANTAGONISTS:

DOXAZOSIN MESYLATE	Cardura
PRAZOSIN HYDROCHLORIDE	Minipress, Various
TERAZOSIN HYDROCHLORIDE	Hytrin

Pharmacology. Doxazosin, prazosin, and terazosin are closely related quinazoline derivatives that selectively block postsynaptic α_1-adrenergic receptors. Total peripheral resistance is reduced through both arterial and venous dilation. Reflex tachycardia that occurs with other vasodilators is infrequent because of the absence of presynaptic, α_2-receptor blockade. The drugs also increase HDL cholesterol and may improve glucose tolerance and reduce left ventricular hypertrophy during long-term therapy. They increase urine flow in BPH by relaxing smooth muscle tone in the bladder neck and prostate.[143,144]

Administration and Adult Dosage. The initial dose, and the first dose of all increased dosage regimens, should be given hs, and the patient observed closely for syncope. **PO for hypertension** (Doxazosin) 1 mg/day initially, double the dose at 1- to 2-week intervals, to a maximum of 16 mg/day in a single dose, although dosages over 4 mg/day are more likely to cause postural side effects. (Prazosin) 1 mg bid or tid initially; increase dosage slowly, based on response, to the usual dosage of 6–15 mg/day; although the maximum effective dosage is usually 20 mg/day, dosages up to 40 mg/day may be effective in some patients who fail to respond to lower dosages. (Terazosin) 1 mg/day initially, increase to 2, 5, or 10 mg/day in 1–2 doses, to a maximum of 20 mg/day. **PO for benign prostatic hypertrophy** (Doxazosin) 1 mg/day initially, double the dose at 1- to 2-week intervals, to a maximum of 8 mg/day. (Terazosin) 1 mg/day initially, increase to 2, 5, and finally 10 mg/day in 1–2 divided doses.

Special Populations. *Pediatric Dosage.* **PO for hypertension** (Prazosin) 0.05–0.4 mg/kg/day in 2–3 divided doses. Do not exceed single doses of 7 mg and a total daily dosage of 15 mg.[145] (Doxazosin, Terazosin) Safety and efficacy not established.

Geriatric Dosage. Same as adult dosage, although the dosage of doxazosin should be increased at longer intervals because of its longer half-life in the elderly.[146]

Dosage Forms. (Doxazosin) **Tab** 1, 2, 4, 8 mg. (Prazosin) **Cap** 1, 2, 5 mg; **Cap** 1, 2, 5 mg with polythiazide 0.5 mg (Minizide). (Terazosin) **Cap** 1, 2, 5, 10 mg.

Patient Instructions. (*See* Antihypertensives Class Instructions.) Take the initial dose of this drug at bedtime. Dizziness or drowsiness may occur with this medication, especially after the first dose or when the dosage is being increased. Do not arise suddenly, stand for long periods, or exercise too vigorously, especially in hot weather. Alcohol may worsen all of these effects.

Pharmacokinetics. *Onset and Duration.* (Doxazosin) onset 1–2 hr, duration 24 hr for hypertension; full effect for BPH may not occur for 1–2 weeks. (Prazosin) onset 1.5 hr after 1.5 mg PO, duration about 10 hr, up to 4–6 weeks may be required for full antihypertensive effect. (Terazosin) onset 1 hr, duration 24 hr, but up to 6–8 weeks may be required for full antihypertensive effect. In BPH, a minimum of 4–6 weeks may be required to fully evaluate response to 10 mg/day dosage.

Serum Levels. No established correlation between serum levels and clinical effect.[9,144,147]

Fate. (Doxazosin) Oral bioavailability is 63 ± 14%; absorption is slowed, but bioavailability is not affected by food; 98–99% is plasma protein bound. V_d is 1.5 ± 0.3 L/kg; Cl is 0.1 ± 0.024 L/kg/hr in young adult patients. Extensively metabolized and excreted primarily in the feces, with only about 9% excreted in urine as unchanged drug and metabolites.[9,144,146] (Prazosin) Bioavailability is 68 ± 17%, 48 ± 16% in the elderly, and lower in patients with CHF; food may delay, but does not affect the extent of absorption. About 95% is plasma protein bound, decreased in cirrhosis and uremia. V_d is 0.63 ± 0.14 L/kg and Cl is 0.24 ± 0.04 L/hr/kg in young patients; V_d is 0.89 ± 0.26 L/kg and Cl is 0.21 ± 0.06 L/hr/kg in the elderly; lower in CHF and pregnancy. Prazosin is metabolized in the liver by demethylation and conjugation; metabolites have about 20% the activity of the drug. It is excreted renally as metabolites and 3.4% or less as unchanged drug.[9,146] (Terazosin) Pharmacokinetics do not appear to be affected by uremia, CHF, or aging. Oral bioavailability is about 90%. From 90–94% is plasma protein bound. V_d is 0.8 ± 0.18 L/kg; Cl is 0.066 ± 0.012 L/hr/kg. It is extensively metabolized, with 20% excreted unchanged in feces, 12% unchanged in urine, and the remainder excreted as metabolites.[9,146]

$t_{1/2}$. (Doxazosin) 10.5 ± 2.4 hr in young adults, 11.9 ± 4.7 hr in the elderly. (Prazosin) 2.1 ± 0.3 hr in young adult, 3.2 ± 0.6 hr in the elderly; also prolonged in CHF and pregnancy. (Terazosin) 13.5 ± 3.5 hr in young adults, 16.2 ± 2.2 hr in the elderly.[146]

Adverse Reactions. The most important adverse effect is first-dose syncope, which is more likely in patients being treated with other antihypertensive drugs, especially diuretics. During long-term treatment, the most frequent reactions are dizziness, headache, drowsiness, lack of energy or weakness, palpitations, or nausea, all of which occur in 5–10% of patients. Occasionally reported are rash, vomiting, diarrhea, edema, orthostatic hypotension, syncope, dyspnea, blurred vision, nasal congestion, or urinary frequency. Rarely allergic reactions, priapism, or impotence occur.[148]

Contraindications. Allergy to a quinazoline derivative.

Precautions. Syncope may occur after the first dose (doxazosin, 2–6 hr; prazosin, 30–90 min; terazosin, 2–3 hr), but may also occur during rapid upward dosage titration or when adding an additional antihypertensive drug. Hold doses of diuretics for one day before starting an α_1-blocker. Increase dosage gradually and reduce dosage when adding another antihypertensive, then retitrate dosage. Use doxazosin with caution in patients with hepatic impairment.

Drug Interactions. β-Blockers and verapamil may enhance postural effects of prazosin; NSAIDs may decrease the hypotensive effect of prazosin. The α_1-blockers may decrease the hypotensive effect of clonidine.

Parameters to Monitor. Monitor blood pressure regularly.

Notes. α_1-Antagonists may be particularly useful for hypertension in men with BPH, in those with hyperlipidemia, in diabetics, in physically active young patients, and in the elderly.[140,143] However, drugs in this class have not been shown to decrease long-term mortality of hypertension.[144] (*See* the α_1-Antagonists Comparison Chart.)

CAPTOPRIL
Capoten, Various

Captopril is an ACE inhibitor (*see* Enalapril). Its oral bioavailability is about 60%. About 30% is plasma protein bound, and its $V_{d\beta}$ is 2 ± 0.09 L/kg; Cl is 0.76 L/hr/kg in normals, 0.31 L/hr/kg in mild renal dysfunction, and 0.096 L/hr/kg in dialysis patients between dialyses. Approximately 50% of a dose is metabolized, primarily to captopril disulfide, which can be converted back to active captopril in vivo. Urinary excretion of unchanged captopril is 24–38% over 24 hr. Its half-life is estimated to be 1.7 ± 0.2 hr in healthy subjects, and is prolonged in renal dysfunction or CHF. Adverse reactions are similar to enalapril, although skin rashes and taste impairment may be more prevalent, whereas cough may be less prevalent. Captopril's rapid onset and short duration of action are advantageous initially to assess patient tolerance to ACE inhibitors, but are inconvenient during long-term use. The adult dosage for hypertension is PO 12.5 mg bid–tid initially, increasing after 1–2 weeks to 50 mg bid–tid, to a maximum of 450 mg/day. The initial dosage for hypertension in neonates is 0.01 mg/kg bid–tid; and in children is 0.3 mg/kg tid. For CHF in adults, give 25 mg tid initially, then increase over several days based on patient tolerance to a dosage of 50 mg tid. Delay further dosage increases, if possible, for at least 2 weeks to evaluate response. Most patients respond to 50–100 mg tid. For hypertension or CHF, reduce initial dosages by 50–75% and increase slowly in patients on diuretic therapy, with sodium restriction, or with renal impairment. For left ventricular dysfunction post-MI give 6.25 mg once at 3 or more days post-MI, then 12.5 mg tid; increase to 25 mg tid over several days to a target of 50 mg tid over several weeks as tolerated. The oral dosage for diabetic nephropathy is 25 mg tid.[149–153] Captopril is available as 12.5-, 25-, 50-, and 100-mg tablets and in 25- or 50-mg tablets in combination with hydrochlorothiazide 15 or 25 mg (Capozide) (*see* ACE Inhibitors Comparison Chart).

CLONIDINE HYDROCHLORIDE
Catapres, Various

Pharmacology. Clonidine stimulates postsynaptic α_2-adrenergic receptors in the CNS, activating inhibitory neurons to produce a decrease in sympathetic outflow. Since clonidine is not a complete agonist, some of its effects may also result from antagonist actions at presynaptic α-receptors.[154] These actions result in a reduction in peripheral vascular resistance, renal vascular resistance, heart rate, and blood pressure.

Administration and Adult Dosage. **PO for hypertension** 0.1 mg bid initially, increasing in 0.1 mg/day increments until the desired response is achieved. The usual maintenance dosage for monotherapy is 0.2–0.6 mg/day, to a maximum of 2.4 mg/day. If rapid blood pressure lowering is desired (eg, hypertensive urgency), give 0.1–0.2 mg initially, then 0.1 mg q 1 hr until desired response is achieved or a total of 0.8 mg has been given. **SR patch for hypertension** initially apply one #1 (0.1 mg/24 hr) patch weekly; dosage may be increased at 1- to 2-week intervals up to a #3 patch that delivers 0.3 mg/24 hr. Dosages in excess of two #3 patches per week do not produce additional efficacy. **PO/SR patch for opiate withdrawal** PO 17 µg/kg/day (usually 0.4–1.2 mg/day) in 3–4 divided doses for 2 days initially, then apply two #2 patches weekly for a total of 14 days of treatment.[155] **PO for smoking cessation** 0.1–0.3 mg/day in divided doses.[156] **SR patch for smoking cessation** apply one #1 (0.1 mg/24 hr) patch weekly.[156] (*See* Notes.)

Special Populations. *Pediatric Dosage.* Safety and efficacy not established.

Geriatric Dosage. Lower oral dosages may be required, but decreased skin permeability may require higher transdermal dosages.[157]

Other Conditions. In renal impairment, lower oral dosages may be required, but decreased skin permeability may require higher transdermal dosages.[157]

Dosage Forms. **Tab** 0.1, 0.2, 0.3 mg; **Tab** 0.1, 0.2, 0.3 mg with chlorthalidone 15 mg (Combipres); **SR Patch** 0.1, 0.2, 0.3 mg/24 hr.

Patient Instructions. (*See* Antihypertensives Class Instructions.) Do not abruptly discontinue this drug or interrupt therapy unless under medical supervision. Apply transdermal patches weekly to a clean, hairless area of the upper arm or torso that is free of irritation, abrasions, or scars. Do not touch the adhesive surface. Apply patch to a different location with each application. If the system loosens during the 7 days, apply the adhesive overlay directly over the system. If a generalized rash or moderate to severe redness or vesicles appear at the site of application, notify the prescriber. Dispose of the patch by folding the sides together and placing in a disposal site inaccessible to children.

Pharmacokinetics. *Onset and Duration.* (Hypertension) PO onset 30–60 min; peak 3–5 hr; duration 6–8 hr.[157] Transdermally, maximal reduction in blood pressure occurs in 2–3 days and persists throughout the 7-day application period. After removal, the blood pressure rapidly increases toward baseline initially, followed by a slower rate of increase, and returns to pretreatment levels over several days.[154] (Opiate withdrawal) PO peak 2 hr; duration 4–6 hr; usefulness in withdrawal appears to be limited to 14–21 days.[155,156]

Serum Levels. (Hypotensive effect) 0.2–2 µg/L (0.9–9 nmol/L); (dry mouth, sedation) 1 µg/L.[9,154]

Fate. Oral bioavailability is 75–95%.[9] Transdermally, maximum serum levels are reached in 3–4 days and remain constant throughout the 7-day application period.[154] Rate of release is a zero-order process and primarily controlled by the delivery system. Serum concentrations remain constant when a patch is removed and another is immediately applied to a different site.[154] Clonidine is 20% plasma protein bound; V_d is 2.1 ± 0.4 L/kg; Cl is 0.186 ± 0.072 L/hr/kg.[9] It is metabolized in the liver, with drug and metabolites excreted primarily in urine; remaining drug may undergo enterohepatic recycling. About 62% is excreted unchanged in urine.[9]

$t_{½}$. (PO) a phase 10.8 ± 4.7 min; ß phase 12 ± 7 hr.[9,157] (Transdermal) 14 hr, but may be up to 26 hr, reflecting continued absorption from a skin depot.[154]

Adverse Reactions. Frequent adverse reactions include dry mouth (40%), drowsiness (33%), dizziness (16%), constipation (10%), weakness (10%), sedation (10%), nausea or vomiting (5%), nervousness and agitation (3%), orthostatic hypotension (3%), and sexual dysfunction (3%). Occasionally rash, weight gain, anorexia, transient abnormalities in liver function tests, insomnia or vivid dreams, palpitations, tachycardia or bradycardia, or urinary retention occur. Rarely hepatitis, parotitis, elevations of blood glucose or CPK, or cardiac conduction disturbances occur. Allergic contact dermatitis occurs in up to 50% of patients treated with patches.[158] Abrupt withdrawal of oral therapy may result in a withdrawal reaction characterized by rapid reversal of antihypertensive effect within 24–48 hr up to or above pretreatment levels, a rise of blood pressure >40 mm Hg systolic or >25 mm Hg diastolic, or a blood pressure >225/125 mm Hg. Subjective symptoms of sweating, palpitations, anxiety, and insomnia may also occur, even in the absence of marked blood pressure changes. The frequency and severity of symptoms appears to be greater in patients treated with high dosages for >3 months and in those with more severe hypertension.[159]

Precautions. Use with caution in patients with severe coronary insufficiency, recent MI, cerebrovascular disease, or chronic renal failure. Patients who develop a rash from the transdermal system may develop a generalized skin rash if oral clonidine is substituted. Inadvertent person-to-person transfer of the patches has been reported; check application site frequently and dispose of patch by folding adhesive sides together and placing in a container inaccessible to children.[158,160]

Drug Interactions. Heterocyclic antidepressants may decrease the hypotensive effect of clonidine. Clonidine may inhibit the antiparkinson effect of levodopa. Clonidine use with propranolol may cause *hyper*tension, especially if clonidine is abruptly discontinued. Direct-acting sympathomimetics may have an exaggerated effect during clonidine use.

Parameters to Monitor. Monitor blood pressure regularly; check patient compliance.

Notes. Clonidine has been used to suppress symptoms of withdrawal of opiates and to reduce craving and other symptoms in alcohol and tobacco withdrawal.[155,156,161] It has also been used in a variety of psychiatric applications including treatment of mania, anxiety, panic disorders, schizophrenia, and in the treatment of antipsychotic-induced tardive dyskinesia.[161] As an aid in the diagnosis of pheochromocytoma, a single 0.3-mg dose has been administered after the determination of baseline catecholamine levels, followed by three subsequent determinations at hourly intervals.[162] Other conditions for which it may be effective include diabetic diarrhea (0.1–0.6 mg q 12 hr), menopausal flushing (0.1–0.2 mg bid), and premenstrual syndrome.[163–165] **Apraclonidine** (Iopidine) is a clonidine derivative for control of intraocular pressure following laser trabeculostomy or iridotomy.

DIAZOXIDE   Hyperstat, Proglycem, Various

Pharmacology. Diazoxide is a nondiuretic thiazide that reduces total peripheral resistance via direct relaxation of arteriolar smooth muscle, it also increases blood glucose by inhibiting insulin release and by inhibiting peripheral utilization.

Administration and Adult Dosage. IV for severe hypertension 1–3 mg/kg, to a maximum single dose of 150 mg administered undiluted over less than 30 sec q 5–15 min, until adequate blood pressure reduction is achieved (*see* Notes). Repeat q 4–24 hr as needed to maintain blood pressure control. A slow infusion of 10–30 mg/min, to a total dosage of 5 mg/kg or until an adequate blood pressure reduction is achieved, is also effective and may avoid excessive reduction in blood pressure.[166] Administration for longer than 10 days is not recommended. **PO for hypoglycemia** 3–8 mg/kg/day in 2–3 equal doses q 8–12 hr, titrated to response.

Special Populations. *Pediatric Dosage.* **IV for severe hypertension** same as adult dosage. **PO for hypoglycemia** (neonates and infants) 8–15 mg/kg/day in 2–3 divided doses q 8–12 hr, titrated to response; (children) same as adult dosage.

Geriatric Dosage. Same as adult dosage.

Other Conditions. Uremic patients may be particularly sensitive to hypotensive effects.

Dosage Forms. Inj 15 mg/mL (Hyperstat); **Cap** 50 mg (Proglycem); **Susp** 50 mg/mL (Proglycem).

Patient Instructions. (*See* Antihypertensives Class Instructions.) Remain in the supine position during and immediately following IV administration.

Pharmacokinetics. *Onset and Duration.* (Hypertension) onset in 1–2 min; peak within 5 min; duration is 3–12 hr. (Hypoglycemia) onset within 1 hr; duration 8 hr.

Serum Levels. 35 mg/L (152 µmol/L) produces a 20–25% reduction in MAP.[9,167] Levels required for the hyperglycemic effect are not known.

Fate. Oral bioavailability is 86–96%; $94 \pm 14\%$ is plasma protein bound at typical concentrations, decreased at higher concentrations and in uremia. V_d is 0.21 ± 0.02 L/kg with normal renal function; Cl is 0.0036 ± 0.0012 L/hr/kg. The drug is metabolized by oxidation and sulfate conjugation and excreted slowly in urine as unchanged drug (20–50%) and metabolites.[9,167]

$t_{1/2}$. ß phase 48 ± 12 hr; prolonged in renal failure in proportion to Cl_{cr}.[9,167,168]

Adverse Reactions. (Hypertension) with the 300-mg bolus dose regimen, hypotension (7%), nausea and vomiting (4%), and dizziness and weakness (2%) are the most frequent reactions. Use of the currently recommended regimen, which has replaced the 300-mg bolus dose, produces similar but less frequent and/or severe adverse effects. Sodium and water retention, and hyperglycemia may occur, especially with repeated administration. Hypotension may lead to cerebral or myocardial ischemia. (Hypoglycemia) Frequent adverse reactions include sodium and fluid retention, which may precipitate CHF; hyperglycemia or glycosuria, which may require dosage reduction; hirsutism of the lanugo type and distribution, which subsides upon drug discontinuation; tachycardia; palpitations; increases in uric acid; thrombocytopenia with or without purpura, which requires discontinuation of the drug; neutropenia, which is transient, is not associated with an increased susceptibility to infection, and usually does not require discontinuation; eosinophilia; decreased hemoglobin and hematocrit; increased AST levels; a reversible nephrotic syndrome; hematuria; and albuminuria. Rarely, diabetic ketoacidosis or hyperosmolar, nonketotic coma may develop rapidly.

Contraindications. Hypersensitivity to thiazides or other sulfonamide derivatives; compensatory hypertension, such as that seen secondary to coarctation of the aorta or arteriovenous shunts; functional hypoglycemia.

Precautions. Avoid extravasation of the IV drug because of its alkalinity. Highly protein bound drugs may be displaced; recent or coadministration of other antihypertensive drugs may produce excessive blood pressure reduction with the IV route. Some patients may attain higher drug levels with the oral suspension than with the capsules; when switching from one oral dosage form to another, it may be necessary to retitrate the dosage.

Drug Interactions. Diazoxide and hydantoins may be mutually antagonistic. Use with a thiazide diuretic may potentiate hyperuricemia and hypotensive effects. Phenothiazines may potentiate the effects of oral diazoxide.

Parameters to Monitor. (Hypertension) Frequent measurements of blood pressure until stable, then hourly; blood glucose and uric acid with repeated doses. Monitor for signs of cerebral or myocardial ischemia. (Hypoglycemia) Frequent blood glucose and urine glucose and ketones initially, and when dosage adjustments or dosage form changes are made, then regularly during stabilization. Because of the long half-life, up to 7 days of monitoring may be required in patients who develop hyperglycemia.

Notes. Previous antihypertensive dosage recommendations used rapid IV push administration to allow for drug effect before extensive protein binding occurred. However, the recognition that diazoxide has a greater affinity for arterial wall binding sites than for serum albumin has led to the use of short infusion regimens.[168]

ENALAPRIL MALEATE	Vasotec
ENALAPRILAT	Vasotec

Pharmacology. Enalapril is a prodrug rapidly converted to its active metabolite, enalaprilat, by ester hydrolysis in the liver. Enalaprilat is a competitive ACE inhibitor. It also reduces serum aldosterone, leading to decreased sodium retention, potentiates the vasodilator kallikrein-kinin system, and may alter prostanoid metabolism, inhibit the sympathetic nervous system, and inhibit the renin-angiotensin system. The net effect is reduction in total peripheral resistance and blood pressure in hypertensive patients, especially those with high pretreatment plasma renin activity and increased renal plasma flow, and reduction of elevated afterload in patients with CHF.[152,169]

Administration and Adult Dosage. PO for hypertension 5 mg/day initially; usual maintenance dosage is 10–40 mg/day in 1–2 doses. If the patient has recently been receiving a diuretic, discontinue the diuretic for 2–3 days or start with a lower initial enalapril dose of 2.5 mg; bid administration may be necessary in some individuals to achieve adequate 24-hr blood pressure control. A diuretic may be added if blood pressure control is inadequate with enalapril monotherapy. **PO for CHF** 2.5 daily, bid initially, using the lower dosage for patients taking a diuretic; the usual maintenance dosage is 5–20 mg/day, to a maximum of 40 mg; bid administration is preferred. **IV for hypertension** 1.25 mg (0.625 mg initially if patient is taking a diuretic) over 5 min q 6 hr. Dosages as high as 5 mg q 6 hr may be tolerated for up to 36 hr, but there is inadequate experience with dosages over 20 mg/day. For patients converting from oral to IV, 5 mg/day orally is about equivalent to 1.25 mg IV q 6 hr.

Special Populations. *Pediatric Dosage.* Safety and efficacy not established.

Geriatric Dosage. No change required necessarily, but observe cautions for impaired renal function.

Other Conditions. For patients with Cl_{cr} ≤30 mL/min, Cr_s >1.6 mg/dL, or a serum sodium <130 mEq/L, use lower initial doses (2.5 mg PO; 0.625 mg IV). For patients on dialysis, the initial dose should be 0.625 mg IV q 6 hr or PO 2.5 mg on dialysis days.[170]

Dosage Forms. **Tab** (enalapril) 2.5, 5, 10, 20 mg; **Tab** 5 mg with hydrochlorothiazide 12.5 mg, 10 mg with hydrochlorothiazide 25 mg (Vaseretic); **SR Tab** 5 mg with diltiazem 180 mg (Teczem); **Inj** (enalaprilat) 1.25 mg/mL.

Patient Instructions. (*See* Antihypertensives Class Instructions.) Use potassium supplements or salt substitutes only under medical supervision. Report any signs or symptoms of the following: infection (eg, sore throat or fever); angioedema (eg, swelling of face, eyes, lips, tongue, larynx, extremities, or hoarseness or difficulty in swallowing); or excessive fluid loss (eg, vomiting, diarrhea, or excessive perspiration). Report any skin rash, taste disturbance, or persistent, dry cough. If you become pregnant while taking this drug, contact your prescriber immediately.

Pharmacokinetics. *Onset and Duration.* PO onset is 1 hr; peak in 4–6 hr; duration is up to 24 hr.[171] The onset of action and maximal hemodynamic response correspond to the appearance of enalaprilat in serum. IV onset is within 15 min; peak is within 1 hr; duration is dose dependent, but is usually 4–6 hr with recommended doses.[171,172]

Serum Levels. (Enalaprilat) 5–20 µg/L (13–52 nmol/L) is the EC_{50} for ACE inhibition; 40 µg/L (104 nmol/L) produces a mean blood pressure reduction of 12 mm Hg.[9,173]

Fate. Oral bioavailability is 41 ± 15%, is not altered by meals, but is decreased in cirrhosis.[9] Peak enalapril and enalaprilat serum levels after a 10-mg oral dose occur at about 1 hr and 4 hr, and range from 40–50 µg/L (104–130 nmol/L) and 30–40 µg/L (78–104 nmol/L), respectively.[173] About 70% of a dose is converted to enalaprilat; conversion may be reduced in patients with cirrhosis.[9,173] Enalapril and enalaprilat levels are increased in renal dysfunction. Less than 50% of enalaprilat is bound to plasma protein.[173] $V_{dß}$ is 1.7 ± 0.7 L/kg; Cl is 0.294 ± 0.09 L/hr/kg.[174] Clearance is decreased in uremia, CHF, the elderly, and neonates.[9] After IV administration, 88% is excreted unchanged in urine;[9] after oral administration, 33% of the dose is recovered in the feces (6% as enalapril, 27% as enalaprilat), and 61% in the urine (18% as enalapril, 43% as enalaprilat).[173,175] Enalapril may be actively secreted into the urine.[175] Fecal recovery may represent unabsorbed drug or biliary excretion.[175]

$t_{1/2}$. (Enalapril) estimated to be 11 hr; (enalaprilat) about 35 hr in normals, increased in CHF and renal dysfunction.[9,171]

Adverse Reactions. ACE inhibitors have a common side effect profile. Most adverse effects are related to dosage and renal function. A dry, nonproductive cough occurs in 1–3% or more (up to 20% in some surveys) of treated patients, most frequently in women and nonsmokers.[152,153] The cough is caused by potentiation of tissue kinins or prostaglandins in the lung. It may be more frequent with longer-acting drugs, but is usually not resolved by switching to another ACE inhibitor. Taste disturbances occur frequently, but may resolve despite continued therapy.[149,152] Skin rashes occur frequently, usually within a few days to weeks after starting. Rashes often resolve with continued therapy and do not appear to cross-react among ACE inhibitors.[153] Angioedema is an occasional serious, potentially fatal reaction, possibly more frequent with longer-acting ACE inhibitors and possibly in blacks.[153,176] Hypotension may occur, especially with the first dose in vigorously diuresed patients, those who are hyponatremic or hypovolemic, those with severe hypertension, and the elderly. In salt-restricted patients with CHF receiving ACE inhibitors and continuous diuretic therapy, up to one-third may experience worsening of renal function, which may improve when sodium is replenished.[153,177] Proteinuria occurs occasionally with normal renal function and frequently with preexisting renal disease,[152] although patients with progressive renal insufficiency tolerate the drug well and many experience a reduction in proteinuria despite transient reductions in renal function.[178] Neutropenia occurs usually in the first 3 months of therapy; it is rare in normal patients, but is more frequent with high doses or in renal impairment.[152] Cholestatic hepatotoxicity is reported rarely and it may cross-react among ACE inhibitors;[153] it is reversible with drug discontinuation, but fatalities have been reported. Serious fetal harm, including renal failure and face or skull abnormalities and increased risk of miscarriage occurs with ACE-inhibitor use during the 2nd and 3rd trimesters of pregnancy.[153]

Contraindications. Angioedema caused by any ACE inhibitor.

Precautions. Pregnancy. It is best to avoid ACE inhibitors in women of childbearing potential who are not actively avoiding pregnancy. Monitor patients on dietary salt restriction, diuretic therapy, or dialysis (salt or volume depletion) for hypotensive episodes following the initial dose. If possible, discontinue these therapies prior to treatment. Titrate dosage slowly to the minimal effective dosage in patients with impaired renal function or collagen vascular disorders, or in patients receiving drugs altering WBC count or immune function.[149,176,178,179] Patients with aortic stenosis may develop decreased coronary perfusion when treated with afterload reducers such as the ACE inhibitors. Elevations in Cr_s and BUN may require dosage reduction or drug discontinuation. Hypotension responsive to volume expansion may occur during surgical procedures.

Drug Interactions. Hyperkalemia may develop with concomitant use of potassium-sparing diuretics, potassium supplements, or potassium-containing salt substitutes, particularly with preexisting renal impairment.[153,180] Sodium and volume depletion because of a loop diuretic may cause postural hypotension when an ACE inhibitor is begun. ACE inhibitors may cause increased lithium levels. ACE inhibitors may potentiate oral hypoglycemic drugs and may increase neutropenia caused by azathioprine and hypotensive reactions when used with IV plasma protein solutions. NSAIDs may antagonize the hypotensive effect of ACE inhibitors.

Parameters to Monitor. Monitor blood pressure regularly. Obtain baseline Cr_s and BUN to assess the potential for adverse effects and titrate dosages accordingly; thereafter, monitor periodically. Obtain WBC count with differential q 2 weeks for the first 3 months, then periodically in renally impaired patients or if signs of infection occur. Obtain baseline serum potassium, then monitor periodically, especially in patients receiving potassium-sparing diuretics, potassium supplements, or salt substitutes. Obtain periodic urinary protein estimates (morning urines) by dipstick in patients with renal impairment.

Notes. ACE inhibitors are considered first-line drugs, along with diuretics, ß-blockers, and calcium-channel blockers for the treatment of hypertension.[166] They are also useful in the management of patients with CHF refractory to digitalis and diuretic therapy or as an alternative to digitalis when they are used in combination with a diuretic in mild to moderate CHF,[181] and there is evidence that their use is associated with prolonged survival in CHF patients.[152,182] Regression or attenuation of left ventricular hypertrophy occurs in patients with hypertension and in post-MI patients.[152,171] Additional advantages of ACE inhibitors are their renal protective effects and improved insulin sensitivity in insulin-dependent diabetics, their lack of adverse effects on serum lipid profile, an improvement in quality of life in hypertensive patients (with one study favoring **captopril** over **enalapril**), and possibly prevention of structural changes in the heart, systemic vasculature, and kidneys.[152,169,171] ACE inhibitors with greater tissue ACE inhibition (eg, **benazepril, quinapril, ramipril**) may be more effective in this latter regard, but studies are lacking.[152] (*See* ACE Inhibitors Comparison Chart.)

GUANABENZ ACETATE   Wytensin, Various

Guanabenz is a central α_2-adrenergic receptor agonist structurally and pharmacologically similar to clonidine. Its onset is within 60 min, peak effect is in 2–4 hr; effect is reduced appreciably by 6–8 hr; and blood pressure approaches baseline within 12 hr after a single dose. It is about 75% orally bioavailable and 90% bound to plasma proteins. Hydroxylation followed by glucuronidation appears to be the major metabolic pathway; the major metabolite is inactive. Renal clearance of unchanged guanabenz is 5.4 and 7.9 L/hr following 16- and 32-mg doses, respectively. Only 1.4% of unchanged drug is recovered in the urine. Its half-life is 6 hr. Adverse reactions and drug interactions are similar to clonidine, with drowsiness or sedation (39%), dry mouth (28%), dizziness (17%), weakness (10%), and headache (5%) being the most frequent side effects. Use with caution in conjunction with other sedating medications and in patients with severe coronary insufficiency, recent MI, cerebrovascular disease, or renal or hepatic dysfunction. The adult oral dosage for hypertension is 4 mg bid initially; dosage may be increased in 4–8 mg/day increments q 1–2 weeks, to a maximum of 32 mg bid.[183,184] Available as 4- and 8-mg tablets.

GUANADREL SULFATE   Hylorel

Guanadrel is a postganglionic adrenergic blocking drug that is structurally and pharmacologically related to guanethidine. Its antihypertensive effect is comparable to guanethidine in mild to moderate hypertension, but it has a faster onset and shorter duration of action. The onset of action of 30–120 min correlates with the appearance of peak serum levels; peak blood pressure lowering occurs in 4–6 hr; the duration of action is approximately 14 hr. The drug is 20% plasma protein bound; 85% is eliminated in the urine in 24 hr, 40% of a dose as unchanged drug. The elimination half-life varies widely but averages 10 hr. Adverse reactions are similar to, but less frequent than, those that occur with guanethidine, and include orthostatic hypotension (20%), diarrhea or increased bowel movements (5–30%), drowsiness (8–20%), fatigue (20–30%), ejaculation disturbances (7–20%), and impotence (1–5%). Peripheral edema, nasal stuffiness, cough, palpitations, and shortness of breath occur in 5–30% of patients; 21–43% of patients report leg cramps and aching limbs. Contraindications, precautions, drug interactions, and patient instructions are the same as for guanethidine. The initial oral dosage is 5 mg bid, increasing in 10–40 mg/day increments at 1- to 4-week intervals to the usual dosage of 20–75 mg/day; dosages in excess of 150 mg/day are rarely needed, but up to 600 mg/day has been used. Higher dosages may require tid or qid administration.[185,186] Available as 10- and 25-mg tablets.

GUANETHIDINE SULFATE
Ismelin

Guanethidine is a postganglionic adrenergic blocking drug that produces a selective block of efferent, peripheral sympathetic pathways. Its long-term antihypertensive effects are caused by a reduction in total peripheral resistance secondary to norepinephrine depletion from adrenergic nerve endings and inhibition of norepinephrine release in response to sympathetic stimulation.[187]

Administration and Adult Dosage. **PO in ambulatory patients** 10 mg/day initially, increased in 10–12.5 mg/day increments at 5- to 7-day intervals based on patient response or an average dosage of 25–50 mg/day. **PO in hospitalized patients** 25–50 mg initially, increased in 25–50 mg/day increments daily or every other day as indicated. The entire dose may be given once daily.

Special Populations. *Pediatric Dosage.* **PO** 0.2 mg/kg/day or 6 mg/m²/day initially as a single dose, increasing q 1–2 weeks in increments equal to the initial dose, to a maximum of 3 mg/kg/day.

Geriatric Dosage. Same as adult dosage, but the elderly may tolerate postural hypotension less well.

Dosage Forms. **Tab** 10, 25 mg; **Tab** 10 mg with hydrochlorothiazide 25 mg (Esimil).

Patient Instructions. (*See* Antihypertensives Class Instructions.) Take this medication exactly as instructed. If a dose is missed, take only the next scheduled dose (without doubling it). Avoid sudden or prolonged standing; arise slowly, especially in the morning, and avoid the use of alcohol to reduce the chance for a sudden drop in blood pressure. Avoid the use of nonprescription products containing ephedrine, phenylpropanolamine, or pseudoephedrine.

Pharmacokinetics. *Onset and Duration.* Maximum hypotensive response may not occur for up to 1–3 weeks after initiating or changing the dosage. Upon discontinuation, blood pressure remains depressed for 3–4 days and gradually returns to pretreatment levels in 1–3 weeks.

Serum Levels. Adrenergic blockade occurs at 8 µg/L (40 nmol/L) or greater.[188]

Fate. Bioavailability is 3–50%; guanethidine is metabolized to inactive metabolites and excreted in urine by glomerular filtration and tubular secretion as unchanged drug (6.4%) and metabolites.[189]

$t_{1/2}$. α phase 1.5 days; β phase 4.1–7.7 days.[189]

Adverse Reactions. Frequently postural or postexercise hypotension manifested as weakness, dizziness, fatigue, and syncope; increased frequency of bowel movements and explosive diarrhea; edema and weight gain, occasionally precipitating CHF; and inhibition of ejaculation (retrograde ejaculation) occur. Occasionally fatigue, anorexia, nausea, vomiting, dermatitis, loss of scalp hair, dry mouth, and increased BUN occur. Rarely myalgia, muscle tremor, mental depression, bradycardia, or complete AV nodal block occur.

Contraindications. Known or suspected pheochromocytoma; frank CHF not caused by hypertension; use of an MAO inhibitor.

Precautions. May potentially aggravate asthma. Use with caution in renal dysfunction (to avoid further worsening caused by a drop in blood pressure), coronary artery disease, recent MI, cerebrovascular disease, encephalopathy, or peptic ulcer disease.

Drug Interactions. With the exception of low-dose doxepin (<150 mg/day), heterocyclic antidepressants and some phenothiazines block the uptake of guanethidine into nerve endings and thus prevent its action. Oral contraceptives, indirect-acting sympathomimetics, drugs with α-blocking properties (eg, phenothiazines, heterocyclic antidepressants, haloperidol), anorexiants (with the exception of fenfluramine), and NSAIDs may decrease the hypotensive effect. Additive hypotensive effects may occur with levodopa and alcohol. Concomitant therapy with minoxidil can result in profound orthostatic hypotension; discontinue guanethidine 1–3 weeks before initiation of oral minoxidil therapy or initiate therapy in the hospital. Consult a comprehensive drug interactions reference before using this drug in combination with any other drug.

Parameters to Monitor. Blood pressure regularly.

Notes. Guanethidine is infrequently used because of poor tolerance and the availability of numerous other drugs. Occasionally useful in patients who are not controlled by, or do not tolerate, other antihypertensives.[187]

GUANFACINE HYDROCHLORIDE   Tenex, Various

Guanfacine is a central α_2-adrenergic receptor agonist pharmacologically similar to clonidine. In equipotent dosages, it is equivalent to clonidine in antihypertensive activity alone or in combination with a diuretic. Bioavailability is about 80%; peak serum levels occur at 1–4 hr (average 2.6); about 70% is bound to plasma proteins; V_d is 6.3 L/kg. Approximately 40–75% of a dose is excreted in the urine as unchanged drug; the remainder is eliminated as conjugates of metabolites. The average elimination half-life is 17 hr, but may be 13–14 hr in younger patients. Dry mouth (30%), sedation (21%), dizziness (11%), constipation (10%), fatigue, headache, and insomnia are the most frequent adverse effects. Rebound hypertension may occur, but may be milder than with clonidine because of guanfacine's longer half-life. Contraindications, precautions, and drug interactions are similar to those for clonidine. Dosage is initiated at 1 mg/day, given hs. The dosage can be increased in 1 mg/day increments at 3- to 4-week intervals. Dosages above 3 mg/day are associated with an increase in adverse effects with no evidence of increased efficacy.[190,191] Available as 1- and 2-mg tablets.

HYDRALAZINE HYDROCHLORIDE   Apresoline, Various

Pharmacology. Hydralazine is a vasodilator that reduces total peripheral resistance by direct action on vascular smooth muscle, with an effect greater on arterioles than on veins (*see* Notes).

Administration and Adult Dosage. **PO for hypertension** 10 mg qid for the first 2–4 days, increasing to 25 mg qid for the remainder of the first week; after the first week, the dosage may be increased to 50 mg qid, to a maximum of 300 mg/day; bid administration may be as effective as qid.[166] **PO for CHF** 50–75 mg bid–qid initially; the usual maintenance dosage is 200–600 mg/day, but dosages as high as 3 g/day have been used.[192] **IM or IV for hypertension and CHF** 10–40 mg prn.

Special Populations. *Pediatric Dosage.* **PO for hypertension and CHF** 0.75 mg/kg/day or 25 mg/m^2/day initially in 4 divided doses; the initial dose should not exceed 25 mg. Increase gradually over 3–4 weeks, to a maximum of 7.5 mg/kg/day or 300 mg/day. **IM or IV for hypertension and CHF** 1.7–3.5 mg/kg/day or 50–100 mg/m^2/day in 4–6 divided doses; initial parenteral dosage should not exceed 20 mg.

Geriatric Dosage. Lower dosage and slower titration is desirable because of longer half-life in the elderly.

Dosage Forms. **Inj** 20 mg/mL; **Tab** 10, 25, 50, 100 mg; **Tab** 25 mg with hydrochlorothiazide 15 mg (Apresazide); **Cap** 25 mg with hydrochlorothiazide (HCTZ) 25 mg, 50 mg with HCTZ 50 mg, 100 mg with HCTZ 50 mg (Apresazide).

Patient Instructions. (*See* Antihypertensives Class Instructions.) This drug may cause headache, dizziness, or palpitations; report if these symptoms are persistent. Report symptoms of drug-induced systemic lupus erythematosus such as fever, joint pains, dermatitis, pleuritic chest pain, and generalized malaise.[193]

Pharmacokinetics. *Onset and Duration.* PO onset is in 1 hr; following 300 mg/day a minimum of 30 hr is required for MAP to return to 50% of baseline value. IV onset is in 10–20 min, peak in 10–80 min; IM onset is in 10–30 min; duration for IV and IM is 2–6 hr.[194]

Serum Levels. 100 µg/L reduces MAP by 10–20 mm Hg.[9]

Fate. Bioavailability is a function of acetylator phenotype and averages 35 ± 4% for slow acetylators and 16 ± 6% for rapid acetylators. Food may enhance the bioavailability; the first-pass effect may be saturable. Plasma protein binding is 87%. V_d is 1.5 ± 1 L/kg; Cl is 3.36 ± 0.78 L/hr/kg, reduced in CHF. The drug is extensively metabolized by acetylation to multiple metabolites, principally hydrazones, at a rate that is genetically determined; only 1–15% of unchanged drug, as well as metabolites, is excreted in the urine.[9]

$t_{1/2}$. β phase 0.96 ± 0.28 hr, longer in CHF.[9]

Adverse Reactions. Frequently headache, anorexia, nausea, vomiting, diarrhea, palpitations, tachycardia, and angina occur. Occasionally hypotension, edema, peripheral neuritis, dizziness, tremors, muscle cramps, urinary retention, nasal congestion, and flushing occur. A syndrome similar to SLE with joint pain and skin rash (only rarely with cerebritis and nephritis) has been reported at an overall frequency of 6.7% in 281 patients over 51 months; daily dosage affects the frequency, with none at 50 mg/day, 5.4% at 100 mg/day, and 10.4% at 200 mg/day. Women had a higher overall frequency than men (11.6 and 2.8%, respectively), and women taking 200 mg/day had a 19.4% rate;[193] slow acetylator phenotype may also increase the risk; the syndrome is reversible upon drug discontinuation.[193] An immune complex glomerulonephritis has been reported in patients with hydralazine-induced SLE.[195]

Contraindications. Coronary artery disease; mitral valvular rheumatic disease.

Precautions. Reflex tachycardia may precipitate anginal attacks or ECG evidence of myocardial ischemia.

Drug Interactions. NSAIDs may antagonize the hypotensive effect of hydralazine.

Parameters to Monitor. Blood pressure and heart rate regularly. Baseline and periodic CBC. ANA titers may become positive after several months of therapy; routine monitoring is generally not warranted because the symptoms of hydralazine-induced SLE are characteristic and reversible upon drug discontinuation.

Notes. Reflex increases in heart rate, cardiac output, and stroke volume, as well as increases in plasma renin activity and retention of sodium and water, can attenuate hydralazine's antihypertensive action; therefore, long-term regimens for hypertension should include a diuretic and a sympatholytic drug. When hydralazine is used as an afterload reducing drug in the treatment of CHF in patients on maintenance diuretics, the increase in cardiac output usually prevents the development of reflex tachycardia; likewise, hypotension is usually prevented by the increased cardiac output, but may occur if myocardial reserves are inadequate or if the heart cannot respond by increasing output (eg, severe cardiomyopathy or aortic stenosis).[192]

LABELTALOL HYDROCHLORIDE   Normodyne, Trandate

Pharmacology. Labetalol is an adrenergic receptor blocking drug that has both selective α_1- and nonselective β-adrenergic receptor blocking action. Although its pharmacologic profile resembles that of other β-blockers and the postsynaptic α_1-adrenergic blocking action of prazosin, its β-blocking activity is approximately 3 times greater than the α-blocking activity following oral administration and 7 times greater following IV administration. During long-term treatment there is a further reduction in relative α-blocking activity.[196,197]

Administration and Adult Dosage. PO for hypertension 100 mg bid initially, increasing at 2- to 3-day intervals in 100-mg bid increments until blood pressure is controlled. Usual maintenance dosage is 200–400 mg bid, to a maximum of 1.2–2.4 g/day for severe hypertension. **IV for hypertension** 20 mg by slow (2 min) injection, followed by 40–80 mg at 10-min intervals until blood pressure is controlled or to a total of 300 mg. Alternatively, administer a dilute solution by continuous infusion at a rate of 2 mg/min, to a maximum of 300 mg; the usual dosage is 50–300 mg, which may be repeated q 6–8 hr.[166,196,197]

Special Populations. *Pediatric Dosage.* Safety and efficacy not established.

Geriatric Dosage. Same as adult dosage.

Other Conditions. Titrate dosage to blood pressure control. In patients with severe renal dysfunction (Cl_{cr} <10 mL/min), once daily administration may be adequate. Patients with hepatic dysfunction may require lower than usual dosages.

Dosage Forms. **Tab** 100, 200, 300 mg; **Tab** 100, 200, 300 mg with hydrochlorothiazide 25 mg (Normozide, Trandate HCT); **Inj** 5 mg/mL.

Patient Instructions. (*See* Antihypertensives Class Instructions.) Do not discontinue medication abruptly except under medical supervision. Do not sit up or stand for 3 hours after IV administration.

Pharmacokinetics. *Onset and Duration.* PO onset within 2 hr, peak 3 hr, duration 8–12 hr; may be longer with higher dosages. IV injection onset within 5 min, peak in 5–15 min, duration 2–4 hr.[197]

Fate. Almost completely absorbed, but bioavailability is only 18 ± 5% because of extensive first-pass metabolism, with the higher values reported in the elderly and patients with cirrhosis.[9,198] Peak serum levels occur within 1–2 hr after oral administration; food delays the time to peak, but may increase bioavailability.[196,197] Plasma protein binding averages 50%. There is little distribution into the brain because of low lipid solubility. V_d is 9.4 ± 3.4 L/kg; Cl is 1.5 ± 0.6 L/hr/kg, lower in young hypertensive patients and the elderly, and unchanged in cirrhosis. The drug is extensively metabolized, primarily in the liver and possibly gut wall to inactive compounds. Unchanged drug (<5%) and metabolites are excreted in urine and feces.[9,196–198]

$t_{1/2}$. β phase 4.9 ± 2 hr, independent of route of administration, increased in the elderly.[9,196,198]

Adverse Reactions. These are generally related to α- and β-adrenergic blockade and usually occur during the first few weeks of therapy. Frequently dizziness, fatigue, headache, scalp tingling, nausea, dyspepsia, and nasal congestion occur. Occasionally postural hypotension, edema, taste disturbance, impotence, rash, and blurred vision occur.

Contraindications. Bronchial asthma; overt cardiac failure; greater than first-degree heart block; cardiogenic shock; bradycardia.

Precautions. Lower dosages may be required in patients with impaired hepatic function.

Drug Interactions. Cimetidine may increase bioavailability of oral labetalol. Glutethimide may decrease the effect of labetalol by inducing hepatic enzymes. Concurrent use with halothane can produce myocardial depression. Labetalol decreases the reflex tachycardia induced by nitroglycerin and the bronchodilator effects of β2-agonist bronchodilators.

Parameters to Monitor. Monitor blood pressure regularly.

Notes. Labetalol injection is incompatible with 5% sodium bicarbonate.

LOSARTAN POTASSIUM	Cozaar

Losartan and its active metabolite are antagonists of the angiotensin II type I receptor, resulting in a decrease in total peripheral resistance. Losartan has an oral bioavailability of about 36% and undergoes some first-pass metabolism to its active carboxylate metabolite. Metabolism is by CYP2C9 and CYP3A4. In healthy adult males, half-lives are 2.1 ± 0.5 hr for losartan and 6.4 ± 2.3 hr for the metabolite. Excretion of the drug and metabolite is primarily via bile, with about 4% and 6%, respectively, excreted unchanged in urine after an oral dose. Although losartan is generally well tolerated, frequent side effects include dizziness, insomnia, diarrhea, and musculoskeletal pain. It is therapeutically similar to ACE inhibitors in hypertension. Observe similar precautions, particularly the avoidance in pregnancy. However, unlike ACE inhibitors, cough does not occur with losartan. Losartan currently appears to be distinguished clinically primarily as an alternative in patients with ACE inhibitor cough. There is as yet no evidence that it prolongs survival in CHF or post-MI, or that it prevents diabetic nephropathy. The initial oral dosage of losartan for hypertension is 50 mg/day (25 mg/day with volume depletion). Usual maintenance dosage ranges from 25 to 100 mg once daily without regard to meals. No dosage adjustment is necessary in the elderly or in renal failure.[199–201] It is available as 25- and 50-mg tablets, and 50-mg tablets with 12.5 mg of hydrochlorothiazide (Hyzaar). Investigational angiotensin II receptor antaagonists include **eprosartan** (Teneten, SKB), **tasosartan** (Wyeth-Ayerst), and **valsartan** (Diovan, Novartus).

METHYLDOPA	Aldomet, Various

METHYLDOPATE HYDROCHLORIDE	

Pharmacology. The action of methyldopa is thought to be mediated through stimulation of central α-adrenergic receptors in a manner similar to clonidine. Stimulation is primarily caused by the metabolite α-methylnorepinephrine.

Administration and Adult Dosage. PO for hypertension 250 mg bid–tid initially, increasing at intervals of no less than 48 hr to the usual daily dosage of 500 mg–2 g/day in a single daily dose hs or in 2 divided doses. **IV for hypertension** usual dosage is 250–500 mg over 30–60 min in 100 mL D5W q 6 hr, to a maximum of 1 g q 6 hr.

Special Populations. *Pediatric Dosage.* PO 10 mg/kg/day in 2–4 doses initially, to a maximum of 65 mg/kg/day or 3 g/day, whichever is less. IV 20–40 mg/kg/day in divided doses q 6 hr, to a maximum of 65 mg/kg/day or 3 g/day, whichever is less.

Geriatric Dosage. Use lower dosages to avoid causing syncope.

Other Conditions. Patients with renal failure may respond to smaller dosages of methyldopa.

Dosage Forms. Tab 125, 250, 500 mg; **Tab** 250 mg with chlorothiazide 150 or 250 mg (Aldoclor); **Tab** 250 or 500 mg with hydrochlorothiazide 15, 25, 30, or 50 mg (Aldoril, various); **Susp** 50 mg/mL; **IV** 50 mg/mL.

Patient Instructions. *See* Antihypertensives Class Instructions. Report changes in mood (depression), loss of appetite, yellowing of eyes or skin, abdominal pain, or unexplained fever or joint pains.

Pharmacokinetics. *Onset and Duration.* PO onset within hours, peak within 4–6 hr; blood pressure usually returns to baseline within 24–48 hr after long-term use. IV onset 4–6 hr, duration 10–16 hr.

Serum Levels. No correlation between serum levels and therapeutic effect.

Fate. Oral bioavailability is 42 ± 16%.[9] Peak serum levels occur in 2–4 hr, but correlate poorly with the hypotensive effect. IV bioavailability is similar to oral, apparently because a large portion of methyldopa ester is not hydrolyzed to methyldopa. From 10–15% is plasma protein bound. V_d is 0.46 ± 0.15 L/kg; Cl is 0.22 ± 0.06 L/hr/kg and is decreased in uremia. The drug is excreted in the urine as metabolites, sulfate conjugate, and unchanged drug, which averages 64% and 18% after IV and PO administration, respectively.[9,202]

$t_{½}$. α phase 0.21 hr (range 0.16–0.26); β phase 1.8 ± 0.6 hr, increased in uremia and in neonates.[9,202]

Adverse Reactions. Frequently drowsiness, headache, weight gain, nasal stuffiness, postural hypotension, or dry mouth occur. A positive Coombs' test develops in 10–20% of patients, usually between 6 and 12 months of therapy; hemolytic anemia, however, is rare. Occasionally depression, sexual dysfunction, diarrhea, or nightmares are reported. Rarely hepatitis, drug fever, lupuslike syndrome, leukopenia, thrombocytopenia, or granulocytopenia occurs.

Contraindications. Active hepatic disease, such as acute hepatitis and active cirrhosis or liver dysfunction associated with previous methyldopa therapy.

Precautions. Use with caution in patients with a prior history of liver disease. A previously positive Coombs' test does not preclude methyldopa use, but early recognition of hemolytic anemia may be more difficult in such patients.

Drug Interactions. Methyldopa may potentiate the effect of tolbutamide and of lithium. It may also cause confusion or disorientation when used with haloperidol. An increase in norepinephrine's pressor response may occur with concurrent use. Iron products reduce methyldopa absorption. Amphetamines and heterocyclic antidepressants may decrease the efficacy of methyldopa.

Parameters to Monitor. Obtain direct Coombs' test initially and at 6 and 12 months. Obtain baseline and periodic CBC and liver function tests to monitor for hemolytic anemia, blood dyscrasias, and hepatic dysfunction.

Notes. Methyldopa is not a first-line drug because of its frequent side effects; however, it may be useful in those with ischemic heart disease or with diastolic dysfunction, in whom it reduces left ventricular mass.[187]

MINOXIDIL Loniten, Rogaine, Various

Pharmacology. Minoxidil is a potent vasodilator that acts by direct relaxation of arteriolar smooth muscle, resulting in a reduction of total peripheral resistance. The vasodilation and associated reduction in blood pressure leads to reflex sympathetic activation, vagal inhibition, and altered renal homeostatic mechanisms manifested as an increase in heart rate and cardiac output, increase in renin secretion, and salt and water retention. Because these responses may attenuate the hypotensive actions, minoxidil should be administered with a sympatholytic drug and a diuretic. Topically, minoxidil stimulates vertex hair growth by an unknown mechanism.

Administration and Adult Dosage. PO for hypertension 5 mg/day initially as a single daily dose, increased to 10, 20, then 40 mg/day q 3 days in single or divided doses based on blood pressure response, to a maximum of 100 mg/day; usual dosage is 10–40 mg/day. If a single dose reduces supine blood pressure by more than 30 mm Hg, divide the total daily dosage into 2 equal doses. **Top for male pattern baldness or female alopecia androgenetica** 1 mL to affected areas bid.

Special Populations. *Pediatric Dosage.* **PO for hypertension** 0.2 mg/kg as a single daily dose, increased in 50–100% increments q 3 days until optimum blood pressure control or a total daily dosage of 50 mg is achieved; usual dosage is 0.25–1 mg/kg/day.

Geriatric Dosage. Same as adult dosage.

Dosage Forms. **Tab** 2.5, 10 mg (Loniten, various); **Top** 20 mg/mL (2%) (Rogaine, various).

Patient Instructions. (*See* Antihypertensives Class Instructions.) If a dose is missed, wait until the next regularly scheduled dose and continue with your regular dose; do not double the next dose. Report any of the following: increase in resting heart rate of greater than 20 beats/minute, rapid weight gain of more than 5 pounds, or the development of edema, increased difficulty in breathing, new or worsening angina, dizziness, lightheadedness, or fainting.

Pharmacokinetics. *Onset and Duration.* PO single dose onset 30 min; peak 2–3 hr; duration up to 75 hr with a gradual return to baseline at a rate of about 30% per day. Time to maximum effect with repeated administration is a function of dose and averages 7 days at 10 mg/day, 5 days at 20 mg/day, and 3 days at 40 mg/day. Top onset 4 or more months; relapse may occur 3–4 months after drug discontinuation.

Serum Levels. No correlation between serum levels and effects.

Fate. Oral absorption is at least 90%, but bioavailability is probably lower. Protein binding is negligible. V_d is 2.7 ± 0.7 L/kg; Cl is 1.4 ± 0.4 L/hr/kg. The drug is primarily metabolized and renally excreted, with about 20% unchanged drug in the urine. The major metabolite, a glucuronide conjugate, is active and may contribute to the drug's effect.[9,203]

$t_{1/2}$. 3.1 ± 0.6 hr.[9]

Adverse Reactions. Frequently hypertrichosis (elongation, thickening, and enhanced pigmentation) (80%), transient ECG T-wave changes (60%), temporary edema (7%), or tachycardia occur. Occasionally pericardial effusion with or without tamponade (3%), CHF, or angina occur. Rarely breast tenderness and rashes (including Stevens-Johnson syndrome) occur. Minor dermatologic reactions occur occasionally after topical application.

Contraindications. (Oral) pheochromocytoma, caused by possible stimulation of catecholamine release from the tumor.

Precautions. For hypertension, minoxidil must usually be administered with a diuretic to prevent fluid retention; a loop diuretic is almost always required. Drugs or regimens that provide around-the-clock sympathetic suppression are usually required to prevent tachycardia, which may precipitate or worsen existing angina. Degenerative myocardial lesions reported in animal studies have yet to be confirmed in humans.

Drug Interactions. Concomitant therapy with guanethidine can result in profound orthostatic hypotension; discontinue guanethidine 1–3 weeks before initiation of oral minoxidil therapy or initiate therapy in the hospital.

Parameters to Monitor. Blood pressure, pulse rate, body weight, cardiac and pulmonary function regularly.

Notes. Minoxidil is reserved for use in severe hypertension in combination with other drugs, usually a diuretic and a sympatholytic drug (eg, β-blocker).[187]

NITROPRUSSIDE SODIUM   Nipride, Various

Pharmacology. Nitroprusside is a potent vasodilator that has direct action on vascular smooth muscle to reduce arterial pressure and produce a slight increase in heart rate, a mild decrease in cardiac output, and a moderate reduction in total peripheral resistance (TPR). The decrease in TPR suggests arteriolar dilation (afterload reduction), whereas the reduction in cardiac output may be caused by peripheral pooling of blood (preload reduction). Nitroprusside is somewhat more active on veins than on arteries. The active component of sodium nitroprusside is the free nitroso (NO^-) group.

Administration and Adult Dosage. IV 0.3 μg/kg/min by continuous infusion initially, increasing to an average rate of 3 μg/kg/min based on blood pressure response with a range of 0.5–10 μg/kg/min. Infusion at the maximum rate should never exceed 10 min. Patients receiving other antihypertensives can usually be controlled with a smaller dosage. Control administration rates carefully using a microdrip regulator or an infusion pump; avoid too rapid reduction in blood pressure. Infusion rates greater than 2 μg/kg/min generate more cyanide ion (CN^-) than the body can metabolize or eliminate. Maintain infusions at the lowest possible dosage, for the shortest possible duration to avoid toxicity.[24,204–206] (*See* Adverse Reactions.)

Special Populations. *Pediatric Dosage.* IV same as adult dosage.

Geriatric Dosage. Initiate therapy with low infusion rates and titrate the rate and degree of blood pressure lowering carefully to avoid coronary and cerebral hypoperfusion.

Other Conditions. Patients with CHF, stroke victims, and patients receiving other antihypertensive drugs may be particularly sensitive to the blood-pressure-lowering effects of sodium nitroprusside; initiate therapy with low infusion rates and titrate the rate and degree of blood pressure lowering carefully to avoid coronary and cerebral hypoperfusion. Limit the total dosage in renal failure to avoid accumulation of thiocyanate.

Dosage Forms. **Inj** 50 mg.

Pharmacokinetics. *Onset and Duration.* Onset within 1 min; peak 1–2 min; blood pressure usually returns to pretreatment levels in 2–10 min.[166,204,206]

Serum Levels. Therapeutic and toxic levels are not established for nitroprusside because of rapid metabolism to cyanide and thiocyanate. Thiocyanate levels >60 mg/L (1 mmol/L) are associated with toxicity.[204,206]

Fate. Nitroprusside is distributed in a volume that approximates the extravascular space, from which it is rapidly metabolized by a reaction with hemoglobin, yielding cyanmethemoglobin and an unstable intermediate that dissociates, releasing cyanide ion. CN^- is converted to thiocyanate by the enzyme thiosulfate-cyanide sulfur transferase (rhodanese) in the liver and the kidney. The rate of conversion is principally determined by the availability of sulfur, usually as thiosulfate. Thiocyanate is largely excreted by the kidneys and may accumulate with high infusion rates for prolonged periods or in the presence of renal dysfunction.

$t_{\frac{1}{2}}$. (Nitroprusside) 2 min; (thiocyanate) 2.7 days, up to 9 days in patients with renal dysfunction.[206,207]

Adverse Reactions. Most adverse reactions are related to excessive or too rapid reduction of blood pressure and include nausea, retching, diaphoresis, apprehension, restlessness, headache, retrosternal discomfort, palpitations, dizziness, and abdominal pain, all of which resolve when the infusion rate is reduced or the infusion is temporarily discontinued. Thiocyanate is not particularly toxic and usually accumulates to toxic levels only with prolonged (>48 hr) or high-dosage (>10 µg/kg/min) infusions, when cyanide elimination is increased by the administration of thiosulfate, or in the presence of renal dysfunction. Manifestations of thiocyanate toxicity include fatigue, anorexia, nausea, disorientation, toxic psychosis, and hallucinations.[204,206] Cyanide toxicity usually occurs only when large dosages (>10 µg/kg/min) are infused rapidly or for periods >1 hr. Since an early manifestation of cyanide toxicity can be apparent nitroprusside resistance, the need for increasing dosages to achieve the same level of blood pressure control should prompt the clinician to look for metabolic acidosis, an indicator of cyanide toxicity, but one that may not be evident for more than 1 hour after accumulation of dangerous cyanide levels. Other symptoms of cyanide toxicity include dyspnea, vomiting, dizziness, loss of consciousness, weak pulse, distant heart sounds, areflexia, dilated pupils, shallow breathing, convulsions, and the occasional smell of bitter almonds on the breath. In patients with impaired liver function, **hydroxocobalamin** (25 mg/hr by continuous infusion) may facilitate the conversion of cyanide to cyanocobalamin;[208] however, an appropriate hydroxocobalamin dosage form is unavailable. Concurrent sodium thiosulfate administration can also prevent cyanide toxicity, but thiocyanate levels may increase.[206,209] Management of cyanide toxicity includes immediate discontinuation of nitroprusside and the administration of sodium nitrite (0.2 mL/kg of a 3% solution IV over 2–4 min), followed by 12.5 g of sodium thiosulfate infused over 10 min. Methemoglobinemia may develop in patients congenitally unable to convert nitroprusside-induced methemoglobin back to hemoglobin. Management consists of IV administration of **methylene blue** 1–2 mg/kg over several min.[206]

Contraindications. Compensatory hypertension (eg, arteriovenous shunt or coarctation of the aorta); controlled hypotension during surgery in patients with inadequate cerebral circulation; congenital (Leber's) optic atrophy.

Precautions. If an adequate hypotensive response is not achieved after the maximum recommended infusion rate of 10 µg/kg/min for a maximum of 10 min, stop the infusion because higher dosages increase the risk of toxicity. Use with caution in renal, hepatic, or thyroid disease, and in vitamin B_{12} deficiency.

Drug Interactions. Use during general anesthesia may impair the capacity to compensate for hypovolemia and anemia, and cause abnormal perfusion/ventilation ratio.

Parameters to Monitor. Monitor blood pressure frequently (eg, every few minutes) because of the rapid onset and offset of effects. Monitor thiocyanate levels after 24–48 hr in patients with normal renal function and daily in patients with impaired renal function or those receiving large dosages. However, these levels are of no value in detecting cyanide toxicity. Monitoring of serum cyanide concentrations has been recommended, but the assay is technically difficult and not readily interpretable if fluids other than packed RBCs are analyzed.[206] Frequent monitoring of acid-base balance, particularly in patients with hepatic dysfunction, is considered by most clinicians to be adequate.

Notes. Protect from light and discard solution after 24 hr or if the color changes from the usual faint brownish tint to blue, green, or dark red. Do not administer IV push medications through the same line or use the solution for the simultaneous administration of any other drug.

RESERPINE   Various

Reserpine is a hypotensive drug that acts primarily by depleting norepinephrine from postganglionic adrenergic neurons. It is a weak antihypertensive that is most effective when used in combination with a diuretic or as an adjunct to other drugs, permitting lower dosages of each drug and possibly minimizing side effects. Full effects are usually delayed for 2–3 weeks; the duration of action is up to 24 hr; CNS and cardiac effects may persist longer. The drug is extensively metabolized. Dose-related mental depression can occur, but this adverse effect is rare at dosages less than 0.25 mg/day. Drowsiness, weakness, GI disturbances (eg, abdominal pain, activation of peptic ulcer disease, diarrhea, epigastric distress), nasal congestion, sexual dysfunction, and bradycardia occur occasionally. Reserpine is contraindicated in patients with a history of mental depression (especially those with suicidal tendencies), active peptic ulcer, or ulcerative colitis, and during electroconvulsive therapy. Advantages include proven efficacy, relatively good patient tolerance in low dosages, once-daily administration, and very low cost. The adult oral dosage is 0.5 mg/day for 1–2 weeks, followed by a maintenance dosage of 0.1–0.25 mg/day in a single dose.[166,187] Available as 0.1-, 0.25-, and 1-mg tablets, and in combination with diuretics, vasodilators, and other rauwolfia alkaloids.

ACE INHIBITORS COMPARISON CHART

DRUG	DOSAGE FORMS	DAILY ADULT DOSAGE (MG)*	PRODRUG	PEAK (HR)	DURATION (HR)	HALF-LIFE (HR)	ELIMINATION ROUTES
Alacepril Cetapril (Investigational, Bristol-Myers Squibb)	—	5–10	Yes	—	6–10	26†	Renal.
Benazepril Lotensin	Tab 5, 10, 20, 40 mg.	10–40	Yes	2–4	24+	22‡	Renal. Hepatic.
Captopril Capoten Various	Tab 12.5, 25, 50, 100 mg.	25–150	No	1	6–10	1.7	Renal. Hepatic
Cilazapril Inhibace	Cap 1, 2.5, 5 mg.	5–20	Yes	3–7	—	2–4	Renal.
Delapril (Investigational, Rorer)	—	30–60	Yes	4–6	24+	1.5†	Renal. Hepatic.
Enalapril Vasotec	Tab 2.5, 5, 10, 20 mg. Inj 1.25 mg/mL.	PO 10–40; IV 1.25–5 mg q 6 hr.	Yes	4–6	24 (PO)	11† (enalaprilat-35)	Renal.
Fosinopril Monopril	Tab 10, 20 mg.	20–80	Yes	3–6	24	12–15‡	Hepatic, Renal
Lisinopril Prinivil Zestril	Tab 2.5, 5, 10, 20, 40 mg.	10–40	No	2–6	24	13‡	Renal.

(continued)

ACE INHIBITORS COMPARISON CHART (continued)

DRUG	DOSAGE FORMS	DAILY ADULT DOSAGE (MG)*	PRODRUG	PEAK (HR)	DURATION (HR)	HALF-LIFE (HR)	ELIMINATION ROUTES
Moexipril Univasc	Tab 7.5, 15 mg.	7.5–30	Yes	3–8	24	2–9[‡]	Hepatic, Renal.
Perindopril Aceon	Tab 2, 4, 8 mg.	4–8	Yes	4–8	24+	9[‡]	Renal.
Quinapril Accupril	Tab 5, 10, 20, 40 mg.	20–80	Yes	2–4	24+	2–3[‡]	Renal.
Ramipril Altace	Cap 1.25, 2.5, 5, 10 mg.	2.5–20	Yes	3–8	24+	11–17[‡]	Renal, Hepatic.
Spirapril (Investigational, Schering)	—	12.5–100	Yes	4–8	24+	30[‡]	Renal, Hepatic.
Trandolapril Mavik	Tab 1, 2, 4 mg.	1–4	Yes	6	24+	24[‡]	Hepatic, Renal.
Zofenopril Zoprace (Investigational, Bristol-Myers Squibb)	—	5–10	Yes	2	24	5.5[‡]	Renal, Hepatic.

*Usual maintenance dosage range. Initial dosage is often lower, and higher dosages are sometimes effective.
[†]Half-life of prodrug; active form longer.
[‡]Half-life of active drug.
From references 171, 176, 210–213.

α₁-ANTAGONISTS COMPARISON CHART

DRUG	DOSAGE FORMS	DAILY ADULT DOSAGE (MG)*	PEAK (HR)	DURATION (HR)	HALF-LIFE (HR)	ELIMINATION ROUTES
Doxazosin Cardura	Tab 1, 2, 4, 8 mg.	1–16	6	18–36	11	Hepatic.
Prazosin Minipress Various	Cap 1, 2, 5 mg.	2–20	1.5	8–10	2	Hepatic.
Terazosin Hytrin	Tab 1, 2, 5, 10 mg.	1–20	2	24	14	Hepatic, Renal.
Trimazosin (Investigational, Pfizer)	—	100–900	3–6	3–6	3	Hepatic.

*Usual maintenance dosage range; higher dosages are sometimes effective. Dosage is the same in the elderly.
From references 143, 146, 214–217.

DRUGS FOR HYPERTENSIVE URGENCIES AND EMERGENCIES COMPARISON CHART

DRUG	DOSAGE RANGE	ONSET (MIN)	DURATION	COMMENTS*
ORAL DRUGS FOR HYPERTENSIVE URGENCIES				
Captopril Capoten Various	PO, SL 12.5–25 mg.	10–30	2–6 hr	Hypotensive effect is particularly large in patients on a diuretic or in hypertensive crisis. Subsequent doses may be less effective unless given with a diuretic. Acute renal failure may occur.
Clonidine Catapres	PO 0.1–0.2 mg initially, then 0.1 mg/hr, to a maximum total dosage of 0.8 mg.	30–60	6–8 hr	Rate of onset slower after a meal; drowsiness or dry mouth can occur. Rebound hypertension is possible.
Labetalol Normodyne Trandate	PO 200–400 mg, may repeat q 2–3 hr.	30–120	6–12 hr	Orthostatic hypotension, bronchoconstriction, heart block can occur. Avoid in COPD, asthma.
Nifedipine Adalat Procardia	PO 10–20 mg, may repeat in 20 min.	5–20	2–6 hr	Bite and swallow capsule. Precipitous drops in blood pressure may occur. Increases cardiac output; mild flushing, headaches, and palpitations may occur; use with caution in patients with severe arteriosclerotic stenosis because it may precipitate cerebral ischemic symptoms.
Prazosin Minipress Various	PO 1–2 mg, may repeat q 1 hr.	30–90	1–10 hr	Useful in presence of increased circulating catecholamines. First-dose syncope, palpitations, tachycardia, headache reported.

(continued)

277

DRUGS FOR HYPERTENSIVE URGENCIES AND EMERGENCIES COMPARISON CHART (continued)

DRUG	DOSAGE RANGE	ONSET (MIN)	DURATION	COMMENTS*
INTRAVENOUS DRUGS FOR HYPERTENSIVE EMERGENCIES				
Diazoxide Hyperstat I.V.	IV 1–3 mg/kg (up to 150 mg) over 30 sec, may repeat q 5–15 min. Alternatively, IV infusion 10–30 mg/min. After 300 mg given, give furosemide IV 40 mg before subsequent doses.	1–2	3–12 hr	Useful in hypertensive encephalopathy, malignant hypertension, and eclampsia. Increases cardiac output; requires blood pressure monitoring at hourly intervals. Avoid with ischemic heart disease or intracranial hemorrhage.
Enalaprilat Vasotec	IV 0.625–1.25 mg (see monograph).	15	4–6 hr	Useful in CHF and those at risk for cerebral hypotension. Avoid in severe renal impairment. Blacks may respond poorly. Hypotension may occur.
Hydralazine Apresoline	IM or IV 10–40 mg q 3–6 hr.	10–20	2–6 hr	Limited to treatment of severe preeclampsia and eclampsia. Increases cardiac output; many patients sensitive to parenteral doses, resulting in excessive hypotension.
Labetalol Normodyne Trandate	IV push 20 mg initially, then 40–80 mg q 10 min until desired response achieved or a total dose of 300 mg. Alternatively, IV infusion 2 mg/min.	<5	2–4 hr	Hypotensive effect is predictable; contra-indicated in CHF, head trauma, intracranial hemorrhage; often causes marked postural hypotension. Avoid use in patients with COPD, CHF, or bradycardia.
Nicardipine Cardene	IV infusion 5–15 mg/hr.	<5–15	30–40 min	Predictable effect. Useful in coronary, cerebral, or peripheral artery disease and in surgical patients. Tachycardia may occur.

(continued)

DRUGS FOR HYPERTENSIVE URGENCIES AND EMERGENCIES COMPARISON CHART (continued)

DRUG	DOSAGE RANGE	ONSET (MIN)	DURATION	COMMENTS*
Nitroglycerin Various	IV 0.3–6 mg/hr by continuous infusion.	1–5	5–15 min	Useful in myocardial ischemia and hypertension associated with MI. Hypotension, headache, tachycardia, and tachyphylaxis occur. Avoid in constrictive pericarditis, pericardial tamponade, or intracranial hypertension.
Nitroprusside Sodium Nipride Various	IV infusion 100 mg/L at a rate of 0.3–10 µg/kg/min by continuous infusion using infusion pump. Average dosage is 3 µg/kg/min.	0.5–1	2–5 min	Especially useful in ischemic heart disease. Continuous monitoring required; arterial pressure response adjusted by changing infusion rate; hypotensive effect enhanced by elevating head of patient's bed. Decreases cardiac output; cyanide toxicity with prolonged, high infusion rates.

*Reduction of arterial pressure may lead to sodium and fluid retention, thus reducing the antihypertensive effectiveness of these drugs; therefore, administer diuretic drugs concomitantly during therapy. Consult the drug monograph or product literature for additional information.
Adapted from references 166, 204, 218–220.

ß-Adrenergic Blocking Drugs

ESMOLOL HYDROCHLORIDE   Brevibloc

Esmolol is an ultra-short-acting, cardioselective, β_1-adrenergic blocking drug. It is effective in controlling ventricular response in patients with atrial fibrillation and other supraventricular tachycardias, and in slowing heart rate in patients with sinus tachycardia associated with acute MI or cardiac surgery. The drug may also be effective in perioperative hypertension. The α half-life is about 2 min; V_d is 3.5 $\pm$ 1.5 L/kg. It is rapidly hydrolyzed by plasma and blood esterases, resulting in an elimination half-life of about 9 min in adults and 3 min in children. Esmolol is metabolized to a metabolite with weak, clinically unimportant β-blocking activity and small amounts of methanol. No unchanged esmolol appears in the urine. Effective serum levels are about 1–1.5 mg/L (3.4–5.1 μmol/L); concurrent IV morphine may increase serum levels by 46%. The side effect profile is similar to that of other β_1-selective β-blockers. Particularly frequent is dose-related hypotension; IV site phlebitis occurs occasionally. Esmolol is contraindicated in sinus bradycardia, second- or third-degree heart block, cardiogenic shock, or overt heart failure. Dilute injection to a final concentration of 10 mg/mL. The IV loading dose is 500 μg/kg/min for 1 min, then 50 μg/kg/min. IV loading dose may be repeated as often as q 5 min with a concomitant increase of infusion rate in 50 μg/kg/min increments, titrated to ventricular response, heart rate, and/or blood pressure. Most patients respond to infusions of 100–200 μg/kg/min. Once the desired end point is obtained, the infusion rate may be decreased in 25–50 μg/kg/min increments at 5- to 10-min intervals. Infusions up to 48 hr in duration are well tolerated.[221,222] Available as 10 and 250 mg/mL injection.

PROPRANOLOL HYDROCHLORIDE   Inderal, Various

Pharmacology. Propranolol is a nonselective ß-adrenergic blocker used in arrhythmias, hypertension, and angina pectoris. It is also effective in decreasing mortality after MI. The antiarrhythmic mechanism is caused by decreased AV nodal conduction in supraventricular tachycardias and blockade of catecholamine-induced dysrhythmias. The antihypertensive mechanism is unknown, but contributing factors are a CNS mechanism, renin blockade, and decreases in myocardial contractility and cardiac output. Propranolol also lowers myocardial oxygen demand by decreasing contractility and heart rate, which symptomatically alleviates anginal pain and increases exercise tolerance in coronary artery disease. (*See* ß-Adrenergic Blocking Drugs Comparison Chart.)

Administration and Adult Dosage. **PO** 10–20 mg q 6 hr initially, increasing gradually to desired effects. In hypertension, over 1 g/day has been used; however, consider adding another drug if 480 mg/day is ineffective.[223] In angina pectoris, the dosage is titrated to pain relief and exercise evidence of ß-blockade (bradycardia). The end point for dosage escalation in acute arrhythmias is the return to sinus rhythm or, in atrial fibrillation or flutter, to a ventricular rate <100 beats a min with hemodynamic stability. Twice-daily administration is effective in angina pectoris and hypertension. Administer SR Cap in the same daily dosage once or twice daily (not indicated post-MI). **PO for post-MI prophylaxis (non-SR)** 180–240 mg/day in 2–3 divided doses. **IV slow push** 1 mg q 5 min, to a maximum of 0.15 mg/kg; some authors recommend that the first dose be given over 2–10 min.

Special Populations. *Pediatric Dosage.* **PO for hypertension** 0.5 mg/kg/day in 2–4 divided doses, increasing to a maximum of 2 mg/kg/day. **IV slow push** 0.01–0.1 mg/kg/dose over 10 min up to 1 mg, may repeat in 6–8 hr.[99]

Geriatric Dosage. Bioavailability is increased in the elderly, necessitating lower initial doses.

Other Conditions. Therapeutic end points may be achieved with lower dosages in hypothyroidism or liver disease. Begin with lower dosages and titrate to clinical response. Patients with thyrotoxicosis require higher dosages to achieve the desired effect.[224]

Dosage Forms. **Soln** 4, 8, 80 mg/mL; **Tab** 10, 20, 40, 60, 80, 90 mg; **SR Cap** 60, 80, 120, 160 mg; **Inj** 1 mg/mL.

Patient Instructions. Report any symptoms such as shortness of breath, swelling, wheezing, fatigue, depression, nightmares, or inability to concentrate. Do not stop therapy abruptly. Do not crush or chew SR capsule. The SR capsule core may appear in the stool, but this does not mean there was a lack of absorption.

Pharmacokinetics. *Onset and Duration.* PO onset is variable; the duration varies from 6 to >12 hr.[224]

Serum Levels. No definite relationship has been established between serum concentrations and therapeutic effect in the treatment of arrhythmias, angina pectoris, or hypertension. ß-Blockade is associated with serum concentrations >100 µg/L (340 nmol/L).[225]

Fate. Propranolol is rapidly and completely absorbed after oral administration; however, a large hepatic first-pass effect occurs, limiting systemic availability to 26 ± 10%. First-pass elimination is saturable with an oral dose greater than about 30 mg.[225] The drug is 87 ± 6% bound to α_1-acid glycoprotein and other plasma proteins.[9,224] V_d is 4.3 ± 0.6 L/kg; Cl is 0.96 ± 0.3 L/hr/kg. Unlike most other drugs, displacement from plasma proteins increases elimination half-life and V_d because of high tissue affinity (nonrestrictive elimination). An active metabolite, 4-hydroxypropranolol, is formed after oral, but not IV, administration. Less than 0.5% of a dose is excreted unchanged in urine.[9]

$t_{1/2}$. α phase is about 10 min;[224] β phase after a single PO dose is 3.9 ± 0.4 hr.[9] With long-term oral therapy, β phase is 4–6 hr; however, it may be as long as 10–20 hr in patients with liver disease.[226]

Adverse Reactions. Adverse effects are often not dose related. Depression, nightmares, insomnia, fatigue, and lethargy occur frequently, and, less often, psychotic changes have been reported. CNS side effects probably occur more often with the lipophilic β-blockers (eg, propranolol). The drug may cause occasional life-threatening reactions when therapy (especially IV) is initiated, and acute CHF with pulmonary edema and hypotension or symptomatic bradycardia and heart block may occur.[227] Acute drug cessation in patients with coronary artery disease may precipitate unstable angina pectoris or MI. The drug may precipitate hypoglycemia, but probably more important in diabetics is its ability to mask hypoglycemic symptoms (except for sweating). It may exacerbate symptoms of peripheral vascular disease or Raynaud's disease. β-Blockers may exacerbate previously stable asthma or chronic airway obstruction by causing bronchospasm,[227] or renal dysfunction by further depressing GFR.[228]

Contraindications. Severe obstructive pulmonary disease, asthma or active allergic rhinitis; cardiogenic shock or severe CHF; second- or third-degree heart block; severe sinus node disease.

Precautions. In coronary artery disease, discontinue drug by tapering the dosage over 4–7 days. Use cautiously in patients with Prinzmetal's vasospastic angina to prevent worsening of chest pain.[229] Use caution in peripheral vascular disease or CHF and in patients with brittle diabetes or a history of hypoglycemic episodes. May worsen atrial fibrillation associated with accessory AV pathway.

Drug Interactions. Concurrent digitalis therapy may lessen the β-blocker exacerbation of CHF. When taken with oral hypoglycemics, nonselective β-blockers such as propranolol prolong hypoglycemic episodes and inhibit tachycardia and tremors, which are signs of hypoglycemia (sweating is not inhibited); hypertension may occur during hypoglycemia. Epinephrine may produce hypertensive reactions in patients on propranolol (and probably other nonselective ß-blockers); this may also occur with other sympathomimetics such as phenylephrine and phenylpropanolamine. Barbiturates and rifampin may increase metabolism of hepatically eliminated β-blockers such as propranolol. Cimetidine may increase propranolol effects. Combined use of clonidine and propranolol may result in *hyper*tensive reactions, especially if clonidine is abruptly discontinued. β-Blockers may increase the first-dose hypotensive effect of prazosin and similar drugs. NSAIDs may blunt the hypotensive response of ß-blockers.

Parameters to Monitor. During IV administration, blood pressure and pulse must be taken q 5 min with constant ECG monitoring for signs of AV nodal block (lengthened PR interval) or bradycardia. Evaluate vital signs routinely for hemodynamic end points (eg, blood pressure in hypertension and heart rate or pressure-rate product in angina pectoris). Question the patient about subjective complaints such as nightmares or fatigue. When a patient at risk for adverse reactions is first given propranolol, signs and symptoms of toxicity must be evaluated (eg, CHF, shortness of breath or edema; bronchospasm, wheezing or shortness of breath; diabetes, blood glucose; peripheral vascular disease, painful or cold extremities).

Notes. Propranolol may be beneficial for treatment of symptomatic hypertrophic obstructive cardiomyopathy by increasing end-diastolic volume, producing ventricular relaxation and relieving ventricular outflow obstruction. If a ß-blocker must be used in lung disease, ß₁-selective drugs (eg, **acebutolol, atenolol,** or **metoprolol**) cause alterations in pulmonary function that are more easily reversed by bronchodilators; these drugs are probably a better choice than propranolol or other nonselective ß-blockers. (*See* ß-Adrenergic Blocking Drugs Comparison Chart.)

β-ADRENERGIC BLOCKING DRUGS COMPARISON CHART

DRUG	DOSAGE FORMS	CARDIO-SELECTIVITY	β HALF-LIFE (HR)	EXCRETED UNCHANGED IN URINE	PROTEIN BINDING	LABELED USES	STARTING DOSAGE	MAXIMUM DOSAGE
Acebutolol [a] Sectral Various	Cap 200, 400 mg.	+	3–4 (diacetolol) 8–13	30–40%	25%	Hypertension, arrhythmias.	PO 400 mg/day.	PO 1.2 g/day.
Atenolol Tenormin Various	Tab 25, 50, 100 mg Inj 0.5 mg/mL.	+ (up to 100 mg)	6–7	85%	10%	Hypertension. Post-MI prophylaxis.	PO 50 mg/day. IV 5 mg × 2, then PO 100 mg/day.	PO 200 mg/day.
Betaxolol [b] Kerlone	Tab 10, 20 mg.	+	14–20	15%	50%	Hypertension.	PO 10 mg/day.	PO 40 mg/day.
Bevantolol Vantol (Investigational, Parke-Davis)	—	+	1–3	<10%	95%	—	PO 150 mg/day.	PO 400 mg/day.
Bisoprolol Zebeta	Tab 5, 10 mg.	+	9–12	50%	30%	Hypertension.	PO 2–5 mg/day.	PO 20 mg/day.
Bopindolol [a] (Investigational, SKB)	—	0	9–12	—	—	—	PO 0.5–1 mg/day.	PO 40 mg/day.
Carteolol [a] Cartrol	Tab 2.5, 5 mg.	0	6–11	60%	15%	Hypertension.	PO 2.5 mg/day.	PO 10 mg/day.
Carvedilol [c] Coreg	Tab 6.25, 12.5, 25 mg.	0	6–8	1%	95%	Hypertension, CHF.	PO 25–50 mg/day. PO 3.125 mg bid.	PO 200 mg/day. PO 25 mg bid.

(continued)

283

B-ADRENERGIC BLOCKING DRUGS COMPARISON CHART (continued)

DRUG	DOSAGE FORMS	CARDIO-SELECTIVITY	β HALF-LIFE (HR)	EXCRETED UNCHANGED IN URINE	PROTEIN BINDING	LABELED USES	STARTING DOSAGE	MAXIMUM DOSAGE
Celiprolol [a,c] (Investigational, Rhone-Poulenc Rorer)	—	+	4–8	10–20%	25%	—	PO 200 mg/day.	PO 600 mg/day.
Esmolol Brevibloc	Inj 10, 250 mg/mL.	+	9 min	0%	55%	Supraventricular tachycardia.	IV 25–50 µg/kg/min.	IV 200 µg/kg/min.
Labetalol[c] Trandate Normodyne	Tab 100, 200, 300 mg Inj 5 mg/mL.	0	4–9	5%	50%	Hypertension.	PO 100 mg/day. IV 20 mg, then 40–80 mg q 10 min.	PO 2.4 g/day. IV 300 mg.
Metoprolol Lopressor	Tab 50, 100 mg SR Tab 50, 100, 200 mg Inj 1 mg/mL.	+ (up to 100 mg)	3–7	39%	10%	Hypertension. Hypertension, angina pectoris. Acute MI.	PO 100 mg/day. PO SR 50–100 mg/day. IV 5 mg × 3, then PO 50 mg q 6 hr × 48 hr.	PO 450 mg/day. PO SR 400 mg/day.
Toprol XL								
Nadolol Corgard Various	Tab 20, 40, 80, 120, 160 mg.	0	17–24	70%	25%	Hypertension, angina pectoris.	PO 40 mg/day.	PO 320 mg/day.
Penbutolol[a] Levatol	Tab 20 mg.	0	4–8	5%	80–90%	Hypertension.	PO 20 mg/day.	PO 80 mg/day.
Pindolol[a] Visken	Tab 5, 10 mg.	0	3–4	40%	57%	Hypertension.	PO 10 mg/day.	PO 60 mg/day.

(continued)

β-ADRENERGIC BLOCKING DRUGS COMPARISON CHART (continued)

DRUG	DOSAGE FORMS	CARDIO-SELECTIVITY	β HALF-LIFE (HR)	EXCRETED UNCHANGED IN URINE	PROTEIN BINDING	LABELED USES	STARTING DOSAGE	MAXIMUM DOSAGE
Propranolol Inderal Various	See monograph.	0	4–6	<0.5%	87%	Hypertension, angina pectoris, arrhythmias. Post-MI prophylaxis.	PO 40–80 mg/day.	PO 480 mg/day.
Sotalol[d] Betapace	Tab 80, 160, 240 mg.	0	7–15	80–90%	0%	Life-threatening ventricular arrhythmias.	PO 180 mg/day. PO 160 mg/day.	PO 240 mg/day. PO 640 mg/day.
Timolol[b] Blocadren	Tab 5, 10, 20 mg.	0	4–5	20%	<10%	Hypertension. Post-MI prophylaxis.	PO 20 mg/day. PO 20 mg/day.	PO 60 mg/day. PO 20 mg/day.

[a]Acebutolol, bopindolol, carteolol, celiprolol, penbutolol, and pindolol have intrinsic agonist (sympathomimetic) activity (ISA).

[b]Betaxolol is also available as Betoptic ophthalmic drops 0.5%; carteolol is also available as Ocupress 1%, and timolol is also available as Timoptic ophthalmic drops 0.25% and 0.5% for treatment of glaucoma.

[c]Carvedilol has α-blocking actions; and celiprolol has weak α₂-blocking actions. Labetalol has potent α₁-blocking actions (ratio of α- to β-blockade 1:3 and 1:7 with PO and IV, respectively).

[d]Sotalol also has type III antiarrhythmic properties.

From references 124, 221, 230–240.

285

Calcium-Channel Blocking Drugs

DILTIAZEM HYDROCHLORIDE   Cardizem, Dilacor XR, Tiazac, Various

Pharmacology. Diltiazem is a calcium-channel blocking drug that decreases heart rate, prolongs AV nodal conduction, and decreases arteriolar and coronary vascular tone. It also has negative inotropic properties. Diltiazem is effective in symptomatic angina pectoris, essential hypertension, and supraventricular tachycardias. It may also reduce early reinfarction rates in patients with non-Q-wave MI and normal left ventricular function. (*See* Calcium-Channel Blocking Drugs Comparison Chart.)

Administration and Adult Dosage. **IV loading dose** 0.25 mg/kg (about 20 mg) over 2 min, may repeat in 15 min with 0.35 mg/kg (about 25 mg). **IV infusion** 5–15 mg/hr, titrated to ventricular response. **PO for angina** 30–60 mg q 6–8 hr initially; dosages up to 480 mg/day may be required for symptomatic relief of angina;[241,242] 180–300 mg once daily with Cardizem CD. **PO for hypertension** 120–240 mg/day initially, in 2 divided doses using Cardizem SR, or 180–300 mg once daily using Cardizem CD or Dilacor XR, titrated to clinical response; **maintenance dosages** of 180–480 mg/day are usually necessary.

Special Populations. *Pediatric Dosage.* Safety and efficacy are not established.

Geriatric Dosage. Same as adult dosage, but titrate dosage slowly.

Other Conditions. Patients with liver disease may require lower dosages; titrate to clinical response.

Dosage Forms. **Tab** 30, 60, 90, 120 mg; **SR Cap** (12-hr; Cardizem SR, various) 60, 90, 120 mg; **SR Cap** (24-hr; Cardizem CD) 120, 180, 240, 300 mg; (24-hr; Dilacor XR) 120, 180, 240 mg; (24-hr; Tiazac) 120, 180, 240, 300, 360 mg; **SR Tab** 120, 180, 240 mg (Tiamete); **Inj** 5 mg/mL; **SR Tab** 180 mg with enalapril 5 mg (Teczem).

Patient Instructions. Report dizziness, leg swelling, or shortness of breath. (For angina) Maintain a diary to document the numbers of episodes of chest pain and sublingual nitroglycerin tablets used.

Pharmacokinetics. *Onset and Duration.* PO onset 0.5–3 hr, duration 6–10 hr;[243,244] 12–24 hr with SR cap, depending on the product.

Serum Levels. Levels over 95 µg/L (230 nmol/L) are necessary to cause hemodynamic changes, but their clinical usefulness is questionable.[245] Levels of desacetyldiltiazem are similar to diltiazem.[246]

Fate. Oral bioavailability is 38 ± 11% with the first dose, but 90 ± 21% during long-term therapy.[246] The drug is 78 ± 3% plasma protein bound; V_d is 5.3 ± 1.7 L/kg;[246] Cl is 0.72 ± 0.3 L/hr/kg.[9] Enterohepatic recycling occurs.[247] The drug is almost entirely metabolized by the liver, with only 1–3% excreted unchanged in urine. One metabolite, desacetyldiltiazem, has 40–50% the activity of diltiazem. Metabolites are excreted primarily in the feces.

$t_{½}$. α phase 2–5 min; β phase 4.9 ± 0.4 hr,[243,244,246] longer in the elderly.[242] β phase for desacetyldiltiazem 6.1 ± 1.2 hr.[246]

Adverse Reactions. Frequency of side effects is dose related.[247] Headache, flushing, dizziness, and edema occur frequently. Sinus bradycardia and AV block occur frequently, often in association with concomitant β-blockers.[242,247] Worsening of CHF may occur in patients with underlying left ventricular dysfunction. A variety of skin reactions have been occasionally reported.[242] Hepatitis occurs rarely.

Contraindications. Second- or third-degree block or sick sinus syndrome in the absence of a ventricular pacemaker; symptomatic hypotension or severe CHF, acute MI, or pulmonary congestion; atrial fibrillation with accessory AV pathway.

Precautions. Use caution with concomitant use of β-blockers in patients with underlying CHF, especially those with poor left ventricular function.[242,247]

Drug Interactions. Cimetidine and propranolol increase diltiazem serum levels.[242,248] Diltiazem inhibits the CYP3A metabolism of many drugs, including carbamazepine, cyclosporine, and theophylline.[242]

Parameters to Monitor. Blood pressure, heart rate, and ECG, especially when initiating therapy. Observe for symptoms of hypotension and CHF. Serial treadmill exercise tests can be performed to assess efficacy in angina. Monitor the number of episodes of chest pain and SL nitroglycerin used.

NIFEDIPINE
Adalat, Procardia

Pharmacology. Nifedipine is a dihydropyridine calcium-channel blocking drug with potent arterial and coronary vasodilating properties. A reflex increase in sympathetic tone (in response to vasodilation) counteracts the direct depressant effects on SA and AV nodal conduction. This renders nifedipine ineffective in the treatment of supraventricular tachycardias. It is used for vasospastic and chronic stable angina and in the treatment of hypertension. (*See* Calcium-Channel Blocking Drugs Comparison Chart.)

Administration and Adult Dosage. **PO for angina** (Cap) 10 mg tid initially, increasing to a usual maximum of 20–30 mg tid or qid; dosages over 180 mg/day are not recommended. **PO for hypertension** (SR Tab only) 30–60 mg/day initially, increasing up to 120 mg/day prn. **PO for severe hypertension** (non-SR) 10 mg, may repeat prn in 20 min. The capsule may be punctured or bitten and swallowed, usually resulting in a more rapid onset than SL administration.[249]

Special Populations. *Pediatric Dosage.* Safety and efficacy not established. **PO for hypertensive crisis** 0.25–0.5 mg/kg q 6–8 hr.[99]

Geriatric Dosage. Same as adult dosage.

Other Conditions. Patients with liver disease may require lower dosages;[250] titrate to clinical response.

Dosage Forms. **Cap** 10, 20 mg; **SR Tab** 30, 60, 90 mg.

Patient Instructions. Report flushing, edema, dizziness, or increased frequency of chest discomfort. Do not split, chew, or crush sustained-release tablets. The SR tablet core may appear in the stool, but this does not mean there was a lack of absorption. Maintain a diary to document the number of episodes of chest pain and sublingual nitroglycerin tablets used.

Pharmacokinetics. *Onset and Duration.* PO onset 0.5–2 hr; duration (Cap) 4–8 hr; (SR Tab) 12–24 hr. PO (punctured capsule) onset 10–20 min; duration 3–4 hr.

Serum Levels. (Therapeutic) above 90 µg/L (260 nmol/L), although clinical utility is questionable.[251]

Fate. Bioavailability is 52 ± 37% in normals and 91 ± 26% in cirrhosis because of extensive and variable first-pass hepatic elimination.[250] It is 96 ± 1% plasma protein bound; V_d is 0.8 ± 0.2 L/kg.[251,252] Cl is 0.42 ± 0.12 L/hr/kg.[9] Nifedipine is almost all eliminated by hepatic metabolism via the CYP3A4 isozyme, which is present in variable amounts (but is not a true polymorphism).[253] Only traces of drug are excreted unchanged in urine.[251]

$t_{1/2}$. α phase 4–7 min; β phase 2 ± 0.4 hr.[251,252]

Adverse Reactions. Most side effects relate to vasodilatory actions and occur frequently; symptoms include dizziness (with or without hypotension), flushing, and headache. These types of side effects seem less frequent with SR dosage forms.[254] Immediate-release products may increase mortality when used to treat hypertension.[247] Edema occurs frequently and is related to venous pooling and usually not exacerbation of CHF. Nifedipine can paradoxically worsen anginal chest pain, possibly because of a reflex increase in sympathetic tone or redistribution of coronary blood flow away from ischemic areas. Acute, reversible renal failure may occur in patients with chronic renal insufficiency;[247,255] rare reactions include hepatitis and hyperglycemia.

Contraindications. Symptomatic hypotension.

Precautions. Use with caution in unstable angina pectoris when used alone (ie, without a β-blocker) and in patients with CHF caused by systolic dysfunction, because mortality may be increased.[247,256] Do not use immediate-release products to treat hypertension. Nifedipine has an antiplatelet action and may increase bleeding time.[257] Nifedipine may worsen symptoms of obstructive cardiomyopathy.

Drug Interactions. Barbiturates increase nifedipine metabolism. Cimetidine may increase nifedipine serum levels. Nifedipine occasionally increases PT in patients on oral anticoagulants. Nifedipine and IV magnesium sulfate may cause neuromuscular blockade and hypotension.

Parameters to Monitor. Blood pressure and heart rate, especially when initiating therapy. Observe for symptoms of hypotension and edema. Serial treadmill exercise tests can be performed to assess efficacy.

Notes. Other potential uses for nifedipine include migraine prophylaxis, achalasia, and Raynaud's phenomenon.

VERAPAMIL HYDROCHLORIDE   Calan, Covera-HS, Isoptin, Verelan, Various

Pharmacology. Verapamil is a calcium-channel blocking drug that prolongs AV nodal conduction. It is used to convert reentrant supraventricular tachycardias and to slow ventricular rate in atrial fibrillation or flutter. Because it decreases contractility and arteriolar resistance, it is used in angina caused by coronary obstruction or vasospasm. Verapamil is also effective in the treatment of hypertension and hypertrophic obstructive cardiomyopathy, and in migraine prophylaxis. (*See* Calcium-Channel Blocking Drugs Comparison Chart.)

Administration and Adult Dosage. PO for angina 80–120 mg tid initially, increasing at daily (for unstable angina) or weekly intervals, to a maximum of 480 mg/day. Covera-HS is designed to be taken hs. **PO for hypertension** usually 240 mg/day using SR tablet; SR dosages of 120 mg/day to 240 mg bid have been used. Covera-HS is designed to be taken hs. **PO for migraine prophylaxis** 160–320 mg/day. **IV for supraventricular arrhythmias** 5–10 mg (0.075–0.15 mg/kg) over at least 2 min (3 min in elderly), may repeat with 10 mg (0.15 mg/kg) in 30 min if arrhythmia is not terminated or desired end point is not achieved. **IV constant infusion** 5–10 mg/hr.[258]

Special Populations. *Pediatric Dosage.* PO 4–8 mg/kg/day in 3 divided doses. **IV** (<1 yr) 0.1–0.2 mg/kg; (1–15 yr) 0.1–0.3 mg/kg, to a maximum of 5 mg over 2–3 min initially, may repeat with same dose in 30 min if initial response inadequate.[99]

Geriatric Dosage. Same as adult dosage, but administer over 3 min.

Other Conditions. Dosage may need to be decreased in patients with liver disease; titrate to clinical response.[259,260]

Dosage Forms. **Tab** 40, 80, 120 mg; **SR Tab** 120, 180, 240 mg; **SR Cap** 120, 180, 240 mg; **Inj** 2.5 mg/mL; **SR Tab** 180 mg with trandolapril 2 mg, 240 mg with trandolapril 4 mg (Tarka).

Patient Instructions. Report any dizziness, shortness of breath, or edema. Constipation occurs often. Maintain a diary to document the number of episodes of chest pain and sublingual nitroglycerin used.

Pharmacokinetics. *Onset and Duration.* IV onset immediate; duration 2–6 hr, up to 12 hr with long-term use.[259,260]

Serum Levels. 50–400 μg/L (100–800 nmol/L), although therapeutic range is not well established.

Fate. Although the drug is well absorbed orally, only 22 ± 8% is bioavailable because of extensive first-pass elimination; bioavailability increases in liver disease.[259,261] Covera-HS provides a 4- to 5-hr delay before releasing the drug. Verapamil has stereospecific pharmacology and pharmacokinetics; l-verapamil is a more potent AV nodal blocking drug, but it undergoes greater first-pass metabolism.[262] Norverapamil is an active metabolite. Verapamil is about 90 ± 2% plasma protein bound, with the more active l-isomer having a greater unbound fraction.[261,263] V_d is 5 ± 2 L/kg and increases in liver disease;[9,264] Cl is 0.9 ± 0.36 L/hr/kg. About 1% is excreted unchanged in urine.[9]

$t_{1/2}$. (Verapamil) α phase 5–30 min; ß phase 4 ± 1.5 hr;[9,261,264] may increase during long-term use;[264] 13.6 ± 3.9 hr in severe liver disease;[261] (norverapamil) 8 ± 1.9 hr.[261,263]

Adverse Reactions. Constipation occurs frequently (5–40%), particularly in elderly patients.[247,263] CHF may occur in patients with left ventricular dysfunction. Serious hemodynamic side effects (eg, severe hypotension) and conduction abnormalities (eg, symptomatic bradycardia or asystole) have been reported; these reactions usually occur when the patient is concurrently receiving a ß-blocker or has underlying conduction disease.[265] Infants appear to be particularly susceptible to arrhythmias.[247] IV **calcium** (gluconate or chloride salts, 10–20 mL of a 10% solution) and/or **isoproterenol** may, in part, reverse these adverse effects.[265] The administration of IV calcium prior to verapamil may prevent hypotension without abolishing the antiarrhythmic actions.[266]

Contraindications. Shock or severely hypotensive states; second- or third-degree AV nodal block; sick sinus syndrome, unless functioning ventricular pacemaker is in place; hypotension or CHF unless caused by supraventricular tachyarrhythmias amenable to verapamil therapy; atrial fibrillation and an accessory AV pathway.

Precautions. Use caution with any wide-QRS tachycardia; severe hypotension and shock may ensue if the tachycardia is ventricular in origin. Use with caution in combination with oral ß-blockers and poor left ventricular function.

Drug Interactions. Verapamil may increase serum levels of several drugs, including carbamazepine, cyclosporine, digoxin, and theophylline. Barbiturates and rifampin may increase verapamil metabolism.

Parameters to Monitor. Blood pressure and constant ECG monitoring during IV administration. Pay particular attention to signs and symptoms of CHF and hypotension. Also, monitor the ECG for PR prolongation and bradycardia.

CALCIUM CHANNEL BLOCKING DRUGS COMPARISON CHART

DRUG	DOSAGE FORMS	ADULT DOSAGE	CONTRACTILITY	HEART RATE	AV NODAL CONDUCTION	VASCULAR RESISTANCE
Amlodipine[a] Norvasc	Tab 2.5, 5, 10 mg.	PO 5–10 mg/day.	0	0	0	→
Bepridil[b] Vasocor	Tab 200, 300, 400 mg.	PO for angina 200–400 mg/day.	0/↓	0/↓	0/↓	→
Cinnarizine[c] (Investigation, Janssen)	—	PO 25–75 mg/day.	0	0	0	→
Diltiazem[d] Cardizem Dilacor XR	See monograph.	See monograph.	→	→	→	→
Felodipine[a] Plendil	SR Tab 2.5, 5 10 mg.	PO for hypertension 5–20 mg once daily.	0/↑	0/↑	0/↑	↓↓
Flunarizine[c] (Investigation, Janssen)	—	PO 5–10 mg once daily.	0	0	0	→
Gallopamil[d] (Investigational)	—	PO 50 mg tid–100 mg bid.	→	→	→	→
Isradipine[a] DynaCirc	Cap 2.5, 5 mg.	PO for hypertension 2.5–10 mg bid.	0/↑	0/↑	0/↑	↓↓
Nicardipine[a] Cardene	Cap 20, 30 mg SR Cap 30, 45, 60 mg Inj 2.5 mg/mL.	PO for angina or hypertension 20–40 mg tid or SR 30–60 mg q 12 hr.	0/↑	0/↑	0/↑	↓↓

(continued)

291

CALCIUM CHANNEL BLOCKING DRUGS COMPARISON CHART (continued)

DRUG	DOSAGE FORMS	ADULT DOSAGE	CONTRACTILITY	HEART RATE	AV NODAL CONDUCTION	VASCULAR RESISTANCE
Nifedipine[a] Adalat Procardia	Cap 10, 20 mg SR Tab 30, 60, 90 mg.	*See monograph.*	0/↑	0/↑	0/↑	↓↓
Nimodipine[a] Nimotop	Cap 30 mg.	PO post-subarachnoid hemorrhage 60 mg q 4 hr for 21 days.	0/↑	0/↑	0/↑	↓↓
Nisoldipine[a] Sular	SR Tab 10, 20, 30, 40 mg.	PO for hypertension SR 20–40 mg once daily.	0/↑	0/↑	0/↑	↓↓
Verapamil[d] Calan Isoptin Verelan	*See monograph.*	*See monograph.*	↓↓	→	↓↓	→

KEY: ↑ = increase; ↓ = decrease, 0 = no change.
[a]Predominantly vascular actions.
[b]Complex pharmacology with probable sodium and potassium channel blockade (quinidinelike).
[c]Selective vascular actions.
[d]Vascular and electrophysiologic actions.
From reference 267 in part.

Hypolipidemic Drugs

Class Instructions: Hypolipidemics. There is a strong relationship between elevated serum cholesterol and death caused by coronary heart disease (CHD). Cholesterol lowering has been demonstrated to decrease events related to CHD and may slow or even reverse atherosclerosis. These effects are associated with a decrease in CHD mortality. Generally, each 1% decrease in serum cholesterol results in a 2% decrease in the risk of coronary events. Hypolipidemic drugs must be taken daily to achieve these results. Drug therapy does not eliminate the need for appropriate diet and other measures such as weight reduction (if appropriate), smoking cessation, and physical activity. Hypolipidemic drug therapy (with the exception of niacin) has been associated with an increase in cancer in animals, but it is not known if they have this effect in humans.

CHOLESTYRAMINE RESIN
Questran, Various

Pharmacology. Cholestyramine is a bile acid sequestrant that acts as an anion exchange resin, releasing chloride ions and adsorbing bile acids in the intestine to form a nonabsorbable complex that is excreted in the feces. The resulting increase in activity of hepatic low-density lipoprotein cholesterol (LDL-c) receptors leads to the oxidation of cholesterol to form new bile acids. Despite a compensatory increase in hepatic cholesterol synthesis, total serum cholesterol and LDL-c levels are reduced by 15–30%. The increase in cholesterol synthesis sometimes results in an increase in very low-density lipoprotein (VLDL) cholesterol levels, which may increase triglyceride levels by 10–50%.[268,269] Cardioprotective high-density lipoprotein (HDL) cholesterol levels may increase by 3–8%.[269]

Administration and Adult Dosage. **PO for hyperlipidemia** 4 g daily–bid initially, increasing slowly to a maintenance dosage of 8–16 g/day in 1–6 (usually 2) divided doses, to a maximum of 24 g/day. Compliance appears to be best in the range of 8–10 g/day in 1–2 divided doses. **PO for treatment of cholestatic pruritus** 4–8 g/day is usual. **PO for treatment of relapsing enterocolitis caused by** *Clostridium difficile* 4 g tid or qid (with or without vancomycin) has been used.

Special Populations. *Pediatric Dosage.* Limited data are available, especially concerning long-term use. Drug therapy is generally reserved for children 10 yr or older, initiated at the lowest possible dosage, and gradually increased until the desired response is achieved. Base initial dosage on serum LDL-c level rather than body weight, and adjust dosage based on response: **PO for hyperlipidemia** (LDL-c <195 mg/dL) 4 g/day; (LDL-c 195–235 mg/dL) 8 g/day; (LDL-c 236–280 mg/dL) 12 g/day; (LDL-c >280 mg/dL) 16 g/day.[270,271] (*See* Precautions.)

Geriatric Dosage. Initiate therapy at lowest possible dosage, and slowly titrate to desired effect. Maximum dosage may not be required or tolerated.

Other Conditions. In patients with a history of constipation, start at the low end of the dosage range. In patients with GI intolerance, reduce dosage and increase gradually (*see* Adverse Reactions).

Dosage Forms. Pwdr 4 g resin/9 g powder (Questran); 4 g resin/5 g powder (Questran Light).

Patient Instructions. (*See* Hypolipidemics Class Instructions.) It is preferable to take this drug before meals, but you may adjust the time of the dosages around the scheduling of other oral medications. Take other oral medications at least 1 hour before or 4–6 hours after cholestyramine. Do not take dry; mix each packet or level scoopful with at least 60–180 mL (2–6 fl oz) of water or noncarbonated beverage, highly fluid soup, or pulpy fruit such as applesauce or crushed pineapple. You may need to experiment with different products and vehicles to determine your preference based on taste, cost, and caloric restrictions. Mixtures may be refrigerated to improve palatability, but do not cook because the drug may be inactivated.[268] This drug frequently causes constipation. If this becomes a problem, contact your physician or pharmacist to discuss measures to potentially minimize constipation. It may cause other gastrointestinal symptoms, which usually decrease over time.

Pharmacokinetics. *Onset and Duration.* Reduction in cholesterol begins in the first month.

Fate. It is not absorbed from the GI tract. Resin and complex are excreted in the feces.

Adverse Reactions. Almost 70% of patients experience at least one GI side effect.[272] Constipation frequently occurs, especially with higher dosages, in the elderly, and in patients with previous constipation; fecal impaction is rare. Nausea, heartburn, abdominal pain, bloating, steatorrhea, and belching also occur frequently, but tend to decrease over time.[268] GI side effects tend to be milder in children than in adults. Hemorrhoids may be aggravated or develop. Rash may occur. Chloride absorption in place of bicarbonate may lead to hyperchloremic acidosis, especially in children, and calcium excretion may be increased. Absorption of vitamins D and K may be impaired, leading to osteomalacia and bleeding, respectively. Absorption of folic acid may also be impaired, especially in children. Alimentary cancers in rats are somewhat more prevalent with cholestyramine treatment because of enhancement of other carcinogens, but the importance of this in humans is unknown.[273]

Contraindications. Complete biliary obstruction.

Precautions. Pregnancy and lactation, caused by possible malabsorption of fat-soluble vitamins. Avoid constipation in patients with symptomatic coronary artery disease. Constipation may be controlled by reducing dosage, slowly titrating dosage, increasing dietary fiber, or using stool softeners. Avoid use in the presence of diverticular disease and local intestinal tract lesions because constipation may be a problem.[274] Discontinue if a clinically important elevation in serum triglycerides occurs. Vitamin supplementation may be needed with high dosage or long-term therapy. Children particularly may need multivitamins with folate and iron.[271] Patients with osteoporosis may need to restrict dietary chloride to limit calcium excretion.[275] Phenylketonurics should avoid Questran Light because it contains aspartame.

Drug Interactions. Absorption of many drugs may be delayed or reduced, including acetaminophen, coumarin anticoagulants, digitoxin (affected to a greater extent than digoxin), digoxin, furosemide, gemfibrozil, hydrocortisone, oral hypo-glycemic drugs,[276] iron, loperamide, methotrexate, naproxen, penicillin G, pheno-barbital, oral phosphate supplements, pravastatin, propranolol, tetracyclines, thy-roid hormones, thiazides, and vancomycin. Monitor for concurrent drug therapy effects when initiating and altering sequestrant therapy, particularly for drugs with a narrow therapeutic index.

Parameters to Monitor. Monitor LDL-c and triglycerides 4 weeks and 3 months after initiation of therapy. If therapy goals are achieved, monitor q 4 months un-less adverse effects are suspected. Periodically monitor hemoglobin and serum folic acid during long-term therapy. Monitor efficacy of and appropriate tests for concurrent drug therapy that may be affected by cholestyramine. In children, mon-itor serum concentrations of vitamins A, D, and E and erythrocyte folate, liver function tests, and CBC annually.[271]

Notes. Bile acid sequestering resins are indicated as an adjunct to diet for primary hypercholesterolemia (type IIa and IIb) in patients for whom hypertriglyceridemia is not a primary concern (triglyceride levels <300 mg/dL).[275] Bile acid seques-trants produce moderate lowering of LDL-c relative to some of the other hypolipi-demic drugs, but are considered to be safer because they are not absorbed. These drugs may be particularly useful with moderately elevated LDL-c and in situations of lower risk of CHD when long-term safety is of concern (eg, primary prevention and in young men and premenopausal women).[268,277] They may be used in combi-nation with other hypolipidemic drugs for additive effects when a larger decrease in LDL-c is required. Long-term use reduces cardiovascular morbidity and mor-tality, including the incidence of first heart attacks. Because over one-third of pa-tients discontinue bile acid sequestrants in the first year, primarily because of ad-verse effects, conservative dosage titration as well as education and support is required to manage and avoid adverse effects.[272,278] Maximum dosage is rarely needed.[269] Low-dose therapy (8–10 g/day) appears to be best tolerated[268] and the most cost-effective, either alone or in combination therapy.[279] Increased dosage may increase adverse effects without meaningful increases in cholesterol lower-ing. Resins are not effective in patients with homozygous familial hypercholes-terolemia.[269] (*See* Recommendations for Initiation of Drug Therapy in Hypercho-lesterolemia Chart.)

The resins are also used for reduction of pruritus caused by dermal deposition of bile acids in patients with partial biliary obstruction, and cholestyramine has been used to treat relapsing *Clostridium difficile* colitis.[280–282] Interference with digoxin and digitoxin absorption suggests a possible role in managing mild intoxi-cation caused by these drugs; however, do not rely on cholestyramine alone in cases of severe digitalis toxicity.[276] Questran contains 14 kcal/9 g packet or scoop; Questran Light is flavored with aspartame and contains 1.6 kcal and 16.8 mg of phenylalanine/5 g packet or scoop.

COLESTIPOL HYDROCHLORIDE
Colestid

Colestipol is a bile acid sequestrant similar to cholestyramine. Its lipid-lowering effects are equivalent to cholestyramine in most patients. Selection of a bile acid sequestrant is generally based on patient preference and cost. Cholestyramine-vehicle combinations are often more palatable than colestipol granules, although colestipol tablets are well tolerated. Patients with moderate hypercholesteremia who are unable to tolerate colestipol because of GI side effects may benefit from a trial of one-half the colestipol dose mixed with 2.5 g of psyllium. One study showed this combination was better tolerated and had similar efficacy. LDL-c reduction is proportionally greater in moderate hypercholesterolemia than in severe hypercholesterolemia. Adverse effects, precautions, monitoring instructions, and drug interactions are similar to cholestyramine. A 5-g dose of colestipol provides a degree of cholesterol lowering equivalent to 4 g of cholestyramine; a 4-g dose of the tablet formulation is approximately equivalent to 5 g of the granules. Dosage of the granules is 5 g bid initially, increasing in 5 g/day increments at 1- to 2-month intervals, to a maximum of 30 g/day in 1–4 doses. For tablets, dosage is 2 g bid, increased in 2 g/day increments at 1- to 2-month intervals, to a maximum of 16 g/day. For treatment of relapsing enterocolitis caused by *Clostridium difficile* 5 g q 12 hr has been used with vancomycin; avoid coadministration with vancomycin to prevent vancomycin binding.[283–289] Available as granules in 5-g packets and bulk containers or as 1-g tablets. (*See* Hypolipidemic Drugs Comparison Chart, and Recommendations for Initiation of Drug Therapy in Hypercholesterolemia Chart.)

GEMFIBROZIL   Lopid, Various

Pharmacology. Gemfibrozil is a fibric acid derivative that decreases triglyceride and VLDL-c concentrations and increases HDL-c concentrations. Effects on LDL-c are variable. LDL-c may increase in some patients, especially those with type IV hyperlipoproteinemia. Its exact mechanism is unclear; however, it appears to act through multiple mechanisms.[290] There is an increased secretion of cholesterol into bile, increased affinity of LDL receptors for LDL particles, activation of lipoprotein lipase, inhibition of triglyceride synthesis, suppression of free fatty acid release from adipose tissue, and a change in LDL-c toward a potentially less atherosclerotic form.[269,290]

Administration and Adult Dosage. PO as an hypolipidemic 600 mg bid.

Special Populations. *Pediatric Dosage.* Safety and efficacy not established.

Geriatric Dosage. Initiate therapy at lowest possible dosage, and slowly titrate to desired effect. Maximum dosage may not be required or tolerated.

Other Conditions. Some advise decreasing dose by one-half with Cl_{cr} of 20–50 mL/min.

Dosage Forms. Tab 600 mg.

Patient Instructions. Take doses 30 minutes prior to morning and evening meals. Gemfibrozil may cause a slightly increased risk of cancer and is similar to another medication that has been found to increase the risk of cancer, gallstones, and pancreatitis. You and your physician may decide the benefit of reducing the risk of coronary heart disease may be worth these other risks. Report any muscle pain, tenderness, or weakness promptly, especially if you are also taking lovastatin or a similar drug.

Pharmacokinetics. *Onset and Duration.* The maximum decrease in serum triglyceride and total cholesterol occurs within 4–12 weeks; lipids return to pretreatment levels after drug discontinuation.

Fate. The drug is rapidly and completely absorbed after oral administration. Mean peak serum concentrations of 15–25 mg/L (60–100 μmol/L) occur within 1–2 hr after administration of 600 mg bid.[291] Serum concentrations are directly proportional to dose. The drug is 97–98.6% bound to albumin. Cl appears to be independent of renal function, but further study may be needed. Gemfibrozil is metabolized in the liver to a number of compounds. Approximately 70% of a dose is excreted in the urine, primarily as the glucuronide conjugates of the drug and metabolites; less than 2% is excreted renally as unchanged drug.[291-293]

$t_{1/2}$. Reportedly 1.5–2 hr, but may be longer allowing for complete distribution.[291]

Adverse Reactions. Dyspepsia (20%), abdominal pain (10%), diarrhea (7%), fatigue (3%), and nausea and vomiting (3%) are frequent; acute appendicitis, dizziness, eczema, rash, vertigo, constipation, headache, paresthesia (all between 1 and 2%) also occur. Occasional side effects include atrial fibrillation and elevations in liver function tests (AST, ALT, LDH, bilirubin, alkaline phosphatase), which return to normal upon drug discontinuation. Occasional mild decreases in WBCs, hematocrit, and hemoglobin occur, but usually stabilize. However, there are rare reports of severe blood dyscrasias. Serum glucose may be slightly elevated, as may LDL-c in some patients with high triglyceride levels. Gemfibrozil may increase biliary lipogenicity and possibly increase long-term risk of cholelithiasis.[269] Cholelithiasis requiring gallbladder surgery developed in 0.9% of gemfibrozil-treated patients, compared to 0.5% of patients in a placebo group. This excess was similar to that which occurs with clofibrate (*see* Notes.) An acute infectionlike syndrome characterized by arthralgias, myalgia, and myositis has occurred during therapy. Rhabdomyolysis with elevated creatine kinase levels may precipitate acute renal failure, especially with the combination of gemfibrozil and lovastatin.[274] This has occurred as early as after several weeks to months of therapy. Routine monitoring of creatine kinase may not detect rhabdomyolysis in a timely manner. Many recommend avoiding the combination of gemfibrozil and any HMG-CoA reductase inhibitor.[276] Worsening of renal insufficiency has been reported with an initial Cr_s over 2 mg/dL. Carcinogenesis, impairment of fertility, and development of cataracts occur in rats (*see* Precautions and Notes.)

Contraindications. Hepatic or severe renal dysfunction; primary biliary cirrhosis; preexisting gallbladder disease.

Precautions. Pregnancy, lactation. Evaluate any reports of muscle pain, tenderness, or weakness for myositis, including a determination of serum creatine kinase. Discontinue if an adequate effect does not occur after 3 months, if cholelithiasis is suspected, or if liver function tests remain elevated.

Drug Interactions. Gemfibrozil may potentiate the effect of oral anticoagulants. Cholesterol-binding resins may decrease absorption of gemfibrozil. Insulin or an oral hypoglycemic may be required.[291,293] Displacement of glyburide from plasma protein binding sites, producing hypoglycemia, has been reported.[294] Gemfibrozil and lovastatin (and possibly other HMG-CoA reductase inhibitors) together may have an increased risk of myotoxicity (*see* Adverse Reactions).

Parameters to Monitor. Serum lipids, initially every few weeks, then approximately q 3 months.[277] Liver function tests and CBC q 3–6 months. Monitor serum glucose if patient is receiving insulin or an oral hypoglycemic and prothrombin time if patient is taking an oral anticoagulant.

Notes. Gemfibrozil is not considered a major treatment for hypercholesteremia because of its effects on LDL-c, but it does increase HDL-c and decrease triglycerides, so it is useful in some patients.[268] Gemfibrozil is indicated for the treatment of types IV and V hyperlipidemias with very high serum triglycerides (usually >2000 mg/dL) in patients at risk for pancreatitis and not responding to diet. It is also indicated in type IIb patients (only those without a history or symptoms of CHD) with low HDL-c and an inadequate response to weight loss, diet, exercise, and other drugs that raise HDL-c (eg, bile acid sequestrants, niacin), but is not indicated in type I or IIa hyperlipidemias or in those patients who have a low HDL-c only. The Helsinki Heart Study showed a 34% reduction in the incidence of CHD in middle-aged men (initially without CHD symptoms) treated with gemfibrozil in a 5-yr study, although total death rate was no different between treated and placebo groups.[295,296] A substudy of the Helsinki Heart Study showed an increase in gallstone and gallbladder surgery in gemfibrozil-treated patients. After a 3.5-yr extension of this study, all-cause mortality was slightly higher in the original gemfibrozil group, primarily because of cancer deaths.[296] An ancillary study of the Helsinki Heart Study investigated the use of gemfibrozil in patients with signs or symptoms of CHD.[297] The rate of serious adverse cardiac advents and total mortality with gemfibrozil treatment did not significantly differ from placebo; however, information on key prognostic indicators and their distribution was not known.[297] Gemfibrozil is chemically and pharmacologically similar to **clofibrate.** A 44% relative increase in age-adjusted, all-cause mortality occurred in a study of long-term clofibrate use related to an 33% increase in noncardiovascular disease such as malignancy, gall bladder disease, and pancreatitis. Because of the smaller size of the gemfibrozil studies, the increase in mortality in the gemfibrozil group relative to placebo may not be statistically significantly different from the excess mortality associated with clofibrate use.

HMG-CoA REDUCTASE INHIBITORS:	
FLUVASTATIN	Lescol
LOVASTATIN	Mevacor
PRAVASTATIN	Pravachol
SIMVASTATIN	Zocor

Pharmacology. Hydroxymethylglutaryl-CoA (HMG-CoA) reductase inhibitors competitively inhibit conversion of HMG-CoA to mevalonate, an early, rate-limiting step in cholesterol synthesis. A compensatory increase in LDL receptors, which bind and remove circulating LDL-c, results. Production of LDL-c may also be decreased because of decreased production of VLDL or increased VLDL removal by LDL receptors. These drugs produce dose-dependent, maximum reductions in LDL of 30–40% and triglycerides of 10–30%, and increases in HDL levels of 2–15%.[269,298,299] Drug effects are dose dependent until the following doses are reached: 20 mg for fluvastatin and simvastatin, 40 mg for lovastatin and pravastatin. Fluvastatin is about 30% less effective in lowering lipids than the other drugs.[269,300]

Administration and Adult Dosage. Adjust dosage at no less than 4-week intervals. **PO for hyperlipidemia** (Fluvastatin) 20 mg hs initially, increasing to 40 mg/day; a slight increase in fluvastatin LDL-c lowering occurs with a bid schedule. (Lovastatin) 20 mg (40 mg with serum cholesterol >300 mg/dL) with the evening meal initially. Start with 10 mg/day in patients requiring <20% decrease in LDL-c or when concurrent use with cyclosporine is unavoidable. Increase to a maintenance dosage of 20–80 mg/day. Do not exceed a lovastatin dosage of 20 mg/day when used with cyclosporine. (Pravastatin) 10–20 mg hs initially, increasing to 10–40 mg/day hs. (Simvastatin) 5–10 mg/day in the evening initially, increasing to 5–40 mg/day in the evening.

Special Populations. *Pediatric Dosage.* Safety and efficacy not established.

Geriatric Dosage. PO (Pravastatin) 10 mg/day initially; (Simvastatin) 5 mg/day initially; the elderly may achieve maximal reductions in LDL-c at doses ≤20 mg/day. Maximum dosage may not be required or tolerated.

Other Conditions. (Lovastatin) start with 10 mg/day when concurrent use with cyclosporine is unavoidable; maximum dosage is 20 mg/day with concurrent immunosuppressant therapy. (Pravastatin) start with 10 mg/day with renal or hepatic impairment and in patients concurrently taking cyclosporine; do not exceed a dose of 20 mg/day in the latter case. (Simvastatin) start with 5 mg/day in patients requiring <20% reductions in LDL-c and with severe renal insufficiency. Use dosages >20 mg/day only with extreme caution in patients with a Cl_{cr} <30 mL/min.

Dosage Forms. (*See* Hypolipidemic Drugs Comparison Chart.)

Patient Instructions. (See Hypolipidemics Class Instructions.) Take the dose in the evening for the best effect. Take lovastatin with the evening meal to increase its absorption; other drugs can be taken without regard to meals. Take pravastatin 1 hour before or 4 hours after a dose of a cholesterol-binding resin. Promptly report any unexplained muscle pain or tenderness, especially if accompanied by malaise or fever. Avoid excessive concurrent use of alcohol, but abstinence is not required. Do not take these drugs during pregnancy because of possible harm to the fetus. Inform your physician if you become or intend to become pregnant.

Pharmacokinetics. *Onset and Duration.* Onset is within 2 weeks; peak effect is within 4–6 weeks; cholesterol levels return to baseline after drug discontinuation.

Fate. Absorption is rapid. Lovastatin and simvastatin are prodrugs that undergo extensive first-pass metabolism to active metabolites. Serum concentrations of the active lovastatin metabolite when taken under fasting conditions are two-thirds of that when taken with food. Absorption of other drugs is unaffected by food. Systemic bioavailability of all drugs is low because of extensive (>60%) first-pass extraction. Peak serum concentrations of active inhibitors are achieved in 1–4 hr for all drugs. Protein binding is 55–60% for pravastatin, 95% for simvastatin, >95% for lovastatin, and 98% for fluvastatin. Lovastatin and simvastatin are lipophilic and cross the blood-brain barrier; fluvastatin and pravastatin are hydrophilic and do not. All the drugs are primarily (>70%) hepatically metabolized to active and inactive metabolites, which then undergo extensive fecal elimination. Renal elimination accounts for 5% of fluvastatin, 10% of lovastatin, 13% of simvastatin, and 20% of pravastatin. Severe renal insufficiency (Cl_{cr} 10–30 mL/min) results in a twofold increase in serum concentrations of lovastatin inhibitors.[268,299–305]

$t_{1/2}$. <2 hr for all drugs.[299,300]

Adverse Reactions. The drugs are generally well tolerated, with discontinuation rates less than other hypolipidemic drugs.[278] The frequency of side effects appears to be similar for all drugs.[299–306] GI complaints such as diarrhea, constipation, flatulence, abdominal pain, and nausea occur in about 5% of patients. Headache (4–9%), rash (3–5%), dizziness (3–5%), and blurred vision (1–2%) are other frequent side effects. Myopathy and myositis occur rarely with single therapy and may be associated with mild elevations of CPK. Rhabdomyolysis leading to acute renal failure is a rare complication, but occurs more frequently in combination with gemfibrozil, cyclosporine, or ≥1 g/day of niacin. Pravastatin may cause less myopathy than lovastatin with cyclosporine.[300] Increases in liver function tests >3 times normal occur in up to 2% of patients, but most are asymptomatic and reverse with discontinuation.[269] Anomalies have been reported with intrauterine exposure. Carcinogenicity occurs in mice and rats at higher than human doses, but the clinical implications are unclear.[273,307]

Contraindications. Pregnancy; lactation; active liver disease; unexplained persistent elevations of serum transaminases.

Precautions. Administer to women of childbearing age only when possibility of becoming pregnant is unlikely. Use with caution in patients who consume substantial quantities of alcohol and/or have a history of liver disease. Discontinue therapy if liver function tests are >3 times normal. Consider withholding the drug in any patient with risk factors for renal failure secondary to rhabdomyolysis, such as severe acute infection; hypotension; major surgery or trauma; severe electrolyte, endocrine, or metabolic abnormalities; or uncontrolled seizures.

Drug Interactions. Myositis and rhabdomyolysis may be more common in combination with cyclosporine (lovastatin levels are quadrupled), erythromycin, gemfibrozil, itraconazole, ketoconazole (and possibly other inhibitors of CYP3A4), or lipid-lowering dosages of niacin (>1 g/day).[300] HMG-CoA reductase inhibitors may increase the effect of warfarin. Bile acid sequestrants may markedly decrease pravastatin oral bioavailability when taken together; take pravastatin 1 hr before or 4 hr after resin doses.

Parameters to Monitor. Obtain serum lipid and liver function tests on initiation, 6 and 12 weeks after initiation, after dosage increases, and at least semiannually thereafter. Others recommend more frequent monitoring.[268,269] Increase the frequency of monitoring if adverse effects are suspected. Routine monitoring of muscle enzymes may not adequately identify patients at risk for rhabdomyolysis, but may be warranted in patients with skeletal muscle complaints and risk factors.

Notes. The HMG-CoA reductase inhibitors are indicated for the treatment of type IIa and IIb hyperlipoproteinemias. They are the most effective in decreasing

LDL-c, and their effect on decreasing coronary morbidity and mortality is proven.[300] The choice of drug depends on cost, amount of cholesterol lowering desired, and risk factors for CHD.[300] Lovastatin, pravastatin, and simvastatin are more effective than fluvastatin and are therefore preferable when a >25% reduction in LDL-c is required.[300,308,309] They may have additive effects with the bile acid sequestrants and have been used in combination with niacin and gemfibrozil (*see* Adverse Reactions and Drug Interactions). **Atorvastatin,** (Lipitor) has shown the greatest decrease in LDL-c of any single drug (25–61%) and appears promising in patients requiring large decreases in cholesterol, which are now only achieved with combination therapy. It has also produced decreases in triglycerides of up to 43% and is being investigated for type IV hyperlipidemias. Atorvastatin may also have a greater effect on VLDL than other HMG-CoA inhibitors.[310–312] Available as 10, 20, and 40 mg tablets.

NIACIN   Various

Pharmacology. Niacin (nicotinic acid), in dosages of 1 g/day or more, decreases serum total cholesterol, low-density and very low-density lipoprotein (LDL and VLDL) cholesterol, and triglycerides, and increases high-density lipopotein (HDL) cholesterol. Mean serum cholesterol and triglyceride levels are reduced by 10% and 26%, respectively. The mechanism for these effects is not entirely known, but may involve inhibition of lipolysis, reduced LDL and VLDL synthesis, and increased lipoprotein lipase activity.[313,314] Niacin consistently decreases lipoprotein (a).[268] **Niacinamide** (nicotinamide) does not have hypolipidemic effects and cannot be substituted for niacin.

Administration and Adult Dosage. PO as an hypolipidemic 250 mg/day with evening meal initially, increasing at 4- to 7-day intervals to 1.5–2 g/day in 3 divided doses. Continue this dosage for 2 months. If necessary, the dosage can then be increased at 2- to 4-week intervals to 1 g tid; the dose can be further increased if necessary to reach the desired clinical effect or the maximum tolerated dosage to a usual maximum of 2 g tid. Use of >3–4 g/day does not appear to increase efficacy appreciably and is associated with increased side effects.[314] If an **SR product** is substituted for an immediate-release form, reduce the dosage by one-half. Risk of hepatotoxicity increases at SR doses >1.5–3 g/day, and these are not recommended.[269]

Special Populations. *Pediatric Dosage.* Safety and efficacy not established. Although niacin is effective in reducing triglycerides and cholesterol in children and adolescents, adverse effects are common and can be severe. Some authors recommend niacin use be avoided in children or used only under close supervision by a lipid specialist if diet and bile acid sequestrants have failed.[270,315] In these cases, niacin should generally be used in combination with diet and a bile acid sequestrant if tolerated.[270] Close monitoring is necessary (*see* Adverse Reactions and Precautions).

Geriatric Dosage. Initiate therapy at lowest possible dosage, and slowly titrate to desired effect. Maximum dosage may not be required or tolerated.

Patient Instructions. Use only under medical supervision. Effects may differ with different preparations. Almost everyone experiences some flushing. Tolerance to flushing generally occurs with time. Taking 325 mg of aspirin or 200 mg of ibuprofen (or an equivalent dose of another nonsteroidal antiinflammatory drug) 30–60 minutes before each niacin dose may reduce flushing. Taking niacin with meals may also help minimize flushing and reduce GI upset. Avoid hot liquids or alcohol after taking a dose. Avoid interruptions in therapy; tolerance may be lost if therapy is interrupted, so slow resumuption of the usual dosage is recommended. Avoid sudden changes in posture if you are also taking medicine for high blood pressure. Report any persistent nausea.

Dosage Forms. **Tab** 25, 50, 100, 250, 500 mg; **Elxr** 10 mg/mL; **SR Cap** 125, 250, 300, 400, 500 mg; **SR Tab** 250, 500, 750 mg; **Inj** 100 mg/mL.

Pharmacokinetics. *Onset and Duration.* The onset of triglyceride and cholesterol reductions usually occurs within several days, although some studies have demonstrated a response after a single dose.[313] A return to pretreatment lipid levels occurs 2–6 weeks after drug discontinuation.

Fate. The drug is almost completely absorbed from standard formulations; peak serum levels 30–60 min after 1-g standard formulations are 15–30 µg/L (120–240 µmol/L). Niacin is largely metabolized in the liver to niacinamide (nicotinamide) and its derivatives (eg, nicotinuric acid), which may contribute to the lipid-lowering activity, especially after long-term use. The majority is excreted as unchanged drug or metabolites in urine.[313]

$t_{1/2}$. 20–48 min.[313]

Adverse Reactions. Dose-related flushing of the neck and face (usually in "blush" areas) occurs in almost all patients and is related to the rate of rise of serum levels rather than the absolute serum concentrations.[316] Tolerance may develop, but may be lost if therapy is interrupted. Administration with food, gradual upward dosage titration, use of an SR formulation, or premedication with 325 mg of aspirin or 200 mg of ibuprofen (or equivalent dose of another NSAID) 30–60 min before each dose may reduce flushing. Postural hypotension may occur, especially when niacin is used with antihypertensive drugs or when it is taken with alcohol or hot liquids. Vasodilatory effects may precipitate or aggravate angina. Rash, pruritus, and stomach discomfort also occur frequently; the latter may occur more commonly with SR preparations. Increases in AST, ALT, bilirubin, and LDH concentrations occur frequently and may be related to increasing the daily dosage by more than 2.5 g/month. Severe hepatotoxicity (hepatic necrosis) is rare and tends to occur with abrupt dosage increases, SR forms substituted for immediate-release products without dosage reduction, or brand interchange.[314] Hepatotoxicity can occur at low dosages (≤3 g/day) of SR products and as soon as 2 days after initiation.[317] Discontinue therapy if liver function tests remain over three times pretreatment values.[314]

Contraindications. Arterial hemorrhage; severe hypotension; hepatic dysfunction; unexplained elevations of transaminases, active peptic ulcer disease.

Precautions. Pregnancy; lactation. Use with caution in patients with gallbladder disease or a history of liver disease, unstable angina, gout, gouty arthritis, glaucoma, or diabetes.[269,318] Nausea may be a presenting sign of hepatotoxicity.[269] If the SR form is substituted for the immediate-release form, reduce dosage by about one-half. If use with an HMG-CoA reductase inhibitor is unavoidable, use with extreme caution. Some formulations contain tartrazine dye, which may cause allergic reactions in sensitive patients.

Drug Interactions. Concurrent use with HMG-CoA reductase inhibitors may increase the risk of rhabdomyolysis. Concurrent therapy with α-adrenergic blocking antihypertensives may result in hypotension. Diet and/or dosage of oral hypoglycemic drugs or insulin may require adjustment with concurrent niacin use. Hepatotoxic drugs may have additive effects.[268]

Parameters to Monitor. Monitor serum lipids q 2 weeks initially, then q 1–3 months. Periodic liver function tests, blood glucose, and serum uric acid levels are recommended, especially at dosages >1.5 g/day.[268] Obtain liver function tests at baseline and q 6–12 weeks for the first year, then semiannually unless hepatotoxicity is suspected.

Notes. Indicated for types II_a, II_b, III, IV, and V hyperlipoproteinemias. A reduction in sudden cardiac deaths and fatal and nonfatal MI occurs, as well as an 11% decrease in mortality (compared to placebo) in patients treated with niacin.[306] The cost of standard niacin formulations can be much lower than alternative drugs; the cost of SR products may be higher. SR products appear to have equal efficacy at lowering LDL-c at one-half the dosage of standard products, but the SR form may be less effective in lowering triglycerides or raising HDL at dosages equal to standard forms.[268,314, 319] Some advocate avoidance of SR preparations altogether for treatment of hyperlipidemia because of their potentially greater hepatotoxicity.[317, 319]

HYPOLIPIDEMIC DRUGS COMPARISON CHART

DRUG	DOSAGE FORMS	ADULT ORAL DOSAGE[a] INITIAL (I) MAINTENANCE (M)	RELATIVE EFFECT ON LIPIDS[b] LDL	HDL	TG	INDICATIONS BY WHO CATEGORY TYPE[c]	COMMENTS
BILE ACID SEQUESTRANTS							
Cholestyramine Questran Questran Light Various	Pwdr 4 g resin/9 g drug packet or scoop Pwdr 4 g resin/5 g packet or scoop.	(I) 4 g daily–bid. (M) 8–16 g/day in 1–6 doses, to a maximum of 24 g/day.[d]	↓↓	↑	↑	IIa	Constipation frequent. May be used in children. Numerous interactions. Decrease in mortality demonstrated. Take before meals.
Colestipol HCl Colestid	Gran 5 g resin/7.5 g packet or scoop Tab 1 g.	(I) (gran) 5 g daily–bid. (M) 15–30 g/day in 1–4 doses.[e]	↓↓	↑	↑	IIa	Similar to cholestyramine. *See* above.
FIBRIC ACID DERIVATIVES							
Gemfibrozil Lopid Various	Tab 600 mg.	(M) 600 mg bid.	↑↓	↑↑	↓↓↓	IIb, IV, V	Overall mortality rate with long- term therapy is increased. Take 30 min prior to A.M. and P.M. meals.
Clofibrate	Not recommended because of a large increase in overall mortality.						
NICOTINIC ACID							
Niacin Various	Tab 25, 50, 100, 250, 500 mg Inj 100 mg/mL Elxr 10 mg/mL SR Cap 125, 250, 300, 400, 500 mg[e] SR Tab 250, 500, 750 mg.[e]	(I) Titrate slowly. *See* monograph. (M) 1.5–3 g/day, to a maximum of 6 g/day.	↓↓	↑↑	↓↓↓	IIa, IIb, III, IV, V	Frequent flushing and GI side effects. Must titrate dosage slowly. Decrease in mortality demonstrated. Avoid SR products. Low cost. Take with food or milk.

(continued)

HYPOLIPIDEMIC DRUGS COMPARISON CHART (continued)

DRUG	DOSAGE FORMS	ADULT ORAL DOSAGE[a] INITIAL (I) MAINTENANCE (M)	RELATIVE EFFECT ON LIPIDS[b] LDL	HDL	TG	INDICATIONS BY WHO CATEGORY TYPE[c]	COMMENTS
HMG-CoA REDUCTASE INHIBITORS							
Atorvastatin Lipitor	Tab 10, 20, 40 mg.	10–80 mg/day.	↓↓↓↓↓	↑	↓↓↓	IIa, IIb	Most potent in homozygous lipidemia.
Fluvastatin Lescol	Cap 20, 40 mg.	(I) 20 mg q hs. (M) 20–40 mg q hs.	↓↓	↑	↓	IIa, IIb	Take without regard to meals. Monitor for myositis and hepatic dysfunction. Important drug interactions.
Lovastatin Mevacor	Tab 10, 20, 40 mg.	(I) 20 mg/day. (M) 20–80 mg/day in 1–2 divided doses.	↓↓↓	↑	↓↓	IIa, IIb	Take with evening meal. See Fluvastatin.
Pravastatin Pravachol	Tab 10, 20, 40 mg.	(I) 10–20 mg q hs. (M) 10–40 mg q hs.	↓↓↓	↑	↓↓	IIa, IIb	Take without regard to meals. See Fluvastatin.
Simvastatin Zocor	Tab 5, 10, 20, 40 mg.	(I) 5–10 mg q hs. (M) 5–40 mg/day.	↓↓↓	↑	↓↓	IIa, IIb	Take without regard to meals. See Fluvastatin.

LDL = serum low-density lipoprotein cholesterol, shown to have a graded, positive relationship with coronary heart disease (CHD); HDL = serum high-density lipoprotein, shown to have a cardioprotective effect against CHD; TG = serum triglycerides, which have a positive relationship to CHD.

[a]Clinical trials in the elderly are limited, but the drugs are considered effective. Base decision on drug treatment on life expectancy, concomitant disease, potential adverse effects, patient desire for treatment, quality of life, assessment of coronary heart disease risk, and cost. A conservative approach is recommended, generally initiating therapy at lowest possible dosage, slowly titrating to desired effect while closely monitoring possible side effects. Maximum dosage may not be required or tolerated.

[b]Arrows represent approximate relative effects based on results achieved with usual dosage. Study results vary because of differences in patient groups, administration schedules, dosage, and degree of hypercholesterolemia.

[c]World Health Organization (WHO) classification by characteristics of dyslipidemia.

[d]All dosages are expressed in terms of anhydrous resin.

[e]Do not substitute SR niacin products for an equal dosage of immediate-release products; use one-half the dosage of immediate-release products.

From references 277, 280–282, 293, 310–312, 320, 321.

RECOMMENDATIONS FOR INITIATION OF DRUG THERAPY IN HYPERCHOLESTEROLEMIA

Evaluate and treat other conditions that may contribute to hyperlipidemia prior to initiation of drug therapy. If possible, avoid drug therapy that may contribute to hyperlipidemia (eg, corticosteroids, isotretinoin, thiazides, anabolic steroids, some β-blockers, cyclosporine, and progestins). Patients should generally also receive an adequate trial of diet and other nonpharmacologic measures such as an increase in physical activity and weight reduction (if appropriate). If these methods fail, then drug therapy may be considered based on the patient's age, serum low-density lipoprotein cholesterol (LDL-c) concentrations, and risk factors for coronary heart disease (CHD) according to the following tables.

ADULT

PRIMARY PREVENTION (Patient currently without signs or symptoms of CHD) Consider drug therapy in men ≥35 yr and postmenopausal women[a] with the following LDL-c levels *and* risk factors:[c,b]

LDL-c	RISK FACTORS[d]	GOAL OF THERAPY
LDL-c ≥190 mg/dL (4.9 mmol/L)	Without any two other risk factors	LDL-c ≤160 mg/dL (4.1 mmol/L)
LDL-c ≥160 mg/dL (4.1 mmol/L)	With any two other risk factors	LDL-c ≤130 mg/dL (3.4 mmol/L)

SECONDARY PREVENTION (Patient currently with signs or symptoms of CHD)[e] Consider drug therapy in patients with the following LDL-c levels *and* risk factors:[c]

LDL-c	RISK FACTORS	GOAL OF THERAPY
LDL-c ≥130 mg/dL (3.4 mmol/L)	Established CHD/atherosclerotic disease	LDL-c ≤100 mg/dL (2.5 mmol/L)

(continued)

RECOMMENDATIONS FOR INITIATION OF DRUG THERAPY IN HYPERCHOLESTEROLEMIA (continued)

PEDIATRIC (Children and adolescents ≥10 yr)[f] Consider drug therapy in patients with the following LDL-c levels and risk factors:[g]

LDL-c	RISK FACTORS	MINIMUM GOAL OF THERAPY	IDEAL GOAL OF THERAPY
LDL-c ≥190 mg/dL (4.9 mmol/L)	Any or none	LDL-c ≤130 mg/dL (3.4 mmol/L)	LDL-c ≤110 mg/dL (2.9 mmol/L)
LDL-c ≥160 mg/dL (4.1 mmol/L)	Family history of CVD before age 55, or with two other risk factors[h]	LDL-c ≤130 mg/dL (3.4 mmol/L)	LDL-c ≤110 mg/dL (2.9 mmol/L)

[a]Estrogen replacement therapy can be an alternative or addition to hypolipidemic drug therapy in postmenopausal women.

[b]In men under 35 yr and premenopausal women without other risk factors, drug therapy can be delayed if LDL-c is 190–220 mg/dL (4.9–5.7 mmol/L).

[c]Use clinical judgment to individualize drug therapy in patients who do not meet the upper LDL-c criteria for drug therapy and have not achieved goal LDL-c levels after maximal efforts to decrease cholesterol (with diet, physical activity, and reduction of other risk factors). Consider potential benefit, side effects, degree of LDL-c elevation above goal, and cost. Low-dose bile acid sequestrant therapy may be useful in these patients.

[d]Risk factors for CHD include age, family history, smoking history, hypertension, diabetes, and HDL-c <35 mg/dL.

[e]Also screen family members of patients with severe hypercholesterolemia.

[f]Use clinical judgment regarding initiation of drug therapy in children <10 yr if cholesterol is extremely high.

[g]Complete a 6 month–1 yr trial of diet therapy before initiating drug therapy. Continue diet therapy even if drug therapy is initiated. Bile acid sequestrants are considered the drugs of choice due to their relative safety (see Cholestyramine).

[h]Before initiating drug therapy, make rigorous attempts to control risk factors.

From the National Cholesterol Education Program (NCEP), references 270 and 277.

Inotropic Drugs

AMRINONE LACTATE
Various, Inocor

Pharmacology. Amrinone increases cyclic AMP and calcium availability via the inhibition of phosphodiesterase III, which improves cardiac output through vasodilatory and positive inotropic actions.[322]

Administration and Adult Dosage. IV loading dose 0.5–1 mg/kg (usually 0.75 mg/kg) over 2–3 min, may repeat in 30 min based on response. **IV maintenance dosage by continuous infusion** 5–10 µg/kg/min.

Special Populations. *Pediatric Dosage.* Safety and efficacy not established;[323] however, the following dosage has been suggested.[145] **IV loading dosage** (neonates and infants) 3–4.5 mg/kg. **IV maintenance dosage by continuous infusion** (neonates) 3–5 µg/kg/min; (infants) 10 µg/kg/min.

Geriatric Dosage. Same as adult dosage.

Dosage Forms. Inj 5 mg/mL.

Pharmacokinetics. *Onset and Duration.* IV onset 2–5 min after bolus, peak 10 min, duration 60–90 min.[322]

Serum Levels. A level of 1.5–4 mg/L (8–21.3 µmol/L) is associated with therapeutic response. Although a correlation exists between amrinone levels and increased cardiac output, the clinical usefulness of serum level monitoring is questionable.[324,325]

Fate. Bioavailability is 93 ± 12%. The drug is 20–50% plasma protein bound; V_d is 1.8 ± 0.9 L/kg; Cl is 0.28 ± 0.1 L/hr/kg.[324] The drug is eliminated primarily by hepatic metabolism, with 30 ± 20% excreted in urine unchanged.[324]

$t_{1/2}$. α phase 1–5 min; β phase 4.3 ± 1.3 hr in normals, 7.3 ± 4.6 hr in CHF.[324,325]

Adverse Reactions. Dose-dependent, asymptomatic thrombocytopenia occurs frequently. Platelet counts return to normal within 2–4 days of discontinuing therapy; in some cases, this side effect may be reversible when dosage is maintained or reduced. Thrombocytopenia may be caused primarily by the metabolite N-acetylamrinone.[326] Nausea and vomiting are unusual with IV use.[322] Occasional side effects include nephrogenic diabetes insipidus, liver enzyme elevation, fever, taste disturbances, flulike syndrome, rash, and aggravation of underlying arrhythmias.[327,328]

Precautions. Caution in hypertrophic obstructive cardiomyopathy. One study suggests a decreased survival rate in patients on long-term amrinone therapy.[328] Use concomitant antiplatelet drugs with caution.

Drug Interactions. None known.

Parameters to Monitor. Continuous ECG and frequent vital signs. Invasive hemodynamic monitoring is necessary in seriously ill patients for adequate dosage titration.

Notes. Do not dilute with dextrose-containing solutions, but may infuse through dextrose-containing IV lines.

DOBUTAMINE HYDROCHLORIDE
Dobutrex, Various

Pharmacology. Dobutamine is a synthetic sympathomimetic amine that exists as the racemic mixture of an l-isomer with predominantly α-adrenergic agonist actions and a d-isomer that has β_1- and β_2-adrenergic agonist actions. The net clinical effect is typically that of a potent β_1-agonist with mild vasodilatory properties. At low dosages, it increases myocardial contractility without markedly increasing heart rate; this specificity is dose dependent and is lost at high dosages. Unlike dopamine, dobutamine does not release stored catecholamines, nor does it have any effect on dopaminergic receptors.[329–331]

Administration and Adult Dosage. IV for inotropic support, by infusion only (in any *non*alkaline IV fluid) 2.5 µg/kg/min initially, increasing gradually in 2.5 µg/kg/min increments up to 20 µg/kg/min, adjusting dosage to desired response. Maintenance dosages are typically 2–10 µg/kg/min.[332] Although dosages up to 40 µg/kg/min have been used, use dosages over 20 µg/kg/min with caution because of increased risks of tachycardia, arrhythmias, and myocardial ischemia.[333]

Special Populations. *Pediatric Dosage.* Safety and efficacy not established. However, **IV infusion** 2 µg/kg/min initially, followed by adjustment to desired hemodynamic response, up to 20 µg/kg/min, has been used.[334]

Geriatric Dosage. Same as adult dosage.

Dosage Forms. Inj 12.5 mg/mL.

Pharmacokinetics. *Onset and Duration.* Onset <2 min; peak within 10 min; duration <10 min.[335]

Fate. Wide interpatient variability exists, especially between adult and pediatric patients.[330] V_d in CHF is 0.2 ± 0.08 L/kg; Cl in CHF is 3.5 ± 1.3 L/hr/kg.[336] The drug is eliminated primarily in the liver to inactive glucuronide conjugates and 3-O-methyldobutamine.[329,336]

$t_{1/2}$. 2.4 ± 0.7 min.[336]

Adverse Reactions. Precipitation or exacerbation of ventricular ectopy occurs frequently; ventricular arrhythmias may occur (although these are less likely than with other sympathomimetics).[330] Modest increases in heart rate or systolic blood pressure occur frequently; dosage reduction usually reverses these effects rapidly. Occasionally, nausea, headache, angina, nonspecific chest pain, palpitations, and shortness of breath are noted. Patients with atrial fibrillation may be at risk of developing rapid ventricular responses because dobutamine facilitates AV conduction.

Contraindications. Idiopathic hypertrophic subaortic stenosis.

Precautions. Correct hypovolemia before using in patients who are hypotensive. Although most cases of extravasation cause no signs of tissue damage, at least one case of dermal necrosis following extravasation of a 2.5 µg/kg/min infusion has been reported. Dobutamine contains a sulfite preservative, which may be problematic in sensitive individuals, especially asthmatics.

Drug Interactions. Bretylium, guanethidine, and heterocyclic antidepressants may potentiate the pressor response to direct-acting vasopressors. Oxytocics used in obstetrics may cause severe, persistent hypertension when used with vasopressors.

Halogenated hydrocarbon anesthetics may predispose patients to serious arrhythmias.

Parameters to Monitor. Monitor heart rate, arterial blood pressure, urine output, pulmonary capillary wedge pressure, cardiac index, ECG for ectopic activity, and infusion rate of solution continuously in the acute care setting and during periods of dosage titration or adjustment.

Notes. The drug is physically incompatible with sodium bicarbonate and other alkaline solutions. Use the reconstituted solution within 24 hr. (*See* Sympathomimetic Drugs for Hemodynamic Support Comparison Chart.)

DOBUTAMINE DILUTION GUIDE

AMOUNT ADDED		VOLUME OF	FINAL
(mg)	*Volume (reconstituted)*	DILUENT	CONCENTRATION*
250	1 vial (20 mL)	1000 mL	250 mg/L
250	1 vial (20 mL)	500 mL	500 mg/L
250	1 vial (20 mL)	250 mL	1 g/L

*Recommended concentrations, but concentrations up to 5 g/L have been used.

DOPAMINE HYDROCHLORIDE   Dopastat, Intropin, Various

Pharmacology. Dopamine is a catecholamine that acts directly, in a dose-dependent fashion, on postsynaptic dopaminergic (DA_1) receptors to produce renal and mesenteric vasodilation as well as on postsynaptic α_1-, α_2-, and β_1-adrenergic receptors. Additionally, it acts indirectly by releasing norepinephrine from sympathetic nerve storage sites. Clinical response varies depending on the patient's clinical condition and baseline sympathetic nervous system activity.[337] Approximate ranges follow: dopaminergic, 0.5–2 µg/kg/min; β_1, 5–10 µg/kg/min; mixed α and β, 10–20 µg/kg/min; predominantly α, >20 µg/kg/min.[330]

Administration and Adult Dosage. **IV for shock, by infusion only** (in any nonalkaline IV fluid) 2.5 µg/kg/min initially, increasing gradually in 5–10 µg/kg/min increments up to 20–50 µg/kg/min, adjusting dosage to desired response. If a dosage over 20 µg/kg/min is required, consider other pressors.[333] Use dosages over 50 µg/kg/min only with careful monitoring of hemodynamic parameters and urine output. **IV for chronic refractory CHF** 2–3 µg/kg/min initially, increasing gradually until desired increases in urine flow, diastolic blood pressure, or heart rate are observed.[338] Dosages over 20 µg/kg/min are rarely used in CHF.[332,337,338]

Special Populations. *Pediatric Dosage.* Safety and efficacy not established. However, **IV for shock** (PALS recommendations) 2–5 µg/kg/min initially, increased to 10–20 µg/kg/min to improve blood pressure, perfusion, and urine output.[334]

Geriatric Dosage. Same as adult dosage.

Dosage Forms. **Inj** 40, 80, 160 mg/mL.

Pharmacokinetics. *Onset and Duration.* Onset within 5 min, duration <10 min.

Fate. There is large interpatient variability.[330] One evaluation in adult surgery patients derived a V_d of 0.89 ± 0.25 L/kg.[339] Cl is usually 3–4.2 L/hr/kg and was 4.48 ± 0.94 L/hr/kg in adult surgery patients.[330,339] The drug is primarily metabolized to homovanillic acid (HVA) and related metabolites; the remainder is metabolized to norepinephrine and excreted in urine as HVA and metabolites of both HVA and norepinephrine; very little is excreted as unchanged dopamine.[330,340]

$t_{1/2}$. α phase 1–2 min, β phase 6–9 min.[330,335]

Adverse Reactions. Increases in ventricular ectopy and ventricular arrhythmias may occur, particularly at high dosages (although this is less likely than with other sympathomimetics); reduce dosage if increased number of ventricular ectopic beats occurs. Hypertension may occur at high infusion rates. Nausea, vomiting, headache, anxiety, and angina pectoris have also been observed. Gangrene of the extremities has occurred in patients given large dosages of dopamine for long periods of time or in patients with occlusive vascular disease given low dosages.[330,341]

Contraindications. Pheochromocytoma; presence of uncorrected tachyarrhythmias or ventricular fibrillation.

Precautions. Correct hypovolemia before using in patients with shock. If increased diastolic pressure, decreased pulse pressure, or decreased urine flow occurs, decrease infusion rate and observe patient for signs of excessive vasoconstriction. Use with caution in patients with occlusive vascular disease, and extreme caution in patients receiving halogenated hydrocarbon anesthesia. Avoid extravasation of solution; however, if it occurs, the area may be infiltrated with 5–10 mg of phentolamine diluted in 10–15 mL of NS. Dopamine contains a sulfite preservative, which may be problematic in sensitive individuals, especially asthmatics.

Drug Interactions. MAOIs (including furazolidone) may increase the pressor response to dopamine by up to 20-fold; avoid these combinations. Bretylium, guanethidine, and heterocyclic antidepressants may potentiate the pressor response to direct-acting vasopressors. Oxytocics used in obstetrics may cause severe, persistent hypertension when used with vasopressors. IV phenytoin may produce hypotension in severely ill patients receiving IV dopamine. Halogenated hydrocarbon anesthetics may predispose patients to serious arrhythmias.

Parameters to Monitor. In shock, closely monitor heart rate, ECG, pulmonary capillary wedge pressure, cardiac index, arterial blood pressure, arterial blood gases, acid-base balance, toe temperature, urine output, and infusion rate of solution, and watch for signs of vasoconstriction or extravasation (eg, blanching). With low dosages for dopaminergic effects, monitor urine output and ECG.

Notes. The drug is physically incompatible with sodium bicarbonate or other alkaline solutions. (*See* Sympathomimetic Drugs for Hemodynamic Support Comparison Chart.)

DOPAMINE DILUTION GUIDE			
AMOUNT ADDED		VOLUME OF	FINAL
(mg)	*Volume (reconstituted)*	DILUENT	CONCENTRATION*
200	5 mL (1 amp, 40 mg/mL)	250 mL	800 mg/L
200	5 mL (1 amp, 40 mg/mL)	500 mL	400 mg/L
400	5 mL (1 amp, 80 mg/mL)	500 mL	800 mg/L
800	5 mL (1 amp, 160 mg/mL)	500 mL	1.6 g/L

*Recommended concentrations, but concentrations up to 3.2 g/L have been used.

EPINEPHRINE AND SALTS
Adrenalin, Sus-Phrine, Various

Pharmacology. Epinephtine stimulates α_1-, α_2- (vasoconstriction, pressor effects), β_1- (increased myocardial contractility and conduction), and β_2-adrenergic (bronchodilation and vasodilation) receptors. It is used for reversible bronchospasm, anaphylactic reactions, laryngeal edema (croup), open-angle glaucoma, and cardiac arrest (*see* Medical Emergencies).

Administration and Adult Dosage. **SC for anaphylaxis** 0.2–0.5 mg (0.2–0.5 mL of 1:1000 aqueous soln), may repeat q 10–15 min prn; if SC is ineffective, then **IV** 0.1–0.25 mg (1–2.5 mL of 1:10,000) q 5–15 min may be given and followed by an IV infusion if necessary. **SC for asthma** same dosage as SC for anaphylaxis; may repeat q 20 min to 4 hr as needed.[145] **SC aqueous suspension for asthma** 0.5–1.5 mg (0.1–0.3 mL of 1:200), may repeat with 0.5–1.5 mg no sooner than q 6 hr. **IV infusion for hemodynamic support** 1 µg/min (1 mg in 500 mL NS or D5W) initially, adjust to hemodynamic response (usually 2–10 µg/min).[333] (*See also* Chapter 5 for regular and high-dose epinephrine guidelines.) **Inhal (metered dose) not recommended** because of low efficacy and ultrashort duration of action.

Special Populations. *Pediatric Dosage.* **SC for anaphylaxis or asthma** 0.01 mL/kg/dose of 1:1000 aqueous soln, to a maximum of 0.5 mL; may repeat q 15–20 min for 2 doses, then q 4 hr prn. **SC aqueous suspension for asthma** (1 month–12 yr) 0.005 mL/kg/dose of 1:200, to a maximum of 0.15 mL/dose for children ≤30 kg, may repeat no sooner than q 6 hr.[145] **Inhal for croup** 0.25–0.5 mL of 2.25% racemic aqueous solution diluted in 1.5–4.5 mL of NS q 1–2 hr prn by nebulizer.[342,343] Alternatively, 5 mL of prediluted l-epinephrine in NS (1:1000) has been used.[343] **IV for hemodynamic support** 0.05–0.3 µg/kg/min initially, adjusted to desired hemodynamic response; avoid dosages >0.3 µg/kg/min if possible, because they are associated with marked vasoconstrictor effects.[334,344]

Geriatric Dosage. Same as adult dosage (*see* Precautions.)

Dosage Forms. **Inhal Pwdr** 200, 220, 250 µg/spray; **Inhal Pwdr** (bitartrate) 160 µg/spray; **Inhal Soln** (HCl) 1% (1:100); **Inhal Soln** (racepinephrine) 2, 2.25%; **Inj** (aqueous solution as HCl) 0.01 mg/mL (1:100,000), 0.1 mg/mL (1:10,000), 0.5 mg/mL (1:2000), 1 mg/mL (1:1000); **Inj** (aqueous suspension as free base) 5 mg/mL (1:200).

Patient Instructions. (Autoinjectors) Periodically familiarize yourself with instructions for use so you maintain an adequate comfort level. Obtain new kit by expiration date, or earlier if precipitate or color change is noted in solution.

Pharmacokinetics. *Onset and Duration.* Onset SC (aqueous soln or susp) 3–10 min; inhal peak 3–5 min. Duration SC (aqueous soln) 0.5–2 hr, (aqueous susp) up to 6–10 hr; inhal 15–60 min.[341,345]

Fate. Parenteral action is terminated by uptake into adrenergic neurons. Metabolism is by MAO and COMT.[330,341] Cl ranges from 2.1–5.3 L/hr/kg.[330]

$t_{1/2}$. About 1 min.[145]

Adverse Reactions. Dose-related restlessness, anxiety, tremor, cardiac arrhythmias, palpitations, hypertension, weakness, dizziness, and headache occur. Cerebral hemorrhage may be caused by a sharp rise in blood pressure from overdosage. Angina may be precipitated when coronary insufficiency is present, and elevation of blood glucose has been reported. Local necrosis from repeated injections and tolerance with prolonged use may also occur.[330,341]

Contraindications. Intra-arterial administration is not recommended because of marked vasoconstriction. Do not use with local anesthetics in fingers or toes, or during general anesthesia with halogenated hydrocarbons. Other contraindications include α-adrenergic blocker-induced (including phenothiazines) hypotension; cerebral arteriosclerosis; organic heart disease; narrow-angle glaucoma; shock; labor.

Precautions. Use with caution in patients with cardiovascular disease, hypertension, diabetes, or hyperthyroidism, and in psychoneurotic patients. Caution is usually recommended in the elderly, because of a higher frequency of cardiovascular intolerance. However, one evaluation of patients suffering from acute asthma attacks found no difference in hemodynamic alterations or arrhythmias between those >40 yr and those <40 yr in response to SC epinephrine.[346] IM injection may produce local tissue necrosis. Epinephrine infusions are preferably administered through a central venous line. Extravasation can cause necrosis; if extravasation occurs, infiltrate the area with **phentolamine** 5–10 mg diluted in 10–15 mL of NS.

Drug Interactions. Bretylium, guanethidine, and heterocyclic antidepressants may potentiate the pressor response to epinephrine. Oxytocics used in obstetrics may cause severe, persistent hypertension when used with vasopressors. Halogenated hydrocarbon anesthetics may predispose patients to serious arrhythmias. A hypertensive reaction may occur when epinephrine is given with nonselective ß-adrenergic blockers (eg, propranolol, nadolol).

Parameters to Monitor. (IV infusion) ECG, infusion rate and site; (in the elderly) ECG; (asthma or allergy) blood pressure, heart rate, relief of symptoms.

Notes. Do not use solution if it is brown in color or contains a precipitate. Protect solution from light. Suspension provides a sustained effect; shake suspension well prior to use. Nonprescription inhalers have only a transient effect because of their low dosage.[345] They should be used only by patients who have infrequent symptoms (less than once a week) and obtain total relief of symptoms from administration of two inhalations. Parenteral administration offers no advantage over inhalation for the treatment of acute bronchospasm.[347] (*See* Sympathomimetic Drugs for Hemodynamic Support Comparison Chart.)

MILRINONE LACTATE	Primacor

Milrinone is a phosphodiesterase inhibitor, a positive inotropic drug, and a vasodilator similar to amrinone, but 10–15 times more potent on a weight basis. Although well absorbed orally, milrinone is only available for IV use. It is 70% bound to plasma proteins; V_d is 0.47 ± 0.3 L/kg. It is 88–90% eliminated as unchanged drug by renal excretion. Elimination half-life in patients with CHF is 2.3 ± 0.1 hr, longer than in normal volunteers. Thrombocytopenia is less frequent (0.4%) with milrinone than with amrinone. Milrinone can cause or worsen existing ventricular and supraventricular arrhythmias. Hypotension and headaches occur frequently. Long-term oral or IV milrinone may lead to increased mortality in patients with CHF. Milrinone is labeled for temporary use in patients with severe left ventricular dysfunction and CHF. It has also been used for postoperative hemodynamic support and for those awaiting cardiac transplantation. Begin with a loading dose of 50 µg/kg over 10 min followed by a continuous infusion of 0.375–0.5 µg/kg/min; adjust dosage, depending upon patient response and hemodynamic variables, to a maximum of 0.75 µg/kg/min. In renal impairment, reduce dosage as follows: Cl_{cr} 50 mL/min, 0.43 µg/kg/min; 40 mL/min, 0.38 µg/kg/min; 30 mL/min, 0.33 µg/kg/min; 20 mL/min, 0.28 µg/kg/min; 10 mL/min, 0.23 µg/kg/min; 5 mL/min, 0.2 µg/kg/min.[348,349] Available as 1 mg/mL injection.

NOREPINEPHRINE BITARTRATE   Levophed

Pharmacology. Norepinephrine is a catecholamine that directly stimulates β_1-, α_1- and α_2-adrenergic receptors. It has little action on β_2-receptors.[331]

Administration and Adult Dosage. IV for shock, by infusion only (in any nonalkaline IV fluid) 8–12 µg of base/min initially, adjusting rate to maintain a systolic blood pressure of about 80–100 mm Hg or to a specific hemodynamic response; average maintenance dosage ranges from 2–4 µg of base/min. Very large dosages (up to 1.5 µg/kg/min) have been used in patients with septic shock.[330,350]

Special Populations. *Pediatric Dosage.* Safety and efficacy not established. **IV for shock, by infusion only** 0.05–0.1 µg/kg/min of base initially, adjust dosage to blood pressure response, to a maximum of 1.5 µg/kg/min.[330]

Geriatric Dosage. Same as adult dosage (*see* Precautions).

Dosage Forms. Inj 1 mg (of base)/mL.

Pharmacokinetics. *Onset and Duration.* Onset 1–2 min; duration 1–2 min after discontinuing infusion.[341]

Fate. Action is primarily terminated by uptake into adrenergic neurons. Free drug is metabolized primarily by COMT, and to a lesser extent by MAO, to inactive metabolites and their conjugates.

$t_{1/2}$. 2–2.5 min.[330]

Adverse Reactions. Dose-related hypertension (sometimes indicated by headache), reflex bradycardia, increased peripheral vascular resistance, and decreased cardiac output occur. Volume depletion may occur if fluid is not replaced. Arrhythmias may occur in extreme hypoxia or hypercarbia.

Contraindications. Hypotension secondary to uncorrected blood volume deficit; severe visceral or peripheral vasoconstriction; mesenteric or peripheral vascular thrombosis, unless drug is life-saving; halogenated hydrocarbon anesthesia.

Precautions. Use with caution in patients receiving MAO inhibitors or heterocyclic antidepressants. Administer into a large vein (antecubital preferred) to avoid necrosis secondary to vasoconstriction; avoid the leg veins whenever possible, especially in the elderly or in those with occlusive vascular diseases. Avoid extravasation of solution; however, if it occurs, the area may be infiltrated with 5–10 mg of **phentolamine** diluted in 10–15 mL of NS.

Drug Interactions. Bretylium, guanethidine, MAOIs, methyldopa, and heterocyclic antidepressants may potentiate the pressor response to direct-acting vasopressors. Oxytocics used in obstetrics may cause severe, persistent hypertension when used with vasopressors. Halogenated hydrocarbon anesthetics may predispose patients to serious arrhythmias.

Parameters to Monitor. In shock, closely monitor heart rate, pulmonary capillary wedge pressure, cardiac index, arterial blood pressure, arterial blood gases, acid-base balance, urine output, and infusion rate of solution, and watch for signs of vasoconstriction or extravasation (eg, blanching).

Notes. Do not use solution if it has a brown color or precipitate. 2 mg of norepinephrine bitartrate = 1 mg norepinephrine base. (*See* Sympathomimetic Drugs for Hemodynamic Support Comparison Chart.)

NOREPINEPHRINE DILUTION GUIDE			
AMOUNT ADDED		VOLUME OF	FINAL
(mg base)	*Volume*	5% DEXTROSE	CONCENTRATION
2 mg	2 mL	500 mL	4 mg/L*
4 mg	4 mL	500 mL	8 mg/L
8 mg	8 mL	500 mL	16 mg/L

*Recommended pediatric concentration.[351]

SYMPATHOMIMETIC DRUGS FOR HEMODYNAMIC SUPPORT COMPARISON CHART[a]

DRUG	Inotropic Activity (B_1)	Chronotropic Activity (B_1)	Vasodilation (B_2)	Vasoconstriction (α)	Renal/ Mesenteric Vasodilation (DA_1)	TOTAL PERIPHERAL RESISTANCE	CARDIAC OUTPUT
Dobutamine Dobutrex Various	++	0/+[b]	+	0/+[b]	0	→	↑
Dopamine Intropin Various	++	+/++[b,c]	++	+/++	+++	↓/↑[b]	↑
Epinephrine Adrenalin Various	+++	+++	++	++++	0	→	↑
Isoproterenol Isuprel Various	++++	++++	+++++	0	0	→	↑
Norepinephrine[d] Levophed Various	++	++[e]	0	++++	0	↑	↑
Phentolamine[f] Regitine	0	g	0	0	0	→	↑

ADRENERGIC RECEPTOR SELECTIVITY

(continued)

SYMPATHOMIMETIC DRUGS FOR HEMODYNAMIC SUPPORT COMPARISON CHART[a] (continued)

DRUG	ADRENERGIC RECEPTOR SELECTIVITY					TOTAL PERIPHERAL RESISTANCE	CARDIAC OUTPUT
	Inotropic Activity (B_1)	Chronotropic Activity (B_1)	Vasodilation (B_2)	Vasoconstriction (α)	Renal/ Mesenteric Vasodilation (DA_1)		
Phenylephrine[h] Neo-Synephrine	0	0[a]	0	+++++	0	↑	↓

+++++ = Pronounced effect; + = Minimal effect; 0 = No effect; ↓ = Decreased; ↑ = Increased.

[a] This table compares only a few of the many factors important in the treatment of shock. Consult references 330, 332, 352–354 for clinical use. Cross-table comparisons of the adrenergic selectivity properties between this table and the Sympathomimetic Bronchodilators Comparison Chart cannot be made for the following reasons: (1) the rating scale of this table reflects a finer degree of differentiation of effects (hence 0–5+ vs. 0–4+); (2) the routes of administration are different; and (3) vascular B_2-receptors appear to respond slightly differently from bronchiolar B_2-receptors.

[b] Dose dependent.

[a] Releases stored norepinephrine via tyraminelike mechanism.

[d] Primarily used to increase peripheral vascular resistance in volume-repleted hypotensive patients.

[e] Decrease in heart rate may result from reflex mechanisms.

[f] α-Adrenergic blocking drug; useful in severe vasoconstriction (eg, extravasation of norepinephrine or dopamine).

[g] Increase in heart rate may result from reflex and direct mechanisms.

[h] Primary use is to increase BP to reflexly increase vagal tone in paroxysmal supraventricular tachycardias. Other pressors are preferred in most shock states because they also have positive inotropic activity. Phenylephrine has no inotropic activity and with its strong α-agonist properties functions as a pure vasopressor (afterload increaser).

317

Nitrates

Class Instructions: Nitrates. This drug may cause headache, dizziness, and/or flushing; alcohol may worsen these side effects. Tolerance to side effects of long-acting nitrates such as headache may occur with continued therapy. If necessary, a mild analgesic may be used until tolerance to side effects occurs. During an acute angina attack, discontinue activity, assume a sitting position, and dissolve one sublingual tablet under the tongue. If chest discomfort does not improve after use of the tablets, seek medical attention. Keep tablets in the original container, tightly closed. If you have been taking this medication for a long time, do not discontinue it abruptly.

ISOSORBIDE DINITRATE
Isordil, Sorbitrate, Various

Pharmacology. (*See* Nitroglycerin.)

Administration and Adult Dosage. **SL tab for acute anginal attack** 2.5–10 mg q 2–3 hr prn;[355,356] **Chew Tab for acute anginal attack** 5 mg initially, then 5–10 mg q 2–3 hr prn.[356] **PO for prophylaxis of angina and for CHF** 10–60 mg q 4–6 hr; individual doses up to 120 mg have been used.[355,357] (*See* Vasodilators in Heart Failure Comparison Chart.) **SR products for prophylaxis of angina** 40–80 mg q 8–12 hr (once daily–bid at 8 A.M. and 2 P.M. preferred). Start the dosage low and adjust upward slowly over a period of several days to weeks to patient tolerance or to the desired therapeutic effect. A daily nitrate-free period of at least 12 hr is desirable in order to minimize tolerance.[357]

Special Populations. *Pediatric Dosage.* Safety and efficacy not established.

Geriatric Dosage. Same as adult dosage. However, some clinicians recommend lower doses, and that initial SL doses be given under medical observation because of an increased likelihood of postural hypotension.[358]

Dosage Forms. **Chew Tab** 5, 10 mg; **SL Tab** 2.5, 5, 10 mg; **SR Cap** 40 mg; **SR Tab** 40 mg; **Tab** 2.5, 5, 10, 20, 30, 40 mg.

Patient Instructions. (*See* Nitrates Class Instructions.) Do not crush or chew sustained-release preparations.

Pharmacokinetics. *Onset and Duration.* Onset is 5–20 min after SL and Chew Tab administration, 15–45 min after PO tab administration, up to 4 hr in rare cases or with SR products; peak occurs 15–60 min after SL administration, 45–120 min after PO tab administration.[355,356] Duration is 1–3 hr after SL or Chew Tab, 2–6 hr after PO tab, up to 8 hr after SR.[355,359] Although PO administration may improve exercise tolerance for 4–8 hr after the first dose, with long-term, around-the-clock administration, the duration of action declines to 2–3 hr, probably because of nitrate tolerance.[359]

Fate. Oral bioavailability is $22 \pm 14\%$. There is extensive first-pass metabolism by liver after oral administration to less active isosorbide mononitrate metabolites (2-ISMN, 5-ISMN). Larger doses and long-term administration saturate metabolic processes, with appreciable increases in serum concentrations of the parent compound and metabolites.[360] The drug is 28 ± 12% bound to plasma proteins; V_d is 1.5 ± 0.8 L/kg; Cl is 2.7 ± 1.2 L/hr/kg.[9] *See* Isosorbide Mononitrate Fate.

$t_{1/2}$. (Isosorbide dinitrate) 50 ± 20 min; (2-ISMN) 1.9 ± 0.5 hr; (5-ISMN) 4.6 ±0.7 hr.[9,361]

Adverse Reactions. (*See* Nitroglycerin.)

Contraindications. (*See* Nitroglycerin.)

Precautions. (*See* Nitroglycerin.)

Drug Interactions. Nitrates can produce additive vasodilation and severe postural hypotension when combined with alcohol or hypotensive drugs.

Parameters to Monitor. Observe for headache, orthostatic hypotension, and dizziness. In angina, monitor frequency of angina. In CHF, monitor hemodynamic and functional measurements.

Notes. Because of their slower onset of action, reserve SL and chewable isosorbide dinitrate (ISDN) for acute anginal attacks only in patients intolerant of or unresponsive to nitroglycerin. ISDN is a mainstay of antianginal and CHF therapy because of its long record of efficacy in these disorders. It is also less expensive than other long-term nitrate preparations. However, patients must take multiple doses daily on an eccentric schedule to achieve and maintain efficacy.

ISOSORBIDE MONONITRATE   Imdur, ISMO, Monoket

Pharmacology. Isosorbide mononitrate (ISMN) is the active 5-mononitrate metabolite of isosorbide dinitrate. (*See* Nitroglycerin.)

Administration and Adult Dosage. **PO for prophylaxis of angina** (ISMO, Monoket) 20 mg bid, doses 7 hr apart. **SR for prophylaxis of angina** (Imdur) 30–60 mg once daily in the morning, may increase to 120 mg once daily, to a maximum (rarely) of 240 mg once daily. There may be some attenuation of antianginal efficacy after 6 weeks of therapy with the 30- and 60-mg doses, but not with the 120-mg dose.[359,362]

Special Populations. *Pediatric Dosage.* Safety and efficacy not established.

Geriatric Dosage. Same as adult dosage.

Other Conditions. For persons of particularly small stature, the manufacturer of Monoket recommends an alternative initial dosage of 5 mg bid, but to increase it to at least 10 mg bid by the second or third day of therapy.

Dosage Forms. **SR Tab** (Imdur) 30, 60, 120 mg; **Tab** (ISMO, Monoket) 10, 20 mg.

Patient Instructions. (*See* Nitrates Class Instructions.) Follow the prescribed administration schedule closely. Do not crush the sustained-release product.

Pharmacokinetics. *Onset and Duration.* Non-SR tablet onset 30–60 min;[362] peak 1–2 hr, duration 12–14 hr with bid administration.[359] SR Tab onset within 4 hr; peak 4 hr; duration about 12 hr.[359,362]

Fate. The tablet is rapidly absorbed and essentially 100% bioavailable; SR Tab bioavailability is 78–86%.[362] The drug is distributed into total body water with negligible plasma protein binding and a V_d of 0.62 ± 0.05 L/kg.[361,363] Cl is 0.094

$\pm$ 0.005 L/hr/kg.[361] It is primarily hepatically metabolized by denitration and glucuronidation to inactive products that are renally eliminated; less than 2% of a dose is excreted unchanged in urine.[363]

$t_{1/2}$. 4.6 $\pm$ 0.7 hr.[361]

Adverse Reactions. (*See* Nitroglycerin.)

Contraindications. (*See* Nitroglycerin.)

Precautions. (*See* Nitroglycerin.)

Drug Interactions. Nitrates can produce additive vasodilation and severe postural hypotension when combined with alcohol or hypotensive drugs.

Parameters to Monitor. Observe for headache, orthostatic hypotension, and dizziness; antianginal efficacy; and compliance with 7-hr dosage regimen for non-SR tablet.

Notes. ISMN is an effective nitrate with dosage schedules proven to avoid tolerance. Patient compliance is favored with the use of ISMN because the products are administered once (Imdur) or twice (ISMO, Monoket) daily. Although the available preparations are comparable to each other in cost at relatively low dosages (ie, 20 mg bid for the immediate-release products and 60 mg/day or less of the SR products), they are much more expensive than generic ISDN, which is also effective when taken properly. Compliance and cost factors must be carefully assessed in the individual patient when choosing an oral nitrate product.

NITROGLYCERIN   Various

Pharmacology. Nitroglycerin and other organic nitrates are believed to be converted to nitric oxide (NO) by vascular endothelium. NO activates guanylate cyclase, increasing cyclic GMP, which in turn decreases intracellular calcium, resulting in direct relaxation of vascular smooth muscle.[355,357,364] The venous (capacitance) system is affected to a greater degree than the arterial (resistance) system. Venous pooling, decreased venous return to the heart (preload), and decreased arterial resistance (afterload) reduce intracardiac pressures and left ventricular size, thereby decreasing myocardial oxygen consumption and ischemia. In myocardial ischemia, nitrates dilate large epicardial vessels, enhance collateral size and flow, and reduce coronary vasoconstriction.[355] The various organic nitrate preparations have the same pharmacologic effects and differ only in bioavailability and pharmacokinetics.[338]

Administration and Adult Dosage. **SL Tab for acute anginal attack** 150–600 µg prn, up to 3 doses in 15 min; **SL aerosol for acute anginal attack** 400–800 µg prn, up to 1200 µg/15 min; **Buccal for acute anginal attack and/or prophylaxis and treatment of angina pectoris or CHF** 1–3 mg q 4–6 hr; **PO SR for prophylaxis of angina or CHF** 2.5–19.5 mg bid or tid;[355,359] **Top ointment for prophylaxis and treatment of angina pectoris or CHF** 1.3–5 cm (0.5–2 in.) q 6–8 hr.[355,359] Start the dosage low and adjust slowly upward over a period of several days to weeks to patient tolerance or to the desired therapeutic effect. **SR Patch for prophylaxis and treatment of angina pectoris** 0.2–0.8 mg/hr, patch applied once daily, dosage adjusted to patient response.[355] Greater antianginal efficacy has been noted with patches delivering 0.4 mg/hr or greater.[355,365] A daily nitrate-free period of 12 hr is desirable in order to minimize nitrate tolerance.[357,359] **IV for CHF post-MI, angina pectoris, perioperative blood pressure control, or hypotensive anesthesia** 5 µg/min initially by constant infusion using an infusion pump. Dosage must be adjusted to the individual patient's response. Increase dosage initially in 5 µg/min increments q 3–5 min until response noted. If no response occurs at 20 µg/min, increments of 10 µg/min, and later, 20 µg/min can be used. Once partial blood pressure response occurs, decrease incremental increases and increase intervals (*see* Notes).

Special Populations. *Pediatric Dosage.* Safety and efficacy not established. **IV** 0.5–20 µg/kg/min has been suggested.[366]

Geriatric Dosage. Same as adult dosage. However, some clinicians recommend lower doses, and that initial SL doses be given under medical observation because of an increased likelihood of postural hypotension.[358]

Dosage Forms. **Buccal Tab** 1, 2, 3 mg; **Oint** 2%; **SL Aerosol** 400 µg/spray; **SL Tab** 300, 400, 600 µg; **SR Cap** 2.6, 6.5, 9 mg; **SR Tab** 2.5, 6.5, 9, 13 mg; **SR Patch** 0.1, 0.2, 0.3, 0.4, 0.6, 0.8 mg/hr; **Inj** 0.5, 5 mg/mL.

Patient Instructions. (*See* Nitrates Class Instructions.)

Pharmacokinetics. *Onset and Duration.* Onset immediate after IV, 2–5 min after SL or buccal, 20–45 min after SR Cap or Tab, 15–60 min after topical ointment, and 30–60 min after transdermal administration.[355] Peak 4–8 min after SL, 4–10 min after buccal, 45–120 min after SR Cap or Tab, 30–120 min after topical ointment, and 1–3 hr after transdermal administration.[355] Duration 10–30 min after IV and SL, 0.5–5 hr after buccal, 2–6 hr after oral, 4–8 hr after SR, and 3–8 hr after topical administration.[355,359] Although the SR patch may act for a longer duration after the first application, long-term continuous therapy limits the duration of action to 4 hr or less, probably because of tolerance.[367] With sustained intermittent therapy (removal of patch after 12 hr), duration is 8–12 hr.[359]

Fate. Bioavailability of SL and Top are 38 ± 26% and 72 ± 20%, respectively.[9,368] Extensive first-pass metabolism occurs after oral administration. The drug is 87 ± 1% plasma protein bound. V_d is 3.3 ± 1.2 L/kg; Cl is 13.8 ± 5.4 L/hr/kg.[9,368] It is metabolized in the liver to less active dinitro and inactive mononitro metabolites. Larger doses and long-term administration may saturate metabolism and result in increased serum concentrations of drug and metabolites.[368]

$t_{½}$. β phase estimated to be 2.3 ± 0.6 min.[9]

Adverse Reactions. Headache occurs very frequently; dizziness occurs frequently, especially with oral or topical administration. Occasionally flushing, weakness, nausea, vomiting, palpitations, tachycardia, and postural hypotension occur. Many of these effects are dose related and may be minimized by increasing the dosage slowly. Tolerance and dependence may occur with prolonged use. Contact dermatitis occurs in up to 40% of patients using transdermal patches.[369]

Contraindications. Severe anemia; severe hypotension or uncompensated hypovolemia; increased intracranial pressure; purported hypersensitivity or idiosyncrasy to nitroglycerin, nitrates, or nitrites. Constrictive pericarditis, pericardial tamponade, and inadequate cerebral circulation are also considered contraindications by some authors.[359]

Precautions. Some tolerance and cross-tolerance with other nitrates may occur with long-term or excessive use.[359] Use with caution in patients with severe renal or hepatic disease, those with low or normal pulmonary capillary wedge pressure, and those receiving drugs that lower blood pressure. With intermittent therapy, anginal episodes may increase during the nitrate-free interval.[370]

Drug Interactions. Nitrates can produce additive vasodilation and severe postural hypotension when combined with alcohol or hypotensive drugs.

Parameters to Monitor. Observe for headache, dizziness and other side effects. Monitor for orthostatic hypotension, especially with first SL dose in elderly. (Angina) Monitor frequency of angina. (CHF) Obtain hemodynamic and functional measurements. (IV use) Monitor blood pressure and heart rate constantly in all patients; pulmonary capillary wedge pressure may also be useful in some patients.

Notes. Large and unpredictable amounts of nitroglycerin are lost through PVC containers, most IV administration sets and tubing, and certain IV filters.[371,372] The manufacturers recommend IV nitroglycerin infusions be prepared and stored in glass bottles and infused via special non-PVC tubing, avoiding the use of in-line filters. However, because nitroglycerin infusion rate is usually adjusted to response rather than by a μg/kg dosage, the need for special tubing has been questioned.[355] Some institutions have discontinued use of nitroglycerin tubing as part of cost-savings efforts, and have achieved good results clinically when using PVC tubing to infuse nitroglycerin.[373,374] However, because substantial amounts of nitroglycerin are adsorbed onto PVC tubing, special attention to patient response is advisable at the time of IV tubing changes. Stored in glass containers, the diluted injection is stable for 48 hr at room temperature and 7 days under refrigeration. When administration sets with large dead spaces are used, flush the line whenever the concentration of solution is changed. (*See* Vasodilators in Heart Failure Comparison Chart.)

APPROXIMATE EQUIVALENT DOSAGES OF NITRATES

PRODUCT	LOW DOSAGE	HIGH DOSAGE
Nitroglycerin Ointment	≤1 inch q 6 hr	1–2 inches q 6 hr
Nitroglycerin Patch	0.4 mg/hr	0.4–0.6 mg/hr
Isosorbide Dinitrate	20 mg tid	20–40 mg tid
Isosorbide Mononitrate		
Immediate-Release	10–20 mg bid	20 mg bid
Sustained-Release	30–60 mg/day	60 mg/day

VASODILATORS IN HEART FAILURE COMPARISON CHART

DRUG	DOSAGE*	DURATION	SITE OF ACTION†	HR	MAP	PCWP	CI	SVR
ACE INHIBITORS								
Captopril	PO 25–100 mg tid.	hours	A,V	0/↓	↓	↓	↑	↓
Capoten								
Enalapril	PO 2.5–10 mg bid;							
Vasotec	IV 0.625–5 mg q 6–12 hr.							
Lisinopril	PO 5–20 mg/day.							
Prinivil								
Zestril								
Quinapril	PO 5–20 mg q 12 hr.							
Accupril								
Hydralazine	PO 50–75 mg	hours	A	0/↑	sl↓	sl↓	↑	↓
Apresoline	q 6–8 hr; usual							
Various	maintenance 200–600 mg/day.							
Isosorbide	PO 10–60 mg	hours	V,(A)	sl↑/↓	↓	↓	↑/↓	sl↓
Dinitrate	q 4–6 hr.							
Isordil								
Sorbitrate								
Various								
Nitroglycerin	See monograph.	minutes	V,(A)	sl↑/↓	↓	↓	↑/↓	sl↓
Various								

(continued)

323

VASODILATORS IN HEART FAILURE COMPARISON CHART[a] (continued)

DRUG	DOSAGE*	DURATION	SITE OF ACTION[†]	HR	MAP	PCWP	CI	SVR
Nitroprusside Sodium Various	IV 0.1–3 µg/kg/min.	minutes	A,V	0	sl↓	↓	↑	↓

A = arterial; V = venous; HR = heart rate; MAP = mean arterial pressure; PCWP = pulmonary capillary wedge pressure; CI = cardiac index; SVR = systemic vascular resistance; ↑ = increase; ↓ = decrease; sl = slight; 0 = no change

*Start with low dosages of these drugs and increase gradually with continuous hemodynamic monitoring. To avoid adverse rebound effects, carefully taper the dosages of these drugs if they are to be discontinued (see Nitroglycerin Notes).

[†]Predominant site of action. Parentheses denote lesser activity.

From references 338, 375–379 and product information.

■ REFERENCES

1. Parker RB, McCollam PL. Adenosine in the episodic treatment of paroxysmal supraventricular tachycardia. *Clin Pharm* 1990;9:261–71.
2. Camm AJ, Garratt CJ. Adenosine and supraventricular tachycardia. *N Engl J Med* 1991;325:1621–9.
3. DiMarco JP et al. Adenosine for paroxysmal supraventricular tachycardia: dose ranging and comparison with verapamil. *Ann Intern Med* 1990;113:104–10.
4. McIntosh-Yellin NL et al. Safety and efficacy of central intravenous bolus administration of adenosine for termination of supraventricular tachycardia. *J Am Coll Cardiol* 1993;22:741–5.
5. Pedrid PJ. Amiodarone: reevaluation of an old drug. *Ann Intern Med* 1995;122:689–700.
6. Gilette PC et al. Amiodarone for children. *Clin Prog Electrophysiol Pacing* 1986;4:328–30.
7. Roden DM. Pharmacokinetics of amiodarone: implications for drug therapy. *Am J Cardiol* 1993;72:45–50F.
8. Rotmensch HH et al. Steady-state serum amiodarone concentrations: relationship with antiarrhythmic efficacy and toxicity. *Ann Intern Med* 1984;101:462–9.
9. Benet LZ et al. Design and optimization of dosage regimens; pharmacokinetic data. In Hardman JG et al., eds. *Goodman and Gilman's the pharmacological basis of therapeutics*, 9th ed. New York: McGraw-Hill; 1996:1707–92.
10. Gill J et al. Amiodarone. An overview of its pharmacologic properties, and review of its therapeutic use in cardiac arrhythmias. *Drugs* 1992;43:69–110.
11. Rigas B et al. Amiodarone hepatotoxicity. A clinicopathologic study of five patients. *Ann Intern Med* 1986;104:348–51.
12. Figge HL, Figge J. The effects of amiodarone on thyroid hormone function: a review of the physiology and clinical manifestations. *J Clin Pharmacol* 1990;30:588–95.
13. Dusman RE et al. Clinical features of amiodarone-induced pulmonary toxicity. *Circulation* 1990;82:51–9.
14. Hohnloser SH et al. Amiodarone-associated proarrhythmic effects. A review with special reference to torsade de pointes tachycardia. *Ann Intern Med* 1994;121:529–35.
15. Roberts SA et al. Invasive and noninvasive methods to predict the long-term efficacy of amiodarone: a compilation of clinical observations using meta-analysis. *PACE Pacing Clin Electrophysiol* 1994;17:1590–602.
16. Echt DS et al. Mortality and morbidity in patients receiving encainide, flecainide, or placebo. The Cardiac Arrhythmia Suppression Trial. *N Engl J Med* 1991;324:781–8.
17. Rapeport WG. Clinical pharmacokinetics of bretylium. *Clin Pharmacokinet* 1985;10:248–56.
18. Adir J et al. Nomogram for bretylium dosing in renal impairment. *Ther Drug Monit* 1985;7:265–8.
19. Anderson JL et al. Kinetics of antifibrillatory effects of bretylium: correlation with myocardial drug concentrations. *Am J Cardiol* 1980;46:583–92.
20. Anderson JL et al. Oral and intravenous bretylium disposition. *Clin Pharmacol Ther* 1980;28:468–78.
21. Narang PK et al. Pharmacokinetics of bretylium in man after intravenous administration. *J Pharmacokinet Biopharm* 1980;8:363–73.
22. Anderson JL et al. Clinical pharmacokinetics of intravenous and oral bretylium tosylate in survivors of ventricular tachycardia or fibrillation: clinical application of a new assay for bretylium. *J Cardiovasc Pharmacol* 1981;3:485–99.
23. Jelliffe RW et al. An improved method of digitoxin therapy. *Ann Intern Med* 1970;72:453–64.
24. Rasmussen K et al. Digitoxin kinetics in patients with impaired renal function. *Clin Pharmacol Ther* 1972;13:6–14.
25. Smith TW, Haber B. Digitalis (3rd of 4 parts). *N Engl J Med* 1973;289:1063–72.
26. Perrier D et al. Clinical pharmacokinetics of digitoxin. *Clin Pharmacokinet* 1977;2:292–311.
27. Jelliffe RW. An improved method of digoxin therapy. *Ann Intern Med* 1968;69:703–17.
28. Jelliffe RW, Brooker G. A nomogram for digoxin therapy. *Am J Med* 1974;57:63–8.
29. Mooradian AD, Wynn EM. Pharmacokinetic prediction of serum digoxin concentration in the elderly. *Arch Intern Med* 1987;147:650–3.
30. Cusack B et al. Digoxin in the elderly: pharmacokinetic consequences of old age. *Clin Pharmacol Ther* 1979;25:772–6.
31. Doherty JE et al. Clinical pharmacokinetics of digitalis glycosides. *Prog Cardiovasc Dis* 1978;21:141–58.
32. Soldin SJ. Digoxin—issues and controversies. *Clin Chem* 1986;32:5–12.
33. Iisalo E. Clinical pharmacokinetics of digoxin. *Clin Pharmacokinet* 1977;2:1–16.
34. Caldwell JH, Cline CT. Biliary excretion of digoxin in man. *Clin Pharmacol Ther* 1976;19:410–5.
35. Ewy GA et al. Digitalis intoxication—diagnosis, management and prevention. *Cardiol Clin* 1974;6:153–74.
36. Mann DL et al. Absence of cardioversion-induced ventricular arrhythmias in patients with therapeutic digoxin levels. *J Am Coll Cardiol* 1985;5:882–8.
37. Green LH, Smith TW. The use of digitalis in patients with pulmonary disease. *Ann Intern Med* 1977;87:459–65.

38. Slaughter RL et al. Appropriateness of the use of serum digoxin and digitoxin assays. *Am J Hosp Pharm* 1978;35:1376–9.
39. Weintraub M. Interpretation of the serum digoxin concentration. *Clin Pharmacokinet* 1977;2:205–19.
40. Podrid PJ et al. Congestive heart failure caused by oral disopyramide. *N Engl J Med* 1980;302:614–7.
41. Lima JJ et al. Antiarrhythmic activity and unbound concentrations of disopyramide enantiomers in patients. *Ther Drug Monit* 1990;12:23–8.
42. Lima JJ. Disopyramide. In Taylor WJ, Caviness MHD, eds. *A textbook for the clinical application of therapeutic drug monitoring.* Irving, TX: Abbott Diagnostics; 1986:97–108.
43. Bauman JL et al. Practical optimisation of antiarrhythmic drug therapy using pharmacokinetic principles. *Clin Pharmacokinet* 1991;20:151–66.
44. Latini R et al. Therapeutic drug monitoring of antiarrhythmic drugs: rationale and current status. *Clin Pharmacokinetic* 1990;18:91–103.
45. Piscitelli DA et al. Bioavailability of total and unbound disopyramide: implications for clinical use of the immediate and controlled-release forms. *J Clin Pharmacol* 1994;34:823–8.
46. Siddoway LA, Woosley RL. Clinical pharmacokinetics of disopyramide. *Clin Pharmacokinet* 1986;11:214–22.
47. Hasselstrom J et al. Enantioselective steady-state kinetics of unbound disopyramide and its dealkylated metabolite in man. *Eur J Clin Pharmacol* 1991;41:481–4.
48. Bauman JL et al. Long-term therapy with disopyramide phosphate: side effects and effectiveness. *Am Heart J* 1986;111:654–60
49. Wald RW et al. Torsade de pointes ventricular tachycardia. A complication of disopyramide shared with quinidine. *J Electrocardiol* 1981;14:301–8.
50. Perry JC, Garson A. Flecainide acetate for treatment of tachyarrhythmias in children: review of world literature on efficacy, safety and dosing. *Am Heart J* 1992;124:1614–21.
51. Holmes B, Heel RC. Flecainide. A preliminary review of its pharmacodynamic properties and therapeutic efficacy. *Drugs* 1985;29:1–33.
52. Conrad GJ, Ober RE. Metabolism of flecainide. *Am J Cardiol* 1984;53:41B–51.
53. Gross AS et al. Polymorphic flecainide disposition under conditions of uncontrolled urine flow and pH. *Eur J Clin Pharmacol* 1991;40:155–62.
54. Forland SC et al. Flecainide pharmacokinetics after multiple dosing in patients with impaired renal function. *J Clin Pharmacol* 1988;28:727–35.
55. McCollam P et al. Proarrhythmia: a paradoxical response to antiarrhythmic drugs. *Pharmacotherapy* 1989;9:144–53.
56. Tworek DA et al. Interference by antiarrhythmic agents with function of electrical cardiac devices. *Clin Pharm* 1992;11:48–56.
57. Anon. Ibutilide. *Med Lett Drugs Ther* 1996;38:38.
58. Roden DM. Current status of class III antiarrhythmic drug therapy. *Am J Cardiol* 1993;72:44B–9.
59. Benowitz NL, Meister W. Clinical pharmacokinetics of lignocaine. *Clin Pharmacokinet* 1978;3:177–201.
60. Galer BS et al. Response to intravenous lidocaine infusion differs based on clinical diagnosis and site of nervous system injury. *Neurology* 1993;43:1233–5.
61. Routledge PA et al. Control of lidocaine therapy: new perspectives. *Ther Drug Monit* 1982;4:265–70.
62. Rowland M et al. Disposition kinetics of lidocaine in normal subjects. *Ann N Y Acad Sci* 1971;179:383–98.
63. Boyes RN et al. Pharmacokinetics of lidocaine in man. *Clin Pharmacol Ther* 1971;12:105–16.
64. Thomson PD et al. Lidocaine pharmacokinetics in advanced heart failure, liver disease, and renal failure in humans. *Ann Intern Med* 1973;78:499–508.
65. Bauer LA et al. Influence of long-term infusions on lidocaine kinetics. *Clin Pharmacol Ther* 1982;31:433–7.
66. Blumer J et al. The convulsant potency of lidocaine and its N-dealkylated metabolites. *J Pharmacol Exp Ther* 1973;186:31–6.
67. Burney RG et al. Anti-arrhythmic effects of lidocaine metabolites. *Am Heart J* 1974;88:765–9.
68. LeLorier J et al. Pharmacokinetics of lidocaine after prolonged intravenous infusions in uncomplicated myocardial infarction. *Ann Intern Med* 1977;87:700–2.
69. Routledge PA et al. Increased alpha-1-acid glycoprotein and lidocaine disposition in myocardial infarction. *Ann Intern Med* 1980;93:701–4.
70. Gupta PK et al. Lidocaine-induced heart block in patients with bundle branch block. *Am J Cardiol* 1974;33:187–92.
71. Singh BN. Routine prophylactic lidocaine administration in acute myocardial infarction. An idea whose time is all but gone? *Circulation* 1992;86:1033–5. Editorial.
72. Berk SI et al. The effect of oral cimetidine on total and unbound serum lidocaine concentrations in patients with suspected myocardial infarction. *Int J Cardiol* 1987;14:91–4.
73. Jonsson A et al. Inhibition of burn pain by intravenous lignocaine infusion. *Lancet* 1991;338:151–2.
74. Stracke H et al. Mexiletine in the treatment of diabetic neuropathy. *Diabetes Care* 1992;15:1550–5.

75. Awerbuch GI, Sandyk R. Mexiletine for thalamic pain syndrome. *Int J Neurosci* 1990;55:129–33.

76. Bauman JL. Mexiletine. In Taylor WJ, Caviness MHD, eds. *A textbook for the clinical application of therapeutic drug monitoring*. Irving, TX: Abbott Diagnostics; 1986:125–30.

77. Allaf D et al. Pharmacokinetics of mexiletine in renal insufficiency. *Br J Clin Pharmacol* 1982;14:431–5.

78. Schrader BJ, Bauman JL. Mexiletine: a new type I antiarrhythmic agent. *Drug Intell Clin Pharm* 1986;20:255–60.

79. Woosley RL et al. Pharmacology, electrophysiology, and pharmacokinetics of mexiletine. *Am Heart J* 1984;107:1058–65.

80. Lledo P et al. Influence of debrisoquine hydroxylation phenotype on the pharmacokinetics of mexiletine. *Eur J Clin Pharmacol* 1993;44:63–7.

81. Campbell NPS et al. The clinical pharmacology of mexiletine. *Br J Clin Pharmacol* 1978;6:103–8.

82. Leahey EB et al. Effect of ventricular failure on steady state kinetics of mexiletine. *Clin Res* 1982;31:239A. Abstract.

83. Pentikainen PJ et al. Pharmacokinetics of oral mexiletine in patients with acute myocardial infarction. *Eur J Clin Pharmacol* 1983;25:773–7.

84. Campbell NPS et al. Long-term oral antiarrhythmic therapy with mexiletine. *Br Heart J* 1978;40:796–801.

85. Duff HJ et al. Molecular basis for the antigenicity of lidocaine analogs: tocainide and mexiletine. *Am Heart J* 1984;107:585–9.

86. Hurwitz A et al. Mexiletine effects on theophylline disposition. *Clin Pharmacol Ther* 1991;50:299–307.

87. Duff HJ et al. Mexiletine in the treatment of resistant ventricular arrhythmias: enhancement of efficacy and reduction of dose-related side effects by combination with quinidine. *Circulation* 1983;67:1124–8.

88. Vaughan Williams EM. Classification of the antiarrhythmic action of moricizine. *J Clin Pharmacol* 1991;31:216–21.

89. Moak JP et al. Newer antiarrhythmic drugs in children. *Am Heart J* 1987;61:179–85.

90. Morganroth J. Dose effect of moricizine on suppression of ventricular arrhythmias. *Am J Cardiol* 1990;65:26D–31.

91. Giardina EG et al. Moricizine concentration to guide arrhythmia treatment with attention to elderly patients. *J Clin Pharmacol* 1994;34:725–33.

92. Yang JM et al. Distribution of moricizine in human blood: binding to plasma proteins and erythrocytes. *Ther Drug Monit* 1990;12:59–64.

93. Siddoway LA et al. Clinical pharmacokinetics of moricizine. *Am J Cardiol* 1990;65:21D–5.

94. Carnes CA, Coyle JD. Moricizine: a novel antiarrhythmic agent. *DICP* 1990;24:745–53.

95. Miura DS et al. Ethmozine toxicity: fever of unknown origin. *J Clin Pharmacol* 1986;26:153–5.

96. The Cardiac Arrhythmia Suppression Trial II Investigators. Effect of the antiarrhythmic agent moricizine on survival after myocardial infarction. *N Engl J Med* 1992;327:227–33.

97. Hoffman BF et al. Electrophysiology and pharmacology of cardiac arrhythmias. VII. Cardiac effects of quinidine and procaine amide. A. *Am Heart J* 1975;89:804–8.

98. Greenspan AM et al. Large dose procainamide therapy for ventricular tachyarrhythmia. *Am J Cardiol* 1980;46:453–62.

99. Johnson KB, ed. *The Harriet Lane handbook*, 13th ed. Mosby-Year Book: St. Louis; 1993.

100. Kessler KM et al. Procainamide pharmacokinetics in patients with acute myocardial infarction or congestive heart failure. *J Am Coll Cardiol* 1986;7:1131–9.

101. Koch-Weser J. Serum procainamide levels as therapeutic guides. *Clin Pharmacokinet* 1977;2:389–402.

102. Connolly SJ, Kates RE. Clinical pharmacokinetics of N-acetylprocainamide. *Clin Pharmacokinet* 1982;7:206–20.

103. Karlsson E. Clinical pharmacokinetics of procainamide. *Clin Pharmacokinet* 1978;3:97–107.

104. Henningsen NC et al. Effects of long-term treatment with procaine amide. A prospective study with special regard to ANF and SLE in fast and slow acetylators. *Acta Med Scand* 1975;198:475–82.

105. Strasberg B et al. Procainamide-induced polymorphous ventricular tachycardia. *Am J Cardiol* 1981;47:1309–14.

106. Meyers DG et al. Severe neutropenia associated with procainamide: comparison of sustained release and conventional preparations. *Am Heart J* 1985;109:1393–5.

107. Lee JT et al. The role of genetically determined polymorphic drug metabolism in the beta-blockade produced by propafenone. *N Engl J Med* 1990;322:1764–8.

108. Funck-Brentano C et al. Propafenone. *N Engl J Med* 1990;322:518–25.

109. Musto B et al. Electrophysiological effects and clinical efficacy of propafenone in children with recurrent paroxysmal supraventricular tachycardia. *Circulation* 1988;78:863–9.

110. Hii JTY et al. Clinical pharmacokinetics of propafenone. *Clin Pharmacokinet* 1991;21:1–10.

111. Lee JT et al. Influence of hepatic dysfunction on the pharmacokinetics of propafenone. *J Clin Pharmacol* 1987;27:384–9.

112. Capucci A et al. Minimal effective concentration values of propafenone and 5-hydroxy-propafenone in acute and chronic therapy. *Cardiovasc Drugs Ther* 1990;4:281–7.
113. Siddoway LA et al. Polymorphism of propafenone metabolism and disposition in man: clinical and pharmacokinetic consequences. *Circulation* 1987;75:785–91.
114. Parker RB et al. Propafenone: a novel type Ic antiarrhythmic agent. *DICP* 1989;23:196–202.
115. Bryson HM et al. Propafenone. A reappraisal of its pharmacology, pharmacokinetics and therapeutic use in cardiac arrhythmias. *Drugs* 1993;45:85–130.
116. Mondardini A et al. Propafenone-induced liver injury: report of a case and review of the literature. *Gastroenterology* 1993;104:1524–6.
117. Verme CN et al. Pharmacokinetics of quinidine in male patients. A population analysis. *Clin Pharmacokinet* 1992;22:468–80.
118. Greenblatt DJ et al. Pharmacokinetics of quinidine in humans after intravenous, intramuscular and oral administration. *J Pharmacol Exp Ther* 1977;202:365–78.
119. Ueda CT, Dzindzio BS. Quinidine kinetics in congestive heart failure. *Clin Pharmacol Ther* 1978;23:158–64.
120. Kessler KM et al. Quinidine pharmacokinetics in patients with cirrhosis or receiving propranolol. *Am Heart J* 1978;96:627–35.
121. Bauman JL et al. Torsade de pointes due to quinidine: observations in 31 patients. *Am Heart J* 1984;107:425–30.
122. Coplen SE et al. Efficacy and safety of quinidine therapy for maintenance of sinus rhythm after cardioversion. *Circulation* 1990;82:1106–16.
123. Oberg KC et al. "Late" proarrhythmia due to quinidine. *Am J Cardiol* 1994;74:192–4.
124. Nappi JM, McCollam PL. Sotalol: a breakthrough antiarrhythmic? *Ann Pharmacother* 1993;27:1359–68.
125. Hanyok JJ. Clinical pharmacokinetics of sotalol. *Am J Cardiol* 1993;72:19A–26A.
126. Fiset C et al. Stereoselective disposition of (±)-sotalol at steady-state conditions. *Br J Clin Pharmacol* 1993;36:75–7.
127. Poirer M et al. The pharmacokinetics of d-sotalol and d,l-sotalol in healthy volunteers. *Br J Clin Pharmacol* 1990;38:579–82.
128. Dumas M et al. Variations of sotalol kinetics in renal insufficiency. *Int J Clin Pharmacol Ther Toxicol* 1989;27:486–9.
129. MacNeil D et al. Clinical safety profile of sotalol in the treatment of arrhythmias. *Am J Cardiol* 1993;72:44A–50.
130. Campbell RWF, Furniss SS. Practical considerations in the use of sotalol for ventricular tachycardia and ventricular fibrillation. *Am J Cardiol* 1993;72:80A–5.
131. Kehoe RF et al. Safety and efficacy of oral sotalol for sustained ventricular tachyarrhythmias refractory to other antiarrhythmic agents. *Am J Cardiol* 1993;72:56A–66.
132. Winkle RA et al. Tocainide for drug-resistant ventricular arrhythmias: efficacy, side effects, and lidocaine responsiveness for predicting tocainide success. *Am Heart J* 1980;100:1031–6.
133. Kutalek SP et al. Tocainide: a new oral antiarrhythmic agent. *Ann Intern Med* 1985;103:387–91.
134. Routledge PA. Tocainide. In Taylor WJ, Caviness MHD, eds. *A textbook for the clinical application of therapeutic drug monitoring.* Irving, TX: Abbott Diagnostics; 1986:175–80.
135. Mohiuddin SM et al. Tocainide kinetics in congestive heart failure. *Clin Pharmacol Ther* 1983;34:596–603.
136. Roden DM, Woosley RL. Tocainide. *N Engl J Med* 1986;315:41–5.
137. Holmes B et al. Tocainide. A review of its pharmacological properties and therapeutic efficacy. *Drugs* 1983;26:93–123.
138. Hoffmann K-J et al. Analysis and stereoselective metabolism after separate oral doses of tocainide enantiomers to healthy volunteers. *Biopharm Drug Dispos* 1990;11:351–63.
139. Braun J et al. Pharmacokinetics of tocainide in patients with severe renal failure. *Eur J Clin Pharmacol* 1985;28:665–70.
140. Forrence E et al. A seizure induced by concurrent lidocaine-tocainide therapy—is it just a case of additive toxicity? *Drug Intell Clin Pharm* 1986;20:56–9.
141. Vaughan Williams ED. A classification of antiarrhythmic actions reassessed after a decade of new drugs. *J Clin Pharmacol* 1984;24:129–47.
142. Task Force of the Working Group on Arrhythmias of the European Society of Cardiology. The Sicilian gambit. A new approach to the classification of antiarrhythmic drugs based on their actions on arrhythmogenic mechanisms. *Circulation* 1991;84:1831–51.
143. Rosenthal J, Kyncl JJ, eds. Clinical applications of alpha₁-receptor blockade: terazosin in the management of hypertension. *J Clin Pharmacol* 1993;33:866–99.
144. Fulton B et al. Doxazosin. An update of its clinical pharmacology and therapeutic applications in hypertension and benign prostatic hypertrophy. *Drugs* 1995;49:295–320.
145. Advice for the patient, Vol II. In, *USP DI*, 15th ed. Rockville, MD: US Pharmacopeal Convention; 1995.

146. Studer JA, Piepho RW. Antihypertensive therapy in the geriatric patient: II. A review of the alpha$_1$-adrenergic blocking agents. *J Clin Pharmacol* 1993;33:2–13.

147. McVeigh GE et al. Goals of antihypertensive therapy. *Drugs* 1995;49:161–75.

148. Carruthers SG. Adverse effects of α_1-adrenergic blocking drugs. *Drug Saf* 1994;11:12–20.

149. Brogden RN et al. Captopril: an update of its pharmacodynamic and pharmacokinetic properties, and therapeutic use in hypertension and congestive heart failure. *Drugs* 1988;36:540–600.

150. O'Dea RF et al. Treatment of neonatal hypertension with captopril. *J Pediatr* 1988;113:403–6.

151. Duchin KL et al. Pharmacokinetics of captopril in healthy subjects and in patients with cardiovascular diseases. *Clin Pharmacokinet* 1988;14:241–59.

152. Burris JF. The expanding role of angiotensin converting enzyme inhibitors in the management of hypertension. *J Clin Pharmacol* 1995;35:337–42.

153. Alderman CP. Adverse effects of the angiotensin-converting enzyme inhibitors. *Ann Pharmacother* 1996;30:55–61.

154. Langley MS, Heel RC. Transdermal clonidine: a preliminary review of its pharmacodynamic properties and therapeutic efficacy. *Drugs* 1988;35:123–42.

155. Guthrie SK. Pharmacologic interventions for the treatment of opioid dependence and withdrawal. *DICP* 1990;24:721–34.

156. Nunn-Thompson CL, Simon PA. Pharmacotherapy for smoking cessation. *Clin Pharm* 1989;8:710–20.

157. Lowenthal DT et al. Clinical pharmacokinetics of clonidine. *Clin Pharmacokinet* 1988;14:287–310.

158. Holdiness MR. A review of contact dermatitis associated with transdermal therapeutic systems. *Contact Dermatitis* 1989;20:3–9.

159. Reid JL et al. Withdrawal reactions following cessation of central α-adrenergic receptor agonist. *Hypertension* 1984;6:(suppl II):71II–5II.

160. Harris JM. Clonidine patch toxicity. *DICP* 1990;24:1191–4.

161. Bond WS. Psychiatric indications for clonidine: the neuropharmacologic and clinical basis. *J Clin Psychopharmacol* 1986;6:81–7.

162. Bravo EL et al. Clonidine-suppression test: a useful aid in the diagnosis of pheochromocytoma. *N Engl J Med* 1981;305:623–6.

163. Fedorak RN. Treatment of diabetic diarrhea with clonidine. *Ann Intern Med* 1985;102:197–9.

164. Hammer M, Berg G. Clonidine in the treatment of menopausal flushing. *Acta Obstet Gynecol Scand Suppl* 1985;132:29–31.

165. Nilsson LC et al. Clonidine for the relief of premenstrual syndrome. *Lancet* 1985;2:549–50.

166. 1988 Joint National Committee. The 1988 report of the Joint National Committee on Detection, Evaluation, and Treatment of High Blood Pressure. *Arch Intern Med* 1988;148:1023–38.

167. Ogilvie RI et al. Diazoxide concentration-response relation in hypertension. *Hypertension* 1982;4:167–73.

168. Andreasen F et al. The biological relevance of the protein binding of diazoxide. *Acta Pharmacol Toxicol (Copenh)* 1985;57:30–5.

169. Schmieder RE. Nephroprotection by antihypertensive agents. *J Cardiovasc Pharmacol* 1994;24(suppl 2):S55–64.

170. Cleland JGF et al. Severe hypotension after first dose of enalapril in heart failure. *Br Med J* 1985;291:1309–12.

171. Leonetti G, Cuspidi C. Choosing the right ACE inhibitor. A guide to selection. *Drugs* 1995;49:516–35.

172. DiPette DJ et al. Enalaprilat, an intravenous angiotensin-converting enzyme inhibitor, in hypertensive crisis. *Clin Pharmacol Ther* 1985;38:199–204.

173. Todd PA, Heel RC. Enalapril: a review of its pharmacodynamic and pharmacokinetic properties and therapeutic use in hypertension and congestive heart failure. *Drugs* 1986;31:198–248.

174. Till AE et al. Pharmacokinetics of repeated oral doses of enalapril maleate (MK-421) in normal volunteers. *Biopharm Drug Dispos* 1984;5:273–80.

175. Ulm EH et al. Enalapril maleate and a lysine analogue (MK-521): disposition in man. *Br J Clin Pharmacol* 1982;14:357–62.

176. Williams GH. Converting-enzyme inhibitors in the treatment of hypertension. *N Engl J Med* 1988;319:1517–25.

177. Packer M et al. Functional renal insufficiency during long-term therapy with captopril and enalapril in severe congestive heart failure. *Ann Intern Med* 1987;106:346–54.

178. Keane WF et al. Angiotensin converting enzyme inhibitors and progressive renal insufficiency; current experience and future directions. *Ann Intern Med* 1989;111:503–16.

179. Cooper RA. Captopril-associated neutropenia: who is at risk? *Arch Intern Med* 1983;143:659–60.

180. Tatro DS, ed. *Drug interaction facts*. St. Louis: Facts and Comparisons; 1996.

181. The Captopril-Digoxin Multicenter Research Group. Comparative effects of therapy with captopril and digoxin in patients with mild to moderate heart failure. *JAMA* 1988;259:539–44.

182. CONSENSUS Trial Study Group. Effects of enalapril on mortality in severe congestive heart failure. *N Engl J Med* 1987;316:1430–5.

183. Holmes B et al. Guanabenz: a review of its pharmacodynamic properties and therapeutic efficacy in hypertension. *Drugs* 1983;26:212–29.

184. Meacham RH et al. Disposition of ^{14}C guanabenz in patients with essential hypertension. *Clin Pharmacol Ther* 1980;27:44–52.

185. Palmer JD, Nugent CA. Guanadrel sulfate: a postganglionic sympathetic inhibitor for the treatment of mild to moderate hypertension. *Pharmacotherapy* 1983;3:220–9.

186. Finnerty FA, Brogden RN. Guanadrel: a review of its pharmacodynamic and pharmacokinetic properties and therapeutic use in hypertension. *Drugs* 1985;30:22–31.

187. Oates JA. Antihypertensive agents and drug therapy of hypertension. In Hardman JG et al., eds. *Goodman and Gilman's the pharmacological basis of therapeutics*, 9th ed. New York: McGraw-Hill; 1996:780–808.

188. Walter IE et al. The relationship of plasma guanethidine levels to adrenergic blockade. *Clin Pharmacol Ther* 1975;18:571–80.

189. Hengstmann JH, Falkner FC. Disposition of guanethidine during chronic oral therapy. *Eur J Clin Pharmacol* 1979;15:121–5.

190. Jerie P. Clinical experience with guanfacine in long-term treatment of hypertension. Part I: efficacy and dosage. *Br J Clin Pharmacol* 1980;10:37S–47.

191. Sorkin EM, Heel RC. Guanfacine: a review of its pharmacodynamic and pharmacokinetic properties, and therapeutic efficacy in the treatment of hypertension. *Drugs* 1986;31:301–36.

192. Mulrow JP, Crawford MH. Clinical pharmacokinetics and therapeutic use of hydralazine in congestive heart failure. *Clin Pharmacokinet* 1989;16:86–99.

193. Cameron HA, Ramsay LE. The lupus syndrome induced by hydralazine: a common complication with low-dose treatment. *Br Med J* 1984;289:410–2.

194. O'Malley K et al. Duration of hydralazine action in hypertension. *Clin Pharmacol Ther* 1975;18:581–6.

195. Shapiro KS et al. Immune complex glomerulonephritis in hydralazine-induced SLE. *Am J Kidney Dis* 1984;3:270–4.

196. Goa KL et al. Labetalol: a reappraisal of its pharmacology, pharmacokinetics and therapeutic use in hypertension and ischaemic heart disease. *Drugs* 1989;37:583–627.

197. MacCarthy EP, Bloomfield SS. Labetalol: a review of its pharmacology, pharmacokinetics, clinical uses and adverse effects. *Pharmacotherapy* 1983;3:193–219.

198. McNeil JJ, Louis WJ. Clinical pharmacokinetics of labetalol. *Clin Pharmacokinet* 1984;9:157–67.

199. Bauer JH, Reams GP. The angiotensin II type 1 receptor antagonists. A new class of antihypertensive drugs. *Arch Intern Med* 1995;155:1361–8.

200. Lo M-W et al. Pharmacokinetics of losartan, an angiotensin II receptor antagonist, and its active metabolite EXP3174 in humans. *Clin Pharmacol Ther* 1995;58:641–9.

201. Carr AA, Prisant LM. Losartan: first of a new class of angiotensin antagonists for the management of hypertension. *J Clin Pharmacol* 1996;36:3–12.

202. Myhre E et al. Clinical pharmacokinetics of methyldopa. *Clin Pharmacokinet* 1982;7:221–33.

203. Fleishaker JC et al. The pharmacokinetics of 2.5 to 10 mg oral doses of minoxidil in healthy volunteers. *J Clin Pharmacol* 1989;29:162–7.

204. Garcia JY, Vidt DG. Current management of hypertensive emergencies. *Drugs* 1987;34:263–78.

205. Vesey CJ, Cole PV. Blood cyanide and thiocyanate concentrations produced by long-term therapy with sodium nitroprusside. *Br J Anaesth* 1985;57:148–55.

206. Nitropress product information. Abbott Laboratories. Abbott Park, IL. Sept. 1990.

207. Schultz V et al. Kinetics of elimination of thiocyanate in 7 healthy subjects and in 8 subjects with renal failure. *Klin Wochenschr* 1979;57:243–7.

208. Cottrell JE et al. Prevention of nitroprusside induced cyanide toxicity with hydroxocobalamin. *N Engl J Med* 1978;298:809–11.

209. Pasch TH et al. Nitroprusside-induced formation of cyanide and its detoxification with thiosulphate during deliberate hypotension. *J Cardiovasc Pharmacol* 1983;5:77–82.

210. McAreavey D, Robertson JI. Angiotensin-converting enzyme inhibitors and moderate hypertension. *Drugs* 1990;40:326–45.

211. Frank GJ et al. Overview of quinapril, a new ACE inhibitor. *J Cardiovasc Pharmacol* 1990;15(suppl 2):S14–23.

212. Salvetti A. Newer ACE inhibitors: a look at the future. *Drugs* 1990;40:800–28.

213. Anon. Moexipril: another ACE inhibitor for hypertension. *Med Lett Drugs Ther* 1995;37:75–6.

214. Cubeddu LX. New alpha₁-adrenergic receptor antagonists for the treatment of hypertension: role of vascular alpha receptors in the control of peripheral resistance. *Am Heart J* 1988;116:133–62.

215. Anon. Doxazosin mesylate. *Hosp Pharm* 1989;24:963–4.

216. Donnelly R et al. Pharmacokinetic-pharmacodynamic relationships of α-adrenoreceptor antagonists. *Clin Pharmacokinet* 1989;17:264–74.

217. Frishman WH et al. Terazosin: a new long-acting α_1-adrenergic antagonist for hypertension. *Med Clin North Am* 1988;72:441–8.

218. Stumpf JL. Drug therapy of hypertensive crises. *Clin Pharm* 1988;7:582–91.

219. Hirschl MM. Guidelines for the drug treatment of hypertensive crisis. *Drugs* 1995;50:991–1000.

220. Abdelwahab W et al. Management of hypertensive urgencies and emergencies. *J Clin Pharmacol* 1995;35:747–62.

221. Angaran DM et al. Esmolol hydrochloride: an ultrashort-acting ß-adrenergic blocking agent. *Clin Pharm* 1986;5:288–303.

222. Cuneo BF et al. Pharmacodynamics and pharmacokinetics of esmolol, a short-acting ß-blocking agent, in children. *Pediatr Cardiol* 1994;15:296–301.

223. Frishman W, Silverman R. Clinical pharmacology of the newer beta-adrenergic blocking drugs. Part 2. Physiologic and metabolic effects. *Am Heart J* 1979;97:797–807.

224. Routledge PA, Shand DG. Clinical pharmacokinetics of propranolol. *Clin Pharmacokinet* 1979;4:73–90.

225. Nies AS, Shand DG. Clinical pharmacology of propranolol. *Circulation* 1975;52:6–15.

226. Johnsson G, Regardh CG. Clinical pharmacokinetics of ß-adrenoreceptor blocking drugs. *Clin Pharmacokinet* 1976;1:233–63.

227. Greenblatt DJ, Koch-Weser J. Adverse reactions to ß-adrenergic receptor blocking drugs: a report from the Boston Collaborative Drug Surveillance Program. *Drugs* 1974;7:118–29.

228. Bauer JH, Brooks CS. The long-term effect of propranolol therapy on renal function. *Am J Med* 1979;66:405–10.

229. Luchi RJ et al. Coronary artery spasm. *Ann Intern Med* 1979;91:441–9.

230. Frishman W. Clinical pharmacology of the new beta-adrenergic blocking drugs. Part 9. Nadolol: a new long-acting beta-adrenoceptor blocking drug. *Am Heart J* 1980;99:124–8.

231. Blanford MF. Nadolol (Corgard-Squibb). *Drug Intell Clin Pharm* 1980;14:825–30.

232. McTavish D et al. Carvedilol. A review of its pharmacodynamic and pharmacokinetic properties, and therapeutic efficacy. *Drugs* 1993;45:232–58.

233. Heel RC et al. Atenolol: a review of its pharmacological properties and therapeutic efficacy in angina pectoris and hypertension. *Drugs* 1979;17:425–60.

234. Milne RJ, Buckley MM-T. Celiprolol. An updated review of its pharmacodynamic and pharmacokinetic properties, and therapeutic efficacy in cardiovascular disease. *Drugs* 1991;41:941–69.

235. MacCarthy EP, Bloomfield SS. Labetalol. A review of its pharmacology, pharmacokinetics, clinical uses and adverse effects. *Pharmacotherapy* 1983;3:193–219.

236. Ryan JR. Clinical pharmacology of acebutolol. *Am Heart J* 1985;109:1131–6.

237. Harron DWG et al. Bopindolol. A review of its pharmacodynamic and pharmacokinetic properties and therapeutic efficacy. *Drugs* 1991;41:130–49.

238. Frishman WH, Covey S. Penbutolol and carteolol: two new beta-adrenergic blockers with partial agonism. *J Clin Pharmacol* 1990;30:412–21.

239. Frishman WH et al. Bevantolol. A preliminary review of its pharmacodynamic and pharmacokinetic properties, and therapeutic efficacy in hypertension and angina pectoris. *Drugs* 1988;35:1–21.

240. Lancaster SG, Sorkin EM. Bisoprolol. A preliminary review of its pharmacodynamic and pharmacokinetic properties, therapeutic efficacy in hypertension and angina pectoris. *Drugs* 1988;36:256–85.

241. Petru MA et al. Long-term efficacy of high-dose diltiazem for chronic stable angina pectoris: 16-month serial studies with placebo controls. *Am Heart J* 1985;109:99–103.

242. Markham A, Brogden RN. Diltiazem. A review of its pharmacology and therapeutic use in older patients. *Drugs Aging* 1993;3:363–90.

243. Zelis RF, Kinney EL. The pharmacokinetics of diltiazem in healthy American men. *Am J Cardiol* 1982;49:529–32.

244. Kinney EL et al. The pharmacokinetics and pharmacology of oral diltiazem in normal volunteers. *J Clin Pharmacol* 1981;21:337–42.

245. Joyal M et al. Pharmacodynamic aspects of intravenous diltiazem administration. *Am Heart J* 1986;111:54–60.

246. Smith MS et al. Pharmacokinetic and pharmacodynamic effects of diltiazem. *Am J Cardiol* 1983;51:1369–74.

247. McAuley BJ, Schroeder JS. The use of diltiazem hydrochloride in cardiovascular disorders. *Pharmacotherapy* 1982;2:121–33.

248. Winship LC et al. The effect of ranitidine and cimetidine on single-dose diltiazem pharmacokinetics. *Pharmacotherapy* 1985;5:16–9.

249. McAllister RG. Kinetics and dynamics of nifedipine after oral and sublingual doses. *Am J Med* 1986;81(suppl 6A):2–5.

250. Kleinbloesem CH et al. Nifedipine: kinetics and hemodynamic effects in patients with liver cirrhosis after intravenous and oral administration. *Clin Pharmacol Ther* 1986;40:21–8.

251. Sorkin EM et al. Nifedipine. A review of its pharmacodynamic and pharmacokinetic properties, and therapeutic efficacy, in ischemic heart disease, hypertension and related cardiovascular disorders. *Drugs* 1985;30:182–274.

252. Kleinbloesem CH et al. Nifedipine: kinetics and dynamics in healthy subjects. *Clin Pharmacol Ther* 1984;36:742–9.

253. Breimer DD et al. Nifedipine: variability in its kinetics and metabolism in man. *Pharmacol Ther* 1989;44:445–54.

254. Vetrovec GW et al. Comparative dosing and efficacy of continuous release nifedipine versus standard nifedipine for angina pectoris: clinical response, exercise performance and plasma nifedipine levels. *Am Heart J* 1988;115:793–8.

255. Diamond JR et al. Nifedipine-induced renal dysfunction. Alterations in renal hemodynamics. *Am J Med* 1984;77:905–9.

256. Elkayam U et al. A prospective, randomized, double-blind, crossover study to compare the efficacy and safety of chronic nifedipine therapy with that of isosorbide dinitrate and their combination in the treatment of chronic congestive heart failure. *Circulation* 1990;82:1954–61.

257. Dale J et al. The effects of nifedipine, a calcium antagonist, on platelet function. *Am Heart J* 1983;105:103–5.

258. Barbarash RA et al. Verapamil infusions in the treatment of atrial tachyarrhythmias. *Crit Care Med* 1986;14:886–8.

259. Kates RE. Calcium antagonists: pharmacokinetic properties. *Drugs* 1983;25:113–24.

260. Schwartz JB et al. Prolongation of verapamil elimination kinetics during chronic oral administration. *Am Heart J* 1982;104:198–203.

261. Hamann SR et al. Clinical pharmacokinetics of verapamil. *Clin Pharmacokinet* 1984;9:26–41.

262. Hoon TJ et al. The pharmacodynamic and pharmacokinetic differences of the D- and L-isomers of verapamil: implications in the treatment of paroxysmal supraventricular tachycardia. *Am Heart J* 1986;112:396–403.

263. McTavish D, Sorkin EM. Verapamil. An updated review of its pharmacodynamic and pharmacokinetic properties, and therapeutic use in hypertension. *Drugs* 1989;38:19–76.

264. McAllister RG, Kirsten EB. The pharmacology of verapamil. IV. Kinetic and dynamic effects after single intravenous and oral doses. *Clin Pharmacol Ther* 1982;31:418–26.

265. Singh BN et al. New perspectives in the pharmacologic therapy of cardiac arrhythmias. *Prog Cardiovasc Dis* 1980;22:243–301.

266. Schoen MD et al. Evaluation of the pharmacokinetics and electrocardiographic effects of intravenous verapamil with intravenous calcium chloride pretreatment in normal subjects. *Am J Cardiol* 1991;67:300–4.

267. Singh BN et al. Second generation calcium antagonists: search for greater selectivity and versatility. *Am J Cardiol* 1985;55:214B–21.

268. Bays HE, Dujovne CA. Drugs for treatment of patients with high cholesterol blood levels and other dyslipidemias. *Prog Drug Res* 1994;43:9–41.

269. Larsen ML, Illingworth DR. Drug treatment of dyslipoproteinemia. *Med Clin North Am* 1994;78:225–45.

270. National Cholesterol Education Program. Report of the Expert Panel on Blood Cholesterol Levels in Children and Adolescents. *Pediatrics* 1992;89:S525–70.

271. Kwiterovich PO. Diagnosis and management of familial dyslipoproteinemia in children and adolescents. *Pediatr Clin North Am* 1990;37:1489–521.

272. Lipid Research Clinics Program. Lipid research clinics coronary primary prevention trial results. I. Reduction in incidence of coronary heart disease. *JAMA* 1984;251:351–64.

273. Newman TB, Hulley SB. Carcinogenicity of lipid-lowering drugs. *JAMA* 1996;275:55–60.

274. Smellie WAS, Lorimer AR. Adverse effects of the lipid-lowering drugs. *Adverse Drug React Toxicol Rev* 1992;11:71–92.

275. Ast M, Frishman WH. Bile acid sequestrants. *J Clin Pharmacol* 1990;30:99–106.

276. Farmer JA, Gotto AM Jr. Antihyperlipidaemic agents. Drug interactions of clinical significance. *Drug Saf* 1994;11:301–9.

277. Expert Panel on Detection, Evaluation and Treatment of High Blood Cholesterol in Adults. Summary of the second report of the National Cholesterol Education Program (NCEP) Expert Panel on Detection, Evaluation, and Treatment of High Blood Cholesterol in Adults (Adult Treatment Panel II). *JAMA* 1993;269:3015–23.

278. Andrade SE et al. Discontinuation rates of antihyperlipidemic drugs—do rates reported in clinical trials reflect rates in primary care settings? *N Engl J Med* 1995;332:1125–31.

279. Hilleman DE et al. Comparative cost-effectiveness of bile acid sequestering resins, HMG Co-A reductase inhibitors, and their combination in patients with hypercholesterolemia. *J Managed Care Pharm* 1995;1:188–92.

280. Shwed JA, Rodvold KA. Anion-exchange resins and oral vancomycin in pseudomembranous colitis. *DICP* 1989;23:70–1. Letter.

281. Bartlett JG. Antibiotic-associated diarrhea. *Clin Infect Dis* 1992;15:573–81.

282. Kelly CP et al. *Clostridium difficile* colitis. *N Engl J Med* 1994:330:257–62.

283. Jungnickel PW et al. Blind comparison of patient preference for flavored Colestid granules and Questran Light. *Ann Pharmacother* 1993;27:700–3.

284. Shaefer MS et al. Acceptability of cholestyramine or colestipol combinations with six vehicles. *Clin Pharm* 1987;6:51–4.

285. Shaefer MS et al. Sensory/mixability preference evaluation of cholestyramine powder formulations. *DICP* 1990;24:472–4.

286. Ito MK, Morreale AP. Acceptability of cholestyramine and colestipol formulations in three common vehicles. *Clin Pharm* 1991;10:138–40.

287. Insull W Jr et al. The effects of colestipol tablets compared with colestipol granules on plasma cholesterol and other lipids in moderately hypercholesterolemic patients. *Atherosclerosis* 1995;112:223–35.

288. Spence JD et al. Combination therapy with colestipol and psyllium mucilloid in patients with hyperlipidemia. *Ann Intern Med* 1995;123:493–9.

289. Superko HR et al. Effectiveness of low-dose colestipol therapy in patients with moderate hypercholesterolemia. *Am J Cardiol* 1992;70:135–40.

290. Shepherd J. Mechanism of action of fibrates. *Postgrad Med J* 1993;69:S34–41.

291. Todd PA, Ward A. Gemfibrozil. A review of its pharmacodynamic and pharmacokinetic properties, and therapeutic use in dyslipidemia. *Drugs* 1988;36:314–39.

292. Evans JR et al. Effect of renal function on the pharmacokinetics of gemfibrozil. *J Clin Pharmacol* 1987;27:994–1000.

293. Shen D et al. Effect of gemfibrozil treatment in sulfonylurea-treated patients with noninsulin-dependent diabetes mellitus. *J Clin Endocrinol Metab* 1991;73:503–10.

294. Lozada A, Dujovne CA. Drug interactions with fibric acids. *Pharmacol Ther* 1994;63:163–76.

295. Frick MH et al. Helsinki heart study: primary prevention trial with gemfibrozil in middle-aged men with dyslipidemia. *N Engl J Med* 1987;317:1237–45.

296. Heinonen OP et al. Helsinki heart study: coronary heart disease incidence during an extended follow-up. *J Intern Med* 1994;235:41–9.

297. Frick MH et al. Efficacy of gemfibrozil in dyslipidaemic subjects with suspected heart disease. An ancillary study in the Helsinki heart study frame population. *Ann Med* 1993;25:41–5.

298 Furberg CD et al. Effect of lovastatin on early carotid atherosclerosis and cardiovascular events. *Circulation* 1994;90:1679–87.

299. Davignon J et al. HMG-CoA reductase inhibitors: a look back and a look ahead. *Can J Cardiol* 1992;8:843–64.

300. Hsu I et al. Comparative evaluation of the safety and efficacy of HMG-CoA reductase inhibitor monotherapy in the treatment of primary hypercholesterolemia. *Ann Pharmacother* 1995;29:743–59.

301. Henwood JM, Heel RC. Lovastatin. A preliminary review of its pharmacodynamic properties and therapeutic use in hyperlipidaemia. *Drugs* 1988:429–54.

302. McTavish D, Sorkin EM. Pravastatin. A review of its pharmacological properties and therapeutic potential in hypercholesterolemia. *Drugs* 1991;65–89.

303. Todd PA, Goa KL. Simvastatin. A review of its pharmacological properties and therapeutic potential in hypercholesterolemia. *Drugs* 1990;40:583–607.

304. Mauro VF, MacDonald JL. Simvastatin: a review of its pharmacology and clinical use. *DICP* 1991;25:257–64.

305. Jungnickel PW et al. Pravastatin: a new drug for the treatment of hypercholesterolemia. *Clin Pharm* 1992;11:677–89.

306. Canner PL et al. Fifteen year mortality in coronary drug project patients: long-term benefit with niacin. *J Am Coll Cardiol* 1986;8:1245–55.

307. Dalen JE, Dalton WS. Does lowering cholesterol cause cancer? *JAMA* 1996;275:67–9. Commentary.

308. Scandinavian Simvastatin Survival Study Group. Randomised trial of cholesterol lowering in 4444 patients with coronary artery disease: the Scandinavian Simvastatin Survival Study (4S). *Lancet* 1994;344:1383–9.

309. Jukema JW et al. Effects of lipid lowering by pravastatin on progression and regression of coronary artery disease in symptomatic men with normal to moderately elevated serum cholesterol levels. *Circulation* 1995;91:2528–40.

310. Nawrocki JW et al. Reduction of LDL cholesterol by 25% to 60% in patients with primary hypercholesterolemia by atorvastatin, a new HMG-CoA reductase inhibitor. *Arterioscler Thromb Vasc Biol* 1995;15:678–82.

311. Black DM. Atorvastatin: a step ahead for HMG-CoA reductase inhibitors. *Atherosclerosis* 1995;10:307–10.

312. Bakker-Arkema RG et al. Efficacy and safety of a new HMG-CoA reductase inhibitor, atorvastatin, in patients with hypertriglyceridemia. *JAMA* 1996;275:128–33.

313. Figge HL et al. Nicotinic acid: a review of its clinical use in the treatment of lipid disorders. *Pharmacotherapy* 1988;8:287–94.

314. Brown WV. Niacin for lipid disorders. *Postgrad Med* 1995;98:185–92.

315. Colletti RB et al. Niacin treatment of hypercholesterolemia in children. *Pediatrics* 1993;92:78–82.

316. Weiner M. Clinical pharmacology and pharmacokinetics of nicotinic acid. *Drug Metab Rev* 1979;9:99–106.
317. Etchason JA et al. Niacin-induced hepatitis: a potential side effect with low-dose time-release niacin. *Mayo Clin Proc* 1991;66:23–8.
318. Hunninghake DB. Diagnosis and treatment of lipid disorders. *Med Clin North Am* 1994;78:247–57.
319. McKenney JM et al. A comparison of the efficacy and toxic effects of sustained- vs immediate-release niacin in hypercholesterolemic patients. *JAMA* 1994;271:672–7.
320. Leaf DA. Lipid disorders: applying new guidelines to your older patients. *Geriatrics* 1994;49:35–41.
321. Deedwania PC. Clinical perspectives on primary and secondary prevention of coronary atherosclerosis. *Med Clin North Am* 1995;79:973–95.
322. Wynne J, Braunwald E. New treatment for congestive heart failure: amrinone and milrinone. *J Cardiovasc Med* 1984;9:393–405.
323. Lawless ST et al. The acute pharmacokinetics and pharmacodynamics of amrinone in pediatric patients. *J Clin Pharmacol* 1991;31:800–3.
324. Rocci ML, Wilson H. The pharmacokinetics and pharmacodynamics of newer inotropic agents. *Clin Pharmacokinet* 1987;13:91–109.
325. Edelson J et al. Relationship between amrinone plasma concentration and cardiac index. *Clin Pharmacol Ther* 1981;29:723–8.
326. Ross MP et al. Amrinone-associated thrombocytopenia: pharmacokinetic analysis. *Clin Pharmacol Ther* 1993;53:661–7.
327. Dunkman WB et al. Adverse effects of long-term amrinone administration in congestive heart failure. *Am Heart J* 1983;105:861–3.
328. Packer M et al. Hemodynamic and clinical limitations of long-term inotropic therapy with amrinone in patients with severe chronic heart failure. *Circulation* 1984;70:1038–47.
329. Majerus TC et al. Dobutamine: ten years later. *Pharmacotherapy* 1989;9:245–59.
330. Zaritsky AL. Catecholamines, inotropic medications, and vasopressor agents. In Chernow B et al., eds. *The pharmacologic approach to the critically ill patient,* 3rd ed. Baltimore: Williams & Wilkins; 1994:387–404.
331. Kulka PJ, Tryba M. Inotropic support of the critically ill patient. A review of the agents. *Drugs* 1993;45:654–67.
332. Trujillo MH, Bellorin-Font E. Drugs commonly administered by intravenous infusion in intensive care units: a practical guide. *Crit Care Med* 1990;18:232–8.
333. American College of Cardiology, American Heart Association Task Force. Adult advanced cardiac life support. *JAMA* 1992;268:2199–241.
334. American College of Cardiology, American Heart Association Task Force. Pediatric advanced life support. *JAMA* 1992;268:2262–75.
335. Bhatt-Mehta V, Nahata MC. Dopamine and dobutamine in pediatric therapy. *Pharmacotherapy* 1989;9:303–14.
336. Benet LZ, Williams RL. Design and optimization of dosage regimens: pharmacokinetic data. In Gilman AG et al., eds. *Goodman and Gilman's the pharmacological basis of therapeutics,* 8th ed. New York: Pergamon Press; 1990:1650–735.
337. Murphy MB, Elliott WJ. Dopamine and dopamine receptor agonists in cardiovascular therapy. *Crit Care Med* 1990;18:S14–8.
338. Geraci SA. Pharmacologic approach in patients with heart failure. In, Chernow B et al., eds. *The pharmacologic approach to the critically ill patient.* 3rd ed. Baltimore: Williams & Wilkins; 1994:80–94.
339. Jarnberg P-O et al. Dopamine infusion in man. Plasma catecholamine levels and pharmacokinetics. *Acta Anaesthesiol Scand* 1981;25:328–31.
340. Cedarbaum JM, Schleifer LS. Drugs for Parkinson's disease, spasticity, and acute muscle spasms. In Gilman AG et al., eds. *Goodman and Gilman's the pharmacological basis of therapeutics,* 8th ed. New York: Pergamon Press; 1990:463–84.
341. Hoffman BB, Lefkowitz RJ. Catecholamines and sympathomimetic drugs. In Gilman AG et al., eds. *Goodman and Gilman's the pharmacological basis of therapeutics,* 8th ed. New York: Pergamon Press; 1990:187–220.
342. Skolnik NS. Treatment of croup. A critical review. *Am J Dis Child* 1989;143:1045–9.
343. Waisman Y et al. Prospective randomized double-blind study comparing L-epinephrine and racemic epinephrine aerosols in the treatment of laryngotracheitis (croup). *Pediatrics* 1992;89:302–6.
344. Zaritsky A, Chernow B. Use of catecholamines in pediatrics. *J Pediatr* 1984;105:341–50.
345. Tashkin DP, Jenne JW. Alpha and beta adrenergic agonists. In Weiss EB et al., eds. *Bronchial asthma: mechanisms and therapeutics,* 2nd ed. Boston: Little, Brown; 1985:604–39.
346. Cydulka R et al. The use of epinephrine in the treatment of older adult asthmatics. *Ann Emerg Med* 1988;17:322–6.
347. Kelly HW. New B_2-adrenergic agonist aerosols. *Clin Pharm* 1985;4:393–403.

348. Edelson J et al. Pharmacokinetics of the bipyridines amrinone and milrinone. *Circulation* 1986;73(suppl III): 145-III-52-III.

349. Young RA, Ward A. Milrinone. A preliminary review of its pharmacological properties and therapeutic use. *Drugs* 1988;36:158–92.

350. Martin C et al. Norepinephrine or dopamine for the treatment of hyperdynamic septic shock? *Chest* 1993;103:1826–31.

351. Notterman DA. Pediatric pharmacotherapy. In Chernow B et al., eds. *The pharmacologic approach to the critically ill patient,* 3rd ed. Baltimore: Williams & Wilkins; 1994:139–55.

352. Neugebauer E et al. Pharmacotherapy of shock. In, Chernow B et al., eds. *The pharmacologic approach to the critically ill patient,* 3rd ed. Baltimore: Williams & Wilkins; 1994:1104–21.

353. Rackow EC, Astiz ME. Mechanisms and management of septic shock. *Crit Care Clin* 1993;9(2):219–37.

354. Zaloga GP et al. Pharmacologic cardiovascular support. *Crit Care Clin* 1993;9:335–62.

355. Abrams J. Nitroglycerin and long-acting nitrates. *P&T* 1992;59–64, 67–9.

356. Parker JO. Nitrate therapy in stable angina pectoris. *N Engl J Med* 1987;316:1635–42.

357. Elkayam U. Tolerance to organic nitrates: evidence, mechanisms, clinical relevance, and strategies for prevention. *Ann Intern Med* 1991;114:667–77.

358. Cannon LA, Marshall JM. Cardiac disease in the elderly population. *Clin Geriatr Med* 1993;9:499–525.

359. Thadani U, Opie LH. Nitrates. In Opie LH ed. *Drugs for the heart,* 4th ed. Philadelphia: WB Saunders; 1995:31–48.

360. Sporl-Radun S et al. Effects and pharmacokinetics of isosorbide dinitrate in normal man. *Eur J Clin Pharmacol* 1980;18:237–44.

361. Abshagen WWP et al. Pharmacokinetics of intravenous and oral isosorbide-5-mononitrate. *Eur J Clin Pharmacol* 1981;20:269–75.

362. Frishman WH et al. Mononitrates: defining the ideal long-acting nitrate. *Clin Ther* 1994;16:130–9.

363. Abshagen WWP. Pharmacokinetics of isosorbide mononitrate. *Am J Cardiol* 1992;70:61G–6.

364. Fung H-L. Clinical pharmacology of organic nitrates. *Am J Cardiol* 1993;72:9C–15.

365. Fletcher A. Transdermal nitroglycerin. Does it really work in the treatment of angina? *Drugs Aging* 1991;1:6–16.

366. Friedman WF, George BL. New concepts and drugs in the treatment of congestive heart failure. *Pediatr Clin North Am* 1984;31:1197–226.

367. Anon. Nitroglycerin patches—do they work? *Med Lett Drugs Ther* 1989;31:65–6.

368. Abrams J. Pharmacology of nitroglycerin and long-acting nitrates and their usefulness in the treatment of chronic congestive heart failure. In Gould L, Reddy CVR, eds. *Vasodilator therapy for cardiac disorders.* Mount Kisco, NY: Futura Publishing; 1979:129–67.

369. Schrader BJ et al. Acceptance of transcutaneous nitroglycerin patches by patients with angina pectoris. *Pharmacotherapy* 1986;6:83–6.

370. DeMots H, Glasser SPP. Intermittent transdermal nitroglycerin therapy in the treatment of chronic stable angina. *J Am Coll Cardiol* 1989;13:786–93.

371. Baaske DM et al. Nitroglycerin compatibility with intravenous fluid filters, containers, and administration sets. *Am J Hosp Pharm* 1980;37:201–5.

372. Amann AH et al. Plastic I.V. container for nitroglycerin. *Am J Hosp Pharm* 1980;37:618. Letter.

373. Haas CE et al. Effect of using a standard polyvinyl chloride intravenous infusion set on patient response to nitroglycerin. *Am J Hosp Pharm* 1992;49:1135–7.

374. Altavela JL et al. Clinical response to intravenous nitroglycerin infused through polyethylene or polyvinyl chloride tubing. *Am J Hosp Pharm* 1994;51:490–4.

375. Mulrow CD et al. Relative efficacy of vasodilator therapy in chronic congestive heart failure. Implications of randomized trials. *JAMA* 1988;259:3422–6.

376. Chaterjee K et al. Vasodilator therapy in chronic congestive heart failure. *Am J Cardiol* 1988;62:46A–54.

377. Cohn JN et al. A comparison of enalapril with hydralazine-isosorbide dinitrate in the treatment of chronic congestive heart failure. *N Engl J Med* 1991;325:303–10.

378. Parillo JE. Vasodilator therapy. In Chernow B et al., eds. *The pharmacological approach to the critically ill patient,* 3rd ed. Baltimore: Williams & Wilkins; 1994:470–83.

379. Johnson JA, Lalonde RL. Congestive heart failure. In DiPiro JT et al., eds. *Pharmacotherapy: a pathophysiologic approach,* 2nd ed. East Norwalk, CT: Appleton & Lange; 1993:160–93.

Central Nervous System Drugs

Anticonvulsants

Class Instructions: Anticonvulsants. It is important to take this medication as prescribed to control seizures; stopping it suddenly may cause an increase in seizures. This medication may cause drowsiness. Until the extent of this effect is known, use caution when driving, operating machinery, or performing other tasks requiring mental alertness. Avoid concurrent use of alcohol or other drugs that cause drowsiness. Report unusual or bothersome side effects. Always use an effective contraceptive; contact your physician if you plan to become or become pregnant.

CARBAMAZEPINE
Tegretol, Various

Pharmacology. Carbamazepine is an iminostilbene compound related structurally to the tricyclic antidepressants. In animals, carbamazepine acts presynaptically to block firing of action potentials, which decreases the release of excitatory neurotransmitters, and postsynaptically by blocking high-frequency repetitive discharge initiated at cell bodies.

Administration and Adult Dosage. PO for epilepsy 100–200 mg bid with meals initially, increase in increments of up to 200 mg/day at weekly intervals to effective dosage. Usual maintenance dosage is 10–30 mg/kg/day or 600–1600 mg/day in 2–4 divided doses;[1,2] tid or qid administration is recommended when enzyme-inducing antiepileptic drugs are administered concurrently. **SR** product may be given bid. **PO for trigeminal neuralgia** 100 mg bid initially; increasing in 200 mg/day increments until relief of pain, to a maximum of 1.2 g/day. Usual maintenance dosage is 400–800 mg/day in 2–3 divided doses. **Rectal administration** has been reported (see Fate).

Special Populations. *Pediatric Dosage.* PO for epilepsy (<6 yr) 10–20 mg/kg/day in 3–4 divided doses with the chewable tablets or in 4 divided doses with the suspension; (6–12 yr) 10–20 mg/kg/day with meals initially, increasing weekly in 100 mg/day increments as needed to achieve optimal clinical response. Usual maintenance dosage is 15–35 mg/kg/day or 400–800 mg/day in 3–4 divided doses. (>12 yr) same as adult dosage.[2]

Geriatric Dosage. Clearance of carbamazepine is reduced in some elderly patients; therefore, a lower maintenance dosage may be required.[3]

Other Conditions. During pregnancy, increases in carbamazepine clearance may occur; dosage increases guided by serum levels and patient status may be necessary.[2]

Dosage Forms. **Chew Tab** 100 mg; **Susp** 20 mg/mL; **Tab** 200 mg; **SR Tab** 100, 200, 400 mg (Tegretol XR).

Patient Instructions. *See* Anticonvulsants Class Instructions. Sore throat, fever, mouth ulcers, or easy bruising may be an early sign of a severe, but rare, blood disorder and should be reported immediately.

Pharmacokinetics. *Onset and Duration.* Steady-state serum levels are attained within 2–4 days and may subsequently decline because of autoinduction of metabolism (*see* Fate).[2]

Serum Levels. (Anticonvulsant) 4–12 mg/L (17–50 µmol/L). Variability exists in the relationship between serum levels and CNS side effects (*see* Notes).

Fate. Absorption from tablets is slow and erratic, with a bioavailability of 75–85%; peak serum levels occur 4–8 hr after dose.[2] Absorption is rapid with the suspension, with a peak serum level of 7.9 ± 1.9 mg/L at 1.6 ± 1.3 hr in the fasting state or 3.4 ± 3.4 hr with concomitant enteral tube feeding after a 500-mg oral dose.[4] A peak serum level of 5.1 ± 1.6 mg/L occurs 6.3 ± 1.5 hr after rectal administration of 6 mg/kg oral suspension (100 mg/5 mL) diluted with an equal volume of water.[5] The drug is 75–78% plasma protein bound.[2,6] V_d is 0.88 ± 0.06 L/kg in adults[4] and 1.2 ± 0.2 L/kg in children.[7] Large differences in Cl occur because of autoinduction of liver enzymes; autoinduction is completed within 1–2 weeks of monotherapy; Cl is 0.052 ± 0.04 L/hr/kg at end of week 1, 0.04 ± 0.02 L/hr/kg at week 2, and 0.054 ± 0.04 L/hr/kg at week 4.[8] Carbamazepine is metabolized to pharmacologically active carbamazepine-10,11-epoxide; the epoxide metabolite to carbamazepine serum level ratio at steady state is 0.19 ± 0.06 at a carbamazepine level of 6.9 ± 1.5 mg/L and 0.28 ± 1.4 at a carbamazepine level of 10.5 ± 2.6 mg/L.[9] (*See* Notes.) Only about 2% of drug is excreted unchanged in the urine.[2,6]

$t_{1/2}$. There are large interindividual differences because of autoinduction of liver enzymes. (Adults) 31.3 ± 5.9 hr after a single dose,[4] 14.5 ± 5.3 hr after 2 months;[9] (children) 29.4 ± 3.6 hr after a single dose, 15.2 ± 5.2 hr after 5 months.[7]

Adverse Reactions. Dizziness, drowsiness, headache, diplopia, nausea, and vomiting occur frequently with initiation of therapy and are minimized by slow titration of dosage. Mild, transient, morbilliform rash and thrombocytopenia also occur frequently. Occasionally, confusion, stomatitis, or rash occur. Hyponatremia and water intoxication occur, and risk factors include carbamazepine monotherapy, elevated serum levels, patient age >25 yr, vomiting, or diarrhea.[2] Transient leukopenia has been observed in 10–20% of patients; persistent leukopenia occurs in 2% of patients.[2] Discontinue drug if leukopenia (absolute neutrophil count less than 1500/µL) persists or any evidence of bone marrow depression develops. Rare effects include aplastic anemia, agranulocytosis, hepatitis, lenticular opacities, and arrhythmias.

Contraindications. History of bone marrow depression; hypersensitivity to tricyclic antidepressants.

Precautions. Pregnancy; history of liver disease. Abrupt withdrawal of the drug in patients with epilepsy may precipitate status epilepticus. Exacerbation of atypical absence seizures may occur in children receiving carbamazepine for mixed seizure disorders.[2] Use carbamazepine cautiously in patients with a history of severe hypersensitivity reactions to phenytoin or phenobarbital.

Drug Interactions. Because of structural similarities to tricyclic antidepressants, discontinue MAOIs for a minimum of 14 days before carbamazepine is begun. Carbamazepine can stimulate the metabolism of many drugs metabolized by CYP3A4, including oral anticoagulants, oral contraceptives, corticosteroids, cyclosporine, doxycycline, haloperidol, heterocyclic antidepressants, and theophylline. Many drugs inhibit carbamazepine metabolism, including cimetidine, clarithromycin, danazol, erythromycin, fluoxetine, isoniazid, propoxyphene, quinine, troleandomycin, verapamil, and diltiazem.

Parameters to Monitor. Baseline CBC and platelet counts; monitor more frequently if a decrease in WBC or platelet counts occurs. Monitor liver function tests periodically during long-term therapy. Monitor serum levels at least weekly during the first month of therapy because of autoinduction. Periodic serum level monitoring is useful in evaluating therapeutic efficacy or potential for adverse effects.[2]

Notes. The contribution of the carbamazepine-10,11-epoxide (CBZ-E) metabolite to the therapeutic or adverse effects of carbamazepine (CBZ) is uncertain. In one study, there was no significant correlation between toxicity score or seizure frequency and serum levels of CBZ, CBZ-E, or their sum in patients receiving CBZ monotherapy, or combination therapy with phenytoin or valproic acid.[9] (*See* Anticonvulsants Comparison Chart.) **Oxcarbazepine,** the 10-keto analogue of CBZ, is an investigational anticonvulsant.

CLONAZEPAM   Klonopin

Pharmacology. Clonazepam is a benzodiazepine anticonvulsant that limits the spread of seizure activity, possibly by enhancing the postsynaptic effect of the inhibitory neurotransmitter, γ-aminobutyric acid (GABA).

Administration and Adult Dosage. PO for epilepsy initial dosage should not exceed 0.5 mg tid; increase in 0.5–1 mg/day increments q 3 days to effective dosage, or to a maximum of 20 mg/day. Usual maintenance dosage is 4–8 mg/day.[1] **PO as an antipanic agent** 1–3 mg/day in 2 divided doses.[10,11] (*See* Notes.) **Rectal administration** has been reported (*see* Fate).

Special Populations. *Pediatric Dosage.* PO for epilepsy (up to 10 yr or 30 kg) 0.01–0.03 mg/kg/day initially in 2–3 divided doses; increase in 0.25–0.5 mg/day increments q 3 days to effective dosage, to a maximum of 0.2 mg/kg/day in 3 divided doses. Rectal administration has been reported (*see* Fate).

Geriatric Dosage. **PO for epilepsy** and as antipanic agent same as adult dosage initially. Maintenance dosage requirements may be lower in elderly patients because of reduced drug clearance and enhanced pharmacodynamic response.[12]

Dosage Forms. **Tab** 0.5, 1, 2 mg.

Patient Instructions. (*See* Anticonvulsants Class Instructions.)

Pharmacokinetics. *Onset and Duration.* Steady-state serum levels are attained in 4–8 days.[2] (*See* Notes.)

Serum Levels. 13–72 µg/L (40–230 nmol/L); however, some patients controlled with clonazepam may have levels below this range. There is a poor correlation between serum levels and efficacy or adverse effects.[2]

Fate. Rapidly absorbed orally; peak serum levels occur 1–3 hr after a dose. Serum levels of 18–40 µg/L occur 20–120 min following rectal administration of a 0.1 mg/kg dose of clonazepam suspension.[13] The drug is 86 ± 0.5% plasma protein bound;[2] V_d is 3.1 ± 1.2 L/kg; Cl is 0.059 ± 0.011 L/hr/kg.[14] The principal metabolite, 7-aminoclonazepam, is inactive. Less than 0.5% of clonazepam is excreted unchanged in urine.[2]

$t_{1/2}$. 34.1 ± 7.5 hr.[14]

Adverse Reactions. Drowsiness, ataxia, behavior disturbances, and personality changes (hyperactivity, restlessness, irritability; especially in children) occur frequently and require dosage reduction.[2] Occasionally, hypersalivation and bronchial hypersecretion occur and may cause respiratory difficulties. Rarely, anemia, leukopenia, thrombocytopenia, and respiratory depression occur. Nearly 50% of patients receiving long-term clonazepam may experience transient exacerbations of seizures, dysphoria, restlessness, or autonomic signs during clonazepam withdrawal.[15] An increased seizure frequency and status epilepticus occur rarely, possibly associated with supratherapeutic serum levels.[2]

Contraindications. Severe liver disease; acute narrow-angle glaucoma.

Precautions. Pregnancy; lactation; patients with chronic respiratory disease. May increase frequency of generalized tonic-clonic seizures in patients with mixed seizure types. Abrupt withdrawal of the drug in patients with epilepsy may precipitate status epilepticus. Absence status has been reported in patients receiving valproic acid concurrently.

Drug Interactions. Concurrent use with other CNS depressants may potentiate the sedation caused by clonazepam.

Parameters to Monitor. Periodic serum level monitoring is of limited value. Close attention to changes in patient's seizure frequency is necessary to monitor for the development of tolerance to the therapeutic effect (*see* Notes).

Notes. Tolerance to the anticonvulsant effect of clonazepam occurs in approximately one-third of patients within 3–6 months of starting the drug. Taper and discontinue clonazepam if therapeutic benefit cannot be demonstrated. Because of prominent CNS adverse effects and the development of tolerance, it is considered an alternative to **valproic acid** for myoclonic seizures and an alternative to **ethosuximide** or **valproic acid** for absence seizures.[1,6] *See* Anticonvulsants Comparison Chart. Clonazepam has also become an alternative to **alprazolam** for treatment of panic disorder. For patients who experience interdose symptom recurrence or morning rebound with alprazolam, clonazepam offers an equally effective alternative with the benefit of a longer duration of effect. When switching a patient from alprazolam to clonazepam, an equivalent dosage of clonazepam is one-half that of alprazolam.[10,11,16]

ETHOSUXIMIDE   Zarontin

Pharmacology. Ethosuximide is a succinimide that produces an anticonvulsant effect by direct modification of membrane function in excitable cells and/or alteration of inhibitory neurotransmitters. In humans, it suppresses three cycle per second spike and wave activity. (*See* Notes.)

Administration and Adult Dosage. PO for epilepsy 250 mg bid initially; increase in 250 mg/day increments at 4- to 7-day intervals to an effective dosage, to a maximum of 1.5 g/day. Usual maintenance dosage is 750–1250 mg/day in 1–2 doses.[1,2]

Special Populations. *Pediatric Dosage.* PO for epilepsy (3–6 yr) 250 mg/day initially; increase in 250 mg/day increments q 4–7 days to effective dosage, to a maximum of 1 g/day. Usual maintenance dosage is 20–40 mg/kg/day in 1–2 doses.[1,2] (>6 yr) same as adult dosage.

Geriatric Dosage. Same as adult dosage.

Dosage Forms. **Cap** 250 mg; **Syrup** 50 mg/mL.

Patient Instructions. (*See* Anticonvulsants Class Instructions.) This drug may be taken with food or milk to minimize stomach upset.

Pharmacokinetics. *Onset and Duration.* Steady-state serum levels are attained in 7–12 days.[2]

Serum Levels. 40–100 mg/L (280–710 µmol/L).[2]

Fate. The drug is well absorbed orally, with peak serum level in 3–7 hr in adults and children. Plasma protein binding is less than 10%. V_d is 0.69 L/kg;[17] Cl is 0.01 ± 0.04 L/hr/kg, greater in children.[2] Ethosuximide is metabolized to three inactive metabolites. About 20% of drug is excreted unchanged in the urine.[2,6]

$t_{1/2}$. (Adults) 52.6 hr;[18] (children) 31.6 ± 5.4 hr.[17]

Adverse Reactions. Nausea, vomiting, drowsiness, headache, hiccups, and dizziness occur frequently during initiation of therapy and usually are dose related. Occasionally, behavior changes or rashes occur. Rarely, SLE, leukopenia, aplastic anemia, or Stevens-Johnson syndrome occur.

Precautions. Pregnancy; patients with known liver or renal disease. Generalized tonic-clonic seizures may occur in patients with mixed seizure types who are treated with ethosuximide alone. Abrupt withdrawal of the drug may precipitate absence status epilepticus.

Contraindications. None known.

Drug Interactions. Ethosuximide may increase phenytoin serum levels and decrease levels of primidone (and its phenobarbital metabolite).

Parameters to Monitor. Periodic serum level monitoring, after attaining steady state (7–12 days), is useful in evaluating therapeutic efficacy or potential adverse effects.[2] Periodically monitor CBC, urinalysis, and liver function tests.

Notes. Ethosuximide is only indicated for treatment of absence seizures. Because of the drug's low potential for serious or long-term toxicity and its proven efficacy, it is considered the drug of choice for absence seizures. (*See* Anticonvulsants Comparison Chart.)

FELBAMATE   Felbatol

Pharmacology. Felbamate is a dicarbamate structurally related to meprobamate; its mechanism of action is not known, but may involve inhibition of N-methyl-d-aspartate responses and potentiation of γ-aminobutyric acid-a (GABA_a) receptor chloride currents.[19]

Administration and Adult Dosage. PO for epilepsy 1.2 g/day initially in 3–4 divided doses while reducing the dosage of concomitant antiepileptic drugs (phenytoin, carbamazepine, valproic acid, or phenobarbital) by 20–30%. Increase in 1200 mg/day increments at weekly intervals to a maximum of 3.6 g/day. Further reduction in the dosage of concomitant antiepileptic drugs may be required during felbamate titration.

Special Populations. *Pediatric Dosage.* **PO for epilepsy** 15 mg/kg/day initially in 3–4 divided doses while reducing the dosage of concomitant antiepileptic drugs (phenytoin, carbamazepine, valproic acid, or phenobarbital) by 20–30%. Increase in 15 mg/kg/day increments at weekly intervals to a maximum of 45 mg/kg/day. Further reduction in the dosage of concomitant antiepileptic drugs may be required during felbamate titration.

Geriatric Dosage. Dosage reduction may be required in patients with reduced hepatic or renal function and should be guided by clinical response.

Dosage Forms. Tab 400, 600 mg; **Susp** 120 mg/mL.

Patient Instructions. (*See* Anticonvulsants Class Instructions.) Felbamate has been associated with severe blood and liver disorders that can be fatal. Report signs of infection, bleeding, easy bruising, or signs of anemia (fatigue, weakness) immediately; also report abdominal pain or yellowing of the skin immediately. Give the patient the information/consent section of the Felbatol prescribing information and obtain informed consent at the time of initial prescribing.

Pharmacokinetics. *Onset and Duration.* Steady-state serum levels are attained in 2–3 days.[2]

Serum Levels. A therapeutic range has not been established. Serum concentrations reported in clinical studies range from 20–137 mg/L.[20,21]

Fate. Rapidly absorbed with over 90% bioavailability; peak serum levels occur 1–4 hr after an oral dose.[22] Food and antacids have no appreciable effect on absorption.[2] The drug is 22–25% plasma protein bound, primarily to albumin. V_d is 0.76 ± 0.08 L/kg; Cl is 0.030 ± 0.008 L/hr/kg in adults. From 40–50% is excreted unchanged in urine; 5% is excreted unchanged in feces; the remainder is excreted as inactive metabolites.[2]

$t_{1/2}$. 20.2 hr in normal volunteers;[22] 14.7 ± 2.8 hr in epileptic patients on concomitant enzyme-inducing antiepileptic drugs.[23]

Adverse Reactions. Anorexia, vomiting, insomnia, nausea, headache, weight loss, dizziness, and somnolence occur frequently. Adverse reaction frequency is lower when felbamate is used as monotherapy, and reactions often resolve during long-term therapy. Adverse reactions during adjunctive therapy may be the result of drug interactions. Felbamate is occasionally associated with aplastic anemia and hepatic failure (*see* Precautions), with fatality rates of 20–30%. It is not known whether the risks of aplastic anemia and hepatic failure are related to the duration of felbamate exposure.

Contraindications. History of any blood dyscrasia or hepatic dysfunction.

Precautions. Do not use felbamate as a first-line antiepileptic drug. Because of the risk of aplastic anemia and hepatic failure, use felbamate only in patients whose seizures cannot be controlled with other antiepileptic drugs and in patients whose epilepsy is so severe that the risks are deemed acceptable. Fully inform patients of the risks of felbamate therapy (see Patient Instructions).

Drug Interactions. Felbamate increases serum concentrations of phenytoin, carbamazepine epoxide (the active metabolite of carbamazepine), and valproate; therefore, reduce the dosage of these antiepileptics by 20–30% when felbamate is initiated.

Parameters to Monitor. Close monitoring of CBC, platelets, liver function tests, and clinical signs or symptoms of infection, bruising, bleeding, or hepatitis is essential. Monitor liver function tests (AST, ALT, bilirubin) q 1–2 weeks while treatment continues. The acceptable frequency of hematologic monitoring is not established. Routine monitoring of serum levels is of limited value because of the lack of a well-defined therapeutic range.

Notes. Felbamate is effective for the treatment of partial and secondarily generalized seizures in adults and for partial and generalized seizures associated with the Lennox-Gastaut syndrome in children.

FOSPHENYTOIN   Cerebyx

Fosphenytoin is a phosphate ester prodrug that is rapidly and completely converted to phenytoin in vivo by phosphatases after parenteral administration. Fosphenytoin appears to have no pharmacologic activity prior to its conversion to phenytoin. Unlike phenytoin, which is relatively water insoluble, fosphenytoin is highly soluble in aqueous solutions (including solutions containing dextrose). Fosphenytoin is effective for short-term use (up to 14 days) in the acute treatment of status epilepticus, for the treatment or prophylaxis of seizures in patients with epilepsy or in neurosurgery patients, and as a substitute for oral phenytoin. Fosphenytoin is extensively bound to plasma proteins (>90%), primarily albumin, and the binding increases nonlinearly with increasing fosphenytoin concentration. Correspondingly, V_d of fosphenytoin varies with concentration: 2.5 L after 100 mg and 8 L after 1200 mg in adults. In healthy subjects, fosphenytoin is converted to phenytoin with a half-life of 8.1 ± 1.5 min after IV administration; the conversion rate is not affected by renal or hepatic disease; 150 mg fosphenytoin yields 100 mg phenytoin. Peak phenytoin concentrations occur approximately 3 hr after IM injection. Fluorescence polarization (eg, TDx) and enzyme multiplied (Emit) immunoassays overestimate phenytoin concentrations when fosphenytoin is present. Consider this when monitoring phenytoin concentrations, especially after IM administration. Adverse effects associated with fosphenytoin are similar to those of phenytoin. In addition, fosphenytoin commonly causes transient pruritus during IV administration that is alleviated by slowing or stopping the infusion. Fosphenytoin is less likely than phenytoin to cause venous irritation after IV administration, and injection site reactions after IM administration are no more frequent than after placebo. Fosphenytoin can be administered by the IV or IM routes. The usual dosage of fosphenytoin for status epilepticus is 22.5–30 mg/kg fosphenytoin (equivalent to 15–20 mg/kg of phenytoin) given IV at a rate of 150–225 mg/min fosphenytoin (100–150 mg/min phenytoin equivalents). A loading dose of 15–30 mg/kg fosphenytoin (10–20 mg/kg phenytoin equivalents) can be given IM or IV for the treatment or prophylaxis of seizures. IM injections of up to 20 (twenty) mL

have been well tolerated when administered at a single site. When used as a substitute for oral phenytoin, fosphenytoin can be administered at the same pheny-
toin-equivalent dosage and frequency.[24–27] Available as 50 mg/mL phenytoin
equivalent injection.

GABAPENTIN   Neurontin

Pharmacology. Gabapentin is a cyclohexane compound structurally related to
γ-aminobutyric acid (GABA); its mechanism of action is not known. Gabapentin
does not interact with GABA receptors, nor does it alter the formation, release,
degradation, or reuptake of GABA.

Administration and Adult Dosage. **PO for epilepsy** 300 mg hs on day 1; 300 mg
bid on day 2; 300 mg tid on day 3. Dosage may be increased further according to
clinical response. Usual maintenance dosage is 900–2400 mg/day in 3 divided
doses.[1] Dosages of 3.6–4.8 g/day have been well tolerated in some patients.[28]

Special Populations. *Pediatric Dosage.* (<12 yr) Safety and efficacy not established.

Geriatric Dosage. Lower dosages may be required due to normal age-related decreases in renal function.

Other Conditions. Reduce dosage in patients with compromised renal function as
indicated below:

CL_{CR} (ML/MIN)	TOTAL DAILY DOSAGE	DOSAGE REGIMEN
>60	1200 mg	400 mg tid
30–60	600 mg	300 mg bid
15–30	300 mg	300 mg daily
<15	150 mg	300 mg every other day
Hemodialysis	—	200–300 mg after dialysis

Dosage Forms. **Cap** 100, 300, 400 mg.

Patient Instructions. (*See* Anticonvulsants Class Instructions.) Do not take this
drug with antacids.

Pharmacokinetics. *Onset and Duration.* Steady-state serum levels are attained in
1–2 days in patients with normal renal function.[29]

Serum Levels. A therapeutic range has not been established. In one study, a therapeutic effect correlated with serum concentrations greater than 2 mg/L.[30]

Fate. Rapidly absorbed and food has no effect on absorption. Absorption occurs
via a saturable transport mechanism; therefore, bioavailability decreases with
dosages greater than 1.8 g/day. At this dosage it is 60%, but at a dosage of 4.8
g/day, bioavailability is 35%.[29] The drug is not bound to plasma proteins. V_d is 58
± 6 L in adults; Cl is 0.17 ± 0.05 L/kg/hr in adults.[31] Gabapentin is not appreciably metabolized, but is eliminated unchanged in urine.

$t_{1/2}$. 4.8 ± 1.4 hr in adults with epilepsy.[31] Clearance is linearly related to creatinine clearance.

Adverse Reactions. Somnolence, dizziness, ataxia, nystagmus, and headache occur frequently. Symptoms are of mild to moderate severity and resolve within 2 weeks with continued treatment.[32] Weight gain (mean, 4.9% of body weight) and peripheral edema also occur frequently.[33] Occasionally rash occurs. Rarely behavioral changes in children occur.[34]

Contraindications. None known.

Precautions. Abrupt withdrawal of gabapentin in patients with epilepsy may precipitate status epilepticus. In vivo carcinogenicity studies demonstrate a high incidence of pancreatic acinar cell tumors in male rats; however, the relevance of this observation to humans is not known.

Drug Interactions. Gabapentin does not induce or inhibit hepatic microsomal enzymes and does not affect the metabolism of other antiepileptic drugs or oral contraceptives. Antacids decrease the oral bioavailability of gabapentin by about 20%.

Parameters to Monitor. Serum level monitoring is of limited value because of the lack of a well-defined therapeutic range. Routine monitoring of clinical laboratory parameters during gabapentin therapy is not indicated.

Notes. Gabapentin is indicated as adjunctive treatment for partial and secondarily generalized seizures in adults. Preliminary studies indicate that the drug may be efficacious as an adjunct in children with refractory partial seizures.[35]

LAMOTRIGINE   Lamictal

Pharmacology. Lamotrigine is a phenyltriazine derivative unrelated to other marketed antiepileptic drugs. Lamotrigine inhibits voltage-dependent sodium channels, thereby stabilizing neuronal membranes and reducing the release of excitatory neurotransmitters such as glutamate and aspartate.

Administration and Adult Dosage. Adjust starting dosages, titration schedules, and maintenance dosage based on concomitant therapy. **PO for epilepsy in patients receiving enzyme-inducing antiepileptic drugs** (eg, carbamazepine, phenytoin, phenobarbital, and primidone) 50 mg/day for 2 weeks, then increase to 50 mg bid for 2 more weeks. Thereafter, increase dosage in 100 mg/day increments at weekly intervals to a maintenance dosage of 300–500 mg/day in 2 divided doses. **PO for epilepsy in patients receiving enzyme-inducing antiepileptic drugs with valproic acid** 25 mg every other day for 2 weeks, then increase to 25 mg/day for 2 more weeks. Thereafter, increase dosage in 25–50 mg/day increments at 1- to 2-week intervals to a maintenance dosage of 100-200 mg/day in 2 divided doses. Dosage recommendations are not available for patients receiving valproic acid alone, but dosages are expected to be lower due to prolonged half-life.

Special Populations. *Pediatric Dosage.* (<16 yr) Safety and efficacy not established.

Geriatric Dosage. Dosage reduction may be required in patients with reduced hepatic or renal function and should be guided by clinical response.

Other Conditions. Patients with chronic renal failure or liver disease may require lower dosages of lamotrigine; however, specific dosage guidelines are not available.

Dosage Forms. **Tab** 25, 100, 150, 200 mg.

Patient Instructions. (*See* Anticonvulsants Class Instructions.) Inform your physician if a skin rash develops.

Pharmacokinetics. *Onset and Duration.* Steady-state serum levels are attained in 2–3 days.[2]

Serum Levels. A therapeutic range has not been established. In most clinical trials, trough serum concentrations of lamotrigine ranged from 1–3 mg/L.[36]

Fate. The drug is rapidly absorbed, with a bioavailability of 98 ± 5%; peak serum levels occur 2.8 ± 1.3 hr after an oral dose. Food does not affect absorption. Lamotrigine is 56% bound to plasma proteins. V_d is 1.2 ± 0.12 L/kg;[37] Cl is 0.049 ± 0.028 L/hr/kg in adults.[38] From 7–30% is excreted unchanged in urine; 80–90% is excreted as the inactive glucuronide conjugate.[37]

$t_{1/2}$. 24.1 ± 5.7 hr in normal volunteers taking no other medications;[37] 14.3 ± 6.9 hr in patients taking enzyme-inducing antiepileptic drugs; 29.6 ± 10 hr in patients taking enzyme-inducing antiepileptic drugs with valproic acid;[38] 59 hr in patients taking valproic acid alone.[37]

Adverse Reactions. Dose-related dizziness, ataxia, somnolence, headache, diplopia, nausea, vomiting, and rash occur frequently. Rash occurs in about 10% of patients, usually within 4–6 weeks of treatment initiation. The rash is usually maculopapular and erythematous; serious rash with systemic involvement (eg, Stevens-Johnson syndrome) occurs rarely. Risk factors for rash include concomitant valproic acid therapy, high initial dosage of lamotrigine, and rapid escalation of lamotrigine dosage. After resolution of mild rash, patients may be rechallenged with a lower dosage or slower titration schedule.

Contraindications. None known.

Precautions. Initiate lamotrigine cautiously in patients taking valproic acid because of a higher risk of rash (*see* Administration and Adult Dosage).

Drug Interactions. Dizziness, diplopia, and ataxia are more common in patients taking carbamazepine concomitantly and may reflect a pharmacodynamic interaction. Lamotrigine has no significant effect on blood levels of phenytoin and carbamazepine. Conflicting data exist regarding the effect of lamotrigine on carbamazepine-10,11-epoxide. Lamotrigine reduces steady-state valproic acid levels by 25%. Valproic acid increases lamotrigine levels by about twofold, and carbamazepine, phenobarbital, primidone, and phenytoin each decrease lamotrigine serum levels.

Parameters to Monitor. Serum level monitoring is of limited value because of the lack of a well-defined therapeutic range. Routine monitoring of clinical laboratory parameters during lamotrigine therapy is not necessary.

Notes. Lamotrigine is indicated as adjunctive treatment for partial and secondarily generalized seizures in adults. It may be an effective treatment for refractory epilepsy in children.[39] Lamotrigine may be effective as monotherapy and appears to be better tolerated than carbamazepine monotherapy at dosages that are equally effective for the treatment of partial epilepsy.[40] (*See* Anticonvulsants Comparison Chart.)

PHENOBARBITAL   Various

Pharmacology. Phenobarbital is a barbiturate that exerts an anticonvulsant effect by depressing excitatory postsynaptic seizure discharge and increasing the convulsive threshold for electric and chemical stimulation.

Administration and Adult Dosage. **PO or IM for epilepsy** 60–90 mg/day initially, increase in 30–60 mg/day increments q 7–14 days to an effective dosage. Usual maintenance dosage is 90–240 mg/day or 1–3 mg/kg/day hs.[1] **IV for status epilepticus** 20 mg/kg at a rate of 100 mg/min.[41] **Rectal administration** has been reported (*see* Fate). (*See also* Adverse Reactions and Notes.)

Special Populations. *Pediatric Dosage.* **PO or IM for epilepsy** initially, titrate dosage to minimize sedation. Usual maintenance dosage is 2–5 mg/kg/day or 125 mg/m²/day given at bedtime.[2] **IV for status epilepticus** 20 mg/kg at a rate of 50–100 mg/min.[42] *See* Adverse Reactions and Notes.

Geriatric Dosage. Clearance of phenobarbital is reduced in the elderly, so lower maintenance dosages may be required.[3]

Other Conditions. During pregnancy, phenobarbital clearance may increase. Dosage increases may be necessary and should be guided by serum levels and patient status.[2]

Dosage Forms. **Cap** 16 mg; **Tab** 15, 16, 30, 60, 100 mg; **Elxr** 3, 4 mg/mL; **Inj** 30, 60, 65, 130 mg/mL.

Patient Instructions. (*See* Anticonvulsants Class Instructions.)

Pharmacokinetics. *Onset and Duration.* Steady-state serum levels are attained in about 21 days.[2]

Serum Levels. (Anticonvulsant) 15–35 mg/L (65–150 μmol/L); dysarthria, ataxia, and nystagmus appear as serum level approaches 40 mg/L (172 μmol/L).[1,2,43]

Fate. The drug is slowly absorbed orally with 95–100% bioavailability; peak serum level occurs 2–4 hr after a PO or IM dose.[2] Rectal bioavailability is 90%, with a peak of 7.2 ± 0.8 mg/L (31 ± 3.4 μmol/L) 4.4 ± 0.6 hr after rectal administration of a 5 mg/kg dose of parenteral phenobarbital sodium soln.[44] The drug is 45–60% plasma protein bound. V_d is 0.61 ± 0.05 L/kg; Cl is 0.004 ± 0.0008 L/hr/kg in adults,[45] with 50–80% metabolized in liver to p-hydroxyphenobarbital (inactive). The drug is 20–50% excreted unchanged in urine; alkalinization of urine increases renal phenobarbital clearance.[2,6]

$t_{1/2}$. (Adults) 100 ± 17 hr;[46] (cirrhosis) 130 ± 15 hr;[45] (children 1–5 yr) 69 ± 3.2 hr.[47]

Adverse Reactions. (*See* Serum Levels.) Sedation is frequent and dose related; tolerance usually develops with long-term administration. In adults, phenobarbital can impair cognition, reaction time, and motor performance.[48] Loss of concentration, mental dulling, depression of affect, insomnia, and hyperkinetic activity occur frequently with long-term therapy in children and the elderly.[43] Connective tissue disorders associated with barbiturates occur in 6% of patients, usually within the first year of treatment.[49] Occasionally, skin rashes or folate deficiency occur. Rarely, megaloblastic anemia, hepatitis, exfoliative dermatitis, or Stevens-Johnson syndrome are reported. Patients may be at risk for similar hypersensitivity reactions if rechallenged with phenytoin or carbamazepine.[50] Neonatal hemorrhage has been reported in newborns whose mothers were taking phenobarbital. SC or intra-arterial injection may produce tissue necrosis. IV administration, especially when given after IV benzodiazepines, may produce severe respiratory depression and provision for respiratory support should be made.

Contraindications. History of porphyria or severe respiratory disease where dyspnea or obstruction is present.

Precautions. Pregnancy; lactation. Use with caution in patients with marked liver or renal disease because drug clearance is slowed. Abrupt withdrawal of the drug in patients with epilepsy may precipitate status epilepticus.

Drug Interactions. Concurrent use with other CNS depressants may potentiate the sedation caused by phenobarbital. Numerous drugs may increase phenobarbital serum levels, possibly requiring phenobarbital dosage reduction; phenobarbital may stimulate CYP2B6 and CYP3A, and increase metabolism of many drugs (see Part II, Chapter 1).

Parameters to Monitor. Periodic serum level monitoring, after attaining steady state (about 21 days), is useful in guiding dosage changes or evaluating adverse effects.[2] Monitor CBC and liver function tests periodically during long-term therapy.

Notes. In tonic-clonic status epilepticus, phenobarbital is usually considered a third agent after IV phenytoin plus IV diazepam or lorazepam have failed to control seizures.[41] Considering clinical efficacy and patient tolerance, phenobarbital is a third- or fourth-line choice for single drug therapy of partial or generalized tonic-clonic seizures compared to the drugs of first choice: carbamazepine, phenytoin, or valproic acid.[2] (*See* Anticonvulsants Comparison Chart.)

PHENYTOIN Dilantin, Various

Pharmacology. Phenytoin is a hydantoin that suppresses the spread of seizure activity mainly by inhibiting synaptic posttetanic potentiation and blocking the propagation of electric discharge. Phenytoin may decrease sodium transport and block calcium channels at the cellular level to produce these actions.

Administration and Adult Dosage. PO maintenance dosage 300 mg/day in 1–3 doses initially. Using serum levels as a guide, increase in 30–100 mg/day increments q 10–21 days to effective dosage.[2] Because of dose-dependent, saturable metabolism, small increases in dosage may produce disproportionate increases in serum levels. **Usual maintenance dosage** is 300–400 mg/day or 4–8 mg/kg/day in 1 or 2 doses.[1] Only extended-release phenytoin sodium capsules are approved for once-daily administration. **PO loading dosage** 15 mg/kg in 3 divided doses, administered at 2-hr intervals. Using serum levels as a guide, a maintenance dosage can be initiated within 24 hr of starting the loading dosage. **IV loading dose** 15–20 mg/kg by direct IV injection, at a rate not greater than 50 mg/min or

0.75 mg/kg/min in adults.[43] Therapeutic serum levels persist for 12–24 hr in most patients.[51] Alternatively, dilute the loading dose in 50–150 mL of 0.45% or 0.9% NaCl and infuse through an IV volume control set with an in-line filter at a rate not greater than 50 mg/min.[2,52] In nonemergency situations, an IV dose of 5 mg/kg q 2 hr for 3 doses at a rate of 50 mg/min results in phenytoin serum levels of 10–20 mg/L 12 hr after the third dose.[53] *See* Adverse Reactions and Notes. **IM administration** is painful and results in slow, but complete, absorption because of deposition of phenytoin crystals in muscle.[2] The IM route is not recommended. The IV route is preferred in patients unable to take phenytoin by mouth.

Special Populations. *Pediatric Dosage.* **PO maintenance dosage** 5 mg/kg/day initially in 2–3 divided doses. Increase initial dosage in small increments q 7–10 days to effective dosage.[2] Because of dose-dependent metabolism, small increases in dosage may produce disproportionate increases in serum levels. Usual maintenance dosage is 4–8 mg/kg/day in 2–3 divided doses.[1] **IV loading dose** (neonates) 1–3 mg/kg/min; (older infants and children) same as adult dosage.

Geriatric Dosage. **PO maintenance dosage** 200–300 mg/day in 1–3 doses. Advanced age may be associated with a decrease in phenytoin clearance and a reduction in albumin concentration.[54] Dosage adjustment should be guided by phenytoin levels and patient status (*see* Serum Levels).

Other Conditions. During pregnancy or febrile illness, or following acute traumatic injury, phenytoin clearance may increase; dosage adjustment may be necessary and should be guided by serum levels and patient status.[55–57] Renal disease and hypoalbuminemia can alter phenytoin binding to plasma proteins, resulting in a change in the usual ratio of free to total phenytoin levels; renal disease alters phenytoin protein binding because of decreased affinity of plasma proteins. Increases in fraction unbound are most pronounced in patients with Cl_{cr} <25 mL/min. Ideally, dosage adjustment should be guided by patient status and actual measurement of unbound and total phenytoin levels (*see* Serum Levels).

Dosage Forms. (Phenytoin) **Chew Tab** 50 mg; **Susp** 6, 25 mg/mL. (Phenytoin sodium) **Cap** (extended or prompt) 30, 100 mg; **Inj** 50 mg/mL. Phenytoin sodium is 92% phenytoin.

Patient Instructions. (*See* Anticonvulsants Class Instructions.) Good dental hygiene and regular dental visits may minimize gum tenderness, bleeding, or enlargement (especially in children). Shake oral suspension well prior to each dose and use a calibrated measuring device (*see* Notes). Call physician if skin rash develops.

Pharmacokinetics. *Onset and Duration.* Time to steady state increases with increasing dosage and serum level. Steady state is usually attained within 7–14 days, but may take as long as 28 days.[2]

Serum Levels. 10–20 mg/L (40–80 μmol/L) in patients with normal renal function and serum albumin concentration. Nystagmus, slurred speech, ataxia, or dizziness appear in most patients as serum level approaches 20 mg/L; drowsiness, diplopia, behavioral changes, and cognitive impairment above 30 mg/L (120 μmol/L).[2] The equation $C_{normal} = C_{observed}/[0.2 \times albumin + 0.1]$ is used to estimate the concentration of phenytoin that would be expected if the albumin concentration were normal (C_{normal}) from the measured total phenytoin concentration in a hypoalbuminemic patient ($C_{observed}$) and the patient's albumin concentration in g/dL (albumin). In patients with end-stage renal disease (Cl_{cr} <10 ml/min), the equation $C_{normal} = C_{observed}/[0.1 \times albumin + 0.1]$ is used.[58] *See also* Special Populations, Other Conditions.

Fate. Oral phenytoin absorption is very slow and incomplete in infants ≤3 months of age.[2] Bioavailability of the suspension is decreased in patients receiving concomitant enteral feedings (*see* Precautions). IM injection is slowly absorbed over several days because of deposition of phenytoin crystals in muscle. Peak serum levels occur 4–8 hr after a single dose of an extended-release capsule;[2] after oral loading given in divided doses, the time to reach a serum level of 10 mg/L is 4.5 ± 2.1 hr for prompt-release capsules and 9.6 ± 2.5 hr for extended-release capsules.[59] Time to peak serum level increases with increasing oral dosages.[60] About 90% is plasma protein bound.[2] Hypoalbuminemia, chronic liver or renal disease, nephrotic syndrome, AIDS, or acute traumatic injury alter protein binding and increase the fraction of unbound phenytoin.[2,55] V_d is 0.83 ± 0.2 L/kg in adults with acute seizures;[52] 0.79 ± 0.25 L/kg in critically ill adults following trauma.[55] Hepatic metabolism is capacity limited, exhibiting Michaelis-Menten pharmacokinetics; therefore, Cl decreases as serum level increases. Mean apparent V_{max} is 0.45 mg/L/hr; mean apparent K_m is 6.2 mg/L in adults.[2] About 70% of phenytoin is excreted in urine as the inactive metabolite, 5-(p-hydroxyphenyl)-5-phenylhydantoin (HPPH). Less than 5% of the parent drug is excreted unchanged in urine.[2,6]

$t_{1/2}$. Phenytoin has no true half-life, but its apparent half-life increases as serum level increases; at phenytoin serum level of 1 mg/L, predicted mean phenytoin half-life is 12.8 hr; 25.8 hr at 10 mg/L; 40.2 hr at 20 mg/L; and 69.1 hr at 40 mg/L.[2,61]

Adverse Reactions. (*See* Serum Levels.) Erythematous morbilliform rash occurs frequently. Do not resume phenytoin if rash is exfoliative, purpuric, bullous or if accompanied by fever. With long-term administration, hirsutism, gingival hypertrophy (especially in children and adolescents), coarsening of facial features, acneiform eruption, osteomalacia, and folate deficiency with mild macrocytosis occur frequently.[2,43] Bradycardia or hypotension caused by rapid IV administration are reported occasionally; slowing the rate of administration may minimize these complications.[41,51] Severe soft tissue injury following IV phenytoin is more likely in elderly (>70 yr) women who receive 2 or more infusions through small (20 gauge or smaller) IV devices.[62] Hepatotoxicity occurs occasionally, usually within the first 6 weeks, and presents with fever, rash, lymphadenopathy, and hepatomegaly.[63] Other idiosyncratic reactions are rare, may occur together within the first 2 months, and include fever, lymphoid hyperplasia, eosinophilia, erythema multiforme, exfoliative dermatitis, Stevens-Johnson syndrome, leukopenia, anemia, thrombocytopenia, serum sickness, and SLE.[2] These patients are at risk for similar hypersensitivity reactions if rechallenged with phenobarbital or carbamazepine.[50] Concurrent cranial irradiation predisposes patients to the development of erythema multiforme.[64] A syndrome of anomalies in infants of phenytoin-exposed mothers has been described (fetal hydantoin syndrome).

Contraindications. None known.

Precautions. Pregnancy; lactation. Use with caution in patients with severe liver disease or diabetes, or those with a history of severe hypersensitivity reactions to carbamazepine or phenobarbital. Abrupt withdrawal of the drug in patients with epilepsy may precipitate status epilepticus. If the patient's nutritional status allows, interrupt tube feeding 2 hr before and after the dose and irrigate the feeding tube to improve absorption; nevertheless, the patient may require an increase in phenytoin dosage. If the feedings are discontinued after the phenytoin dosage is increased, the dosage must be adjusted to prevent toxic serum levels from occurring.[65]

Drug Interactions. Chronic alcohol use, barbiturates, rifampin, and some other drugs may stimulate phenytoin metabolism and increase phenytoin dosage requirements. Numerous drugs may increase phenytoin serum levels, possibly requiring phenytoin dosage reduction; phenytoin may stimulate CYP2B6 and CYP3A, and may increase metabolism of many drugs (*see* Part II, Chapter 1). IV phenytoin may produce hypotension in severely ill patients receiving IV dopamine. The antiparkinson effect of levodopa may be inhibited by phenytoin. Signs of lithium toxicity may occur in the absence of increased serum lithium in patients on phenytoin.

Parameters to Monitor. Serum level monitoring, after attaining steady state (10–21 days), is useful in evaluating therapeutic efficacy or potential for adverse effects.[2] Patient and serum level monitoring are recommended when changing phenytoin dosage form or brand; monitor serum levels q 5–7 days to assess trend in concentrations. Monitor CBC and liver function tests periodically with long-term therapy.

Notes. Agitation or shaking is needed to resuspend phenytoin suspension; settling occurs 5 weeks after resuspension.[66] In tonic-clonic status epilepticus, phenytoin's anticonvulsant effect appears 20–30 min after start of the infusion. Thus, in this situation, concurrent use of phenytoin with a rapid-acting injectable benzodiazepine (**diazepam** or **lorazepam**) is recommended.[41] Phenytoin is recommended, as is **carbamazepine,** as a drug of first choice for single drug therapy of partial or generalized tonic-clonic seizures.[67] (*See* Anticonvulsants Comparison Chart.)

PRIMIDONE
Mysoline, Various

Pharmacology. Primidone (desoxyphenobarbital) is structurally related to the barbiturates. Primidone and its metabolites, phenylethylmalonamide (PEMA) and phenobarbital, all exert anticonvulsant activity. (See Phenobarbital.)

Administration and Adult Dosage. PO for epilepsy 50–100 mg hs initially; increase in 100–125 mg/day increments q 2–3 days to effective dosage, to a maximum of 2 g/day. Usual maintenance dosage is 250–500 mg tid.[1]

Special Populations. *Pediatric Dosage.* **PO for epilepsy** (<8 yr) 50 mg hs initially; increase by 50 mg in 3 days and thereafter in 100–125 mg/day increments q 3 days to effective dosage. Usual maintenance dosage is 125–250 mg tid or 10–20 mg/kg/day in 3 divided doses. (≥8 yr) same as adult dosage.

Geriatric Dosage. Clearance of primidone is unchanged in elderly patients; however, phenobarbital clearance is reduced. Lower maintenance dosages may be required.

Dosage Forms. **Susp** 50 mg/mL; **Tab** 50, 250 mg.

Patient Instructions. (*See* Anticonvulsants Class Instructions.)

Pharmacokinetics. *Onset and Duration.* Steady-state serum levels are attained in about 3 days.[2]

Serum Levels. (Primidone) 6–12 mg/L (28–55 μmol/L).[1,2,43] (*See also* Phenobarbital.) During monotherapy, primidone to phenobarbital serum level ratios are about 1:1.[2] During polytherapy with enzyme-inducing agents, this ratio increases to 4:1.[2] During monotherapy, the PEMA to primidone serum level ratio at steady state is 0.74 ± 0.38 for samples drawn before the first morning dose.[2]

Fate. The drug is rapidly absorbed with 90–100% bioavailability; peak serum levels occur 2–6 hr after an oral dose. The drug is 0–20% plasma protein bound; V_d is 0.86 ± 0.22 L/kg;[68] Cl with monotherapy is 0.035 ± 0.02 L/hr/kg; with concomitant anticonvulsants, it is 0.052 ± 0.02 L/hr/kg;[2] and in monotherapy with concomitant acute viral hepatitis, it is 0.042 ± 0.14 L/hr/kg.[68] Primidone is metabolized in liver to PEMA and phenobarbital; 76% of the drug is excreted into the urine within 5 days after a single dose as 64% primidone, 7% PEMA, 2% phenobarbital, and 3% unidentified products.[2]

$t_{1/2}$. (Primidone) 15.2 ± 4.8 hr (monotherapy); 8.3 ± 2.9 hr (with concomitant enzyme-inducing anticonvulsants); 18 ± 3.1 hr (with acute viral hepatitis).[68] (PEMA) 21 ± 3 hr (primidone monotherapy); 17 ± 4.3 hr (with concomitant anticonvulsants).[69] (*See also* Phenobarbital.)

Adverse Reactions. Drowsiness, ataxia, nausea, weakness, and dizziness occur frequently during first month of therapy and may become tolerable with time. Behavioral disturbances, depression of affect, and cognitive impairment occur frequently with long-term therapy in children and the elderly.[2] Occasionally, skin rashes and rarely, impotence, leukopenia, thrombocytopenia, megaloblastic anemia, or lymphadenopathy occur.[2,43]

Contraindications. History of porphyria; hypersensitivity to phenobarbital.

Precautions. Pregnancy; lactation. Use with caution in patients with severe liver or renal disease. Abrupt withdrawal of the drug in patients with epilepsy may precipitate status epilepticus. (*See* Phenobarbital Notes.)

Drug Interactions. Concurrent use with other CNS depressants may potentiate the sedation caused by phenobarbital. Primidone levels may be decreased by concurrent acetazolamide, carbamazepine, or succimides. Primidone levels may be increased by concurrent hydantoins, isoniazid, or niacinamide.

Parameters to Monitor. Periodic serum level monitoring of primidone and phenobarbital after attaining steady state (primidone, 3 days; phenobarbital, 21 days) is useful in guiding dosage changes, detecting noncompliance, or evaluating adverse effects.[2] Monitor CBC, electrolytes, and liver function tests periodically during long-term therapy.

Notes. Considering comparative efficacy and good patient tolerance of **carbamazepine, phenytoin,** and **valproic acid,** primidone is a fourth- or fifth-line choice for single drug therapy of generalized tonic-clonic seizures. In a large, multicenter trial comparing carbamazepine, phenytoin, phenobarbital, and primidone, primidone was least successful in controlling seizures with acceptable adverse effects.[67]

TOPIRAMATE   Topamax

Topiramate, a derivative of the naturally occurring monosaccharide d-fructose, reduces the frequency of action potentials elicited by depolarizing currents in a manner similar to phenytoin and carbamazepine. Topiramate also increases γ-aminobutyric acid (GABA)-induced chloride flux, although the drug has no direct effect on GABA binding sites. Its mechanism of action appears to be distinct from other antiepileptic drugs. It is effective as adjunctive therapy for medically refractory partial seizures: about 50% of patients treated with topiramate have a 50% or greater reduction in the frequency of partial seizures. It is rapidly absorbed after oral administration, with peak concentrations occurring within 4 hr. Food has little effect on the rate or extent of topiramate absorption. Topiramate is about 15% bound to plasma proteins. V_d is about 0.7 L/kg; Cl is 1.3–2.2 L/hr in adults. Topiramate is 50–80% excreted unchanged in urine; the remainder is metabolized. The half-life is 20–30 hr during monotherapy and 12–15 hr during concomitant therapy with enzyme-induced antiepileptic drugs. A therapeutic range of topiramate serum concentrations has not been defined. The drug has no effect on the clearance of **carbamazepine** and **valproic acid;** however, **phenytoin** clearance is reduced by approximately 20%. Common adverse effects during topiramate therapy include somnolence, dizziness, fatigue, impaired concentration, nervousness, and confusion. These effects occur during the dosage titration period and often resolve during maintenance therapy. A higher frequency of renal stones has been noted in topiramate-treated patients, although the risk is not related to dosage or duration of therapy. The usual oral dosage is 400 mg/day in 2 divided doses.[2,70,71] Available as 25-, 100-, and 200-mg tablets.

VALPROIC ACID   Depakene, Depacon, Various

DIVALPROEX SODIUM   Depakote

Pharmacology. Valproic acid is a carboxylic acid compound whose anticonvulsant activity may be mediated by an inhibitory neurotransmitter, γ-aminobutyric acid (GABA). Valproic acid may increase GABA levels by inhibiting GABA metabolism or by enhancing postsynaptic GABA activity. Valproic acid also limits repetitive neuronal firing through voltage- and usage-dependent sodium channels. Divalproex is comprised of sodium valproate and valproic acid (*see* Notes).

Administration and Adult Dosage. PO for epilepsy (valproic acid) 15 mg/kg/day initially in 2–3 divided doses, increasing in 5–10 mg/kg/day increments at weekly intervals to an effective dosage, to a maximum of 60 mg/kg/day. Usual maintenance dosage is 15–40 mg/kg/day in 3 divided doses.[72] In patients receiving valproic acid, divalproex can be substituted at the same daily dosage, and in selected patients, it can be given bid. **PO for migraine prophylaxis** (divalproex) 250 mg bid, to a maximum of 1 g/day. **PO for mania** (divalproex) 750 mg/day in divided doses, increasing as rapidly as possible to the lowest dosage that produces the desired effect, to a maximum of 60 mg/kg/day (*see* Serum Levels). Long-term experience with this use is minimal and characterized by a high drop-out rate. **IV for epilepsy** (valproic acid) same as oral dosage. **Rectal administration** has been reported (*see* Fate).

Special Populations. *Pediatric Dosage.* Same as adult dosage.

Geriatric Dosage. Reduce the starting dosage in the elderly. Protein binding and unbound clearance of valproic acid are reduced in the elderly, and the desired clinical response may be achieved with a lower dosage than in younger adults. Dosage adjustments should be guided by valproic acid levels (preferably free levels in patients with low serum albumin) and patient status.[3]

Dosage Forms. (Valproic acid) **Cap** 250 mg; **Syrup** 50 mg/mL; **Inj** 100 mg/mL; (divalproex) **EC Tab** 125, 250, 500 mg; **Cap** (EC granules) 125 mg.

Patient Instructions. (*See* Anticonvulsants Class Instructions). This drug may be taken with food or milk to minimize stomach upset. Do not chew, break, or crush the tablet or capsule, because this may irritate your mouth or throat. Sprinkle capsule may be swallowed whole or administered by sprinkling the entire contents on small amount (1 teaspoonful) of soft food such as pudding or applesauce; swallow the drug/food mixture immediately (avoid chewing). Polymer from the sprinkles may appear in the stools, but does not indicate a lack of absorption. Weakness, tiredness, repeated vomiting, or loss of seizure control may be an early sign of severe, but rare, liver disorder and should be reported immediately.

Pharmacokinetics. *Onset and Duration.* Steady-state serum levels are attained in 2–4 days.[2] Several weeks may be required for attainment of maximal therapeutic effect.[72] For mania, levels should be above 45 mg/L for efficacy and below 125 mg/L to minimize adverse effects.

Serum Levels. 50–120 mg/L (350–830 μmol/L) for epilepsy and mania. Some patients require and can tolerate serum levels up to 150 mg/L.[72] Tremor, irritability, confusion, and restlessness may be observed with levels >100–150 mg/L.[2]

Fate. The bioavailability of the oral capsule is 93 ± 13%, with peak levels occurring 1–2 hr after dose. The bioavailability of the EC divalproex tablet is 90 ± 14%, with peak levels in 4 hr.[2,73] The peak time of both is delayed by food: (cap) 5.2 ± 1.7 hr; (EC divalproex tab) 8.1 ± 3.6 hr.[74] Bioavailability is 80 ± 7% after a 250-mg suppository.[75] Peak serum levels of 40–50 mg/L (280–350 μmol/L) occur 2–4 hr after a 15–20 mg/kg dose of syrup diluted 1:1 with water as a retention enema.[13] V_d is 0.19 ± 0.05 L/kg in adults and 0.26 ± 0.09 L/kg in children.[2] Plasma protein binding is about 90%.[73] Increasing serum concentrations, hypoalbuminemia, severe liver disease, renal disease, or pregnancy reportedly increase the unbound fraction and may alter clearance. Cl is (healthy adults) 0.0066 ± 0.0005 L/hr/kg; (epileptic adults) 0.018 ± 0.011 L/hr/kg; (children) 0.027 ± 0.015 L/hr/kg.[2] Over 96% is metabolized to at least 10 metabolites. Only 1.8–3.2% of drug is excreted unchanged in urine.[2]

$t_{1/2}$. (Healthy adults) 13.9 ± 3.4 hr; (epileptic adults) 8.5 ± 3.3 hr; (children) 7.2 ± 2.3 hr.[2]

Adverse Effects. (*See* Serum Levels.) Nausea, vomiting, diarrhea, and abdominal cramps occur frequently during initiation of therapy and are minimized by slow titration of valproic acid or substitution of EC divalproex for valproic acid. Transient elevations in liver function tests occur frequently. The risk of valproate-exposed women having children with spina bifida is approximately 1–2%. Drowsiness, ataxia, tremor, behavioral disturbances, transient hair loss, asymptomatic hyperammonemia, or weight gain occur occasionally. Drowsiness and ataxia are more prominent in patients taking valproic acid together with other anticonvulsants.[2] Rarely, thrombocytopenia, acute pancreatitis, abnormal coagulation parameters, or hyperglycinemia occur. Liver failure occurs rarely; the greatest risk is during the first 6 months of therapy and in children <2 yr who receive multiple anticonvulsants.[76]

Contraindications. Hepatic dysfunction or disease.

Precautions. Pregnancy; lactation. The drug may alter results of urine ketone test.

Drug Interactions. Valproate levels may be decreased by concurrent carbamazepine, lamotrigine, phenytoin, or rifampin. Valproate levels may be increased by concurrent aspirin, chlorpromazine, cimetidine, or felbamate. Lamotrigine and phenobarbital levels may be increased by valproate.

Parameters to Monitor. Baseline liver function tests (LFTs) and platelets; repeat LFTs frequently, especially during the first 6 months. Monitor coagulation tests prior to surgery. Periodic serum level monitoring is useful for guiding dosage changes and evaluating potential adverse effects. Serum levels fluctuate considerably during a 24-hr period, making a single random measurement of limited value. Predose blood sampling at standard times is recommended.[2,73]

Notes. Valproic acid and ethosuximide are equally effective for treating absence seizures, although **ethosuximide** is sometimes preferred as a first-line agent because of its lower risk of serious toxicity. Valproic acid is preferred for patients with both absence and generalized tonic-clonic seizures. Many clinicians in the United States use valproic acid as a second-line agent (after **phenytoin** or **carbamazepine**) for the treatment of partial seizures. Valproic acid is as effective as phenytoin and carbamazepine for tonic-clonic seizures and is a drug of choice for atonic and myoclonic seizures. [2,72,77] *See* Anticonvulsants Comparison Chart.

Divalproex is the treatment of choice for bipolar patients who are unresponsive to or cannot tolerate **lithium.** It is more effective than lithium for rapid-cycling bipolar patients (4 or more episodes in 1 yr) and comorbid substance abuse. Carbamazepine is more effective as an adjunctive treatment with lithium to enhance partial efficacy with lithium alone.[78–80]

For migraine prophylaxis, divalproex is effective and well tolerated. It may be more effective in those having frequent migraines than in those characterized as having tension headaches.[81,82]

VIGABATRIN (Investigational, Hoechst Marion Roussel)   Sabril

Vigabatrin, a synthetic amino acid, is a γ-vinyl analogue of γ-aminobutyric acid (GABA), an inhibitory neurotransmitter. Vigabatrin irreversibly inhibits GABA transaminase, the primary degradative enzyme for GABA, resulting in increases in GABA in the cerebrospinal fluid. Vigabatrin is effective as adjunctive therapy for medically refractory partial seizures. In clinical trials, 33–66% of patients had a 50% or greater reduction in the frequency of seizures. Vigabatrin also appears to be effective as monotherapy in patients with newly diagnosed epilepsy. The S(+)-enantiomer of vigabatrin is pharmacologically active, although the drug is administered as a racemate. The inactive R(−)-enantiomer is not converted to the S(+) form, nor does it influence the pharmacokinetics of the S(+)-enantiomer. Vigabatrin is rapidly absorbed after oral administration, with peak concentrations reached within 2 hr. However, because of vigabatrin's mechanism of action, there is no correlation between serum levels and therapeutic effect. Food has little effect on the rate of absorption. Vigabatrin does not bind to plasma proteins. V_d is 0.81 L/kg; renal Cl is 0.076 ± 0.019 L/hr/kg. Vigabatrin is not metabolized. In healthy volunteers, the half-life of the S(+)-enantiomer is 7.5 ± 2.2 hr; the half-life is increased to 13.2 ± 8.4 hr in the elderly, probably reflecting the age-related reduction in Cl_{cr}. The duration of therapeutic effect outlasts the presence of the drug in serum and is affected by the rate of resynthesis of GABA transaminase. CSF levels of GABA return to baseline within 2 weeks after drug discontinuation. Vigabatrin has no effect on serum concentrations of carbamazepine or valproic acid, but phenytoin concentrations are reduced by 20% during vigabatrin therapy. In 1983, clinical trials of vigabatrin in the United States were suspended because of reports of microscopic vacuoles in the brain white matter of rats, mice, and dogs. However, neuropathologic evaluation of surgery and autopsy specimens uncovered no evidence of similar changes in humans, and clinical trials have resumed. Common adverse effects include drowsiness, fatigue, dizziness, tremor, and weight gain. Behavioral changes including anxiety, depression, and psychosis are reported, and are more common in patients with a history of psychiatric disturbance. The usual oral dosage is 2–4 g/day in 1–2 divided doses. Dosage reduction is recommended in patients with a $Cl_{cr} <60$ mL/min.[2,83–87]

ANTICONVULSANTS COMPARISON CHART

CHOICE OF ANTICONVULSANT FOR CLINICAL SEIZURE TYPE*

ANTICONVULSANT DOSAGE RANGE AND SERUM LEVELS

DRUG	Tonic-Clonic	Generalized Seizures — Absence	Generalized Seizures — Myoclonic	Generalized Seizures — Atonic	Partial Seizures†	Dosage Range (mg/kg/day) — Adult	Dosage Range (mg/kg/day) — Pediatric	Therapeutic Serum Levels (mg/L)	Therapeutic Serum Levels (µmol/L)
Carbamazepine	1	W	—	—	1	10–30	15–35	4–12	17–50
Clonazepam	W	3	2	1	—	0.01–0.2	0.01–0.2	13–72 µg/L	40–230 nmol/L
Ethosuximide	—	1	—	—	—	10–30	20–40	40–100	280–710
Gabapentin	—	—	—	—	4	15–35	—	—	—
Lamotrigine	—	—	—	—	4	1.5–7	—	—	—
Phenytoin	1	—	—	—	1	4–8	4–8	10–20	40–80
Valproic Acid‡	1	2	1	1	2	15–60	15–60	50–120	350–830

1 = Drug of first choice; initial agent; given as monotherapy.

2 = Drug of second choice; alternative to first choice; given as monotherapy or in combination with agent of first choice.

3 = Drug of third choice; alternative to first or second choice; given as monotherapy or in combination with another agent.

4 = Useful as adjunctive therapy after failure of monotherapy with preferred agents.

W = May worsen clinical seizure type.

*Choice of anticonvulsant based on relative and comparative efficacy and potential for adverse effects. Choice of agent should consider individual patient factors. *See* references 1, 67, 72, and 77.

†Includes simple-partial, complex-partial, and secondarily generalized tonic-clonic seizures.

‡Drug of first choice when both generalized tonic-clonic and absence seizures are present.

Antidepressants

Class Instructions: Antidepressants. This drug may cause drowsiness. Until the extent of this effect is known, use caution when driving, operating machinery, or performing other tasks requiring mental alertness. Avoid excessive concurrent use of alcohol or other drugs that cause drowsiness.

BUPROPION   Wellbutrin

Bupropion is a monocyclic antidepressant, unique as a dopamine uptake inhibitor with no direct effect on norepinephrine or serotonin receptors, or on MAO, and it is essentially devoid of anticholinergic, antihistaminic, and adrenergic effects. Elimination half-life is 11–14 hr, but an active hydroxy metabolite has a half-life of greater than 24 hr. In contrast with **heterocyclic antidepressants,** bupropion produces no clinically important effect on cardiac conduction, no orthostatic hypotension, and minimal anticholinergic effects, and it is not associated with weight gain. Frequent adverse effects include insomnia, agitation, headache, and nausea. Its lack of sedation and its activating effect may be advantageous for patients with decreased psychomotor activity and lethargy. Compared to **serotonin reuptake inhibitors (SSRIs),** bupropion offers a similar side effect profile without sexual dysfunction. Disadvantages of bupropion include seizures and the necessity of multiple daily doses. With dosages of 450 mg/day or less, seizures occur in 0.4% of patients, with a 1-yr cumulative incidence of 0.5%. Bupropion is contraindicated in patients with psychotic disorders (its dopamine agonist effect may cause increased psychotic symptoms), seizure disorders, anorexia, or bulimia, and in those receiving MAOIs. Bupropion may increase levodopa side effects; phenelzine may increase bupropion's acute adverse reactions. Although still too early to assess, bupropion seems to offer better safety in overdose than the **heterocyclic antidepressants.** The initial dosage is 100 mg bid, increasing to 100 mg tid no sooner than 3 days after the start of therapy. Bupropion must be administered in a divided schedule, with a maximum single dose of 150 mg. After several weeks, the dosage in nonresponding patients may be increased to a maximum of 450 mg/day in divided doses.[88–91] Available as 75 and 100 mg tablets and 50-, 100-, and 150-mg SR tablets (Wellbutrin SR). (*See* Antidepressants Comparison Chart.)

CLOMIPRAMINE   Anafranil

Clomipramine, a 3-chloro analogue of imipramine, has a specific indication for treatment of obsessive-compulsive disorder (OCD). It is a potent inhibitor of serotonin reuptake and, unlike other TCAs, also antagonizes dopaminergic neurotransmission. Clomipramine is a highly lipophilic drug with a large first-pass effect and oral bioavailability of 36–62%. The major route of elimination is metabolism by demethylation, then hydroxylation and conjugation, with an elimination half-life of 20–24 hr. Clomipramine's adverse effect profile is similar to amitriptyline's (ie, frequent sedation, anticholinergic effects, orthostatic hypotension, tremor, nausea, and sweating), but it has a much higher prevalence of sexual dysfunction and seizures. In controlled studies, 42% of patients experienced ejaculatory failure and

20% were impotent. Seizures occur in 0.5% of patients receiving 250 mg/day or less, and 2% of patients experience seizures with dosages above 250 mg/day. Although it is an effective antidepressant, its adverse effect profile makes other antidepressants preferred. Antiobsessional effects are first seen at week 4, with maximum effects between weeks 10–18. Few patients experience complete symptom relief; typically, about 40–50% of patients have marked improvement in obsessive-compulsive symptoms. Drug interactions are the same as other TCAs. Clomipramine is contraindicated in patients who have received MAOIs within the past 14 days. Use with caution in patients with cardiovascular disease (CHF, arrhythmias, angina, recent MI). Initial dosage for OCD is 25 mg/day, increasing to 100 mg/day during the first 2 weeks, then gradually increasing over several weeks to a maximum of 250 mg/day. An effective antidepressant dosage range is 100–150 mg/day. Clomipramine can be given safely once daily at bedtime.[92–94] Available as 25-, 50-, and 75-mg capsules. (*See* Antidepressants Comparison Chart.)

FLUOXETINE   Prozac

Pharmacology. Fluoxetine is a bicyclic antidepressant that is a specific and potent inhibitor of presynaptic reuptake of serotonin (an SSRI). It does not affect reuptake of norepinephrine or dopamine, and has a relative lack of affinity for muscarinic, histamine, α_1- and α_2-adrenergic, and serotonin receptors.[95]

Administration and Adult Dosage. (*See* Antidepressants Comparison Chart.) **PO initial and maintenance dosage** 20 mg/day, administered in the morning. Increase dosage no more frequently than q 3–5 weeks. Divide higher dosages, with the last dose given in early afternoon. Although the maximum labeled dosage is 80 mg/day, 20 mg is equal in efficacy for major depression to higher dosages with the benefit of fewer adverse effects.[96,97]

Special Populations. *Pediatric Dosage.* (<18 yr) safety and efficacy not established.

Geriatric Dosage. Reduce initial dosage and rate of dosage increase in the elderly. Single-dose studies suggest no difference in maintenance dosage in the elderly, but data from multiple-dose studies are needed. (*See* Notes.)

Other Conditions. Reduce initial dosage and rate of dosage increase in patients with hepatic impairment. Dosage adjustment in renal impairment is unnecessary.[96]

Dosage Forms. **Cap** 10, 20 mg; **Soln** 4 mg/mL.

Patient Instructions. This drug requires at least 2 weeks for a noticeable response in mood, and up to 4 weeks for full therapeutic benefit. Take fluoxetine in the morning or early afternoon. Inform your physician of any other medications you are taking.

Pharmacokinetics. *Onset and Duration.* Onset is delayed 2–4 weeks, which is similar to other antidepressants.

Serum Levels. Not established.

Fate. Oral bioavailability is 95%. It is 94% plasma protein bound with a V_d of 35 ± 21 L/kg; Cl is 0.58 ± 0.41 L/hr/kg, decreasing with repeated administration.

The primary active metabolite is norfluoxetine; the metabolic rate may be under polygenic control.

$t_{\frac{1}{2}}$. (Fluoxetine) 1–3 days after a single oral dose, increasing with multiple doses to 4–5 days; (norfluoxetine) 7–15 days. Half-lives do not appear to be altered in the elderly or in patients with renal impairment. Patients with alcohol-induced cirrhosis have fluoxetine half-life increased by 100% and norfluoxetine half-life increased by 60% compared to controls.[96,98]

Adverse Reactions. Nausea, anxiety, insomnia, nervousness, diarrhea, anorexia, dry mouth, headache, and tremor occur with a frequency of over 10%. Anorgasmia or delayed orgasm has been reported in 8% of patients.[99] Unlike TCAs, which typically cause weight gain, fluoxetine dosages over 40 mg/day cause a weight loss of 1–2 kg within the first 6 weeks of treatment.[100] Fluoxetine rarely causes sedation except at dosages over 40 mg/day, and has no adverse cardiovascular or anticholinergic effects.[101] Initial case reports of patients developing new and intense suicidal preoccupation, agitation, and impulsiveness after several weeks of fluoxetine therapy have been adequately evaluated and found not to be directly drug related.[102]

Contraindications. Pregnancy. Concurrent use of an MAOI; 5 weeks must elapse between discontinuation of fluoxetine and starting an MAOI.[103]

Precautions. Use cautiously in the elderly and patients with hepatic impairment. Use fluoxetine with caution in depressed patients with psychomotor agitation and anxiety, or anorexia and weight loss.

Drug Interactions. Fluoxetine is the most potent inhibitor of CYP2D6 of the SSRIs, causing decreased metabolism and increased serum levels and adverse effects of many drugs, including most other antidepressants, antipsychotics, β-blockers, and type Ic antiarrhythmics. Fluoxetine's effect on other CYP isoenzymes has not yet been well defined.

Parameters to Monitor. Monitor liver function tests periodically during long-term therapy.

Notes. Fluoxetine is a useful alternative to TCAs because of its greater safety in overdose and relative lack of anticholinergic and cardiovascular effects. For severely depressed elderly patients, fluoxetine has been shown to be less effective than **nortriptyline**.[104] Fluoxetine and other SSRIs have demonstrated efficacy for obsessive-compulsive disorder and panic disorder. (*See* Antidepressants Comparison Chart.)

FLUVOXAMINE
Luvox

Fluvoxamine has a selective and potent inhibitory effect on serotonergic presynaptic reuptake similar to fluoxetine. Although it is also an effective antidepressant, fluvoxamine has been marketed for use in obsessive-compulsive disorder (OCD). It is the least protein bound of the SSRIs (77%), and bioavailability is not affected by food. Elimination half-life is about 16 hr in adults, but 26 hr in the elderly. On the same dosage, elderly patients have 40% higher serum levels than younger patients. Fluvoxamine is metabolized to inactive metabolites. Frequent adverse effects include nausea, somnolence or insomnia, dry mouth, and sexual dysfunction. Unlike other SSRIs, fluvoxamine is a potent inhibitor of CYP1A2, so increased levels and adverse effects are possible with warfarin, propranolol, metoprolol, caffeine, and theophylline. As with all SSRIs, do not administer fluvoxamine with MAOIs. Fluvoxamine is equal in efficacy to **clomipramine** in OCD, causing fewer anticholinergic effects and sexual dysfunction, but more headache and insomnia. The initial dosage is 50 mg/day, with a dosage of 100–300 mg/day effective for both uses. Give dosages over 100 mg/day in 2 divided doses. Available as 50 and 100 mg tablets.[94,105,106] (*See* Antidepressants Comparison Chart.)

HETEROCYCLIC ANTIDEPRESSANTS

Pharmacology. Heterocyclic antidepressants (**tricyclic antidepressants [TCAs], amoxapine,** and **maprotiline**) are not general CNS stimulants, but rather have a very specific effect on neurotransmitters and receptor sensitivity. The primary pharmacologic effect of heterocyclic antidepressants is blockade of presynaptic reuptake of norepinephrine, with subsequent down-regulation of adrenergic receptors. Amoxapine, a metabolite of **loxapine,** retains some postsynaptic dopamine reuptake inhibition. Heterocyclic antidepressants have less effect on serotonergic activity than on other neurotransmitters.[107,108]

Administration and Adult Dosage. (*See* Antidepressants Comparison Chart for dosage ranges.) **PO for depression** initiate dosage at lower limit of range. Administer in divided doses to assess tolerance to side effects, then once daily hs can be used.[107,109] Maintenance dosage should be the same as the dosage necessary to treat the acute depressive episode.[110] **IM** rarely used (eg, surgical patient NPO for 1–2 days). **PO for chronic pain (amitriptyline** or **imipramine)** 10–25 mg/day initially; most patients respond to a dosage of 25–75 mg/day, although dosages up to 200 mg/day have been used.[111,112] (*See* Notes.)

Special Populations. *Pediatric Dosage.* Not recommended under 12 yr except for childhood enuresis. **PO for enuresis (imipramine)** (<12 yr) 25–50 mg/day; (≥12 yr) up to 75 mg/day.[113] Imipramine maximum dosage in children is 2.5 mg/kg/day; however, use in prepubertal major depression disorder often requires up to 5 mg/kg/day with serum levels over 150 μg/L.[114]

Geriatric Dosage. (>65 yr) reduce initial dosage by at least 50% of adult dosage, and increase the dosage slowly.[115]

Other Conditions. Reduce initial dosage and rate of titration in patients with cardiovascular or hepatic disease.[116] During the last trimester of pregnancy, the mean dosage of TCAs required is 1.6 times that of nonpregnant women.[117]

Dosage Forms. (*See* Antidepressants Comparison Chart.)

Patient Instructions. (*See* Antidepressants Class Instructions.) These drugs usually take 2 weeks for a noticeable response in mood and up to 4 weeks for full therapeutic benefit. If you have small children, be sure to keep this medication in a secure place.

Pharmacokinetics. *Onset and Duration.* Physiologic symptoms of depression (eg, sleep and appetite disturbance, decreased energy) should show some improvement after 1 week, but mood (pessimism, hopelessness, anhedonia) often requires 2–4 weeks for response.

Serum Levels. **Nortriptyline** has a well-established therapeutic range and a curvilinear relationship of serum levels and response ("therapeutic window"). Other antidepressants show a linear response relationship.[118] (*See* Antidepressants Comparison Chart.)

Fate. Bioavailability is variable (30–70%) because of first-pass metabolism. Major metabolites for TCAs are desmethyl (for tertiary amines) and hydroxy compounds; rate may be genetically determined and result in 30-fold variation in steady-state levels in patients given the same dosage.[119]

$t_{1/2}$. (Tertiary amine TCAs) 10–25 hr; (secondary amine TCAs) 12–44 hr.[118]

Adverse Reactions. Sedation, postural hypotension, anticholinergic effects (dry mouth, blurred near vision, constipation, urinary retention, aggravation of narrow-angle glaucoma, and prostatic hypertrophy), weight gain, and cardiac effects (ECG changes and slowed AV conduction) are frequent. **Nortriptyline** is least likely to cause postural hypotension among the TCAs. *See* Antidepressants Comparison Chart for relative differences in frequency of common adverse reactions. Occasionally, fine hand tremor, seizures, cardiac arrhythmia, or cholestasis occur, as well as hypomanic or manic episodes in bipolar patients. Seizures and blood dyscrasias are rare.[120,121]

Contraindications. Cardiac arrhythmias, especially bundle-branch block.

Precautions. Use with caution in the elderly, in pregnancy, or in patients with CHF and angina pectoris, epilepsy, glaucoma, prostatic hypertrophy, or renal or liver disease. When discontinuing therapy, taper the heterocyclic antidepressant dosage to prevent cholinergic rebound. Cases of sudden cardiac death have been reported in children with attention deficit disorder who received **desipramine** in therapeutic or subtherapeutic dosages.[122] Ingestion of 1 g of a heterocyclic antidepressant constitutes a life-threatening medical emergency. Limit the quantities dispensed to depressed patients with suicidal ideation. **Maprotiline** has an increased frequency of seizures at dosages >225 mg/day. **Amoxapine** has a metabolite with dopamine-blocking activity, resulting in possible extrapyramidal effects, tardive dyskinesia, endocrine effects, and neuroleptic malignant syndrome. Neither amoxapine nor maprotiline offers greater efficacy or safety in overdose than TCAs.

Drug Interactions. Many drug interactions occur (*see* Part II, Chapter 2). Use with caution with MAOIs. The antihypertensive effect of guanethidine, clonidine, and closely related drugs may be reduced.

Parameters to Monitor. Monitor hepatic and renal function tests periodically during long-term therapy. Obtain ECG in the elderly, children, and those with preexisting heart disease. With **amoxapine,** monitor carefully for signs of tardive dyskinesia.

Notes. TCAs are commonly used in treating pain associated with diabetic neuropathy and postherpetic neuralgia. **Amitriptyline, desipramine,** and **nortriptyline** have proven efficacy, but **specific serotonin reuptake inhibitors (SSRIs)** are less effective.[111,112] (*See* Antidepressants Comparison Chart.)

MONOAMINE OXIDASE INHIBITORS

Pharmacology. MAOIs are thought to exert their antidepressant action because of alterations in adrenergic and serotonergic receptor sensitivity. The most consistent findings during long-term MAOI therapy include down-regulation of ß-adrenergic and adenyl cyclase activity. **Phenelzine** is a hydrazine derivative; **tranylcypromine** is a nonhydrazine.

Administration and Adult Dosage. PO (phenelzine) 45–90 mg/day; (tranylcypromine) 30–60 mg/day. Initiate dosage at the lower limit and titrate upward depending on tolerance to side effects. Dosage schedule should remain divided, usually bid or tid. Avoid bedtime administration because MAOIs can delay onset of sleep.

Special Populations. *Pediatric Dosage.* (<16 yr) not recommended.

Geriatric Dosage. Limited information, but decrease initial dosage by 50% because of orthostatic hypotension. Contraindicated in patients >60 yr.

Other Conditions. Reduce the initial dosage and rate of upward titration if the patient has taken a heterocyclic antidepressant within 7–10 days.

Dosage Forms. (Phenelzine) **Tab** 15 mg; (tranylcypromine) **Tab** 10 mg.

Patient Instructions. (*See* Antidepressants Class Instructions.) This drug usually takes 2 weeks for noticeable response in mood and up to 4 weeks for full therapeutic benefit to occur. This drug may cause faintness or dizziness, especially after rising suddenly or standing for prolonged periods, or after exertion or alcohol intake. Nausea, vomiting, sweating, severe occipital headache, and stiff neck may be signs of a serious adverse effect and should be reported immediately. Avoid concurrent use of diet pills and cough and cold remedies, and restrict consumption of aged foods high in tyramine (*see* Foods That Interact with MAO Inhibitors Chart).

Pharmacokinetics. *Onset and Duration.* Onset 2 weeks; maximum improvement occurs after 3–4 weeks.[123]

Serum Levels. Not used clinically.

Fate. Termination of drug action is dependent upon MAO regeneration, because the drugs or their active metabolites chemically combine with the MAO enzyme.

Adverse Reactions. Autonomic effects are frequent and not necessarily dose dependent; these include postural hypotension, dry mouth, and constipation. Drowsiness is more frequent with phenelzine; while overstimulation and agitation are more likely with tranylcypromine. Occasionally delayed ejaculation, edema, skin rash, urinary retention, and blurred vision occur. MAOIs are much less likely than TCAs to cause weight gain, with tranylcypromine the least likely.[124]

Contraindications. Patients >60 yr; patients with confirmed or suspected cerebrovascular defect; cardiovascular disease; pheochromocytoma; history of liver disease or abnormal liver function tests.

Precautions. Always consider the possibility of suicide in depressed patients and take adequate precautions. Like other antidepressant drugs, MAOIs may switch bipolar patients to a hypomanic or manic state.

Drug Interactions. Postural hypotension may be increased with coadministration of antipsychotic, heterocyclic antidepressant, or antihypertensive drugs, and in patients with CHF. Avoid concurrent use with buspirone, heterocyclic antidepressants, meperidine, sympathomimetic drugs, SSRIs, and other MAOIs. A 1- to 2-week drug-free interval is necessary when switching from an MAOI to a TCA, but a drug-free interval is not necessary when switching from a TCA to an MAOI.[125] Although uncommon, hypertensive crisis may result from concurrent use of sympathomimetic amines or ingestion of high-tyramine-content food and drinks.[126,127] Avoid diets high in tyramine content (*see* Foods That Interact with MAO Inhibitors Chart).

Parameters to Monitor. Monitor blood pressure frequently.

Notes. MAOIs are excellent alternatives to heterocyclic antidepressants in major depressive disorder, are very effective in panic disorder, and are drugs of choice for atypical depression.[126,128]

FOODS THAT INTERACT WITH MAO INHIBITORS

Many fermented foods contain tyramine as a byproduct formed by the bacterial breakdown of the amino acid tyrosine; it can also be formed by parahydroxylation of phenylethylamine or dehydroxylation of DOPA and dopamine. Tyramine and some other amines found in food can cause hypertensive reactions in patients taking MAO inhibitors. MAO found in the GI tract inactivates tyramine; when drugs prevent this, exogenous tyramine and other monoamines are absorbed and release norepinephrine from sympathetic nerve endings and epinephrine from the adrenal gland. If sufficient quantities of these pressor compounds are released, palpitations, severe headache, and hypertensive crisis can result.

FOOD CONTAINING TYRAMINE

Avocados	Particularly if overripe.
Bananas	Reactions can occur if eaten in large amounts; tyramine levels high in peel.
Bean curd	Fermented bean curd, fermented soya bean, soya bean pastes, soy sauces, and miso soup, prepared from fermented bean curd, all contain tyramine in large amounts; miso soup has caused reactions.
Beer and ale	Major domestic brands do not contain appreciable amounts; some imported brands have had high levels. Nonalcoholic beer may contain tyramine and should be avoided.
Caviar	Safe if vacuum-packed and eaten fresh or refrigerated only briefly.
Cheese	Reactions possible with most, except unfermented varieties such as cottage cheese. In others, tyramine concentration is higher near rind and close to fermentation holes.
Figs	Particularly if overripe.
Fish	Safe if fresh; dried products should not be eaten. Caution required in restaurants. Vacuum-packed products are safe if eaten promptly or refrigerated only briefly.
Liver	Safe if very fresh, but rapidly accumulates tyramine; caution required in restaurants.
Meat	Safe if known to be fresh; caution required in restaurants.
Milk products	Milk and yogurt appear to be safe.
Protein extracts	See also soups; avoid liquid and powdered protein dietary supplements.
Sausage	Fermented varieties such as bologna, pepperoni, and salami have a high tyramine content.

(*continued*)

FOODS THAT INTERACT WITH MAO INHIBITORS (continued)

Shrimp paste	Contains large amounts of tyramine.
Soups	May contain protein extracts and should be avoided.
Soy sauce	Contains large amounts of tyramine; reactions have occurred with teriyaki.
Wines	Generally do not contain tyramine, but many reactions have been reported with Chianti, champagne, and other wines.
Yeast extracts	Dietary supplements (eg, Marmite) contain large amounts. Yeast in baked goods, however, is safe.

FOOD NOT CONTAINING TYRAMINE

Caffeine	A weak pressor agent; large amounts may cause reactions.
Chocolate	Contains phenylethylamine, a pressor agent that can cause reactions in large amounts.
Fava beans	(Broad beans, "Italian" green beans) Contain dopamine, a pressor amine, particularly when overripe.
Ginseng	Some preparations have caused headache, tremulousness, and maniclike symptoms.
Liqueurs	Reactions reported with some (eg, Chartreuse, Drambuie); cause unknown.
New Zealand prickly spinach	Single case report; patient ate large amounts.
Whiskey	Reactions have occurred; cause unknown.

For further information, consult Lippman SB, Nash K. Monoamine oxidase inhibitor update. Potential adverse food and drug interactions. *Drug Saf* 1990;5:195–204.
Anon. Foods interacting with MAO inhibitors. Med Lett Drugs Ther *1989;31:11–2, reproduced with permission.*

MIRTAZAPINE Remeron

Mirtazapine is an antidepressant that antagonizes presynaptic α_2-adrenergic auto- and heteroreceptors that are responsible for controlling release of norepinephrine and serotonin (5-HT). It is also a potent antagonist of postsynaptic 5-HT$_2$ and 5-HT$_3$ receptors. The net outcome of these effects is increased noradrenergic activity and enhanced 5-HT activity, especially at 5-HT$_{1A}$ receptors. This unique mechanism of action preserves antidepressant efficacy, but minimizes many of the adverse effects common to both tricyclic antidepressants and selective serotonin reuptake inhibitors. Mirtazapine is effective in both moderate and severe major depression. It has an onset of clinical effect in 2–4 weeks, similar to other antidepressants. It has an elimination half-life of 20–40 hr, allowing once-daily administration at bedtime. Mirtazapine has minimal cardiovascular and anticholinergic effects, and essentially lacks adverse GI effects, insomnia, and sexual dysfunction. Sedation, increased appetite, and weight gain are the most frequent side effects; agranulocytosis occurs rarely. It should not be used within 14 days of an MAOI. Cases of overdose up to 975 mg in combination with a benzodiazepine caused marked sedation, but no difficulty with cardiovascular or respiratory effects. Initial dosage is 15 mg/day at bedtime, increasing at 1–2-week intervals to a maximum of 45 mg/day.[129,130] Available as 15- and 30-mg tablets.

NEFAZODONE Serzone

Nefazodone is a postsynaptic serotonin 5-HT$_{2A}$ antagonist and presynaptic serotonin reuptake inhibitor. These two serotonergic effects make it different from

SSRIs and TCAs. Nefazodone has an oral bioavailability of about 20% and is highly protein bound (>99%). It is extensively metabolized, with a dose-dependent elimination half-life ranging from about 1–2.3 hr in young patients, modestly prolonged in the elderly and 2–3 times longer in hepatic disease; the major active metabolite, hydroxynefazodone, has a half-life ranging from 1.2–1.6 hr in young and elderly patients, increasing to 2–4 hr with hepatic disease. Single-dose studies in the elderly show a 100% larger AUC, and with multiple doses, the AUC differences decrease to 10–20% above younger populations. Renal impairment does not markedly affect nefazodone pharmacokinetics. Although chemically similar to trazodone, it causes less sedation and orthostatic hypotension, and its lower α-adrenergic blockade makes priapism much less likely (no cases reported). Frequent adverse effects include sedation, dry mouth, nausea, and dizziness. Unlike SSRIs, nefazodone's effects on sexual function, agitation, tremor, insomnia, and weight change are no different from placebo. Nefazodone is a potent inhibitor of the CYP3A4 isoenzyme and a weak inhibitor of the CYP2D6 isoenzyme. Drug interactions of concern thus include astemizole, terfenadine, and the triazolobenzodiazepines (ie, alprazolam, triazolam, midazolam). A 1- to 2-week washout period is recommended when converting a patient to or from a MAOI and nefazodone. Initial dosage is 100 mg bid (50 mg bid in the elderly), increased q 4–7 days to the effective dosage range of 150–300 mg bid.[131–134] Available as 100-, 150-, 200- and 250-mg tablets. (*See* Antidepressants Comparison Chart.)

PAROXETINE   Paxil

Paroxetine is a highly selective and potent inhibitor of serotonin reuptake (an SSRI) similar to fluoxetine. Unlike fluoxetine, it is metabolized to inactive metabolites and has an elimination half-life of 24 hr. Paroxetine causes the typical SSRI adverse effects of nausea, sexual dysfunction, and headache, but is more likely to cause sedation than insomnia. Like the other SSRIs, it is much safer in overdose than TCAs. Paroxetine is a potent inhibitor of the CYP2D6 isoenzyme, so most other antidepressants, antipsychotics, ß-blockers, and type Ic antiarrhythmics may have increased serum levels and adverse effects when paroxetine is combined with these drugs. Do not use paroxetine together with MAOI. The effective dosage for depression is 20 mg/day, with a few patients needing 30–50 mg/day for full efficacy. The initial dosage for panic disorder is 10 mg/day and for obsessive-compulsive disorder is 20 mg/day; the maintenance dosage for both panic and obsessive-compulsive disorder is 20 mg/day; the maintenance dosage for both panic and obsessive-compulsive disorders is 40 mg/day, to a maximum of 60 mg/day. The starting dosage for all uses in elderly patients and those with marked renal or hepatic impairment should begin at 10 mg/day. Once-daily administration is preferred, either in the morning or evening.[105,135–137] Paroxetine is available as 20- and 30-mg tablets. (*See* Antidepressants Comparison Chart.)

SERTRALINE   Zoloft

Sertraline is a highly selective and potent inhibitor of serotonin reuptake (an SSRI) similar to fluoxetine, which indirectly results in a down-regulation of ß-adrenergic receptors. It has no clinically important effect on noradrenergic or histamine receptors and no effect on MAO. It lacks stimulant, cardiovascular, anticholinergic, and convulsant effects. Sertraline has an oral bioavailability of 36%, and, when it is taken with food, both peak serum levels and total absorption increase by 30–40%. Peak serum levels are reached in 6–8 hr. Cl is decreased by up to 40% in the elderly; mean steady-state half-life is 27 hr. Its primary metabolite is N-desmethylsertraline, which has 5–10 times less activity than sertraline as an SSRI and has no demonstrated antidepressant activity. Frequent adverse effects include nausea, diarrhea, ejaculatory delay, tremor, and increased sweating. Sertraline thus far has demonstrated antidepressant effects equal to TCAs and may have anorectic effects and efficacy in obsessive-compulsive disorder. Compared to fluoxetine, sertraline is equal in efficacy; causes less agitation, anxiety, and insomnia; and is a less potent inhibitor of the CYP2D6 isoenzyme at a dosage of 50 mg/day. Use the drug with caution in patients with renal or hepatic impairment, and do not use it within 14 days of using an MAOI. Adult dosage is 50 mg/day initially, increasing if necessary at weekly intervals to a maximum of 200 mg/day in a single dose in the morning or evening.[108,138–140] Sertraline is available as 50- and 100-mg tablets. (*See* Antidepressants Comparison Chart.)

TRAZODONE HYDROCHLORIDE   Desyrel, Various

Pharmacology. Trazodone shares some effects with other antidepressants, but it causes selective inhibition of serotonin reuptake and blocks postsynaptic serotonin-5HT$_2$ and α-adrenergic receptors.

Administration and Adult Dosage. PO as an antidepressant 150 mg/day initially, increasing in 50 mg/day increments q 3–4 days. Trazodone is less potent than most antidepressants; therefore, do not abandon a trial of trazodone without reaching a dosage of 400–600 mg/day for inpatients. Maximum dosage in outpatients is 400 mg/day. Administration after meals minimizes sedation and postural hypotension.[141,142] **PO as a hypnotic** 50–100 mg is commonly used, often in combination with an SSRI.[143]

Special Populations. *Pediatric Dosage.* (<18 yr) safety and efficacy not established.

Geriatric Dosage. Sedation and orthostatic hypotension require initial dosage reduction by 33–50% and slower rate of titration.

Other Conditions. Dosage adjustments in patients with hepatic or renal impairment may be prudent, although limited experience, thus far, does not suggest that major dosage adjustments are necessary.[119,142] Base dosage on ideal body weight in obese patients.

Dosage Forms. Tab 50, 100, 150, 300 mg.

Patient Instructions. (*See* Antidepressants Class Instructions.) Take trazodone after a meal.

Pharmacokinetics. *Onset and Duration.* Onset is delayed, similar to heterocyclic antidepressant drugs.

Serum Levels. Not established.

Fate. The drug is well absorbed after oral administration; relative bioavailability 72–91%. The rate of absorption is decreased with food, but the total amount absorbed is unchanged. V_d is 1–2 L/kg; Cl is 0.13 ± 0.04 L/hr/kg. V_d is larger and

Cl lower in the elderly and in obesity. Metabolism is extensive, with one active metabolite.[98,118]

$t_½$. 5.9 ± 1.9 hr, prolonged in the elderly and obesity.[98]

Adverse Reactions. Sedation and postural hypotension are frequent. Trazodone does not affect AV conduction, nor does it cause tachycardia as do heterocyclic antidepressants. Rarely, trazodone may aggravate ventricular arrhythmias[101] and cause nonsexual penile tumescence and priapism. Priapism can be treated with an α-adrenergic agonist; surgery is not required.[144]

Contraindications. Pregnancy; cardiac ventricular arrhythmia; initial recovery phase of myocardial infarction.

Precautions. Always consider the possibility of suicide in depressed patients and take adequate precautions. Use with caution or avoid in patients immediately post-MI, or with preexisting cardiac disease.

Drug Interactions. Concurrent use with other CNS depressants may potentiate the sedation caused by trazodone. Use with MAOIs is not well studied, so the combination is best avoided.

Parameters to Monitor. Obtain WBC count and differential in any patient who develops fever, sore throat, or other sign of infection.

Notes. Trazodone is much safer in overdose than heterocyclic antidepressants; overdoses of 9 g of trazodone alone have been survived without medical sequelae. Trazodone is also a useful choice for patients who cannot tolerate anticholinergic effects or who have CHF, angina pectoris, or bundle-branch block in which heterocyclic antidepressants are contraindicated. (*See* Antidepressants Comparison Chart.)

VENLAFAXINE   Effexor

Venlafaxine is a potent reuptake inhibitor of both serotonin and norepinephrine like many of the TCAs, but lacks effects on muscarinic, α-adrenergic, or histamine receptors. Unlike SSRIs, it has minimal protein binding (27–30%). Venlafaxine has an elimination half-life of 5 hr, and one major metabolite with an 11-hr half-life is active. Venlafaxine exhibits linear pharmacokinetics over the recommended dosage range, and steady state is reached in 3 days. Serum concentrations in elderly patients are no different from those in younger patients. Frequent adverse effects include expected serotonin-related effects (eg, nausea, headache, insomnia or somnolence, and sexual dysfunction). At higher dosages (375 mg/day), venlafaxine is unique in causing a consistent but mild elevation in diastolic blood pressure (6 mm Hg). Regular blood pressure monitoring is required for all patients. Venlafaxine is not a potent inhibitor of the cytochrome P450 enzyme system, making it different from most of the SSRIs. Initial dosage is 75 mg bid or tid, increasing q 4–7 days to an effective antidepressant dosage of 225–375 mg/day. Patients with renal impairment or on hemodialysis require a 25–50% dosage reduction. Thus far, studies support use of either bid or tid administration, but not a once-daily schedule.[145–147] Available as 25-, 37.5-, 50-, 75-, and 100-mg tablets. (*See* Antidepressants Comparison Chart.)

ANTIDEPRESSANTS COMPARISON CHART

CLASS AND DRUG	DOSAGE FORMS	USUAL DAILY ADULT DOSAGE RANGE (MG)	THERAPEUTIC SERUM LEVELS (µG/L)	RELATIVE FREQUENCY OF SIDE EFFECTS		
				Sedation	*Anticholinergic*	*Orthostatic Hypotension*
α₂-ADRENERGIC BLOCKERS						
Mirtazapine Remeron	Tab 15, 30 mg.	15–45	a	Moderate	None	None
CHLOROPROPIOPHENONES						
Bupropion Wellbutrin	Tab 75, 100 mg.	300–450	a	None	None	None
DIBENZOXAZEPINES[b]						
Amoxapine Asendin Various	Tab 25, 50, 100, 150 mg.	300–600	a	Low	Low	Low
MONOAMINE OXIDASE INHIBITORS (MAOIs)						
Phenelzine Nardil	Tab 15 mg.	45–90	a	Moderate	Low	Very High
Tranylcypromine Parnate	Tab 10 mg.	30–60	a	Low	Low	Very High
SPECIFIC SEROTONIN REUPTAKE INHIBITORS (SSRIs)						
Fluoxetine Prozac	Cap 10, 20 mg Soln 4 mg/mL.	10–80	a	None	Very Low	None

(continued)

ANTIDEPRESSANTS COMPARISON CHART (continued)

CLASS AND DRUG	DOSAGE FORMS	USUAL DAILY ADULT DOSAGE RANGE (MG)	THERAPEUTIC SERUM LEVELS (μG/L)	RELATIVE FREQUENCY OF SIDE EFFECTS		
				Sedation	Anticholinergic	Orthostatic Hypotension
Fluvoxamine Luvox	Tab 50, 100 mg.	100–300[c]	a	None	None	None
Paroxetine Paxil	Tab 20, 30 mg.	20–50	a	Very Low	Very Low	Very Low
Sertraline Zoloft	Tab 50, 100 mg.	50–200	a	None	None	None
SEROTONIN NOREPINEPHRINE REUPTAKE INHIBITORS (SNRIs)						
Venlafaxine Effexor	Tab 25, 37.5, 50, 75, 100 mg.	225–375	a	Very Low	Very Low	Very Low
TETRACYCLICS[b]						
Maprotiline Ludiomil Various	Tab 25, 50, 75 mg.	150–225	200–300[a]	Moderate	Moderate	Moderate
TRIAZOLOPYRIDINES						
Trazodone Desyrel Various	Tab 50, 100, 150, 300 mg.	200–600	a	High	Very Low	High
Nefazodone Serzone	Tab 100, 150, 200, 250 mg.	300–600	a	Moderate	Very Low	Moderate

(continued)

369

ANTIDEPRESSANTS COMPARISON CHART (continued)

CLASS AND DRUG	DOSAGE FORMS	USUAL DAILY ADULT DOSAGE RANGE (MG)	THERAPEUTIC SERUM LEVELS (μG/L)	RELATIVE FREQUENCY OF SIDE EFFECTS		
				Sedation	Anticholinergic	Orthostatic Hypotension
TRICYCLICS (TCAs)[c]						
Amitriptyline Elavil Endep Various	Tab 10, 25, 50, 75, 100, 150 mg Inj 10 mg/mL.	150–300	75–175[d]	High	High	High
Clomipramine Anafranil	Cap 25, 50, 75 mg.	100–250[c] 100–150[e]	a	High	High	High
Desipramine Norpramin Various	Cap 25, 50 mg Tab 10, 25, 50, 75, 100, 150 mg.	150–300	100–160	Low	Low	Moderate
Doxepin Adapin Sinequan Various	Cap 10, 25, 50, 75, 100, 150 mg Soln 10 mg/mL.	150–300	110–250[d]	High	Moderate	High
Imipramine Tofranil Janimine Various	Tab 10, 25, 50 mg Inj 12.5 mg/mL Cap (as pamoate) 75, 100, 125, 150 mg.	150–300	>200[d]	Moderate	Moderate	High

(continued)

ANTIDEPRESSANTS COMPARISON CHART (continued)

CLASS AND DRUG	DOSAGE FORMS	USUAL DAILY ADULT DOSAGE RANGE (MG)	THERAPEUTIC SERUM LEVELS (µG/L)	RELATIVE FREQUENCY OF SIDE EFFECTS		
				Sedation	Anticholinergic	Orthostatic Hypotension
Nortriptyline	Cap 10, 25, 50, 75 mg	100–200	50–150	Moderate	Moderate	Low
Aventyl						
Pamelor	Soln 2 mg/mL.					
Various						
Protriptyline	Tab 5, 10 mg.	30–60	70–260[a]	Very Low	Moderate	Moderate
Vivactil						
Various						
Trimipramine	Cap 25, 50, 100 mg.	150–300	a	Moderate	Moderate	High
Surmontil						

[a] Not well established.
[b] Amoxapine, maprotiline, and the tricyclic antidepressants are categorized together here as heterocyclic antidepressants because their therapeutic and side effect profiles are similar.
[c] For obsessive-compulsive disorder.
[d] Includes active metabolites.
[e] Major depression.
From references 88, 93, 96, 101, 105, 106, 118, 119, 124, 129–131, 136, 137, 141, and 146.

Antipsychotic Drugs

Class Instructions: Antipsychotics. This drug may cause drowsiness. Until the extent of this effect is known, use caution when driving, operating machinery, or performing other tasks requiring mental alertness. Avoid excessive concurrent use of alcohol or other drugs which cause drowsiness.

ANTIPSYCHOTIC DRUGS

Pharmacology. Antipsychotic efficacy is most likely related to blockade of post-synaptic dopaminergic receptors in the mesolimbic and prefrontal cortex of the brain, although other neurotransmitter systems are also involved.[148]

Administration and Adult Dosage. (*See* Antipsychotic Drugs Comparison Chart for oral dosage ranges.) Initiate therapy with divided doses until therapeutic dosage is found, then, for most patients, once-daily hs administration is preferred. For maintenance therapy, decrease acute dosage by 25% q 3 months, with a target maintenance dosage being 50–67% of the acute treatment dosage.[149] Recent concern has focused on the need to establish a minimum effective dosage for antipsychotic drugs, and treatment regimens at the low end of the dosage range are preferred. Oral dosages of high-potency antipsychotics (eg, **fluphenazine, haloperidol**) in the range of 5–20 mg/day are better tolerated and equal in efficacy to dosages above 20 mg/day.[150] Most patients can be given a maintenance dosage of one-half the acute dosage by the end of 1 yr, although 10–15% of chronically ill patients require a maintenance dosage of more than 15 mg/day of **haloperidol** or its equivalent.[151,152] For manic episodes, no additional benefit is achieved with dosages over 10 mg/day of haloperidol.[153]

Special Populations. *Pediatric Dosage.* As with adults, dosage is determined primarily by titration to individual response. No precise dosage range exists, but in general, the initial dosage is lower and should be increased more gradually in children.

Geriatric Dosage. Initial dosage is 20–25% of the dosage used in younger adults. Typical starting dosages in the elderly are **haloperidol** 0.5–2 mg/day, or **thioridazine** 10–50 mg/day. Dosage adjustments must also be done more slowly than in younger adults.[154]

Other Conditions. Dosages in the lower range are sufficient for most elderly patients, and the rate of dosage titration should be slower.

Dosage Forms. (*See* Antipsychotic Drugs Comparison Chart.)

Patient Instructions. (*See* Antipsychotics Class Instructions.) These drugs usually take several weeks for clinical response and up to 8 weeks for full therapeutic response.

Pharmacokinetics. *Onset and Duration.* Onset of antipsychotic activity is variable, with noticeable response requiring days to weeks.

Serum Levels. Correlation of serum levels with clinical response is not yet consistently established. The best evidence exists for **haloperidol**, with serum concentrations of 5–15 µg/L (13–40 nmol/L) correlating well with therapeutic effects in adult psychotic patients, and an increasing risk of adverse effects and decreased efficacy when steady-state concentrations exceed 15 μg/L.[155,156]

Fate. **Haloperidol** is well absorbed; peak serum levels are achieved 2–6 hr after liquid or tablets, and within 30 min after IM. Oral bioavailability of haloperidol is 60–70%. Haloperidol is extensively metabolized, with one active hydroxy metabolite. **Chlorpromazine** and other phenothiazines are well absorbed, but undergo extensive and variable presystemic metabolism in the gut wall and liver; over 20 chlorpromazine metabolites with varying activity have been identified in human plasma.

$t_{1/2}$. Serum half-lives have no clinical correlation with biologic half-lives for antipsychotic drugs. **Chlorpromazine** serum half-life is 30 hr, **thioridazine** 4–10 hr, **thiothixene** 34 hr, and **haloperidol** 12–24 hr. Of more clinical importance is that steady-state CNS levels and tissue saturation allow once-daily administration of all antipsychotic drugs.[119]

Adverse Reactions. (*See* Antipsychotic Drugs Comparison Chart for relative frequency of common adverse reactions.) Frequently, sedation, extrapyramidal effects (eg, parkinsonism, dystonic reactions, akathisia), tardive dyskinesia, anticholinergic effects (eg, dry mouth, blurred vision, constipation, urinary retention), photosensitivity, and postural hypotension occur. Occasionally weight gain, amenorrhea, galactorrhea, ejaculatory disturbance, neuroleptic malignant syndrome, agranulocytosis, skin rash, cholestatic jaundice, and skin or eye pigmentation occur. Rarely seizures, thermoregulatory impairment, and slowed AV conduction occur. Low-potency drugs are more likely to cause sedation, anticholinergic effects, and orthostatic hypotension, whereas high-potency drugs cause more extrapyramidal effects. Tardive dyskinesia is a long-term adverse effect, untreatable, and sometimes irreversible. Tardive dyskinesia occurs at a 4% yearly incidence for at least the first 5–6 yr of treatment. Neuroleptic malignant syndrome (ie, fever, extrapyramidal rigidity, autonomic instability, alterations in consciousness) occurs more frequently with high-potency antipsychotics, with a prevalence of 1.4% and a fatality rate of 4%.[150,157,158]

Contraindications. Coma; circulatory collapse or severe hypotension; bone marrow depression; history of blood dyscrasia.

Precautions. Use cautiously in patients with myasthenia gravis, Parkinson's disease, seizure disorders, or hepatic disease.

Drug Interactions. Barbiturates may enhance phenothiazine metabolism; carbamazepine may enhance haloperidol metabolism. Phenothiazines may decrease efficacy of guanethidine or guanadrel or may have additive hypotensive effects with hypotensive drugs. Phenothiazines may inhibit the antiparkinson activity of levodopa. Haloperidol may increase the CNS toxicity of lithium. Combined use of haloperidol and methyldopa may result in dementia.

Notes. (*See also* Prochlorperazine Salts in the Antiemetics section for antiemetic uses.)

CLOZAPINE   Clozaril

Clozapine is an atypical antipsychotic drug that is chemically similar to loxapine and has unique pharmacologic effects and indications, as well as very serious adverse effects. Whereas typical antipsychotic drugs exert their effects primarily via blockade of dopamine-D_2 receptors, clozapine has effects on several dopamine and serotonin receptors. Its high serotonin-5HT_2 to dopamine-D_2 ratio is the likely explanation for its unique efficacy. Compared to traditional antipsychotic drugs, clozapine is more effective for negative symptoms of schizophrenia, is more effective in treatment-resistant patients, and rarely causes extrapyramidal effects. Clozapine is nearly completely absorbed after oral administration, with about 30% oral bioavailability because of extensive first-pass metabolism. Clozapine is 95% plasma protein bound; with multiple doses its elimination half-life is 12 hr. Frequent adverse effects include sedation, orthostatic hypotension, anticholinergic effects, fever, and excessive salivation. Seizures are dose related, with a frequency up to 5% in the therapeutic dosage range and a 1-yr cumulative incidence of 10%. Agranulocytosis is the major adverse effect of concern, occurring in 0.8% of patients after 1 yr. Most cases of agranulocytosis occur within the first 3 months of therapy. Patients must have a baseline WBC count and differential before initiating therapy, and mandatory weekly WBC monitoring throughout treatment and for 4 weeks after discontinuation. Substantial weight gain has been reported in most patients receiving clozapine. A dosage of 100–200 mg tid is effective for most patients, but some may require up to 900 mg/day. A therapeutic trial of 12–24 weeks is required for the full therapeutic effect to become apparent.[159–164] Available as 25- and 100-mg tablets. (*See* Antipsychotic Drugs Comparison Chart.)

HALOPERIDOL DECANOATE · Haldol Decanoate

Haloperidol decanoate (HD) is the preferred long-acting depot antipsychotic drug. Depot antipsychotics are indicated only for patients who demonstrate good response, but who are consistently drug-noncompliant with resultant frequent psychotic relapse. Depot antipsychotics provide fewer relapses and hospitalizations, stable serum drug levels, and fewer side effects compared to oral antipsychotic drugs. HD can be given q 4 weeks; **fluphenazine decanoate** (FD) is similar in efficacy and adverse effects, but it must be administered q 2 weeks. Do not use HD or FD to treat acute psychotic symptoms, but rather, only after a patient is stabilized on an oral antipsychotic drug. After IM administration of HD, esterases cleave the decanoate chain to release the active drug. Peak serum concentrations of haloperidol occur in 3–9 days, with an apparent half-life of 3 weeks; steady-state levels are reached after 12–16 weeks. There is no evidence that HD causes adverse effects with a frequency different from oral haloperidol. Do not exceed an initial HD dosage of 100 mg IM, with a target monthly dosage 20 times the oral haloperidol daily dosage. An IM loading dose technique has been described that gives 20 times the daily oral dosage, using 100–200 mg of depot q 3–7 days to reach the calculated amount, with a maximum of 450 mg. In geriatric or hepatically impaired patients, use a monthly HD dose of 15 times the oral haloperidol dosage. Experience with HD doses greater than 500 mg is limited, and injections over 5 mL should be divided into two equal portions given at two sites. Oral haloperidol supplementation may be necessary between monthly injections to treat reemergence of psychotic symptoms until steady-state concentrations are reached.[165–169] Available as a 50 and 100 mg/mL IM injection.

PIMOZIDE   Orap

Pimozide is indicated for the treatment of Tourette's disorder. Although structurally different from other antipsychotic drugs, pimozide shares their ability to block dopaminergic receptors. Its lack of effect on norepinephrine receptors led to the hope that pimozide would have a more favorable adverse effect profile than other antipsychotic drugs. **Haloperidol** is the drug of choice for Tourette's disorder. Thus far, the relative frequency of adverse effects of these two drugs is similar, and pimozide remains an alternative to haloperidol for Tourette's disorder. Initial oral dosage is 1–2 mg/day in divided doses, with dosage increased every other day up to a maximum of 20 mg/day. Most patients who respond require 10 mg/day or less. Periodically attempt to decrease the dosage and withdraw treatment.[170,171] Available as 2-mg tablets.

RISPERIDONE   Risperdal

Risperidone is a potent serotonin-5HT$_2$ antagonist with dopamine-D$_2$ antagonism. Whereas typical antipsychotics are dopamine antagonists, the additional serotonin antagonism increases efficacy for negative symptoms of schizophrenia and reduces the likelihood of extrapyramidal symptoms. Initial evidence also suggests that risperidone is more effective than traditional antipsychotic drugs for treatment-resistant schizophrenic patients. Risperidone is metabolized by CYP2D6, so inhibitors can increase risperidone levels and adverse effects. Risperidone's elimination half-life is 3 hr; its active metabolite has a half-life of 24 hr. The half-lives of one or both are prolonged in patients with renal disease and free fraction of risperidone in serum increases in hepatic disease, necessitating lower dosages in both conditions. Frequent dose-related adverse effects include extrapyramidal effects, orthostatic hypotension, headache, rhinitis, and insomnia. Because of orthostatic hypotension, the initial dosage is 1 mg bid (0.5 mg bid in the elderly or patients with severe renal or hepatic impairment); titrate q 2–4 days to the usual effective dosage of 4–6 mg/day. Occasionally, dosages above 6 mg/day may be necessary, but adverse effects increase and efficacy can be less.[172–176] Available as 1-, 2-, 3-, and 4-mg tablets and 1 mg/mL solution. (*See* Antipsychotic Drugs Comparison Chart.)

ANTIPSYCHOTIC DRUGS COMPARISON CHART

| DRUG AND CLASS | DOSAGE FORMS | ADULT ORAL DOSAGE RANGE (MG/DAY) | ORAL EQUIVALENT ANTIPSYCHOTIC DOSE (MG) | RELATIVE FREQUENCY OF SIDE EFFECTS | | | |
				Sedation	Anticholinergic	Extra-Pyramidal	Orthostatic Hypotension
LOW POTENCY							
Chlorpromazine Thorazine Various	Soln 30, 100 mg/mL Syrup 2 mg/mL Tab 10, 25, 50, 100, 200 mg Inj 25 mg/mL Supp 25, 100 mg SR Cap not recommended.	50–1200	100	High	Moderate	Moderate	High
Thioridazine Mellaril Various	Soln 30, 100 mg/mL Susp 5, 20 mg/mL Tab 10, 15, 25, 50, 100, 150, 200 mg.	50–800	100	High	High	Low	High
INTERMEDIATE POTENCY							
Loxapine Loxitane	Cap 5, 10, 25, 50 mg Soln 25 mg/mL Inj 50 mg/mL.	20–250	10	Low	Low	Moderate	Low

(continued)

ANTIPSYCHOTIC DRUGS COMPARISON CHART (continued)

DRUG AND CLASS	DOSAGE FORMS	ADULT ORAL DOSAGE RANGE (MG/DAY)	ORAL EQUIVALENT ANTIPSYCHOTIC DOSE (MG)	RELATIVE FREQUENCY OF SIDE EFFECTS			
				Sedation	Anticholinergic	Extra-Pyramidal	Orthostatic Hypotension
Molindone Moban	Tab 5, 10, 25, 50, 100 mg Soln 20 mg/mL	25–225	10	Very Low	Low	Moderate	Low
ATYPICAL							
Clozapine Clozaril	Tab 25, 100 mg.	300–900	50	High	High	Very Low	High
Risperidone Risperdal	Tab 1, 2, 3, 4 mg Soln 1 mg/mL	4–6 mg*	—	Very Low	Very Low	Low*	Moderate
HIGH POTENCY							
Fluphenazine Permitil Prolixin Various	Elxr 0.5 mg/mL Soln 5 mg/mL Tab 1, 2.5, 5, 10 mg Inj 2.5 mg/mL.	2–40	2	Low	Low	Very High	Low
Fluphenazine Decanoate Prolixin Various	Inj 25 mg/mL.	12.5–75 (IM) q 2 weeks	—	Low	Low	Very High	Low

(continued)

377

ANTIPSYCHOTIC DRUGS COMPARISON CHART (continued)

DRUG AND CLASS	DOSAGE FORMS	ADULT ORAL DOSAGE RANGE (MG/DAY)	ORAL EQUIVALENT ANTIPSYCHOTIC DOSE (MG)	RELATIVE FREQUENCY OF SIDE EFFECTS			
				Sedation	Anticholinergic	Extra-Pyramidal	Orthostatic Hypotension
Haloperidol Haldol Various	Soln 2 mg/mL Tab 0.5, 1, 2, 5, 10, 20 mg Inj 5 mg/mL.	2–100	2	Very Low	Very Low	Very High	Very Low
Haloperidol Decanoate Haldol Decanoate	Inj 50, 100 mg/mL.	50–450 (IM) monthly	—	Very Low	Very Low	Very High	Very Low
Perphenazine Trilafon Various	Soln 3.2 mg/mL Tab 2, 4, 8, 16 mg Inj 5 mg/mL.	12–64	8	Low	Low	High	Low
Trifluoperazine Stelazine Various	Soln 10 mg/mL Tab 1, 2, 5, 10 mg Inj 2 mg/mL.	5–40	5	Low	Low	High	Low
Thiothixene Navane Various	Cap 1, 2, 5, 10, 20 mg Soln 5 mg/mL Inj 2, 5 mg/mL.	5–60	4	Low	Low	High	Low

*At dosages over 6 mg/day, nausea and insomnia are limiting side effects; extrapyramidal symptoms markedly increase at dosages over 6 mg/day.
From references 148–150, 159, 162, 166, 167, and 174.

Anxiolytics, Sedatives, and Hypnotics

Class Instructions: Sedatives and Hypnotics. This drug causes drowsiness and may produce sleep. Do not exceed prescribed dosage, and use caution when driving, operating machinery, or performing other tasks requiring mental alertness. Avoid concurrent use of alcohol or other drugs that cause drowsiness or sleep. Do not abruptly stop taking this medication; the dosage must be slowly decreased.

ALPRAZOLAM   Xanax, Various

Alprazolam is a triazolobenzodiazepine that is equal in efficacy to other benzodiazepines for generalized anxiety disorder, but more effective in the treatment of panic disorder. Although alprazolam has some efficacy in major depression, it is less effective than heterocyclic antidepressants. Like diazepam, alprazolam has a rapid onset of effect after oral administration, but its shorter half-life requires tid administration. The half-life is 11 hr in adults; the elderly may have a decreased clearance and an increased half-life of 21 hr. Patients do not show complete cross-tolerance between triazolobenzodiazepines and other benzodiazepines, but **clonazepam** has been shown to be an effective long-half-life substitute drug for use in alprazolam withdrawal. Alprazolam tablets can be administered SL with no difference from oral administration in onset, peak serum levels, clearance, or half-life. Initial oral dosage for generalized anxiety disorder is 0.25 mg tid, which may be gradually increased to 4 mg/day. An initial dosage of 0.5 mg tid is recommended for panic disorder; most panic patients require 5–6 mg/day, and occasionally 10 mg/day may be needed for full response. To discontinue alprazolam, decrease the daily dosage by no more than 0.5 mg/day q 3 days until the daily dosage reaches 2 mg, then decrease dosage in 0.25 mg/day increments q 3 days.[177–181] Available as 0.25-, 0.5-, 1-, and 2-mg tablets. (*See also* Clonazepam, and the Benzodiazepines and Related Drugs Comparison Chart.)

BENZODIAZEPINES

Pharmacology. Benzodiazepines have a more specific anxiolytic effect than other sedatives. Benzodiazepines facilitate the inhibitory effect of γ-aminobutyric acid (GABA) on neuronal excitability by increasing membrane permeability to chloride ions.[182]

Administration and Adult Dosage. (*See* Benzodiazepines and Related Drugs Comparison Chart.) Optimal oral use requires individual dosage titration to clinical response. The long-acting drugs can be administered once daily hs; the short-acting drugs require multiple daily doses (*see* Benzodiazepines and Related Drugs Comparison Chart). Determine the dosage schedule by the individual patient's relative degree of dysfunction from daytime anxiety compared to insomnia. Despite physiologic dependence, benzodiazepines may need to be used for months and sometimes years for treatment of panic disorder and generalized anxiety disorder; situational anxiety, adjustment disorders, and anxiety secondary to other causes require only days to weeks of drug treatment.[183] **PO for alcohol withdrawal** evidence suggests no superiority of any benzodiazepine in alcohol withdrawal, although chlordiazepoxide has been most adequately studied; (chlordiazepoxide) 25–100 mg for agitation, anxiety, and tremor; on the first day, up to 400 mg may be given in divided doses with gradual dosage reductions over 4 days; (diazepam) 5–20 mg for agitation, anxiety, and tremor; alternatively, it may be given in 20 mg doses q 2 hr until complete suppression of signs and symptoms is achieved. After this loading dose, further administration is unnecessary;[184] (oxazepam) 15–60 mg q 4–6 hr for agitation, anxiety, and tremor. Oxazepam is preferred in patients with severe liver disease. IM **chlordiazepoxide is not recommended** because of slow, erratic absorption; however, **lorazepam** is suitable for IM administration.[119,184] **Diazepam** injectable solution (Valium, various) can be administered **IM or IV;** the injectable emulsion (Dizac) is for **IV use only** (do not administer IM or SC); neither the solution nor the emulsion should be administered faster than 5 mg/min into a peripheral vein, and small veins should be avoided; neither product is recommended to be added to other drugs or solutions. (*See* Fate.)

Special Populations. *Pediatric Dosage.* PO (**diazepam,** >6 months) 1–2.5 mg tid or qid. Most benzodiazepines are not recommended in children because of insufficient clinical experience and concern about the stimulating and paradoxical effects that occur because of disinhibition. **Midazolam** is commonly used in children for preanesthetic sedation (*see* Midazolam).

Geriatric Dosage. Elderly may have reduced clearance and enhanced CNS sensitivity, which requires initial dosage to be reduced by 33–50%.[185]

Other Conditions. Higher dosages may be needed in heavy smokers. Patients with liver disease may have reduced clearance and/or enhanced CNS sensitivity, which requires reduction of initial and subsequent doses. Alcoholic patients with reduced plasma proteins may require a lower dosage because of decreased protein binding.

Dosage Forms. (*See* Benzodiazepines and Related Drugs Comparison Chart.)

Patient Instructions. (*See* Sedatives and Hypnotics Class Instructions.)

Pharmacokinetics. *Serum Levels.* Not used clinically.

Fate. Diazepam and chlordiazepoxide are absorbed faster and more completely orally than intramuscularly. Lorazepam and midazolam have rapid and reliable IM absorption.[119,186] (*See* Benzodiazepines and Related Drugs Comparison Chart.)

Adverse Reactions. Frequent effects include drowsiness, dizziness, ataxia, and disorientation; these effects rarely require drug discontinuation and are easily managed by dosage reduction. Anterograde amnesia is frequent.[119] Occasionally, agitation and excitement may occur.[187] With parenteral therapy, hypotension and respiratory depression occur occasionally. Rarely, hepatotoxicity or blood dyscrasias occur. Diazepam emulsion is associated with less venous thrombosis and phlebitis than the solution, which can be very irritating to veins.

Contraindications. Acute narrow-angle glaucoma; (diazepam emulsion injection) hypersensitivity to soy protein.

Precautions. Pregnancy; impaired hepatic function. Abrupt drug withdrawal may result in rebound insomnia, abstinence syndrome similar to barbiturate withdrawal, seizures, or, rarely, psychosis. Patients do not show complete cross-tolerance between triazolobenzodiazepines and other benzodiazepines. Past history of substance abuse may indicate an increased likelihood of benzodiazepine misuse.[182]

Drug Interactions. Concurrent use with other CNS depressants may potentiate the sedation caused by benzodiazepines. Nefazodone inhibits alprazolam and triazolam metabolism; fluoxetine and fluvoxamine increase levels of alprazolam and diazepam; omeprazole increases serum diazepam levels.

Parameters to Monitor. Periodically reassess the need for therapy during long-term use.

BUSPIRONE HYDROCHLORIDE   BuSpar

Pharmacology. Buspirone is the first of a new class of selective serotonin-$5HT_{1A}$-receptor partial agonists. It also has some effect on dopamine-D_2 autoreceptors and, like antidepressants, can down-regulate ß-adrenergic receptors. Unlike benzodiazepines, it lacks amnestic, anticonvulsant, muscle relaxant, and hypnotic effects. Its exact anxiolytic mechanism of action is complex and not yet clearly defined.[188,189]

Administration and Adult Dosage. **PO for anxiety** 5 mg tid for 3 weeks, increasing in 5 mg/day increments q 2–3 days to a maximum of 60 mg/day. Most patients require 15–30 mg/day in divided doses.

Special Populations. *Pediatric Dosage.* Safety and efficacy not established.

Geriatric Dosage. Same as adult dosage.

Other Conditions. Decrease the initial dose to 5 mg bid in patients with hepatic or renal impairment.[188,190]

Dosage Forms. **Tab** 5, 10 mg.

Patient Instructions. This drug requires several weeks of continuous use for therapeutic effect and is not effective when used intermittently.

Pharmacokinetics. *Onset and Duration.* Onset of anxiolytic effect several weeks.

Fate. The drug is well absorbed; oral bioavailability is 3.9 ± 4.3%. Administration after meals increases bioavailability by 80%. It is extensively metabolized by oxidative dealkylation pathways.[191]

$t_{1/2}$. 2.1 ± 1.2 hr.[191]

Adverse Reactions. Dosages 60 mg/day may cause dysphoria.[182] Frequent nausea, dizziness, headache, and insomnia occur. Unlike benzodiazepines, buspirone does not cause dependence or withdrawal effects.[188,192]

Contraindications. None known.

Precautions. Buspirone has no cross-tolerance with benzodiazepines, so patients being switched from a benzodiazepine should have their dosage of the benzodiazepine decreased slowly.

Drug Interactions. Unlike benzodiazepines, buspirone does not interact with alcohol.[188,192] Buspirone may increase haloperidol serum levels. Avoid concurrent buspirone and a MAOI because the combination may cause hypertension.

Parameters to Monitor. Monitor renal and hepatic function initially and periodically during long-term therapy.

Notes. Buspirone is indicated only for the treatment of generalized anxiety disorder and is not effective as a prn medication or hypnotic. Buspirone's anxiolytic effect without sedation or respiratory depression has led to its use in agitation and anxiety, in dementia, mental retardation, and spinal cord injury. Its unique effect on the $5HT_{1A}$ receptor has led to uncontrolled studies and clinical use for premenstrual tension syndrome and to decrease craving in smoking cessation.[193]

CHLORAL HYDRATE   Noctec, Various

Chloral hydrate is a chlorinated aliphatic alcohol that is a useful alternative hypnotic to benzodiazepines for prn use or for brief treatment of situational insomnia; hypnotic efficacy is lost by the second week of continuous use. It is rapidly reduced to the active hypnotic, trichloroethanol. Onset of hypnotic effect is 30–60 min, and trichloroethanol's half-life is 8 hr. Instruct patients to take the capsule with a full glass of liquid, and to mix the syrup in at least one-half glass of water or juice. (See also Sedatives and Hypnotics Class Instructions.) Frequent adverse effects include gastric irritation and nausea; rarely, excitement, delirium, disorientation, and erythematous and urticarial allergic reactions may occur. Chloral hydrate is genotoxic and a potential carcinogen, so some investigators caution against its routine use. The drug is contraindicated in marked hepatic or renal impairment and must be used with caution in pregnancy and in patients with gastritis or ulcers. Unlike barbiturates, chloral hydrate causes no enzyme induction or effect on REM sleep or REM rebound. In adults, the oral hypnotic dose is 500–1500 mg. In children, the hypnotic dose is 50 mg/kg to a maximum of 1 g, and the sedative dosage is 25 mg/kg/day up to 500 mg as a single dose.[118,194,195] (See Sedatives and Hypnotics Comparison Chart.)

FLUMAZENIL   Romazicon

Flumazenil is a selective inhibitor of the CNS effects of benzodiazepine sedatives. It competitively blocks the effect of benzodiazepines and zolpidem on GABA-mediated inhibitory pathways within the CNS. Flumazenil finds its greatest use in the management of benzodiazepine overdose and the reversal of benzodiazepine sedation following medical and surgical procedures. First-pass hepatic metabolism limits the bioavailability of oral flumazenil, so the drug is administered by IV injection. It is rapidly hydroxylated in the liver to inactive metabolites, and its elimination half-life is 0.7–1.3 hr. V_d is 0.6–1.6 L/kg. Reversal of benzodiazepine coma may occur within 1–2 min and last 1–5 hr, depending on the dosages of the benzodiazepine and flumazenil. Frequent side effects have been minimal and are usually limited to nausea and vomiting, anxiety, and agitation. However, seizures have occurred, most often in patients on long-term benzodiazepine therapy or following overdose with heterocyclic antidepressants or other potentially convulsant drugs (eg, buproprion, cocaine, cyclosporine, isoniazid, lithium, methylxanthines, MAOIs, propoxyphene). Be prepared to manage seizures before giving flumazenil. Flumazenil does not consistently reverse benzodiazepine amnesia, so patients should be given written instructions to avoid operation of motor vehicles or hazardous equipment, or ingestion of alcohol or nonprescription medications for 18–24 hr, or longer if benzodiazepine effects persist. The adult dose for reversal of conscious sedation is 0.2 mg over 15 sec; this dose may be repeated after 45 sec and every minute thereafter prn, to a total dosage of 1 mg. In benzodiazepine overdose, give 0.2 mg over 30 sec, followed, if necessary, by 0.3 mg after 30 sec. Further doses of 0.5 mg over 30 sec may be given at 1-min intervals to a cumulative dosage of 3 mg. Rarely, patients who respond partially to 3 mg respond more completely to a dosage of 5 mg. If resedation occurs after either use, additional doses of up to 1 mg can be given at 20-min intervals to a maximum of 3 mg/hr.[267–270] Available as 0.1 mg/mL injection.

MIDAZOLAM HYDROCHLORIDE   Versed

Midazolam is a short-acting triazolobenzodiazepine for use in anesthesia. It is unique in its physicochemical properties; at a pH under 4 the drug exists as a highly water-soluble, stable compound, but at physiologic pH it becomes lipophilic. This allows IV administration of a water-soluble, rapidly acting drug with a very low frequency of venous irritation. Midazolam is given IM for preoperative sedation and IV for induction of anesthesia or for conscious sedation for endoscopy and other procedures. The usual adult IM dose for preoperative sedation is 0.07–0.08 mg/kg (about 5 mg) 1 hr before surgery. For endoscopy and other conscious sedation procedures, IV dosage must be individualized and *not* administered by rapid bolus. Titrate *slowly* to desired effect; some patients may respond to as little as 1 mg. Give no more than 2.5 mg over at least 2 min as the 1 mg/mL (or more dilute) solution; in elderly, debilitated, or chronically ill patients, limit the initial dose to 1.5 mg. Further small doses may be given after waiting at least 2 min. See product information for anesthesia induction dosage. Do not give the drug IV without oxygen and resuscitation equipment immediately available. Rectal administration of a solution of 0.3 mg/kg diluted in 5 mL of saline solution in children for preanesthetic sedation is a safe and effective alternative to IM administration.[196–200] Available as 1 and 5 mg/mL injection.

TRIAZOLAM   Halcion, Various

Pharmacology. Triazolam is a triazolobenzodiazepine hypnotic whose effect is likely related to its facilitation of γ-aminobutyric acid (GABA)-mediated neurotransmission, but its exact mechanism is unknown.

Administration and Adult Dosage. (*See* Benzodiazepines and Related Drugs Comparison Chart.) **PO as a hypnotic** 0.25 mg hs initially; do not exceed 0.5 mg.

Special Populations. *Pediatric Dosage.* (<18 yr) safety and efficacy not established.

Geriatric Dosage. **PO** Decrease initial dose to 0.125 mg, increase if necessary to 0.25 mg hs.[201,202]

Other Conditions. **PO** 0.125 mg initially in debilitated patients and those with a low body weight or with hepatic impairment.

Dosage Forms. Tab 0.125, 0.25 mg.

Patient Instructions. (*See* Sedative-Hypnotics Class Instructions.)

Pharmacokinetics. *Onset and Duration.* Onset of hypnotic effect is 0.5–1 hr, with peak serum levels achieved within 2 hr.

Fate. Oral bioavailability 44%, SL 53%, because of nonhepatic presystemic metabolism. V_d is 1.2 ± 0.5 L/kg; Cl is 0.34 ± 0.2 L/hr/kg. Cl is decreased with increasing age (attributed to reduced hepatic oxidizing capacity in the elderly). Triazolam undergoes hydroxylation and rapid conjugation. Smoking does not affect elimination.[98,203] Accumulation does not occur with multiple doses.

$t_{1/2}$. 2.6 ± 1 hr. Half-life is not affected by end-stage renal disease or liver disease.[98,203,204]

Adverse Reactions. Frequently anterograde amnesia,[205] daytime anxiety, and ataxia may occur. Occasionally agitation, confusion, or mood disturbance occur. Rarely respiratory depression, depersonalization, and derealization, or psychosis occur. Unlike other benzodiazepines, several fatalities have been reported in elderly patients who overdosed on triazolam.[206,207]

Contraindications. Pregnancy.

Precautions. Pregnancy; impaired hepatic function. Abrupt drug withdrawal may result in rebound insomnia, abstinence syndrome similar to barbiturate withdrawal, seizures, or, rarely, psychosis. Patients do not show complete cross-tolerance between triazolam and other benzodiazepines. Past history of substance abuse may indicate an increased likelihood of triazolam misuse.[182] Do not prescribe the drug for more than 7–10 days of consecutive therapy or in quantities greater than a 30-day supply.

Drug Interactions. Concurrent use with other CNS depressants may potentiate the sedation caused by benzodiazepines. Nefazodone inhibits triazolam metabolism.

Notes. Compared to other benzodiazepine hypnotics, triazolam is equally effective in reducing sleep latency and less likely to cause daytime sedation; however, it is less likely to prevent early morning awakening and more likely to cause rebound insomnia. Hypnotic drugs are most effective when used to treat transient situational insomnia (1–3 days) and short-term insomnia (1–3 weeks maximum).[207,208]

ZOLPIDEM TARTRATE   Ambien

Zolpidem is the first in a class of short-acting nonbenzodiazepine hypnotics indicated for the short-term treatment of insomnia. Most benzodiazepines bind to all γ-aminobutyric acid (GABA)-benzodiazepine (omega) receptor complexes, but zolpidem selectively binds only to the omega-1 receptor. This difference suggests a more selective sedative-hypnotic effect without anxiolytic, anticonvulsant, or muscle relaxant effects. After oral administration, zolpidem reaches peak serum concentrations in 1.6 hr, is highly protein bound (93%), has no active metabolites, and has an elimination half-life of 1.5–4 hr (average 2.5). Half-life is increased by one-third in elderly, and greatly increased in patients with hepatic impairment (9.9 hr). Dose-related side effects include daytime drowsiness, dizziness, and diarrhea. Clinical trials with 20-mg doses report headache, nausea, memory problems, and CNS stimulation. Tolerance has not been reported, nor has rebound insomnia following therapeutic doses. Psychomotor performance is impaired when zolpidem is combined with alcohol. Efficacy has been demonstrated for 35 nights at doses of 10 mg without affecting sleep stages or psychomotor performance. A dose of 10 mg is recommended immediately before bedtime. In the elderly, patients with hepatic impairment, or patients taking other CNS depressants, the dose is 5 mg.[209–211] Zolpidem is available as 5- and 10-mg tablets. (*See* Benzodiazepines and Related Drugs Comparison Chart.)

BENZODIAZEPINES AND RELATED DRUGS COMPARISON CHART

DRUG AND SCHEDULE[a]	DOSAGE FORMS	ADULT ORAL DOSAGE RANGE	PEAK ORAL SERUM LEVELS (HR)	HALF-LIFE (HR)
ANXIOLYTICS				
SHORT-ACTING				
Alprazolam (C-IV) Xanax Various	Tab 0.25, 0.5, 1, 2 mg.	0.75–4 mg/day[c] 5–10 mg/day[d]	0.7–1.6	11–21
Lorazepam[e] (C-IV) Ativan Various	Tab 0.5, 1, 2 mg Soln 2 mg/mL Inj 2, 4 mg/mL.	2–10 mg/day	2	10–20
Oxazepam (C-IV) Serax Various	Cap 10, 15, 30 mg Tab 15 mg.	30–120 mg/day	1–2	5–15
LONG-ACTING				
Chlordiazepoxide (C-IV) Librium Libritabs Various	Cap 5, 10, 25 mg Tab 5, 10, 25 mg Inj 100 mg.	15–100 mg/day	2–4	>24
Clorazepate (C-IV) Tranxene Various	Cap 3.75, 7.5, 15 mg Tab 3.75, 7.5, 15 SR Tab 11.25, 22.5 mg.	15–60 mg/day	1–2[f]	>24
Diazepam (C-IV) Dizac Valium Various	SR Cap 15 mg Tab 2, 5, 10 mg Soln 1, 5 mg/mL Inj 5 mg/mL.	6–40 mg/day	1–2	>24
Halazepam (C-IV) Paxipam	Tab 20, 40 mg.	60–160 mg/day	1–3	>24
Prazepam (C-IV) Various	Cap 5, 10, 20 mg Tab 10 mg.	20–60 mg/day	6	>24
HYPNOTICS				
SHORT-ACTING				
Midazolam[e] (C-IV) Versed	Inj 1, 5 mg/mL.	—	0.4–0.7	1.5–3
Triazolam (C-IV) Halcion Various	Tab 0.125, 0.25 mg.	0.125–0.25 mg	0.5–2	1.5–3.6
Zolpidem[g] (C-IV) Ambien	Tab 5, 10 mg.	5–20 mg	2	1.5–4
INTERMEDIATE-ACTING				
Estazolam (C-IV) Pro-Som	Tab 1, 2 mg.	1–2 mg	1–2	12–15

(continued)

		ADULT ORAL DOSAGE RANGE	PEAK ORAL SERUM LEVELS (HR)	HALF-LIFE (HR)[b]
BENZODIAZEPINES AND RELATED DRUGS COMPARISON CHART (continued)				
DRUG AND SCHEDULE[a]	DOSAGE FORMS			
Temazepam (C-IV) Restoril Various	Cap 15, 30 mg.	7.5–30 mg	2–3	10–15
LONG-ACTING				
Flurazepam (C-IV) Dalmane Various	Cap 15, 30 mg.	15–30 mg	h	>24[b]
Quazepam (C-IV) Doral	Tab 7.5, 15 mg.	7.5–15 mg	1–2	>24[b]

[a]Controlled substance schedule designated after each drug (in parentheses).
[b]Parent drug plus active metabolites.
[c]For generalized anxiety disorder.
[d]For panic disorder.
[e]Also used as an IV anesthetic; well absorbed IM.
[f]Hydrolyzed to nordazepam (desmethyldiazepam) before absorption.
[g]Not a benzodiazepine chemically, but an imidazopyridine, which is a selective benzodiazepine-1 receptor agonist.
[h]Rapidly and completely metabolized to desalkylflurazepam.
From references 178, 180, 182, 186, 196, 203, 205, and 211–214.

SEDATIVES AND HYPNOTICS COMPARISON CHART

DRUG AND SCHEDULE*	DOSAGE FORMS	ADULT ORAL DOSAGE	HALF-LIFE (HR)
SEDATIVES			
BARBITURATES			
Phenobarbital (C-IV)	Cap 16 mg	15–30 mg bid or qid	48–120
Various	Elxr 3, 4 mg/mL		
	Tab 8, 15, 30, 60, 100 mg		
	Inj 30, 60, 65, 130 mg/mL		
	Pwdr for Inj 120 mg.		
PROPANEDIOLS			
Meprobamate (C-IV)	Tab 200, 400, 600 mg	400 mg tid or qid	6–16
Equanil	SR Cap 200, 400 mg.	or 600 mg bid	
Miltown			
Various			
HYPNOTICS			
BARBITURATES			
Pentobarbital (C-II)	Cap 50, 100 mg	100–200 mg	21–42
Nembutal	Exlr 4 mg /mL		
Various	Supp 30, 60, 120, 200 mg (C-III)		
	Inj 50 mg/mL.		
Secobarbital (C-II)	Cap 100 mg	100–200 mg	19–34
Seconal	Inj 50 mg/mL.		
Various			
CHLORAL DERIVATIVES			
Chloral Hydrate (C-IV)	Cap 250, 325, 500, 650 mg	500 mg–1.5 g	8
Noctec	Supp 325, 500, 650 mg		(Trichloroethanol)
Various	Syrup 50, 100 mg/mL.		
PIPERIDINEDIONES			
Glutethimide (C-II)	Tab 250 mg.	250–500 mg	5–22
Various			
ACETYLINIC ALCOHOLS			
Ethchlorvynol (C-IV)	Cap 200, 500, 750 mg.	500 mg–1 g	6
Placidyl			
Various			

*Controlled Substance Schedule designated after each drug (in parentheses).
From references 207, 208, and 215.

Lithium

LITHIUM CARBONATE	Various
LITHIUM CITRATE	Cibalith-S, Lithonate-S

Pharmacology. Lithium's mechanism of antimanic effect is unknown; it alters actions of several second messenger systems (eg, adenylate cyclase and phosphoinositol).[216,217]

Administration and Adult Dosage. Individualize dosage according to serum levels and clinical response. Acute manic episodes typically require **PO** 1.2–2.4 g/day; maintenance therapy requires 900 mg–1.5 g/day. A loading dose of 30 mg/kg, in 3 divided doses, can be given to achieve the desired serum level within 12 hr.[218] A number of predictive dosage techniques have been developed based on estimated steady state after one serum level.[219,220]

Special Populations. *Pediatric Dosage.* (<12 yr) **PO** 15–20 mg (0.4–0.5 mEq)/kg/day in 2–3 divided doses; (12–18 yr) same as adult dosage.[221]

Geriatric Dosage. (>65 yr) decrease adult dosage by 33–50%.[222]

Other Conditions. Adjust the dosage more carefully in patients with decreased renal function and in patients receiving thiazide diuretics or NSAIDs.

Dosage Forms. **Cap** 150, 300, 600 mg; **Tab** 300 mg; **SR Tab** 300, 450 mg; **Syrup** 1.6 mEq/mL (as citrate).

Patient Instructions. This drug may be taken with food, milk, or antacid to minimize stomach upset. Report immediately if signs of toxicity occur, such as persistent diarrhea, vomiting, coarse hand tremor, drowsiness, or slurred speech, or prior to beginning any diet. In hot weather, ensure adequate water and salt intake.

Pharmacokinetics. *Onset and Duration.* Onset 7–10 days for therapeutic effect.[119]

Serum Levels. (Acute mania or hypomania) 0.8–1.5 mEq/L; (prophylaxis) 0.6–1.2 mEq/L, although concern about long-term renal effects suggests most patients should be maintained below 0.9 mEq/L. Levels above 1.5 mEq/L are regularly associated with some signs of toxicity, and levels above 2 mEq/L result in serious toxicity.[223] *See* Adverse Reactions.

Fate. Absorption is virtually complete within 8 hr after oral administration, with peak levels occurring in 2–4 hr. Distribution is throughout total body water, but tissue uptake is not uniform. The drug is not protein bound or metabolized, but freely filtered through the glomerulus, with about 80% being reabsorbed.

$t_{1/2}$. 18–20 hr; up to 36 hr in the elderly.[119]

Adverse Reactions. Frequent, dose-related effects with therapeutic serum levels include nausea, diarrhea, polyuria, polydipsia, fine hand tremor, and muscle weakness. Signs of toxicity include coarse hand tremor, persistent GI effects, muscle hyperirritability, slurred speech, confusion, stupor, seizures, increased deep tendon reflexes, irregular pulse, and coma. Frequent, non–dose-related effects include nontoxic goiter, hypothyroidism, nephrogenic diabetes insipidus–like syndrome, folliculitis, aggravation of acne or psoriasis, leukocytosis, hypercalcemia, and weight gain.[224,225]

Contraindications. Pregnancy; fluctuating renal function; severe renal or cardiovascular disease.

Precautions. Use with caution in patients with cardiac disease, dehydration, sodium depletion, diuretic therapy, or dementia, in nursing mothers, and in the elderly. (*See* Special Populations.)

Drug Interactions. ACE inhibitors may increase serum lithium concentrations. Theophylline or excess sodium enhance renal lithium clearance; sodium deficiency may promote lithium retention and increase risk of toxicity. Long-term diuretic or NSAID use may result in decreased lithium elimination. Haloperidol may increase the CNS toxicity of lithium; with methyldopa or phenytoin, signs of lithium toxicity may occur in the absence of increased serum lithium.

Parameters to Monitor. Prelithium workup should include thyroid function tests, Cr_s, BUN, CBC (for baseline WBC count), urinalysis (for baseline specific gravity), electrolytes, and ECG (if >40 yr). During therapy, obtain serum lithium levels (drawn 12 hr after last dose) weekly during initiation and monthly during maintenance.[226,227]

Notes. Divalproex sodium is the treatment of choice for bipolar patients who are unresponsive to or cannot tolerate lithium. (*See* Divalproex/Valproic Acid.)

Parkinsonism Drugs

AMANTADINE
Symmetrel, Various

Pharmacology. Amantadine is an antiviral compound that appears to prevent the release of viral nucleic acid into the host cell. In Parkinson's disease, the drug increases presynaptic dopamine release, blocks the reuptake of dopamine into the presynaptic neurons, and exerts anticholinergic effects.

Administration and Adult Dosage. **PO for Parkinson's disease** usual maintenance dosage is 100 mg bid. In patients with serious medical illnesses or who are receiving other antiparkinson drugs, give 100 mg/day initially, increasing in 100 mg/day increments q 7–14 days to effective dosage, or to a maximum of 400 mg/day in 2 divided doses. **PO for extrapyramidal reactions** 100 mg bid, to a maximum of 300 mg/day in 3 divided doses. **PO for prophylaxis of influenza A** 200 mg/day in 1–2 divided doses continuing for at least 10 days following exposure, for 2–3 weeks after giving influenza A vaccine, or for up to 90 days when vaccine is unavailable or contraindicated. **PO for treatment of influenza A** 200 mg/day in 1–2 divided doses starting within 24–48 hr after onset of illness and continuing for 24–48 hr after symptoms disappear.

Special Populations. *Pediatric Dosage.* **PO for prophylaxis or treatment of influenza A** (<1 yr) safety and efficacy not established; (1–9 yr) 4.4–8.8 mg/kg/day in 2 divided doses, to a maximum of 150 mg/day; (9–12 yr) 100 mg bid. For prophylaxis, continue therapy for at least 10 days following exposure, for 2–3 days after giving influenza A vaccine, or for up to 90 days when vaccine is unavailable or contraindicated. For treatment, continue for 24–48 hr after symptoms disappear.

Geriatric Dosage. **PO for influenza prophylaxis or treatment** (>65 yr) 100 mg/day. **PO for Parkinson's Disease** same as adult dosage, adjusting for renal impairment.

Other Conditions. Reduce dosage in renal impairment as follows: with Cl_{cr} of 30–50 mL/min give 200 mg first day, then 100 mg/day; with Cl_{cr} of 15–29 mL/min give 200 mg first day, then 100 mg every other day; with Cl_{cr} <15 mL/min or for patients on hemodialysis give 200 mg q 7 days.

Dosage Forms. **Cap** 100 mg; **Syrup** 10 mg/mL.

Patient Instructions. This medication may cause dizziness, confusion, or difficulty in concentrating. Until the extent of these effects is known, use caution when driving, operating machinery, or performing other tasks requiring mental alertness. Avoid excessive concurrent use of alcohol. **Parkinson's disease.** Stopping this medication suddenly may cause your Parkinson's disease to worsen.

Pharmacokinetics. *Onset and Duration.* Loss of antiparkinson effects occurs in most patients after 6–12 weeks of therapy.[228]

Serum Levels. (Therapeutic trough, antiviral) 300 µg/L (2 µmol/L). Neurotoxicity above 1 mg/L (6.6 µmol/L).[229]

Fate. Peak serum levels occur in 1–4 hr in young adults, 4.5–7 hr in older adults. Steady-state serum levels occur in healthy volunteers and Parkinson's patients within 4–7 days;[230] V_d is 6.6 ± 1.5 L/kg; Cl is 0.39 ± 0.13 L/hr/kg in normal renal function. From 78–88% is excreted unchanged in urine.[229]

$t_{½}$. (Healthy young adults) 11.8 ± 2.1 hr;[231] (elderly adults) 31 ± 7.2 hr;[232] (during chronic hemodialysis) 8.3 ± 1.5 days.[231]

Adverse Reactions. Nausea, dizziness, insomnia, confusion, hallucinations, anxiety, restlessness, depression, irritability, peripheral edema, orthostatic hypotension, or livedo reticularis occur frequently. Occasionally, CHF, psychosis, urinary retention, or reversible elevation of liver enzymes may occur. Rarely, seizures, corneal opacities, or leukopenia are reported.

Drug Interactions. Amantadine can potentiate the CNS effects of anticholinergic agents.

Precautions. Pregnancy; lactation. Use with caution in patients with CHF, seizures, renal or hepatic disease, peripheral edema, orthostatic hypotension, psychosis, or a history of eczematoid rash, or in those receiving CNS stimulants. Abrupt drug discontinuation in patients with Parkinson's disease may result in rapid clinical deterioration.

Parameters to Monitor. Monitor renal function and disease symptoms impairment periodically in Parkinsonian patients.

Notes. In Parkinson's disease, amantadine is indicated as initial treatment alone or in combination with **levodopa.** Amantadine produces clinical improvements in akinesia and rigidity, but to a lesser degree than levodopa.[228] There is no evidence that amantadine alters the course of Parkinson's disease. **Anticholinergics** appear to reduce tremor to a greater degree than amantadine.[233] Concomitant administration of anticholinergics and amantadine may worsen side effects. **Rimantadine** (Flumadine) is an antiviral compound with efficacy similar to amantadine against influenza A. It appears to be slightly better tolerated than amantadine. Dosage is

100 mg bid in adults and 5 mg/kg/day in one dose for children under 10 yr.[234,235] Available as 100-mg tablets and 10 mg/mL syrup.

BENZTROPINE MESYLATE   Cogentin

Pharmacology. Benztropine is a synthetic competitive antagonist of acetylcholine. In Parkinson's disease, the drug reduces the relative excess of cholinergic activity in the basal ganglia that develops because of absolute dopamine deficiency in this area.

Administration and Adult Dosage. PO, IM, or IV for Parkinson's disease 0.5–1 mg/day initially; increase in 0.5 mg/day increments q 5–6 days to effective dosage, to a maximum of 6 mg/day. Usual maintenance dosage is 1–2 mg/day in 2–3 divided doses. When used concurrently with levodopa, the dosages of both drugs may require reduction. **PO, IM, or IV for drug-induced extrapyramidal disorders** 1–4 mg/day in 1–2 doses.

Special Populations. *Pediatric Dosage.* (<3 yr) contraindicated; (>3 yr) 0.02–0.05 mg/kg/dose once or twice daily.

Geriatric Dosage. Same as adult dosage, although older patients can often be controlled with 1–2 mg/day.

Dosage Forms. Tab 0.5, 1, 2 mg; **Inj** 1 mg/mL.

Patient Instructions. This drug may cause constipation, difficult or painful urination, dry mouth, blurred vision, or drowsiness. Until the extent of the latter two effects is known, use caution when driving, operating machinery, or performing other tasks requiring mental alertness. Avoid excessive concurrent use of alcohol and other drugs that cause drowsiness. Becoming overheated during exercise or hot weather while taking this drug may result in heat stroke.

Pharmacokinetics. *Onset and Duration.* Onset of resolution of drug-induced extrapyramidal symptoms is within minutes following IV or IM administration, and 1–2 hr after oral administration. Duration is 24 hr.[221]

Fate. Benztropine pharmacokinetics are not well studied, but the drug apparently is hepatically metabolized to conjugates and may undergo enterohepatic recycling.[236]

Adverse Reactions. Frequent adverse effects are dose related and include dry mouth, blurred vision, nausea, dizziness, constipation, nervousness, and urinary retention. Confusional states, impairment of recent memory, and hallucinations occur with use of high doses and in patients with advanced age and underlying dementia. Rarely, paralytic ileus, parotitis, hyperthermia, or skin rash occur.

Contraindications. Children <3 yr; narrow angle glaucoma.

Precautions. Pregnancy. Use with caution in hot weather or during exercise and in patients with tachycardia, prostatic hypertrophy, open-angle glaucoma, or obstructive diseases of the GI tract.

Drug Interactions. Anticholinergics may decrease the effectiveness of phenothiazines. Use with amantadine may result in increased CNS anticholinergic effects. Anticholinergics may decrease digoxin absorption from digoxin tablets.

Parameters to Monitor. Intraocular pressure monitoring and gonioscope evaluation periodically. Monitor for Parkinson's disease symptoms periodically.

Notes. Anticholinergic agents are considered useful for the initial treatment of parkinsonism in patients >60 yr with a resting tremor and who do not require treatment for akinesia. Improvements of 20–25% in parkinsonian symptoms are reported.[228] The drug does not alleviate the symptoms of tardive dyskinesia.

BROMOCRIPTINE MESYLATE   Parlodel

Pharmacology. Bromocriptine is an ergot alkaloid that directly stimulates dopamine-D_2 receptors and is a partial antagonist at D_1 receptors.[237,238] This results in reduction of prolactin and growth hormone release from the pituitary gland and improves motor function in Parkinson's disease.

Administration and Adult Dosage. **PO for Parkinson's disease** 1.25 mg bid initially with food, increasing in 2.5 mg/day increments q 14–28 days to effective dosage, to a maximum of 100 mg/day. When given to patients concurrently receiving carbidopa/levodopa, usual maintenance dosage is 10–40 mg/day in 2–3 divided doses (*see* Notes). **PO for amenorrhea with or without galactorrhea or infertility** 1.25 mg/day or bid initially with food, increase in 2.5 mg/day increments q 3–7 days to effective dosage. Usual maintenance dosage is 2.5 mg bid or tid. **PO for acromegaly** 1.25 mg/day or bid initially with food, increasing in 1.25–2.5 mg/day increments q 3–7 days to effective dosage, to a maximum of 100 mg/day. Usual maintenance dosage is 20–30 mg/day in 2–3 divided doses.[239]

Special Populations. *Pediatric Dosage.* (<15 yr) safety and efficacy not established.

Geriatric Dosage. Same as adult dosage.

Dosage Forms. **Cap** 5 mg; **Tab** 2.5 mg.

Patient Instructions. This drug may cause dizziness, drowsiness, or fainting, especially after the initial dose. Until the extent of these effects is known, use caution when driving, operating machinery, or performing tasks requiring mental alertness. Mental disturbances, including vivid dreams, paranoid delusion, and confusion, can occur even with low doses, especially when added to levodopa therapy. Take this drug with food to minimize stomach upset. Avoid concurrent use of alcohol. Use a barrier contraceptive in women taking this drug to induce ovulation. Report persistent watery nasal discharge after transphenoidal surgery.

Pharmacokinetics. *Onset and Duration.* (Parkinsonism) Onset of pharmacologic action 30–90 min; duration 3–5 hr.[230] (Amenorrhea) Normal menstrual function may return within 6–8 weeks.

Fate. About 29% is orally absorbed with peak serum levels in 1.2 ± 0.4 hr, and detectable levels are found for up to 12 hr following discontinuation of drug.[240] About 90–96% is bound to albumin; Cl is 4.4 ± 2.6 L/hr/kg.[241] The majority (98%) is metabolized and excreted in the feces via bile.[240]

$t_{1/2}$. 3 ± 0.5 hr.[240]

Adverse Reactions. Nausea, headache, hallucinations, dyskinesias, vomiting, symptomatic hypotension, dizziness, fatigue, constipation, and lightheadedness occur frequently. Patient intolerance is greater with dosages >30 mg/day. Occasionally, abdominal cramps, diarrhea, drowsiness, or syncope may occur. Rarely, hypertension, stroke, seizures (mostly in postpartum patients), CSF rhinorrhea, or erythromelalgia are reported. Pleuropulmonary disease is rare and usually occurs in men, especially in smokers receiving 20–100 mg/day for 3–6 months; it presents with dyspnea and improves with drug discontinuation.[242]

Contraindications. Pregnancy; lactation; uncontrolled hypertension; preeclampsia; concurrent use of other ergot alkaloids; hypersensitivity to ergot alkaloids.

Precautions. Use a barrier contraceptive in women with amenorrhea, galactorrhea, or infertility, If pregnancy is detected, discontinue drug. Use with caution in patients with symptoms of peptic ulcer disease, history of pulmonary disease, MI, liver disease, severe angina, or psychiatric disease. Capsules contain sulfite.

Drug Interactions. Erythromycin may increase bromocriptine serum levels.

Parameters to Monitor. Monitor blood pressure frequently during the first few days of therapy and periodically thereafter. Periodically evaluate hepatic, hematopoietic, cardiovascular, and renal function during long-term therapy. Monitor symptoms of Parkinson's disease periodically.

Notes. Bromocriptine is not recommended for the treatment of newly diagnosed Parkinson's disease alone or with levodopa. As an adjunct to **levodopa** in Parkinson's disease, greatest improvement occurs in patients with mild to moderate disease. Bromocriptine may improve motor fluctuations in disease by increasing "on" time, allowing a decrease in levodopa dosage.[243,244] Most patients require a 20–30% reduction in levodopa dosage.

CARBIDOPA AND LEVODOPA   Sinemet

Pharmacology. Levodopa is centrally converted to dopamine by DOPA decarboxylase, replenishing dopamine, which is deficient in the basal ganglia of patients with Parkinson's disease. Carbidopa, which does not cross the blood-brain barrier, inhibits peripheral DOPA decarboxylase, thereby increasing the amount of levodopa available to the brain for conversion to dopamine while limiting peripheral side effects. Addition of carbidopa decreases levodopa-induced nausea and vomiting, but does not decrease adverse reactions caused by the central effects of levodopa.

Administration and Adult Dosage. PO for Parkinson's disease in patients not receiving levodopa (standard formulation) (combination with bromocriptine, pergolide, or selegiline may permit lower dosages) 25 mg carbidopa/100 mg levodopa tid initially, increasing in 1 tablet/day increments q 1–2 days to effective dosage, to a maximum of 8 tablets/day. Alternatively, 10 mg carbidopa/100 mg levodopa tid or qid initially, to a maximum of 8 tablets/day. Initial use of 10 mg carbidopa/100 mg levodopa may result in more nausea and vomiting, because 70–100 mg/day of carbidopa is needed to saturate peripheral DOPA decarboxylase. If initial dosage maximum is reached with 10/100 tablets and further titration is necessary, substitute 25 mg carbidopa/250 mg levodopa tid or qid, increase in 0.5–1 tablet/day increments q 1–2 days to effective dosage, to a maximum of 8 tablets/day. **SR Tab** in patients already taking non-SR tablets, start with a dosage that provides 10% more levodopa daily. Initially, divide dosage bid or tid with an interval of 4–8 hr between doses while awake. Ultimately, dosages up to 30%

greater may be needed, depending on patient response. In patients not receiving carbidopa/levodopa, give 1 tablet bid initially, at least 6 hr apart, and allow 3 days between dosage adjustments. Usual dosage is 2–8 tablets/day. **PO for Parkinson's disease in patients receiving levodopa** discontinue levodopa at least 8 hr before starting carbidopa/levodopa. Daily dosage of carbidopa/levodopa should provide approximately 25% of the previous levodopa daily dosage. Start patients taking less than 1.5 g/day of levodopa on 25 mg carbidopa/100 mg levodopa tid or qid; start those taking more than 1.5 g/day of levodopa on 25 mg carbidopa/250 mg levodopa tid or qid.

Special Populations. *Pediatric Dosage.* (<18 yr) safety and efficacy not established.

Geriatric Dosage. Same as adult dosage.

Dosage Forms. **Tab** 10 mg carbidopa/100 mg levodopa, 25 mg carbidopa/100 mg levodopa, 25 mg carbidopa/250 mg levodopa; **SR Tab** 25 mg carbidopa/100 mg levodopa, 50 mg carbidopa/200 mg levodopa. (*See* Notes.)

Patient Instructions. Stopping this medication suddenly may cause Parkinson's disease to worsen quickly. Report bothersome or unexpected side effects. Unless prescribed, do not take levodopa in addition to this drug. Avoid pyridoxine (vitamin B_6) if you are taking levodopa alone, but it may be taken with carbidopa/levodopa. Avoid high-protein meals for maximum absorption. If you are taking the sustained-release tablet, swallow a whole or half tablet without chewing or crushing it.

Pharmacokinetics. *Onset and Duration.* Up to 67% of patients experience a reduction in efficacy after 5 yr.[230] (*See* Notes.)

Fate. Carbidopa's inhibition of peripheral levodopa decarboxylation doubles the oral bioavailability of levodopa and decreases its clearance by one-half.[245] Dietary proteins compete with levodopa for intestinal absorption and decrease its effectiveness.[230] (Rapid-release 50 mg carbidopa/200 mg levodopa) levodopa bioavailability is 99 ± 21%. A peak of 3.2 ± 1.1 mg/L occurs in 0.7 ± 0.3 hr.[246] (SR 50 mg carbidopa/200 mg levodopa) levodopa bioavailability is 71 ± 24%, increased in the presence of food. A peak of 1.14 ± 0.42 mg/L occurs in 2.4 ± 1.2 hr.[246] Levodopa V_d is 1.09 ± 0.59 L/kg; Cl is 0.28 ± 0.06 L/hr/kg; 90% of clearance is nonrenal.[245]

$t_{1/2}$. (Carbidopa) 2.1 ± 0.6 hr;[246] (levodopa) 2 ± 1.3 hr.[245]

Adverse Reactions. Anorexia, nausea, vomiting, and involuntary muscle movements (dyskinesias) occur frequently and are generally reversible with dosage reduction. Occasionally mental changes, depression, dementia, palpitations, or orthostatic hypotensive episodes occur. Rarely, psychosis, hemolytic anemia, leukopenia, or agranulocytosis are reported. Compared to levodopa alone, carbidopa/levodopa has markedly reduced GI and cardiovascular side effects. However, mental disturbances are not eliminated and dyskinesias may appear earlier in therapy.[247] These dyskinesias may require a decrease in dosage or dosage interval.[248] Side effects may be more pronounced in patients receiving **selegiline** or a dopamine agonist as adjunctive therapy.

Contraindications. Lactation; nonselective MAO inhibitors concurrently or 2 weeks prior to carbidopa/levodopa; narrow-angle glaucoma; undiagnosed skin lesions; history of melanoma.

Precautions. Pregnancy. Use with caution in patients with history of MI complicated by arrhythmias; peptic ulcer disease; severe cardiovascular, pulmonary, renal, hepatic, or endocrine disease; open-angle glaucoma; bronchial asthma; urinary retention; or psychosis. Also, use caution in patients receiving antihypertensives. Symptoms resembling neuroleptic malignant syndrome have been reported when carbidopa/levodopa in combination with other antiparkinson agents was reduced abruptly or discontinued.

Drug Interactions. Hydantoins (eg, phenytoin) may decrease levodopa efficacy. Administration of the sustained-release product with food increases its bioavailability. Selegiline may increase levodopa side effects and levodopa/carbidopa dosage may need to be reduced 10–30% when selegiline is started.

Parameters to Monitor. Monitor CBC, renal, cardiovascular, and liver function periodically during long-term therapy. Monitor symptoms of Parkinson's disease periodically. In patients with open-angle glaucoma, monitor intraocular pressure.

Notes. Levodopa produces sustained improvement in rigidity and bradykinesia in 50–60% of patients.[249] Tremor is variably affected, and postural stability is unresponsive.[250] Loss of therapeutic effect is manifested by fluctuations in motor performance. Patients may experience periods of lack of drug effect ("off" periods) alternating with periods of therapeutic efficacy ("on" periods). Response may be predictable where the effect fades before the next dose ("wearing-off" or "end-of-dose"), or unpredictable ("yo-yo") where there is no relationship to the time of dose.[251] SR carbidopa/levodopa reduces "off" time an average of 30–40 min/day and allows a mean 33% reduction in the frequency of administration; the lower bioavailability of the SR product necessitates a 25% median increase in the daily dosage of levodopa compared with non-SR carbidopa/levodopa.[252] With disease progression, adjunctive therapy with an MAO-B inhibitor or a dopamine agonist may be required to decrease the frequency of fluctuations caused by dyskinesia or dystonia.

PERGOLIDE MESYLATE   Permax

Pergolide is a synthetic ergoline dopamine receptor agonist with an affinity for dopamine-D_1 and D_2 receptors; its greatest activity is at D_2 receptors. This action improves motor function in patients with Parkinson's disease. The drug is rapidly absorbed, with peak serum concentrations in 1–2 hr; 90% is bound to plasma proteins. About 40–50% of the dose is excreted in feces over 7 days as at least 10 metabolites. Elimination half-life is 27 ± 13.7 hr. Pergolide is contraindicated in patients hypersensitive to ergot alkaloids. Adverse reactions such as GI disturbances and dyskinesias are similar in nature to those of **bromocriptine** and may require dosage reduction. Pergolide can also cause symptomatic orthostatic and/or sustained hypotension during initial treatment, atrial premature contractions, sinus tachycardia, or hallucinosis of sufficient severity to require discontinuation. Pergolide is indicated as adjunctive treatment with carbidopa/levodopa in Parkinson's disease. In Parkinson's patients with motor fluctuations, pergolide use results in reductions in **levodopa** dosage by an average of 44%, median levodopa dosage frequency from 7.5 to 5 doses/day, and median "off" time decreases from 5 to 2.2 hr/day. In adults and adolescents, pergolide is initiated with an oral dosage of 0.05 mg/day for 2 days, then increased in 0.1 or 0.15 mg/day increments q 3 days over the next 12 days. Then, increase dosage in 0.25 mg/day increments q 3 days to optimal dosage, not to exceed a maximum dosage of 5 mg/day. Optimal dosage is usually is 2–4 mg/day, administered in 3 divided doses.[253–256] Available as 0.05-, 0.25-, and 1-mg tablets.

SELEGILINE HYDROCHLORIDE   Eldepryl

Pharmacology. Selegiline (formerly l-deprenyl) is a selective irreversible MAO-B inhibitor used as adjunctive therapy in the management of Parkinson's disease. MAO-B is found in the brain and plays a role in the catabolism of dopamine. By preventing the breakdown of dopamine by MAO-B, selegiline increases the net amount of dopamine available in the brain. Selegiline also inhibits the uptake of dopamine and noradrenaline into the presynaptic neuron, and may exert a protective effect by preventing the accumulation of neurotoxic free radicals generated by dopamine metabolism.[257–259]

Administration and Adult Dosage. **PO for Parkinson's disease** 5 mg bid taken at breakfast and lunch. Alternatively, give an initial dosage of 2.5 mg/day and slowly increase to 10 mg/day over several weeks to minimize side effects.[258] There is no evidence that dosages over 10 mg/day increase efficacy.

Special Populations. *Pediatric Dosage.* Safety and efficacy not established.

Geriatric Dosage. Same as adult dosage.

Dosage Forms. **Cap** 5 mg; **Tab** 5 mg.

Patient Instructions. Take this medication with morning and midday meals to minimize nausea and nighttime insomnia. At a dosage of 10 mg per day or less, tyramine-containing foods and medications containing amines are safe to consume. Initiation of selegiline may require a reduction of carbidopa/levodopa dosage. Report immediately any severe headache or other atypical or unexpected symptoms.

Pharmacokinetics. *Onset and Duration.* Recovery of platelet MAO-B activity after a single oral dose is 2–4 days; after long-term treatment, over 90% of platelet MAO-B remains inhibited after 5 days.[260] With continued use, clinical efficacy lasts 6–12 months in most patients, to a maximum of 12–24 months.[255,261]

Fate. Selegiline is readily absorbed from the GI tract, with a peak at 0.5–2 hr; 94% is plasma protein bound.[260] It is metabolized by the liver to N-desmethylselegiline, l-amphetamine, and l-methamphetamine; these isomers, however, are 10 times less potent than the d-isomers. After long-term therapy with 10 mg/day in 2 divided doses, mean trough serum levels of selegiline and N-desmethylselegiline are undetectable, l-amphetamine is 5.9 ± 2.7 μg/L (22 ± 10 nmol/L), and l-methamphetamine is 14.9 ± 6.8 μg/L (100 ± 45 nmol/L). The concentrations of these metabolites are probably too low to contribute to the drug's clinical efficacy, but may contribute to adverse effects. About 86% is excreted in urine as inactive metabolites.[262,263]

$t_{1/2}$. (N-desmethylselegiline) 2 ± 1.2 hr; (l-amphetamine) 17.7 ± 16.3 hr; (l-methamphetamine) 20.5 ± 11.4 hr.[263]

Adverse Reactions. Nausea, abdominal pain, dry mouth, confusion, hallucinations, dizziness, insomnia, lightheadedness, and/or fainting occur frequently. Occasionally vivid dreams, dyskinesias, and headache occur. In decreasing order of frequency, nausea, hallucinations, confusion, depression, loss of balance, and insomnia may lead to discontinuation of the drug. Mild, asymptomatic elevations in liver function tests were observed in one long-term study.[261]

Precautions. Pregnancy; lactation. Concurrent use with meperidine, because experience with selegiline is limited. Do not use at dosages exceeding 10 mg/day.

Drug Interactions. Concurrent administration of selegiline and serotonin reuptake inhibitors (eg, SSRIs, nefazodone, venlafaxine) may cause serotonin syndrome; they should not be given concurrently within 1–2 weeks of each other (5 weeks after stopping fluoxetine).

Parameters to Monitor. Evaluate clinical status and monitor liver function tests periodically.

Notes. Selegiline is indicated as adjunctive treatment with **carbidopa/levodopa** in Parkinson's disease. Although selegiline's efficacy has not been shown to be superior to other adjunctive drugs such as **bromocriptine** or an **anticholinergic**, it appears to be better tolerated.[264] Approximately 50–70% of patients who receive selegiline experience a modest (10% or less) reduction in "off" periods and are able to reduce their levodopa dosage by 10–30%.[265] A role for the drug as an initial agent in patients with mild disease is supported by results of a study comparing selegiline 10 mg/day to placebo in patients with early (<5 yr) untreated Parkinson's disease; selegiline delayed the onset of disease-related disability by nearly 1 yr.[266]

TRIHEXYPHENIDYL HYDROCHLORIDE   Artane, Various

Trihexyphenidyl, like benztropine, is a competitive antagonist of acetylcholine at central muscarinic receptors. In Parkinson's disease, it is an adjunctive treatment that balances cholinergic activity in cerebral synapses. The onset of action is within 1 hr, and the peak effect lasts 2–3 hr; the duration of action is 6–12 hr. The majority of the drug is excreted in the urine probably unchanged, and the elimination half-life is 10.2 ± 4.7 hr. Precautions, contraindications, drug interactions, and adverse reactions are the same as for benztropine. The dosage for Parkinson's disease is 1 mg/day PO initially, increasing in 2 mg/day increments q 3–5 days to an effective dosage, to a maximum of 12–15 mg/day. The usual maintenance dosage is 6–10 mg/day in 3 divided doses or 3–6 mg/day in 3 divided doses concurrent with levodopa. SR caps may be given bid, once the maintenance dosage is determined. When trihexyphenidyl is used concurrently with levodopa, the dosages of both drugs may require reduction. For drug-induced extrapyramidal disorders give 1 mg initially, increasing in 1-mg increments every few hours until symptoms are controlled, usually 5–15 mg/day in 3–4 divided doses. Available as 0.4 mg/mL elixir, 2- and 5-mg tablets, and 5-mg SR capsules.

■ REFERENCES

1. Anon. Drugs for epilepsy. *Med Lett Drugs Ther* 1995;37:37–40.
2. Levy RH et al., eds. *Antiepileptic drugs*, 4th ed. New York: Raven Press; 1995.
3. Cloyd JC et al. Antiepileptics in the elderly: pharmacoepidemiology and pharmacokinetics. *Arch Fam Med* 1994;3:589–98.
4. Bass J et al. Effects of enteral tube feedings on the absorption and pharmacokinetic profile of carbamazepine suspension. *Epilepsia* 1989;30:364–9

5. Graves NM et al. Relative bioavailability of rectally administered carbamazepine suspension in humans. *Epilepsia* 1985;26:429–33.
6. Morrow JI, Richens A. Disposition of anticonvulsants in childhood. *Clin Pharmacokinet* 1989;17(suppl 1):89–104.
7. Bertilsson L et al. Autoinduction of carbamazepine metabolism in children examined by a stable isotope technique. *Clin Pharmacol Ther* 1980;27:83–8.
8. Mikati MA et al. Time course of carbamazepine autoinduction. *Neurology* 1989;39:592–4.
9. Theodore WH et al. Carbamazepine and its epoxide: relation of plasma levels to toxicity and seizure control. *Ann Neurol* 1989;25:194–6.
10. Pollack MH et al. Long-term outcome after acute treatment with alprazolam or clonazepam for panic disorder. *J Clin Psychopharmacol* 1993;13:257–63.
11. Herman JB et al. The alprazolam to clonazepam switch for the treatment of panic disorder. *J Clin Psychopharmacol* 1987;7:175–8.
12. Greenblatt DJ et al. Clinical pharmacokinetics of anxiolytics and hypnotics in the elderly: therapeutic considerations (Part I). *Clin Pharmacokinet* 1991;21:165–77.
13. Graves NM, Kriel RL. Rectal administration of antiepileptic drugs in children. *Pediatr Neurol* 1987;3:321–6.
14. Berlin A, Dahlstrom H. Pharmacokinetics of the anticonvulsant drug clonazepam evaluated from single oral and intravenous doses and by repeated oral administration. *Eur J Clin Pharmacol* 1975;9:155–9.
15. Specht U et al. Discontinuation of clonazepam after long-term treatment. *Epilepsia* 1989;30:458–63.
16. Beauclair L et al. Clonazepam in the treatment of panic disorder: a double-blind, placebo-controlled trial investigating the correlation between clonazepam concentrations in plasma and clinical response. *J Clin Psychopharmacol* 1994;14:111–8.
17. Buchanan RA et al. Absorption and elimination of ethosuximide in children. *J Clin Pharmacol* 1969;9:393–8.
18. Goulet JR et al. Metabolism of ethosuximide. *Clin Pharmacol Ther* 1976;20:213–8.
19. Rho JM et al. Mechanism of action of the anticonvulsant felbamate: opposing effects on N-methyl-D-aspartate and γ-aminobutyric acid$_A$ receptors. *Ann Neurol* 1994;35:229–34.
20. Sachdeo R et al. Felbamate monotherapy: controlled trial in patients with partial onset seizures. *Ann Neurol* 1992;32:386–92.
21. Espe-Lillo J et al. Safety and efficacy of felbamate in treatment of infantile spasms. *Epilepsia* 1993;34:110.
22. Perhach JL et al. Felbamate. In Meldrum BS, Porter RJ, eds. *New anticonvulsant drugs*. London: John Libby; 1986:117–23.
23. Wilensky AJ et al. Pharmacokinetics of W-554 (ADD 03055) in epileptic patients. *Epilepsia* 1985;26:602–6.
24. Gerber N et al. Safety, tolerance and pharmacokinetics of intravenous doses of the phosphate ester of 3-hydroxymethyl-5,5-diphenylhydantoin: a new prodrug of phenytoin. *J Clin Pharmacol* 1988;28:1023–32.
25. Leppik IE et al. Pharmacokinetics and safety of a phenytoin prodrug given IV or IM in patients. *Neurology* 1990;40:456–60.
26. Jamerson BD et al. Venous irritation related to intravenous administration of phenytoin versus fosphenytoin. *Pharmacotherapy* 1994;14:47–52.
27. Aweeka F et al. Conversion of ACC-9653 to phenytoin in patients with renal or hepatic diseases. *Clin Pharmacol Ther* 1989;45:152. Abstract.
28. Crockett JG et al. Open-label follow-on study of gabapentin (GBP; Neurontin) monotherapy in patients with refractory epilepsy. *Epilepsia* 1995;36:69. Abstract.
29. McLean MJ. Clinical pharmacokinetics of gabapentin. *Neurology* 1994;44(suppl 5):S17–22.
30. Sivenius J et al. Double-blind study of gabapentin in the treatment of partial seizures. *Epilepsia* 1991;32:539–42.
31. Hooper WD et al. Lack of a pharmacokinetic interaction between phenobarbitone and gabapentin. *Br J Clin Pharmacol* 1991;31:171–4.
32. Ramsay RE. Clinical efficacy and safety of gabapentin. *Neurology* 1994;44(suppl 5):S23–30.
33. Asconape J, Collins T. Weight gain associated with the use of gabapentin. *Epilepsia* 1994;36(suppl 4):72. Abstract.
34. Wolf SM et al. Gabapentin toxicity in children manifesting as behavioral changes. *Epilepsia* 1996;36:1203–5.
35. Mikati M et al. Efficacy of gabapentin in children with refractory partial seizures. *Neurology* 1995;45(suppl 4):A201–2. Abstract.
36. Btaiche IF, Woster PS. Gabapentin and lamotrigine: novel antiepileptic drugs. *Am J Health-Syst Pharm* 1995;52:61–9.
37. Rambeck B, Wolf P. Lamotrigine clinical pharmacokinetics. *Clin Pharmacokinet* 1993;25:433–43.
38. Jawad S et al. Lamotrigine: single-dose pharmacokinetics and initial 1 week experience in refractory epilepsy. *Epilepsy Res* 1987;1:194–201.
39. Timmings PL, Richens A. Lamotrigine as an add-on drug in the management of Lennox-Gastaut syndrome. *Eur Neurol* 1992;32:305–7.

40. Brodie MJ et al. Double-blind comparison of lamotrigine and carbamazepine in newly diagnosed epilepsy. *Lancet* 1995;345:476–9.

41. Working Group on Status Epilepticus. Treatment of convulsive status epilepticus. *JAMA* 1993;270:854–9.

42. Dunn DW. Status epilepticus in infancy and childhood. *Neurol Clin* 1990;8:647–57.

43. Scheuer ML, Pedley TA. The evaluation and treatment of seizures. *N Engl J Med* 1990;323:1468–74.

44. Graves NM et al. Relative bioavailability of rectally administered phenobarbital sodium parenteral solution. *DICP* 1989;23:565–8.

45. Alvin J et al. The effect of liver disease in man on the disposition of phenobarbital. *J Pharmacol Exp Ther* 1975;192:224–35.

46. Wilensky AJ et al. Kinetics of phenobarbital in normal subjects and epileptic patients. *Eur J Clin Pharmacol* 1982;23:87–92.

47. Heimann G, Gladtke E. Pharmacokinetics of phenobarbital in childhood. *Eur J Clin Pharmacol* 1977;12:305–10.

48. Meador KJ et al. Comparative cognitive effects of phenobarbital, phenytoin, and valproate in healthy adults. *Neurology* 1995;45:1494–99.

49. Mattson RH et al. Barbiturate-related connective tissue disorders. *Arch Intern Med* 1989;149:911–4.

50. Alldredge BK et al. Anticonvulsant hypersensitivity syndrome: in vitro and clinical observations. *Pediatr Neurol* 1994;10:169–71.

51. Ramsay RE. Pharmacokinetics and clinical use of parenteral phenytoin, phenobarbital, and paraldehyde. *Epilepsia* 1989;30(suppl 2):S1–3.

52. Dela Cruz FG et al. Efficacy of individualized phenytoin sodium loading doses administered by intravenous infusion. *Clin Pharm* 1988;7:219–24.

53. Blaser KU et al. Intravenous phenytoin: a loading scheme for desired concentrations. *Ann Intern Med* 1989;110:1029–31.

54. Bauer LA, Blouin RA. Age and phenytoin kinetics in adult epileptics. *Clin Pharmacol Ther* 1982;31:301–4.

55. Boucher BA et al. Phenytoin pharmacokinetics in critically ill trauma patients. *Clin Pharmacol Ther* 1988;44:675–83.

56. Levy RH, Yerby MS. Effects of pregnancy on antiepileptic drug utilization. *Epilepsia* 1985;26(suppl 1): S52–7.

57. Leppik IE et al. Altered phenytoin clearance with febrile illness. *Neurology* 1986;36:1367–70.

58. Tozer TN, Winter ME. Phenytoin. In Evans WE et al., eds. *Applied pharmacokinetics: principles of therapeutic drug monitoring*, 3rd ed. Vancouver: Applied Therapeutics; 1992.

59. Goff DA et al. Absorption characteristics of three phenytoin sodium products after administration of oral loading doses. *Clin Pharm* 1984;3:634–8.

60. McCauley DL et al. Time for phenytoin concentration to peak: consequences of first-order and zero-order absorption. *Ther Drug Monit* 1989;11:540–42.

61. Browne TR et el. Estimation of the elimination half-life of a drug at any serum concentration when the K_m and V_{max} of the drug are known: calculations and validation with phenytoin. *J Clin Pharmacol* 1987;27:318–20.

62. Spengler RF et al. Severe soft-tissue injury following intravenous infusion of phenytoin—patient and drug administration risk factors. *Arch Intern Med* 1988;148:1329–33.

63. Smythe MA, Umstead GS. Phenytoin hepatotoxicity: a review of the literature. *DICP* 1989;23:13–8.

64. Delattre JY et al. Erythema multiforme and Stevens-Johnson syndrome in patients receiving cranial irradiation and phenytoin. *Neurology* 1988;38:194–8.

65. Haley CJ, Nelson J. Phenytoin-enteral feeding interaction. *DICP* 1989;23:796–8.

66. Sarkar MA et al. The effects of storage and shaking on the settling properties of phenytoin suspension. *Neurology* 1989;39:207–9.

67. Mattson RH et al. Comparison of carbamazepine, phenobarbital, phenytoin and primidone in partial and secondarily generalized tonic-clonic seizures. *N Engl J Med* 1985;313:145–51.

68. Pisani F et al. Single dose kinetics of primidone in acute viral hepatitis. *Eur J Clin Pharmacol* 1984;27:465–9.

69. Cottrell PR et al. Pharmacokinetics of phenylethylmalonamide (PEMA) in normal subjects and in patients treated with antiepileptic drugs. *Epilepsia* 1982;23:307–13.

70. Shank RP et al. Topiramate: preclinical evaluation of a structurally novel anticonvulsant. *Epilepsia* 1994;35:450–60.

71. Giscion LG et al. The steady-state pharmacokinetics of phenytoin (Dilantin) and topiramate (Topamax) in epileptic patients on monotherapy, and during combination therapy. *Epilepsia* 1994;35:54. Abstract.

72. Brodie MJ, Dichter MA. Antiepileptic drugs. *N Engl J Med* 1996;334:168–75.

73. Zaccara G et al. Clinical pharmacokinetics of valproic acid—1988. *Clin Pharmacokinet* 1988;15:367–89.

74. Fischer JH et al. Effect of food on the serum concentration profile on enteric-coated valproic acid. *Neurology* 1988;38:1319–22.

75. Holmes GB et al. Absorption of valproic acid suppositories in human volunteers. *Arch Neurol* 1989;46:906–9.

76. Dreifuss FE et al. Valproic acid hepatic fatalities—II. US experience since 1984. *Neurology* 1989;39:201–7.
77. Mattson RH et al. A comparison of valproic acid with carbamazepine for the treatment of complex partial seizures and secondarily generalized tonic-clonic seizures in adults. *N Engl J Med* 1992;327:765–71.
78. APA Practice Guideline for the Treatment of Patients with Bipolar Disorder. *Am J Psychiatry* 1994;12(suppl):1–36.
79. Bowden CL et al. Efficacy of divalproex vs lithium and placebo in the treatment of mania. *JAMA* 1994;271:918–24.
80. Bowden CL. Predictors of response to divalproex and lithium. *J Clin Psychiatry* 1995;56(suppl 3):25–30.
81. Rothrock JF et al. A differential response to treatment with divalproex sodium in patients with intractable headache. *Cephalalgia* 1994;14:241–4.
82. Mathew NT et al. Migraine prophylaxis with divalproex. *Arch Neurol* 1995;52:281–6.
83. Browne TR et al. Multicenter long-term safety and efficacy study of vigabatrin for refractory complex partial seizures: an update. *Neurology* 1991;41:363–4.
84. Kalviainen R et al. Vigabatrin vs carbamazepine monotherapy in patients with newly diagnosed epilepsy. *Arch Neurol* 1995;52:989–96.
85. Connelly JF. Vigabatrin. *Ann Pharmacother* 1993;27:197–204.
86. Haegele KD, Schechter PJ. Kinetics of the enantiomers of vigabatrin after an oral dose of the racemate or the active S-enantiomer. *Clin Pharmacol Ther* 1986;40:581–6.
87. Haegele KD et al. Pharmacokinetics of vigabatrin: implications of creatinine clearance. *Clin Pharmacol Ther* 1988;44:558–65.
88. Preskorn SH, Othmer SC. Evaluation of bupropion hydrochloride: the first of a new class of atypical antidepressants. *Pharmacotherapy* 1984;4:20–34.
89. Davidson J. Seizures and bupropion: a review. *J Clin Psychiatry* 1989;50:256–61.
90. Lineberry CG et al. A fixed-dose (300 mg) efficacy study of bupropion and placebo in depressed outpatients. *J Clin Psychiatry* 1990;51:194–9.
91. Walker PW et al. Improvement in fluoxetine-associated sexual dysfunction in patients switched to bupropion. *J Clin Psychiatry* 1993;54:459–65.
92. Jermain DM et al. Pharmacotherapy of obsessive-compulsive disorder. *Pharmacotherapy* 1990;10:175–98.
93. Peters MD et al. Clomipramine: an antiobsessional tricyclic antidepressant. *Clin Pharm* 1990;9:165–78.
94. Freeman CPL et al. Fluvoxamine versus clomipramine in the treatment of obsessive-compulsive disorder: a multi-center, randomized, double-blind, parallel group comparison. *J Clin Psychiatry* 1994;55:301–5.
95. Stokes PE. Fluoxetine: a five-year review. *Clin Ther* 1993;15:216–43.
96. Sommi RW et al. Fluoxetine: a serotonin-specific second-generation antidepressant. *Pharmacotherapy* 1987;7:1–15.
97. Schweizer E et al. What constitutes an adequate antidepressant trial for fluoxetine? *J Clin Psychiatry* 1990;51:8–11.
98. Benet LZ et al. Design and optimization of dosage regimens: pharmacokinetic data. In Hardman JG et al., eds. *Goodman and Gilman's the pharmacological basis of therapeutics*, 9th ed. New York: McGraw-Hill; 1996: 1707–92.
99. Herman JB et al. Fluoxetine-induced sexual dysfunction. *J Clin Psychiatry* 1990;51:25–7.
100. Kinney-Parker JL et al. Fluoxetine and weight: something lost and something gained? *Clin Pharm* 1989;8:727–33.
101. Jefferson JW. Cardiovascular effects and toxicity of anxiolytics and antidepressants. *J Clin Psychiatry* 1989; 50:368–78.
102. Tollefson GD et al. Absence of a relationship between adverse events and suicidality during pharmacotherapy for depression. *J Clin Psychopharmacol* 1994;14:163–9.
103. Feighner JP et al. Adverse consequences of fluoxetine-MAOI combination therapy. *J Clin Psychiatry* 1990;51:222–5.
104. Roose SP et al. Comparative efficacy of selective serotonin reuptake inhibitors and tricyclics in the treatment of melancholia. *Am J Psychiatry* 1994;151:1735–9.
105. Grimsley SR, Jann MW. Paroxetine, sertraline, and fluvoxamine: new selective serotonin reuptake inhibitors. *Clin Pharm* 1992;11:930–57.
106. Wilde MI et al. Fluvoxamine. an updated review of its pharmacology and therapeutic use in depressive illness. *Drugs* 1993;46:895–924.
107. Potter WZ et al. The pharmacologic treatment of depression. *N Engl J Med* 1991;325:633–42.
108. Preskorn SH. Recent pharmacologic advances in antidepressant therapy for the elderly. *Am J Med* 1993;94(suppl 5A):2S–12S.
109. Baldessarini RJ. Current status of antidepressants: clinical pharmacology and therapy. *J Clin Psychiatry* 1989;50:117–26.
110. Frank E et al. Comparison of full-dose versus half-dose pharmacotherapy in the maintenance treatment of recurrent depression. *J Affect Disord* 1993;27:139–45.

111. Wright JM. Review of the symptomatic treatment of diabetic neuropathy. *Pharmacotherapy* 1994;14:689–97.

112. Max MB. Treatment of post-herpetic neuralgia: antidepressants. *Ann Neurol* 1994;35:S50–3.

113. Rappoport JL et al. Childhood enuresis II. Psychopathology, tricyclic concentration in plasma, and antienuretic effect. *Arch Gen Psychiatry* 1980;37:1146–52.

114. Puig-Antich J et al. Imipramine in prepubertal major depressive disorders. *Arch Gen Psychiatry* 1987;44:81–9.

115. Salzman C. Pharmacologic treatment of depression in the elderly. *J Clin Psychiatry* 1993;54(suppl 2):23–8.

116. Salzman C. Practical considerations in the pharmacologic treatment of depression and anxiety in the elderly. *J Clin Psychiatry* 1990;51(suppl 1):40–3.

117. Wisner KL, et al. Tricyclic dose requirements across pregnancy. *Am J Psychiatry* 1993;150:1541–2.

118. Preskorn SH. Pharmacokinetics of antidepressants. *J Clin Psychiatry* 1993;54(suppl 9):14–34.

119. DeVane CL. *Fundamentals of monitoring psychoactive drug therapy.* Baltimore: Williams & Wilkins; 1990.

120. Cole JO, Bodkin A. Antidepressant drug side effects. *J Clin Psychiatry* 1990;51(suppl 1):21–6.

121. Rosenstein DL et al. Seizures associated with antidepressants: a review. *J Clin Psychiatry* 1993;54:289–99.

122. Anon. Sudden death in children treated with a tricyclic antidepressant. *Med Lett Drugs Ther* 1990;32:53.

123. Goodman WK, Charney DS. Therapeutic applications and mechanisms of action of monoamine oxidase inhibitors and heterocyclic antidepressant drugs. *J Clin Psychiatry* 1985; 46(10, sec 2):6–22.

124. Cantú TG, Korek JS. Monoamine oxidase inhibitors and weight gain. *Drug Intell Clin Pharm* 1988;22:755–9.

125. Kahn D et al. The safety of switching rapidly from tricyclic antidepressants to monoamine oxidase inhibitors. *J Clin Psychopharmacol* 1989;9:198–202.

126. Brown CS, Bryant SG. Monoamine oxidase inhibitors: safety and efficacy issues. *Drug Intell Clin Pharm* 1988;22:232–5.

127. Shulman KI et al. Dietary restriction, tyramine, and the use of monoamine oxidase inhibitors. *J Clin Psychopharmacol* 1989;9:397–402.

128. Nierenberg AA, Amsterdam JD. Treatment-resistant depression: definition and treatment approaches. *J Clin Psychiatry* 1990;51(suppl 6):39–47.

129. Stimmel GL et al. Mirtazapine: an antidepressant with selective α_2-adrenoreceptor antagonist effects. *Pharmacotherapy* (in press).

130. Sambunaris A et al. Development of new antidepressants. *J Clin Psychiatr* (in press).

131. Dopheide JA et al. Focus on nefazodone: a serotonergic drug for major depression. *Hosp Formul* 1995;30:205–12.

132. Fontaine R et al. A double-blind comparison of nefazodone, imipramine, and placebo in major depression. *J Clin Psychiatry* 1994;55:234–41.

133. Barbhaiya RH et al. Single-dose pharmacokinetics of nefazodone in healthy young and elderly subjects and in subjects with renal or hepatic impairment. *Eur J Clin Pharmacol* 1995;49:221–8.

134. Barbhaiya RH et al. Steady-state pharmacokinetics of nefazodone in subjects normal and impaired renal function. *Eur J Clin Pharmacol* 1995;49:229–35.

135. DeWilde J et al. A double-blind, comparative, multicentre study comparing paroxetine with fluoxetine in depressed patients. *Acta Psychiatr Scand* 1993;87:141–5.

136. Dechant KL, Clissold SPP. Paroxetine. *Drugs* 1991;41:225–53.

137. DeVane CL. Pharmacokinetics of the selective serotonin reuptake inhibitors. *J Clin Psychiatry* 1992;53(suppl 2):13–20.

138. Heym J, Koe BK. Pharmacology of sertraline: a review. *J Clin Psychiatry* 1988;49(suppl 8):40–5.

139. Doogan DP, Caillard V. Sertraline: a new antidepressant. *J Clin Psychiatry* 1988;49(suppl 8):46–51.

140. Aguglia E et al. Double-blind study of the efficacy and safety of sertraline versus fluoxetine in major depression. *Int Clin Psychopharmacol* 1993;8:197–202.

141. Bryant SG, Ereshefsky L. Antidepressant properties of trazodone. *Clin Pharm* 1982;1:406–17.

142. Georgotas A et al. Trazodone hydrochloride: a wide spectrum antidepressant with a unique pharmacological profile. *Pharmacotherapy* 1982;2:255–65.

143. Nierenberg AA et al. Trazodone for antidepressant-associated insomnia. *Am J Psychiatry* 1994;151:1069–72.

144. Dittrich A et al. Treatment of pharmacological priapism with phenylephrine. *J Urol* 1991;146:323–4.

145. Schweizer E et al. Placebo-controlled trial of venlafaxine for the treatment of major depression. *J Clin Psychopharmacol* 1991;11:233–236.

146. Montgomery SA. Venlafaxine: a new dimension in antidepressant pharmacotherapy. *J Clin Psychiatry* 1993;54:119–26.

147. Cunningham LA et al. A comparison of venlafaxine, trazodone, and placebo in major depression. *J Clin Psychopharmacol* 1994;14:99–106.

148. Ereshefsky L et al. Pathophysiologic basis for schizophrenia and the efficacy of antipsychotics. *Clin Pharm* 1990;9:682–707.

149. Coyle JT. The clinical use of antipsychotic medications. *Med Clin North Am* 1982;66:993–1009.

150. Kane JM. The current status of neuroleptic therapy. *J Clin Psychiatry* 1989;50:322–8.

151. Heresco-Levy U et al. Trial of maintenance neuroleptic dose reduction in schizophrenic outpatients: two year outcome. *J Clin Psychiatry* 1993;54:59–62.

152. Brotman AW et al. A role for high-dose antipsychotics. *J Clin Psychiatry* 1990;51:164–6.

153. Rifkin A et al. Dosage of haloperidol for mania. *Br J Psychiatry* 1994;165:113–6.

154. Zaleon CR, Guthrie SK. Antipsychotic drug use in older adults. *Am J Hosp Pharm* 1994;51:2917–43.

155. Palao DJ et al. Haloperidol: therapeutic window in schizophrenia. *J Clin Psychopharmacol* 1994;14:303–10.

156. Khot V et al. The assessment and clinical implications of haloperidol acute-dose, steady-state, and withdrawal pharmacokinetics. *J Clin Psychopharmacol* 1993;13:120–7.

157. Pearlman CA. Neuroleptic malignant syndrome: a review of the literature. *J Clin Psychopharmacol* 1986;6:257–73.

158. Gardos G et al. Ten year outcome of tardive dyskinesia. *Am J Psychiatry* 1994;151:836–41.

159. Ereshefsky L et al. Clozapine: an atypical antipsychotic agent. *Clin Pharm* 1989;8:691–709.

160. Lieberman JA et al. Clozapine: guidelines for clinical management. *J Clin Psychiatry* 1989;50:329–38.

161. Meltzer HY. An overview of the mechanism of action of clozapine. *J Clin Psychiatry* 1994;55(suppl 9):47–52.

162. Jann MW et al. Pharmacokinetics and pharmacodynamics of clozapine. *Clin Pharmacokinet* 1993;24:161–76.

163. Alvir JMJ, Lieberman JA. Agranulocytosis: incidence and risk factors. *J Clin Psychiatry* 1994;55(suppl 9):137–8.

164. Lieberman JA et al. Clinical effects of clozapine in chronic schizophrenia: response to treatment and predictors of outcome. *Am J Psychiatry* 1994;151:1744–52.

165. Chouinard G et al. A randomized clinical trial of haloperidol decanoate and fluphenazine decanoate in the outpatient treatment of schizophrenia. *J Clin Psychopharmacol* 1989; 9:247–53.

166. Hemstrom CA et al. Haloperidol decanoate: a depot antipsychotic. *Drug Intell Clin Pharm* 1988;22:290–5.

167. Gerlach J. Oral versus depot administration of neuroleptics in relapse prevention. *Acta Psychiatr Scand* 1994;89(suppl 382):28–32.

168. Inderbitzin LB et al. A double-blind dose-reduction trial of fluphenazine decanoate for chronic, unstable schizophrenic patients. *Am J Psychiatry* 1994;151:1753–9.

169. Ereshefsky L et al. A loading-dose strategy for converting from oral to depot haloperidol. *Hosp Community Psychiatry* 1993;44:1155–61.

170. Colvin CL, Tankanow RM. Pimozide: use in Tourette's syndrome. *Drug Intell Clin Pharm* 1985;19:421–4.

171. Tueth MJ, Cheong JA. Clinical uses of pimozide. *South Med J* 1993;86:344–9.

172. Heykants J et al. The pharmacokinetics of risperidone in humans: a summary. *J Clin Psychiatr* 1994;55:(suppl 5):13–7.

173. Ereshefsky L, Lacomb S. Pharmacological profile of risperidone. *Can J Psychiatry* 1993;38(suppl 3):S80–8.

174. Cohen LJ. Risperidone. *Pharmacotherapy* 1994;14:253–65.

175. Livingston MG. Risperidone. *Lancet* 1994;343:457–60.

176. Marder SR, Meibach RC. Risperidone in the treatment of schizophrenia. *Am J Psychiatry* 1994;151:825–35.

177. Patterson JF. Alprazolam dependency: use of clonazepam for withdrawal. *South Med J* 1988;81:830–2.

178. Scavone JM et al. Alprazolam kinetics following sublingual and oral administration. *J Clin Psychopharmacol* 1987;7:332–4.

179. Kroboth et al. Alprazolam in the elderly: pharmacokinetics and pharmacodynamics during multiple dosing. *Psychopharmacology* 1990;100:477–84.

180. Fawcett JA, Kravitz HM. Alprazolam: pharmacokinetics, clinical efficacy, and mechanism of action. *Pharmacotherapy* 1982;2:243- 54.

181. Jonas JM, Cohon MS. A comparison of the safety and efficacy of alprazolam versus other agents in the treatment of anxiety, panic, and depression: a review of the literature. *J Clin Psychiatry* 1993;54(suppl 10):25–45.

182. Dubovsky SL. Generalized anxiety disorder: new concepts and psychopharmacologic therapies. *J Clin Psychiatry* 1990; 51(suppl 1):3–10.

183. Gorman JM, Papp LA. Chronic anxiety: deciding the length of treatment. *J Clin Psychiatry* 1990;51(suppl 1):11–5.

184. Kranzler HR, Orrok B. The pharmacotherapy of alcoholism. In Tasman A et al., eds. *Review of psychiatry,* vol. 8. Washington DC: American Psychiatric Press; 1989:359–80.

185. Roy-Byrne PP, Cowley DS. *Benzodiazepines in clinical practice: risks and benefits.* Washington DC: American Psychiatric Press; 1991:213–27.

186. Greenblatt DJ et al. Benzodiazepines: a summary of pharmacokinetic properties. *Br J Clin Pharmacol* 1981;11:11S–6.

187. Dietch JT, Jennings RK. Aggressive dyscontrol in patients treated with benzodiazepines. *J Clin Psychiatry* 1988;49:184–8.

188. Jann MW. Buspirone: an update on a unique anxiolytic agent. *Pharmacotherapy* 1988;8:100–16.

189. Sussman N. The uses of buspirone in psychiatry. *J Clin Psychiatry Monogr* 1994;12:3–19.

190. Gammans RE et al. Pharmacokinetics of buspirone in elderly subjects. *J Clin Pharmacol* 1989;29:72–8.

191. Gammans RE et al. Metabolism and disposition of buspirone. *Am J Med* 1986;80(suppl 3B):41–51.

192. Newton RE et al. Review of the side-effect profile of buspirone. *Am J Med* 1986;80(suppl 3B):17–21.

193. Schweizer E, Rickels K. New and emerging clinical uses for buspirone. *J Clin Psychiatry Monogr* 1994;12:46–54.

194. Kales A et al. Comparative effectiveness of nine hypnotic drugs: sleep laboratory studies. *J Clin Pharmacol* 1977;17:207–13.

195. Salmon AG et al. Potential carcinogenicity of chloral hydrate—a review. *J Toxicol Clin Toxicol* 1995;33:115–21.

196. Kanto JH. Midazolam: the first water-soluble benzodiazepine. *Pharmacotherapy* 1985;5:138–55.

197. Anon. Midazolam—is antagonism justified? *Lancet* 1988;1:140–2. Editorial.

198. Bell GD et al. Intravenous midazolam for upper gastrointestinal endoscopy: a study of 800 consecutive cases relating dose to age and sex of patient. *Br J Clin Pharmacol* 1987;23:241–3.

199. Daneshmend TK, Logan RFA. Midazolam. *Lancet* 1988;1:389. Letter.

200. Saint-Maurice C et al. The pharmacokinetics of rectal midazolam for premedication in children. *Anesthesiology* 1986;65:536–8.

201. Yakabowich MR. Hypnotics in the elderly: appropriate usage guidelines. *J Geriatr Drug Ther* 1992;6:5–21.

202. Weiss KJ. Management of anxiety and depression syndromes in the elderly. *J Clin Psychiatry* 1994;55(suppl 2):5–12.

203. Garzone PD, Kroboth PD. Pharmacokinetics of the newer benzodiazepines. *Clin Pharmacokinet* 1989;16:337–64.

204. Robin DW et al. Triazolam in cirrhosis: pharmacokinetics and pharmacodynamics. *Clin Pharmacol Ther* 1993;54:630–7.

205. Scharf MB et al. Comparative amnestic effects of benzodiazepine hypnotic agents. *J Clin Psychiatry* 1988;49:134–7.

206. Roth T et al. Pharmacology and hypnotic efficacy of triazolam. *Pharmacotherapy* 1983;3:137–48.

207. Gillin JC, Byerley W. The diagnosis and management of insomnia. *N Engl J Med* 1990;322:239–48.

208. Treatment of sleep disorders of older people. *NIH Consensus Dev Conf Consens Statement* 1990;8(March):26–8.

209. Scharf MB et al. A multi-center placebo-controlled study evaluating zolpidem in the treatment of chronic insomnia. *J Clin Psychiatry* 1994;55:192–9.

210. Jonas JM et al. Comparative clinical profiles of triazolam versus other shorter-acting hypnotics. *J Clin Psychiatry* 1992;53(suppl 12):19–31.

211. Langtry HD, Benfield P. Zolpidem: a review of its pharmacodynamic and pharmacokinetic properties and therapeutic potential. *Drugs* 1990;40:291–313.

212. Mitler MM. Evaluation of temazepam as a hypnotic. *Pharmacotherapy* 1981;1:3–13.

213. Kales A. Quazepam: hypnotic efficacy and side effects. *Pharmacotherapy* 1990;10:1–12.

214. Scherf MB et al. Estazolam and flurazepam: a multicenter, placebo-controlled comparative study in outpatients with insomnia. *J Clin Pharmacol* 1990;30:461–7.

215. Breimer DD. Clinical pharmacokinetics of hypnotics. *Clin Pharmacokinet* 1977;2:93–109.

216. Post RM, Weiss SRB, Chuang DM. Mechanisms of action of anticonvulsants in affective disorders: comparisons with lithium. *J Clin Psychopharmacol* 1992;12:23S–35S.

217. Baldessarini RJ. Drugs and the treatment of psychiatric disorders. In Hardman JG et al., eds. *Goodman and Gilman's the pharmacological basis of therapeutics*, 9th ed. New York: McGraw-Hill; 1996:431–59.

218. Kook KA et al. Accuracy and safety of a priori lithium loading. *J Clin Psychiatry* 1985;46:49–51.

219. Lobeck F. A review of lithium dosing methods. *Pharmacotherapy* 1988;8:248–55.

220. Gutierrez MA et al. Evaluation of a new steady-state lithium prediction method. *Lithium* 1991;2:57–9.

221. *USP-DI*, Vol I. Rockville, MD. The United States Pharmacopoeal Convention. 1996.

222. Hardy BG et al. Pharmacokinetics of lithium in the elderly. *J Clin Psychopharmacol* 1987;7:153–8.

223. Jefferson JW. Lithium: a therapeutic magic wand. *J Clin Psychiatry* 1989;50:81–6.

224. Jefferson JW. Lithium: the present and the future. *J Clin Psychiatry* 1990;51(suppl 8):4–8.

225. Gitlin MJ et al. Maintenance lithium treatment: side effects and compliance. *J Clin Psychiatry* 1989;50:127–31.

226. Salem RB. Recommendations for monitoring lithium therapy. *Drug Intell Clin Pharm* 1983;17:346–50.

227. Gitlin MJ. Lithium-induced renal insufficiency. *J Clin Psychopharmacol* 1993;13:276–9.

228. Erwin WG, Turco TF. Current concepts in clinical therapeutics: Parkinson's disease. *Clin Pharm* 1986;5:742–53.

229. Aoki FY, Sitar DA. Clinical pharmacokinetics of amantadine hydrochloride. *Clin Pharmacokinet* 1988;14:35–51.

230. Cedarbaum JM. Clinical pharmacokinetics of anti-parkinsonian drugs. *Clin Pharmacokinet* 1987;13:141–78.

231. Hordam VW et al. Pharmacokinetics of amantadine hydrochloride in subjects with normal and impaired renal function. *Ann Intern Med* 1981;94(part 1):454–8.

232. Aoki FY, Sitar DS. Amantadine kinetics in healthy elderly men: implications for influenza prevention. *Clin Pharmacol Ther* 1985;37:137–44.

233. Koller WC. Pharmacologic treatment of parkinsonian tremor. *Arch Neurol* 1986;43:126–7.

234. Brady MT et al. Safety and prophylactic efficacy of low-dose rimantadine in adults during an influenza A epidemic. *Antimicrob Agents Chemother* 1990;34:1633–6.

235. Tominack RL, Hayden FG. Rimantadine hydrochloride and amantadine hydrochloride use in influenza A virus infections. *Infect Dis Clin North Am* 1987;1:459–78.

236. He H et al. Development of a sensitive and specific radioimmunoassay for benztropine. *J Pharm Sci* 1993;82:1027–32.

237. Jenner P. The rationale for the use of dopamine agonists in the treatment of Parkinson's disease. *Neurology* 1995;45(suppl 3):S6–12.

238. Wolters EC et al. Dopamine agonists in Parkinson's disease. *Neurology* 1995;45(suppl 3):S28–34.

239. Anon. Drugs for parkinsonism. *Med Lett Drugs Ther* 1988;30:113–6.

240. Schran HF et al. The pharmacokinetics of bromocriptine in man. In Goldstein M et al., eds. *Ergot compounds and brain function*. New York: Raven Press; 1980:125–39.

241. Friis ML et al. Pharmacokinetics of bromocriptine during continuous oral treatment of Parkinson's disease. *Eur J Clin Pharmacol* 1979;15:275–80.

242. McElvaney NG et al. Pleuropulmonary disease during bromocriptine treatment of Parkinson's disease. *Arch Intern Med* 1988;148:2231–6.

243. Montastruc JL et al. Current status of dopamine agonists in Parkinson's disease management. *Drugs* 1993;46:384–93.

244. Olsson JE et al. Early treatment with a combination of bromocriptine and levodopa compared with levodopa monotherapy in the treatment of Parkinson's disease. *Curr Ther Res* 1989;46:1002–14.

245. Nutt JG et al. The effect of carbidopa on the pharmacokinetics of intravenously administered levodopa: the mechanism of action in the treatment of parkinsonism. *Ann Neurol* 1985;18:537–43.

246. Yeh KC et al. Pharmacokinetics and bioavailability of Sinemet CR: a summary of human studies. *Neurology* 1989;39(suppl 2):S25–38.

247. Bodagh IYO, Robertson DRC. A risk-benefit assessment of drugs used in the management of Parkinson's disease. *Drug Saf* 1994;11:94–103.

248. LeWitt PA. Treatment strategies for extension of levodopa effect. *Neurol Clin* 1992;10:511–26.

249. Juncos JL. Levodopa: pharmacology, pharmacokinetics, and pharmacodynamics. *Neurol Clin* 1992;10: 487–509.

250. Koller WC, Hubble JP. Levodopa therapy in Parkinson's disease. *Neurology* 1990;40(suppl 3):S40–7.

251. Cedarbaum JM. Pharmacokinetic and pharmacodynamic considerations in management of motor response fluctuations in Parkinson's disease. *Neurol Clin* 1990;8:31–49.

252. Hutton JT et al. Multicenter controlled study of Sinemet CR vs Sinemet (25/100) in advanced Parkinson's disease. *Neurology* 1989;39(suppl 2):S67–72.

253. Langtry HD, Clissold SPP. Pergolide. A review of its pharmacological properties and therapeutic potential in Parkinson's disease. *Drugs* 1990;39:491–506.

254. Mizuno Y et al. Pergolide in the treatment of Parkinson's disease. *Neurology* 1995;45(suppl 3):S13–21.

255. Anon. Pergolide and selegiline for Parkinson's disease. *Med Lett Drugs Ther* 1989;31:81–3.

256. Rubin A et al. Physiologic disposition of pergolide. *Clin Pharmacol Ther* 1981;30:258–65.

257. The Parkinson Study Group. Effects of tocopherol and deprenyl on the progression of disability in early Parkinson's disease. *N Engl J Med* 1993;328:176–83.

258. Saint-Hilaire M et al. Deprenyl for the treatment of early Parkinson's disease. *N Engl J Med* 1990;322:1527. Letter.

259. Golbe LI et al. Selegiline and Parkinson's disease. Protective and symptomatic considerations. *Drugs* 1990;39:646–51.

260. Heinonen EH et al. Pharmacokinetics and metabolism of selegiline. *Acta Neurol Scand* 1989;80(suppl 126):93–9.

261. Golbe LI. Long-term efficacy and safety of deprenyl (selegiline) in advanced Parkinson's disease. *Neurology* 1989;39:1109–11.

262. Youdim MBH, Finberg JPM. Pharmacological actions of l-deprenyl (selegiline) and other selective monoamine oxidase B inhibitors. *Clin Pharmacol Ther* 1994;56:725–33.

263. Eldepryl (selegiline hydrochloride) NDA. Data on file, Somerset Pharmaceuticals. Denville, NJ.

264. Fuller MA, Tolbert SR. Selegiline: initial or adjunctive therapy of Parkinson's disease? *DICP* 1991;25:36–40.

265. Lieberman A. Long-term experience with selegiline and levodopa in Parkinson's disease. *Neurology* 1992;(suppl A2):32–6.

266. The Parkinson Study Group. Effect of deprenyl on the progression of disability in early Parkinson's disease. *N Engl J Med* 1989;321:1364–71.

267. Brogden RN, Goa KL. Flumazenil. A preliminary review of its benzodiazepine antagonist properties, intrinsic activity and therapeutic use. *Drugs* 1988;35:448–67.

268. Longmire AW, Seger DL. Topics in clinical pharmacology: flumazenil, a benzodiazepine antagonist. *Am J Med Sci* 1993;306:49–52.

269. Hoffman EJ, Warren EW. Flumazenil: a benzodiazepine antagonist. *Clin Pharm* 1993;12:641–56.

270. Spivey WH. Flumazenil and seizures: analysis of 43 cases. *Clin Ther* 1992;14:292–305.

Gastrointestinal Drugs

ANTACIDS

Pharmacology. Antacids are weakly basic inorganic salts whose primary action is to neutralize gastric acid; pH 4 inhibits the proteolytic activity of pepsin. Aluminum-containing antacids suppress, but do not eradicate, *Helicobacter pylori* and may promote ulcer healing in peptic ulcer disease by enhancing mucosal defense mechanisms.[1,2] Aluminum salts also bind phosphate and bile salts in the GI tract, decreasing serum phosphate and serum bile salt levels. Antacids may increase urine pH.

Administration and Adult Dosage. **PO for symptomatic relief of indigestion, nonulcer dyspepsia, epigastric pain in peptic ulcer disease (PUD) or heartburn in gastroesophageal reflux disease (GERD)** 10–30 mL prn or 1 and 3 hr after meals and hs.[1,2] **PO for treatment of PUD** 100–160 mEq of acid-neutralizing capacity per dose, given 1 and 3 hr after meals and hs for 4–8 weeks or until healing is complete. Additional doses may be taken if epigastric pain persists. There is evidence that lower dosages may heal peptic ulcers.[1,2] **PO or NG for prevention or treatment of upper GI bleeding in critically ill patients** titrate to maintain intragastric pH above 4.0.[2,3] **PO for phosphate binding in renal failure** (aluminum hydroxide) 1.9–4.8 g tid or qid, or (calcium carbonate) 8–12 g/day; titrate dosage based on serum phosphate.[1]

Special Populations. *Pediatric Dosage.* **PO for treatment of PUD or GERD** (≤12 yr) at least 5–15 mL up to q 1 hr; (>12 yr) same as adult dosage.

Geriatric Dosage. Avoid using magnesium-containing antacids in renal impairment.

Other Conditions. Avoid using magnesium-containing antacids in patients with Cl_{cr} <30 mL/min.

Dosage Forms. (*See* Antacid Products Comparison Chart.)

Patient Instructions. If antacids do not relieve symptoms of indigestion, upset stomach, or heartburn within 2 weeks, contact your healthcare provider. When antacids are used to treat symptomatic PUD or GERD, epigastric pain or heartburn may be relieved initially; however, it may be necessary to continue taking antacids for the duration of therapy. Diarrhea may occur with magnesium-containing antacids; decrease the daily dosage, alternate doses with, or switch to, an aluminum- or calcium-containing antacid. Constipation may occur with aluminum-containing antacids; decrease the daily dosage, alternate doses with, or switch to, a magnesium-containing antacid. Refrigerating liquid antacids may improve their palatability. Antacids may interfere with other medications; take other medications 1–2 hours before or after antacids unless otherwise directed. If tablets are used, chew thoroughly before swallowing and follow with a glass of water.

Pharmacokinetics. *Onset and Duration.* Onset of acid neutralizing is immediate; duration is 30 ± 10 min in the fasted state and 1–3 hr if ingested after meals.[1,2]

Fate. Antacid cations are absorbed to varying degrees. Sodium is highly soluble and readily absorbed; calcium absorption is generally less than 30%, but may decrease with increasing age, intake, achlorhydria, and estrogen loss at menopause; magnesium is generally about 30% absorbed, but absorption may vary inversely with intake; aluminum is slightly absorbed. Calcium, magnesium, and aluminum are excreted renally with normal renal function.[1,2,4,5] The unabsorbed portion is excreted in the feces.

Adverse Reactions. Long-term use of sodium- or calcium-containing antacids can cause systemic alkalosis. Hypercalcemia may occur with ingestion of large amounts of calcium; soluble antacids plus a diet high in milk products may result in milk-alkali syndrome, which can lead to nephrolithiasis.[1,2] Magnesium-containing antacids cause a dose-related laxative effect; hypermagnesemia occurs in patients with renal impairment.[1] Aluminum-containing antacids cause dose-related constipation, especially in the elderly. Prolonged administration or large dosages of aluminum hydroxide or carbonate can result in hypophosphatemia, particularly in the elderly and in alcoholics; encephalopathy has been reported in dialysis patients receiving aluminum-containing antacids alone or with sucralfate.[1–3]

Precautions. Use with caution in patients with chronic renal failure, edema, hypertension, or CHF. Because antacids are particulate and elevate intragastric pH, they may predispose critically ill patients to nosocomial pneumonia.[2,3]

Drug Interactions. Antacids reduce the absorption of numerous drugs, the most important of which are digoxin, oral iron (calcium carbonate, sodium bicarbonate, and possibly magnesium trisilicate), isoniazid (aluminum-containing), ketoconazole, oral quinolones, and oral tetracyclines (di- and trivalent cations). Antacids may reduce salicylate levels and increase quinidine levels because of urinary pH changes. Large dosages of calcium antacids may produce hypercalcemia in the presence of thiazides. Sodium polystyrene sulfonate resin can bind magnesium and calcium ions from the antacid in the gut, resulting in systemic alkalosis.

Parameters to Monitor. Monitor for relief of epigastric pain or heartburn and diarrhea or constipation. Monitor serum magnesium levels periodically in patients with renal impairment and serum phosphate during long-term use of aluminum-containing products. Monitor for drug interactions.

Notes. Aggressive antacid therapy is at least as effective as the H_2-receptor antagonists or sucralfate when treating PUD or preventing stress-related mucosal bleeding; however, do not use antacids as first-line agents because high, frequent doses are inconvenient and associated with an increased risk of adverse effects.[1–3] Magaldrate is a chemical mixture of magnesium and aluminum hydroxides. Alginic acid has foaming and floating properties that are of benefit in GERD. Most antacid products have been reformulated to contain low amounts of sodium; some antacid products contain considerable amounts of sugar or artificial sweetener. Antacid tablets, if chewed and swallowed, may be as effective as equivalent doses of liquid formulations. Although gastrin is stimulated by calcium, gastric acid rebound with calcium-containing antacids is of questionable clinical importance.[1]

BISMUTH PREPARATIONS	Pepto-Bismol, Various

Bismuth salts are used to treat nausea, indigestion, diarrhea, gastritis, and peptic ulcers. The precise method by which bismuth heals gastritis and ulcers is uncertain, but possible mechanisms include a local gastroprotective effect, stimulation of endogenous prostaglandins, and antimicrobial activity against *Helicobacter pylori*. When *H. pylori* exists, duodenal and gastric ulcer recurrence rates following short-term treatment with **colloidal bismuth subcitrate** (CBC) or **tripotassium dicitrato bismuthate** (TDB) are lower than those with other ulcer-healing regimens. Given alone, bismuth salts suppress *H. pylori*, but long-term eradication requires combination therapy with antibiotics. **Bismuth subsalicylate** (BSS; Pepto-Bismol, various) is the bismuth salt used most frequently in the United States. Given alone, BSS may not have the same antiulcer effects as CBC or TDB. Following oral administration, BSS (58% bismuth, 42% salicylate) is converted in the GI tract to bismuth oxide and salicylic acid. Bismuth is less than 0.2% absorbed, with more than 99% of an oral dose excreted in the feces. Over 90% of the salicylate dose is absorbed and excreted in urine. Bacterially produced hydrogen sulfide in the mouth and colon convert bismuth oxide to bismuth sulfide, which imparts a gray-black color to the tongue and stool. Use BSS with caution in children, in the elderly, in patients with renal impairment, salicylate sensitivity, or bleeding disorders, in those receiving high-dosage salicylate therapy, or when potentially interacting medications are taken. Salicylic acid is less likely than aspirin to cause gastric mucosal damage and blood loss. Prolonged BSS therapy and the use of other salts (subgallate and subnitrate) have been associated with neurotoxicity. Bismuth subsalicylate 525 mg (305 mg elemental bismuth) PO qid is used in adults for the control of nausea, abdominal cramps, and diarrhea. Do not exceed a BSS dosage of 4.2 g/day. When given with antibiotics to eradicate *H. pylori*, BSS treatment is usually limited to 1–2 weeks.[1,2,6,7] Bismuth subsalicylate is available as 17.5 and 35 mg/mL suspensions, and 262-mg chewable tablets. Ranitidine bismuth citrate (Tritec) tablets 400 mg contain ranitidine 150 mg and bismuth citrate 240 mg/tablet. (*See also* Treatment of *Helicobacter pylori* in Peptic Ulcer Disease Comparison Chart.)

HISTAMINE H₂-RECEPTOR ANTAGONISTS:	
CIMETIDINE	Tagamet, Various
FAMOTIDINE	Pepcid
NIZATIDINE	Axid
RANITIDINE	Zantac

Pharmacology. Histamine H_2-receptor antagonists competitively inhibit the action of histamine at the H_2 receptors of the parietal cell and reduce basal, nocturnal, pentagastrin-, and food-stimulated gastric acid.

ANTACID PRODUCTS COMPARISON CHART[a]

ANTACID	ACID NEUTRALIZING CAPACITY		SODIUM CONTENT			
	mEq/5 mL	mEq/Tablet	mEq/5 mL	mg/5 mL	mEq/Tablet	mg/Tablet
Aluminum Carbonate, Basic						
Basalgel	11.5	12.5 (Cap/Tab)	0.13	3	0.12	2.8
Aluminum Hydroxide						
ALternaGEL	16	—	0.109	<2.5	—	—
Amphojel	10	8 (300-mg Tab) 16 (600-mg Tab)	0.10	<2.3	0.08 0.13	1.8 3
Aluminum Hydroxide with Magnesium Carbonate						
Gaviscon[b]	3.3–4.3	—	0.57	13	—	—
Gaviscon Extra Strength[b]	14.3	5–7.5	0.9	20.7	1.3	29.9
Maalox Heartburn Relief[b]	8.5	7.4	0.11	2.5	0.13	3
Aluminum Hydroxide with Magnesium Hydroxide						
Maalox	13.3	9.7 (Original) 10.7 (Regular)	0.04	1	0.04 0.03	1 0.8
Maalox Therapeutic Concentrate	27.2	—	0.03	0.8	—	—
Aluminum Hydroxide with Magnesium Hydroxide and Simethicone						
Di-Gel	9	—	0.07	1.5	—	—
Gelusil	—	11	—	—	<0.22	<5
Maalox Plus[d]	—	10.7	—	—	0.04	<1
Maalox Plus,[d] Extra Strength	29.1	18.6	0.04	<1	0.07	<1.7
Mylanta	12.7	11.5	0.03	0.68	0.03	0.77
Mylanta Double Strength	25.4	23	0.05	1.14	0.06	1.3

(continued)

409

ANTACID PRODUCTS COMPARISON CHART[a] (continued)

ANTACID	ACID NEUTRALIZING CAPACITY		SODIUM CONTENT			
	mEq/5 mL	mEq/Tablet	mEq/5 mL	mg/5 mL	mEq/Tablet	mg/Tablet
Aluminum Hydroxide with Magnesium Trisilicate and Sodium Bicarbonate						
Gaviscon[b]	—	0.5	—	—	0.8	18.4
Gaviscon-2[b]	—	1	—	—	1.6	36.8
Calcium Carbonate						
Di-Gel[c]	—	10	—	—	0.05	1.25
Titralac	—	8.5	—	—	0.01	0.3
Titralac Extra Strength	—	15.1	—	—	0.03	0.6
Titralac Plus[d]	11	8.5	0.01	0.25	0.04	1
Tums	—	10	—	—	0.09	2
Tums E-X	—	15	—	—	0.13	3
Tums ULTRA	—	20	—	—	0.17	4
Magaldrate						
Riopan	15	13.5	0.013	0.3	0.004	0.1
Riopan Plus[d]	15	13.5	0.013	0.3	0.004	0.1
Riopan Plus Double Strength[d]	30	30	0.013	0.3	0.022	0.5

[a]The product brands listed are representative of numerous brand and generic products on the market. Product formulations, and hence neutralizing capacity and sodium content, are subject to change by the manufacturer.
[b]Contains alginate.
[c]Tablet contains calcium carbonate, magnesium hydroxide, and simethicone.
[d]Contains simethicone.

	CIMETIDINE	FAMOTIDINE	NIZATIDINE	RANITIDINE
Ring Structure	Imidazole	Thiazole	Thiazole	Furan
Relative Potency	1	20–50	4–10	4–10

Administration and Adult Dosage.

INDICATION	CIMETIDINE	FAMOTIDINE	NIZATIDINE	RANITIDINE
PO for symptomatic relief of heartburn or indigestion (OTC)	200 mg/day or 200 mg bid.	10 mg/day or 10 mg bid.	75 mg/day or 75 mg bid.[a]	75 mg/day or 75 mg bid[a]
PO for short-term treatment of duodenal ulcer (4–8 weeks)	300 mg qid, 400 mg bid, 800 mg hs, or 1600 mg hs.[b]	20 mg bid or 40 mg hs.	150 mg bid or 300 mg hs.	150 mg bid or 300 mg hs.
PO for maintenance of healing of duodenal ulcer	400 mg hs.	20 mg hs.	150 mg hs.	150 mg hs.
PO for short-term treatment of active benign gastric ulcer (6–8 weeks)	300 mg qid or 800 mg hs.	20 mg bid[a] or 40 mg hs.	150 mg bid or 300 mg hs.	150 mg bid or 300 mg hs.[a]
PO for maintenance of healing of gastric ulcer	400 mg hs.[a]	20 mg hs.[a]	150 mg hs.[a]	150 mg hs.
PO for symptomatic gastroesophageal reflux disease (6–12 weeks)	300 mg qid[a] or 400 mg bid.[a]	20 mg bid.	150 mg bid.	150 mg bid.
PO for healing of erosive esophagitis (6–12 weeks)	400 mg qid or 800 mg bid.	20 or 40 mg bid.	150 mg bid[a] or 300 mg bid.[a]	150 mg qid or 300 mg bid.[a]
PO for maintenance of healing of erosive esophagitis	300 mg qid,[a] 400 mg qid,[a] or 800 mg bid.[a]	20 mg bid[a] or 40 mg bid.[a]	150 mg bid or 300 mg bid.[a]	150 or 300 mg bid.[a]
PO for pathological hypersecretory conditions	300 mg qid, up to 2.4 g/day; or adjust to patient needs.	20 mg q 6 hr, up to 160 mg q 6 hr; or adjust to patient needs.	a	150 mg bid, up to 6 g/day; or adjust to patient needs.

(*continued*)

INDICATION	CIMETIDINE	FAMOTIDINE	NIZATIDINE	RANITIDINE
IM	300 mg q 6–8 hr.[c]	d	d	50 mg q 6–8 hr.[c]
IV Intermittent	300 q 6–8 hr, up to 2.4 g/day.[c]	20 mg q 12 hr.[c]	d	50 mg q 6–8 hr, up to 400 mg/day.[c]
IV Intermittent Bolus	Dilute to 20 mL; inject over not less than 5 min.[c]	Dilute to 5–10 mL; inject over not less than 2 min.[c]	d	Dilute to 20 mL; inject over not less than 5 min.[c]
IV Intermittent Infusion	Dilute to 50 mL; infuse over 15–20 min.[c]	Dilute to 100 mL; infuse over 15–30 min.[c]	d	Dilute to 100 mL; infuse over 15–20 min.[c]
IV Continuous Infusion	37.5 mg/hr (900 mg/day); adjust to patient needs; up to 600 mg/hr has been given.[c,e]	1.67 mg/hr[a] (40 mg/day); adjust to patient needs.[c,e]	d	6.25 mg/hr (150 mg/day), adjust to patient needs; up to 220 mg/hr has been given.[c,e]

IV for prevention of upper GI bleeding in critically ill patients (cimetidine) 50 mg/hr by continuous infusion;[e] (cimetidine, famotidine, or ranitidine) use standard dosages given by intermittent or continuous infusion.[a,e] In high-risk surgical patients, adjust the dose and/or frequency of intermittent IV therapy or the rate of continuous infusion to maintain the intragastric pH above 4.0.

[a]Nonlabeled indication and dosage.
[b]Heavy smokers with ulcer larger than 1 cm in diameter.
[c]Pathologic hypersecretory states, intractable ulcers, or patients unable to take oral medication.
[d]Nonlabeled route of administration.
[e]Loading dose may be given, but appears to offer little advantage.
From references 2, 3, and 8–12.

Special Populations. *Pediatric Dosage.* Safety and efficacy not well established.

	CIMETIDINE	FAMOTIDINE	NIZATIDINE	RANITIDINE
Neonates	10–20 mg/kg/day.	Unknown.	Unknown.	Unknown.
Children (3–16 yr)	20–40 mg/kg/day.	0.4–1.6 mg/kg/day.	Unknown.	1–3 mg/kg/day.

From references 8 and 13–15.

Geriatric Dosage. Reduce dosage based upon renal function.

Other Conditions.

	CIMETIDINE	FAMOTIDINE	NIZATIDINE	RANITIDINE
Renal Impairment*	Cl_{cr} 15–30 mL/min: 600 mg/day; <15 mL/min: 300–400 mg/day.	Cl_{cr} under 10 mL/min: 20 mg/day or 20 mg every other day.	Cl_{cr} 20–50 mL/min: 150 mg/day; <20 mL/min: 150 mg every other day.	Cl_{cr} <50 mL/min: PO 150 mg/day or IM/IV 50 mg q 12–24 hr.

*Use the lowest dosage that permits an adequate response; further dosage reduction of cimetidine, famotidine, or ranitidine may be necessary with concomitant severe liver disease. Because only small amounts of H_2-receptor antagonists are removed by hemodialysis and peritoneal dialysis, additional doses may not be necessary; adjust dosage schedule so that the time of the scheduled dose coincides with the end of dialysis.
From references 8, 10, and 16.

Dosage Forms.

	CIMETIDINE	FAMOTIDINE	NIZATIDINE	RANITIDINE
	Tab 100, 200, 300, 400, 800 mg.	Tab 10, 20, 40 mg.	Cap 150, 300 mg.	Tab 150, 300 mg Tab (chewable) 150 mg Tab (effervescent) 150 mg* Granules (effervescent) 150 mg* Cap 150, 300 mg
	Soln 60 mg/mL Inj 150 mg/mL.	Susp 8 mg/mL† Inj 10 mg/mL.‡		Syrup 15 mg/mL Inj 25 mg/mL.

*Dissolve dose in approximately 180–240 mL (6–8 fl oz) of water before drinking.
†Discard reconstituted suspension after 30 days.
‡Store at 2–8°C (36–46°F).

Patient Instructions. The effectiveness of H_2-receptor antagonists in peptic ulcer disease may be decreased by cigarette smoking. Discontinue or decrease smoking, or avoid smoking after the last dose of the day. Antacids may be used as needed for relief of epigastric pain. Even though symptoms may improve, continue treatment for the duration of therapy unless instructed otherwise.

Pharmacokinetics.

	CIMETIDINE	FAMOTIDINE	NIZATIDINE	RANITIDINE
Onset.				
All agents have an oral onset of 1 hr and an IV onset of 15 min.				
Serum Levels.				
EC_{50}*	625 ± 375 µg/L	11 ± 2 µg/L	167 ± 13 µg/L	112 ± 52 µg/L
Fate.				
Oral Bio-availability	60 ± 20%	41 ± 4%	95 ± 5%; 75% in renal failure.	55 ± 25%
V_d	1 ± 0.2 L/kg	1.2 ± 0.3 L/kg	1.4 ± 0.2 L/kg	1.6 ± 0.4 L/kg
Protein Binding	20 ± 6%	16%	30 ± 5%	15%
Excreted Unchanged in Urine	75%	70 ± 5%	70 ± 5%	70%
$t_{1/2}$.				
Normal	1.9 ± 0.4 hr	3 ± 0.5 hr	1.4 ± 0.2 hr	2 ± 0.4 hr
Anuric	4.5 ± 0.5 hr	20+ hr	7.2 ± 1.3 hr	7 ± 3 hr

*EC_{50} is the serum concentration necessary to inhibit pentagastrin-stimulated secretion of acid by 50%.
From references 2, 8, 10, and 16–18.

Adverse Reactions. Adverse reactions are generally mild. The most frequent adverse events occur in 1–7% of patients and include headache, diarrhea, constipation, dizziness, drowsiness, and fatigue.[2,8,10,19] Reversible confusional states, depression, agitation, and other CNS manifestations may occur occasionally with all H2-receptor antagonists, predominantly in severely ill patients or those with renal and/or hepatic disease.[2,3,8,19] Reversible dose-dependent increases in ALT have been reported with IV cimetidine and IV ranitidine. Rare cases of fatal hepatic disease with and without jaundice have been reported with cimetidine and ranitidine.[8,19] H2-receptor antagonists do not markedly decrease hepatic blood flow.[8,19] Cardiac arrhythmias, tachycardia, and hypotension may occur following rapid IV bolus administration of cimetidine or ranitidine; bradycardia has been reported with both IV and oral administration of cimetidine and ranitidine. Although a negative inotropic effect has been noted following oral administration of famotidine in healthy subjects and patients with CHF, refined hemodynamic monitoring has failed to demonstrate a clinically important effect;[8,19] IV famotidine has been given safely to patients undergoing cardiac surgery.[20] Hematologic reactions occur occasionally with all H2-receptor antagonists and include leukopenia, neutropenia, thrombocytopenia, and pancytopenia; agranulocytosis and aplastic anemia occur rarely.[2,8,19] Gynecomastia develops in less than 1% of all men receiving cimetidine, but in 4% of men treated for pathologic hypersecretory states. Dose-dependent increases in serum prolactin concentrations have been reported with cimetidine and ranitidine.[8] Hyperuricemia has been reported with nizatidine. All

H_2-receptor antagonists may cause a mild, but reversible, increase in fasting serum gastrin.[21] The effects of H_2-receptor antagonist therapy on gastric emptying are unclear.

Precautions. Pregnancy; lactation. Dosage adjustment may be required in severe renal and/or hepatic failure. Symptomatic response to therapy does not preclude the possibility of gastric malignancy.

Drug Interactions. Cimetidine inhibits hepatic CYP1A2, CYP2C8–10, CYP2D6, and CYP3A3–5; ranitidine inhibits CYP2D6 and CYP3A3–5 to a much lesser extent. Clinically important interactions with drugs metabolized by these isoenzymes may occur (the most important of which are carbamazepine, chlordiazepoxide, clozapine, diazepam, glipizide, lidocaine, phenytoin, propranolol, theophylline, tolbutamide, tricyclic antidepressants, quinidine, tacrine, and warfarin). Hepatic micosomal enzyme interactions with cimetidine are dose dependent.[19,22] Controversy remains about interactions with ranitidine, although in general they seem less likely and less severe than with cimetidine.[8,19,22] Cimetidine may inhibit the elimination of certain drugs secreted by renal tubules (eg, procainamide).[19,22] Nizatidine has been reported to increase serum salicylate concentrations in patients on high aspirin doses (3.9 g/day). Cimetidine, ranitidine, and nizatidine (but not famotidine) inhibit gastric mucosal alcohol dehydrogenase; the clinical importance of this interaction is uncertain. Elevations in gastric pH could alter the rate or extent of absorption of ketoconazole, itraconazole, and other drugs whose dissolution and absorption are pH dependent.[19,22]

Parameters to Monitor. Improvement in epigastric pain or heartburn. However, pain relief in peptic ulcer disease (PUD) and gastroesophageal reflux disease (GERD) does not correlate directly with endoscopic evidence of healing. Monitor Cr_s, CBC, AST, ALT, and CNS status periodically. In patients receiving IV doses of cimetidine ($\geq$2.4 g/day) or ranitidine ($\geq$400 mg/day), it is advisable to monitor serum transaminases routinely throughout the duration of IV therapy. When the drug is used to prevent upper GI bleeding in critically ill patients, measure the intragastric pH periodically. Monitor for potential drug and alcohol interactions.

Notes. In general, the H_2-receptor antagonists are similar in efficacy when conventional dosages are prescribed for the treatment of gastric and duodenal ulcer and for maintenance of healing of duodenal ulcer. Ulcer healing rates are similar to **sucralfate** or aggressive **antacid** therapy.[2,9,10] The H_2-receptor antagonists are often used in combination with a number of antibiotics to eradicate *Helicobacter pylori* in peptic ulcer disease (*see* Treatment of *Helicobacter pylori* in Peptic Ulcer Disease). Usual dosages of H_2-receptor antagonists are less effective than **misoprostol** in preventing NSAID-induced gastric ulcer. However, high-dose H_2-receptor antagonists may be as effective as misoprostol in preventing NSAID-induced gastric and duodenal ulcers[23] and they appear effective in preventing NSAID-induced duodenal ulcer and in healing NSAID-induced gastric and duodenal ulcers.[2,24] Although all H_2-receptor antagonists provide symptomatic relief and esophageal healing, higher dosages are required in patients with moderate to severe esophagitis than those used in patients with mild GERD symptoms.[9,25] Intermittent administration or continuous infusion of IV cimetidine, ranitidine, or famotidine is more effective than placebo in preventing upper GI bleeding in critically ill patients.[2,3,11] The maintenance of intragastric pH above 4.0 does not conclusively prevent upper GI bleeding.[3,11] Although it is easier to maintain the intragastric pH above 4.0 by continuous infusion, the superiority of continuous infusion of the H_2-receptor antagonists in preventing upper GI bleeding in the critically ill has not been established; both intermittent administration and continuous infusion are at least as effective as **sucralfate** or aggressive **antacid** therapy.[2,3,11] Combination of an H_2-receptor antagonist with sucralfate provides two different mechanisms of drug action and may be of possible benefit. However, enhanced efficacy of two drugs compared to single-drug therapy has not been substantiated in controlled trials in patients with duodenal ulcer, gastric ulcer, or GERD, or when used to prevent or treat upper GI bleeding or NSAID-induced ulcers.[2,3] Coadministration of an H_2-receptor antagonist with a proton pump inhibitor is without established benefit and may compromise the action of the proton pump inhibitor.[2] Controlled trials have not demonstrated that H_2-receptor antagonists are of benefit in patients with active upper GI bleeding.[2,8] The relationship of H_2-receptor antagonist therapy to the development of nosocomial pneumonia in critically ill patients is inconclusive.[2,3,11] Cimetidine may augment cell-mediated immunity by blockade of H_2 receptors on suppressor T-lymphocytes; it remains difficult to determine whether this effect is clinically useful or whether it is potentially dangerous, especially following organ transplantation and in autoimmune disorders.[19] Although it is not certain whether this immune system action is class specific or drug specific, it appears to be related to the cimetidine molecule. All H_2-receptor antagonists are stable in D5W, D10W, NS, LR, TPN, or 5% sodium bicarbonate for 48 hr at room temperature.

LANSOPRAZOLE   Prevacid

Lansoprazole is an H^+/K^+-ATPase inhibitor structurally, pharmacologically, and pharmacokinetically similar to omeprazole. Lansoprazole has uses similar to those of omeprazole; combination therapy with antibiotics (eg, amoxicillin, clarithromycin, and/or metronidazole) eradicates *Helicobacter pylori* and heals peptic ulcers; however, the optimal drug treatment regimen has not been determined. The short- and long-term safety of lansoprazole appears to be similar to that of omeprazole. Although lansoprazole selectively inhibits hepatic CYP2C, there have been no reports of clinically important interactions with warfarin, phenytoin, diazepam, propranolol, theophylline, or prednisone in healthy subjects. Lansoprazole elimination is prolonged in patients with severe hepatic disease, but not in severe renal impairment. Consider dosage reduction in severe hepatic disease. Although the clearance of lansoprazole is slightly prolonged in older patients, dosage reduction does not appear necessary. The adult oral dosage for healing duodenal and gastric ulcer is 15 mg/day before a meal for 4 weeks. The recommended dosage for the treatment of erosive esophagitis is 30 mg/day for up to 8 weeks. An additional 8 weeks of therapy may be required for patients whose esophagitis does not heal. Lansoprazole 15 mg/day provides ulcer healing rates and symptomatic relief that are similar to those provided by omeprazole 20 mg/day. In most patients, lansoprazole 30 mg/day heals erosive esophagitis and relieves GERD symptoms similarly to omeprazole 20 mg/day. Lansoprazole

30–60 mg/day generally heals peptic ulcer disease and gastroesophageal reflux disease refractory to H_2-receptor antagonists. Lansoprazole 15 mg/day prevents recurrence of duodenal ulcer, and a dosage of 15 mg/day is used as maintenance therapy of erosive esophagitis. In patients with Zollinger-Ellison syndrome, lansoprazole 15–180 mg/day appears to be as effective as omeprazole 20–160 mg/day.[26,27] Available as 30-mg capsules containing EC granules. Granules may be sprinkled on applesauce and swallowed immediately without chewing. (*See* Treatment of *Helicobacter pylori* in Peptic Ulcer Disease).

OMEPRAZOLE   Prilosec

Pharmacology. Omeprazole is an inactive drug that, when protonated in the secretory canaliculus of the parietal cell, covalently binds to H^+/K^+-ATPase. It produces a profound and prolonged antisecretory effect, and inhibits basal and stimulated gastric acid secretion by irreversibly blocking the proton pump at the terminal stage of acid secretion. Serum gastrin levels increase during treatment but return to pretreatment levels within 1–2 weeks of discontinuing therapy.

Administration and Adult Dosage. **PO for erosive esophagitis or poorly responsive symptomatic gastroesophageal reflux disease (GERD)** 20 mg/day for 4–8 weeks. In patients not responding to 8 weeks of treatment, treat for an additional 4 weeks or increase the dosage to 40 mg/day and treat for as long as clinically necessary. **PO for maintenance of healing of erosive esophagitis** 20 mg/day.[25,28–30] **PO for short-term treatment of duodenal ulcer** 20 mg/day for 4 weeks; some patients may require 4 additional weeks. **PO for short-term treatment of active benign gastric ulcer** 40 mg/day for 4–8 weeks.[2,28–30] **PO for treatment of refractory duodenal or gastric ulcer** 40–80 mg/day.[28–30] When used as a single agent in peptic ulcer disease, omeprazole is usually given in the morning before breakfast; the optimal administration time for patients with erosive esophagitis should be based on the patient's symptoms. **PO for maintenance of healing of duodenal or gastric ulcer** 10–20 mg/day or 20 mg on alternate days or weekend days (Friday, Saturday, and Sunday).[2,28–30] **PO for pathological hypersecretory conditions** 60 mg/day initially, increasing prn; up to 120 mg tid has been administered to patients with severe Zollinger-Ellison syndrome (ZES);[28–31] give dosages over 80 mg/day as divided doses. Some patients with ZES have been treated continuously for up to 8 yr.[28] *See* Notes.

Special Populations. *Pediatric Dosage.* Safety and efficacy not established.

Geriatric Dosage. Dosage reduction is usually unnecessary; reduce dosage only if not well tolerated.[28]

Other Conditions. Dosage reduction is unnecessary in renal impairment, but should be considered in chronic hepatic disease and in Asian patients.

Dosage Forms. **Cap** (EC granules) 20 mg.

Patient Instructions. Swallow capsules whole and take the drug before meals. Do not open, chew, or crush the capsule. Antacids may be used as needed for relief of epigastric pain or heartburn. The effectiveness of omeprazole in peptic ulcer disease may be decreased by cigarette smoking. Even though symptoms may decrease, continue treatment for the duration of therapy unless instructed otherwise.

Pharmacokinetics. *Onset and Duration.* (Antisecretory effect) PO onset within 1 hr; duration with doses of 20 mg is up to 72 hr. Gastric acid inhibition increases with repeated daily doses, reaching a plateau after 4 days. Gastric secretory activity gradually returns to pretreatment levels 3–5 days after discontinuation; rebound hypersecretion does not occur.[30]

Serum Levels. Antisecretory effect correlates with AUC rather than serum levels.[30] Inhibition of gastric acid secretion continues after serum drug concentrations have decreased below the limit of detection, apparently caused by prolonged drug binding to parietal cell H^+/K^+-ATPase.[28,30]

Fate. Absorption of omeprazole from enteric-coated granules begins only after granules leave the stomach. Oral absorption is rapid, with peak serum levels occurring within 2 ± 1.5 hr. Bioavailability is $35 \pm 5\%$ with doses of 20–40 mg and may increase slightly with repeated administration and more extensively in the elderly or in chronic hepatic impairment. Peak serum concentrations and AUC are dose dependent up to 40 mg, but because of a saturable first-pass effect, a greater response occurs with higher doses. In single-dose studies, Asians had an AUC about 4 times as great as Caucasians. Protein binding of omeprazole is about 95%. Three inactive metabolites (hydroxyomeprazole and the sulfide and sulfone derivatives of omeprazole) have been identified in plasma. Following oral administration, 77% is eliminated as metabolites in urine; the remainder is recovered in the feces as metabolites. Little drug is excreted unchanged in urine.

$t_{1/2}$. 0.75 ± 0.25 hr in healthy young adults; 1 hr in healthy elderly; 3 hr in chronic hepatic disease.

Adverse Reactions. Headache, dizziness, nausea, diarrhea, constipation, and skin rash occur frequently.[19,28,30] Fatigue, malaise, muscle cramps, joint pain, myalgia, anxiety, and taste perversion occur occasionally. Rarely interstitial nephritis, gynecomastia, thrombocytopenia, hemolytic anemia, severe skin reactions (eg, Stevens-Johnson syndrome), and psychic disturbances have been reported. Rare cases (some fatal) of overt hepatic failure, liver necrosis, pancreatitis, and agranulocytosis have occurred.[28,30] Rarely, gastric polyposis occurs in patients receiving 20–40 mg of omeprazole for 12 months or longer.[29] Long-term omeprazole use may reduce the absorption of protein-bound vitamin B_{12}.[21] Long-term studies indicate that the adverse effects are similar to the H_2-receptor antagonists. Atrophic gastritis has been observed during long-term omeprazole use. Adverse effects in patients over 65 yr are similar to those in younger patients.

Precautions. Pregnancy, because of sporadic reports of congenital abnormalities. Symptomatic response to therapy does not preclude the possibility of gastric malignancy.

Drug Interactions. Omeprazole interacts selectively with hepatic CYP2C and may inhibit the metabolism of drugs, such as some benzodiazepines (eg, diazepam), carbamazepine, cyclosporine, phenytoin, and (R)-warfarin, but not lidocaine, propranolol, quinidine, or theophylline.[19,28,32] Elevations in gastric pH could alter the rate or extent of absorption of ampicillin esters, digoxin, itraconazole, iron salts, ketoconazole, and other drugs or dosage forms that are pH dependent.[19,25,28–30] Omeprazole induces CYP1A, which could theoretically potentiate the hepatotoxicity of acetaminophen or increase the cancer risk in smokers.[2,19,28] Omeprazole may inhibit the renal elimination of methotrexate.

Parameters to Monitor. Improvement in epigastric pain or heartburn; however, pain relief in peptic ulcer disease and GERD does not correlate directly with endoscopic evidence of healing. Monitor for potential drug interactions and adverse effects. Assess the indication, dosage, and duration of omeprazole therapy, especially the need for treatment beyond 12 weeks. Consider monitoring serum vitamin B_{12} concentration every several years in patients on long-term omeprazole therapy.

Notes. Omeprazole is the drug of choice in erosive esophagitis and Zollinger-Ellison syndrome.[2,25–31] Omeprazole 20 mg/day produces more rapid relief of symptoms and duodenal ulcer healing than standard dosages of **H₂-receptor antagonists;** however, the longer treatment is continued, the smaller the difference.[2,28–30] Gastric ulcer healing rates are generally similar to those with standard doses of the H₂-receptor antagonists.[2,28–30] Patients with gastric or duodenal ulcers or esophagitis refractory to H₂-antagonists are likely to respond to omeprazole, but the rate of recurrence following discontinuation is similar.[2,25,28–30] Omeprazole appears to be effective in preventing **NSAID**-induced gastroduodenal injury, but well-controlled comparisons with **misoprostol** are lacking; stronger evidence exists for the use of omeprazole 20–40 mg/day to heal duodenal or gastric ulcer during continued NSAID therapy.[2,28–30] *See* Treatment of *Helicobacter pylori* in Peptic Ulcer Disease.

Omeprazole is formulated in pH-sensitive granules that release the drug at a pH above 6.[28–30,33] Crushing the granules destroys the protective coating and decreases the drug's bioavailability; however, the capsule may be opened and the granules administered through a nasogastric tube or mixed with acidic juices.[28,29,33] Coadministration of omeprazole with an **H₂-receptor antagonist** or **sucralfate** is without established benefit; the action of omeprazole may be compromised if administered with an H₂-receptor antagonist or **octreotide.**[2]

SUCRALFATE Carafate, Various

Pharmacology. Sucralfate is an aluminum hydroxide salt of a sulfated disaccharide. Its exact mechanism of action is not known; however, it forms an ulcer-adherent complex with proteinaceous exudates at the ulcer site, thereby protecting against further attack by acid, pepsin, and bile salts. Adherence to the ulcer crater is enhanced at a pH below 3.5. Sucralfate inhibits pepsin activity; a 1-g dose has approximately 14–16 mEq of acid-neutralizing capacity. The aluminum moiety stimulates endogenous prostaglandins and binds bile salts and phosphate in the GI tract.[2,34,35]

Administration and Adult Dosage. **PO for short-term treatment of duodenal ulcer** 1 g qid on an empty stomach, 1 hr before meals and at bedtime or 2 g bid for 4–8 weeks.[2,34,35] **PO for maintenance of healing of duodenal ulcer** 1 g bid. **PO for short-term treatment of active benign gastric ulcer** 1 g qid.[2,34,35] **PO for treatment of symptomatic gastroesophageal reflux disease (GERD) or erosive esophagitis** 1 g qid.[34,35] **PO or NG for prevention of upper GI bleeding in criti-**

cally ill patients 1 g q 4–6 hr.[2,11,34–36] **PO or NG for phosphate binding in renal failure** titrate dosage based on serum phosphate.[2,34]

Special Populations. *Pediatric Dosage.* Safety and efficacy not well established. **PO** 500 mg bid has been used.[37]

Geriatric Dosage. Dosage reduction usually not necessary.

Dosage Forms. Tab 1 g; **Susp** 100 mg/mL.

Patient Instructions. Take this drug with water on an empty stomach, 1 hour before each meal and at bedtime. Antacids may be used as needed for pain relief, but do not take them within 30 minutes before or after sucralfate. Take potentially interacting drugs 2 hours before sucralfate in order to avoid or minimize drug interactions. Even though symptoms may decrease, continue treatment for the duration of therapy unless instructed otherwise.

Pharmacokinetics. *Onset and Duration.* Onset (attachment of sucralfate to ulcer site) is within 1 hr; duration is about 6 hr.

Fate. Sucralfate is only minimally absorbed from the GI tract and is excreted primarily in the feces. About 3–5% (primarily aluminum) is absorbed and excreted in urine.[2,34] Aluminum excretion is decreased in uremia.[2]

Adverse Reactions. Adverse reactions are usually minor and occur in about 5% of patients. Constipation occurs in about 2% of patients. Other effects, including diarrhea, nausea, gastric discomfort, indigestion, dry mouth, rash, pruritus, backache, dizziness, drowsiness, vertigo, and a metallic taste occur occasionally.[2,34,35] Aluminum accumulation and toxicity, including osteodystrophy, osteomalacia, encephalopathy, and seizures, have been reported in patients with chronic renal failure.[2,34] Hypophosphatemia may develop in critically ill patients and those on prolonged sucralfate therapy.[2,34] Bezoar formation has been reported.[34]

Precautions. Use with caution in patients receiving other aluminum-containing drugs or in chronic renal failure and dialysis.

Drug Interactions. Sucralfate may inhibit the absorption of drugs including digoxin, ketoconazole, levothyroxine, phenytoin, quinidine, oral quinolones, tetracyclines, theophylline, and warfarin.[22] In most cases, these interactions can be avoided if the drug is given 2 hr before sucralfate administration.

Parameters to Monitor. Improvement in epigastric pain or heartburn; however, pain relief in peptic ulcer disease and GERD does not correlate directly with endoscopic evidence of healing. Observe for constipation and signs of aluminum toxicity in the elderly, in chronic renal failure, or in patients receiving other aluminum-containing drugs. Obtain serum phosphate periodically in patients receiving concurrent aluminum-containing drugs or with prolonged use. Monitor for potential drug interactions.

Notes. Sucralfate is as effective as standard doses of the **H$_2$-receptor antagonists** in the short-term treatment and maintenance of duodenal ulcer.[2,34,35] Sucralfate may overcome the negative effect of cigarette smoking on duodenal ulcer healing and recurrence.[34] Its efficacy in healing erosive esophagitis and in maintenance of esophageal healing is generally inferior to the H$_2$-receptor antagonists or proton pump inhibitors. Sucralfate is effective in preventing **NSAID**-induced duodenal ulcer and stress-related mucosal bleeding.[2,3,11,23,24,34,36] Its efficacy as a single agent in preventing NSAID-induced gastric ulcer, chemotherapy-induced stomatitis, and stress-related bleeding in high-risk critically ill surgical patients requires further documentation.[2,3,11,22-24,34,35] Whether sucralfate is associated with a lower frequency of nosocomial pneumonia in critically ill patients than H_2-receptor antagonists is inconclusive.[2,3,11,34,36] The value of topical sucralfate after sclerotherapy or in treating proctitis, inflammatory bowel disease, or decubitus ulcers is questionable.[34] Although therapy with sucralfate and an **H_2-receptor antagonist** or **proton pump inhibitor** provides two different mechanisms of drug action, enhanced efficacy of two drugs has not been substantiated for any indication.[2,3,34,35] (*See also* Antacids.)

MISOPROSTOL   Cytotec

Misoprostol is a synthetic prostaglandin E_1 analogue that inhibits gastric acid secretion and enhances gastric mucosal defense. Antisecretory effects are dose dependent with single doses of 50–200 µg; cytoprotective effects occur with single doses of 200 µg or more. Misoprostol also produces uterine contractions that may endanger pregnancy. After oral administration, misoprostol is extensively absorbed and rapidly deesterified to the active drug, misoprostol acid. Peak serum concentrations of misoprostol acid are reduced when the drug is taken with food. Plasma protein binding of misoprostol acid is less than 90%. Misoprostol acid undergoes further metabolism, but about 80% is excreted unchanged in urine. In most trials in patients who were receiving long-term NSAID therapy for rheumatoid arthritis, misoprostol 200 µg qid was superior to the **H_2-receptor antagonists** or **sucralfate** in preventing NSAID-induced gastric and duodenal ulcers; however, misoprostol does not relieve GI pain or discomfort associated with NSAID use. Recent evidence suggests that misoprostol reduces the frequency of NSAID-induced complications, including GI perforation, obstruction, and bleeding, but its cost-effectiveness remains controversial. Abdominal pain is reported in 13–20% of patients on NSAIDs receiving misoprostol 800 µg/day, but there is no consistent difference from placebo. Antacids (except those containing magnesium) may be used for abdominal pain relief. Diarrhea is reported to occur within 2 weeks of initiating therapy in 14–40% of patients on NSAIDs receiving 800 µg/day and less frequently with 400–600 µg/day. Diarrhea is usually self-limiting and resolves in about 1 week with continued treatment; rarely, profound diarrhea occurs in patients with inflammatory bowel disease. Nausea, flatulence, headache, dyspepsia, vomiting, and constipation occur occasionally. Women who receive misoprostol occasionally develop gynecologic disorders including cramps or vaginal bleeding. Misoprostol is contraindicated in pregnancy because of the risk of abortion. Women of childbearing potential should have a negative serum pregnancy test within 2 weeks prior to beginning therapy, should begin treatment on the second or third day of the next menstrual period, should comply with effective contraceptive measures, and should receive both oral and written warnings of the hazards of misoprostol therapy and the risk of contraceptive failure. Warn patients not to give misoprostol to others. Misoprostol does not affect the hepatic cytochrome P450 microsomal enzyme system, nor does it interfere with the beneficial effects of

NSAIDs in rheumatoid arthritis. Misoprostol, 200 μg bid or tid, offers substantial protection against gastric and duodenal ulcers in patients at high risk of developing NSAID-induced ulcers and complications. These regimens appear to be similar in efficacy and are better tolerated than the initially approved dosage of 200 μg qid. The gastric ulcer protective effect of misoprostol appears to plateau between 200 μg bid and 200 μg tid, but no dose-response effect is apparent in preventing duodenal ulcers. Take misoprostol with meals and for the duration of NSAID therapy. Dosage reduction is not required in renal impairment or hepatic failure, or in the elderly. A dosage of 200 μg qid or 400 μg bid for 4–8 weeks is as effective as H_2-receptor antagonists in the treatment of duodenal ulcer; but its efficacy in healing gastric ulcer is not as well established.[23,38–41] Available as 100- and 200-μg tablets.

TREATMENT OF *HELICOBACTER PYLORI* IN PEPTIC ULCER DISEASE

Virtually all patients with gastric or duodenal ulcers who are not taking an NSAID have evidence of *H. pylori* infection and antral gastritis. An epidemiologic association between *H. pylori* and gastric cancer exists, but a causal relationship is uncertain. Drug regimens to eradicate *H. pylori* infections are considered first-line therapy for *H. pylori*–associated gastric and duodenal ulcers. Eradication of *H. pylori* heals ulcers, reduces recurrence to less than 10%, and is more cost-beneficial than conventional antiulcer treatments. Conventional antiulcer drugs, bismuth salts, and antibiotics are generally ineffective as single agents in eradicating *H. pylori*. The discrepancy between high in vitro and low in vivo antibiotic efficacy may be caused by degradation of the antibiotic in gastric acid, insufficient penetration through gastric mucus, or microbial resistance. *H. pylori* resistance has been reported with nitroimidazoles (eg, metronidazole), macrolides, and fluoroquinolones. The value of *H. pylori* eradication to treat nonulcer dyspepsia or to prevent gastric cancer remains controversial.

Although the optimal regimen to eradicate *H. pylori* and cure peptic ulcer disease has not been established, a number of antibiotic combinations are effective. An antisecretory drug is often added to achieve more rapid relief of ulcer symptoms and ulcer healing, although omeprazole use immediately before treatment has been reported to decrease the efficacy of the omeprazole-amoxicillin regimen. If initial treatment fails, consider a different antibiotic regimen. Do not use antibiotics for longer than 2 weeks.

Erythromycin may be substituted for amoxicillin in penicillin-allergic patients. Do not substitute azithromycin for clarithromycin or metronidazole. Do not substitute doxycycline for tetracycline, nor ampicillin for amoxicillin. Although lansoprazole-antibiotic regimens appear to provide eradication rates similar to omeprazole-antibiotic regimens, data are limited as to their equivalence for this use.

Regimens of bismuth, metronidazole, and either tetracycline or amoxicillin plus an antisecretory agent are associated with up to 30% diarrhea, occasional antibiotic-associated colitis, and other drug-specific adverse effects. Noncompliance with drug regimens is an important problem and increases with the number of drugs used, higher dosages, and longer duration of therapy. Selection of an initial treatment regimen should take into consideration factors such as efficacy, compliance, adverse effects, drug resistance, and cost.[27,42–52]

TREATMENT OF *HELICOBACTER PYLORI* INFECTION IN PEPTIC ULCER DISEASE[a]

DRUG	ADMINISTRATION AND ADULT DOSAGE	DURATION OF THERAPY	SUCCESS RATE (%)
BISMUTH-CONTAINING REGIMENS			
Bismuth subsalicylate	525 mg qid	2 weeks	>90 (with tetracycline)
Tetracycline or amoxicillin	500 mg qid	2 weeks	or 80 (with amoxicillin)
Metronidazole	250–500 mg tid or qid	2 weeks	
H₂-receptor antagonist	Standard dosage[b]	4–6 weeks	
Bismuth subsalicylate	525 mg qid	2 weeks	85–95
Tetracycline or amoxicillin	500 mg qid	2 weeks	
Clarithromycin	500 mg tid	2 weeks	
H₂-receptor antagonist	Standard dosage[b]	4–6 weeks	
Bismuth subsalicylate	525 mg qid	1 week	>95
Tetracycline or amoxicillin	500 mg qid	1 week	
Metronidazole	500 mg qid	1 week	
Omeprazole	20 mg bid[c]	1–4 weeks	
Clarithromycin[d]	500 mg tid	2 weeks	70–90
Ranitidine bismuth citrate[d]	400 mg bid	4 weeks	
BISMUTH-FREE REGIMENS			
Amoxicillin	750 mg tid	12–14 days	>90
Metronidazole	500 mg tid	12–14 days	
H₂-receptor antagonist	Standard dosage[b]	6–10 weeks	
Clarithromycin[d]	500 mg tid	2 weeks	70–90
Omeprazole[d]	20 mg bid[c]	2 weeks	
Amoxicillin[e]	500 mg qid or 1 g bid	2 weeks	30–90
Omeprazole	40 mg/day	4 weeks	
	20 mg/day	2 weeks	
Metronidazole	500 mg bid	1 week	>95
Clarithromycin	250–500 mg bid	1 week	
Omeprazole	20 mg bid[c]	1 week	
Clarithromycin	250–500 mg bid	1 week	85–90
Amoxicillin	1 g bid–tid	1 week	
Omeprazole[c]	20 mg bid	1 week	
Metronidazole	250–500 mg qid	1 week	>95
Amoxicillin	1 g bid or tid	1 week	
Omeprazole	20 mg bid[c]	1 week	

[a]All drug regimens are oral and begin concurrently.
[b]Standard ulcer-healing dosage (not maintenance dosage). Standard ulcer-healing dosage regimen of a proton pump inhibitor may be substituted for the histamine H₂-receptor antagonist.
[c]Omeprazole daily dosage may be reduced by one-half after completion of antibiotic(s). Equivalent antisecretory dosage of lansoprazole may be substituted for omeprazole.[27]
[d]FDA-approved indication.
[e]No longer advocated in the United States because eradication rate varies widely.
From references 27 and 42–51.

Antiemetics

DRONABINOL   Marinol

Pharmacology. Dronabinol (delta-9-tetrahydrocannabinol [THC]) is the most active antinauseant component of *Cannabis*. Its mechanism of action as an antiemetic is complex and poorly understood, but probably includes inhibition of the chemoreceptor trigger zone in the medulla.

Administration and Adult Dosage. **PO as an antiemetic** 5 mg/m^2 1–3 hr before chemotherapy, then q 2–4 hr after chemotherapy for a total of 4–6 doses/day. Dosage may be increased in 2.5 mg/m^2 increments, to a maximum of 15 mg/m^2/dose. **PO for appetite stimulation** 2.5 mg before lunch and dinner.

Special Populations. *Pediatric Dosage.* **PO as an antiemetic during cancer chemotherapy** same as adult dosage in mg/m^2.

Geriatric Dosage. Same as adult dosage.

Dosage Forms. **Cap** 2.5, 5, 10 mg.

Patient Instructions. This drug may cause drowsiness. Until the extent of this effect is known, use caution when driving, operating machinery, or performing other tasks requiring mental alertness. Avoid excessive concurrent use of alcohol or other drugs that cause drowsiness.

Pharmacokinetics. *Onset and Duration.* Oral onset 30–60 min; peak 2–4 hr; duration is 4–6 hr, but may be longer in those who have not previously used the drug.[53,54]

Fate. Bioavailability is 4–12% orally, 2–50% by smoking. About 95% plasma protein bound. V_d is 8.9 ± 4.2 L/kg; Cl is 0.21 ± 0.054 L/hr/kg. Primarily metabolized by hydroxylation to active and inactive metabolites. Ultimately, 35% of metabolites are found in feces and 15% in urine, with less than 1% excreted unchanged in urine.[55-57]

t½. Terminal phase 32 ± 12 hr, although time course of effects more closely parallels initial distribution phase.[55]

Adverse Reactions. Drowsiness occurs frequently. It may be accompanied by dizziness, ataxia, loss of balance, and disorientation to the point of being disabling. Other frequent side effects include dry mouth, orthostatic hypotension, and conjunctival injection.[58] The cannabis "high" experienced by some is not always well tolerated, especially by older patients.[59]

Contraindications. Allergy to dronabinol, marijuana, or sesame oil.

Precautions. Avoid during lactation. Use with caution in patients with hypertension or heart disease.

Drug Interactions. Not well studied, but some apparent interactions have been reported following marijuana use. These include additive or supraadditive sedation with alcohol and other CNS depressants; additive hypertension and/or tachycardia with anticholinergics, antihistamines, sympathomimetics, or TCAs; and hypomania with disulfiram or fluoxetine.

Parameters to Monitor. Observe for frequency of emesis, drowsiness, or disorientation.

Notes. Dronabinol is at least as effective as **phenothiazines** for chemotherapy-induced nausea and vomiting,[60] but is not as effective as **serotonin antagonists** or IV **metoclopramide.**[61] It is not particularly effective for cisplatin-induced nausea and vomiting. It may not be as effective as smoking cannabis, which is easier to titrate. (*See* Antiemetic Drugs Comparison Chart.)

GRANISETRON   Kytril

Granisetron is a selective antagonist at the 5-HT$_3$ (serotonin-S$_3$) receptor used for the prevention of nausea and vomiting associated with cancer chemotherapy. Its use in cancer chemotherapy is similar to that of ondansetron, and its efficacy and side effects are comparable to those of ondansetron. Oral absorption is approximately 60%; V$_d$ is 30 $\pm$ 1.5 L/kg; Cl is 0.060 $\pm$ 0.54 L/hr/kg; and half-life is 5.3 $\pm$ 3.5 hr (may be longer in cancer patients than in normals). Elimination is mostly by hepatic metabolism, with 16 $\pm$ 14% appearing in the urine as unchanged drug. The metabolism of ondansetron may be changed by inducers or inhibitors of the cytochrome P450 system, but dosage adjustment is not recommended. The IV dose for nausea and vomiting caused by cancer chemotherapy for adults and children >2 yr is 10 μg/kg administered in 20–50 mL NS or D5W over 5 min, 30 min before the start of chemotherapy. The oral dosage for adults is 1 mg up to 1 hr before chemotherapy and additional 1-mg doses at 12-hr intervals thereafter while receiving chemotherapy. Available as 1 mg/mL injection and 1-mg tablets.[62–64] (*See* Antiemetic Drugs Comparison Chart.)

ONDANSETRON HYDROCHLORIDE   Zofran

Pharmacology. Ondansetron is a selective antagonist at the 5-HT$_3$ (serotonin-S$_3$) receptor used for the prevention of nausea and vomiting associated with cancer chemotherapy, especially cisplatin, and for postoperative nausea and vomiting. It may also be useful for radiation-induced nausea and vomiting. It is not a dopamine receptor antagonist, so it has no extrapyramidal side effects. (*See* Notes.)

Administration and Adult Dosage. **IV for chemotherapy-induced nausea or vomiting** 0.15 mg/kg for 3 doses (30 min before chemotherapy, then 4 and 8 hr after) or 0.45 mg/kg, to a maximum of 32 mg as a single dose.[64] Infuse slowly over 15 min in 50 mL D5W or NS. **IV bolus for postoperative nausea or vomiting** 4 mg over 2–5 min before induction or postoperatively. **PO for chemotherapy- or radiotherapy-induced nausea or vomiting** 8 mg q 8 hr. **PO for postoperative nausea or vomiting** 16 mg 1 hr before surgery.

Special Populations. *Pediatric Dosage.* **IV for chemotherapy-induced nausea or vomiting** (<4 yr) safety and efficacy not established; (4–18 yr) same as adult dosage. **PO for chemotherapy-induced nausea and vomiting** (4–12 yr) 4 mg q 8 hr.

Geriatric Dosage. Same as adult dosage.

Other Conditions. In hepatic function impairment, do not exceed a single oral dose of 8 mg or a total daily IV dosage of 8 mg.

Dosage Forms. **Inj** 2 mg/mL; **Tab** 4, 8 mg; **Soln** 1.25 mg/mL.

Pharmacokinetics. *Fate.* Oral absorption is 62 ± 15%.[55] V_d is 1.9 ± 0.5 L/kg; Cl is 0.35 ± 0.16 L/hr/kg in adults and may be higher in children.[55,62] The drug is extensively metabolized to glucuronide and sulfate conjugates.[63] About 5% appears in urine as unchanged ondansetron.[55]

$t_{1/2}$. 2.8 ± 0.6 hr in normal adults;[62] about 5 hr in the elderly.[63]

Adverse Reactions. Headache, dizziness, and sedation occur frequently. Transient increased serum levels of hepatic enzymes also occur frequently, but these are probably caused by chemotherapy rather than by ondansetron.[64-67]

Contraindications. None known.

Precautions. Pregnancy; lactation; suspected ileus.

Drug Interactions. The metabolism of ondansetron may be changed by inducers or inhibitors of the cytochrome P450 system, but dosage adjustment is not recommended.

Parameters to Monitor. Frequency of vomiting.

Notes. Protect vials from light; inspect for discoloration and particulate matter before using. Ondansetron appears to be more effective than **metoclopramide** for cisplatin-induced vomiting, without the risk of extrapyramidal reactions.[68,69] **Dexamethasone** enhances the antiemetic effect of ondansetron (*see* Dexamethasone). (*See* Antiemetic Drugs Comparison Chart.)

PROCHLORPERAZINE SALTS   Compazine, Various

Pharmacology. Prochlorperazine is a phenothiazine tranquilizer having antidopaminergic and weak anticholinergic activity. It suppresses the chemoreceptor trigger zone in the CNS and is used mainly for its antiemetic properties. It is not effective for the treatment of motion sickness or vertigo.

Administration and Adult Dosage. **PO as an antiemetic** 5–10 mg tid or qid; **PR as an antiemetic** 25 mg bid; **IM as an antiemetic** (deep in upper outer quadrant of buttock) 5–10 mg q 4–6 hr, to a maximum of 40 mg/day. **IM presurgically** (deep in upper outer quadrant of buttock) 5–10 mg 1–2 hr before induction, may repeat once before or after surgery; **IV presurgically** 2.5–10 mg 15–30 min before induction or as infusion (20 mg/L) started 15–30 min before induction. **SC not recommended.**

Special Populations. *Pediatric Dosage.* Not to be used in surgery, or in patients <9 kg or 2 yr. **PO or PR as an antiemetic** (9–13 kg) 2.5 mg daily–bid; (14–18 kg) 2.5 mg bid–tid; (19–39 kg) 2.5 mg tid–5 mg bid. **IM as an antiemetic** (deep in upper outer quadrant of buttock) 0.13 mg/kg. **SC not recommended.**

Geriatric Dosage. Use the lower end of the recommended dosage range in elderly patients.

Dosage Forms. **Inj** 5 mg/mL; **Supp** 2.5, 5, 25 mg; **Syrup** 1 mg/mL; **Tab** 5, 10, 25 mg. Larger dose tablets are available for psychiatric use. **SR Cap** not recommended.

Patient Instructions. This drug may cause drowsiness. Until the extent of this effect is known, use caution when driving, operating machinery, or performing other tasks requiring mental alertness. Avoid excessive concurrent use of alcohol or other drugs that cause drowsiness.

Pharmacokinetics. *Onset and Duration.* PO onset 30–40 min; PR onset 60 min; IM onset 10–20 min. Duration for all routes 3–4 hr.

Fate. The drug is well absorbed, but extensive and variable presystemic metabolism in the gut wall and liver limits bioavailability. Primarily eliminated by hepatic metabolism and biliary excretion.

$t_{1/2}$. 23 hr.[70]

Adverse Reactions. Extrapyramidal reactions, especially dystonias and dyskinesias, occur occasionally in adults and frequently in children (other extrapyramidal reactions are less likely because of the short duration of therapy when used as an antiemetic). Anticholinergic effects such as dry mouth, mydriasis, cycloplegia, urinary retention, decreased GI motility, and tachycardia occur occasionally. SC administration can cause local reactions at injection site.

Contraindications. Pediatric surgery; children <9 kg or 2 yr; comatose or greatly depressed state caused by CNS depressants.

Precautions. Antiemetic action may mask signs and symptoms of overdose with other drugs and may mask the diagnosis and treatment of other conditions such as intestinal obstruction, brain tumor, or Reye's syndrome. Use with caution in conditions in which the drug's anticholinergic effects might be detrimental, in children with acute illnesses or dehydration, or in patients with a history of allergy to phenothiazine derivatives (eg, blood dyscrasias, jaundice). Avoid getting the concentrate or injectable solutions on hands or clothing because of the possibility of contact dermatitis.

Drug Interactions. Phenothiazines may decrease the efficacy of guanethidine or guanadrel or may have additive hypotensive effects with hypotensive drugs. Phenothiazines may inhibit the antiparkinson activity of levodopa.

Parameters to Monitor. Observe for extrapyramidal side effects and drug efficacy.

Notes. Protect the solution from light; a slight yellowish discoloration does not indicate altered potency, but markedly discolored solution should be discarded. Protect suppositories from heat. (*See* Antiemetic Drugs Comparison Chart.)

ANTIEMETIC DRUGS COMPARISON CHART

DRUG	DOSAGE FORMS	INITIAL DOSE[a] Adult	INITIAL DOSE[a] Pediatric	Nausea and Vomiting	Motion Sickness	Vertigo
ANTIHISTAMINES						
Buclizine Bucladin-S	Chew Tab 50 mg.	PO 50 mg.	—		X	
Cyclizine Marezine	Tab 50 mg Inj 50 mg/mL.	PO, IM 50 mg.	PO (6–12 yr) 25 mg.		X	
Dimenhydrinate Dramamine Various	Cap 50 mg Tab 50 mg Chew Tab 50 mg Liquid 3.1 mg/mL Inj 50 mg/mL.	PO 50–100 mg IM, IV 50 mg.	PO (2–6 yr) 12.5–25 mg. (6–12 yr) 25–50 mg IM (>2 yr) 1.25 mg/kg.		X	X
Diphenhydramine Benadryl Various	Cap 25, 50 mg Tab 25, 50 mg Elxr 2.5 mg/mL Syrup 2.5 mg/mL Inj 10, 50 mg/mL.	PO 50 mg IM, IV 10–50 mg.	PO (>9 kg) 12.5–25 mg IM, IV (> 9 kg) 1.25 mg/kg.		X	
Meclizine Antivert Bonine Various	Cap 25, 30 mg Tab 12.5, 25, 50 mg Chew Tab 25 mg.	PO 25–50 mg.	—		X	b
CANNABINOIDS						
Dronabinol Marinol	Cap 2.5, 5, 10 mg.	PO 5 mg/m².	PO 5 mg/m².	X		

(continued)

ANTIEMETIC DRUGS COMPARISON CHART (continued)

		INITIAL DOSE[a]			INDICATIONS	
				Nausea and	Motion	
DRUG	DOSAGE FORMS	Adult	Pediatric	Vomiting	Sickness	Vertigo

PHENOTHIAZINES

Chlorpromazine
Thorazine
Various
- Tab 10, 25, 50 mg
- Liquid 30, 100 mg/mL
- Syrup 2 mg/mL
- Supp 25, 100 mg
- Inj 25 mg/mL.

Adult: PO 10–25 mg; PR 100 mg; IM 25 mg.
Pediatric: PO, IM (> 6 months) 0.55 mg/kg; PR (> 6 months) 1.1 mg/kg.
Nausea and Vomiting: X

Perphenazine
Trilafon
- Tab 2, 4, 8, 16 mg
- Liquid 3.2 mg/mL
- Inj 5 mg/mL.

Adult: PO 2–4 mg; IM 5 mg.
Pediatric: —
Nausea and Vomiting: X

Prochlorperazine
Compazine
Various
- Tab 5, 10, 25 mg
- Syrup 1 mg/mL
- Supp 2.5, 5, 25 mg
- Inj 5 mg/mL.

Adult: PO, IM 5–10 mg; IV 2.5–10 mg; PR 25 mg.
Pediatric: PO, PR (>9 kg or 2 yr) 2.5 mg; IM (>9 kg or 2 yr) 0.13 mg/kg.
Nausea and Vomiting: X

Promethazine
Phenergan
Various
- Syrup 1.25, 5 mg/mL
- Tab 12.5, 25, 50 mg
- Supp 12.5, 25, 50 mg
- Inj 25, 50 mg/mL.

Adult: PO, PR 25 mg; IM, IV 12.5–25 mg.
Pediatric: PO, PR, IM (>2 yr) 0.25–0.5 mg/kg.
Nausea and Vomiting: X
Motion Sickness: X

Thiethylperazine
Norzine
Torecan
- Tab 10 mg
- Supp 10 mg
- Inj 5 mg/mL.

Adult: PO, PR, IM 10 mg.
Pediatric: —
Nausea and Vomiting: X

(continued)

429

ANTIEMETIC DRUGS COMPARISON CHART (continued)

| | | INITIAL DOSE[a] | | INDICATIONS | | |
DRUG	DOSAGE FORMS	Adult	Pediatric	Nausea and Vomiting	Motion Sickness	Vertigo
Trifluoperazine Vesprin	Inj 10, 20 mg/mL.	IM 5–15 mg IM (elderly) 2.5 mg IV 1 mg.	IM (>2.5 yr) 0.2–0.25 mg/kg.	X		
SEROTONIN 5-HT₃ ANTAGONISTS						
Granisetron Kytril	Tab 1 mg Inj 1 mg/mL.	PO 1 mg IV 10 µg/kg.	IV (>2 yr) 10 µg/kg.	X		
Ondansetron Zofran	Tab 4, 8 mg Inj 2 mg/mL.	PO 8 or 16 mg IV 0.15 mg/kg.	PO (>4 yr) 4 mg IV (>4 yr) 0.15 mg/kg.	X		
MISCELLANEOUS						
Benzquinamide Emete-Con	Inj 50 mg/mL.	IM 50 mg IV 25 mg.	—	X		
Dexamethasone Decadron Various	Tab 0.25, 0.5, 0.75, 1, 1.5, 2 mg Inj 4, 10, 20, 24 mg/mL.	PO 10–20 mg IV 10–20 mg.	—	c		
Droperidol Inapsine	Inj 2.5 mg/mL.	IM, IV 2.5 mg.	—	d		
Lorazepam Ativan Various	Tab 0.5, 1, 2 mg Soln 2, 4 mg/mL.	PO 1–2 mg.	PO 0.05 mg/kg.	c		

(continued)

ANTIEMETIC DRUGS COMPARISON CHART (continued)

DRUG	DOSAGE FORMS	INITIAL DOSE[a] Adult	INITIAL DOSE[a] Pediatric	INDICATIONS Nausea and Vomiting	INDICATIONS Motion Sickness	INDICATIONS Vertigo
Methylprednisolone Solu-Medrol Various	Inj 40, 125, 500 mg.	IV up to 100 mg.	IV 2–4 mg/kg.	c		
Metoclopramide Reglan	Inj 5 mg/mL.	IV 1–2 mg/kg.	IV 1–2 mg/kg.	X		
Trimethobenzamide Tigan Various	Cap 100, 250 mg Supp 100, 200 mg Inj 100 mg/mL.	PO 250 mg PR 200 mg IM 200 mg.	PO (14–40 kg) 100–200 mg PR (<14 kg) 100 mg, (14–40 kg) 100–200 mg.	X		

aInitial dose only; check prescribing information for subsequent dosage.

bPossibly effective.

cNot labeled for this use; used as adjunctive for cancer chemotherapy-induced nausea and vomiting.

dEffective, but not labeled for this use.

Gastrointestinal Motility

BISACODYL

Pharmacology. Bisacodyl is a stimulant cathartic structurally similar to phenolphthalein that produces its effect by direct contact with colonic mucosa. It may stimulate water and electrolyte secretion in the colon.[71]

Administration and Adult Dosage. PO as a laxative/cathartic 10–30 mg; **PR** 10 mg. Adjust dosage based on response.

Special Populations. *Pediatric Dosage.* **PO** (>6 yr) 5–10 mg or 0.3 mg/kg hs or before breakfast; **PR** (<2 yr) 5 mg; (>2 yr) 10 mg.

Geriatric Dosage. Same as adult dosage.

Dosage Forms. EC Tab 5 mg; **Enema** (adult) 10 mg; **Supp** 10 mg.

Patient Instructions. Swallow tablets whole (not chewed or crushed) and do not take within 1 hour of antacids or dairy products. Do not use oral products in children <6 years of age.

Pharmacokinetics. *Onset and Duration.* Onset PO 6–12 hr; PR 15 min–1 hr.[72,73]

Fate. Absorption is less than 5% by oral or rectal route with subsequent conversion to the glucuronide salt and excretion in urine and bile. Rapidly converted in the gut by intestinal and bacterial enzymes to its active, but nonabsorbed, desacetyl metabolite.[74]

Adverse Reactions. Abdominal cramps occur frequently; with long-term use, metabolic acidosis or alkalosis, hypocalcemia, tetany, loss of enteric protein, and malabsorption occur occasionally; suppositories can cause proctitis and rectal inflammation.

Drug Interactions. Antacids or milk can dissolve the enteric coating of oral bisacodyl tablets, causing drug release in the stomach and gastric irritation.

Contraindications. Acute surgical abdomen; nausea, vomiting, or other symptoms of appendicitis; fecal impaction; intestinal or biliary tract obstruction; abdominal pain of unknown origin.

Notes. Useful for preoperative or preradiographic bowel preparation.[71,72] Bisacodyl has been used in combination with PEG electrolyte lavage solution to decrease the amount of solution required.[71,75] (*See* PEG Electrolyte Lavage Solution.)

CISAPRIDE

Pharmacology. Cisapride is a prokinetic drug chemically related to metoclopramide. It acts primarily by facilitating the release of acetylcholine from postganglionic nerve endings of the myenteric plexus in GI smooth muscle and appears to be a serotonin $5HT_3$-receptor antagonist and a serotonin $5HT_4$-receptor agonist. Unlike metoclopramide, cisapride does not have direct cholinergic, antidopaminergic, or antiemetic effects and has no effect on serum prolactin or gastric secretion. Cisapride increases lower esophageal sphincter pressure and, unlike metoclopramide, it stimulates motility in all portions of the GI tract, including the esophagus and large intestine. It has no effect on normal gastric function and does not override normal homeostatic mechanisms.[76–78]

Administration and Adult Dosage. **PO for the treatment of symptomatic nocturnal heartburn or esophagitis related to gastroesophageal reflux disease (GERD)** 10 mg qid 15 min before meals and hs; may be increased to 20 mg qid if needed;[76–78] **PO for maintenance of healing of esophagitis related to GERD** 10–20 mg bid (before breakfast and hs) depending on initial severity of esophagitis or 20 mg hs;[76] **PO for functional dyspepsia or chronic constipation** 5–10 mg tid; **PO for symptomatic gastroparesis** 10 mg tid-qid.[76–78]

Special Populations. *Pediatric Dosage.* (<18 yr) safety and efficacy not established. **PO** (infants and children) 0.15–0.3 mg/kg tid or qid has been used.[76–78]

Geriatric Dosage. Same as adult dosage.

Other Conditions. In severe hepatic failure, reduce the daily dosage by 50% initially.[77] Dosage reduction in severe renal impairment does not appear necessary; however, some investigators recommend a 50% dosage reduction because of the accumulation of cisapride and/or norcisapride.[76,77] Administration of an extra dose after hemodialysis does not appear necessary.[79]

Dosage Forms. **Tab** 10, 20 mg; **Susp** 1 mg/mL.

Patient Instructions. Take this drug at least 15 minutes before meals. Cisapride may initially cause diarrhea or abdominal cramping, which usually disappears with continued use. Until the degree of drowsiness is known, use caution when driving, operating machinery, or performing other tasks that require mental alertness. Concomitant use of cisapride and alcohol has been shown to increase blood alcohol concentrations.[76,78] Other drugs that cause drowsiness, anticoagulants, or drugs that affect gastrointestinal motility (eg, antidepressants, antihistamines, anticholinergics) may interact with cisapride; report any unusual symptoms.

Pharmacokinetics. *Onset and Duration.* PO onset 45 ± 15 min.

Fate. Oral bioavailability is 37.5 ± 2.5% because of first-pass metabolism in the liver and/or gut. Food increases the bioavailability, but not the rate of absorption.[77] Cisapride is 98% plasma protein bound, primarily to albumin.[77] V_d is about 2.4 L/kg;[76] Cl is 6 L/hr. Cisapride is extensively metabolized by CYP3A4, primarily to norcisapride, which is about one-sixth as active as the parent drug.[77,79] Less than 1% of cisapride is excreted unchanged in urine.[79] Norcisapride is eliminated renally and appears to accumulate in severe renal failure.[74,79] Steady-state serum concentrations are higher in the elderly because of a moderate prolongation of the half-life of cisapride and/or norcisapride.

$t_{1/2}$. 8.5 ± 1.5 hr in healthy subjects, prolonged in patients with severe hepatic failure, but not substantially increased in renal impairment.[76,78]

Adverse Reactions. Diarrhea, abdominal pain, constipation, flatulence, and rhinitis occur frequently and appear to be dose related. Diarrhea and abdominal cramping tend to subside after several days of continuous therapy.[77] Headache, fatigue, depression, and dizziness occur frequently and are not dose related. Urinary disorders, including incontinence, frequency, hesitancy, retention, and cystitis, are also reported frequently.[80] Seizures have been reported in patients with a prior history of seizures who were treated with cisapride, but a causal relationship has not been established. Extrapyramidal reactions and sinus tachycardia (with relapse upon rechallenge in some cases) occur rarely.

Contraindications. Mechanical obstruction; GI hemorrhage, perforation or other situations in which an increase in GI motility could be harmful; concurrent use of clarithromycin, erythromycin, fluconazole, ketoconazole, itraconazole, IV miconazole, or troleandomycin.

Precautions. Pregnancy; lactation.

Drug Interactions. Sedative effects of benzodiazepines and of alcohol may be exaggerated by cisapride. Acceleration of gastric emptying may affect the rate of absorption (increase or decrease) of other orally administered drugs. In some patients receiving oral anticoagulants, cisapride may result in prolonged coagulation times. Drugs that inhibit hepatic CYP3A4 may markedly increase the serum cisapride concentration and lead to a prolongation of the QT interval, resulting in ventricular arrhythmias, including torsades de pointes and even death (*see* Contraindications).

Parameters to Monitor. Symptomatic relief of GERD, dyspepsia, chronic constipation, or gastroparesis. Monitor for adverse effects, especially diarrhea and abdominal cramping. Monitor for potential drug interactions. Serum concentrations of drugs with a narrow therapeutic index may require reassessment after initiation and discontinuation of cisapride therapy. In patients receiving oral anticoagulants, measure the PT/INR within the first few days of the start or discontinuation of cisapride.

Notes. The combination of cisapride with an **H$_2$-receptor antagonist** may improve esophageal healing and symptomatic response in severe erosive esophagitis.[76] In some studies, cisapride remained an effective gastrokinetic for up to 3 yr of treatment.[76] When cisapride is used to treat constipation, optimal effects may require 2–3 months of therapy. Unlike **metoclopramide,** cisapride has relatively few CNS side effects associated with its use.[76]

DIPHENOXYLATE HYDROCHLORIDE AND ATROPINE SULFATE

Lomotil, Various

Pharmacology. Diphenoxylate is a synthetic meperidine congener lacking analgesic activity that slows GI motility; atropine is added in subtherapeutic amounts to decrease abuse potential.

Administration and Adult Dosage. PO for diarrhea 2 tablets or 10 mL qid initially, then, if control is achieved (usually within 48 hr), decrease to a maintenance dosage as low as 2 tablets or 10 mL daily prn. If chronic diarrhea is not controlled in 10 days at the full dosage, then symptoms are unlikely to be controlled by further administration.

Special Populations. *Pediatric Dosage.* **Use liquid only.** Not recommended <2 yr. **PO for diarrhea** 0.3–0.4 mg/kg/day of diphenoxylate in 4 divided doses initially, not to exceed adult dosage. Reduce dosage once diarrhea is controlled.

Geriatric Dosage. Same as adult dosage.

Dosage Forms. Syrup 500 μg diphenoxylate and 5 μg atropine/mL; **Tab** 2.5 mg diphenoxylate and 25 μg atropine.

Patient Instructions. This drug may cause dry mouth, blurred vision, drowsiness, or dizziness; use caution while driving or performing other tasks requiring alertness, coordination, or physical dexterity. Avoid alcohol and other CNS depressants. Seek medical attention if diarrhea persists or if fever, palpitations, or abdominal distention occurs.

Pharmacokinetics. *Onset and Duration.* Onset 45–60 min; duration 3–4 hr.

Fate. Diphenoxylate is well absorbed from the GI tract and metabolized to an active metabolite, diphenoxylic acid. Both drug and metabolite attain peak serum levels in 2 hr. Diphenoxylate V_d is 3.8 ± 1.1 L/kg; Cl is 1.04 ± 0.14 L/hr/kg.[81] Conjugates of the drug and metabolite are excreted primarily in the urine.

$t_{1/2}$. (Diphenoxylate) 2.5 ± 0.6 hr; (diphenoxylic acid) 7.2 ± 0.7 hr.[82]

Adverse Reactions. Anticholinergic symptoms such as dry mouth, urinary retention, blurred vision, fever, or tachycardia may occur frequently with high daily dosages, or occasionally with usual dosages in children.[83] Drowsiness, dizziness, and headache occur occasionally.

Contraindications. Children <2 yr; obstructive jaundice; diarrhea associated with pseudomembranous enterocolitis or enterotoxin-producing bacteria. *See* Notes.

Precautions. Use with caution in children because of variable response and potential for toxicity (atropinism) with recommended dosages (particularly in Down's syndrome patients), and in patients with acute ulcerative colitis, hepatic dysfunction, or cirrhosis (*see* Notes).

Drug Interactions. Because of its chemical similarity to meperidine, avoid diphenoxylate use with MAOIs. Use with caution in combination with CNS depressants.

Parameters to Monitor. Frequency and volume of bowel movements; body temperature. Observe for signs of atropine toxicity. Monitor for abdominal distention.

Notes. In chronic diarrhea, diphenoxylate 5 mg is about equipotent with **loperamide** 2 mg or **codeine** 30–45 mg. It may provide temporary symptomatic relief of infectious traveler's diarrhea if used cautiously with an antibiotic, but discontinue it if fever occurs, symptoms persist beyond 48 hr, or blood or mucus appears in the stool.[84,85]

DOCUSATE SALTS   Various

Pharmacology. Docusate is an anionic surfactant that lowers the surface tension of the oil-water interface of the stool, allowing fecal material to be penetrated by water and fat, thereby softening the stool. The emulsifying action also enhances the absorption of many fat-soluble drugs and mineral oil.[71,72,86]

Administration and Adult Dosage. PO as a stool softener (sodium salt) 50–500 mg/day in single or divided doses (give soln/syrup in milk or fruit juice to mask taste); begin therapy with up to 500 mg/day and adjust after maximal effects occur (about 3 days);[74] (calcium salt) 240 mg/day; (potassium salt) 100–300 mg/day. Use of 200 mg/day or less of the sodium salt in the hospital setting may be ineffective in altering the prevalence of constipation.[86,87] **PR as enema** 50–100 mg in water.

Special Populations. *Pediatric Dosage.* PO (sodium salt) (<3 yr) 10–40 mg/day; (3–6 yr) 20–60 mg/day; (6–12 yr) 40–120 mg/day; (>12 yr) same as adult dosage;

give soln/syrup in milk, fruit juice, or formula to mask taste; (**calcium salt**) (≥ 6 yr) 50–150 mg/day; (**potassium salt**) (≥ 6 yr) 100 mg/day.

Geriatric Dosage. Same as adult dosage (*see* Notes).

Dosage Forms. (Sodium salt: Colace, various) **Cap** 50, 100, 240, 250 mg; **Soln** 10, 50 mg/mL; **Syrup** 3.3, 4 mg/mL; **Tab** 100 mg. (Calcium salt: Surfak, various) **Cap** 50, 240 mg. (Potassium salt: Dialose, various) **Cap** 240 mg; **Tab** 100 mg.

Patient Instructions. Take this with a full glass of fluid; take the liquid or solution forms in milk, fruit juice, or infant formula to mask the bitter taste.

Pharmacokinetics. *Onset and Duration.* Onset of effect on stools is 2–3 days after first dose with continuous use.

Fate. Drug action is local in the gut, but docusate may be partially absorbed in the duodenum and jejunum, and secreted in the bile.[83,86]

Adverse Reactions. Bitter taste, throat irritation, and nausea (more common with syrup and liquid) occur frequently, abdominal cramps occasionally. Docusate may change intestinal morphology and cellular function, and may cause fluid and electrolyte accumulation in the colon.[86,87]

Contraindications. Undiagnosed abdominal pain; intestinal obstruction; concomitant use with mineral oil.

Precautions. Rectal bleeding or failure to respond to therapy may indicate a serious condition and the need for medical attention.

Drug Interactions. Concomitant use with mineral oil may enhance mineral oil absorption.[71,72]

Parameters to Monitor. Frequency and consistency of stools; ease of defecation.

Notes. Surfactant stool softeners are useful for softening hard, dry stools, in painful anorectal conditions, and in cardiac and other conditions to lessen the strain of defecation. They are more useful in preventing constipation rather than treating it; however, they may not be effective for long-term prevention of constipation in institutionalized elderly patients.[71,88]

LACTULOSE
Cephulac, Chronulac

Pharmacology. Lactulose is a synthetic disaccharide analogue of lactose that contains galactose and fructose and is metabolized by colonic bacteria to lactic and small amounts of acetic and formic acids. These acids result in acidification of colonic contents, decreased ammonia absorption, diffusion of ammonia from plasma to GI tract, and an osmotic catharsis.[89,90]

Administration and Adult Dosage. PO as a cathartic 15–30 mL (10–20 g), to a maximum of 60 mL; **PO for hepatic encephalopathy** 30–45 mL (20–30 g) q 1 hr until laxation, then 30–45 mL tid or qid, titrated to produce about 2 or 3 soft stools per day. **PR for hepatic encephalopathy as an enema** 300 mL with 700 mL water or NS retained for 30–60 min, may repeat q 4–6 hr. Repeat immediately if evacuated too promptly.

Special Populations. *Pediatric Dosage.* **PO for hepatic encephalopathy** (infants) 2.5–10 mL/day in divided doses; (older children and adolescents) 40–90 mL/day in divided doses, titrated to produce 2 or 3 soft stools daily. If initial dose causes diarrhea, reduce dose immediately; if diarrhea persists, discontinue.

Geriatric Dosage. Same as adult dosage (*see* Notes).

Dosage Forms. **Syrup** 667 mg/mL.

Patient Instructions. This syrup may be mixed with fruit juice, water, or milk to improve its palatability. In the treatment of hepatic encephalopathy, 2–3 loose stools per day are common, but report any worsening of diarrhea. Report belching, flatulence, or abdominal cramps if they are bothersome.

Pharmacokinetics. *Onset and Duration.* (Catharsis) onset 24–48 hr; duration 24–48 hr. (Hepatic encephalopathy) onset and duration variable; however, reversal of coma may occur within 2 hr of the first enema.

Fate. After oral administration, less than 3% is absorbed and most reaches the colon unabsorbed and unchanged. Unabsorbed drug is metabolized in the colon by bacteria to low molecular weight acids and carbon dioxide. The small amount of absorbed drug is excreted in the urine unchanged.[89,90]

Adverse Reactions. Flatulence, belching, and abdominal discomfort are frequent initially. Colonic dilation occurs occasionally.[91] Excessive diarrhea and fecal water loss may result in hypernatremia.[92]

Contraindications. Patients who require a low galactose diet.

Precautions. Use with caution in diabetics because of small amounts of free lactose and galactose in the drug. Rectal bleeding or failure to respond to therapy may indicate a serious condition and the need for medical attention.

Drug Interactions. Do not use other laxatives concomitantly, because their induction of loose stools may confound proper lactulose dosage titration for hepatic encephalopathy. Nonabsorbable antacids may interfere with the colonic acidification of lactulose. Theoretically, some antibacterials might interfere with the intestinal bacteria that metabolize lactulose; however, oral neomycin has been used concurrently in hepatic encephalopathy.[90]

Parameters to Monitor. (Hepatic encephalopathy) observe for changes in hepatic encephalopathy and number of stools per day. Periodically obtain serum sodium, chloride, potassium, and bicarbonate levels during prolonged use, especially in elderly or debilitated patients.

Notes. Lactulose is effective in hepatic encephalopathy, but as a general laxative it offers no advantage over less expensive drugs.[91,93] One study of constipation in the elderly found that up to 60 mL/day of 70% **sorbitol** was equivalent in laxative effects and caused less nausea than the same dosage of lactulose syrup.[94]

LOPERAMIDE   Imodium

Pharmacology. Loperamide is a synthetic antidiarrheal structurally similar to haloperidol and without appreciable opiate activity that causes a dose-related inhibition of colonic motility and affects water and electrolyte movement through the bowel. Tolerance has not been observed.

Administration and Adult Dosage. **PO for acute diarrhea** (℞) **or traveler's diarrhea (OTC)** 4 mg initially, then 2 mg after each unformed stool, to a maximum of 16 mg/day (8 mg/day for no more than 2 days OTC product). **PO for chronic diarrhea** (℞) initiate therapy as above, then individualize dosage; usual maintenance dosage is 4–8 mg/day in single or divided doses. If clinical improvement does not occur after treatment with 16 mg/day for a minimum of 10 days, symptoms are unlikely to be controlled by further use.

Special Populations. *Pediatric Dosage.* (<2 yr) not recommended. **PO for acute diarrhea** (℞) (2–5 yr) up to 1 mg tid as liquid; (6–8 yr) 2 mg bid; (8–12 yr) 2 mg tid. After first day of therapy, give 1 mg/10 kg after each loose stool, to a maximum daily dosage equal to the initial daily dosage. **PO for acute or traveler's diarrhea** (OTC) (2–5 yr) not recommended; (6–8 yr) 1 mg initially, then 1 mg after each loose stool, to a maximum of 4 mg/day for 2 days; (9–11 yr) 2 mg initially, then 1 mg after each loose stool, to a maximum of 6 mg/day for 2 days. **PO for chronic diarrhea** dosage not established.

Geriatric Dosage. Same as adult dosage.

Dosage Forms. **Cap** 2 mg; **Tab** 2 mg; **Tab** (chewable) 2 mg; **Liquid** 0.2, 1 mg/mL; **Tab** (chewable) 2 mg plus simethicone (Imodium Advanced).

Patient Instructions. This drug may cause drowsiness or dizziness. Until the severity of these reactions is known, use caution when performing tasks that require mental alertness. It may cause dry mouth. If diarrhea does not stop after a few days, or if abdominal pain, distention, or fever occurs, seek medical attention.

Pharmacokinetics. *Onset and Duration.* Onset 45–60 min; duration 4–6 hr.

Fate. GI absorption is approximately 40%; 25% or more is excreted in the stool unchanged; less than 2% of a dose is recovered in the urine.[18,95]

$t_{1/2}$. 10.8 ± 1.7 hr.[18,95]

Adverse Reactions. Abdominal cramping, constipation, distention, headache, rash, tiredness, drowsiness, dizziness, and dry mouth occur frequently.[96]

Contraindications. (℞, OTC) Patients who must avoid constipation; children <2 yr. (OTC) bloody diarrhea; body temperature over 38°C (101°F); diarrhea associated with pseudomembranous colitis; or enterotoxin-producing bacteria (*see* Notes).

Precautions. Use with caution in patients with ulcerative colitis. Discontinue if improvement is not observed in 48 hr. Use cautiously in patients with hepatic dysfunction.

Drug Interactions. Absorption of loperamide may be decreased by cholesterol-binding resins.

Parameters to Monitor. Frequency and volume of bowel movements; body temperature. Monitor for abdominal distention.

Notes. Adverse reactions may be less frequent and efficacy may be greater than with **diphenoxylate** with atropine.[96] Loperamide may provide temporary symptomatic relief of infectious traveler's diarrhea if used cautiously with an antibiotic, but discontinue if fever occurs or other symptoms persist beyond 48 hr, or blood or mucus in stool develops.[84,85,96]

MAGNESIUM SALTS   Various

Pharmacology. Magnesium salts act as saline cathartics that inhibit fluid and elec-trolyte absorption by increasing osmotic forces in the gut lumen. Part of the action may be caused by cholecystokinin release, which stimulates small bowel motility and inhibits fluid and electrolyte absorption from the small intestine.[71]

Administration and Adult Dosage. PO as a laxative/cathartic (citrate) 240 mL; (sulfate) 20–30 mL of 50% solution (10–15 g) in a full glass of water; (hydroxide; milk of magnesia) 30–60 mL with liquid; (concentrate) 10–30 mL (*see* Notes).

Special Populations. *Pediatric Dosage.* **PO** (citrate) one-half the adult dosage; (sulfate) (2–5 yr) 2.5–5 g, (≥6 yr) 5–10 g in one-half glass or more of water; (hy-droxide; milk of magnesia) 0.5 mL/kg.[71]

Geriatric Dosage. Same as adult dosage.

Other Conditions. Avoid use in patients with impaired renal function.[71]

Dosage Forms. Soln (citrate) 77 mEq/dL magnesium, 300 mL; (sulfate) 50%; **Susp** (hydroxide; milk of magnesia) 7–8.5%, many sizes, *see* Notes (also avail-able as concentrates with 10 mL equivalent to 20 or 30 mL of susp); **Tab** (hydrox-ide; milk of magnesia) 311 mg; **Pwdr** (sulfate) 150, 240, 454 g, 1.8 kg.

Patient Instructions. Take milk of magnesia or magnesium sulfate with at least one full glass of liquid. You may take magnesium sulfate with fruit juice to partially mask its bitter taste. Refrigerating magnesium citrate improves its palatability.

Pharmacokinetics. *Onset and Duration.* Onset is dose dependent: (high end of dosage range) 0.5–3 hr; (low end of dosage range) 6–8 hr.[74]

Fate. Slow absorption of 15–30% of a dose from the GI tract. Absorbed magne-sium is rapidly excreted in the urine in normal renal function.[71,74]

Adverse Reactions. Abdominal cramping, excessive diuresis, nausea, vomiting, and diarrhea occur frequently. Excessive use can lead to electrolyte abnormalities; dehydration may occur if taken with insufficient fluids. Use in patients with renal impairment may lead to hypermagnesemia, CNS depression, and hypotension.[71]

Contraindications. Acute surgical abdomen; fecal impaction; intestinal obstruc-tion; abdominal pain of unknown origin; nausea; vomiting.

Precautions. Rectal bleeding or failure to respond to therapy may indicate a seri-ous condition and the need for medical attention. Avoid use in patients with im-paired renal function.[71]

Drug Interactions. None known.

Parameters to Monitor. Periodic serum magnesium levels in patients with im-paired renal function who are receiving long-term daily administration.

Notes. Magnesium salts are useful for preparing the bowel for radiologic exami-nation and surgical procedures. The following amounts of various magnesium salts are approximately equivalent to 80 mEq of magnesium: 100 mL citrate; 2.4 g (30 mL) milk of magnesia; and 10 g sulfate. The sulfate salt is the most potent cathartic, but is the least palatable. (*See also* Magnesium Salts in the Renal and Electrolyte sections.)

METOCLOPRAMIDE   Reglan, Various

Pharmacology. Metoclopramide antagonizes central and peripheral dopamine activity, sensitizes receptors in the GI tract to acetylcholine, and exerts a direct effect on smooth muscle. It increases peristalsis of the gastric antrum, duodenum, and jejunum, with little effect on the colon or gallbladder. In patients with gastroesophageal reflux disease (GERD), metoclopramide produces a dose-dependent increase in lower esophageal sphincter pressure. Its antiemetic action results from a direct antidopaminergic effect on the chemoreceptor trigger zone and vomiting center, and antagonistic effect on serotonin-$5HT_3$ receptors.[97–99] Metoclopramide also increases prolactin secretion and serum prolactin.[100]

Administration and Adult Dosage. **PO for short-term treatment of symptomatic GERD in patients who fail to respond to conventional therapy** up to 15 mg qid 30 min before each meal and hs for 4–12 weeks or intermittent single doses of up to 20 mg; **PO for symptomatic diabetic gastroparesis** 10 mg qid 30 min before each meal and hs for 2–8 weeks; **IM or IV for severe symptoms associated with gastroparesis** 10 mg qid for up to 10 days; **IV to facilitate small bowel intubation or to aid in radiologic examination** 10 mg over 1–2 min; **PO to increase maternal milk supply** 10 mg tid for 10–14 days.[100] **PO, IM, or IV for treatment of hiccups PO** 10 mg q 6 hr, or **IM, IV** 5–10 mg q 8 hr, continue treatment for 10 days after resolution;[101] **IV for prevention of cancer chemotherapy-induced emesis** (drugs with high emetic potential) 2 mg/kg 30 min before chemotherapy, then q 2 hr for 2 doses, and then q 3 hr for 3 more doses; (drugs with low emetic potential) 1 mg/kg may be adequate; **IM for prevention of postoperative nausea and vomiting** 10–20 mg near the end of surgery. Dilute IV doses over 10 mg to 50 mL and infuse over at least 15 min (*see* Notes).

Special Populations. *Pediatric Dosage.* **IV to facilitate small bowel intubation or to aid radiologic examination** (<6 yr) 0.1 mg/kg; (6–14 yr) 2.5–5 mg; (>14 yr) same as adult dosage.

Geriatric Dosage. Begin at one-half the initial dose (usually 5 mg) and increase or decrease based on efficacy and side effects.

Other Conditions. With Cl_{cr} <40 mL/min, begin at one-half the initial dose (usually 5 mg) and increase or decrease based on efficacy and side effects.

Dosage Forms. **Tab** 5, 10 mg; **Soln** 10 mg/mL; **Syrup** 1 mg/mL; **Inj** 5 mg/mL.

Patient Instructions. Take each dose 30 min before meals and at bedtime. This drug may cause drowsiness. Until the degree of drowsiness is known, use caution when driving, operating machinery, or performing other tasks requiring mental alertness. Avoid excessive concurrent use of alcohol or other drugs that cause drowsiness. Report any involuntary movements (eg, muscle spasms and jerky movements of the head and face) that may occur, especially in children and the elderly.

Pharmacokinetics. *Onset and Duration.* (GI effects) PO onset 45 ± 15 min, IM 12.5 ± 2.5 min, IV 2 ± 1 min; duration 1–2 hr.

Fate. Bioavailability is 80 ± 15.5% PO, and 85 ± 11% IM. Peak serum concentration after a PO dose occurs in 1–2 hr, but may be delayed with impaired gastric emptying. The drug is about 30% plasma protein bound. V_d is 3.4 ± 1.3 L/kg, increased in uremia and in cirrhosis; Cl is 0.37 ± 0.08 L/hr/kg, decreased in uremia and in cirrhosis. About 85% of orally administered drug is recovered in the urine after 72 hr as unchanged and conjugated drug; 20% of an IV dose is excreted unchanged in urine.[55,102]

$t_{1/2}$. α phase 5 min; ß phase 5.5 ± 0.5 hr, increasing to about 14 hr in severe renal failure. Half-life may also be prolonged in cirrhosis.[55,102]

Adverse Reactions. Most side effects are dose related.[97] Drowsiness, restlessness, fatigue, and lassitude occur in 10% of patients with a dosage of 10 mg qid, and in 70% with IV doses of 1–2 mg/kg. Acute dystonic reactions occur in 0.2% of patients receiving 30–40 mg/day, 2% in cancer chemotherapy-treated patients >35 yr receiving doses of 1–2 mg/kg, and 25% in cancer chemotherapy-treated children without prior diphenhydramine treatment. Parkinsonian symptoms, tardive dyskinesia, and akathisia occur less frequently. Rapid IV push produces transient, intense anxiety, and restlessness followed by drowsiness. Transient flushing of the face and/or diarrhea occur frequently following large IV doses. Hyperprolactinemia may occur, resulting in gynecomastia and impotence in males, and galactorrhea and amenorrhea in females. Fluid retention may result from transient elevations of aldosterone. Diarrhea, hypertension, and mental depression have been reported.

Contraindications. GI hemorrhage; mechanical obstruction or perforation; pheochromocytoma; epilepsy; concurrent use of drugs that cause extrapyramidal effects.

Precautions. Pregnancy; lactation. Use with caution in the elderly and in patients with hypertension, renal failure, or Parkinson's disease, a prior history of depression or attempted suicide and following gut anastomosis. In patients with diabetic gastroparesis, insulin dosage or timing may require adjustment.

Drug Interactions. Absorption of drugs from the stomach or small bowel may be altered by metoclopramide (eg, digoxin and cimetidine absorption is decreased; cyclosporine absorption is increased). Anticholinergics and narcotics may antagonize GI effects of metoclopramide. Use with an MAOI may result in hypertension and the combination should be avoided. Additive sedation can occur with alcohol or other CNS depressants.

Parameters to Monitor. Monitor periodically for CNS effects, extrapyramidal reactions, and changes in Cr_s, blood glucose, or blood pressure. (GERD or diabetic gastroparesis) Observe for symptomatic relief.

Notes. Tolerance to the drug's gastrokinetic effect may develop with long-term therapy;[97] however, this remains controversial.[102] Metoclopramide has been used in the treatment of neurogenic bladder, orthostatic hypotension, Tourette's syndrome, adynamic or chemotherapy-induced ileus, anorexia, and complications of scleroderma.[103] If extrapyramidal symptoms occur, administer **diphenhydramine** 50 mg IM or **benztropine** 1–2 mg IM.

Domperidone, a peripheral dopamine antagonist unavailable in the United States, is a prokinetic drug that dose dependently stimulates antroduodenal coordination and has antiemetic properties;[98,104] however, it does not appear to be effective in diseases of delayed colonic transit.[104] Domperidone does not readily cross the blood-brain barrier; therefore, CNS side effects are minimal.[97,98] Doses of 10–20 mg qid appear to provide symptomatic relief in gastroparesis, but adequate studies are lacking.[97,99]

Erythromycin in low doses binds to motilin receptors in the GI tract to stimulate gastric emptying.[97,104] In gastroparesis, doses of 200 mg IV of the lactobionate salt, 250 mg PO of the ethylsuccinate salt, or 500 mg PO of the base 15–120 min before meals and at hs appear to be effective.[105] Differences in efficacy between the various salts of erythromycin have not been established.[105] Erythromycin has also been used in other GI motility disorders.[105-107]

PEG ELECTROLYTE LAVAGE SOLUTION   GoLYTELY, Various

Polyethylene glycol (PEG) electrolyte lavage solution is an isosmotic solution containing approximately 5.69 g/L sodium sulfate, 1.68 g/L sodium bicarbonate, 1.46 g/L sodium chloride, 745 mg/L potassium chloride, and 60 g/L PEG 3350 used for total bowel cleansing prior to GI examination. A solution lacking sodium sulfate, with a slight variation in other salts and PEG (NuLYTELY), and flavored solutions are available with improved palatability. PEG acts as an osmotic cathartic, and the electrolyte concentrations are such that there is little net fluid or electrolyte movement into or out of the bowel. This method of bowel cleansing is well suited for colonoscopy, but because of some residual lavage fluid retained in the colon, other cleansing methods may be preferred prior to barium enema. Use the solution at least 4 hr before the examination, allowing the patient 3 hr for drinking and a 1-hr waiting period to complete bowel evacuation. Another method is to give the solution the evening before the examination. Withhold solid food for 2 hr and medication for 1 hr before the solution is administered. The first bowel movement usually occurs after 1 hr, with total bowel cleansing 3–4 hr after starting. Frequent side effects include nausea, abdominal fullness, bloating (in up to 50% of patients), cramps, anal irritation, and vomiting. Urticaria, rhinorrhea, and dermatitis are reported occasionally. Do not use PEG electrolyte lavage solution in patients with GI obstruction, gastric retention, toxic colitis, toxic megacolon, ileus, or bowel perforation; however, the solution appears safe for patients with liver, kidney, or heart disease. The usual adult dosage is 200–300 mL orally q 10 min or by NG tube at a rate of 20–30 mL/min until about 4 L are consumed or the rectal effluent is clear. Give a 1-L trial before the full dosage in patients suspected of having bowel obstruction. These solutions appear safe and useful for bowel evacuation in children using 25–40 mL/kg/hr for 4–10 hr. Chilling the solution may improve its palatability, but do not add any additional ingredients. Colonic cleansing with bisacodyl 15 mg orally followed by 2 L of PEG lavage solution 8 hr later has been found to be equally effective and more acceptable to patients than 4 L of solution used alone. The drug may be useful as a GI evacuant in ingestions and overdoses with iron and some enteric-coated and SR drug products.[75,108-111] It is available as powder for reconstitution and oral solution.

PSYLLIUM HUSK   Konsyl, Metamucil, Various

Pharmacology. Psyllium is a bulk-forming cathartic that absorbs water and provides an emollient mass.

Administration and Adult Dosage. PO for constipation 2.5–12 g daily–tid, stirred in a full glass of fluid, followed by an additional glass of liquid. **PO for mild diarrhea** usual doses titrated to effect may be used to "firm up" effluent. **PO to lower cholesterol** 10–30 g/day in divided doses in combination with diet may decrease cholesterol in patients with mild to moderate hypercholesterolemia.[112,113]

Special Populations. *Pediatric Dosage.* **PO for constipation** (6–12 yr) 2.5–3 g (psyllium) daily–tid, with fluid as above.

Geriatric Dosage. Same as adult dosage.

Dosage Forms. Pwdr Metamucil, Sugar Free Orange Flavor (containing 65% or 92% psyllium), Konsyl (sugar-free, containing 100% psyllium) 3.7, 5.2 g packet, 111–621 g; **Pwdr** Metamucil Orange Flavor (containing 50% or 65% sucrose) 7, 11 g packet, 210, 420, 630, 960 g; **Pwdr** (effervescent, sugar-free, containing 63% psyllium) 5.4 g packet; **Wafer** Metamucil (containing 4.5 g fat) 1.7 g of psyllium per wafer, Fiberall (containing 78 kcal of carbohydrate) 3.4 g psyllium per wafer.

Patient Instructions. Mix with a full glass of fluid before taking and follow with another glass of liquid.

Pharmacokinetics. *Onset and Duration.* Onset 12–24 hr, but 2–3 days may be required for full effect.[71,114]

Fate. Not absorbed from GI tract.

Adverse Reactions. Flatulence occurs frequently. Serious side effects are rare, but esophageal, gastric, intestinal, and rectal obstruction have been reported. Allergic reactions and bronchospasm have occurred following inhalation of dry powder.[71,115]

Contraindications. Acute surgical abdomen; fecal impaction; intestinal obstruction; abdominal pain of unknown origin; nausea, vomiting.

Precautions. Rectal bleeding or failure to respond to therapy may indicate a serious condition and the need for medical attention. Use with caution in patients who require fluid restriction, because constipation may occur unless fluid intake is adequate. Psyllium may be hazardous in patients with intestinal ulcerations, stenosis, or disabling adhesions. Use effervescent Metamucil formulations (packet) with caution in patients who require potassium restriction (7.4 and 7.9 mEq potassium/packet). Use the noneffervescent formulations of Metamucil cautiously in diabetics, because they contain 50% or 65% sucrose. Sugar-free preparations include Konsyl and Metamucil Sugar Free.

Drug Interactions. None known.

Notes. Psyllium is useful in lessening the strain of defecation and for inpatients who are on low-residue diets or constipating medications. It is safe to use in pregnancy.[71]

Miscellaneous Gastrointestinal Drugs

ACTIVATED CHARCOAL

Pharmacology. Activated charcoal is a nonspecific GI adsorbent with a surface area of 900–2000 m^2/g used primarily in the management of acute poisonings.[116]

Administration and Adult Dosage. PO or via gastric tube 50–120 g dispersed in liquid as soon as possible after ingestion of poison (the FDA suggests 240 mL diluent/30 g activated charcoal). Repeat administration of activated charcoal after gastric lavage (*see* Notes).

Special Populations. *Pediatric Dosage.* **PO or via gastric tube** (≤12 yr) 25–50 g or 1–2 g/kg dispersed in liquid; (>12 yr) same as adult dosage.[117]

Geriatric Dosage. Same as adult dosage.

Dosage Forms. Pwdr (plain, or dispersed in water or sorbitol-water).

Patient Instructions. This drug causes the stools to turn black.

Pharmacokinetics. *Onset and Duration.* Onset is immediate; duration is continual while it remains in the GI tract.

Fate. Eliminated unchanged in the feces.

Adverse Reactions. Black stools; gritty consistency may cause emesis in some patients.

Precautions. Insufficient hydration or use in patients with decreased bowel motility may result in intestinal bezoars.

Drug Interactions. Activated charcoal may decrease the oral absorption and efficacy of many drugs (*see* Notes).

Parameters to Monitor. Passage of activated charcoal in the stools. If sorbitol or other cathartics are administered, limit their dosages to prevent excessive fluid and electrolyte losses.

Notes. A suspension of activated charcoal in 25–35% **sorbitol** may increase palatability of the drug; total dosage of sorbitol should not exceed 1 g/kg. Substances *not* adsorbed by activated charcoal include mineral acids, alkalis, iron, cyanide, lithium and other small ions, and alcohols. Repeated oral doses of activated charcoal (eg, 15–30 g q 4–6 hr) have been used to enhance the elimination of some drugs, most notably **carbamazepine, phenobarbital, salicylates,** and **theophylline.**

CHOLELITHOLYTIC DRUGS

The oral bile acids, **chenodiol** (chenodeoxycholic acid; Chenix) and **ursodiol** (ursodeoxycholic acid; Actigall), are used to dissolve small (<20 mm), radiolucent cholesterol gallstones in mildly symptomatic patients with a functioning gallbladder who are unable to undergo a cholecystectomy. Radiopaque gallstones, which consist primarily of calcium, do not respond to bile acid therapy. The exact mechanism by which these drugs dissolve cholesterol gallstones is unclear. Chenodiol expands the bile acid pool, inhibits synthesis of cholesterol and bile acids, and reduces biliary cholesterol saturation, allowing solubilization of cholesterol. Ursodiol does not appear to inhibit the synthesis of bile acids, but it does suppress the synthesis, secretion, and intestinal absorption of cholesterol, and it promotes nonmicellar mechanisms of cholesterol solubilization. Complete gallstone dissolution usually requires 6–24 months of treatment. Cessation of oral bile acid therapy results in gallstone recurrence in approximately 50% of patients within 5 yr. The combination of chenodiol or ursodiol with extracorporeal shock-wave lithotripsy (ECSWL) is more effective than ECSWL alone and may decrease the time to stone dissolution compared with either drug alone or with ECSWL alone. Stone fragmentation via ECSWL with subsequent oral bile acid therapy is the norm; however, some clinicians begin oral therapy 2 weeks prior to ECSWL. Although similar in efficacy, chenodiol is not widely used because of its dose-related side effects: diarrhea (50%), increased AST and ALT (40%), usually reversible hepatitis (3%), and a 10% or greater increase in LDL cholesterol. Ursodiol has fewer and less severe adverse effects, but the safety of ursodiol beyond 24 months has not been established. The dosage of chenodiol is 13–16 mg/kg/day, and the dosage of ursodiol is 8–10 mg/kg/day; higher dosages do not provide additional efficacy. Oral bile acids are not recommended during pregnancy. Although studies conflict, a single bedtime dose may be more effective than multiple daily doses in reducing cholesterol saturation of bile. Continue treatment for at least 3 months after stones or sludge are not apparent on ultrasonography because of the possible presence of microscopic stones and/or crystals. Maintenance therapy (300 mg/day) with ursodiol may decrease the recurrence rate by one-half, especially in patients <50 yr; maintenance therapy with chenodiol appears to be ineffective. Combination therapy of the two drugs is no longer recommended. Ursodiol has also been used as prophylaxis against gallstone formation during weight loss (600 mg/day) and in biliary disorders associated with cystic fibrosis (15–20 mg/kg/day), primary biliary cirrhosis (8–15 mg/kg/day), and other cholestatic diseases. Ursodiol is available as a 300-mg capsule and can be formulated into a suspension. Chenodiol is available as a 250-mg tablet from the manufacturer as an orphan drug.[118–127]

MESALAMINE AND ITS DERIVATIVES

Pharmacology. Mesalamine (5-aminosalicylic acid, 5-ASA) is thought to be the active moiety of sulfasalazine. Each molecule of olsalazine that reaches the colon is converted to 2 molecules of mesalamine. The mechanism of action of mesalamine in inflammatory bowel disease (IBD) is unknown, but appears to be topical rather than systemic.[128–133] Mucosal production of arachidonic acid metabolites, through both the cyclooxygenase and lipoxygenase pathways, are increased in patients with chronic IBD. Mesalamine may block cyclooxygenase in the arachidonic cascade and down-regulate production of inflammatory prostaglandins in the large bowel. Modulation of the lipoxygenase pathway may inhibit formation of chemotactically active leukotrienes and hydroxyeicosatetraenoic acids.[128,129] Mesalamine inhibits macrophage and neutrophil chemotaxis, reduces intestinal mononuclear cell production of IgA and IgG antibodies, and is a scavenger of oxygen-derived free radicals, which are increased during active IBD.[128]

Administration and Adult Dosage.

INDICATION	ASACOL *Mesalamine*	DIPENTUM *Olsalazine*	PENTASA *Mesalamine*	ROWASA *Mesalamine*
Short-term treatment of active mild to moderate ulcerative colitis, and proctosigmoiditis.	PO 800 mg tid, or 1.6 g tid[a] for 6 weeks.	PO 500 mg tid,[a] 1 g bid,[a] or 1 g tid[b] for 3–6 weeks.	PO 1 g qid for 6–8 weeks.	PR 2 g hs,[a,b] or 4 g hs[b] for 3–6 weeks (enema).
Maintenance of ulcerative colitis remission.	PO 800 mg tid.[a]	PO 500 mg bid.[c]	PO 1 g bid[a] or 1 g qid.[a]	PR 1–2 g hs.[a,b] (enema).
Short-term treatment of active mild to moderate Crohn's disease.	PO 800 mg tid[a] or 1.6 g tid[a] for 8–16 weeks.	a	PO 1 g qid[a] for 8–16 weeks.	a
Maintenance of Crohn's disease remission.	PO 800 mg–1.6 g tid.[a]	a	PO 1 g bid–qid.[a]	a
Treatment of active proctitis.	PO 800 mg tid.	a	PO 1 g qid.	PR 1–2 g hs,[a,b] 4 g hs[b] (enema); 500 mg bid or tid[d] (suppository).

[a]Nonlabeled indication and dosage; optimal dosage regimen has not been determined.
[b]Retain enema for approximately 8 hr.
[c]Patients intolerant to sulfasalazine.
[d]Retain suppository for 1–3 hr or longer.
From references 128–132.

Special Populations. *Pediatric Dosage.* Safety and efficacy not established.

Geriatric Dosage. No dosage reduction is necessary. However, older patients are more likely to have renal impairment (*see* Precautions).

Other Conditions. Dosage reduction may be considered in severe renal and/or hepatic impairment.[128] (*See* Precautions.)

Dosage Forms.

Drug	ASACOL *Mesalamine*	DIPENTUM *Olsalazine**	PENTASA *Mesalamine*	ROWASA *Mesalamine*
Formulation.	Tablet enteric-coated pH-dependent (pH 7), delayed release.	Capsule containing 5-ASA diamer; diazo bond is degraded by bacteria in colon.	Capsule containing ethylcellulose-coated microgranules, controlled release.	Rectal suspension, suppository.
Site of Action.	Distal ileum-colon	Colon	Duodenum-colon	Rectum-splenic flexure (enema); rectum (suppository)
Dosage Forms.	EC Tab 400 mg.	Cap 250 mg.	SR Cap 250 mg.	Enema 4 g/60 mL; Supp 500 mg.

*Each molecule of olsalazine that reaches the colon is converted to 2 molecules of mesalamine.

Patient Instructions. (Oral) Take mesalamine with food and a full glass of water. Swallow tablets or capsules whole without breaking or chewing. The tablet core (Asacol) or small beads (Pentasa) may appear in the stool after mesalamine is released, but this does not mean there was a lack of effect. Report intact or partially intact, tablets in the stool (Asacol), because this may indicate that the expected amount of mesalamine was not released from the tablet. Report nausea, vomiting, abrupt change in character or volume of stools, or skin rashes. (Rectal) Empty bowel immediately prior to insertion of enema or suppository. Use enema at bedtime and retain for 8 hours, if possible. Retain suppository for 1 to 3 hours or longer. Report signs of anal or rectal irritation.

Pharmacokinetics. *Onset and Duration.* The onset of action of Asacol, Dipentum, and Pentasa is delayed because of the release characteristics of their dosage forms; duration of action varies depending on intestinal transit time.[128,129]

Fate. About 70 ± 10% of oral mesalamine is absorbed in the proximal small bowel when administered in an uncoated product or unbound to a carrier molecule; some absorption may occur in the distal small bowel, but mesalamine is poorly absorbed from the colon. Various oral dosage forms have been formulated to deliver mesalamine topically to the more distal sites of inflammation.[128-133] *See* Dosage Forms and Notes. After oral administration, about 50% of mesalamine from Pentasa is released in the small bowel and 50% is released in the colon, although the amount released may vary and is patient specific. About 25 ± 10% of released mesalamine is absorbed following oral administration of Asacol or Pentasa; the remainder is excreted in the feces. About 98% of an oral olsalazine dose reaches the large bowel; less than 2% is absorbed. Mesalamine absorption from the enema is pH dependent; neutral solutions are better absorbed than acidic solutions.[128] Rowasa (at pH 4.5) is less than 15% rectally absorbed. Plasma protein binding: mesalamine (55 ± 15%); N-acetylmesalamine (80%); olsalazine and olsalazine-O-sulfate (greater than 99%).[128,129] Absorbed mesalamine is rapidly acetylated to N-acetyl-5-aminosalicylate (N-acetylmesalamine) in the intestinal mucosal wall and the liver. Absorbed olsalazine is conjugated in the liver to olsalazine-O-sulfate. N-acetylmesalamine is excreted in urine. Less than 1% of a dose of olsalazine is recovered unchanged in urine.

$t_{1/2}$. (Mesalamine) 1 ± 0.5 hr; (N-acetylmesalamine) 7.5 ± 1.5 hr; (olsalazine-O-sulfate) 7 days.[128,133]

Adverse Reactions. Adverse effects are usually less frequent than those reported with oral sulfasalazine. Headache, flatulence, abdominal pain, diarrhea, dizziness, and fatigue occur frequently with oral or rectal mesalamine. An acute intolerance syndrome develops in 3% of patients taking mesalamine; dose-dependent secretory diarrhea occurs in about 17% of patients receiving olsalazine 1 g/day, although it is sometimes difficult to distinguish these adverse effects from the underlying disease. Oral, esophageal, and duodenal ulceration as well as gastritis and GI bleeding have been reported. Dermatologic reactions, including acne, pruritus, urticaria, alopecia, and photosensitivity, occur occasionally (*see* Contraindications). Rarely, pericarditis, fatal myocarditis, hypersensitivity pneumonitis, pancreatitis, nephrotic syndrome, interstitial nephritis, and hepatitis occur (*see* Precautions). Anal irritation or a hypersensitivity reaction to mesalamine or the sulfite contained in the rectal suspension is rare; however, patients intolerant to sulfasalazine may also be sensitive to rectal mesalamine.

Contraindications. Pyloric stenosis; intestinal obstruction; salicylate hypersensitivity.

Precautions. Pregnancy; lactation. Renal tubular damage caused by absorbed mesalamine or its N-acetylated metabolite may occur, especially in patients with preexisting renal impairment or those on concomitant 5-ASA-liberating medication. Use caution if mesalamine is used in patients with impaired hepatic function. Patients who experience rash or fever with sulfasalazine may have the same reaction to mesalamine or olsalazine, indicating possible cross-sensitivity to salicylates.

Drug Interactions. Increased PT in patients taking warfarin has been reported.

Parameters to Monitor. Improvement in abdominal cramping, diarrhea, and rectal bleeding. Monitor for adverse effects, including diarrhea (olsalazine), acute intolerance syndrome, and hypersensitivity reaction. Monitor BUN, Cr_s, and urinalysis prior to and periodically during therapy. Monitor PT in patients taking concurrent warfarin.

Notes. The release characteristics of Pentasa are primarily time dependent, whereas those of Asacol are pH dependent; consequently, Asacol may not provide reliable site-specific release of mesalamine if intestinal pH is inadequate. In 2–3% of patients taking Asacol, intact or partially intact tablets have been reported in the stool.

There appears to be no therapeutic advantage of one oral mesalamine product over another or over **sulfasalazine,** in treating or maintaining remission of mild to moderate ulcerative colitis.[128,130–132,134] However, the mesalamine preparations may be of benefit in the sulfasalazine-sensitive patient. The enema is as effective as oral sulfasalazine or **hydrocortisone** enema in patients with mild to moderate distal ulcerative colitis.[131] Patients refractory to oral sulfasalazine and oral or rectal hydrocortisone may respond to rectal mesalamine. Rectal mesalamine combined with oral sulfasalazine or a corticosteroid may enhance efficacy, but the risk of adverse effects is increased.

In Crohn's disease with involvement of the ileum or proximal large bowel, oral formulations, which deliver meslamine to the small bowel and colon, are preferable to sulfasalazine or olsalazine. Pentasa, and possibly Asacol, may be effective in treating active Crohn's disease (including ileal or ilealcolonic), maintaining remission, and preventing recurrence after curative surgery.[128,130–132,135] Pentasa may improve the quality of life in Crohn's patients.[136] Rectal mesalamine may be less effective in Crohn's disease.[131] (*See also* Sulfasalazine.)

OCTREOTIDE	Sandostatin

Pharmacology. Octreotide is a long-acting synthetic octapeptide with pharmacologic actions similar to somatostatin. It suppresses the secretion of numerous substances, including serotonin, gastrin, vasoactive intestinal peptide (VIP), insulin, glucagon, secretin, motilin, pancreatic polypeptide, growth hormone (GH), and intrinsic factor. It suppresses the luteinizing hormone (LH) response to gonadotropin releasing hormone (GnRH), the intestinal secretion of water and electrolytes, and the secretion of thyroid stimulating hormone (TSH).[137] It also decreases renal and splanchnic blood flow.

Administration and Adult Dosage. SC administration is recommended for symptom control. **SC for symptomatic treatment of severe diarrhea and facial flushing associated with metastatic carcinoid tumors** 100–600 µg/day in 2–4 divided doses during the first 2 weeks of therapy; maintenance dosages of 50–1500 µg/day (median about 450 µg/day) have been used. **SC for symptomatic treatment of profuse watery diarrhea associated with VIP-secreting tumors (VIPomas)** 200–300 µg/day in 2–4 divided doses for the first 2 weeks (range 150–750 µg/day) to control symptoms, then adjust dosage based on therapeutic response; dosages over 450 µg/day are usually not required. **SC to reduce GH and/or IGF-1 (insulin-like growth factor, somatomedin C) in patients with acromegaly** 50 µg tid initially, increase dosage q 2 weeks based on IGF-1 concentration. The most common dosage is 100 µg tid, with some patients requiring 500 µg tid. A more rapid titration can be obtained by drawing multiple GH concentrations from 0 to 8 hr after the octreotide dose. The goal is to achieve GH <5 µg/L (or IGF-1 concentration <1.9 units/mL in males and <2.2 units/mL in females). Discontinue octreotide for about 4 weeks each year in acromegalics who have received irradiation; if clinical symptoms or abnormal laboratory results recur, resume therapy. **IV** same dosage as SC, diluted in 50–200 mL of NS or D5W and infused over 15–30 min, or given by IV push over 3 min. In emergency situations (eg, carcinoid crisis) give by rapid IV bolus.

Special Populations. *Pediatric Dosage.* SC 1–10 µg/kg are well tolerated in patients 1 month or older. Studies of various GI disorders used widely varying dosages in children 3 days–16 yr.[138] Octreotide has been studied in the treatment of hyperinsulinemic hypoglycemia in neonates in varying dosages.[138] **SC for anti-VIP effects** 3.5 µg/kg/day divided q 8 hr has been used.[139]

Geriatric Dosage. Dosage reduction is recommended because of decreased renal clearance.

Other Conditions. The effect of hepatic disease on the disposition of octreotide is unknown. Reduction of maintenance dosages may be required in patients with renal impairment and those undergoing dialysis.[140]

Dosage Forms. **Inj** 50, 100, 200, 500, 1000 µg/mL.

Patient Instructions. Instruct patient in sterile SC injection technique. Avoid multiple SC injections at the same site within a short period of time. Systematically rotate injection sites. Do not use solution if particulates and/or discoloration are present. Store medication in refrigerator, but do not allow it to freeze; individual ampules can remain at room temperature for up to 24 hours. Pain at injection site can be minimized by bringing solution to room temperature prior to injection, but do not warm artificially. Stop medication and report if symptoms of high or low blood sugar occur.

Pharmacokinetics. *Onset and Duration.* SC peak concentrations occur in 0.4 hr (0.7 hr in acromegaly). Duration is up to 12 hr, depending on tumor type.

Fate. Oral absorption is poor; SC and IV routes are bioequivalent. The drug is 65% protein bound (41.2% in acromegaly), primarily to lipoprotein and, to a lesser extent, albumin. V_d is 0.35 ± 0.22 L/kg; Cl is 0.16 ± 0.08 L/hr/kg. Cl is decreased in the elderly and in those with renal impairment. Octreotide exhibits nonlinear pharmacokinetics at dosages of 600 µg/day or greater. About 11–20% is excreted unchanged in urine.[55]

$t_{1/2}$. 1.5 ± 0.4 hr; increased by 46% in the elderly.

Adverse Reactions. Single doses of octreotide can inhibit gallbladder contractility and decrease bile secretion. About one-half of patients on octreotide for 12 months or longer experience cholesterol gallstones or sludge, unrelated to age, gender, or dosage. About 5–10% of nonacromegalic patients and 30–58% of acromegalics experience diarrhea, loose stools, nausea, and abdominal discomfort. The severity, but not the frequency, is dose dependent; symptoms spontaneously subside in about 14 days.[141] Diabetics appear to be especially susceptible to nausea and abdominal cramping.[137] Octreotide suppresses the secretion of TSH, alters the balance between insulin, glucagon, and GH, and may be responsible for cardiac conduction abnormalities, which are particularly frequent in acromegaly: bradycardia (21%), conduction abnormalities (9%), and arrhythmias (9%). Adverse reactions that occur in 1–10% of patients include vomiting, flatulence, constipation, and headache. Adverse GI effects often diminish with time.[142] Pain on injection occurs frequently and can be minimized by warming the solution prior to injection and using the smallest possible drug volume to obtain the appropriate dose. Several cases of pancreatitis have been reported. Abnormal Schilling's tests and decreased vitamin B_{12} levels have been reported.

Precautions. Pregnancy; lactation. Use with caution in patients with diabetic gastroparesis because octreotide slows GI transit time;[137] insulin-dependent diabetics may require a reduction in insulin dosage.

Drug Interactions. In acromegaly, reduction of dosage of medications causing bradycardia (eg, β-blockers) may be required. In all patients, the dosage of calcium-channel blockers, diuretics, insulin, or oral hypoglycemics may require reduction with concurrent octreotide. Octreotide may decrease the absorption of some orally administered nutrients and drugs (eg, fat, cyclosporine).

Parameters to Monitor. Perform ultrasound of the gallbladder periodically during extended therapy. Baseline and periodic total and/or free T_4 during long-term therapy. Monitor closely for hyper- or hypoglycemia, especially in diabetics. Periodically monitor vitamin B_{12} during long-term therapy. Evaluate cardiac function both at baseline and periodically during therapy, especially in acromegalics. Monitor serum concentrations of drugs whose absorption may be affected by octreotide (eg, cyclosporine). In acromegaly, evaluate GH or IGF-1 concentrations q 6 months.

Notes. Octreotide has been investigated for a variety of conditions, including GH-secreting pituitary tumors, insulinomas, thyrotropinomas, hypotension caused by carcinoid crisis or autonomic neuropathy, Zollinger-Ellison syndrome, glucagonomas, diabetes mellitus, variceal and nonvariceal upper GI bleeding, refractory secretory-, diabetic-, AIDS- or ileostomy-related diarrhea, acute and chronic pancreatitis, pancreatic or liver transplantation, GI fistulas, short bowel syndrome, dumping syndrome, psoriasis, resistant hypercalcemia, and intrathecally and intraventricularly for pain management.[137,141,142] Octreotide 200 µg/mL is stable for up to 60 days in polypropylene syringes under refrigeration and protected from light.[143]

SULFASALAZINE
Azulfidine, Various

Pharmacology. Sulfasalazine is a conjugate of sulfapyridine and mesalamine that is thought to be the active moiety. (*See* Mesalamine and Its Derivatives.)

Administration and Adult Dosage. **PO for short-term treatment of active mild to moderate ulcerative colitis or Crohn's disease** 3–4 g/day in equally divided doses; do not exceed an interval of 8 hr between nighttime and morning doses; administer after meals when feasible. A lower initial dosage of 1–2 g/day in evenly divided doses may decrease adverse GI effects.[130–132] **PO for maintenance of remission of ulcerative colitis** 1–2 g/day in divided doses.[130,131] Dosages up to 12 g/day have been used; however, dosages >4 g/day are associated with an increased frequency of adverse effects. Low-dose therapy is not effective in maintaining remission in Crohn's disease.[130,131] **PO for desensitization of allergic patients** reinstitute sulfasalazine at a total daily dosage of 50–250 mg; thereafter, double the daily dosage q 4–7 days until the desired therapeutic effect is achieved. If symptoms of sensitivity recur, discontinue sulfasalazine. Do not attempt desensitization in patients who have a history of agranulocytosis or an anaphylactic reaction during previous sulfasalazine therapy. Consider mesalamine instead of desensitization in sulfasalazine-sensitive patients.

Special Populations. *Pediatric Dosage.* (<2 yr) contraindicated; (≥2 yr) **PO for short-term treatment of active mild to moderate ulcerative colitis or Crohn's disease** 40–60 mg/kg/day in 3–6 equally divided doses. **PO for maintenance of remission of ulcerative colitis** 30 mg/kg/day in 4 equally divided doses.

Geriatric Dosage. No dosage reduction necessary. However, older patients may have renal impairment.

Other Conditions. Consider dosage reduction in severe renal or hepatic impairment.[128]

Dosage Forms. **Tab** 500 mg; **EC Tab** 500 mg; **Susp** 50 mg/mL.

Patient Instructions. Take each dose after meals or with food, and drink at least 1 full glass of water with each dose; drink several additional glasses of water daily. This medication must be taken continually to be effective. It is often necessary to continue medication even when symptoms such as diarrhea and abdominal cramping have been controlled. Report any nausea, vomiting, abrupt change in character or volume of stools, or skin rashes. Sulfasalazine may cause an orange-yellow discoloration of the urine or skin. Reversible infertility may occur in males.

Pharmacokinetics. ***Onset and Duration.*** Maximum effect is in 1–2 weeks; duration is 10 ± 2 hr following an oral dose.[18]

Serum Levels. (Sulfapyridine) levels >50 mg/L (200 μmol/L) are associated with increased toxicity.[18] Therapeutic effect appears to be related to topical mesalamine levels in the bowel.[131,132]

Fate. Sulfasalazine is about 30% absorbed from the small intestine, but the absorbed drug is almost completely secreted unchanged in the bile. It is then metabolized in the large bowel, probably by intestinal bacteria, to sulfapyridine and mesalamine. Most of the sulfapyridine is absorbed from the bowel. Plasma protein binding: sulfasalazine (>99%); sulfapyridine (50%); mesalamine (55 ±15%); N-acetylmesalamine (80%). Sulfapyridine is metabolized by the liver and excreted in the urine; slow acetylators have higher serum sulfapyridine concentrations. After an oral dose of sulfasalazine, about 91% of sulfapyridine is recovered in the urine in 3 days as sulfapyridine, its metabolites, and small amounts of sulfasalazine. Mesalamine is eliminated primarily in the feces; only a small portion is absorbed, metabolized, and excreted in the urine as N-acetylmeslamine.[18]

t½. (Sulfapyridine) 9 ± 4 hr, depending on acetylator phenotype.[18] (*See also* Mesalamine.)

Adverse Reactions. Anorexia, nausea, vomiting, dyspepsia, and headache occur in about one-third of patients and are related to serum sulfapyridine concentrations. Reversible oligospermia and leukopenia occur frequently. Skin rash occurs occasionally. Rare toxic hypersensitivity reactions (caused by sulfapyridine) include neutropenia, agranulocytosis, hepatitis, pancreatitis, pericarditis, pneumonitis, peripheral neuropathy, and severe hemolytic anemia.[130,141,144] Sulfasalazine may cause an orange-yellow discoloration of the urine or skin and may precipitate acute attacks of porphyria.

Contraindications. Intestinal or urinary obstruction; porphyria; infants <2 yr; hypersensitivity to sulfasalazine, its metabolites, sulfonamides, or salicylates.

Precautions. Pregnancy, despite reports of safety; lactation. Use with caution in patients with renal or hepatic impairment, blood dyscrasias, slow acetylators, bronchial asthma, G-6-PD deficiency, or severe allergies.

Drug Interactions. Reduced metabolism of dietary folate has been reported in sulfasalazine-treated patients. Consider folic acid supplementation in patients on long-term therapy.[131] Decreased digoxin bioavailability has been reported when sulfasalazine is concurrently administered.

Parameters to Monitor. Monitor therapeutic response (decrease in degree and frequency of diarrhea, rectal bleeding, abdominal cramping) and adverse effects (headache, anorexia, dyspepsia, nausea, hypersensitivity reactions). Obtain baseline and periodic CBC, reticulocyte counts, and urinalysis. Monitor serum folate periodically in patients on long-term therapy.[18,131] Monitor serum digoxin levels during initiation and after discontinuation of sulfasalazine. Serum sulfapyridine levels may be useful in confirming toxicity.

Notes. There appears to be no clinical advantage of sulfasalazine over oral **mesalamine** when used to treat or maintain remission of ulcerative colitis.[134] Crohn's disease patients with involvement of the ileum may not respond as well to sulfasalazine as those with only large bowel disease.[130-132] Combining sulfasalazine with an oral or rectal **corticosteroid** or with rectal mesalamine may be of benefit in patients with ulcerative colitis who do not respond to single drug therapy.[131] Sulfasalazine has also been used to treat ankylosing spondylitis and rheumatoid arthritis.[144] Occasionally, the enteric-coated tablet may appear whole in the stool; if this occurs, switch the patient to the uncoated form. (*See also* Mesalamine and Its Derivatives.)

■ REFERENCES

1. Pinson JB, Weart CW. Antacid products, H$_2$-receptor antagonists, antireflux and anti-flatulence products. In Covington TR et al., eds. *Handbook of nonprescription drugs,* 11th ed. Washington, DC: American Pharmaceutical Association; 1996.
2. Soll AH. Gastric, duodenal, and stress ulcer. In Sleisenger MH et al., eds. *Gastrointestinal disease. Pathophysiology, diagnosis, management,* 5th ed. Philadelphia: WB Saunders; 1993.
3. Smythe MA, Zarowitz BJ. Changing perspectives of stress gastritis prophylaxis. *Ann Pharmacother* 1994;28:1073–85.
4. Food and Nutrition Board, NRC. *Recommended dietary allowances,* 10th ed. Washington, DC: National Academy Press; 1989.
5. Reinhart RA. Magnesium metabolism: a review with special reference to the relationship between intracellular content and serum levels. *Arch Intern Med* 1988;148:2415–20.
6. Marshall BJ. The use of bismuth in gastroenterology. *Am J Gastroenterol* 1991;86:16–25.
7. Anon. Drugs for treatment of peptic ulcers. *Med Lett Drugs Ther* 1994;36:65–7.
8. Feldman M, Burton ME. Histamine$_2$-receptor antagonists. Standard therapy for acid-peptic diseases (Part I). *N Engl J Med* 1990;323:1672–80.
9. Feldman M, Burton ME. Histamine$_2$-receptor antagonists. Standard therapy for acid-peptic diseases (Part II). *N Engl J Med* 1990;323:1749–55.
10. Lipsy RJ et al. Clinical review of histamine$_2$-receptor antagonists. *Arch Intern Med* 1990;150:745–51.
11. Navab F, Steingrub J. Stress ulcer: is routine prophylaxis necessary? *Am J Gastroenterol* 1995;90:708–12.
12. Amsden GW et al. Pharmacodynamics of bolus famotidine versus infused cimetidine, ranitidine, and famotidine. *J Clin Pharmacol* 1994;34:1191–8.
13. Chhattriwalla Y et al. The use of cimetidine in the newborn. *Pediatrics* 1980;65:301–2.
14. Dimand RJ. Use of H$_2$-receptor antagonists in children. *DICP* 1990;24(suppl):S42–6.
15. Treem WR et al. Suppression of gastric acid secretion by intravenous administration of famotidine in children. *J Pediatr* 1991;118:812–6.
16. Gladziwa U, Klotz U. Pharmacokinetic optimisation of the treatment of peptic ulcer in patients with renal failure. *Clin Pharmacokinet* 1994;27:393–408.
17. Lauritsen K et al. Clinical pharmacokinetics of drugs used in the treatment of gastrointestinal diseases (Part I). *Clin Pharmacokinet* 1990;19:11–31.
18. Lauritsen K et al. Clinical pharmacokinetics of drugs used in the treatment of gastrointestinal disease (Part II). *Clin Pharmacokinet* 1990;19:94–125.
19. Smallwood RA. Safety of acid-suppressing drugs. *Dig Dis Sci* 1995;40(suppl):63S–80.
20. Wagner BKJ et al. Famotidine pharmacokinetics in patients undergoing cardiac surgery. *Drug Invest* 1994;8:271–7.
21. McCloy RF et al. Pathophysiological effects of long-term acid suppression in man. *Dig Dis Sci* 1995;40(suppl):96S–120.

22. Welage LS, Berardi RR. Drug interactions with antiulcer agents: considerations in the treatment of acid-peptic disease. *J Pharm Pract* 1994;7:177–95.

23. Taha AS et al. Famotidine for the prevention of gastric and duodenal ulcers caused by nonsteroidal antiinflammatory drugs. *N Engl J Med* 1996;334:1435–9.

24. Loeb DS et al. Management of gastroduodenopathy associated with use of nonsteroidal anti-inflammatory drugs. *Mayo Clin Proc* 1992;67:354–64.

25. Berardi RR, Dunn-Kucharski VA. Omeprazole: defining its role in gastroesophageal reflux disease. *Hosp Formul* 1995;30:216–25.

26. Spencer CM, Faulds D. Lansoprazole. A reappraisal of its pharmacodynamic and pharmacokinetic properties, and its therapeutic efficacy in acid-related disorders. *Drugs* 1994;48:404–30.

27. Takemoto T, Hunt RH, eds. Suppression of acid secretion by lansoprazole and its effects on *Helicobacter pylori*. *J Clin Gastroenterol* 1995;20(suppl 1):S1–51.

28. Wilde MI, McTavish D. Omeprazole. An update of its pharmacology and therapeutic use in acid-related disorders. *Drugs* 1994;48:91–132.

29. Berardi RR, Welage LS. Current status of gastric proton pump inhibitors in the treatment of acid-peptic disease. *J Pharm Pract* 1994;7:165–76.

30. Maton PN. Omeprazole. *N Engl J Med* 1991;324:965–75.

31. Jensen RT, Fraker DL. Zollinger-Ellison syndrome. Advances in treatment of gastric hypersecretion and the gastrinoma. *JAMA* 1994;271:1429–35.

32. Petersen K-U. Review article: omeprazole and the cytochrome P450 system. *Aliment Pharmacol Ther* 1995;9:1–9.

33. Garnett WR. Efficacy, safety, and cost issues in managing patients with gastroesophageal reflux disease. *Am J Hosp Pharm* 1993;50(suppl 1):S11–8.

34. McCarthy DM. Sucralfate. *N Engl J Med* 1991;325:1017–25.

35. Jensen SL, Jensen PF. Role of sucralfate in peptic disease. *Dig Dis* 1992;10:153–61.

36. Ben-Menachem T et al. Prophylaxis for stress-related gastric hemorrhage in the medical intensive care unit. A randomized, controlled, single-blind study. *Ann Intern Med* 1994;121:568–75.

37. *USP-DI*, Vol I. Rockville, MD. The United States Pharmacopoeal Convention, 1996.

38. Ballinger A. Cytoprotection with misoprostol: use in the treatment and prevention of ulcers. *Dig Dis* 1994;12:37–45.

39. Raskin JB et al. Misoprostol dosage in the prevention of nonsteroidal anti-inflammatory drug-induced gastric and duodenal ulcers: a comparison of three regimens. *Ann Intern Med* 1995;123:344–50.

40. Silverstein FE et al. Misoprostol reduces serious gastrointestinal complications in patients with rheumatoid arthritis receiving nonsteroidal anti-inflammatory drugs: a randomized, double-blind, placebo-controlled trial. *Ann Intern Med* 1995;123:241–9.

41. Stucki G et al. Is misoprostol cost-effective in the prevention of nonsteroidal anti-inflammatory drug-induced gastropathy in patients with chronic arthritis? A review of conflicting economic evaluations. *Arch Intern Med* 1994;154:2020–5.

42. NIH Consensus Development Panel on *Helicobacter pylori* in Peptic Ulcer Disease. *JAMA* 1994;272:65–9.

43. Soll AH. Medical treatment of peptic ulcer disease: practice guidelines. *JAMA* 1996;275:622–9.

44. Graham KS et al. Variability with omeprazole-amoxicillin combinations for treatment of *Helicobacter pylori* infection. *Am J Gastroenterol* 1995;90:1415–7.

45. Walsh JH, Peterson WL. The treatment of *Helicobacter pylori* infection in the management of peptic ulcer disease. *N Engl J Med* 1995;33:984–91.

46. Fennerty MB, Melnyk CS. *Helicobacter pylori*: review of triple, dual, 7-day, and other treatment strategies. *Formulary* 1995;30:682–8.

47. Marshall BJ. *Helicobacter pylori*. *Am J Gastroenterol* 1994;89:S116–28.

48. Markaham A, McTavish D. Clarithromycin and omeprazole: as *Helicobacter pylori* eradication therapy in patients with *H. pylori*–associated gastric disorders. *Drugs* 1996;51:161–78.

49. de Boer WA et al. Randomized study comparing 1 with 2 weeks of quadruple therapy for eradicating *Helicobacter pylori*. *Am J Gastroenterol* 1994;89:1993–7.

50. Bayerdorffer E et al. Double-blind trial of omeprazole and amoxicillin to cure *Helicobacter pylori* infection in patients with duodenal ulcers. *Gastroenterology* 1995;108:1412–7.

51. Al-Assi MT et al. Azithromycin triple therapy for *Helicobacter pylori* infection: azithromycin, tetracycline, and bismuth. *Am J Gastroenterol* 1995;90:403–5.

52. Sonnenberg A, Townsend WF. Costs of duodenal ulcer therapy with antibiotics. *Arch Intern Med* 1995;155:922–8.

53. Lemberger L et al. Delta-9-tetrahydrocannabinol. Temporal correlation of the psychologic effects and blood levels after various routes of administration. *N Engl J Med* 1972;286:685–8.

54. Hollister LE et al. Do plasma concentrations of Δ⁹-tetrahydrocannabinol reflect the degree of intoxication? *J Clin Pharmacol* 1981;21:171S–7S.

55. Benet LZ et al. Design and optimization of dosage regimens; pharmacokinetic data. In Hardman JG et al., eds. *Goodman and Gilman's the pharmacological basis of therapeutics*, 9th ed. New York: McGraw-Hill; 1996:1707–92.

56. Wall ME et al. Metabolism, disposition, and kinetics of delta-9-tetrahydrocannabinol in men and women. *Clin Pharmacol Ther* 1983;34:352–63.

57. Agurell S et al. Pharmacokinetics and metabolism of Δ¹-tetrahydrocannabinol and other cannabinoids with emphasis in man. *Pharmacol Rev* 1986;38:21–43.

58. Devine ML et al. Adverse reactions to delta-9-tetrahydrocannabinol given as an antiemetic in a multicenter study. *Clin Pharm* 1987;6:319–22.

59. Anon. Synthetic marijuana for nausea and vomiting due to cancer chemotherapy. *Med Lett Drugs Ther* 1985;27:97–8.

60. Bakowski MT. Advances in anti-emetic therapy. *Cancer Treat Rev* 1984;11:237–56.

61. Gralla RJ et al. Antiemetic therapy: a review of recent studies and a report of a random assignment trial comparing metoclopramide with delta-9-tetrahydrocannabinol. *Cancer Treat Rep* 1984;68:163–72.

62. Colthup PV, Palmer JL. The determination in plasma and pharmacokinetics of ondansetron. *Eur J Cancer Clin Oncol* 1989;25(suppl 1):S71–4.

63. Adams VR, Valley AW. Granisetron: the second serotonin-receptor antagonist. *Ann Pharmacother* 1995;29:1240–51.

64. Beck TM et al. Stratified, randomized, double-blind comparison of intravenous ondansetron administered as a multiple-dose regimen versus two single-dose regimens in the prevention of cisplatin-induced nausea and vomiting. *J Clin Oncol* 1992;10:1969–75.

65. Blackwell CP, Harding SM. The clinical pharmacology of ondansetron. *Eur J Cancer Clin Oncol* 1989;25(suppl 1):S21–4.

66. Hesketh PJ et al. GR 38032F (GR-C507/75): a novel compound effective in the prevention of acute cisplatin-induced emesis. *J Clin Oncol* 1989;7:700–5.

67. Grunberg SM et al. Dose ranging phase I study of the serotonin antagonist GR38032F for prevention of cisplatin-induced nausea and vomiting. *J Clin Oncol* 1989;7:1137–41.

68. Marty M et al. Comparison of the 5-hydroxytryptamine₃ (serotonin) antagonist ondansetron (GR 38032F) with high-dose metoclopramide in the control of cisplatin-induced emesis. *N Engl J Med* 1990;322:816–21.

69. Chaffee BJ, Tankanow RM. Ondansetron—the first of a new class of antiemetic agents. *Clin Pharm* 1991;10:430–46.

70. Vozeh S et al. Pharmacokinetic drug data. *Clin Pharmacokinet* 1988;15:254–82.

71. Covington TR et al., eds. *Handbook of nonprescription drugs*, 11th ed. Washington, DC: American Pharmaceutical Association; 1996.

72. Jinks MJ, Fuerst RH. Geriatric therapy. In Koda-Kimble MA, Young LY, eds. *Applied therapeutics: the clinical use of drugs*, 5th ed. Vancouver, WA: Applied Therapeutics; 1992:79-1–19.

73. Anon. Laxative drug products for over-the-counter human use; tentative final monograph. *Fed Regist* 1985;50:2124–58.

74. Brunton LL. Agents affecting gastrointestinal water flux and motility; emesis and antiemetics; bile acids and pancreatic enzymes. In Hardman JG et al., eds. *Goodman and Gilman's the pharmacological basis of therapeutics*, 9th ed. New York: McGraw-Hill; 1996:917–36.

75. Adams WJ et al. Bisacodyl reduces the volume of polyethylene glycol solution required for bowel preparation. *Dis Colon Rectum* 1994;37:229–33.

76. Wiseman LR, Faulds D. Cisapride. An updated review of its pharmacology and therapeutic efficacy as a prokinetic agent in gastrointestinal motility disorders. *Drugs* 1994;47:116–52.

77. Barone JA et al. Cisapride: a gastrointestinal prokinetic drug. *Ann Pharmacother* 1994;28:488–500.

78. McCallum RW. Cisapride: a new class of prokinetic agent. *Am J Gastroenterol* 1991;86:135–49.

79. Gladziwa U et al. Pharmacokinetics and pharmacodynamics of cisapride in patients undergoing hemodialysis. *Clin Pharmacol Ther* 1991;50:673–81.

80. Boyd IW, Rohan AP. Urinary disorders associated with cisapride. *Med J Aust* 1994;160:579–80.

81. Karim A et al. Pharmacokinetics and metabolism of diphenoxylate in man. *Clin Pharmacol Ther* 1972;13:407–19.

82. Jackson LS, Stafford JE. The evaluation and application of a radioimmunoassay for the measurement of diphenoxylic acid, the major metabolite of diphenoxylate hydrochloride (Lomotil), in human plasma. *J Pharmacol Methods* 1987;18:189–97.

83. Gattuso JM, Kamm MA. Adverse effects of drugs used in the management of constipation and diarrhoea. *Drug Saf* 1994;10:47–65.

84. Wolfe MS. Acute diarrhea associated with travel. *Am J Med* 1990;88(suppl 6A):34–7.

85. DuPont HL. Travellers' diarrhoea. Which antimicrobial? *Drugs* 1993;45:910–7.

86. Anon. The safety of stool softeners. *Med Lett Drugs Ther* 1977;19:45–6.

87. Pietrusko RG. Use and abuse of laxatives. *Am J Hosp Pharm* 1977;34:291–300.

88. Castle SC et al. Constipation prevention: empiric use of stool softeners questioned. *Geriatrics* 1991;46:84–6.

89. Fraser CL, Arlieff AI. Hepatic encephalopathy. *N Engl J Med* 1985;313:865–73.

90. Crossley IR, Williams R. Progress in the treatment of chronic portasystemic encephalopathy. *Gut* 1984;25:85–98.

91. Kot TV, Pettit-Young NA. Lactulose in the management of constipation: a current review. *Ann Pharmacother* 1992;26:1277–82.

92. Nelson DC et al. Hypernatremia and lactulose therapy. *JAMA* 1983;249:1295–8.

93. Anon. Lactulose (Chronulac) for constipation. *Med Lett Drugs Ther* 1980;22:2–4.

94. Lederle FA et al. Cost-effective treatment of constipation in the elderly: a randomized double-blind comparison of sorbitol and lactulose. *Am J Med* 1990;89:597–601.

95. Killinger JM et al. Human pharmacokinetics and comparative bioavailability of loperamide hydrochloride. *J Clin Pharmacol* 1979;19:211–8.

96. Ericsson CD, Johnson PC. Safety and efficacy of loperamide. *Am J Med* 1990;88(suppl 6A):10–4.

97. Drenth JPH, Engels LGJB. Diabetic gastroparesis. A critical reappraisal of new treatment strategies. *Drugs* 1992;44:537–53.

98. Reynolds JC, Putnam PE. Prokinetic agents. *Gastroenterol Clin North Am* 1992;21:567–96.

99. DuBois A. Gastroparesis, nausea, and vomiting. In Lewis JH, ed. *A pharmacologic approach to gastrointestinal disorders.* Baltimore: Williams & Wilkins; 1994:131–62.

100. Anderson PO, Valdés V. Increasing breast milk supply. *Clin Pharm* 1993;12:479–80.

101. Lewis JH. Hiccups: reasons and remedies. In Lewis JH, ed. *A pharmacologic approach to gastrointestinal disorders.* Baltimore: Williams & Wilkins; 1994:209–27.

102. Brown CK, Khanderia U. Use of metoclopramide, domperidone, and cisapride in the management of diabetic gastroparesis. *Clin Pharm* 1990;9:357–65.

103. Stewart RB et al. Metoclopramide: an analysis of inappropriate long-term use in the elderly. *Ann Pharmacother* 1992;26:977–9.

104. Kreek MJ, Culpepper-Morgan JA. Constipation syndromes. In Lewis JH, ed. *A pharmacologic approach to gastrointestinal disorders.* Baltimore: Williams & Wilkins; 1994:179–208.

105. Weber FH, et al. Erythromycin: a motilin agonist and gastrointestinal prokinetic agent. *Am J Gastroenterol* 1993;88:485–90.

106. Peeters TL. Erythromycin and other macrolides as prokinetic agents. *Gastroenterology* 1993;105:1886–99.

107. Lartey PA et al. New developments in macrolides: structures and antibacterial and prokinetic activities. *Adv Pharmacol* 1994;28:307–43.

108. DiPalma JA, Brady CE. Colon cleansing for diagnostic and surgical procedures: polyethylene glycol-electrolyte lavage solution. *Am J Gastroenterol* 1989;84:1008–16.

109. Goodale EP, Noble TA. Pediatric bowel evacuation with a polyethylene glycol and iso-osmolar electrolyte solution. *DICP* 1990;23:1008–9.

110. Fordtran JS et al. A low-sodium solution for gastrointestinal lavage. *Gastroenterology* 1990;98:11–6.

111. Tenenbein M. Whole bowel irrigation as a gastrointestinal decontamination procedure after acute poisoning. *Med Toxicol Adv Drug Exp* 1988;3:77–84.

112. Glore SR et al. Soluble fiber and serum lipids: a literature review. *J Am Diet Assoc* 1994;94:425–36.

113. Chan EK, Schroeder DJ. Psyllium in hypercholesterolemia. *Ann Pharmacother* 1995;29:625–6.

114. Tedesko FJ et al. Laxative use in constipation. *Am J Gastroenterol* 1985;80:303–9.

115. Freeman GL. Psyllium hypersensitivity. *Ann Allergy* 1994;73:490–2.

116. Cooney DO. *Activated charcoal in medical applications.* New York: Marcel Dekker; 1995.

117. Palatnick W, Tennenbein M. Activated charcoal in the treatment of drug overdose. *Drug Saf* 1992;7:3–7.

118. Paumgartner G et al. Ursodeoxycholic acid treatment of cholesterol gallstone disease. *Scand J Gastroenterol* 1994;29(suppl 204):27–31.

119. Strandvik B, Lindblad A. Cystic fibrosis. Is treatment with ursodeoxycholic acid of value? *Scand J Gastroenterol* 1994;29(suppl 204):65–7.

120. Leuschner U. Ursodeoxycholic acid therapy in primary biliary cirrhosis. *Scand J Gastroenterol* 1994;29(suppl 204):40–6.

121. Krasman ML et al. Biliary tract disease in the aged. *Clin Geriatr Med* 1991;7:347–70.

122. Rubin RA et al. Ursodiol for hepatobiliary disorders. *Ann Intern Med* 1994;121:207–18.

123. Plaisier PW et al. Dissolution of gallstones. *Dig Dis* 1993;11:181–8.

124. Broughton G II. Chenodeoxycholate: the bile acid. The drug. A review. *Am J Med Sci* 1994;307:54–63.

125. Johnson CE, Nesbitt J. Stability of ursodiol in an extemporaneously compounded oral liquid. *Am J Health-Syst Pharm* 1995;52:1798–800.

126. Shiffman ML et al. Prophylaxis against gallstone formation with ursodeoxycholic acid in patients participating in a very-low-calorie diet program. *Ann Intern Med* 1995;122:899–905.

127. Sackmann M et al. The Munich gallbladder lithotripsy study. *Ann Intern Med* 1991;114:290–6.

128. Small RE, Schraa CC. Chemistry, pharmacology, pharmacokinetics, and clinical applications of mesalamine for the treatment of inflammatory bowel disease. *Pharmacotherapy* 1994;14:385–98.

129. Segars LW, Gales BJ. Mesalamine and olsalazine: 5-aminosalicylic acid agents for the treatment of inflammatory bowel disease. *Clin Pharm* 1992;11:514–28.

130. Hanauer SB. Inflammatory bowel disease. *N Engl J Med* 1996;334:841–8.

131. Peppercorn MA. Antiinflammatory agents. In Targan SR, Shanahan F, eds. *Inflammatory bowel disease: from bench to bedside.* Baltimore: Williams & Wilkins; 1994.

132. Zarling EJ, Sedghi S. Current and promising new therapies for inflammatory bowel disease. *Hosp Formul* 1993;28:466–85.

133. Wadworth AN, Fitton A. Olsalazine. A review of its pharmacodynamic and pharmacokinetic properties, and therapeutic potential in inflammatory bowel disease. *Drugs* 1991;41:647–64.

134. Sutherland LR et al. Sulfasalazine revisited: a meta-analysis of 5-aminosalicylic acid in the treatment of ulcerative colitis. *Ann Intern Med* 1993;118:540–9.

135. Brignola C et al. Mesalamine in the prevention of endoscopic recurrence after intestinal resection for Crohn's disease. *Gastroenterology* 1995;108:345–9.

136. Singleton JW et al. Quality-of-life results of double-blind, placebo-controlled trial of mesalamine in patients with Crohn's disease. *Dig Dis Sci* 1995;40:931–5.

137. Mosdell KW, Visconti JA. Emerging indications for octreotide therapy (part 1). *Am J Hosp Pharm* 1994;51:1184–92.

138. Tauber MT et al. Clinical use of the long acting somatostatin analogue octreotide in pediatrics. *Eur J Pediatr* 1994;153:304–10.

139. Colon AR. Drug therapy in pediatric gastrointestinal disease. In Lewis JH, ed. *A pharmacologic approach to gastrointestinal disorders.* Baltimore: Williams & Wilkins; 1994:519–34.

140. Harris AG. Somatostatin and somatostatin analogues: pharmacokinetics and pharmacodynamic effects. *Gut* 1994;35(suppl 3):S1–4.

141. Lamberts SWJ et al. Octreotide. *N Engl J Med* 1996;334:246–54.

142. Mosdell KW, Visconti JA. Emerging indications for octreotide therapy (part 2). *Am J Hosp Pharm* 1994;51:1317–30.

143. Ripley RG et al. Stability of octreotide acetate in polypropylene syringes at 5 and 20°C. *Am J Health-Syst Pharm* 1995;52:1910–1.

144. Laasila K, Leirisalo-Repo M. Side effects of sulphasalazine in patients with rheumatic diseases or inflammatory bowel disease. *Scand J Rheumatol* 1994;23:338–400.

Hematologic Drugs

Coagulants and Anticoagulants

ALTEPLASE
Activase

Pharmacology. Alteplase (recombinant tissue-type plasminogen activator; rt-PA) is a 1-chain tissue plasminogen activator (fibrinolytic) produced by recombinant DNA technology. It has a high affinity for fibrin-bound plasminogen, allowing activation on the fibrin surface. Most plasmin formed remains bound to the fibrin clot, minimizing systemic effects.[1-3]

Administration and Adult Dosage. **Accelerated IV infusion for post-MI clot lysis (preferred)** 15 mg as a bolus, followed by 0.75 mg/kg (up to 50 mg) over 30 min, then 0.5 mg/kg (up to 35 mg) over the next 60 min. Start heparin infusion (to an aPTT of 1.5–2.0 times control) with or upon completion of the alteplase infusion and continue for at least 48 hr.[5] *See* Notes. **Alternatively, IV infusion for post-MI clot lysis** 60 mg over 1 hr (6–10 mg in the first 1–2 min), then 20 mg/hr for 2 hr to a total of 100 mg (for patients <65 kg, administer a dose of 1.25 mg/kg over 3 hr). Begin as soon as possible after acute MI symptoms. Adjunctive heparin is also recommended.[2,4,5] **IV infusion for pulmonary embolism** 100 mg over 2 hr. Institute heparin infusion immediately following alteplase infusion when the aPTT or thrombin time returns to two times normal. Alternatively, 0.6 mg/kg as a single dose over 2 min in addition to heparin infusion has been used successfully.[6] **IV infusion for acute ischemic stroke** 0.9 mg/kg, to a maximum of 90 mg; give 10% initially as a bolus, with the remainder given over the next 60 min. Avoid anticoagulants or antiplatelet drugs for 24 hr after treatment.[7,8]

Special Populations. *Pediatric Dosage.* Safety and efficacy not established.

Geriatric Dosage. Same as adult dosage.

Dosage Forms. Inj 20, 50, 100 mg.

Pharmacokinetics. *Onset and Duration.* Duration is several hours because of binding with fibrin. However, rethrombosis after reperfusion appears to be inversely proportional to serum half-life.[2]

Fate. There is rapid uptake by hepatocytes and fibrin binding. V_c is 3.8–6.6 L and $V_{d\beta}$ is 0.1 ± 0.01 L/kg; Cl is 0.6 ± 0.24 L/hr/kg.[2,9]

$t_{1/2}$. α phase 4.8 ± 2.4 min; β 26 ± 10 min.[9]

Adverse Reactions. Bleeding from GI and GU tracts and ecchymoses occur frequently. Retroperitoneal or gingival bleeding or epistaxis occur occasionally. Superficial bleeding from trauma sites may also occur. The overall risk of intracranial hemorrhage is 0.1–0.75%.[7] In ISIS-3 the rates for definite or possible cerebral bleed were as follows: rt-PA (deuteplase, a two-chain form of alteplase), 0.5%; streptokinase, 0.2%; anistreplase, 0.7%.[10] Independent risk factors for thrombolytic-induced intracranial hemorrhage with alteplase include age >65 yr, body weight <70 kg, and hypertension on hospitalization.[5]

Contraindications. Active internal bleeding; history of CVA; recent (within 2 months) intracranial or intraspinal surgery or trauma; intracranial neoplasm, AV malformation, or aneurysm; bleeding diathesis; severe uncontrolled hypertension.

Precautions. Use with caution in the following: pregnancy; recent (within 10 days) major surgery, trauma, GI or GU bleeding; cerebrovascular disease; systolic blood pressure of 180 mm Hg or above, diastolic of 110 mm Hg or above; high likelihood of left heart thrombus; acute pericarditis; subacute bacterial endocarditis; hemostatic defects; significant liver dysfunction; septic thrombophlebitis; age >75 yr; concurrent oral anticoagulants. Avoid IM injections and noncompressible arterial punctures; minimize arterial and venous punctures and excessive patient handling. Stop immediately if severe bleeding or anaphylactoid reaction occurs.

Drug Interactions. Preliminary data from a nonrandomized study suggest that concurrent IV nitroglycerin therapy may impair the thrombolytic effect of alteplase in acute MI.[11] Anticoagulants or antiplatelet drugs may increase the risk of bleeding.

Parameters to Monitor. For short-term thrombolytic therapy of MI, laboratory monitoring is of little value. No correlation has been made between clotting test results and likelihood of hemorrhage or efficacy.[2]

Notes. Other than cerebral hemorrhage, no clear differences in bleeding risk have been observed with the various thrombolytics.[2,5] Data from the ISIS-3 trial show the 5-week mortality for **duteplase, streptokinase,** and **anistreplase** to be virtually identical.[10] Based on the GUSTO trial, some investigators suggest that the accelerated alteplase regimen be used for patients <75 yr with anterior or large infarctions presenting within 4 hr of symptoms. The absolute survival advantage over streptokinase was 0.9%, representing a 14% risk reduction.[4,13]

ANISTREPLASE
Eminase

Anistreplase (anisoylated plasminogen-streptokinase activator complex; APSAC) is an acylated form of the streptokinase-plasminogen complex that is temporarily inactive. After deacylation, the streptokinase-plasminogen complex promotes thrombolysis by converting plasminogen to the proteolytic enzyme plasmin. Thrombolysis occurs through the action of plasmin on fibrin. Deacylation and thrombolysis begin immediately after injection. Duration of fibrinolytic activity is 4–6 hr. Anistreplase undergoes deacylation and local inactivation in the circulation by inhibitor complex formation and proteolysis, and to a lesser extent is metabolized rapidly by the liver. V_d is 0.084 ± 0.027 L/kg, with a Cl of 0.055 ± 0.02 L/hr/kg and half-life of 1.2 ± 0.4 hr. Data from ISIS-3 indicate that bleeding was slightly more common with anistreplase than with streptokinase or rt-PA; however, major bleeding rates were similar. In ISIS-3 the rates for definite or possible cerebral bleeding were as follows: anistreplase, 0.7%; streptokinase, 0.2%; rt-PA (deutoplase, a two-chain form of alteplase), 0.5%.[10] Allergic reactions similar to those reported with streptokinase include rash, erythema, bronchoconstriction, and, rarely, anaphylaxis. Precautions and monitoring parameters are the same as for streptokinase. Adjunctive IV heparin is associated with higher bleeding rates than aspirin alone in anistreplase-treated patients and offers no additional improvement in outcome. Ease of administration (30 units given over 2–5 minutes as a single IV injection) is a potential advantage of anistreplase for the emergent treatment of acute MI in some settings (eg, in the field). However, anistreplase is more expensive than streptokinase, has the same allergy profile, offers no efficacy advantage, and is potentially associated with a slightly higher bleeding risk.[5,7,9,14–16] Available as a 30-unit lyophilized vial for injection.

ENOXAPARIN SODIUM   Lovenox

Enoxaparin is a low molecular weight heparin (average 3500–5500 daltons) prepared by depolymerization of unfractionated porcine intestinal mucosal heparin. Like unfractionated heparin, enoxaparin binds with antithrombin III, accelerating the rate at which antithrombin III neutralizes several activated clotting factors. However, enoxaparin has many biologic properties that differ from heparin's: enoxaparin has a higher ratio of antifactor Xa to antifactor IIa activity (about 3.3:1 vs 1:1), reduced interactions with platelets, and less lipoprotein-lipase-releasing activity. Enoxaparin also has a lower affinity for heparin cofactor II, platelet factor 4, von Willebrand factor (VIIIR), and vascular endothelium. Mean bioavailability following SC injection is about 92%. V_d is 0.12 ± 0.04 L/kg; Cl is 0.018 ± 0.006 L/hr/kg; half-life is 3.8 ± 1.3 hr, increased in uremia. Activity against factor Xa persists for about 12 hr following a 40-mg SC injection. At recommended doses, single injections do not markedly affect platelet aggregation, prothrombin time, or aPTT. A number of clinical trials indicate that enoxaparin is more effective than placebo or heparin for DVT prophylaxis in patients undergoing hip replacement, and better than placebo in total knee replacement. Enoxaparin and other low molecular weight heparins have also been demonstrated to be safe and effective in the treatment of active DVT. In a large multicenter trial comparing enoxaparin 1 mg/kg SC q 12 hr with standard heparin infusion, recurrent thromboembolic rates were 5.3% and 6.7%, respectively. In hip replacement surgery, major bleeding has occurred in 4% of enoxaparin-treated patients and in 6% of heparin-treated patients. Overall, rates of major and minor bleeding complications in comparative studies with heparin have been similar. Thrombocytopenia, fever, pain on injection, asymptomatic increases in transaminase levels, hypochromic anemia, and edema occur frequently. Skin necrosis is observed occasionally. CBCs, including platelet count and stool for occult blood, are recommended periodically during enoxaparin treatment; aPTT monitoring is not required. Use enoxaparin with extreme caution in patients with a history of heparin-induced thrombocytopenia (in vitro platelet testing is recommended). Enoxaparin is indicated for the prevention of DVT following hip or knee replacement or abdominal surgery. The adult dosage is (hip or knee replacement) 30 mg SC q 12 hr for an average of 7–10 days or (abdominal surgery) 40 mg SC daily.[17–21] Available as 30 mg/0.3 mL and 40 mg/0.4 mL prefilled syringes.

LOW MOLECULAR WEIGHT HEPARINS COMPARISON CHART

DRUG	DOSAGE FORMS	ADULT DOSAGE	AVERAGE MASS (DALTONS)	AF-Xa[a] (IU/MG)	AF-Xa/AF-IIa[b] RATIO	HALF-LIFE (HR)
Ardeparin Normiflo	Inj 5000, 10,000 units.	SC for DVT prophylaxis 50 units/kg q 12 hr.	5500–6500	100	—	3.3
Dalteparin Fragmin	Inj 2500, 5000 IU/ 0.2 mL.	SC for DVT prophylaxis 2500–5000 IU/day SC for DVT treatment 120 IU/kg bid.	4000–6000	160	2:1	2.8–4
Danaparoid[c] Orgaran	Inj 750 units/0.6 mL.	SC for DVT prophylaxis 750 IU SC for DVT treatment 2000 IU q 12 hr.	6500	—	20:1	18.3
Enoxaparin Lovenox	Inj 30 mg/0.3 mL.	SC for DVT prophylaxis 30 mg bid[d] SC for DVT treatment 1 mg/kg q 12 hr.[e]	3500–5500	100	2.7:1	3.5–5.9
Nadroparin Fraxiparin (Investigational, Sanofi)	—	SC for DVT prophylaxis 4400 IU once daily SC for DVT treatment 90–92 IU/kg bid.	4500	85	3.2:1	2.3–5.6

(continued)

LOW MOLECULAR WEIGHT HEPARINS COMPARISON CHART

DRUG	DOSAGE FORMS	ADULT DOSAGE	AVERAGE MASS (DALTONS)	AF-Xa[a] (IU/MG)	AF-Xa/AF-IIa[b] RATIO	HALF-LIFE (HR)
Tinzaparin Logiparin (Investigational, Novo)	—	SC for DVT prophylaxis 50–75 IU/kg once daily SC for DVT treatment 175 IU/kg once daily.	4900	86	1.9:1	1.85

[a]Antifactor Xa activity.
[b]Antifactor Xa to antifactor II ratio.
[c]A heparinoid; mixture of low molecular weight sulfated glycosaminoglycans: heparan sulfate (84%), dermatan sulfate (12%), and chondroitin sulfate (4%).
[d]Equivalent to 30 mg bid SC.
[e]Equivalent to 1 mg/kg q 12 hr SC.
From references 2, 17, 18, 20, 22, and 23.

HEPARIN SODIUM   Various

Pharmacology. A heterogeneous, unfractionated group of mucopolysaccharides derived from the mast cells of animal tissues. It binds with antithrombin III, accelerating the rate at which antithrombin III neutralizes *activated forms* of factors XII, XI, IX, X, VII, and II. It is active in vitro and in vivo.

Administration and Adult Dosage. Express dosage in units only; dosage must be individually titrated to desired effect (usually 1.5–2.5 times aPTT).[1,5,24] Weight-based nomogram and computer-assisted dosage of heparin are effective, safe, and superior to "standard care" or empiric approaches.[25–27] **IV for thrombophlebitis or pulmonary embolus** (continuous infusion) 50–100 units/kg initially, then 15–25 units/hr/kg; alternatively, 5000 units initially, then 1000 units/hr; (intermittent) 75–125 units/kg q 4 hr.[1,5,24,28] Duration of therapy for thrombophlebitis or pulmonary embolus is 7–10 days, followed by oral anticoagulation (preferably initiated during the first 24 hr of heparin therapy).[24,29] A 5-day course of heparin has been shown to be as effective as a 10-day course in treating deep vein thrombosis.[30] **SC for thrombophlebitis or pulmonary embolus** 10,000–20,000 units initially (preceded by a 5000-unit IV loading dose), then 8000–10,000 units q 8 hr or 15,000–20,000 units q 12 hr. **SC for prophylaxis of deep vein thrombosis (low-dose)** 5000 units 2 hr before surgery, repeated q 8–12 hr for 5–7 days or until patient is ambulatory.[31] **IV for heparin lock flush** inject sufficient solution (of 10 or 100 units/mL) into injection hub to fill the entire set after each heparin lock use. Some institutions reserve the 100 units/mL solution for flushing triple lumen central catheters and use NS for all other catheters.

Special Populations. *Pediatric Dosage.* Same as adult dosage in units/kg.

Geriatric Dosage. Same as adult dosage.

Other Conditions. Patients with pulmonary embolus may require larger heparin doses than patients with thrombophlebitis (*see* Administration and Adult Dosage).[28] Patients with severe renal dysfunction may require lower dosages.[2] There is no good evidence that liver disease markedly affects dosage requirements.

Dosage Forms. **Inj** 1000, 2500, 5000, 7500, 10,000, 15,000, 20,000, 40,000 units/mL; 2, 40, 50, 100 units/mL (prediluted); **Heparin Lock Flush** 10, 100 units/mL.

Patient Instructions. This drug is potentially harmful when taken with nonprescription or prescription drugs. Consult your physician or pharmacist when considering the use of other medications, particularly aspirin-containing products.

Pharmacokinetics. *Onset and Duration.* Onset immediate after IV administration.

Serum Levels. The relationship between heparin serum concentrations and aPTT response may vary between reagents and reagent lots. It is recommended that each laboratory establish a therapeutic aPTT range corresponding to heparin serum concentrations of 0.2–0.4 units/mL using protamine titration.[2] Circadian variation in heparin activity may occur, and aPTT response may vary during the day at a given infusion rate.[32]

Fate. SC bioavailability is 20–40% and is dose dependent.[2] There is no biotransformation in plasma or liver; transfer and storage in reticuloendothelial cells has been suggested.[24,33] V_d is 0.058 ± 0.011 L/kg (approximates plasma volume).[9] Cl is dose dependent; Cl may be increased in pulmonary embolus, but this has not been a consistent finding.[24]

$t_{1/2}$. (Pharmacologic) 90 ± 60 min, dose-related; higher doses lead to increased half-life; half-life may be decreased in pulmonary embolus, but this has not been a consistent finding.[24,28,33,34] Shorter half-life is also reported in smokers than in nonsmokers.[2]

Adverse Reactions. Bleeding occurs in 3–20% of patients receiving short-term, high-dose therapy.[24,35] Bleeding risk is increased by threefold when the aPTT is 2.0–2.9 and by eightfold when the aPTT is >3.0 times control.[24] Heparin administration by continuous IV infusion may cause a lower frequency of bleeding complications than intermittent IV administration.[24] Renal dysfunction, liver disease, and other factors (serious cardiac illness, malignancy, age >60 yr, and maximum aPTT greater than 2.2 times control) may increase bleeding risk.[2,33,35] (*See* Precautions.) Thrombocytopenia occurs frequently (usually 1–5%, although up to 30% is reported) and may be more common with heparin derived from bovine lung. However, recent studies suggest little difference and an overall decline in prevalence.[24,36,37] The decline may be related to improved manufacturing techniques and reduced therapy duration.[36] Osteoporosis and bone fractures occur rarely with doses of 15,000 units/day or more for longer than 5 months.[24] Rarely patients receiving prolonged therapy or with diabetes or renal dysfunction may develop marked hyperkalemia.[38]

Contraindications. Active bleeding; thrombocytopenia; threatened abortion; subacute bacterial endocarditis; suspected intracranial hemorrhage; regional or lumbar block anesthesia; severe hypotension; shock; and after eye, brain, or spinal cord surgery.

Precautions. Risk factors for hemorrhage may include IM injections, trauma, recent surgery, age >60 yr, malignancy, peptic ulcer disease, potential bleeding sites, and acquired or congenital hemostatic defects.[24]

Drug Interactions. Anticoagulants or antiplatelet drugs may increase risk of bleeding. Concurrent use with aspirin and other NSAIDs may increase the risk of bleeding.

Parameters to Monitor. Baseline aPTT, PT/INR, hematocrit, and platelet count. Obtain aPTT (therapeutic range 1.5–2.5 times control) 3 or 4 times (or until therapeutic range is achieved) on day 1, and at least daily thereafter. Monitor platelets and hematocrit every other day and signs of bleeding (melena, hematuria, ecchymoses, hematemesis, epistaxis) daily.[1,5,24]

PHYTONADIONE AquaMephyton, Konakion, Mephyton

Pharmacology. Vitamin K is a required cofactor for the hepatic microsomal enzyme system that carboxylates glutamyl residues in precursor proteins to γ-carboxyglutamyl residues. These proteins are present in vitamin K–dependent clotting factors (II, VII, IX, and X) and anticoagulation proteins (protein C and protein S), as well as bone (osteocalin), some plasma proteins (protein Z), and the protein of several organs (kidney, lung, and testicular tissue).[39–41]

Administration and Adult Dosage. The normal daily nutritional requirement is about 0.03–1.5 µg/kg.[40,42,43] The adult RDA is 70 µg/day for males 19–24 yr and 80 µg/day for males >25 yr; it is 60 µg/day for women 19–24 yr and 65 µg/day for women >25 yr.[44] **PO, SC, or IM to reverse bleeding** (Konakion may only be given IM) 2.5–10 mg up to 25 mg initially. A single dose of 1–5 mg is usually sufficient to normalize PT during anticoagulant therapy, but in the presence of severe bleeding, 20–50 mg may be needed.[40,44] The initial dose may be repeated, based on PT and clinical response, after 12–48 hr if given PO and 6–8 hr if given parenterally. Use the smallest dosage possible to reverse anticoagulants, to obviate possible refractoriness to further anticoagulant therapy.[40,46] Do not give AquaMephyton intravenously unless it is absolutely essential, and do not exceed an infusion rate of 1 mg/min. The drug may be diluted in preservative-free dextrose or saline solution just prior to use.

Special Populations. *Pediatric Dosage.* RDAs are (<6 months) 5 µg/day; (6 months–1 yr) 10 µg/day; (1–3 yr) 15 µg/day; (4–6 yr) 20 µg/day; (7–10 yr) 30 µg/day; (11–14 yr) 45 µg/day; (15–18 yr) 55 µg/day for females, 65 µg/day for males.[44] **IM for prophylaxis of hemorrhagic disease of the newborn** 0.5–1 mg within 1 hr of birth. **SC or IM for treatment of hemorrhagic disease of the newborn** 1 mg; more if mother has been receiving an oral anticoagulant.

Geriatric Dosage. (>55 yr) the RDA is 65 µg/day for females and 80 µg/day for males.[44]

Other Conditions. **PO for antenatal use in pregnant women receiving anticonvulsants** 20 mg/day throughout the last 4 weeks of pregnancy.[41]

Dosage Forms. **Tab** (Mephyton) 5 mg; **Inj** (AquaMephyton, Konakion) 2, 10 mg/mL.

Pharmacokinetics. *Onset and Duration.* Reversal of anticoagulant effect is variable among individuals; parenteral onset is often within 6 hr; peak and duration is variable among individuals and with dose. A 5-mg IV dose usually returns PT to normal in 24–48 hr.[45] Large doses may cause prolonged refractoriness to oral anticoagulants.[40,46]

Fate. Absorbed from the GI tract via intestinal lymphatics only in the presence of bile; well absorbed after parenteral administration. Metabolized in the liver to hydroquinone form, and epoxide form which are interconvertible with the quinone.[39] Little storage occurs in the body. In the absence of bile, hypoprothrombinemia develops over a period of several weeks.[40,46,47]

Adverse Reactions. The drug itself appears to be nontoxic; however, severe reactions (eg, flushing, dyspnea, chest pain) and occasionally deaths have occurred after IV administration of AquaMephyton, possibly caused by the emulsifying agents.[40,43,48] This product should rarely be used IV, and only when other routes of administration are not feasible. A transient flushing sensation, peculiar taste, and pain and swelling at the injection site may occur. Large parenteral doses in neonates have caused hyperbilirubinemia.

Contraindications. Konakion is contraindicated for other than IM use.

Precautions. Temporary refractoriness to oral anticoagulants may occur, especially with large doses of vitamin K. Reversal of anticoagulant activity may restore previous thromboembolic conditions. Either no effect or worsening of hypoprothrombinemia may occur in severe liver disease, and repeated doses are not warranted if response to the initial dose is unsatisfactory.[40,48]

Drug Interactions. Mineral oil and cholesterol-binding resins may impair phytonadione absorption.

Parameters to Monitor. Monitor PT before, and at intervals after, administration of the drug; the interval depends on the route of administration, the condition being treated, and the patient's status (*see* Administration and Adult Dosage).

Notes. Protect drug from the light at all times. Phytonadione reverses the effects of oral anticoagulant therapy, but has no antagonist activity against heparin.

RETEPLASE   Retavase

Reteplase (recombinant plasminogen activator; r-PA) is a nonglycosylated mutant of wild-type tissue plasminogen activator. In animals, this modification results in less high-affinity fibrin binding, longer half-life, and greater thrombolytic potency than rt-PA (alteplase). In the Reteplase Angiographic Phase II International Dose-finding study (RAPID) open-label MI trial, reteplase achieved more rapid, complete, and sustained thrombolysis than standard-dose rt-PA with comparable bleeding risk. The RAPID trial did not, however, have sufficient power to detect differences in mortality among the groups. Comparative mortality rates between reteplase and rt-PA will be reported in the results of the GUSTO-3 trial. The International Joint Efficacy Comparison of Thrombolytics (INJECT) trial suggests that reteplase mortality rates are similar to those observed with streptokinase. (*See* Alteplase Contraindications, Precautions, and Parameters to Monitor.) Reteplase is given as two 10 IU IV bolus doses 30 min apart, with adjunctive IV heparin given as a 5000-unit bolus followed by 1000 units/hr (aPTT target 1.5–2.0 times control) for at least 24 hr. Available as 10.8 IU injection.

STREPTOKINASE   Kabikinase, Streptase

Pharmacology. A bacterial protein derived from group C ß-hemolytic streptococci. It acts indirectly, forming a streptokinase-plasminogen activator complex that activates other plasminogen, converting it to the proteolytic enzyme plasmin. Plasmin then hydrolyzes fibrin, fibrinogen, factors V, VIII, II, complement, and kallikreinogen.

Administration and Adult Dosage. **IV for post-MI clot lysis** 1.5 million IU over 60 min. **IV for pulmonary embolism, DVT, arterial thrombosis, or embolism** 250,000 IU over 30 min, followed by 100,000 IU/hr for 24–72 hr (72 hr if DVT suspected).[49] Institute heparin therapy (*see* Parameters to Monitor). **For arteriovenous cannula occlusion** slowly instill 250,000 IU in 2-mL solution into each occluded limb of cannula; clamp for 2 hr, aspirate contents, and flush with NS. **Selective intra-arterial infusion** (investigational) 5000 IU/hr for 5–48 hr.[50,51] (*See* Notes.)

Special Populations. *Pediatric Dosage.* Safety and efficacy not established.

Geriatric Dosage. Same as adult dosage.

Dosage Forms. **Inj** 250,000, 600,000, 750,000, 1.5 million IU.

Pharmacokinetics. *Onset and Duration.* Onset of fibrinolytic activity immediately following IV administration; duration 8–24 hr following discontinuation of the infusion.[52]

Fate. V_d is 0.08 ± 0.04 L/kg; Cl is 0.1 ± 0.04 L/hr/kg.[9] Clearance results, in part, from formation of an antigen-antibody complex that remains soluble and is rapidly removed.[2] Local inactivation in the circulation by inhibitor complex formation and proteolysis occurs.[15] It is postulated that the reticuloendothelial system also contributes to clearance.[53]

t½. α phase averages 18–23 min and is related to antigen-antibody formation; β phase averages 83 min and appears to be related to clearance by the reticuloendothelial system.[2,53]

Adverse Reactions. Surface bleeding complications occur frequently and are primarily related to invasive procedures (eg, venous cutdowns, arterial punctures, and sites of surgical intervention). Severe internal bleeding is reported occasionally; however, its prevalence is no greater than with other thrombolytics or standard anticoagulant therapy. Transient hypotension occurs occasionally. In ISIS-3 the rates for definite or possible cerebral bleeding were as follows: streptokinase, 0.2%; rt-PA (deuteplase, a two-chain form of alteplase), 0.5%; anistreplase, 0.7%.[10] Occasional allergic reactions include fever, urticaria, itching, flushing, and musculoskeletal pain. Anaphylactoid reactions occur rarely with preparations now in use.[2,54]

Contraindications. (*See* Alteplase.)

Precautions. (*See* Alteplase.) Prior exposure to anistreplase or streptokinase within the last 12 months.

Drug Interactions. Anticoagulants or antiplatelet drugs may increase risk of bleeding.

Parameters to Monitor. For short-term thrombolytic therapy of MI, laboratory monitoring is of little value. For IV continuous infusion, monitor thrombin time, aPTT, or PT to detect activation of the fibrinolytic system, performed 3–4 hr after initiating therapy and q 12 hr throughout treatment.[54] No correlation has been made between clotting test results and likelihood of hemorrhage or efficacy; however, prolongation of the thrombin time to 2–5 times normal control value has been recommended.

Notes. In addition to post-MI clot lysis, streptokinase is recommended only for treatment of thrombosis involving the axillary-subclavian system or the popliteal vein or deep veins of the thigh and pelvis, and for patients in whom massive pulmonary emboli have caused obstruction of blood flow to one or more lung segments or when clinical shock is present.[54] The risk of stroke and intracranial bleeding appears to be less with streptokinase (by a difference of ≤ 0.5%) than with other thrombolytic agents.[55] Thrombolytic therapy may help prevent venous valvular damage and the development of venous or pulmonary hypertension.[56] The recommended fixed dosage schedule results in sufficient activation of plasminogen in 95% of patients.[57] However, consider using alteplase in those patients with exposure to streptokinase or anistreplase in the last 12 months.[5] The benefits of instituting anticoagulant therapy with heparin after completion of the thrombolytic infusion are not clear. However, it is recommended that heparin infusion (to an aPTT of 1.5–2.0 times control) be given only in the presence of high risk for systemic or venous thromboembolism (eg, anterior MI, CHF, previous embolus, atrial fibrillation). Heparin is initiated without a bolus 4 hr after the start of streptokinase infusion (or when aPTT is less than twice control) and continued for at least 48 hr.[5,7]

TICLOPIDINE
Ticlid

Ticlopidine is an antiplatelet agent that inhibits most known stimuli (eg, ADP, collagen, epinephrine) for platelet aggregation. It prolongs bleeding time, normalizes shortened platelet survival, suppresses platelet growth factor release, and may block von Willebrand factor and fibrinogen interactions with platelets. The onset of clinical effect is delayed, with maximum efficacy being achieved in 3–8 days. Approximately 80% of the drug is absorbed orally, with peak serum concentrations occurring in about 2 hr. Ticlopidine undergoes extensive liver metabolism to possibly active metabolites, with only 2% excreted unchanged in urine. The Ticlopidine Aspirin Stroke Study (TASS) trial found a 12% risk reduction in nonfatal stroke or cardiovascular death with ticlopidine (250 mg bid) compared to aspirin (650 mg bid) in high-risk (previous TIA or minor stroke) males and females. For secondary stroke prevention, the Canadian American Ticlopidine Study (CATS) trial found that the risk of stroke, MI, or cardiovascular death was reduced by 23% with ticlopidine (250 mg bid) over placebo. Ticlopidine 250 mg bid has also been shown to markedly reduce MI, cardiovascular death, and ECG evidence of ischemia in patients with unstable angina. Diarrhea and rash occurs frequently. Minor bleeding such as bruising, petechiae, epistaxis, and hematuria occurs occasionally. Severe neutropenia occurs in about 0.8% of patients and mild to moderate neutropenia in about 1.6% of patients during the first 3 months of therapy; neutropenia usually resolves within 3 weeks of discontinuation, although sepsis and death are reported. Thrombocytopenia and cholestasis occur rarely. Obtain CBC and differential counts q 2 weeks during the first 3 months of therapy; more frequent monitoring is recommended if the absolute neutrophil count is consistently declining or is less than 30% of the baseline value. Because of the risk of neutropenia, reserve ticlopidine for patients who are intolerant to aspirin therapy. Ticlopidine may increase the effect of aspirin on platelet aggregation and decrease theophylline clearance; cimetidine may reduce ticlopidine clearance. Ticlopidine is indicated for reduction of the risk of thrombotic stroke in patients who have had stroke precursors or a completed thrombotic stroke. Ticlopidine has also been recommended as an alternative to aspirin in patients with unstable angina or undergoing coronary bypass graft or coronary angioplasty. The adult dosage is 250 mg bid with food.[58–62] Available as 250-mg tablets.

UROKINASE
Abbokinase

Urokinase is a proteolytic enzyme produced by renal parenchymal cells that acts to directly convert plasminogen to plasmin with effects similar to streptokinase. The drug's half-life is about 10–20 min. Side effects, contraindications, and precautions are similar to streptokinase, although allergic reactions occur much less frequently. It is administered IV for pulmonary emboli as a 4400 IU/kg loading dose over 10 min, followed by 4400 IU/kg/hr for 12 hr. Heparin therapy is initiated without a loading dose after discontinuation of the thrombolytic, when the thrombin time or other coagulation test no longer exceeds twice normal control. It may be given by selective intracoronary infusion 6000 IU/min for up to 2 hr. For IV catheter clearance, attach a 1-mL tuberculin syringe filled with 5000 IU reconstituted solution (Open-Cath) and slowly inject an amount equal to the catheter volume; aspirate and repeat q 5 min as necessary. If not successful, allow urokinase to remain in the catheter for 30–60 min before attempting to aspirate. For central venous catheters whose function has not been restored by the bolus method, a 6- or 12-hr infusion of 40,000 IU/hr (5000 IU/mL at 8 mL/hr) in adults may be useful.[2,64] Available as injection 5000-, 9000-, and 250,000-IU vials.

WARFARIN SODIUM
Coumadin, Panwarfin

Pharmacology. Warfarin prevents the conversion of vitamin K back to its active form from vitamin K epoxide. This impairs formation of the vitamin K–dependent clotting factors VII, IX, X, II (prothrombin) and proteins C and S (physiologic anticoagulants). The (S)-warfarin enantiomer is approximately fourfold more potent an anticoagulant than (R)-warfarin.[2,65]

Administration and Adult Dosage. PO or IV 5–7.5 mg/day (range 2–10 mg/day), titrating dosage to an INR of 2.0–3.0 for treatment or prophylaxis of venous thrombosis, pulmonary embolism, systemic embolism, tissue heart valves, valvular heart disease, atrial fibrillation (except patients <60 yr with "lone AF"), and recurrent systemic embolism. Adjust dosage to an INR of 2.5–3.5 for management of mechanical prosthetic valves (upper end of range for caged-ball, tilting-disk, and mitral position valves);[66] adding aspirin 100 mg/day offers additional protection, but increases the risk of mild bleeding.[5,24] For postmyocardial infarction patients who are at increased risk of systemic or pulmonary embolism, maintain a warfarin dose that achieves an INR of 2.5–3.5 for up to 3 months. Low-dose warfarin (1 mg/day) without measurable changes in PT/INR begun 3 days before central venous catheter placement and continued while the catheter remains in place is recommended to reduce the risk of axillary-subclavian venous thrombosis.[5,67] (*See* Notes.)

Special Populations. *Pediatric Dosage.* (<18 yr) safety and efficacy not established. However, when used, dosage is titrated based on INR as in adult dosage.

Geriatric Dosage. Same as adult dosage (*see also* Precautions).

Other Conditions. Large variability in response requires that dosage be carefully individualized in all patients. Patients with liver disease, CHF, hyperthyroidism, or fever may be particularly sensitive to warfarin. Renal failure does not enhance the hypoprothrombinemic response to warfarin; however, these patients may have compromised hemostatic mechanisms that predispose to bleeding.[68]

Dosage Forms. Tab 1, 2, 2.5, 5, 7.5, 10 mg.

Patient Instructions. This drug is potentially harmful when taken with nonprescription or prescription drugs. Consult your physician or pharmacist when considering the use of other medications, particularly aspirin-containing products.

Pharmacokinetics. *Onset and Duration.* Peak PT effect is in 36–72 hr;[69] at least 4–6 days of warfarin therapy are required before full therapeutic effect is achieved.[1,24] Duration after discontinuation depends on resynthesis of vitamin K–dependent clotting factors II, VII, IX, and X (which requires about 4–5 days).

Fate. Completely absorbed orally; well absorbed following small bowel resection;[70] 99 ± 1% is plasma protein bound.[9] V_d (racemic) is 0.14 ± 0.06 L/kg; Cl (racemic) is 0.0027 ± 0.0014 L/hr/kg.[9] It undergoes oxidative P450 enzyme biotransformation in the liver (R)-warfarin, CYP1A2; (S)-warfarin, CYP2C subfamily),[71] producing warfarin alcohols, which have minor anticoagulant activity.[72,73] Less than 2% is excreted unchanged in urine.[9]

$t_{1/2}$. 37 ± 15 hr,[9,74] unchanged in acute hepatic disease.[75] Enantiomer half-lives: (R)-warfarin 43 ± 14 hr; (S)-32 ± 12 hr.[9]

Adverse Reactions. Bleeding (major and minor) occurs frequently (6–29%); fatal or life-threatening hemorrhage has been reported in 1–8%. Risk factors for increased bleeding include prothrombin-time ratio greater than 2.0, age >60 yr, and other comorbid conditions. Rarely, skin necrosis (occurring early in therapy and involving the breast, buttocks, thigh, or penis), purple-toe syndrome (occurring after 3–8 weeks of therapy), and alopecia may occur.[1,24,35,76,77]

Contraindications. Pregnancy; threatened abortion; blood dyscrasias; bleeding tendencies; unsupervised patients with senility, alcoholism, psychosis, or lack of cooperation; anticipated spinal puncture procedure; regional or lumbar anesthesia.

Precautions. Avoid all IM injections because of the risk of hematoma. Several other factors may influence response: diet, travel, and environment. Monitor patients with liver disease, CHF, atrial fibrillation, hyperthyroidism, or fever especially carefully. The elderly have a higher risk of major trauma (eg, hip fractures) and physiologic changes in subcutaneous tissues and joint spaces, which may allow bleeding to expand unchecked.[77]

Drug Interactions. Many important drug interactions (*see* Part II, Chapter 2).

Parameters to Monitor. PT/INR daily while hospitalized, then weekly to monthly to monitor therapeutic effect; hematocrit; stool guaiac; urinalysis (for hematuria) for toxicity. Also observe for ecchymoses, hemoptysis, and epistaxis.

Notes. Loading dose has no therapeutic advantage and may be unsafe because of excessive depression of factor VII.[24,78] Predictive techniques using small loading doses (eg, 10 mg/day for 2–3 days) were developed using desired prothrombin-time ratios of 1.5–2.5. With the current prothrombin-time ratio recommendations of 1.3–1.5, the predictive error of these techniques for this narrow range may be unacceptable.[24,79] **Phytonadione** begins to restore the PT toward normal within 4–8 hr, although large doses may induce a subsequent resistance to anticoagulant effect lasting one or more weeks.[80] A small oral dose (eg, 2.5 mg) or small slow IV injection (0.5–1 mg) of phytonadione may be used to bring an elevated PT/INR back into target range without resulting resistance.[5] Treat the first episode of venous thrombosis for 6 weeks in patients with reversible risk factors and 6 months in others. Consider continuing warfarin for an indefinite period in patients with active cancer or recurrent venous thrombosis.[81]

Hematopoietics

EPOETIN ALFA
Epogen, Procrit

Pharmacology. Epoetin alfa (erythropoietin, EPO) is a recombinant human glycoprotein produced from mammalian cells that stimulates RBC production. The product contains the identical amino acid sequence and produces the same biologic effects as natural erythropoietin.[82–85]

Administration and Adult Dosage. IV or SC for dialysis or nondialysis chronic renal failure patients 50–100 units/kg 3 times/week initially, increased or decreased by 25 units/kg to maintain a target hematocrit of 30–36%. When the target hematocrit is reached (or when there is an increase >4 points in any 2-week period), reduce the dosage to 25 units/kg 3 times/week. If at any time the hematocrit exceeds 36%, discontinue epoetin until the target hematocrit is achieved and then resume at a lower dosage. Individualize the maintenance dosage to maintain the target hematocrit. **IV or SC for zidovudine-treated or HIV-infected patients** 100 units/kg 3 times/week for 8 weeks initially, increased or decreased by 50–100 units/kg based on response; maximum effective dosage is 300 units/kg 3 times/week. If hematocrit exceeds 40%, discontinue epoetin until the hematocrit returns to 36%, then reduce dosage by 25%; adjust dosage to maintain desired hematocrit target. Patients with initial erythropoietin levels >500 units/L are unlikely to respond to epoetin. **SC for chemotherapy-treated cancer patients** 150 units/kg 3 times/week for 8 weeks initially, increasing to 300 units/kg 3 times/week if there is an unsatisfactory reduction in transfusion requirement or an unsatisfactory increase in hematocrit. If hematocrit exceeds 40%, discontinue epoetin until the hematocrit returns to 36%, then reduce dosage by 25%; adjust dosage to maintain desired hematocrit target. **SC for reduction of allogenic blood transfusion in surgery patients** 300 units/kg/day for 10 days before, the day of and 4 days following surgery.

Special Populations. *Pediatric Dosage.* Safety and efficacy not established. **SC for anemia of prematurity** (preterm neonates) 200 units (140 units/kg) every other day for 10 doses;[86] alternatively, 250 units/kg 3 times/week.[85] **SC or IV for anemia of end-stage renal disease** (newborn–18 yr) 50 units/kg 3 times/week has been used.[87,88]

Geriatric Dosage. Same as adult dosage.

Dosage Forms. Inj 2000, 3000, 4000, 10,000 units/mL.

Pharmacokinetics. *Onset and Duration.* In response to administration 3 times/week, reticulocyte count increases within 10 days followed by increases in RBC count, hematocrit, and hemoglobin in about 2–6 weeks.

Fate. Not orally bioavailable. Peak serum levels occur 5–24 hr after SC administration. V_d is 0.033–0.055 L/kg; Cl is about 0.00282 L/hr/kg.[82]

$t_{1/2}$. 9.3 ± 3.3 hr initially; 6.2 ± 1.8 hr during long-term therapy.[82]

Adverse Reactions. Hypertension, headache, tachycardia, nausea, vomiting, clotted vascular access, shortness of breath, hyperkalemia, and diarrhea occur frequently. Occasionally seizures and rarely CVA, TIA, or MI occur.[82–85]

Contraindications. Uncontrolled hypertension. Hypersensitivity to mammalian cell-derived products or albumin.

Precautions. Pregnancy. Use cautiously with a known history of seizure or underlying hematologic disease including sickle cell anemia, myelodysplastic syndromes, or hypercoagulable states.

Drug Interactions. None known.

Parameters to Monitor. Evaluate iron stores prior to and during therapy. Supplemental iron may be required to maintain a transferrin saturation of at least 20% and ferritin levels of at least 100 µg/L. Determine hematocrit twice a week for 2–6 weeks or until stabilized in the target range; monitor at regular intervals thereafter. Monitor CBC with differential, platelet count, BUN, Cr_s, serum uric acid, serum phosphorus, and serum potassium at regular intervals.

FERROUS SALTS   Various

Pharmacology. Ferrous salts are soluble forms of iron, an essential nutrient that functions primarily as the oxygen-binding core of heme in RBCs (as hemoglobin), muscles (as myoglobin), and in the respiratory enzyme cytochrome C.

Administration and Adult Dosage. **PO as dietary supplement** RDA for adult males is 10 mg/day, and for adult females (19–51 yr) is 15 mg/day.[44] **PO for treatment of iron deficiency** 2–3 mg/kg/day of elemental iron in divided doses (*see* Ferrous Salts Comparison Chart for usual dosage ranges for individual salts). Dose-related adverse effects may be decreased by using suboptimal dosages, by increasing the daily dosage gradually, or by administering with a small amount of food (although this latter method reduces absorption). After hemoglobin is normalized, continue oral therapy for 3–6 months to replenish iron stores.

Special Populations. *Pediatric Dosage.* **PO for prophylaxis RDA** (infants) 6 mg/day; (1–10 yr) 10 mg/day; (11–18 yr, males) 12 mg/day; (11–18 yr, females) 15 mg/day.[44] **PO for treatment** (infants) 10–25 mg of elemental iron in 3–4 divided doses; (6 months-2 yr) up to 6 mg/kg/day of elemental iron in 3–4 divided doses; (2–12 yr) 3 mg/kg/day of elemental iron in 3–4 divided doses.

Geriatric Dosage. Same as adult dosage, except dosage in women >51 yr is 10 mg/day of elemental iron.

Other Conditions. Iron requirement during pregnancy is approximately twice that of the normal, nonpregnant woman because of an expanding blood volume and the demands of the fetus and placenta. The RDA in pregnancy is 30 mg/day, and a prophylactic dose of 15–30 mg/day of elemental iron during the second and third trimesters has been recommended to prevent depletion of maternal iron stores. Iron-deficient patients may need higher doses.

Dosage Forms. (*See* Ferrous Salts Comparison Chart.)

Patient Instructions. Take this drug with a full glass of water on an empty stomach (1 hour before or 2 hours after meals) for best absorption. Take liquid preparations in water or juice, and drink with a straw to minimize tooth staining. If gastric distress or nausea occurs, a small quantity of food may be taken with the drug, but do not take with antacids because absorption is decreased. Iron preparations may cause constipation and black stools. Keep all iron products out of the reach of children.

Pharmacokinetics. *Onset and Duration.* Response to equivalent amounts of oral or parenteral therapy is essentially the same. Reticulocytes increase within 4–7 days and reach a peak about the tenth day. An increase in hemoglobin of 2 g/dL or more and a 6% increase in hematocrit should occur in about 3–4 weeks.[89,90] Three to 6 months of therapy are generally required for restoration of iron stores.[89,90]

Serum Levels. Normal is 65–170 µg/dL (12–30 µmol/L) in adult males, 50–170 µg/dL (9–30 µmol/L) in adult females, and 50–120 µg/dL (9–21 µmol/L) in children. A decrease in the transferrin saturation (serum iron ÷ total iron binding capacity × 100) is an indication of preanemic iron deficiency. A transferrin saturation <16% or plasma ferritin concentration <12 µg/L indicates probable iron deficiency.[89,90] In overdosage, toxicity may occur at iron levels >350 µg/dL (63 µmol/L). Chelation therapy is indicated at these levels, especially if the patient is symptomatic.[89]

Fate. Iron is absorbed primarily from the duodenum at a rate dependent on the amount of iron in storage sites. About 10% of dietary iron is absorbed in normal subjects, 20% in iron-deficient patients, and as much as 70% of medicinal iron is absorbed during marked iron deficiency or increased erythropoiesis. In the plasma, iron is oxidized to the ferric state, combined with transferrin, and either used or stored as ferritin (mostly in the reticuloendothelial system and hepatocytes). The average loss in the healthy adult male is about 1 mg/day. GI loss of extravasated red cells, iron in bile, and exfoliated mucosal cells accounts for two-thirds of this iron. The other third is lost in the skin and urine. Menstruating women have an additional loss of about 0.5 mg/day.

Adverse Reactions. Side effects are primarily related to the dose of elemental iron. Frequent GI irritation, constipation, and stained teeth (liquid preparations only—dilute and use a drinking straw). An increased risk of cancer associated with excessive iron stores has been reported.[91]

Contraindications. Hemochromatosis; hemosiderosis; hemolytic anemias in which no true iron deficiency exists.

Precautions. Use with caution in patients with peptic ulcer, regional enteritis, or ulcerative colitis. Serious acute poisoning (which can be fatal) occurs frequently in children: doses as low as 20 mg/kg of elemental iron can cause toxicity, 40 mg/kg is considered serious, and greater than 60 mg/kg is potentially lethal.[92]

Drug Interactions. Food, calcium carbonate, sodium bicarbonate, and possibly magnesium trisilicate can reduce iron absorption. Vitamin E can reduce utilization of iron in iron deficiency anemia. Iron salts can reduce oral absorption of carbidopa/levodopa, methyldopa, penicillamine, quinolones, tetracyclines, and thyroid hormones.

Parameters to Monitor. Periodic reticulocyte count, hemoglobin and hematocrit (*see* Onset and Duration).

Notes. Ferrous salts are used in prevention and treatment of iron deficiency anemias. Such anemias occur most frequently with exceptional blood losses (eg, pathologic bleeding, menstruation) and during periods of rapid growth (eg, infancy, adolescence, pregnancy). Iron is ineffective in hemoglobin disturbances not caused by iron deficiency. Concurrent administration of high doses of ascorbic acid may enhance absorption (particularly when given with SR formulations), but cost/benefit may not warrant its use. Wide variation in dissolution and absorption exists among SR and enteric-coated products, and the frequency of adverse effects, although negligible, probably reflects the small amount of ionic iron available for absorption because of transport of the iron past the duodenum and proximal jejunum.[93]

FILGRASTIM   Neupogen

Pharmacology. Filgrastim is an *Escherichia coli*–derived (nonglycosylated) recombinant human granulocyte colony-stimulating factor (G-CSF). G-CSF is one of many glycoprotein hormones that regulate the proliferation and differentiation of hematopoietic progenitor cells and the function of mature blood cells. Specifically, G-CSF promotes proliferation and maturation, and enhances the function and migration of neutrophil granulocytes. G-CSF also promotes pre-B-cell activation and growth, and acts in synergy with interleukin-3 to support megakaryocyte and platelet production.[83,94]

Administration and Adult Dosage. **SC or IV for myelosuppressive cancer chemotherapy** 5 µg/kg/day as a single injection; continue for up to 2 weeks until absolute neutrophil count (ANC) is 10,000/µL. Discontinue therapy if the ANC becomes greater than 10,000/µL following the expected nadir. Based on severity of ANC nadir, dosage may be increased in 5 µg/kg/day increments for each chemotherapy cycle. **SC continuous infusion for chemotherapy-induced febrile neutropenia** 12 µg/kg/day beginning within 12 hr of empiric antibiotic therapy and continued until neutrophil count is greater than 5000/µL and the patient is afebrile for 4 days.[95] **IV or SC for bone marrow transplant patients** 10 µg/kg/day infused IV over 4 or 24 hr or as a continuous SC infusion, decreasing to 5 µg/kg/day when ANC is greater than 1000/µL for 3 consecutive days. Discontinue therapy if the ANC remains >1000/µL for 3 more consecutive days; resume at a dosage of 5 µg/kg/day when ANC becomes less than 1000/µL. **SC for severe chronic neutropenia** (congenital) 6 µg/kg bid; (idiopathic or cyclic) 5 µg/kg/day. Target ANC range is 1500–10,000/µL; decrease dosage if ANC is persistently >10,000/µL. **SC with erythropoietin to decrease hematologic toxicity from zidovudine** 3.6 µg/kg/day initially, increasing or decreasing weekly by 1 µg/kg/day to maintain a target ANC of 1500–5000/µL.[96]

Special Populations. *Pediatric Dosage.* Safety and efficacy not established. **IV or SC** (3 months–18 yr.) 0.6–120 µg/kg/day for up to 3 yr has been reported to be well tolerated.

Geriatric Dosage. Same as adult dosage.

Dosage Forms. **Inj** 300 µg/mL.

Patient Instructions. Your pharmacist or physician should instruct you on proper dosage, administration, and disposal. Store vials in the refrigerator, but do not freeze. Vials are designed for single use only; discard any unused portion. Bring vial to room temperature before administration; do not shake.

FERROUS SALTS COMPARISON CHART

DRUG	SOLID DOSAGE FORMS*	ADULT DOSAGE (CAP OR TAB/DAY)	ELEMENTAL IRON/CAP OR TAB (%)	(mg Fe)	OTHER DOSAGE FORMS*
Ferrous Fumarate	SR Tab 324 mg	1-2	33	106	Drp 75 mg/mL
	SR Cap 325 mg	1-2	33	106	Susp 20 mg/mL.
	Tab (Chewable) 100 mg	1-4	33	33	
	Tab 63, 195, 200 mg	1-4	33	20, 64, 66	
	Tab 324, 325, 350 mg.	1-2	33	106, 106, 115	
Ferrous Gluconate	Cap 86 mg	3-6	12	10	Elxr 60 mg/mL.
	SR Tab 320 mg	3-6	12	37	
	Tab 300, 320, 325 mg.	3-6	12	35, 37, 38	
Ferrous Sulfate	Cap 190 mg	3	30	60	
Exsiccated	SR Cap 159 mg	1-2	30	50	
	SR Tab 160 mg	1-2	30	50	
	Tab 200 mg.	3-4	30	65	
Ferrous Sulfate	SR Cap/Tab various	—	20	—	Drp 125 mg/mL
Hydrous	Tab 195 mg	3-6	20	39	Elxr 44 mg/mL
	Tab 300, 324 mg.	3	20	60, 65	Syrup 18 mg/mL.
Polysaccharide-Iron	Cap 150 mg iron	1-2	—	150	Elxr 20 mg/mL iron.
Complex	Tab 50 mg iron.	2-4	—	50	

*Doses listed represent total iron salt, not elemental iron, except for polysaccharide-iron complex.

Pharmacokinetics. *Onset and Duration.* Elevation in neutrophilic band forms occurs within about 60 min following administration. With discontinuation of therapy, neutrophil counts return to baseline values in about 4 days.[94]

Fate. Not orally bioavailable. V_d is about 0.15 L/kg; Cl is 0.03–0.042 L/hr/kg. $t_{1/2}$, 3.5–3.85 hr.

Adverse Reactions. Mild to moderate bone pain responsive to nonnarcotic analgesics is reported frequently. Transient decreases in blood pressure occur occasionally. During long-term therapy, splenomegaly occurs frequently; occasional exacerbation of skin disorders, alopecia, hematuria, proteinuria, thrombocytopenia, and osteoporosis were also reported. Other adverse effects occur during administration of filgrastim that are likely the consequence of the underlying malignancy or cytotoxic chemotherapy. Acute reactions to sargramostim (eg, febrile episodes, flushing, hypotension, tachycardia, and hypoxia) appear to be more common than with filgrastim.[83,94,96,97]

Contraindications. History of hypersensitivity to *E. coli*-derived proteins. Do not use within the period of 24 hr before and 24 hr after administration of cytotoxic chemotherapy.

Precautions. Use with caution in any malignancy with myeloid characteristics because of the possibility of tumor growth. The efficacy of filgrastim has not been established in patients receiving nitrosoureas, mitomycin, fluorouracil, or cytarabine.

Drug Interactions. None known.

Parameters to Monitor. Perform a CBC and platelet count prior to chemotherapy and twice a week during filgrastim therapy. Regular monitoring of WBC counts at the time of recovery from the postchemotherapy nadir is recommended to avoid excessive leukocytosis. Discontinue therapy if the ANC >10,000/μL following the expected chemotherapy nadir.

Notes. Other potential uses for filgrastim include AIDS-related neutropenia, myelodysplastic syndromes, and drug-induced neutropenia or aplastic anemia. Further clinical trials are needed to prove that use for these and other indications is beneficial, safe, and cost-effective.

MACROPHAGE COLONY-STIMULATING FACTOR (Investigational)

Macrophage colony-stimulating factor (M-CSF) is a cytokine that promotes proliferation of macrophages and monocytes, enhances macrophage antitumor and antimicrobial activity, and stimulates the release of G-CSF, GM-CSF, interferon, interleukin-1, and tumor necrosis factor. Adverse reactions to M-CSF include fever and ophthalmologic toxicity (conjunctivitis, iritis). Most clinical trials evaluated the antitumor and antimicrobial activities of M-CSF. Phase I dose escalation studies using 10–160 µg/kg/day show increased circulating monocytes (at greater than 30 µg/kg/day) and increased antibody-dependent, monocyte-mediated cytotoxicity (at 50–80 µg/kg/day). Antitumor response has been observed in a limited number of patients. M-CSF is also being evaluated in the treatment of fungal infections following marrow transplant, where macrophage activation may be critical for host defense response. Complete or partial clinical improvement has been observed in some patients. M-CSF is being used investigationally in three forms:

native protein from urine, a glycosylated recombinant form, and a truncated nong-lycosylated form.[83]

IRON DEXTRAN InFeD

Pharmacology. (*See* Ferrous Salts.) The overall response to parenteral iron is no more rapid or complete than the response to orally administered iron, so iron dextran is indicated only when oral iron therapy is determined to be ineffective or impossible.

Administration and Adult Dosage. The total cumulative amount required for restoration of hemoglobin (Hb) in g/dL and body stores of iron can be approximated using lean body weight (LBW) in kg (or actual body weight if less than LBW) from the formula:

$$\text{Total mg Iron} = [0.0442 \times (\text{Desired Hb} - \text{Observed Hb}) \times \text{LBW} + (0.26 \times \text{LBW})] \times 50$$

To calculate dose in mL, divide the result by 50. Usual Hb target for adults is 14.8 g/dL. The dose of iron required secondary to blood loss can be estimated from the formula:

$$\text{Total mg Iron} = \text{Blood Loss (mL)} \times \text{Hematocrit (observed, as decimal fraction)}$$

Deep IM (in upper outer quadrant of buttock only, using Z-track technique) 25-mg (0.5-mL) test dose the first day, then, if no adverse reaction occurs, administer a maximum daily dose of 100 mg (2 mL) until the total calculated amount is reached. **Slow IV** test dose of 25 mg (0.5 mL) over at least 30 sec the first day; if no adverse reaction occurs after a minimum of 1 hr, proceed (until the total calculated amount is reached) by daily increments over 2–3 days, to a maximum dose of 100 mg/day at a rate not to exceed 50 mg/min.[96] **IV in erythropoietin-treated dialysis patients** 100–200 mg/week after dialysis. **Total dose IV infusion** the total calculated dose of iron dextran is diluted in 250–1000 mL of NS (dextrose solutions cause increased local phlebitis) and infused over a period of 2–6 hr after a 25-mg test dose is delivered over 5–10 min.[98] This method is an off-label use and is discouraged by the manufacturer and the FDA.

Special Populations. *Pediatric Dosage.* (<4 months) safety and efficacy not established; (5–15 kg) total cumulative amount required for restoration of hemoglobin ([Hb] in g/dL) and body stores of iron can be estimated using body weight (W) in kg from the formula:

$$\text{Total mg Iron} = [0.0442 \times (\text{Desired Hb} - \text{Observed Hb}) \times \text{W} + (0.26 \times \text{W})] \times 50$$

To calculate dose in mL, divide the result by 50. Usual Hb target for children ≤15 kg is 12 g/dL. Maximum daily dose is (infants <5 kg) 25 mg (0.5 mL), (children <10 kg) 50 mg (1 mL), (children >15 kg) same as adult dosage.

Geriatric Dosage. Same as adult dosage.

Dosage Forms. **Inj** 50 mg elemental iron/mL.

Pharmacokinetics. *Onset and Duration.* Hematologic response is the same as with oral therapy, although total body stores of iron are replaced when the above dosage regimens are used.

Serum Levels. (*See* Ferrous Salts.)

Fate. Following IV administration, the inert complex is gradually cleared from the plasma by the reticuloendothelial cells of the liver, spleen, and bone marrow. With doses >500 mg, the rate of uptake is 10–20 mg/hr. Iron dextran is then dissociated and released as free ferric iron (at a rate controlled by the serum iron level), which combines with transferrin and is incorporated into hemoglobin within the bone marrow.[98–100] Although all iron is eventually released in this manner, many months are often required for this process to be completed.[89]

Adverse Reactions. Hypotension and peripheral vascular flushing occur with too rapid IV administration. Mild, transient reactions including flushing, fever, myalgia, arthralgia, and lymphadenopathy usually occur only occasionally, although they occur in 80–90% of patients with active rheumatoid arthritis or active SLE. Immediate anaphylactoid reactions, which may be life-threatening, occur in 0.1–0.6% of patients.[101] A predictive test for predisposition to anaphylaxis is not available. IM administration has been associated with variable degrees of soreness, sterile abscess formation, tissue staining, and sarcoma formation.[99]

Contraindications. Anemias other than iron deficiency anemia; hemochromatosis; hemosiderosis; SC administration.

Precautions. Pregnancy. Use with extreme caution in the presence of serious liver impairment. Patients with rheumatoid arthritis may have an acute exacerbation or reactivation of joint pain and swelling following administration. History of allergies and/or asthma. Because of the potential for anaphylactoid reactions, have epinephrine, diphenhydramine, and methylprednisolone immediately available during iron dextran administration. Use parenteral iron only in patients in whom an iron deficient state has been clearly established and who are not amenable to oral therapy.

Drug Interactions. None known.

Parameters to Monitor. (*See* Ferrous Salts.)

SARGRAMOSTIM   Leukine

Sargramostim is a yeast-derived (glycosylated) recombinant human granulocyte-macrophage colony-stimulating factor (GM-CSF). GM-CSF is one of many glycoprotein hormones that regulate the proliferation and differentiation of hematopoietic progenitor cells and the function of mature blood cells. Specifically, GM-CSF promotes proliferation, maturation, and function of neutrophils, eosinophils, monocytes, and macrophages. GM-CSF also stimulates production of cytokines including interleukin-1 and tumor necrosis factor. Sargramostim is indicated for myeloid reconstitution after autologous bone marrow transplantation. It has also been used with some success to maintain normal neutrophil counts in AIDS patients receiving ganciclovir. Some data suggest a beneficial effect in AIDS patients with hematologic intolerance to zidovudine. Other potential uses for GM-CSF include AIDS-related neutropenia, myelodysplastic syndromes, and congenital, chronic, or drug-induced neutropenia and aplastic anemia. Controlled clinical trials are needed to prove that use for these and other indications is beneficial, safe, and cost-effective. Clinical and laboratory evidence appears to suggest

GM-CSF enhances the effect of zidovudine against HIV. Acute reactions to sargramostim (eg, febrile episodes, flushing, hypotension, tachycardia, and hypoxia) appear to be more common than with filgrastim. Other adverse reactions that occur frequently with GM-CSF are bone pain, lethargy, rash, and fluid retention. Usual dosage is IV 250 $\mu g/m^2$/day given as a 2-hr infusion beginning 2–4 hr after the autologous bone marrow infusion. Give the first dose no sooner than 24 hr after the last chemotherapy dose or before 12 hr following the last dose of radiotherapy. Continue sargramostim until the ANC >1500/μL for 3 consecutive days. For bone marrow transplantation failure or engraftment delay IV 250 $\mu g/m^2$/day is given for 14 days as a 2-hr infusion repeated in 7 days if engraftment has not occurred. If there is no improvement, a third course with 500 $\mu g/m^2$/day given for 14 days may be tried. Long-term therapy with GM-CSF SC in a dosage of 1–15 μg/kg/day has been used investigationally in AIDS patients receiving ganciclovir.[83,94,97,102–105] Sargramostim is available as a 250- and 500-μg injection.

■ REFERENCES

1. Hyers TM et al. Antithrombotic therapy for venous thromboembolic disease. *Chest* 1995;108:335S–51.
2. Lutomski DM et al. Pharmacokinetic optimisation of the treatment of embolic disorders. *Clin Pharmacokinet* 1995;28:67–92.
3. International Society and Federation of Cardiology and World Health Organization Task Force on Myocardial Reperfusion. Reperfusion in acute myocardial infarction. *Circulation* 1994;90:2091–102.
4. The GUSTO investigators. An international randomized trial comparing four thrombolytic strategies for acute myocardial infarction. *N Engl J Med* 1993;329:673–82.
5. Becker RC, Ansell J. Antithrombotic therapy: an abbreviated reference for clinicians. *Arch Intern Med* 1995;155:149–61.
6. Levine M et al. A randomized trial of a single bolus dosage regimen of recombinant tissue plasminogen activator in patients with acute pulmonary embolism. *Chest* 1990;98:1473–9.
7. Cairns JA et al. Coronary thrombolysis. *Chest* 1995;108:401S–23.
8. The National Institute of Neurological disorders rt-PA Stroke Study Group. tissue plasminogen activator for acute ischemic stroke. *N Engl J Med* 1995;333:1581–7.
9. Benet LZ et al. Design and optimization of dosage regimens; pharmacokinetic data. In Hardman JG et al., eds. *Goodman and Gilman's the pharmacological basis of therapeutics*, 9th ed. New York: McGraw-Hill; 1996:1707–92.
10. Third International Study of Infarct Survival Collaborative Study. ISIS-3: a randomized comparison of streptokinase vs tissue plasminogen activator vs anistreplase and of aspirin plus heparin vs aspirin alone among 41,299 cases of suspected acute myocardial infarct. *Lancet* 1992;339:753–70.
11. Nicolini FA et al. Concurrent nitroglycerin therapy impairs tissue-type plasminogen activator-induced thrombolysis in patients with acute myocardial infarction. *Am J Cardiol* 1994;74:662–6.
12. Smalling RW et al. More rapid, complete, and stable coronary thrombolysis with bolus administration of reteplase compared with alteplase infusion in acute myocardial infarction. *Circulation* 1995;91:2725–32.
13. Fuster V. Coronary thrombolysis—a perspective for the practicing physician. *N Engl J Med* 1993;329:723–4.
14. Munger MA, Forrence EA. Anistreplase: a new thrombolytic for the treatment of acute myocardial infarction. *Clin Pharm* 1990;9:530–40.
15. Fears R. Biochemical pharmacology and therapeutic aspects of thrombolytic agents. *Pharmacol Rev* 1990;42:201–22.
16. O'Connor CM et al. A randomized trial of intravenous heparin in conjunction with anistreplase (anisoylated plasminogen streptokinase activator complex) in acute myocardial infarction: the Duke University clinical cardiology study (DUCCS) 1. *J Am Coll Cardiol* 1994;23:11–8.
17. Cziraky MJ, Spinler SA. Low-molecular-weight heparins for the treatment of deep-vein thrombosis. *Clin Pharm* 1993;12:892–9.
18. Green D et al. Low molecular weight heparin: a critical analysis of clinical trials. *Pharmacol Rev* 1994;46:89–109.
19. Noble S et al. Enoxaparin. A reappraisal of its pharmacology and clinical applications in the prevention and treatment of thromboembolic disease. *Drugs* 1995;49:388–410.

20. Levine M et al. A comparison of low-molecular-weight heparin administered primarily at home with unfractionated heparin administered in the hospital for proximal deep-vein thrombosis. *N Engl J Med* 1996;334:677–81.

21. Lensing AWA et al. Treatment of deep venous thrombosis with low-molecular-weight heparins. A meta-analysis. *Arch Intern Med* 1995;155:601–7.

22. Verstraete M. Pharmacotherapeutic aspects of unfractionated and low molecular weight heparins. *Drugs* 1990;40:498–530.

23. de Valk HW et al. Comparing subcutaneous danaparoid with intravenous unfractionated heparin for the treatment of venous thromboembolism. A randomized controlled trial. *Ann Intern Med* 1995;123:1–9.

24. Carter BL. Therapy of acute thromboembolism with heparin and warfarin. *Clin Pharm* 1991;10:503–18.

25. Raschke RA et al. The weight-based heparin dosing nomogram compared with a "standard care" nomogram. A randomized controlled trial. *Ann Intern Med* 1993;119:874–81.

26. Kershaw B et al. Computer-assisted dosing of heparin. Management with a pharmacy-based anticoagulation service. *Arch Intern Med* 1994;154:1005–11.

27. Gunnarsson PS et al. Appropriate use of heparin. Empiric vs nomogram-based dosing. *Arch Intern Med* 1995;155:526–32.

28. Simon TL et al. Heparin pharmacokinetics: increased requirements in pulmonary embolism. *Br J Haematol* 1978;39:111–20.

29. Kruchoski ME, Emory CE. Initiating heparin and warfarin therapy concurrently. *Hosp Pharm* 1986;21:174.

30. Hull RD et al. Heparin for 5 days as compared with 10 days in the initial treatment of proximal venous thrombosis. *N Engl J Med* 1990;322:1260–4.

31. Melamed AJ, Suarez J. Detection and prevention of deep venous thrombosis. *Drug Intell Clin Pharm* 1988;22:107–14.

32. Cooke HM, Lynch A. Biorhythms and chronotherapy in cardiovascular disease. *Am J Hosp Pharm* 1994;51:2569–80.

33. Estes JW. Clinical pharmacokinetics of heparin. *Clin Pharmacokinet* 1980;5:204–20.

34. Hirsh J et al. Heparin kinetics in venous thrombosis and pulmonary embolism. *Circulation* 1976;53:691–5.

35. Landefeld CS et al. A bleeding risk index for estimating the probability of major bleeding in hospitalized patients starting anticoagulant therapy. *Am J Med* 1990;89:569–78.

36. Bailey RT et al. Heparin-associated thrombocytopenia: a prospective comparison of bovine lung heparin, manufactured by a new process, and porcine intestinal heparin. *Drug Intell Clin Pharm* 1986;20:374–8.

37. Becker PS, Miller VT. Heparin-induced thrombocytopenia. *Stroke* 1989;20:1449–59.

38. Oster JR et al. Heparin-induced aldosterone suppression and hyperkalemia. *Am J Med* 1995;98:575–86.

39. Uotila L. The metabolic functions and mechanism of action of vitamin K. *Scand J Clin Lab Invest* 1990;201(suppl):109–17.

40. Hardman JG et al., eds. *Goodman and Gilman's the pharmacological basis of therapeutics*, 9th ed. New York: McGraw-Hill; 1996:1583–5.

41. Thorp JA et al. Current concepts and controversies in the use of vitamin K. *Drugs* 1995;49:376–87.

42. Frick PG et al. Dose response and minimal daily requirement for vitamin K in man. *J Appl Physiol* 1967;23:387–9.

43. Mattea EJ, Quinn K. Adverse reactions after intravenous phytonadione administration. *Hosp Pharm* 1981;16:224–35.

44. Food and Nutrition Board, NRC. *Recommended dietary allowances*, 10th ed. Washington, DC: National Academy Press; 1989.

45. Zieve PD, Solomon HM. Variation in the response of human beings to vitamin K. *J Lab Clin Med* 1969;73:103–10.

46. Koch-Weser J, Sellers EM. Drug interactions with coumarin anticoagulants (2 parts). *N Engl J Med* 1971;285:487–9, 547–58.

47. Woolf IL, Babior BM. Vitamin K and warfarin. *Am J Med* 1972;53:261–7.

48. Finkel MJ. Vitamin K and the vitamin K analogues. *Clin Pharmacol Ther* 1961;2:794–814.

49. Rogers LQ, Lutcher CL. Streptokinase therapy for deep vein thrombosis: a comprehensive review of the English literature. *Am J Med* 1990;88:389–95.

50. Katzen BT, van Breda A. Low dose streptokinase in the treatment of arterial occlusion. *AJR* 1981;136:1171–8.

51. Belkin M et al. Intra-arterial fibrinolytic therapy. *Arch Surg* 1986;121:769–73.

52. Fletcher AP et al. The maintenance of a sustained thrombolytic state in man. I. Induction and effects. *J Clin Invest* 1959;38:1096–110.

53. Fletcher AP et al. The clearance of heterologous protein from the circulation of normal and immunized man. *J Clin Invest* 1958;37:1306–15.

54. Sherry S et al. Thrombolytic therapy in thrombosis: a National Institutes of Health consensus development conference. *Ann Intern Med* 1980;93:141–4.

55. Levine MN et al. Hemorrhagic complications of thrombolytic therapy in the treatment of myocardial infarction and venous embolism. *Chest* 1995;108:291S–301.

56. Goldhaber SZ. Contemporary pulmonary embolism thrombolysis. *Chest* 1995;107(suppl):45S–51.

57. Marder VJ. The use of thrombolytic agents: choice of patient, drug administration, laboratory monitoring. *Ann Intern Med* 1979;90:802–8.

58. Hass WK et al. A randomized trial comparing ticlopidine hydrochloride with aspirin for the prevention of stroke in high-risk patients. *N Engl J Med* 1989;321:501–7.

59. Gent M et al. The Canadian American ticlopidine study (CATS) in thromboembolic stroke. *Lancet* 1989;1:1215–20.

60. Haynes RB et al. A critical appraisal of ticlopidine, a new antiplatelet agent. Effectiveness and clinical indications for prophylaxis of atherosclerotic events. *Arch Intern Med* 1992;152:1376–80.

61. Matchar DB et al. Medical treatment for stroke prevention. *Ann Intern Med* 1994;121:41–53.

62. Carlson JA, Maesner JE. Fatal neutropenia and thrombocytopenia associated with ticlopidine. *Ann Pharmacother* 1994;28:1236–8.

63. Cassidy LJ et al. Probable ticlopidine-induced cholestatic hepatitis. *Ann Pharmacother* 1995;29:30–2.

64. Haire WD, Lieberman RP. Thrombosed central venous catheters: restoring function with 6-hour urokinase infusion after failure of bolus urokinase. *J Parenter Enteral Nutr* 1992;16:129–32.

65. Breckenridge A et al. Pharmacokinetics and pharmacodynamics of the enantiomers of warfarin in man. *Clin Pharmacol Ther* 1974;15:424–30.

66. Fihn SD. Aiming for safe anticoagulation. *N Engl J Med* 1995;333:54–5. Editorial.

67. Bern MM et al. Very low doses of warfarin can prevent thrombosis in central venous catheters. *Ann Intern Med* 1990;112:423–8.

68. O'Reilly RA, Aggeler PM. Determinants of the response to oral anticoagulant drugs in man. *Pharmacol Rev* 1970;22:35–96.

69. Nagashima R et al. Kinetics of pharmacologic effects in man: the anticoagulant action of warfarin. *Clin Pharmacol Ther* 1969:10:22–35.

70. Lutomski DM et al. Warfarin absorption after massive small bowel resection. *Am J Gastroenterol* 1985;80:99–102.

71. Slaughter RL, Edwards DJ. Recent advances: the cytochrome P450 enzymes. *Ann Pharmacother* 1995;29:619–24.

72. Yacobi A et al. Serum protein binding as a determinant of warfarin body clearance and anticoagulant effect. *Clin Pharmacol Ther* 1976;19:552–8.

73. Lewis RJ et al. Warfarin metabolites: the anticoagulant activity and pharmacology of warfarin alcohols. *J Lab Clin Med* 1973;81:925–31.

74. O'Reilly RA et al. Studies on the coumarin anticoagulant drugs: the pharmacodynamics of warfarin in man. *J Clin Invest* 1963;42:1542–51.

75. Williams RL et al. Influence of acute viral hepatitis on disposition and pharmacologic effect of warfarin. *Clin Pharmacol Ther* 1976;20:90–7.

76. Hirsh J. Drug therapy: oral anticoagulant drugs. *N Engl J Med* 1991;324:1865–75.

77. Landefeld CS, Goldman L. Major bleeding in outpatients treated with warfarin: incidence and prediction by factors known at the start of outpatient therapy. *Am J Med* 1989;87:144–52.

78. O'Reilly RA, Aggeler PM. Studies on coumarin anticoagulant drugs. Initiation of warfarin therapy without a loading dose. *Circulation* 1968;38:169–77.

79. Livengood BH, Maley MB. Lack of relationship between initial response to warfarin and maintenance dose. *Hosp Pharm* 1985;20:529–31.

80. Deykin D. Warfarin therapy (second of two parts). *N Engl J Med* 1970;283:801–3.

81. Hirsh J. The optimal duration of anticoagulant therapy for venous thrombosis. *N Engl J Med* 1995;332:1710–1. Editorial.

82. Schwenk MH, Halstenson CE. Recombinant human erythropoietin. *DICP* 1989;23:528–36.

83. Petersdorf SH, Dale DC. The biology and clinical applications of erythropoietin and the colony-stimulating factors. *Adv Intern Med* 1995;40:395–428.

84. Erslev AJ. Erythropoietin. *N Engl J Med* 1991;324:1339–44.

85. Zachée P. Controversies in selection of epoetin dosages. Issues and answers. *Drugs* 1995;49:536–47.

86. Ohis RK, Christensen RD. Recombinant erythropoietin compared with erythrocyte transfusion in the treatment of anemia of prematurity. *J Pediatr* 1991;119:781–8.

87. Ongkingco JR et al. Use of low-dose subcutaneous recombinant human erythropoietin in end-stage renal disease: experience with children receiving continuous cycling peritoneal dialysis. *Am J Kidney Dis* 1991; 18:446–50.

88. Rigden SP et al. Recombinant human erythropoietin therapy in children maintained by haemodialysis. *Pediatr Nephrol* 1990;4:618–22.

89. Hardman JG et al., eds. *Goodman and Gilman's the pharmacological basis of therapeutics,* 9th ed. New York: McGraw-Hill; 1996.

90. Koeller JM, Van Den Berg C. Anemias. In Koda-Kimble MA, Young LY, eds. *Applied therapeutics: the clinical use of drugs,* 6th ed. Vancouver, WA: Applied Therapeutics; 1995:88.3–88.17

91. Stevens RG. Iron and the risk of cancer. *Med Oncol Tumor Pharmacother* 1990;7:177–81.

92. Olson KR, ed. *Poisoning and drug overdose.* Norwalk, CT: Appleton & Lange; 1990.

93. Middleton EJ et al. Studies on the absorption of orally administered iron from sustained-release preparations. *N Engl J Med* 1966;274:136–9.

94. Anon. G-CSF and GM-CSF: white blood cell growth factors. *Hosp Pharm* 1990;25:881–2.

95. Maher DW et al. Filgrastim in patients with chemotherapy-induced febrile neutropenia. *Ann Intern Med* 1994;121:492–501.

96. Miles SA et al. Combined therapy with recombinant granulocyte colony-stimulating factor and erythropoietin decreases hematologic toxicity zidovudine. *Blood* 1991;77:2109–17.

97. Demuynck H et al. Comparative study of peripheral blood progenitor cell collection in patients with multiple myeloma after single-dose cyclophosphamide combined with rhGM-CSF or rhG-CSF. *Br J Haematol* 1995;90:384–92.

98. Hanson DB, Hendeles L. Guide to total dose intravenous iron dextran therapy. *Am J Hosp Pharm* 1974;31:592–5.

99. Kumpf VJ, Holland EG. Parenteral iron dextran therapy. *DICP* 1990;24:162–6.

100. Wood JK et al. The metabolism of iron-dextran given as a total-dose infusion to iron deficient Jamaican subjects. *Br J Haematol* 1968;14:119–29.

101. Novey HS et al. Immunologic studies of anaphylaxis to iron dextran in patients on renal dialysis. *Ann Allergy* 1994;72:224–8.

102. Hogan KR, Peters MD. Granulocyte-macrophage colony-stimulating factor in neutropenia. *DICP* 1991;25:32–5.

103. Grossberg HS, Bonnem EM. GM-CSF with ganciclovir for the treatment of CMV retinitis in AIDS. *N Engl J Med* 1989;320:1560. Letter.

104. Groopman JE. Granulocyte-macrophage colony-stimulating factor in human immunodeficiency virus disease. *Semin Hematol* 1990;27(suppl 3):8–14.

105. Israel RJ, Levine JD. Granulocyte-macrophage colony-stimulating factor and azidothymidine in patients with acquired immunodeficiency syndrome. *Blood* 1991;77:2085–6. Letter.

Hormonal Drugs

Adrenal Hormones

Class Instructions: Corticosteroids. (Systemic use) These drugs may be taken with food, milk, or an antacid to minimize stomach upset. Take single daily doses or alternate-day doses in the morning prior to 9 AM. Take multiple daily doses at evenly spaced intervals during the day. Report unusual weight gain, lower extremity swelling, muscle weakness, black tarry stools, vomiting of blood, facial swelling, menstrual irregularities, prolonged sore throat, fever, cold, infection, serious injury, fatigue, anorexia, nausea, vomiting, diarrhea, weight loss, dizziness, or low blood sugar. Consult physician during periods of increased stress. If you are diabetic, you may have increased requirements for insulin or oral hypoglycemics. Carry appropriate identification if you are taking long-term corticosteroid therapy. Do not discontinue this medication without medical approval; tell any new health care provider that you are taking a corticosteroid. Avoid immunizations with live vaccines.

COSYNTROPIN
Cortrosyn

Cosyntropin is a synthetic polypeptide containing the first 24 of the 39 amino acids of natural corticotropin (adrenocorticotropic hormone; ACTH) and retaining the full activity of corticotropin with decreased antigenicity. **Corticotropin** and cosyntropin stimulate the adrenal cortex to produce and secrete gluco- and mineralocorticoids and androgens. Cosyntropin 250 μg is equivalent to corticotropin 25 units, and either drug in these doses infused IV over 8 hr elicits maximal adrenocortical secretion. Cosyntropin is used as a diagnostic agent to detect adrenocortical insufficiency, but can also be used therapeutically as a substitute for the more antigenic corticotropin from animal source; however, used therapeutically, both cause salt and water retention and virilization, and neither is preferred over the more reliable glucocorticoids. Adverse reactions of diagnostic cosyntropin are limited to rare reports of hypersensitivity. For diagnostic use, exogenous cortisone or hydrocortisone is held on the test day and, if the patient is not taking spironolactone or an estrogen, a baseline cortisol level (which should exceed 5 μg/dL) is drawn in the morning just before the dose. Then, cosyntropin 250 μg in 1 mL of NS is given IM, or 250 μg in 2–5 mL NS is given IV push over 2 min (use one-half dose for those ≤2 yr). Normal cortisol levels are >18 μg/dL (500 nmol/L) 30 min after the injection and ≥7 μg/dL (190 nmol/L) above baseline. If the cortisol level is drawn 60 min postadministration, then an approximate doubling of the baseline cortisol value indicates a normal response. Alternatively, give an infusion of 250 μg in D5W or NS over 6 hr in the morning with serum cortisol levels drawn before and after. The second cortisol level should be >18 μg/dL (500 nmol/L) and ≥7 μg/dL (190 nmol/L) above baseline.[1-4] Available as injection 250-μg vial.

DEXAMETHASONE

Decadron, Hexadrol, Various

Pharmacology. Dexamethasone is a potent, long-acting glucocorticoid lacking sodium-retaining activity with low to moderate doses (*see* Prednisone and the Oral Corticosteroids Comparison Chart).

Administration and Adult Dosage. Total daily dosage is variable depending on the clinical disorder and patient response. **PO for acute, self-limited allergic disorders or exacerbation of chronic allergic disorders** 0.75–9 mg/day in 2 divided doses on the first day, then tapered over 7 days and discontinued. **IV for cerebral edema** 10 mg (as the sodium phosphate) initially, followed by 4 mg IM or IV q 6 hr for several days until maximal response occurs; then decrease the dosage over 5–7 days and discontinue. **PO or IV as an antiemetic with cancer chemotherapy** (usually in combination with other antiemetics) 10–20 mg immediately prior to therapy; optionally, up to 40 mg may be given after chemotherapy.[5–8] **PO or IV for acute exacerbations of multiple sclerosis** (after 200 mg/day prednisolone given for 1 week) 4–8 mg dexamethasone every other day for 1 month. **PO as the dexamethasone suppression test to screen for Cushing's disease** 1 mg at 11 PM; a measured serum cortisol at 8 AM the next morning <5 μg/dL (140 nmol/L) indicates a normal response.[9] Alternatively, PO 0.5 mg q 6 hr for 48 hr (8 doses), with a 24-hr urine collected for 17-hydroxycorticosteroids (17-OHCs) during the second 24-hr period. A normal response is 2.5 mg (6.9 μmol) or less of 17-OHCs during the second 24-hr period.[9] **PO as a Cushing's syndrome test to distinguish pituitary origin from other causes** 2 mg q 6 hr for 48 hr (8 doses). A normal response is a 24-hr urine concentration of less than 2.5 mg (6.9 μmol) of 17-OHCs.[9] *See* Notes. **IM (aqueous) in the mother for antenatal prevention of neonatal distress syndrome** starting 24 hr or more before premature delivery, give 5 mg q 12 hr for 4 doses, or 12 or 16 mg q 24 hr for 2 doses.[10] **IV for septic shock** not recommended because of a lack of efficacy and a possible increase in mortality.[11,12] **IM (depot) for prolonged systemic effect** 8–16 mg q 1–3 weeks. (*See also* Inhaled Corticosteroids Comparison Chart.)

Special Populations. *Pediatric Dosage.* **PO, IM, or IV for airway edema** 0.25–0.5 mg/kg/dose q 6 hr prn for croup or beginning 24 hr before planned extubation, then for 4–6 doses; **PO, IM, or IV as an antiinflammatory or immunosuppressive** 0.03–0.15 mg/kg/day divided q 6–12 hr; **PO, IM, or IV for cerebral edema** 1.5 mg/kg once, then 1.5 mg/kg/day divided q 4–6 hr for 5 days, then taper over the next 5 days and discontinue. **IV to prevent hearing loss and other neurologic sequelae in** *Haemophilus influenzae* **bacterial meningitis** (>2 months) 0.15 mg/kg q 6 hr, beginning no sooner than 20 min before (or with) the first dose of antibiotics and continued for 4 days.[12–15]

Geriatric Dosage. Consider using a lower dosage for decreased body size.

Patient Instructions. (*See* Corticosteroids Class Instructions.)

Dosage Forms. **Elxr** 0.1 mg/mL; **Soln** 0.1, 1 mg/mL; **Tab** 0.25, 0.5, 0.75, 1, 1.5, 2, 4, 6 mg; **Inj** 4, 10, 20, 24 mg/mL; **Depot Inj** 8, 16 mg/mL (as acetate).

Pharmacokinetics. *Onset and Duration.* (*See* Oral Corticosteroids Comparison Chart.)

Serum Levels. Serum concentration is not directly correlated with therapeutic effect.[2,16]

Fate. After oral administration, 78 ± 14% is absorbed; 68% is plasma protein bound. V_d is 0.82 ± 0.22 L/kg. The drug is eliminated primarily by hepatic metabolism, with about 2.6 ± 0.6% excreted unchanged in urine.[3,7,18]

$t_{\frac{1}{2}}$. (Males) 3.5 ± 0.87 hr; (females) 2.4 ± 0.16 hr.[3,7,18]

Adverse Reactions. (*See* Prednisone Adverse Reactions.) Perineal itching or burning may occur after IV administration.[19]

Contraindications. Systemic fungal infections (except as maintenance therapy in adrenal insufficiency); administration of live virus vaccines to patients receiving an immunosuppressive dosage of dexamethasone; IM use in idiopathic thrombocytopenic purpura.

Precautions. (*See* Prednisone.)

Parameters to Monitor. (*See* Prednisone.)

Notes. The dexamethasone suppression test for diagnosis of depression is of unproven value.[20,21] Variations of the dexamethasone suppression test (for Cushing's disease screening) have been used.[1,9]

METHYLPREDNISOLONE SODIUM SUCCINATE   Solu-Medrol, Various

Methylprednisolone sodium succinate is an injectable glucocorticoid that has about 1.25 times greater antiinflammatory potency than prednisone or prednisolone and a similar duration of biologic activity (*see* Oral Corticosteroids Comparison Chart). It is commonly used when oral therapy is not possible and in situations in which large parenteral doses are necessary. Plasma protein binding is 78 ± 3% and the V_d is 1.2 ± 0.2 L/kg; Cl is 0.37 ± 0.054 L/hr/kg. The serum half-life is 2.2 ± 0.5 hr and is not affected by renal function. The drug is extensively metabolized, with 4.9 ± 2.3% excreted unchanged in urine. Side effects are similar to prednisone in equivalent dosages. Ketoconazole reduces methylprednisolone elimination, possibly leading to excessive corticosteroid effect (*see also* Prednisone Drug Interactions). Evidence of efficacy in improving the outcome of septic shock is lacking, and, because of increased mortality in some patient groups, the use of methylprednisolone in septic shock is not recommended. Patients with acute spinal-cord injury treated with high-dose methylprednisolone within 8 hr may have improved neurologic recovery. Large doses (≥250 mg) should usually be infused slowly (eg, over 1–2 hr), because arrhythmias and sudden death have occurred with rapid infusions. Initial IV adult dosages range from 10–40 mg given over one to several minutes, to 30 mg/kg q 4–6 hr (high-dose therapy) for up to 48–72 hr for severe, acute conditions. Dosage in acute spinal cord injury (begun within 8 hr) is IV 30 mg/kg over 15 min, followed 45 min later by a continuous IV infusion of 5.4 mg/kg/hr for 23 hr. Pediatric dosage as an antiinflammatory or immunosuppressive is IV 0.16–0.8 mg/kg/day in 2–4 divided doses.[3,11–13,18,22–24] Available as injection 40, 125, 500 mg, 1 and 2 g, and as depot injection 20, 40, 80 mg/mL (as acetate). Also available as tablets (nonsuccinate salt) (*see* Oral Corticosteroids Comparison Chart).

PREDNISONE   Deltasone, Orasone, Various

Pharmacology. Prednisone is a synthetic glucocorticoid with less sodium-retaining activity than hydrocortisone. Prednisone is inactive until converted into prednisolone. At the cellular level, glucocorticoids appear to act by controlling the rate of protein synthesis. Clinically, these drugs are used primarily for their antiinflammatory and immunosuppressant effects.

Administration and Adult Dosage. Total daily dosage is variable, depending on the clinical disorder and patient response.[16,25] Daily divided high-dose therapy for initial control of more severe disease states may be necessary until satisfactory control is obtained, usually 4–10 days for many allergic and collagen diseases. Administration of a short- or intermediate-acting preparation given as a single dose in the morning (prior to 9 AM) is likely to produce fewer side effects and less pituitary-adrenal suppression than either a divided dosage regimen with the same agent or an equivalent dosage of a long-acting agent.[16] Alternate-day therapy (ie, total 48-hr dosage administered every other morning) with intermediate-acting agents (eg, prednisone) further reduces the prevalence and degree of side effects. However, it may not be uniformly effective in treating all disease states, unless large doses are used (eg, 40–60 mg every other day for adults requiring long-term corticosteroid therapy for asthma).[16,26,27] Complete adrenal suppression may not occur with single daily doses given either in the morning or evening if the prednisone dose is 15 mg or less, but Cushing's syndrome may still occur and patients should receive supplemental corticosteroids during periods of unusual stress. **In times of stress** (eg, surgery, severe trauma, serious illness), patients on long-term corticosteroid therapy (>5 mg/day prednisone or equivalent) should receive supplemental IV hydrocortisone 100–300 mg/day or PO prednisone 25-75 mg/day in divided doses.[2,3,16,25,28] Guidelines for withdrawal from glucocorticoid therapy have been published.[2,9]

Common initial doses are: **PO for acute asthma exacerbations in adults and adolescents** 40 mg 2–4 times/day for 3–5 days; hospitalized patients may require a parenteral preparation. Reduce dosage to minimum effective maintenance dosage as soon as possible; **PO as an adjunct therapy for** *Pneumocystis carinii* **pneumonia** (with an arterial PO_2 of 70 mm Hg or less, or an arterial-alveolar gradient ≥35 mm Hg) 40 mg bid for 5 days begun with antimicrobial therapy, then 20 mg bid for 5 days, then 20 mg/day for the duration of antimicrobial therapy; **PO for arthritis** 10 mg/day; **PO for collagen diseases** 1 mg/kg/day; **PO for acute gout** 30–50 mg/day, gradually decreased over 10 days; **PO for rheumatic carditis** 40 mg/day; **PO for nephrotic syndrome** 60 mg/day; **PO for skin disorders** 40 mg/day, up to 240 mg/day in pemphigus; **PO for ulcerative colitis** 10–30 mg/day or, if severe, 60–120 mg/day; **PO for thrombocytopenia** 0.5 mg/kg/day; **PO for organ transplantation** (in combination with cyclosporine) 200 mg once, then taper dosage in 40-mg increments daily until reaching a dose of 20 mg/day; continue at 20 mg/day for 60 days, then reduce dosage to 10 mg/day and make further dosage adjustments based on the clinical situation; **PO for acute exacerbations of multiple sclerosis** 200 mg/day for 1 week, then 80 mg every other day for 1 month.[3,12,26–33]

Special Populations. *Pediatric Dosage.* Dosage depends on disease state and patient response. *Common initial doses are:* **PO for acute asthma** 1–2 mg/kg/day in 1–2 divided doses; **PO for inflammation or immunosuppression** 0.2–1 mg/kg/day in 2–4 divided doses.[13]

Dosage Forms. **Soln** 1, 5 mg/mL; **Syrup** 1 mg/mL; **Tab** 1, 2.5, 5, 10, 20, 50 mg.

Patient Instructions. (*See* Corticosteroids Class Instructions.) If a dose is missed and the proper schedule is *every other day*, take it as soon as possible and resume the schedule unless it is past noon. In that case, wait until the next morning and resume every other day administration. If the proper schedule is *once a day*, take the dose as soon as possible. If you do not remember until the next day, do not double that day's dose; skip the missed dose. If the proper schedule is *several times a day*, take the dose as soon as possible and resume the normal schedule. If you do not remember until the next dose is due, then take both the regular dose and the missed dose, and resume the normal dosage schedule.

Pharmacokinetics. *Onset and Duration.* (*See* Oral Corticosteroids Comparison Chart.)

Serum Levels. Serum concentration is not directly correlated with therapeutic effect.[2,16] A timed prednisolone serum drug level may be useful in estimating clearance and identifying abnormalities in absorption, elimination, or patient compliance.[34]

Fate. Bioavailability is 77–99%, with peak levels occurring 1–4 hr postingestion;[18] 90–95% is plasma protein bound, depending on serum concentration. Prednisone is metabolized in the liver to its active form, prednisolone.[2,16] Liver disease does not impair conversion to active metabolite. In fact, patients with liver disease and hypoalbuminemia are more likely to suffer major side effects of prednisone as a result of decreased protein binding and reduced prednisolone clearance.[2,16,35,36] V_d of prednisolone is 1.5 ± 0.2 L/kg. Over 90% of metabolites are excreted in urine; $3 \pm 2\%$ of a dose of prednisone is excreted unchanged in urine with an additional $15 \pm 5\%$ excreted as prednisolone.[3,18,35]

$t_{\frac{1}{2}}$. (Prednisone) 3.4 hr; (prednisolone) 2–5 hr.[18,35] Biologic half-life exceeds serum half-life (*see* Corticosteroids Comparison Chart).

Adverse Reactions. Dose- and duration-related side effects include fluid and electrolyte disturbances (with possible edema and hypertension), hyperglycemia and glycosuria, spread of herpes conjunctivitis, activation of tuberculosis, peptic ulcers (possibly), osteoporosis, bone fractures,[37] myopathy, menstrual irregularities, behavioral disturbances (increasing with dosages >40 mg/day),[38] poor wound healing, ocular cataracts, glaucoma, arrest of growth (in children), hirsutism, pseudotumor cerebri (primarily in children), and Cushing's syndrome (moon face, buffalo hump, central obesity, easy bruising, acne, hirsutism, and striae).[2,16,25] Prolonged therapy may lead to suppression of pituitary-adrenal function. Too rapid withdrawal of long-term therapy can cause acute adrenal insufficiency (eg, fever, myalgia, arthralgia, and malaise); adrenally suppressed patients are also unable to respond to stress.

Contraindications. Systemic fungal infections (except as maintenance therapy in adrenal insufficiency); administration of live virus vaccines in patients receiving immunosuppressive doses of corticosteroids.

Precautions. Pregnancy. Use with caution in diabetes mellitus; osteoporosis; peptic ulcer; esophagitis; tuberculosis; and other acute and chronic bacterial, viral, and fungal infections; hypertension or other cardiovascular diseases; hypothyroidism; immunizations; hypoalbuminemia; psychosis; and liver disease. Suppression of PPD and other skin test reactions may occur.

Drug Interactions. Corticosteroids may increase serum glucose levels, and an increase in the dosage of antidiabetic drugs may be required. Corticosteroids may decrease salicylate serum levels. Amphotericin B and loop and thiazide diuretics may enhance corticosteroid-induced potassium depletion. Carbamazepine, phenobarbital (and possibly other barbiturates), phenytoin (best documented with dexamethasone), rifampin, and possibly aminoglutethimide increase the metabolism of corticosteroids. Ketoconazole reduces methylprednisolone elimination, but its effect on other corticosteroids is not well established.

Parameters to Monitor. Observe for behavioral disturbances and signs or symptoms of Cushing's syndrome. With short-term, high-dose therapy, frequently monitor serum potassium and glucose, and blood pressure. With long-term therapy, monitor these parameters occasionally and perform periodic eye examinations and possibly stool guaiac. Monitor growth in infants and children on prolonged therapy.

Notes. Other, more expensive glucocorticoids offer minimal advantages over prednisone in most clinical situations.[3,39] Dosage ranges for **prednisolone** are the same as those for prednisone. Patients who have received daily glucocorticoid therapy for asthma for less than 2 weeks *do not* require dosage tapering to prevent acute adrenal sufficiency; however, dosage tapering may be required to maintain an adequate clinical response.[25,29] Efficacy in patients with stable COPD is controversial.[40,41]

ORAL CORTICOSTEROIDS COMPARISON CHART

DURATION AND DRUG	DOSAGE FORMS	EQUIVALENT ANTI-INFLAMMATORY DOSE (MG)*	RELATIVE ANTI-INFLAMMATORY POTENCY*	RELATIVE MINERALOCORTICOID ACTIVITY	SERUM HALF-LIFE (HR)	COMMENTS
SHORT-ACTING GLUCOCORTICOIDS (biologic activity 8–12 hr)						
Cortisone Various	Tab 5, 10, 25 mg.	25	0.8	0.8	0.5	Must be metabolized to active form (hydrocortisone).
Hydrocortisone Various	Tab 5, 10, 20 mg Susp (as cypionate) 2 mg/mL.	20	1	1	1.5	Daily secretion in man is 20 mg.
INTERMEDIATE-ACTING GLUCOCORTICOIDS (biologic activity 12–36 hr)						
Methylprednisolone Medrol Various	Tab 2, 4, 8, 16, 24, 32 mg.	4	5	0.5	2.3	Minimal sodium-retaining activity.
Prednisolone Various	Tab 5 mg Syrup 3 mg/mL.	5	4	0.8	2–5	Minimal sodium-retaining activity.
Prednisone Various	Tab 1, 2.5, 5, 10, 20, 50 mg Soln 1, 5 mg/mL Syrup 1 mg/mL.	5	4	0.8	3.4	Must be metabolized to active form (prednisolone).

(continued)

ORAL CORTICOSTEROIDS COMPARISON CHART (continued)

DURATION AND DRUG	DOSAGE FORMS	EQUIVALENT ANTI-INFLAMMATORY DOSE (MG)*	RELATIVE ANTI-INFLAMMATORY POTENCY*	RELATIVE MINERALOCORTICOID ACTIVITY	SERUM HALF-LIFE (HR)	COMMENTS
Triamcinolone Aristocort Kenacort Various	Tab 1, 2, 4, 8 mg Syrup 0.8 mg/mL.	4	5	0	2.6	
LONG-ACTING GLUCOCORTICOIDS (biologic activity 36–54 hr)						
Betamethasone Celestone	Tab 0.6 mg Syrup 0.12 mg/mL.	0.6	25	0	5+	Minimal sodium-retaining activity, but with high doses, retention may occur.
Dexamethasone Decadron Hexadrol Various	Tab 0.25, 0.5, 0.75, 1, 1.5, 2, 4, 6 mg Elxr 0.1 mg/mL Soln 0.1, 1 mg/mL.	0.75	30	0	Males 3.5 Females 2.4	No sodium-retaining activity with low to moderate doses.
MINERALOCORTICOID (biologic activity 18–36 hr)						
Fludrocortisone Florinef	Tab 100 µg.	—	10	125	3.5+	Mineralocorticoid used in Addison's disease.

*Antiinflammatory potency does not correlate with immunosuppressive effects.[43]
From references 2, 3, 17, 18, 25, 35, and 42.

Antidiabetic Drugs

ACARBOSE

Acarbose is an oral α-glucosidase inhibitor indicated for the management of hyperglycemia caused by type II diabetes mellitus or non-insulin-dependent diabetes mellitus (NIDDM). Inhibition of this gut enzyme system effectively reduces the rate of complex carbohydrate digestion and the subsequent absorption of glucose, lowering postprandial glucose excursions in NIDDM. In obese and nonobese patients with NIDDM, acarbose monotherapy is associated with a 0.5–1% decrease in hemoglobin A_{1c} (HbA_{1c}). The drug is poorly absorbed from the GI tract (<2%) and undergoes extensive metabolism in the GI tract via intestinal flora and digestive enzymes. All metabolites and absorbed acarbose are excreted via the kidneys. The half-life of the drug with normal renal function is about 2 hr. It is contraindicated in patients with inflammatory bowel disease, colonic ulceration, obstructive bowel disorders, or insulin-dependent diabetes, or in those with a history of diabetic ketoacidosis. Acarbose is not recommended in patients with a Cr_s >2 mg/dL, because it may accumulate in serum and long-term studies have not been performed in this population. Use the drug with caution in patients with disorders of digestion or absorption or those with a medical condition that might deteriorate with increased intestinal gas formation. The major side effect of acarbose is flatulence. Acarbose monotherapy is not associated with hypoglycemia; however, patients managed with combination therapy (acarbose plus a sulfonylurea or insulin) may have hypoglycemia secondary to the other drug. In this setting, do not manage hypoglycemia with a complex carbohydrate (eg, sucrose), but rather with oral glucose (if the patient is conscious) or IV glucose or glucagon (if the patient is unconscious). Attempting to manage hypoglycemia with oral sugar sources other than glucose is not effective in acarbose-treated patients and may have grave consequences. The recommended initial dosage is 25 mg PO tid just prior to meals. Increase dosage to 50 mg tid after 4–8 weeks, and again to 100 mg tid after 4–8 additional weeks, if necessary. Dosages >100 mg tid are not recommended because of increased risk of hepatotoxicity.[44] Available as 50- and 100-mg tablets.

ALDOSE REDUCTASE INHIBITORS

Prolonged hyperglycemia causes excess flux of glucose into tissues, and glucose is shunted to the polyol pathway, resulting in excess sorbitol production. Excess intracellular sorbitol causes a reduction in the uptake of myoinositol and ultimately a down-regulation in the Na^+/K^+-ATPase system. This process is thought to be one of the biochemical mechanisms leading to the development of neuropathy, collagen disorders, cataracts, and possibly retinopathy in diabetics. Because aldose reductase is the rate-limiting enzyme in this pathway, aldose reductase inhibitors are being studied as a possible means of decreasing the sorbitol-linked sequelae of diabetes. Although this is a promising class of drugs, the side effects, dosage regimens, and long-term benefits are yet to be determined. **Tolrestat** (Alredase, Ayerst) has a serum half-life of 10–13 hr and has been used investigationally in doses of 100 mg bid. In one study, tolrestat was shown to reduce the rate of progression of neuropathy compared to placebo. Other aldose reductase inhibitors, **ponalrestat** (Prodiax, Merck) and **zenarestat** (Warner-Lambert), are also currently under investigation.[45–47]

GLUCAGON

Glucagon is a counterregulatory hormone that increases blood glucose levels by induction of glycogenolysis. It is indicated for the treatment of the unconscious hypoglycemic patient, but it is effective only in patients with hepatic glycogen stores. Glucagon may also be used as a bowel relaxant during diagnostic procedures. Glucagon occasionally causes nausea and vomiting, so position patients given glucagon to prevent aspiration. Administration of glucagon may occasionally result in generalized allergic reactions such as urticaria, respiratory distress, and hypotension. Glucagon may also precipitate hypertensive crisis in the patient with underlying pheochromocytoma (secondary to release of catecholamines). Glucagon may be administered IM, SC, or IV in doses of 0.5–1 mg. Response is usually observed in 10–20 min.[48] Available as 1- and 10-mg injection.

INSULINS

Pharmacology. Insulin promotes cellular uptake of glucose, fatty acids, and amino acids, and their conversion to glycogen, triglycerides, and proteins. Beef and pork insulins are extracted and purified from the animal's pancreas. Human insulin is produced either by recombinant DNA technology or by enzymatic conversion of pork insulin to human. No differences in side effects or long-term control of diabetes have been observed between human insulin and highly purified pork insulin.

Administration and Adult Dosage. **SC for type I diabetes** usual initial dosage ranges from 0.6–0.75 units/kg/day in divided doses.[49] During the first week of therapy, the dosage requirement may escalate to 1 unit/kg/day in divided doses because of insulin resistance and the usual age group (adolescents) being treated. The dosage requirement may temporarily decrease to 0.1–0.5 units/kg/day if the patient experiences a "honeymoon phase." Dosage adjustments are made on the basis of clinical symptoms, blood glucose levels, and hemoglobin A_{1c} values. Insulin may be administered by various methods depending on a number of factors. Single daily SC injections of intermediate-acting insulin are often used, but should not usually be used in the type I patient, because although single daily injections may offer protection from diabetic ketoacidosis, they are not sufficient to prevent long-term complications. Intensive forms of insulin therapy, which may provide better glycemic control, include the split-and-mixed regimen (2 SC injections daily of mixed short- and long-acting insulin), multiple daily SC doses of short-acting insulin in combination with a single injection of long-acting insulin, and insulin pump therapy. **IV, SC, or IM for diabetic ketoacidosis (IV preferred for patients in shock)** 0.1 unit/kg, followed by a continuous infusion of 0.1–0.2 units/hr/kg. If the serum glucose does not decline by 75 mg/dL in 1–2 hr, increase the dosage; dosage is titrated in this manner to reverse ketoacidosis.[50,51] Fluid and electrolyte repletion must accompany insulin therapy. **SC for type II diabetes** those who require insulin (patients unresponsive to oral agent therapy or patients with extreme hyperglycemia [fasting serum glucose >200–225 mg/dL]) may need as little as 5–10 units/day or more than 100 units/day.[52] Patients who require <30 units/day may be well controlled with 1 injection/day of intermediate-acting insulin; patients who require more than 30 units/day should be treated with 2 or more injections per day. Insulin resistance in the type II population is usually associated with obesity. Weight reduction and improved glycemic control usually improve insulin response.

Special Populations. *Pediatric Dosage.* (*See* Administration and Adult Dosage.) Common maintenance dosages are 0.6–0.9 units/kg/day in divided doses in prepubertal children, up to 1.5 units/kg/day during puberty, and <1 unit/kg/day after puberty. Requirements may occasionally be as high as 200 units/day during growth spurts.

Geriatric Dosage. Same as adult dosage.

Other Conditions. Insulin requirements may be decreased in patients with renal or hepatic impairment, or hypothyroidism. Requirements may be increased during pregnancy (especially in the second and third trimesters), in patients with high fever, hyperthyroidism, or severe infections; and following trauma or surgery.

Dosage Forms. (*See* Insulins Comparison Chart.)

Patient Instructions. Instruct patients in the following areas: use of insulin syringes and needles; storage, mixing,[53] and handling of insulin; urine ketone testing; blood glucose testing; adherence to proper diet and regular meals; personal hygiene (especially the feet); and recognition and treatment of hypoglycemia and hyperglycemia (*see* Sulfonylurea Agents).

Pharmacokinetics. *Onset and Duration.* Human insulin is more soluble than animal source insulins and may have a shorter onset and duration of action (*see* Insulins Comparison Chart).

Serum Levels. Diabetics vary widely in their response to insulin, and serum levels are not normally monitored clinically.

Fate. The rate of absorption depends on the insulin type (*see* Insulins Comparison Chart). Serum levels are affected by obesity, diet, degree of activity, pancreatic β-cell activity, growth hormone, and circulating antibodies. Insulin is primarily metabolized in the liver, although the kidneys are responsible for the metabolism of up to 50% of the daily insulin output.[54]

$t_{1/2}$. (Regular insulin) 4–5 min after IV administration.[55]

Adverse Reactions. Hypoglycemia is dose related. Patients being treated with intensive insulin regimens of 3 or more injections/day are more prone to hypoglycemic episodes than are patients treated with the conventional 1–2 injections/day.[56] Local allergic reactions, with an onset of 15 min–4 hr, are usually caused by insulin impurities, and 70% of these patients have a history of interrupted treatment. Immune or nonimmune insulin resistance occurs occasionally. Lipohypertrophy at the injection site may occur, especially with repeated use of the same site. Lipoatrophy may also occur at the injection site and may be less frequent with the highly purified animal or human insulins. Allergy, resistance, and lipoatrophy may be overcome by switching to insulin from another animal source or to a more highly purified product (eg, human insulin). In general, pork insulin is less antigenic than beef-pork or pure beef insulin (no longer available in the United States) because it is more structurally similar to human insulin, which is the least immunogenic.[57]

Contraindications. Hypersensitivity, although desensitization procedures may be warranted in some patients.[58]

Precautions. Use with caution in patients with renal or hepatic disease, or hypothyroidism. Insulin requirements may change with exercise or infection, or when switching animal sources or to more purified products.

Drug Interactions. Alcohol may produce hypoglycemia, especially in fasting patients; moderate increases in blood glucose may occur in nonfasting patients. Oral contraceptives, corticosteroids, furosemide, niacin (large doses), thiazide diuretics, and thyroid hormones (large doses) may increase insulin requirements. Anabolic steroids may decrease the insulin requirement. Avoid MAO inhibitors in diabetics because they may interfere with the normal adrenergic response to hypoglycemia, prolonging the action of antidiabetic agents. β-Blockers prolong hypoglycemic episodes and inhibit tachycardia and tremors, which are signs of hypoglycemia (sweating is not inhibited); hypertension may occur during hypoglycemia; cardioselective β-blockers (eg, atenolol, metoprolol) are less likely to cause problems than nonselective types (eg, nadolol, propranolol).

Parameters to Monitor. Monitor blood glucose routinely (*see* Blood Glucose Monitors Comparison Chart). Long-term diabetic control is best monitored using hemoglobin A$_{1c}$.[49] The patient should continually watch for subjective symptoms of hypoglycemia and hyperglycemia. Observe for signs of lipoatrophy, lipohypertrophy, and allergic reactions.

Notes. Insulin is stable for 1–2 months at constant room temperature and up to 24 months under refrigeration. Insulin is adsorbed by glass and plastic IV infusion equipment, with little difference between glass and plastic; maximal adsorption occurs within 15 sec. Adsorption may be minimized by the addition of small amounts (1–2%) of **albumin** to the infusion container; however, this may be costly and unnecessary because patient response is generally adequate without addition of albumin. Variation can be minimized by flushing all new IV administration equipment with 50 mL of the insulin-containing solution (thereby saturating "binding sites") before it is used.[59]

Pump devices are available to deliver insulin depending on or independent of a measured serum glucose level. "Open-loop" devices can deliver insulin at a constant rate and can be manually controlled. Although the open-loop devices have been used successfully in selected patients, few physicians place patients on the pumps because of concern with infection at the injection site, hypoglycemia, and the relatively high cost. "Closed-loop" devices (the "artificial pancreas") can deliver insulin at variable rates in response to serum glucose, but are used only in the experimental setting.

Human insulin is the insulin of choice for patients with insulin resistance, pregnancy, or allergy, new insulin-dependent patients, or any patient taking insulin intermittently.

INSULIN ANALOGUES

Insulin injected SC does not result in serum insulin concentrations that mimic normal physiologic insulin response. Over 30 human insulin analogues with differing pharmacokinetic profiles have been produced using recombinant DNA technology. The goal of insulin analogue research is to produce a human insulin analogue with a rapid action (to provide bolus postprandial insulin) and a human insulin analogue with a slow, extended release pattern (to provide basal insulin). **Insulin lispro** (Humalog) is a rapid-acting analogue with a pharmacokinetic profile between that of IV and SC regular human insulin. Humalog offers a pharmacokinetic profile that is superior to regular human insulin when used to cover postprandial glycemic excursions. Long-acting analogues are also being evaluated.[60–62] Humalog is available as injection 100 units/mL.

INSULINS COMPARISON CHART*		
PRODUCT	MANUFACTURER	STRENGTH
SHORT-ACTING (onset, 0.5–2 hr; peak, 3–4 hr; duration, 4–8 hr)		
Beef/Pork		
Iletin I Regular	Lilly	U-100
Pork		
Iletin II Regular	Lilly	U-100, U-500
Purified Pork Regular	Novo/Nordisk	U-100
Human		
Humalog	Lilly	U-100
Humulin Regular	Lilly	U-100
Novolin R	Novo/Nordisk	U-100
Velosulin Human R	Novo/Nordisk	U-100
INTERMEDIATE-ACTING (onset, 2–4 hr; peak, 8–14 hr; duration, 14–24 hr)		
Beef/Pork		
Iletin I Lente	Lilly	U-100
Iletin I NPH	Lilly	U-100
Pork		
Iletin II Lente	Lilly	U-100
Iletin II NPH	Lilly	U-100
Purified Pork Lente	Novo/Nordisk	U-100
Purified Pork NPH	Novo/Nordisk	U-100
Human		
Humulin L (Lente)	Lilly	U-100
Humulin N (NPH)	Lilly	U-100
Novolin L (Lente)	Novo/Nordisk	U-100
Novolin N (NPH)	Novo/Nordisk	U-100
LONG-ACTING (onset, 6–14 hr; peak, none; duration, 20–30 hr)		
Human		
Humulin U (Ultralente)	Lilly	U-100

(continued)

INSULINS COMPARISON CHART* (continued)		
PRODUCT	MANUFACTURER	STRENGTH

FIXED COMBINATIONS† (onset, 0.5–1 hr; peak, 3–10 hr; duration, 14–18 hr)

Human

Humulin 70/30†	Lilly	U-100
Novolin 70/30†	Novo/Nordisk	U-100
Humulin 50/50†	Lilly	U-100

*There may be variations within the ranges of onset, peak, and duration among manufacturers. Onset and duration may be prolonged in long-standing diabetes, and large doses may have prolonged duration of action. Site of injection, depth of injection, and whether site is exercised, massaged, or has heat applied to it also affect rate of insulin absorption. Human insulins have a slightly more rapid onset and a shorter duration of action than animal-derived insulins. SCHumalog is more rapidly absorbed and has a shorter duration than other human insulins.
†These products contain isophane and regular insulin in the specified proportions; the first number designates the percentage of isophane insulin and the second designates the percentage of regular insulin.
From references 49, 56, and product information.

METFORMIN   Glucophage

Pharmacology. Metformin is a biguanide antihyperglycemic agent used in the management of type II diabetes mellitus. It does not affect insulin secretion, but rather reduces hepatic glucose production, primarily by a reduction in glycogenolysis.[63] It also enhances glucose utilization by muscle.[63,64] Reported increases in glucose utilization in muscle are 7–35%.[63] In addition to blood glucose reductions (mean 53 mg/dL), metformin may also have beneficial effects on serum lipids.[65] (*See* Notes.)

Administration and Adult Dosage. PO for type II diabetes initiate 500 mg tablets with a dosage of 1 tablet bid with the morning and evening meals. Increase dosage in 500 mg/day increments at weekly intervals, to a maximum of 2.5 g/day. Initiate 850-mg tablets with 1 tablet/day before the morning meal. Increase dosage in 850 mg/day increments q 2 weeks, to a maximum of 850 mg tid. Individualize maintenance dosage based on glycemic response. Give all dosages up to 2 g/day in 2 divided doses; larger dosages require a tid regimen to reduce GI discomfort.

Special Populations. *Pediatric Dosage.* Safety and efficacy not established.

Geriatric Dosage. Initial and maintenance dosages should be low in the elderly. Avoid usual maximum adult dosage.

Dosage Forms. Tab 500, 850 mg.

Patient Instructions. Take metformin just prior to meals in order to reduce gastrointestinal side effects (diarrhea, nausea, and heartburn). Contact your physician if gastrointestinal side effects persist. Do not take metformin if you develop a serious medical condition such as myocardial infarction, stroke, or serious infection; require surgery; consume excessive amounts of alcohol; or require x-ray procedures with contrast dyes.

Pharmacokinetics. *Serum Levels.* Not monitored clinically.

Fate. Absorption half-life is 0.9–2.6 hr; absolute bioavailability is 50–60%.[64] Peak serum levels are 1–2 mg/L in patients with non-insulin-dependent diabetes. Plasma protein binding is negligible; V_d is 654 ± 358 L after a single 850-mg oral dose; Cl is proportionate to renal function. Metformin is excreted in the urine unchanged.

$t_{1/2}$. 1.7–4.5 hr in patients with normal renal function.

Adverse Reactions. Acute side effects may occur in as many as 30% of patients treated with metformin. The side effects include primarily GI complaints, such as diarrhea, abdominal discomfort, nausea, anorexia, and metallic taste. GI side effects are usually transient and dose related, and can be mitigated by giving the drug just prior to meals, initiating therapy with small doses, and increasing the dosage slowly.[65] Metformin reduces serum vitamin B_{12} levels in approximately 7% of patients, but is rarely associated with anemia. If vitamin B_{12} deficiency anemia occurs, it may be treated with vitamin B_{12} supplementation or by discontinuing metformin. Lactic acidosis has been reported; however, almost all cases occur in patients in whom metformin was contraindicated or in patients who attempted suicide by overdose.[65] Lactic acidosis occurs in 0.03 cases/1000 patient-yr, with fatalities in about 50% of cases.

Contraindications. Patients with acute or chronic metabolic acidosis; patients undergoing radiographic studies requiring contrast media (withhold metformin temporarily); abnormal Cl_{cr} or Cr_s >1.5 mg/dL in males or 1.4 mg/dL in females; any disease that can cause hypoxia and could result in accumulation of lactate (eg, myocardial infarction, severe infections, stroke); or hepatic dysfunction.

Precautions. Avoid in pregnancy and lactation.

Drug Interactions. Furosemide and nifedipine increase serum levels of metformin, the clinical relevance of which is unknown. Cimetidine reduces the tubular secretion of metformin and may increase peak serum concentrations by as much as 60%.[25] (*See also* Insulin Drug Interactions.)

Parameters to Monitor. Monitor renal function, hepatic function, and CBC prior to initiation of therapy and at least annually thereafter. Monitor renal function more closely in the elderly because of the age-related changes in renal function and greater risk for acute renal failure (*see* Contraindications). The goal of therapy is to reduce fasting blood glucose and glycosylated hemoglobin levels to normal or near normal using the lowest effective dosage of the drug.

Notes. Because of its effect on weight and lipids, metformin is an appropriate choice for initial monotherapy in obese, new-onset non-insulin-dependent diabetic patients, whereas sulfonylureas are usually a better choice for nonobese patients. In patients who do not respond to metformin monotherapy, combination therapy with a sulfonylurea may be effective.[65] Weight loss has been associated with metformin therapy (mean 0.8 kg); weight gain (mean 2.8 kg) has been found in patients treated with sulfonylureas.[67] Reductions in total cholesterol, LDL cholesterol, and triglycerides of 5, 8, and 16%, respectively, and an increase of 2% in HDL cholesterol have been reported.[65]

SULFONYLUREA AGENTS

Pharmacology. Sulfonylureas acutely enhance insulin secretion from pancreatic β-cells and potentiate insulin action on several extrahepatic tissues. Long-term, sulfonylureas increase peripheral utilization of glucose, suppress hepatic gluconeogenesis, and possibly increase the sensitivity and/or number of peripheral insulin receptors. Second-generation sulfonylureas (eg, **glyburide, glipizide**) are more potent than first-generation agents and are used in much smaller dosages, with lower resultant blood levels. These lower serum concentrations decrease the likelihood of protein-binding displacement and hepatic metabolic interference.

Administration and Adult Dosage. (*See* Sulfonylurea Agents Comparison Chart.)

Special Populations. *Pediatric Dosage.* Not used in children.

Geriatric Dosage. Same as adult dosage, but observe precautions in renal impairment.

Other Conditions. Dosage alterations may be necessary with all sulfonylureas in patients with severe hepatic dysfunction. With renal disease, especially in geriatric patients, there is an increased duration of action with **chlorpropamide, acetohexamide,**[68] and possibly **glyburide.**[69]

Dosage Forms. (*See* Sulfonylurea Agents Comparison Chart.)

Patient Instructions. Eat an approved diet consistently on a day-to-day basis. Take this medication at the same time each day (in the morning for once-daily medications). Report factors that might alter blood glucose levels (eg, infection, fasting states) as well as any side effects.

Pharmacokinetics. (*See* Sulfonylurea Agents Comparison Chart.)

Adverse Reactions. Hypoglycemic reactions (especially with **chlorpropamide**), anorexia, nausea, vomiting, diarrhea, allergic skin reactions, and cholestatic jaundice occur occasionally. Hematologic disorders, mild disulfiramlike reaction to alcohol, hyponatremia (most common with **chlorpropamide,** but may occur with **tolbutamide**), and bone marrow suppression occur rarely.[68,70]

Contraindications. Pregnancy; insulin-dependent diabetes; juvenile, unstable, or brittle diabetes; diabetes complicated by acidosis, ketosis, diabetic coma, major surgery, severe infection, or severe trauma.[57]

Precautions. Displacement from protein occurs with sulfonamides and high-dose salicylates. **Chlorpropamide** may cause hyponatremia, particularly in elderly women taking diuretics.[68] Drugs that impair glucose tolerance include oral contraceptives, corticosteroids, thiazide diuretics, furosemide, thyroid hormones (large doses), and niacin.[71] Acute ingestion of alcohol in combination with sulfonylureas can produce severe hypoglycemia.

Drug Interactions. Drugs that have been reported to enhance sulfonylurea effects include chloramphenicol (chlorpropamide and tolbutamide), dicumarol, fluconazole (glipizide, glyburide, tolbutamide, and possibly others), sulfonamides, and high-dose salicylates. Rifampin stimulates the metabolism of tolbutamide and possible other sulfonylureas. (*See also* Insulin Drug Interactions.)

Parameters to Monitor. Monitor clinical symptoms of hyperglycemia (mainly polyphagia, polyuria, polydipsia, or numbing or tingling of feet) or hypoglycemia (hunger, nervousness, warmth, sweating, palpitations, headaches, confusion, drowsiness, anxiety, blurred vision, or paresthesias of lips). Monitor fasting serum glucose levels frequently at the initiation of therapy to gauge the adequacy of the dosage. Self-monitoring of fasting and selected postprandial blood glucose levels by the patient is also helpful (*see* Blood Glucose Monitors Comparison Chart). Long-term diabetic control may best be monitored using hemoglobin A_{1c}.

Notes. Sulfonylureas are usually an appropriate choice for nonobese, new-onset non-insulin-dependent diabetic (NIDDM) patients, whereas metformin may be more appropriate for obese NIDDM patients.[64] Individualize the choice of sulfonylurea based on the patient's characteristics (eg, renal function, hepatic function, likelihood of hypoglycemia) and the pharmacokinetics of the drugs. Glyburide, glipizide, glimepiride, and chlorpropamide are more effective at lowering blood glucose than acetohexamide, tolazamide, or tolbutamide.[57] **Acetohexamide, tolazamide,** and **tolbutamide** should probably be reserved for mild hyperglycemia or in those likely to develop hypoglycemia (eg, the elderly). In patients who do not respond to sulfonylurea monotherapy, combination therapy with insulin, metformin, or acarbose may be effective.[68,69]

SULFONYLUREA AGENTS COMPARISON CHART

DRUG	DOSAGE FORMS	DAILY DOSAGE	FATE	DURATION (HR)	COMMENTS
FIRST GENERATION					
Acetohexamide Dymelor Various	Tab 250, 500 mg.	250 mg–1.5 g in 2 divided doses.	65% converted to an active metabolite (hydroxyhexamide).	12–18	May be useful in the elderly and others prone to hypoglycemia, but avoid in patients with renal dysfunction.
Chlorpropamide Diabinese Various	Tab 100, 250 mg.	100–500 mg in a single daily dose.	Metabolized, and 20% excreted unchanged.	24–72	Avoid in elderly, patients with renal dysfunction. Causes disulfiramlike reaction in 30% of patients.
Tolazamide Tolinase Various	Tab 100, 250, 500 mg.	100 mg–1 g in 1–2 divided doses.	Converted to weakly active metabolites.	16–24	Delayed onset of action (3–4 hr). May be useful in the elderly and others prone to hypoglycemia.
Tolbutamide Orinase Various	Tab 250, 500 mg.	500 mg–3 g in 2–3 divided doses.	Converted to inactive compounds.	6–12	May be useful in the elderly and others prone to hypoglycemia.
SECOND GENERATION					
Glimepiride Amaryl	Tab 1, 2, 4 mg.	1–8 mg once daily.	Converted to inactive and active metabolites	24	Similar to glyburide.
Glipizide Glucotrol	Tab 5, 10 mg SR Tab 5, 10 mg.	Non-SR 5–40 in 1–2 divided doses. SR 5–20 mg once daily.	Converted to inactive metabolites.	10–24 (non-SR)	Take non-SR product on an empty stomach.

(continued)

SULFONYLUREA AGENTS COMPARISON CHART (continued)

DRUG	DOSAGE FORMS	DAILY DOSAGE	FATE	DURATION (HR)	COMMENTS
Glyburide DiaBeta Glynase Micronase Various	Tab 1.25, 2.5, 5 mg. Tab (micronized) 1.5, 3, 6 mg.	(Nonmicronized) 1.25–20 mg in 1–2 divided doses (Micronized) 0.75–12 mg in 1–2 divided doses.	Converted to inactive and active metabolites.	18–24 (SR)	The micronized product (Glynase) offers no advantage over the nonmicronized products.

From references 57, 68, 70, and product information.

BLOOD GLUCOSE MONITORS COMPARISON CHART

NAME AND MANUFACTURER	TEST STRIP USED	RANGE MG/DL	TEST TIME	FEATURES
Accu-Check Easy (Boehringer Mannheim)	Easy Test Strips	20–500	15–60 sec	Large display; 30-value memory.
Accu-Check III (Boehringer Mannheim)	Chemstrip bG	20–500	2 min	Time and date; 20-value memory; icons to guide tester; test strips may be visually read.
Companion 2 Sensor (Medisense)	Pen 2/Companion 2	20–600	20 sec	Same as for Pen 2 Sensor; credit card size; large display window.
Diascan-S (Home Diagnostics)	Diascan	10–600	90 sec	Does not require hanging drop of blood; confidence strip supplied; 10-value memory.
ExacTech Companion Sensor (Medisense)	ExacTech	40–450	30 sec	Provides same features as ExacTech Pen Sensor in a credit card size; large digital display.
ExacTech Pen Sensor (Medisense)	ExacTech	40–450	30 sec	Simple three-step procedure; no wiping, no blotting, no timing; does not need cleaning; 1-value memory.
Glucometer Elite (Miles)	Glucometer Elite	20–500	60 sec	No buttons; turns on when test strip inserted; no wiping, no blotting, no timing; does not need cleaning; 1 test memory and 3-min shut-off.
Glucometer M+ (Miles)	Glucofilm	20–500	60 sec	300-value memory; stores insulin, exercise, and diet information by date and time.
Glucometer 3 (Miles)	Glucofilm	20–500	60 sec	Automatic shut-off; 10-value memory.

(continued)

BLOOD GLUCOSE MONITORS COMPARISON CHART (continued)

NAME AND MANUFACTURER	TEST STRIP USED	RANGE (MG/DL)	TEST TIME	FEATURES
Glucose Alert (Polymer Technology)	Glucose Alert	30–400	50 sec	100-value memory.
One Touch Basic (LifeScan)	One Touch	0–600	45 sec	No timing or wiping; large display in English or Spanish; detects most sample application errors; notifies you when meter needs cleaning; 1-value memory.
One Touch II (LifeScan)	One Touch	0–600	45 sec	No timing or wiping; large display in English, Spanish, or 7 other languages; detects most sample application errors; notifies you when meter needs cleaning; 250-value memory with date and time, 14-day average.
Pen 2 Sensor (Medisense)	Pen 2/Companion 2	20–600	20 sec	Biosensor technology; no cleaning, wiping, timing; extended memory.
Supreme bG Meter (Supreme Medical)	Supreme bG	40–400	55 sec	No wiping or blotting; timing is automatic.
Tracer II (Boehringer Mannheim)	Tracer bG	40–400	2 min	Small and portable; small blood sample.
ULTRA (Home Diagnostics)	ULTRA	0–600	45 sec	No-wipe system with visual confirmation; large display.

Adapted from reference 72.

BLOOD GLUCOSE TEST STRIPS COMPARISON CHART

NAME AND MANUFACTURER	COLOR CHART INCREMENTS (MG/DL)	PROCEDURE
Chemstrip bG (Boehringer Mannheim)	20, 40, 80, 120, 180, 240.	Wipe after 1 min, read after 2 min.
Diascan (Home Diagnostics)	20, 40, 80, 120, 180, 300, 500, 800.	Wipe after 30 sec, read 60 sec later.
Glucostix Reagent Strips (Miles)	20, 40, 70, 110, 140, 180, 250, 400, 800.	Blot after 30 sec, read 90 sec later.
Supreme Strips (Supreme Medical)	Low, 20, 40, 70, 120, 180, 240, 400, High.	Wait 60 sec, turn strip over and read.
Trend Strips (Supreme Medical)	0, 20, 40, 80, 120, 180, 240, 400, 800.	Wipe after 1 min, read after 2 min. If over 240, wait an additional min and read.

Adapted from reference 72.

Contraceptives

Class Instructions: Oral Contraceptives. Take drug at approximately the same time each day for maximum efficacy. This drug may be taken at bedtime or with food, milk, or an antacid if stomach upset occurs. Use an additional form of contraception concurrently during the first 7 days of the oral progestin-only products or if you do not start your oral contraceptives on day 1 of menses. If spotting occurs and no oral doses have been missed, continue to take tablets even if spotting continues. Report immediately if any of the following occur: new severe or persistent headache; blurred or loss of vision; shortness of breath; severe leg, chest, or abdominal pain; or any abnormal vaginal bleeding. Hormonal contraceptives do not protect against human immunodeficiency virus (HIV) infection or other sexually transmitted diseases.

COMBINATION ORAL CONTRACEPTIVES

Pharmacology. These products contain an estrogen, either ethinyl estradiol or mestranol, and one of several 19-nortestosterone progestins, which are taken in a cyclic fashion, usually 21 of 28 days. As contraceptives, estrogens suppress follicle-stimulating hormone (FSH) and luteinizing hormone (LH) to inhibit ovulation, cause edematous endometrial changes that are hostile to implantation of the fertilized ovum, accelerate ovum transport, and produce degeneration of the corpus luteum (luteolysis). Progestins inhibit ovulation by suppression of LH, inhibit sperm capacitation, slow ovum transport, produce a thinning endometrium that hampers implantation, and cause cervical mucus changes that are hostile to sperm migration. Induction of a pseudopregnancy state and anovulation improves symptoms of endometriosis. Anovulatory dysfunctional uterine bleeding caused by unopposed estrogen or estrogen withdrawal responds to progestins. (*See* Contraception Efficacy, and Risks and Benefits of Oral Contraceptives Comparison Charts.)

Administration and Adult Dosage. PO for contraception (monophasic combinations) 1 tablet daily beginning on the first day of menses and continued for 21 days; stop for 7 days and start the next cycle of 21 tablets. Combination 28-day products (7 inert or iron tablets) are taken 1 tablet daily continuously; (multiphasic combinations) 1 tablet daily beginning on the first day of menses (Triphasil only) or manufacturer states first Sunday following the beginning of menstruation (if menstruation begins on Sunday, take first tablet on that day), although day 1 start is most effective, then 1 tablet daily for 21 or 28 days as above. **PO for contraception postpartum** start 6 weeks postpartum if not breastfeeding; lactation may prolong period of infertility. **PO for contraception postabortion** start immediately if gestation is terminated at 12 weeks or earlier; start in 1 week if gestation is terminated at 13–28 weeks. **PO for emergency postcoital contraception** 2 tablets of Ovral taken as soon as possible after coitus, and 2 more tablets taken 12 hr later, but within 72 hr after coitus.[73–75] (*See* Notes.) **PO for dysfunctional uterine bleeding (anovulatory cycles)** (any combination agent) 1 tablet daily to qid for 5–7 days for acute bleeding, then 1 tablet daily cyclically as for contraception for 3 months to prevent further bleeding.[76] **PO for dysmenorrhea or endometriosis**

(any combination tablet) 1 tablet daily continuously for 15 weeks, followed by 1 drug-free week; repeat 16-week cycle for 6–12 months to induce a pseudopregnant state.[77]

Special Populations. *Geriatric Dosage.* Same as adult dosage.

Other Conditions. Discontinue oral contraceptives at least 2 weeks before elective major surgery and do not reinstitute until at least 2 weeks afterward. Stop immediately in patients undergoing emergency surgery or immobilization for long time periods; institute low-dose SC heparin or other appropriate thromboembolytic prophylaxis in the postoperative period and restart cycle 4 weeks after return to normal activities.[75] Start with an agent containing at least 50 µg estrogen in women receiving rifampin, or any anticonvulsant except clonazepam or valproate.[73,75]

Dosage Forms. (*See* Oral Contraceptive Agents Comparison Chart.)

Patient Instructions. (Contraception) (*See* Oral Contraceptives Class Instructions.) If you miss 1 active dose, take it as soon as you remember it and take the next tablet at the correct time even if you take 2 tablets on the same day or at the same time. If you miss 2 active doses in week 1 or 2, take 2 tablets on the day you remember and 2 tablets the next day. If you miss 2 active doses in week 3 or miss 3 or more active tablets, then either (if you start on day 1) start a new pack the same day, or (if you start on Sunday) take 1 tablet daily until Sunday, then start a new pack that day. Use an alternative form of contraception for the next 7 days after you miss 2 or more active doses in weeks 1, 2, or 3, or abstain from sex for the next 7 days. Any menstrual irregularities and bothersome side effects should diminish after the first 3–4 cycles. Report if no menses occur for 2 months. (Acute anovulatory bleeding) Expect heavy and severely cramping flow 2 to 4 days after stopping therapy, with normal periods thereafter.

Pharmacokinetics. *Onset and Duration.* Onset of contraception after 1 week of oral regimen. Dysfunctional uterine bleeding should decrease within 12–24 hr of starting regimen.[76]

Serum Levels. No correlation of estradiol or mestranol serum levels with pharmacologic activity.

Fate. There is marked intra- and interpatient variability in the pharmacokinetics of all these agents. All are concentrated in body fat and endometrium, and penetrate poorly into breast milk.[78–87] (Desogestrel) Desogestrel is a prodrug that undergoes extensive first-pass and possibly gut-wall metabolism to its active form, 3-ketodesogestrel. Bioavailability is 62.7 ± 7%; 65% bound to albumin and 35% to sex hormone binding globulin (SHBG); SHBG increases by about 200% during long-term use. V_d is 2.4 ± 1.1 L/kg; Cl is 0.2 ± 0.1 L/hr/kg. About 45% is recovered in urine as glucuronides (38–61%), sulfates (23–29%), and unconjugated forms (14–28%); 30.9% is recovered in feces.[78,79,88–90]

(Ethinyl estradiol) Ethinyl estradiol is rapidly absorbed, with peak concentrations in 60 ± 30 min; bioavailability is 59 ± 13%.[78,83,84] It undergoes extensive small intestine and hepatic first-pass metabolism and conjugation to sulfates, and hydroxylation to active 2-hydroxylethinyl estradiol and other hydroxylated metabolites. Ethinyl estradiol is 98.5% bound to albumin and is not bound to

SHBG. V_d is 5 ± 2 L/kg; reported Cl has ranged from 0.4 ± 0.2 to 1 ± 0.3 L/hr/kg. About 23–59% is excreted in urine, 30–53% in feces as glucuronides and sulfates, and 28–43% undergoes enterohepatic circulation with a rebound in estradiol levels 10–14 hr after administration.[75,78,80–84,88,90] (*See* Estradiol and its Esters monograph for estrogen replacement.)

(Ethynodiol diacetate) Ethynodiol diacetate undergoes rapid absorption and hydrolysis to norethindrone and its metabolites in vivo (*see* Norethindrone). (Mestranol) Approximately 54% is demethylated to ethinyl estradiol; serum levels of ethinyl estradiol after oral administration of 50 μg of mestranol are equivalent to those after 35 μg of ethinyl estradiol.[84,87] (Norgestrel/Levonorgestrel) (*See* Progestin-Only Contraceptives.) (Norethindrone and norethindrone acetate) (*See* Norethindrone.) (Norethynodrel) Norethynodrel is rapidly converted to norethindrone in vivo.[80,87] (*See* Norethindrone.) (Norgestimate) Norgestimate undergoes hepatic and gut metabolism to levonorgestrel ($15.4 \pm 5.4\%$), norgestrel acetate ($9.5 \pm 1.7\%$), norgestrel oxime ($10.6 \pm 1.8\%$), and $8.1 \pm 4.5\%$ as other conjugated metabolites.[81] It is not bound to SHBG. From 35 to 49% is excreted in urine (57% conjugated sulfates and glucuronides and 12% unconjugated) and 16–49% in feces.

$t_{\frac{1}{2}}$. (Desogestrel) α phase 1.6 hr, β phase 24 ± 5 hr;[88,89] (ethinyl estradiol) α phase 50 ± 7 min, β phase 15 ± 3 to 33 ± 10 hr;[78–88] (levonorgestrel) α phase 0.3 ± 0.2 hr, β phase 31.4 ± 18.5 hr;[78–83,86,87] (norgestimate) 16 hr, (norethindrone) α phase 0.7 ± 0.3 hr, β phase 7.6 ± 1.9 hr.[78–82,87,91]

Adverse Reactions. The risk of major congenital malformations is not increased if oral contraceptives are taken during pregnancy.[92,93] (*See* Risks and Benefits of Oral Contraceptives, and Hormone Excess and Deficiency Symptomatology Comparison Charts.) Most of the risks due to oral contraceptives are minimal with the lower dosages of estrogens and newer progestins currently available.[75,93–97]

Contraindications. Known or suspected pregnancy; presence or history of thrombophlebitis or thromboembolic disorders; presence or history of carcinoma of breast or genitals, or other estrogen-dependent tumors; cerebral vascular or coronary artery disease; uncontrolled hypertension; focal migraine; markedly impaired liver function; hepatic adenoma or carcinoma; cholestatic jaundice of pregnancy or jaundice with prior pill use; undiagnosed abnormal genital bleeding; malabsorption syndrome, heavy smoking (>15 cigarettes/day) in women ≥35 yr;[75,95] polycythemia vera because of greater tendency for deep vein thrombosis (*see* Notes).

Precautions. Use with caution in patients with hyperlipidemia, diabetes, conditions that may be aggravated by fluid retention (eg, hypertension, convulsions, migraine, and cardiac or renal dysfunction), or severe varicosities, in adolescents in whom regular menses are not established, and during lactation.

Drug Interactions. Oral contraceptives may be less effective, resulting in increased breakthrough bleeding or pregnancy, when given with some antibiotics (eg, ampicillin, griseofulvin, metronidazole, nitrofurantoin, neomycin, penicillin, rifampin, tetracycline), or anticonvulsants (eg, barbiturates, carbamazepine, phenytoin). Administer doses of vitamin C ≥1 g/day at least 4 hr before or after oral contraceptives to avoid increasing the bioavailability of ethinyl estradiol; use caution if long-term vitamin C intake is discontinued.[75,98]

Parameters to Monitor. Complete pretreatment physical examination with special reference to blood pressure, breasts, abdomen, pelvic organs, and Pap smear at least q 1–2 yr.

Notes. The initial oral contraceptive prescribed should be a combined product (eg, Ovcon-35, Ortho-Cept, Desogen, Ortho-Novum 7/7/7, Tri-Norinyl, Ortho-Cyclen) containing the smallest effective dose of estrogen (≤35 µg ethinyl estradiol) and progestin (≤0.15 mg desogestrel or levonorgestrel, ≤1 mg norethindrone, or ≤0.25 mg norgestimate) that provides an acceptable pregnancy rate and minimizes side effects.[73,75] Prescribing oral contraceptives to smokers >35 yr requires adequate informed consent because of a doubled risk of cardiovascular disease.[94,96] The health risks of pregnancy in healthy, nonsmoking women in their forties is greater than the risks of taking sub-50-µg estrogen or progestin-only contraceptives.[93,96] (*See* Risks and Benefits of Oral Contraceptives Comparison Chart.) For emergency postcoital contraception, 2 doses of Ovral is the standard of care, but might be somewhat less effective than high-dose estrogens.[99]

PROGESTIN-ONLY CONTRACEPTIVES:	
LEVONORGESTREL/NORGESTREL	Norplant, Ovrette
MEDROXYPROGESTERONE ACETATE	Depo-Provera
NORETHINDRONE	Micronor, Nor-Q.D.

Pharmacology. Norgestrel and norethindrone are 19-nortestosterone derivatives; only the l-isomer of norgestrel (levonorgestrel) is active. Medroxyprogesterone acetate is a 17α-acetoxyprogesterone derivative with greater progestational activity and oral efficacy than native progesterone. These compounds share the actions of progestins, although progestin-only contraceptives suppress ovulation in only about 50% of cycles (*see* Combination Oral Contraceptives).

Administration and Adult Dosage. **PO** (norethindrone) 0.35 mg/day, or (norgestrel) 0.075 mg/day continuously at the same time each day, starting on the first day of menses or immediately postpartum. **IM** (medroxyprogesterone acetate) 150 mg q 3 months, starting within 5 days of menses or immediately postabortion or postpartum (within 5 days to 6 weeks of delivery). In breastfeeding mothers, the first dose is recommended at 6 weeks postpartum, although some clinicians give it between 3 and 6 weeks postpartum.[73,100–104] **Subdermal** (levonorgestrel) 216 mg (6 Norplant implants) q 5 yr, or 225 mg (3 Norplant II implants) q 3 yr; insert within 7 days of onset of menstruation, immediately postabortion, or no earlier than 6 weeks postpartum if breastfeeding; insertion and removal requires a simple surgical procedure performed by trained personnel.[105] (*See also* Progesterone.)

Dosage Forms. **Tab** (norethindrone) 0.35 mg (Micronor, Nor-Q.D.); (norgestrel) 0.075 mg (Ovrette). **Implant Pellet** (levonorgestrel) kit of 6 capsules each containing 36 mg (Norplant); kit of 3 capsules each containing 75 mg (Norplant II).

Inj (medroxyprogesterone acetate) Use only the 150 mg/mL dosage form of Depo-Provera for contraception.

Patient Instructions. (*See* Oral Contraceptives Class Instructions.) Spotting and breakthrough bleeding occur more frequently than with the combination oral contraceptives during the first few months of use; notify prescriber if this persists through the third month.[73,93,105] (Oral) If you miss a dose, even if it is taken only 3 hours late, use an additional backup method for the next 48 hours. Take the missed dose as soon as you remember. If menses do not occur within 45 days, discontinue the contraceptive, use an alternate nonhormonal method of contraception, and make sure you are not pregnant. Because of the higher risk of failure if 1 tablet is missed every 1–2 cycles, consider changing the time of tablet taking or using a different contraceptive.[93] (Depo-Provera) Use an alternative form of contraception for the first 2 weeks if your first injection is more than 5 days after the start of menses. Cessation of menses is common after 1–2 years.[73,100,101] (Norplant) Use an alternative form of contraception for the first 24 hours if inserted more than 7 days after the start of menses. Irregular bleeding patterns should become more regular 9–12 months after insertion. The implants may be visible under the skin. Removal at 5 years must be done by trained personnel.

Pharmacokinetics. *Onset and Duration.* (Oral) onset after 1 week; duration 24 hr. (Depo-Provera) onset is within 24 hr if given within 5 days of menses; the drug prevents ovulation the first month of use; ovulation is inhibited for at least 14 weeks after 150 mg IM; mean interval before return of ovulation after last injection is 9 months; 70% of former users conceive within first 12 months after stopping.[79,100,101] (Norplant) onset is within 24 hr after subdermal implantation if inserted within 7 days of menses; immediately reversible once removed, normal ovulatory cycles return during first month after removal.

Serum Levels. (Ovulation inhibition) levonorgestrel 0.2 μg/L (0.64 nmol/L); medroxyprogesterone over 0.1 μg/L (0.25 nmol/L);[98–101] norethindrone 0.4 μg/L (1.34 nmol/L).[105]

Fate. (Levonorgestrel) Levonorgestrel is 99.7 ± 16% absorbed orally with no first-pass metabolism.[78–83,86] Peak serum levels occur in 1.1 ± 0.4 hr, are dose dependent, and exhibit considerable interindividual variation. Oral administration of 30 μg yields peak levels of 0.9 ± 0.7 μg/L (2.9 ± 2.2 nmol/L); 150 μg yields 3.6 ± 0.5 μg/L (11.5 ± 1.6 nmol/L); 250 μg yields 5 ± 0.5 μg/L (16 ± 1.6 nmol/L). Within 24 hr after implantation of Norplant, levonorgestrel produces serum levels greater than 0.3 μg/L (0.96 nmol/L). Release of 80 μg/day of levonorgestrel during the first 6–12 months yields levels of 0.4 ± 0.1 μg/L (1.1 ± 0.4 nmol/L); thereafter, release of 25–35 μg/day yields levels that remain above 0.28 ± 0.16 μg/L (0.9 ± 0.5 nmol/L) for the remainder of the 5 yr. Levels are unmeasurable within 48 hr after removal of the implant.[105] Levonorgestrel is concentrated in body fat and endometrium, but penetrates poorly into breast milk (approximately 10% of serum levels); it is bound 69.4% to sex-hormone-binding globulin and 30% to albumin. V_d is 1.5 ± 0.4 L/kg; Cl is 0.05 ± 0.01 L/hr/kg. Conjugated glucuronides, sulfates, and unconjugated levonorgestrel and its metabolites are excreted 45% in urine and 32% in feces.[81,86] (*See* Medroxyprogesterone Acetate and Norethindrone.)

$t_{1/2}$. (Levonorgestrel) α phase 0.3 ± 0.2 hr, β phase 31.4 ± 18.5 hr;[78–83,86,87] (medroxyprogesterone acetate) about 50 days, reflecting slow IM absorption from depot; (norethindrone) α phase 0.7 ± 0.3 hr, β phase 6.4 ± 3 hr.[78–82,87,91]

Adverse Reactions. Menstrual irregularities, including spotting, breakthrough bleeding, prolonged cycles, and amenorrhea are frequent. Because ovulation is suppressed in only about 50% of cycles, functional ovarian cysts may occur. Most resolve spontaneously within 4 weeks, and surgical intervention is usually not necessary. Ectopic pregnancy occurs in 6% of all pregnancies. Low doses of progestins have minimal impact on glucose; insulin levels; liver, coagulation, lipid, hepatic, or thyroid function; blood pressure; or cardiovascular complications.[73,93,100,101,105] (Depo-Provera) Menstrual irregularities, spotting, and breakthrough bleeding are frequent in the first 12 months after IM injection; amenorrhea (after 1 yr), infertility (up to 18 months), and weight gain of 1–1.5 kg also occur. Reversible reduced bone density changes occur with over 5 yr of use as contraceptive, but there is no clinical evidence of fractures. Long-term use (over 5 yr) does not increase the overall risk of ovarian, liver, breast, or cervical cancer, but reduces the risk of endometrial cancer for at least 8 yr after stopping.[93,100,101,106] (Norplant) the most frequent adverse effects include irregular menstrual bleeding, headaches, weight gain, mood changes and depression, premenstrual bilateral mastalgia, galactorrhea (especially upon discontinuation of lactation), acne, outbreaks of genital herpes in patients with a previous history. Rarely, rash, implant expulsions, and local complications (eg, infection, hematoma formation, irritation, allergic reactions to adhesives) occur.[105–108]

Contraindications. Thrombophlebitis or history of deep vein thrombophlebitis or thromboembolic disorders; known or suspected carcinoma of the breast or endometrium, or other estrogen-dependent tumors; undiagnosed abnormal genital bleeding. Known or suspected pregnancy is a contraindication, but the risk of congenital malformations is not increased when progestin-only contraceptives are taken during pregnancy.[93,102] Although acute liver disease, benign or malignant liver tumors, history of cholestatic jaundice of pregnancy, or jaundice with prior hormonal contraceptive use are listed as contraindications by manufacturers, liver disease is not considered by others to be a contraindication to progestin-only contraceptives.[93]

Precautions. Use with caution in patients with a history of depression, diabetes, gestational diabetes, coronary artery disease, cerebrovascular disease, hyperlipidemia, liver disease, or hypertension. Although progestins are not harmful to the fetus during the first 4 months of pregnancy; confirm a negative pregnancy test before reinjecting women more than 2 weeks late for their IM injection.[93,102] Progestin-only contraceptives used during breastfeeding are unlikely to pose any risk to the infant,[93,100–104] and they usually do not decrease breast milk production if begun after 6 weeks postpartum.

Drug Interactions. Rifampin and all anticonvulsants (except clonazepam and valproate) can decrease efficacy. Long-term use of griseofulvin can increase menstrual irregularities.[73,93,100,101,105]

Parameters to Monitor. Complete pretreatment physical examination with special reference to blood pressure, breasts, abdomen, pelvic organs, and Pap smear at least q 1–2 yr.

Notes. Progestin-only contraceptives are the hormonal contraceptives of choice during breastfeeding or in patients with contraindications to estrogen therapy (eg, hypertension, diabetes, hyperlipidemia, smokers).[73,93,100,101] Long-term noncontraceptive benefits of IM medroxyprogesterone acetate include a decreased prevalence of menstrual blood loss, anemia, candidal vulvovaginitis, pelvic inflammatory disease, and endometrial cancer. A 30% reduction in seizure frequency was observed in a small group of women with uncontrolled seizures who became amenorrheic with medroxyprogesterone.[100,101]

CONTRACEPTION EFFICACY COMPARISON CHART

METHOD	AVERAGE PREGNANCY RATES PER 100 WOMAN-YR
Oral Monophasic Combination	
<30 µg ethinyl estradiol (EE)*	0.75
35 to 49 µg EE	0.27
50 µg EE	0.16
>50 µg EE	0.32
Oral Multiphasic Combination	0.33
*Oral Progestin-Only**	
Age 25–30 yr	3.1
Age 30–34 yr	2.0
Age 35–39	1.0
Age >40 yr	0.3
Lactating	0.3
Subdermal Progestin Implant	0.2
Injectable Depot Progestin	0.3
Emergency Postcoital	
(within 72 hr of intercourse)	
Ovral 2 tablets q 12 hr for 2 doses	0.2–2.5‡
Ethinyl estradiol 5 mg/day for 5 days	0.5–1.6‡
Intrauterine Device	
Copper T 380	0.5
Progestasert	2.9
Barrier Method	
Diaphragm	1.9
Condom†	3.6
Vaginal Sponge	10
Cervical Cap	13
Vaginal Spermicide (cream, foam, jelly)	11.9
Other	
Tubal Sterilization	<1
Coitus Interruptus	6.7
Rhythm	15.5
Abstinence Method	70

*Mestranol 50 µg is approximately equal to 35 µg of ethinyl estradiol.
†Protects against most sexually transmitted diseases.
‡Postcoital contraception numbers represent the percentage of women in whom pregnancies occur.
From references 73, 74, 92, 93, 101, 105, and 109–111.

ORAL CONTRACEPTIVE AGENTS COMPARISON CHART

PRODUCT	CYCLE[a]	ESTROGEN[b]	PROGESTIN[c]	POTENCY[d]			BREAKTHROUGH BLEEDING AND SPOTTING (%)[h]
				Estrogenic[e]	Progestational[f]	Androgenic[g]	
MONOPHASIC COMBINATION AGENTS CONTAINING LESS THAN 50 μg OF ESTROGEN							
Loestrin 1/20	21, 28	Ethinyl estradiol 20 μg.	Norethindrone acetate 1 mg.	+	++	++	25.2
Desogen, Ortho-Cept	21, 28	Ethinyl estradiol 30 μg.	Desogestrel 0.15 mg.	+	+	±	3.6
Loestrin 1.5/30	21, 28	Ethinyl estradiol 30 μg.	Norethindrone acetate 1.5 mg.	+	+++	+++	30.9
Levlen, Nordette	21, 28	Ethinyl estradiol 30 μg.	Levonorgestrel 0.15 mg.	+	+	++	14
Lo-Ovral	21, 28	Ethinyl estradiol 30 μg.	Norgestrel 0.3 mg.	+	+	++	9.8
Brevicon, ModiCon, Various	21, 28	Ethinyl estradiol 35 μg.	Norethindrone 0.5 mg.	++	+	+	14.6
Ovcon-35	21, 28	Ethinyl estradiol 35 μg.	Norethindrone 0.4 mg.	++	+	+	19
Demulen 1/35	21, 28	Ethinyl estradiol 35 μg.	Ethynodiol diacetate 1 mg.	+	++	+	37.5
Norinyl 1+35, Ortho-Novum 1/35, Various	21, 28	Ethinyl estradiol 35 μg.	Norethindrone 1 mg.	++	++	+	14.7

(continued)

ORAL CONTRACEPTIVE AGENTS COMPARISON CHART (continued)

PRODUCT	CYCLE[a]	ESTROGEN[b]	PROGESTIN[c]	POTENCY[d] Estrogenic[e]	POTENCY[d] Progestational[f]	POTENCY[d] Androgenic[g]	BREAKTHROUGH BLEEDING AND SPOTTING (%)[h]
Ortho-Cyclen	21, 28	Ethinyl estradiol 35 µg.	Norgestimate 0.25 mg.	++	++	+	11.3
BIPHASIC[c] COMBINATION PRODUCTS CONTAINING LESS THAN 50 µg OF ESTROGEN							
Jenest-28	28	Ethinyl estradiol 35 µg (days 1–21).	Norethindrone 0.5 mg (days 1–7); 1 mg (days 8–21).	++	+	+	6.5
Ortho-Novum 10/11, *Various*	21, 28	Ethinyl estradiol 35 µg (days 1–21).	Norethindrone 0.5 mg (days 1–10); 1 mg (days 11–21).	++	+	+	19.6
TRIPHASIC[c] COMBINATION PRODUCTS CONTAINING LESS THAN 50 µg OF ESTROGEN							
Ortho-Novum 7/7/7	21, 28	Ethinyl estradiol 35 µg (days 1–21).	Norethindrone 0.5 mg (days 1–7); 0.75 mg (days 8–14); 1 mg (days 15–21).	++	+	+	12.2

(continued)

513

ORAL CONTRACEPTIVE AGENTS COMPARISON CHART (continued)

PRODUCT	CYCLE[a]	ESTROGEN[b]	PROGESTIN[c]	POTENCY[d] Estrogenic[e]	Progestational[f]	Androgenic[g]	BREAKTHROUGH BLEEDING AND SPOTTING (%)[h]
Ortho Tri-Cyclen	21, 28	Ethinyl estradiol 35 μg (days 1–21).	Norgestimate 0.18 mg (days 1–7); 0.215 mg (days 8–14); 0.25 mg (days 15–21).	++	+	±	9
Tri-Norinyl	21, 28	Ethinyl estradiol 35 μg (days 1–21).	Norethindrone 0.5 mg (days 1–7); 1 mg (days 8–16); 0.5 mg (days 17–21).	++	+	+	14.7

(continued)

ORAL CONTRACEPTIVE AGENTS COMPARISON CHART (continued)

PRODUCT	CYCLE[a]	ESTROGEN[b]	PROGESTIN[c]	Estrogenic[e]	Progestational[f]	Androgenic[g]	BREAKTHROUGH BLEEDING AND SPOTTING (%)[h]
					POTENCY[d]		
Tri-Levlen *Triphasil*	21, 28	Ethinyl estradiol 30 μg (days 1–6); 40 μg (days 7–11); 30 μg (days 12–21).	Levonorgestrel 0.05 mg (days 1–6); 0.075 mg (days 7–11); 0.125 mg (days 12–21).	+	+	+	15.1
MONOPHASIC COMBINATION AGENTS CONTAINING 50 μg OF ESTROGEN							
Norinyl 1 + 50, *Ortho-Novum 1/50,* *Various*	21, 28	Mestranol 50 μg.	Norethindrone 1 mg.	++	++	+	10.6
Demulen 1/50	21, 28	Ethinyl estradiol 50 μg.	Ethynodiol Diacetate 1 mg.	+	++	+	13.4
Ovcon-50	21, 28	Ethinyl estradiol 50 μg.	Norethindrone 1 mg.	++	++	++	11.9
Ovral	21, 28	Ethinyl estradiol 50 μg.	Norgestrel 0.5 mg.	++	+++	+++	4.5

(continued)

515

ORAL CONTRACEPTIVE AGENTS COMPARISON CHART (continued)

				POTENCY[d]			BREAKTHROUGH BLEEDING AND SPOTTING (%)[h]
PRODUCT	CYCLE[a]	ESTROGEN[b]	PROGESTIN[c]	Estrogenic[e]	Progestational[f]	Androgenic[g]	
PROGESTIN ONLY							
Micronor, Nor-Q.D.	Continuous	None	Norethindrone 0.35 mg.	0	+++	+	42.3
Ovrette	Continuous	None	Norgestrel 0.075 mg.	0	+	+	34.9

+++ = High; + = Low; ± = Very low.

[a]28-day cycles contain 7 inert or iron tablets to complete the 28-day cycle.

[b]Estrogen equivalent potency: ethinyl estradiol is about 1.5 times as potent as mestranol. Inhibition of ovulation requires 50 μg of ethinyl estradiol or 80 μg of mestranol.

[c]Most products contain either norethindrone or norgestrel. Norethindrone may be preferred over norgestrel, which has a marked adverse effect on lipid profile (decreased HDL, increased LDL). Only levonorgestrel is biologically active and exists in newer preparations. Older preparations contain norgestrel, which also has an inactive d-isomer. Desogestrel and norgestimate have positive effects on lipids.

[d]Potency designations are based on laboratory tests of individual components. Applicability of these methods for combination products used clinically has been questioned.

[e]Overall estrogenic effect as modified by antiestrogenic or estrogenic effect of progestational component. Relative estrogenic potency as measured by affinity for estrogen receptor (all are relatively weak): norethynodrel > ethynodiol diacetate > norethindrone acetate > norethindrone > levonorgestrel/norgestimate/desogestrel. Antiestrogenic potency: norethindrone acetate > levonorgestrel > norethindrone > ethynodiol diacetate > norethynodrel > norethindrone > norgestimate > desogestrel.

[f]Progestational potency as measured by delay of menses test. Relative progestogenic potency: norgestimate > desogestrel > levonorgestrel > norethindrone acetate > norethindrone acetate > ethynodiol diacetate > norethynodrel.

[g]Relative androgenic potency (prostate growth in rats): levonorgestrel > norethindrone acetate > ethynodiol diacetate > norethynodrel > norgestimate > desogestrel.

[h]Prevalence of breakthrough bleeding (BTB) decreases from the first cycle to third cycle by 50–66% per cycle; these figures represent data submitted to FDA on prevalence of BTB in the third cycle of use. BTB can result from either estrogen or progestin deficiency. Bleeding decreases after the first 6 months of use regardless of the formulation used.

[i]Bi- and triphasic compounds are overall estrogen dominant.

From references 73, 75, 82, and 94.

RISKS AND BENEFITS OF ORAL CONTRACEPTIVES COMPARISON CHART

CONDITION	CLINICAL INFORMATION	COMMENTS
RISKS		
Breast Cancer	Controversial. Overall, lifetime risk is not increased. A meta-analysis of 27 studies indicates a relative risk of 1.16 after 4–12 yr of use. The relative risk is increased to 3 if started in teenage years and duration is over 10 yr.	Further information required regarding risk with progestin-only contraceptives.
Cerebrovascular Accidents	Risk of hemorrhagic stroke is increased 2.5-fold compared to nonusers; ever-users have a 1.5-fold risk compared to never-users. Risk is mostly in heavy smokers >35 yr and with predisposing risk factors (eg, hypertension, diabetes, hyperlipidemia). Odds ratio is 2.9 with combined OCs containing 50 µg of estrogen, 1.8 for combined OCs with 30–40 µg estrogen, and 0.9 for progestin-only products.	Related to both the estrogen and progestin components. Minimal risk with 35 µg/day and progestin-only preparations.
Cervical Cancer	Increased risk of cervical erosions, eversions, dysplasias, and conversion to cancer in situ. Relative risk is 1.8–2.1 times that of nonusers and increased with duration of use over 5 yr; other risk factors include multiple sexual partners and early sexual activity.	May increase risk of herpes or papillomavirus infection, which accelerate progression of preinvasive lesions.
Gallbladder Disease	Relative risk of 1.36 for gallstones in users compared to nonusers only during the first 4 yr of use, then risk returns to baseline.	Estrogens increase cholesterol saturation.
Hepatic Tumors	Both benign and malignant tumors reported. Relative risk is 2.6 for users; 9.6 with duration of use over 5 yr. Shock can result from rupture of mass. Surgical intervention may be needed, because tumors are not always reversible after discontinuation. Risk is greater in smokers and those with a history of hepatitis B infection or diabetes.	Unknown, although mestranol and higher dosage formulations are implicated. Progestin-only contraceptives not implicated.

(continued)

517

RISKS AND BENEFITS OF ORAL CONTRACEPTIVES COMPARISON CHART (continued)

CONDITION	CLINICAL INFORMATION	COMMENTS
Hyperglycemia	Abnormal glucose tolerance found in predisposed individuals (eg, sub-clinical or gestational diabetes) and rare cases of diabetic ketoacidosis reported. These effects are minimal with combinations containing ≤35 μg/day of ethinyl estradiol or newer progestins. Norgestrel has greatest insulin-antagonizing activity.	Hyperinsulinemia with relative insulin resistance caused by progestins with minimal effect from estrogens.
Hyperlipidemia	Elevated triglycerides; may precipitate pancreatitis in patients with underlying hyperlipidemia; adverse effects on lipids is greatest with progestin-dominant products, especially levonorgestrel and ethynodiol diacetate, and lowest with norgestimate and desogestrel.	Estrogens increase triglycerides and HDL; progestins increase LDL and decrease HDL. Minimal effect with progestin-only products.
Hypertension	Mild BP elevations of 4 mm Hg systolic and 1 mm Hg diastolic, usually reversible upon drug discontinuation, occur in 1–5% of users. Rare with low-dose products. More common in older women and in those with a family history of hypertension.	Related to both estrogen/progestin component. Consider progestin-only contraceptive.
Infertility	Little risk of permanent sterility. Conception rate after discontinuation may temporarily lag behind that of nonusers for a few months.	Risk concentrated in older women with a long history of contraceptive use.
Myocardial Infarction	No increased risk in healthy nonsmokers; risk is increased 2.8 times that of nonusers in smokers >35 yr with presence of other predisposing factors (eg, hyperlipidemia, diabetes, hypertension). Relative risk of 1.9 for current and past users of low-dose products.	Questionably thromboembolic because risk reverses after drug discontinuation.
Postpill Amenorrhea	Prevalence is 0.2–2.6% after use; check for pituitary tumor in presence of galactorrhea.	Risk is increased if menses were irregular prior to starting. Unrelated to duration or dose.

(continued)

RISKS AND BENEFITS OF ORAL CONTRACEPTIVES COMPARISON CHART (continued)

CONDITION	CLINICAL INFORMATION	COMMENTS
Thromboembolism and Thrombophlebitis	Risk is increased 2.8-fold that of nonuser; risk is concentrated in smokers, sedentary females >50 yr, and duration of use >5 yr. Desogestrel-containing products have a twofold risk compared with other progestins and four- to fivefold risk of nonuser. Minimal risk with progestin-only products.	Related to desogestrel and to estrogen dose. Estrogens decrease antithrombin III and increase coagulation factors and platelet aggregation.
Teratogenesis	No increased risk of congenital cardiac, limb, or other malformations if oral or progestin-only contraceptives taken during pregnancy. Reports of masculinization of female genitalia reported when high doses of progestin were used for threatened abortion.	Exhaustive review of 18 prospective studies and meta-analysis of 12 prospective cohorts show relative risk of 0.99–1.04.
BENEFITS* *Breast Disease*	A 50–75% reduction in fibrocystic disease and fibroadenoma with >2 yr of use.	Protection greatest with progestin-dominant products. Does not prevent breast cancer.
Endometrial Cancer	A 54–72% reduction in endometrial cancer with ≥2 yr of continuous use. Benefit persists for as long as 15 yr after drug discontinuation. Greatest effects in nulliparous women.	Progestin component protective against endometrial adenomatous hyperplasia (precursor to adeno cancer) by opposing estrogen effect. Mechanism unknown.
Ovarian Cancer	A 30% risk reduction with duration of use ≤4 yr, 60% risk reduction with >5 yr, 80% risk reduction with >12 yr of use compared to nonusers. Protection persists for 10 yr after drug discontinuation.	
Ovarian Cysts	An 80–90% risk reduction.	Less protection with triphasics and low-dose products.

(continued)

519

RISKS AND BENEFITS OF ORAL CONTRACEPTIVES COMPARISON CHART (continued)

CONDITION	CLINICAL INFORMATION	COMMENTS
Pelvic Inflammatory Disease/Ectopic Pregnancy	Risk reduction of 50–70% with >1 yr of use and beneficial reduction of ectopic pregnancy rate.	Does not protect against gonorrhea or chlamydial cervicitis.
Menstrual Cycle Effects	A 90% improvement in dysmenorrhea and 50% reduced risk of iron deficiency anemia. Reduction in premenstrual symptoms (eg, anxiety, depression, and headache).	Decrease in menstrual flow and menstrual fluid prostaglandins.
Acne	Combined oral contraceptives lower serum testosterone levels with improvement of acne.	Use least androgenic progestins (eg, desogestrel, norgestimate) for greatest effect.
Rheumatoid Arthritis	A 50% reduction in frequency.	Progesterone attenuates immune response.

*Most risks and benefits have been documented with the higher dosage estrogen products (>50 µg/day).
From references 73, 75, 92–97, and 109–114.

HORMONE EXCESS AND DEFICIENCY SYMPTOMATOLOGY COMPARISON CHART

CONDITION	SYMPTOMATOLOGY
Estrogen* Excess	Estrogen excess may also be a result of progestin deficiency. Symptoms include nausea, vomiting, vertigo, leukorrhea, increase in leiomyoma size, uterine cramps, breast tenderness with fluid retention, cystic breast changes, cholasma, edema, and fluid retention resulting in abdominal or leg pain with cyclic weight gain, headaches on pill days, and hypertension.
Estrogen Deficiency	Estrogen deficiency may also be a result of progestin excess. Symptoms include irritability, nervousness, decreased libido, hot flashes, early and midcycle breakthrough bleeding and spotting (days 1–7), atrophic vaginitis, dyspareunia, no withdrawal bleeding with continued contraceptive use, and decreased amount of withdrawal bleeding.
Progestin Excess	Progestin excess may also be a result of estrogen deficiency. Symptoms include increased appetite and weight gain on non-pill days, tiredness, fatigue, weakness, depression, decreased libido, decreased length of menstrual flow, *Candida* vaginitis, headaches on nonpill days, and breast tenderness on nonpill days.
Progestin Deficiency	Progestin deficiency may also be a result of estrogen excess. Symptoms include late breakthrough bleeding (days 8–21), heavy menstrual flow and clots, dysmenorrhea, and delayed onset of menses following last pill.
Androgen Excess	Symptoms include increased appetite and weight gain, oily scalp, acne, and hirsutism.

*Less likely with preparations containing <50 µg/day ethinyl estradiol.
From references 73 and 93–95.

Female Sex Hormones

ESTRADIOL AND ITS ESTERS
Climara, Delestrogen, Estinyl, Estrace, Estraderm, Estring, Vivelle, Various

Pharmacology. Estradiol (17β-estradiol; E_2) is the most potent of the naturally occurring estrogens and is the major estrogen secreted during the reproductive years. Estradiol and other estrogens produce charact eristic effects on specific tissues (such as breast), cause proliferation of vaginal and uterine mucosa, increase calcium deposition in bone, and accelerate epiphyseal closure following initial growth stimulation. Addition of the ethinyl radical results in an orally active compound that is 200 times more potent than estradiol. (*See* Notes.)

Administration and Adult Dosage. For patients with an intact uterus, either continuous daily or monthly (minimum of 10–12 days) administration of a progestin is recommended to induce endometrial sloughing and decrease the risk of endometrial cancer; administration of progestin quarterly (14 days of progestin q 3 months) might also be effective.[115–117] **PO for postmenopausal symptoms and atrophic vaginitis** administer daily or, if uterus is present, continuous daily or in cyclic regimen of 3 weeks on followed by 1 week off, using the smallest effective dosage (micronized estradiol) 0.5–2 mg/day initially, adjusted as necessary to control symptoms; (ethinyl estradiol) 0.02 mg/day or every other day, to a maximum of 0.05 mg/day; severe cases may require 0.05 mg tid initially until improvement, then decrease to 0.05 mg/day; administer as with micronized estradiol. **Top patch for postmenopausal symptoms or osteoporosis** initiate with 50 µg/day patch; patch is changed once (Climara) or twice (Estraderm, Vivelle) weekly and is administered continuously or cyclically (eg, for 3 weeks followed by 1 week without patch). Dosage may be increased to a 75 or 100 µg/day patch if symptoms are not controlled (*see* Notes). **Vag for postmenopausal vasomotor symptoms and atrophic vaginitis** 200–400 µg/day as micronized estradiol cream for 1–2 weeks, then reduce to 100–200 µg/day for 1–2 weeks, then to maintenance of 100 µg 1–3 times/week. **Vag for symptoms of urogenital atrophy** (Estring) insert one 2-mg ring into the upper vagina every 3 months. **PO for prevention of osteoporosis** use minimum effective dosage of 2 mg/day micronized estradiol or 20 µg/day of ethinyl estradiol, or equivalent. **PO for dysfunctional uterine bleeding** 0.05–0.1 mg/day of micronized estradiol or 10–20 µg/day of ethinyl estradiol for 10–20 days with addition of progestin the third week.[76] **PO for palliation of breast cancer in postmenopausal women** (ethinyl estradiol) 1 mg tid, or (micronized estradiol) 10 mg tid for at least 3 months. **PO for palliation of advanced inoperable prostatic cancer** (ethinyl estradiol) 0.15–2 mg/day, or (micronized estradiol) 1–2 mg tid. **IM for postmenopausal symptoms and prevention of osteoporosis** when oral or vaginal therapy does not provide expected response, is poorly tolerated or when noncompliance occurs (estradiol cypionate) 1–5 mg q 3–4 weeks; (estradiol valerate) 10–20 mg q 4 weeks. **IM for dysfunctional uterine bleeding** (estradiol valerate) 20 mg initially, then 5 mg q 2 weeks with addition of progestin. **IM for palliation of advanced inoperable prostatic cancer** (polyestradiol phosphate) 40 mg q 2–4 weeks; (estradiol valerate) 30 mg or more q 1–2 weeks depending on patient response.

Special Populations. *Geriatric Dosage.* Same as adult dosage.

Other Conditions. Because estrogens can increase the risk of postsurgery thromboembolic complications, discontinue estrogens at least 4 weeks before surgery if feasible.

Dosage Forms. **Tab** (micronized estradiol) 0.5, 1, 2 mg; (ethinyl estradiol) 0.02, 0.05, 0.5 mg; **SR Patch** (estradiol) 37.5, 50, 75, 100 µg/day; **Vag Crm** (estradiol) 100 µg/g; **Vag Ring** (estradiol) 2 mg (Estring); **Inj** (estradiol cypionate in oil) 5 mg/mL; 2 mg/mL with testosterone cypionate 50 mg/mL (DepoTestadiol, various); (estradiol valerate in oil) 10, 20, 40 mg/mL; 2 mg/mL with testosterone enanthate 90 mg/mL (Androgyn LA, various); (polyestradiol phosphate) 40 mg/mL.

Patient Instructions. Report immediately if any of the following occur: new severe or persistent headache or vomiting; blurred or loss of vision; speech impairment; calf, chest, or abdominal pain; weakness or numbness of extremities; or any abnormal vaginal bleeding. This (oral) drug may be taken with food, milk, or an antacid to minimize stomach upset. (Patch) discard the protective liner and apply the patch to a clean, dry, and intact area of skin, preferably on the abdomen. Avoid excessively hairy, oily, or irritated areas. Apply immediately after opening and press the patch firmly in place with the palm of your hand for about 10 seconds to ensure good contact, particularly around the edges. Do not apply to the breasts or the waistline. To minimize irritation, rotate sites with an interval of at least 1 week between applications to a particular site.

Pharmacokinetics. *Onset and Duration.* (Menopausal symptoms) Onset of therapeutic E_2 levels after oral or vaginal administration is 0.5–1 hr, with peak levels at 5 hr and progressive decline toward baseline by 12–24 hr. Onset of relief of menopausal symptoms occurs within days of first cycle of therapy. Reductions of LH and FSH levels occur within 3 hr and 6 hr, respectively, with a duration of 24 hr.[88,118] Peak E_2 levels after IM products are (valerate) 2.2 days, (cypionate) 4 days. Duration of depot products is variable following IM injection: (valerate) 14–21 days, (cypionate) 14–28 days, (polyestradiol phosphate) 14–28 days.[118,119] (Cancer) Response to estradiol therapy should be apparent within 3 months after initiation of oral therapy.

Serum Levels. (Relief of menopausal symptoms) E_2 levels: apparent over 40 ng/L (147 pmol/L); 80% relief with 68 ng/L (250 pmol/L); 100% relief with 112 ng/L (411 pmol/L).[79,99,115,116,118,120,121] (Prevention of osteoporosis) 60 ng/L (220 pmol/L).

Fate. (Ethinyl estradiol) PO administration of 20 µg yields ethinyl estradiol levels of 25 ng/L (84 pmol/L); 30 µg yields 60 ng/L (202 pmol/L). (*See* Combination Oral Contraceptives.)

(Estradiol) Oral bioavailability of micronized estradiol (E_2) is 4.9 ± 5% because of extensive and rapid first-pass metabolism.[122] Topical absorption may be affected by skin thickness and site of patch application: 100% (abdomen) and 85% (thigh).[99,121] Oral or vaginal administration results in unphysiologic levels of estrone ($E_1 > E_2$; E_1 is less after Vag than PO administration).[79,99,115,118–122] Patch yields levels of $E_2 > E_1$ (minor E_1 elevations).[99,115,118–122] Steady-state E_2 level after PO administration of 1 mg estradiol is 35 ± 5 ng/L (128 ± 18 pmol/L) or an increase of 25 ng/L (92 pmol/L) over baseline; after 2 mg, 63 ± 11 ng/L (231 ± 40 pmol/L) or 40 ng/L (147 pmol/L) over baseline; after 4 mg, 121 ± 15 ng/L (444 ± 55 pmol/L) or 50 ng/L (183 pmol/L) over baseline; after 6 mg, 207 ± 200 ng/L (760 ± 734 pmol/L).[79,118] Vaginal 0.2-mg estradiol yields 80 ± 19 ng/L (293 ± 7 pmol/L) of E_2.[118] Patch 25 μg yields 25 ng/L (92 pmol/L); 50 μg yields 38 ± 10 ng/L (138 ± 36 pmol/L); 100 μg yields 89 ± 82 ng/L (327 ± 302 pmol/L) of E_2.[99,121] (*See* Notes.)

Estradiol is about 60% bound to albumin and 38% to sex-hormone-binding globulin, 3% unbound. It is widely distributed and concentrated in fat. V_d is 10.9 ± 2.9 L; Cl is 24.2 ± 7 L/hr/m² or 0.77 L/hr/kg.[79,118,119] Estradiol and its esters are converted in the liver, endometrium, and intestine, 15% to estrone (active), 65% to estrone sulfate and its conjugates (primarily sulfates and glucuronides with reconversion of 5% estrone and 1.4% estrone sulfate back to E_2). E_2 is excreted 50% in urine and 10% in feces, with some enterohepatic circulation. Less than 1% is excreted unchanged in urine and 50–80% as conjugates: estrone 20%, estriol 20%, estradiol glucuronide 7%.[79,118,119] (Estradiol valerate and cypionate) These are slowly hydrolyzed to E_2 and their respective free acids. (Polyestradiol phosphate) Slowly hydrolyzed to E_2.

$t_{½}$. (Estradiol) 1 hr;[79,118,119] (ethinyl estradiol) α phase 50 ± 7 min; ß phase 15 ± 3 to 33 ± 10 hr.[78–88]

Adverse Reactions. (*See* Postmenopausal Hormone Replacement Risks and Benefits Comparison Chart.) Nausea, vomiting, bloating, breast tenderness, and spotting occur frequently (*see* Hormone Excess and Deficiency Symptomatology Comparison Chart). Hypercalcemia occurs occasionally in patients with breast cancer. Thromboembolism, thrombophlebitis, diabetes, hypertension, and gall bladder disease are less likely to occur with hormone replacement dosages than with oral contraceptive dosages. Pain at injection site occurs frequently. Occasional redness and irritation at application site with patch; rash rarely.

Contraindications. Pregnancy; history or presence of estrogen-dependent cancer (except in appropriate patients treated for metastatic disease); undiagnosed abnormal genital bleeding; history or presence of thromboembolism or severe thrombophlebitis. A history of breast cancer may not be an absolute contraindication to estrogen therapy in women with severe menopausal symptoms.[115,123] Active or severe chronic liver disease is a contraindication for combinations with testosterone.

Precautions. Use with caution in patients with disease states that may be exacerbated by increased fluid retention (eg, asthma, epilepsy, migraine, and cardiac, hepatic, or renal dysfunction); in women with a strong family history of breast cancer or presence of fibrocystic disease, fibroadenoma, or abnormal mammogram; in women with fibromyomata, cardiovascular disease, diabetes, hypertriglyceridemia, severe liver disease, or history of jaundice during pregnancy; and in young patients in whom bone growth is not complete. Oral estrogen can increase thyroid-binding globulin and cause false elevations in total T_4 and T_3 and false depression of resin T_3 uptake while the thyroid index, thyroid-stimulating hormone (TSH), and the patient remain euthyroid. Estrace 2 mg and Estinyl 0.02 mg both contain tartrazine, which may cause allergic reactions, including bronchospasm, in susceptible individuals.

Drug Interactions. Estrogens may reduce the effects of tricyclic antidepressants and of warfarin, and may increase the effects of corticosteroids by increasing their half-lives. Barbiturates, rifampin, and other enzyme inducers may decrease estrogen levels.

Parameters to Monitor. Signs and symptoms of side effects, especially abnormal bleeding. Pretreatment and physical examination with reference to blood pressure, breasts, abdomen, pelvic organs, and Pap smear. Baseline laboratory tests should include glucose, triglycerides, cholesterol, liver function tests, and calcium. Repeat physical examination annually; repeat laboratory tests only if abnormal at baseline.

Notes. Estradiol has been advocated as the estrogen replacement of choice because it is the principal estrogen of the reproductive years; however, advantages over other estrogens have not been established. Synthetic 17α-alkylated estrogens (eg, ethinyl estradiol) are generally not recommended in menopausal replacement therapy because of their potent hepatic effects. The combination of an **androgen** with estrogen is indicated for moderate to severe vasomotor symptoms in patients not improved by estrogen alone. Potential benefits include increased libido and psychological well-being. An alternative to estrogens for hot flashes is **megestrol** acetate 20 mg bid, which reduced hot flashes by 50% during 4 weeks of use in one study.[124]

Nonoral estradiol administration (eg, patch, vaginal, implant, injection), avoids first-pass effect and theoretically results in a preferable premenopausal physiologic serum level ratio of $E_2 > E_1$. Oral administration results in an unphysiologic ratio of $E_2 < E_1$ (E_1 levels are not directly related to efficacy).[79,99,118,119,121,125] Avoiding the first-pass effect allows a smaller dosage to be used and prevents undesirable changes from liver stimulation (ie, increases in renin substrate, sex-hormone-binding globulin, thyroxin-binding globulin, coagulation factors, transferrin, growth hormone levels, and cortisol-binding globulin, and a reduction in insulinlike growth factor) and their subsequent sequelae (ie, gall bladder disease, hypertension, and hypercoagulable states in some women).[99,121,125,126] Hepatic stimulation varies with oral preparations, with ethinyl estradiol > conjugated estrogens > E_2. Enhanced liver action is also responsible for the cardioprotective effects on lipids, and occurs even with vaginal estrogens.[127] Transdermal administration appears to exert favorable effects on serum lipoproteins (ie, elevation of high-density lipoproteins and depression of low-density lipoproteins) after more than 4 months of use, and protects against bone loss and fractures similarly to oral estrogens.[99,121,125,126] However, one study found no effect on lipid profile,[99] and there are no studies that evaluate long-term estradiol patch use as protection against cardiovascular disease.

Postmenopausal women most likely to develop osteoporosis are whites and Asians, whereas blacks are at less risk.[115,125,128] In women in whom estrogen replacement therapy is intolerable or contraindicated, **alendronate sodium** (Fosamax) 10 mg/day PO has increased bone mass and reduced vertebral fractures, vertebral deformities, and loss of height. It must be taken at least 30 min before the first food, beverage, or medications of the day with a full glass of plain tap water only, and the person must remain in an upright position after taking the tablet because erosive esophagitis has occurred.[129,130] A trend toward reduction in the incidence of nonvertebral fractures also occurs. Concomitant estrogen replacement and alendronate in the treatment of osteoporosis in postmenopausal women is not recommended because of limited clinical experience. **Calcitonin salmon** (Miacalcin) 200 IU/day intranasally has increased bone mass in women >5 yr postmenopausal with low bone mass who cannot take estrogens.[131] Intermittent administration of **etidronate disodium** (Didronel) 400 mg/day PO 2 hr before or after a meal for 14 days, given q 3–3.5 months, can increase bone mass and offers an effective alternative for patients unable to take estrogens. Further studies are required to determine its safety because abnormal mineralization, microfractures, increased bone pain, and increased frequency of nonvertebral fractures have been reported occasionally.[128,132] Slow-release **fluoride** (Slow Fluoride) appears to be useful in a dosage of 25 mg/day for up to 4 years, but immediate-release products are not useful because the drug is irritating to the GI tract and the new bone formed is brittle and subject to fracture.[133]

ESTROGENS, CONJUGATED	Premarin, Various
ESTROGENS, ESTERIFIED	Estratab, Menest, Various

Pharmacology. Conjugated estrogens contain a mixture of 50–65% sodium estrone sulfate, 20–35% sodium equilin sulfate, and other estrogenic substances obtained from the urine of pregnant mares. Esterified estrogens are a combination of 75–85% sodium estrone sulfate and 6.5–15% sodium equilin sulfate prepared from Mexican yams. (*See* Estradiol and its Esters.)

Administration and Adult Dosage. For patients with an intact uterus, continuous daily or monthly (for a minimum of 10–12 days) administration of a progestin is recommended to induce endometrial sloughing and decrease the risk of endometrial cancer; administration of progestin quarterly (14 days of progestin q 3 months) might also be effective.[115–117] **PO for postmenopausal symptoms and atrophic vaginitis** use smallest effective dosage in the range of 0.3–1.25 mg/day continuously or, if uterus is present, in cycles of 21–25 days/month. **PO for prevention of postmenopausal osteoporosis** use minimum effective dosage of 0.625 mg/day continuously, or cyclically if uterus is present, or 0.3 mg/day if 1.5 g/day of elemental calcium is also used;[115] higher dosages of 1.25 mg/day may be necessary following fractures caused by osteoporosis.[115] For women experiencing migraine or other symptoms during the withdrawal period, a 5 day/week regimen or a shorter withdrawal period may be used. **Vaginally for postmenopausal symptoms and/or atrophic vaginitis** 1.25–2.5 mg/day; (atrophic vaginitis) 0.3 mg 3 times a week might be effective.[120] **PO for dysfunctional uterine bleeding** 1.25–2.5 mg/day for 10 days.[76] **IV (preferred) or IM for rapid cessation of dysfunctional uterine bleeding** 25 mg of conjugated estrogens, may repeat in 6–12 hr prn, to a maximum of 3 doses.[76] **IV for bleeding from uremia** 0.6 mg/kg/day diluted in 50 mL of NS and infused over 30–40 min for 5 days; dosages as high as 60 mg/day IV have been used.[134,135] **PO for palliation of breast cancer** (patients should be ≥5 yr postmenopausal) 10 mg tid. **PO for palliation of prostatic cancer** 1.25–2.5 mg tid.

Special Populations. *Geriatric Dosage.* Same as adult dosage.

Dosage Forms. **Tab** (conjugated) 0.3, 0.625, 0.9, 1.25, 2.5 mg; 0.625 mg with medroxyprogesterone acetate 2.5 mg (Prempro); 0.625 mg with medroxyprogesterone acetate 5 mg (Premphase); 0.625 mg with methyltestosterone 5 mg; 1.25 mg with methyltestosterone 10 mg (Premarin with methyltestosterone); (esterified) 0.3, 0.625, 1.25, 2.5 mg; 0.625 mg with testosterone 1.25 mg (Estratest H.S.); 1.25 mg with testosterone 2.5 mg (Estratest); **Inj** (conjugated) 25 mg; **Vag Crm** (conjugated) 0.625 mg/g.

Patient Instructions. Report immediately if any of the following occur: new severe or persistent headache or vomiting; blurred or loss of vision; speech impairment; calf, chest, or abdominal pain; weakness or numbness of extremities; or any abnormal vaginal bleeding. This (oral) drug may be taken with food, milk, or an antacid to minimize stomach upset.

Pharmacokinetics. *Onset and Duration.* (Menopausal symptoms) PO peak onset of equilin sulfate is 4 hr; onset of estrone is 3 hr, with a peak of 5 hr; duration is >24 hr. After vaginal administration, onset of therapeutic estradiol levels is 3 hr and peak occurs in 6 hr, with decline over 24 hr to baseline values. Gonadotropin suppression occurs within 1 month of therapy, although suppression to premenopausal levels may not occur.[121] (Uremia) Improvement in bleeding time occurs within 6 hr after starting estrogens; maximum improvement occurs within 2–5 days after initiation of estrogens; effects last 3–10 days after drug discontinuation.[134,135]

Serum Levels. (*See* Estradiol and its Esters.)

Fate. Both conjugated equilin and estrone sulfate are rapidly absorbed and hydrolyzed to unconjugated forms when given orally or vaginally. Oral administration of 0.3 mg yields steady-state estradiol (E_2) levels of 48 ± 12 ng/L (175 ± 45 pmol/L) or an increase of 20 ng/L (73 pmol/L) over baseline; 0.625 mg yields 103 ± 33 ng/L (378 ± 120 pmol/L) or 50 ng/L (184 pmol/L) over baseline; 1.25 mg yields 125 ± 66 ng/L (460 ± 243 pmol/L) or 70 ng/L (257 pmol/L) over baseline. Vaginal administration of 0.3 mg yields steady-state E_2 levels of −7 ± 22 ng/L (−26 ± 81 pmol/L); 0.625 mg yields 36 ± 16 ng/L (131 ± 57 pmol/L); 1.25 mg yields 94 ± 44 ng/L (344 ± 161 pmol/L).[79,118,119] (Estrone sulfate) V_d is 38 ± 13 L; Cl is 3.9 ± 1.2 L/hr/m². [136,137] Estrone sulfate is rapidly converted to estrone and estradiol. (Equilin sulfate) Cl is 7.3 ± 4 L/hr/m². Approximately 30% of equilin sulfate is metabolized to active 17β-dihydroequilin sulfate and 2% to active 17β-dihydroequilin.[136] Inactivation of estrogens occurs mainly in the liver, with degradation to less active estrogenic products (eg, estrone). Metabolites are conjugated with sulfate and glucuronic acid; urinary recovery is 70–88% within 5 days after oral administration. (*See* Estradiol and its Esters.)

$t_{1/2}$. (Estrone sulfate) α phase 3.2 ± 0.5 min; β phase 4–5 hr. (Equilin) 19–27 min. (Equilin sulfate) 190 min. (17β-dihydroequilin) α phase 5.5 ± 2 min; β phase 45 ± 5 min. (17β-dihydroequilin sulfate) α phase 5 ± 0.5 min; β phase 2.5 ± 0.6 hr.[136]

Adverse Reactions. (*See* Estradiol and its Esters.)

Contraindications. (*See* Estradiol and its Esters.)

Precautions. (*See* Estradiol and its Esters.)

Drug Interactions. (*See* Estradiol and its Esters.)

Parameters to Monitor. (*See* Estradiol and its Esters.)

Notes. Both oral and vaginal administration result in an unphysiologic $E_1 > E_2$ ratio, although higher E_2 levels occur orally than vaginally.[118–121] (*See* Estradiol Notes, and Postmenopausal Hormone Replacement Risks and Benefits Comparison Chart.)

| **ESTRONE AND ITS ESTERS** | Various |
| **ESTROPIPATE** | Ogen, Various |

Pharmacology. Estrone (E_1) is the major estrogen produced in the post-menopausal period. It is one-half as potent as estradiol (E_2) and shares the actions of other estrogens. Estropipate is estrone sulfate stabilized with inert piperazine. (*See* Estradiol and its Esters.)

Administration and Adult Dosage. For patients with intact uterus, either continuous daily or monthly administration (minimum of 10–12 days) of progestin is recommended to induce endometrial sloughing and decrease the risk of endometrial cancer; administration of progestin quarterly (14 days of progestin q 3 months) might also be effective.[115–117] **PO for postmenopausal symptoms and prevention of osteoporosis** (estropipate) use smallest effective dosage in the range of 0.625–5 mg/day continuously or in cycles of 21–25 days/month; administer as with conjugated estrogens. **Vaginally for postmenopausal symptoms and/or atrophic vaginitis** (estropipate) 3–6 mg/day. **IM for postmenopausal symptoms and prevention of osteoporosis** when oral or vaginal therapy does not provide expected response or is poorly tolerated, or when noncompliance occurs (estrone) 0.1–0.5 mg 2–3 times/week. **IM for dysfunctional uterine bleeding** (estrone) 2–5 mg/day for several days. **IM for breast cancer in postmenopausal women** (estrone) 5 mg 3 times/week. **PO for palliation of inoperable advanced prostatic cancer** (estropipate) 3–6 mg tid. **IM for inoperable advanced prostatic cancer** (estrone) 2–4 mg 2–3 times/week.

Special Populations. *Geriatric Dosage.* Same as adult dosage.

Dosage Forms. **Tab** (estropipate, as conjugated estrogens equivalent) 0.625, 1.25, 2.5, 5 mg; **Vag Crm** (estropipate) 1.5 mg/g; **Inj** (estrone) 2, 5 mg/mL.

Patient Instructions. Report immediately if any of the following occur: new severe or persistent headache or vomiting; blurred or loss of vision; speech impairment; calf, chest, or abdominal pain; weakness or numbness of extremities; or any abnormal vaginal bleeding. This (oral) drug may be taken with food, milk, or an antacid to minimize stomach upset.

Pharmacokinetics. *Fate.* Estrone is not orally active because of enzymatic degradation in the gut and liver. Addition of a piperazine moiety increases oral absorption such that E_2 levels are similar to those after administration of estradiol. Oral administration of 0.6 mg estropipate yields E_2 serum levels of 34 ng/L (124 pmol/L); 1.2 mg yields 42 ng/L (154 pmol/L).[79,118,119] Estrone is hydroxylated to α-hydroxyestrone, estriol, and 2-hydroxyestrone.[79,122] (*See* Estradiol and its Esters.)

$t_{1/2}$. (Estrone) estimated to be 12 hr in serum; however, this does not reflect events in peripheral tissues; (estrone sulfate) 4–5 hr.[79,118,119,122]

Adverse Reactions. (*See* Estradiol and its Esters.)

Contraindications. (*See* Estradiol and its Esters.)

Precautions. (*See* Estradiol and its Esters.)

Drug Interactions. (*See* Estradiol and its Esters.)

Parameters to Monitor. (*See* Estradiol and its Esters.)

Notes. (*See* Estradiol and its Esters.)

ESTROGENS COMPARISON CHART

DRUG	DOSAGE FORMS	EQUIPOTENT PHYSIOLOGIC DOSE*†	COMMENTS
STEROIDAL AGENTS			
Conjugated Estrogens			
Premarin	Tab 0.3, 0.625, 0.9, 1.25, 2.5 mg	0.625 mg.	Mixture of 50–65% sodium estrone sulfate,
Various	Vag Crm 0.625 mg/g		20–35% equilin sulfate, and other estrogenic
	Inj 25 mg.		substances from the urine of pregnant mares.
			Expensive; nausea is rare.
Esterified Estrogens			
Estratab	Tab 0.3, 0.625, 1.25, 2.5 mg.	0.625 mg.	Similar to conjugated estrogens. Mixture of 75–85%
Menest			sodium estrone sulfate and 6.5–15% sodium equilin
Various			sulfate obtained from Mexican yams.
Estradiol, Micronized			
Estrace	Tab 0.5, 1, 2 mg	1 mg.	Moderate cost; some nausea with oral; pain at site
	Vag Crm 100 µg/g.		of injection; variable onset with duration of 14–28
			days with depot injections; estradiol is the major
			estrogen secreted during the reproductive years.
Estradiol			
Climara	SR Patch 37.5, 50, 75, 100 µg/day.	50 µg/day.	Estraderm contains alcohol; Climara and Vivelle
Estraderm			do not contain alcohol and may be less irritating.
Vivelle			
Estradiol Cypionate			
Depo-Estradiol	Inj (in oil) 5 mg/mL.	—	
Various			

(continued)

ESTROGENS COMPARISON CHART (continued)

DRUG	DOSAGE FORMS	EQUIPOTENT PHYSIOLOGIC DOSE*,†	COMMENTS
Estradiol Valerate Delestrogen Various	Inj (in oil) 10, 20, 40 mg/mL.	1 mg.	
Ethinyl Estradiol Estinyl Feminone	Tab 0.02, 0.05, 0.5 mg.	5 µg	Not recommended for estrogen replacement because of its potent hepatic effects. *See* Estradiol Notes.
Estrone Various	Inj 2, 5 mg/mL.	0.9 mg.	No advantage over conjugated/esterified estrogens; estrone is the major estrogen of the postmenopausal years.
Estropipate Ogen Various	Tab 0.625, 1.25, 2.5, 5 mg Vag Crm 1.5 mg/g.	0.625 mg.	Ogen 0.625 mg = 0.75 mg estropipate. Ogen 1.25 mg = 1.5 mg estropipate. Ogen 2.5 mg = 3 mg estropipate. Ogen 5 mg = 6 mg estropipate.
Quinestrol Estrovis	Tab 100 mg.	—	Promoted for once-a-week estrogen therapy because it is stored in fat and gradually released.
NONSTEROIDAL AGENTS			
Chlorotrianisene Tace	Cap 12, 25 mg.	12 mg.	Expensive; weak estrogenic activity, metabolized by liver to a more active compound. Infrequently used because of long duration of action because of storage in adipose tissue.

(continued)

ESTROGENS COMPARISON CHART (continued)

DRUG	DOSAGE FORMS	EQUIPOTENT PHYSIOLOGIC DOSE*·†	COMMENTS
Dienestrol Various	Vag Crm 0.01%.	—	
Diethylstilbestrol Various	Tab 1, 5 mg.	0.25 mg.	Antineoplastic agent no longer indicated for estrogen replacement therapy. Inexpensive; frequent nausea.
Diethylstilbestrol Diphosphate Stilphostrol	Tab 50 mg Inj 50 mg/mL.	0.4 mg.	

*Potency of estrogens: estradiol > estrone > estriol. Potency is based on the effects on the liver.
†See monographs or product information for exact dosage regimens for various uses.

POSTMENOPAUSAL HORMONE REPLACEMENT RISKS AND BENEFITS COMPARISON CHART

RISKS/BENEFITS	CLINICAL INFORMATION	COMMENTS
Cancer, Breast	Controversial; no association with <5 yr duration of use to relative risk of 1.25–1.45 among current users with >5 yr duration of use; highest risk of 1.7 reported among long-term users >60 yr. No risk found in past users, regardless of duration of use. Two meta-analyses show minimal risk with >15 yr of use.	Addition of progestin does not reduce risk. Regular mammography is recommended. Consider limiting duration of treatment to <5 yr if risks of cancer outweigh cardioprotective benefits.
Cancer, Colon	A 46% decrease in colon cancer risk; no effect on rectal cancer.	In slender women, risk is reduced by up to 75%.
Cancer, Endometrial	Relative risk of 8.2 with unopposed estrogen use; risk increases with higher dosage and duration >5 yr; 34% risk after 3 yr; 20% lifetime probability of needing a hysterectomy with unopposed estrogen therapy.	Relative risk of 1 with the concurrent addition of a minimum of 10–14 days of progestin. No increased risk of estrogen hyperplasia or need for hysterectomy with concurrent progestin therapy.
Cardiovascular Disease	Three meta-analyses and a cohort study suggest a 40–50% reduction in the risk of coronary and fatal heart disease with unopposed estrogens; benefits may be greater in those with heart disease and >15 yr duration of use. Decreased lifetime probability of developing coronary artery disease. Unknown protection against stroke.	Combination with progestin may be protective, but data are insufficient. May be related to estrogen's effects on lipids or direct effect of relaxing blood vessel walls.
Hypertension	Estrogens can reduce BP.	Hormone replacement is not contraindicated in hypertension.

(continued)

POSTMENOPAUSAL HORMONE REPLACEMENT RISKS AND BENEFITS COMPARISON CHART (continued)

RISKS/BENEFITS	CLINICAL INFORMATION	COMMENTS
Lipids	Unopposed oral estrogens reduce LDL and increase HDL by 10–15%; however, estrogens can increase triglyceride levels.	Progesterone antagonizes beneficial estrogen lipid effects less than medroxyprogesterone. Most favorable effects on lipids occur with estrogen alone. Nonoral estrogens (eg, patch, vaginal) produce less HDL beneficial effects.
Gall Bladder Disease	Estrogen treatment is associated with a 2.1 relative risk (RR). RR of 2.6 with >10 yr of use; RR of 2.4 for users of 1.25 mg or more.	Mortality unaffected; may require cholecystectomy.
Osteoporosis	Inhibits bone resorption and prevents bone loss; 15–50% increase in bone density if begun within 3 yr of menopause. Osteoporosis risk increased in Caucasian and Asian ethnic groups, in sedentary lifestyle, in smokers, with low calcium and vitamin D intake, and excessive alcohol or thyroxine intake.	Alendronate (Fosamax) orally, intranasal calcitonin (Miacalcin), etidronate (Didronel), and slow-release fluoride may also be effective. (See Estradiol Notes.)
Fractures	One-half as many fractures of spinal and hip bones with >5 yr of use: 28% reduction with 10 yr use; 40% with 15 yr use; and 55% with 20 yr. Risk returns near baseline 6 yr or more after cessation of therapy. Decreased lifetime probability of osteoporotic fracture. Risk increases fourfold for each 1 SD decrease in bone density at the hip; 66% of femoral neck fractures occur when bone density is below the lowest quartile.	Bone densitometry can identify women at highest risk.
Vaginal Bleeding	Unpredictable bleeding occurs in 35–40% of women with uteruses yearly.	Amenorrhea usually occurs after 6–8 months of combination estrogen/progestin therapy.

From references 115, 117, 123, 126, 128, and 137–144.

MEDROXYPROGESTERONE ACETATE	Depo-Provera,
	Provera, Various

Pharmacology. Medroxyprogesterone is a 17α-acetoxyprogesterone derivative with greater progestational effects and oral efficacy than progesterone. Progesterone transforms an estrogen-primed proliferative endometrium into a secretory endometrium.

Administration and Adult Dosage. PO for secondary amenorrhea and dysfunctional uterine bleeding, and to induce withdrawal bleeding following postmenopausal estrogen replacement therapy 5–10 mg/day for 5–10 days, depending on degree of endometrial stimulation desired, beginning on the presumed day 1–12 of the cycle (during the first week of estrogen administration). In cases of secondary amenorrhea, therapy can be started at any time. **PO for postmenopausal symptoms and osteoporosis** (combined with continuous estrogen) 2.5–5 mg/day.[145,146] (*See* Notes.) **PO for relief of vasomotor symptoms** 20 mg/day; **IM for relief of vasomotor symptoms** 150 mg/day.[147] (*See* Notes.) **IM for endometrial or renal carcinoma** 400 mg–1 g/week initially for a few weeks, then, if improvement occurs, reduce to maintenance dosage of 400 mg/month. (*See also* Progestin-Only Contraceptives.)

Special Populations. *Geriatric Dosage.* Same as adult dosage.

Dosage Forms. Tab 2.5, 5, 10 mg; **Inj** 150, 400 mg/mL.

Patient Instructions. Report immediately if any of the following occur: new severe or persistent headache; blurred vision; calf, chest, or abdominal pain; or any abnormal vaginal bleeding. This (oral) drug may be taken with food, milk, or an antacid to minimize stomach upset. (Dysfunctional uterine bleeding) Expect heavy and severely cramping flow 2–4 days after stopping therapy; expect a normal period after a few days. The first 48 hours of menses may be excessive, but of normal duration.[76]

Pharmacokinetics. *Onset and Duration.* Withdrawal bleeding (in estrogen-primed endometrium) occurs 3–7 days after last dose.[100,101] Onset of symptomatic relief of hot flashes within 4–7 days; maximum relief after 1 month; duration 8–20 weeks after discontinuation.[147]

Serum Levels. Inhibition of ovulation and tumor response occurs with medroxyprogesterone levels >0.1 μg/L (0.25 nmol/L).[98,100,101,148]

Fate. Medroxyprogesterone acetate (MPA) is rapidly absorbed orally with no first-pass metabolism; oral bioavailability is 5.7 ± 3.8%; IM bioavailability is 2.5 ± 1.7%, with a large interpatient variation in serum levels after oral or IM administration.[79,148] Higher concentration depot formulation is associated with lower serum concentrations, but equivalent bioavailability.[149] Peak concentrations occur in 2–7 hr and are 2–10 times higher after oral than after IM depot injection. PO 10 mg yields peak levels of 3–4 μg/L (7.5–10 nmol/L), declining to 0.3–0.6 μg/L (0.8–1.5 nmol/L) by 24 hr; PO 100 mg yields 13 ± 7 μg/L (34 ± 18 nmol/L), declining to 2 μg/L (5 nmol/L) by 24 hr; PO 500 mg yields 13 ± 8 μg/L (34 ± 21 nmol/L). After 150 mg IM of the 150 mg/mL formulation, peak levels of 8.3 ± 3.2 μg/L (21 ± 8 nmol/L) occur within a few days, declining to levels of 0.8 ± 0.7 μg/L (2 ± 1.8 nmol/L) for 92 ± 44 days. After the 400-mg IM of the 400 mg/mL formulation, peak serum levels of 6.2 ± 2.3 μg/L (16± 6 nmol/L) are achieved after 16.3 ± 15.6 days.[79,91,100,101,149] The drug is stored in fat; over 90% is protein bound to albumin; 83% of a dose is present in serum as the parent drug and conjugated medroxyprogesterone; it is hydroxylated to 6-β-hydroxy-MPA, and 21-hydroxy-MPA, which have unknown activity. From 15–20% of a dose is excreted in urine as glucuronide and sulfate conjugates; 45–80% is excreted in feces.[91]

$t_{1/2}$. About 50 days, reflecting slow IM absorption from depot.

Adverse Reactions. Frequent breast tenderness, weight gain, and depression occur. Adverse lipid effects (increased low-density lipoproteins, decreased high-density lipoproteins) occur with dosages ≥10 mg/day; dosages of 2.5–5 mg/day have negligible effects.[117,145,149] (*See also* Progestin-Only Contraceptives, Postmenopausal Hormone Replacement Risks and Benefits Comparison Chart, and Hormone Excess and Deficiency Symptomatology Comparison Chart.)

Contraindications. Known or suspected pregnancy or as a diagnostic test for pregnancy. Thrombophlebitis, history of deep vein thrombophlebitis, or thromboembolic disorders; known or suspected carcinoma of the breast or endometrium, or other estrogen-dependent tumors; undiagnosed abnormal genital bleeding. Although acute liver disease, benign or malignant liver tumors, and history of cholestatic jaundice of pregnancy or jaundice with prior hormonal contraceptive use are listed as contraindications by manufacturers, liver disease is not considered by others to be a contraindication to progestin-only contraceptives.[93]

Precautions. Use with caution in patients with a history of depression, diabetes, gestational diabetes, coronary artery disease, cerebrovascular disease, hyperlipidemia, liver disease, or hypertension. Although progestins are not harmful to the fetus during the first 4 months of pregnancy; confirm a negative pregnancy test before reinjecting women more than 2 weeks late for their IM injection.[93,102] Progestin-only contraceptives used during breastfeeding are unlikely to pose any risk to the infant,[93,100–104] and they usually do not decrease breast milk production if begun after 6 weeks postpartum.

Drug Interactions. Rifampin and all anticonvulsants (except clonazepam and valproate) can increase progestin metabolism. Long-term use of griseofulvin can increase menstrual irregularities.[73,93,100,101,105]

Parameters to Monitor. Complete pretreatment physical examination with special reference to blood pressure, breasts, abdomen, pelvic organs, and Pap smear yearly.

Notes. Continuous administration of low-dose progestin and estrogen combinations in postmenopausal syndrome causes amenorrhea in more than 50% of women and does not appear to negatively influence blood lipids when compared to cyclic therapy.[117,145,146,150] Concurrent administration of estrogen with progestin for amenorrhea may be associated with less breakthrough bleeding than with progestin alone. There is no evidence that progestins are effective in preventing habitual abortion or treating threatened abortion.

NORETHINDRONE	Norlutin
NORETHINDRONE ACETATE	Aygestin, Norlutate

Pharmacology. Norethindrone and norethindrone acetate are 19-nortestosterone derivatives that share the actions of progestins. They have oral efficacy, increased progestational activity compared to progesterone, and reduced androgenic activity compared to androgens. Norethindrone acetate differs from norethindrone only in potency; the acetate is twice as potent. (*See also* Medroxyprogesterone Acetate, and Progesterone.)

Administration and Adult Dosage. **PO for withdrawal bleeding following post-menopausal estrogen replacement therapy or combined for estrogen replacement therapy** (norethindrone) 5–20 mg/day or (norethindrone acetate) 2.5–10 mg/day starting on day 15–20 of the cycle and continuing for 5–10 days; or (norethindrone) 1–2.5 mg/day or (norethindrone acetate) 0.5–1 mg/day continuously combined with estrogen.[145,146,150] *See* Medroxyprogesterone Acetate Notes. **PO for amenorrhea or abnormal uterine bleeding** (norethindrone) 5–20 mg/day, or (norethindrone acetate) 2.5–10 mg/day starting on day 5 and ending on day 25 of menses. In cases of secondary amenorrhea, therapy can be started at any time.[76] **PO for endometriosis** (norethindrone) 10 mg/day, or (norethindrone acetate) 5 mg/day for 2 weeks, increasing in (norethindrone) 5 mg/day or (norethindrone acetate) 2.5 mg/day increments q 2 weeks until a maintenance dosage of (norethindrone) 30 mg/day or (norethindrone acetate) 15 mg/day is reached.[77]

Special Populations. *Geriatric Dosage.* Same as adult dosage.

Dosage Forms. **Tab** (norethindrone) 5 mg (Norlutin); (norethindrone acetate) 5 mg (Aygestin, Norlutate).

Patient Instructions. Report immediately if any of the following occur: new severe or persistent headache; blurred vision; calf, chest, or abdominal pain; or any abnormal vaginal bleeding. This (oral) drug may be taken with food, milk, or an antacid to minimize stomach upset. (Dysfunctional uterine bleeding) Expect heavy and severely cramping flow 2–4 days after stopping therapy; expect a normal period after a few days. The first 48 hours of menses may be excessive, but of normal duration.[76]

Pharmacokinetics. *Onset and Duration.* (Uterine bleeding) After oral administration, acute bleeding should decrease in 1–2 days and stop in 3–4 days. (Withdrawal bleeding) onset 3–7 days after last oral dose.[76]

Fate. (Norethindrone) marked intra- and interpatient variability in pharmacokinetics. Norethindrone and its acetate are rapidly and completely absorbed with mean bioavailability of 64 ± 16% because of first-pass metabolism.[78–82,91] Norethindrone acetate is rapidly converted to norethindrone in vivo.[78,82,84,87] Oral administration of 1 mg of norethindrone yields peak levels of 4.8 ± 0.3 to 17 ± 8 µg/L (16 ± 0.9 to 57 ± 26 nmol/L), declining to 0.4 µg/L (1.3 nmol/L) after 24 hr; 3 mg yields peak levels of 8.3 ± 0.8 µg/L (27.8 ± 2.5 nmol/L). The drug is 35.5% bound to sex-hormone-binding globulin and 61% bound to albumin; It is concentrated in body fat and endometrium; breast milk levels are 10% of maternal serum levels. V_d is 4.3 ± 9 L/kg; Cl is 0.5 ± 1.5 L/hr/kg. Over 50% is eliminated in urine and 20–40% in feces as conjugated glucuronides and sulfates; less than 5% of norethindrone and its acetate are excreted as unchanged norethindrone.[78–82,87,91]

$t_{1/2}$. (Norethindrone) 6.4 ± 3 hr.[78–82,87,91]

Adverse Reactions. (*See* Medroxyprogesterone Acetate, Postmenopausal Hormone Replacement Risks and Benefits Comparison Chart, and Hormone Excess and Deficiency Symptomatology Comparison Chart.)

Contraindications. (*See* Medroxyprogesterone Acetate, and Postmenopausal Hormone Replacement Risks and Benefits Comparison Chart.)

Precautions. (See Medroxyprogesterone Acetate, Postmenopausal Hormone Replacement Risks and Benefits Comparison Chart, and Hormone Excess and Deficiency Symptomatology Comparison Chart.)

Drug Interactions. (*See* Medroxyprogesterone Acetate.)

Parameters to Monitor. (*See* Medroxyprogesterone Acetate.)

Notes. (*See* Medroxyprogesterone Acetate.)

PROGESTERONE	Progestasert, Various
HYDROXYPROGESTERONE CAPROATE	Duralutin, Various

Pharmacology. Progesterone is the natural hormone that induces secretory changes in the endometrium, relaxes uterine smooth muscle, and maintains pregnancy. Hydroxyprogesterone is a natural progestin with minimal progestational activity; esterification with caproic acid produces a progestational compound more potent than progesterone with a prolonged duration of activity.

Administration and Adult Dosage. **IM for secondary amenorrhea or dysfunctional uterine bleeding** (progesterone) 5–10 mg/day for 6–8 days or (only for amenorrhea) 100–150 mg as a single dose; (hydroxyprogesterone caproate) 375 mg, may repeat in 4 weeks prn. **IM for palliation of metastatic endometrial cancer** (hydroxyprogesterone caproate) 500 mg–1 g 2–3 times/week. **Intrauterine for contraception** (progesterone) 38 mg q 12 months, releases 68 µg/day; insert at any time during menstrual cycle or within 7 days of onset of menses, immediately postabortion, or no earlier than 6 weeks postpartum if breast feeding; insertion and removal are done by trained personnel. **PO to induce withdrawal bleeding following postmenopausal estrogen replacement therapy** (micronized progesterone) 200 mg/day for first 12 days of cycle.[117] (*See* Notes.)

Special Populations. *Geriatric Dosage.* Same as adult dosage.

Dosage Forms. **Inj** (progesterone in oil) 50 mg/mL; (hydroxyprogesterone caproate in oil) 125, 250 mg/mL; **Intrauterine** (progesterone) 38 mg (Progestasert).

Patient Instructions. Report immediately if any of the following occur: new severe or persistent headache; blurred vision; calf, chest or abdominal pain; or any abnormal vaginal bleeding. (Dysfunctional uterine bleeding) Expect heavy flow and severe cramping 2–4 days after injection; expect a normal period after a few days.[76] (Progestasert only) You may experience increased menstrual flow, cramping, and spotting. Check the position of the strings monthly after each period or after abnormal cramping to ensure proper placement of the IUD. Contact your prescriber immediately if the strings are missing, if you miss a menstrual period or if you have fever, pelvic pain, severe cramping, unusual vaginal bleeding, or any signs of infection.[73]

Pharmacokinetics. *Onset and Duration.* (Amenorrhea) Onset of withdrawal bleeding occurs 48–72 hr after last dose of IM progesterone and 2 weeks after IM hydroxyprogesterone caproate; (dysfunctional uterine bleeding) onset within 6 days of IM progesterone.[76] Duration is 12–24 hr with oral progesterone, 9–17 days with IM hydroxyprogesterone caproate. (Contraception) Onset within 24 hr after insertion of Progestasert.

Serum Levels. (Endometrial progestational activity [luteal phase]) 15 µg/L (48 nmol/L) or greater of progesterone.

Fate. (Progesterone) Bioavailability of oral progesterone is incomplete because of first-pass metabolism with wide interpatient variation; investigational micronized forms are somewhat better absorbed.[79,117,150,151] Higher levels of progesterone and active metabolites occur after IM, vaginal, or rectal administration, because first-pass effect is avoided. Serum levels of progesterone after oral and IM increase rapidly to reach luteal phase values within 2.4 ± 1.1 hr and remain elevated for <12 hr after oral administration and for 48 hr after IM administration. PO 100-mg micronized progesterone yields peak progesterone levels of 7 ± 3.4 µg/L (23 ± 11 nmol/L); 200 mg yields 28 ± 19 µg/L (89 ± 59 nmol/L); IM 100 mg yields 60 µg/L (192 nmol/L); Vag 200 mg bid yields 19 ± 2 µg/L (61 ± 7 nmol/L); Vag 400 mg once daily yields 29 ± 53 µg/L (93 ± 188 nmol/L).[79,150,152] Oral progesterone V_d is 850 ± 265 L/kg; Cl is 18.7 ± 38 L/hr/kg.[150] Progesterone circulates 80% bound to albumin and 17% to corticosteroid-binding globulin, and distributes into fat. It undergoes rapid gut and hepatic metabolism, with formation of active metabolites: 20α-dihydroprogesterone (25–50% of the progestational activity of progesterone), 17-hydroxyprogesterone, and 11-deoxycorticosterone (a potent mineralocorticoid).[79,153,154] Hydroxyprogesterone caproate is cleaved to form 17-hydroxyprogesterone in the body; 17-hydroxyprogesterone, whether formed from progesterone or exogenously administered, is further metabolized to 11-deoxycortisol and then cortisol. Urinary excretion of progesterone is 50–60% as 5β-pregnanediol glucuronide and other conjugated glucuronic acid or sulfate metabolites; 5–10% excreted in feces.

$t_{1/2}$. (Progesterone) α phase 5 min; β phase 32.6 ± 9.3 hr.[150]

Adverse Reactions. Local reactions and swelling at the site of progesterone injection. The beneficial effects of estrogen-increased high-density lipoprotein levels are not reversed by progesterone.[117] (*See* Postmenopausal Hormone Replacement Risks and Benefits Comparison Chart, and Hormone Excess and Deficiency Symptomatology Comparison Chart.) (Progestasert) intermenstrual spotting and menstrual bleeding irregularities, expulsion, ectopic pregnancy, uterine perforation, pelvic inflammatory disease, cramping, and pain. Intrauterine administration of contraceptive doses of progesterone has no systemic effects.[73]

Contraindications. (*See* Medroxyprogesterone Acetate. [Progestasert] Pregnancy; active, recent, or recurrent pelvic infections, including gonorrhea or *Chlamydia* infection.)

Precautions. (*See* Medroxyprogesterone Acetate, and Postmenopausal Hormone Replacement Risks and Benefits Comparison Chart, and Hormone Excess and Deficiency Symptomatology Comparison Chart.)

Drug Interactions. (*See* Medroxyprogesterone Acetate.)

Parameters to Monitor. Complete pretreatment and annual physical examination with special reference to blood pressure, breasts, abdomen, pelvic organs, and Pap smear.

Notes. Progesterone is widely used in the treatment of premenstrual syndrome; however, in double-blind, controlled trials, oral micronized and vaginal progesterone were no better than placebo.[155,156]

Thyroid and Antithyroid Drugs

IODIDES   Various

Pharmacology. Iodide inhibits the synthesis and release of thyroid hormone and preoperatively decreases the size and vascularity of the hyperplastic thyroid gland. Large doses block the uptake of radioactive iodine by the thyroid gland.

Administration and Adult Dosage. PO for hyperthyroidism, as an adjunct to antithyroid agents or for preoperative thyroidectomy preparation 50–100 mg q 8 hr diluted in a glass of water, milk, or juice; dosages as high as 500 mg/day have been used. Use for 7–10 days before surgery. **PO for thyroid storm** 200 mg q 6 hr. **PO for prophylaxis in a radiation emergency** 100 mg iodine immediately before or within 1–2 hr after exposure and daily for 3–7 days, to a maximum of 10 days after exposure. However, administration of smaller doses of 30–50 mg iodine and continued suppression with doses of 15–50 mg/day may also be effective.[157]

Special Populations. *Pediatric Dosage.* **PO for thyrotoxicosis** 300 mg (6 drops SSKI) q 8 hr diluted as above. **PO for prophylaxis in a radiation emergency** (<1 yr) 50 mg iodine immediately before or after exposure and daily for 3–7 days, to a maximum of 10 days after exposure; (>1 yr) same as adult dosage.

Geriatric Dosage. Same as adult dosage.

Dosage Forms. Soln (SSKI) 50 mg/drop iodide (1 g/mL); (Lugol's or strong iodine) 8 mg/drop iodide (50 mg/mL iodine plus 100 mg/mL potassium iodide); (potassium iodide) 21 mg/drop iodide; **Tab** 100 mg iodide (130 mg potassium iodide); **EC Tab not recommended.**

Patient Instructions. Dilute solution in 240 mL (8 fl oz) of liquid before taking; it may be taken with food, milk, or an antacid to minimize stomach upset. Do not use if solution turns brownish-yellow. If crystals form in the solution, they may be dissolved by warming the closed container in warm water. Dissolve tablets in one-half glass of water or milk before taking. Do not use if you are breastfeeding; advise your physician if you are pregnant. Discontinue use and report if fever, skin rash, epigastric pain, or joint swelling occur.

Pharmacokinetics. *Onset and Duration.* Onset is in 24–48 hr in hyperthyroidism, with maximum effect in 10–15 days (*see* Notes).

Serum Levels. Iodide levels >50 µg/L (0.4 mmol/L) inhibit iodide binding by thyroid in hyperthyroidism; levels >200 µg/L (1.6 mmol/L) inhibit iodide uptake by normal thyroid.[158]

Fate. Iodide is well absorbed throughout the GI tract and concentrated in the thyroid, stomach, and salivary glands. Renal clearance is 1.8 L/hr/kg; approximately 100 µg of iodine is excreted in urine daily; fecal excretion of iodine is negligible.[158]

Adverse Reactions. Any adverse reaction warrants drug discontinuation. Goiter, hypothyroidism, and hyperthyroidism occur frequently in euthyroid patients with a history of a thyroid disorder.[159–163] Iodism occurs with prolonged use and is indicated by metallic taste, GI upset, soreness of teeth and gums, coryza, frontal headaches, painful swelling of salivary glands, diarrhea, acneiform skin eruptions, and erythema of face and chest. Rarely, hypersensitivity occurs and is manifested by angioedema, cutaneous hemorrhages, and symptoms resembling serum sickness (*see* Precautions).

Contraindications. Pulmonary tuberculosis; pulmonary edema.

Precautions. Pregnancy, because fetal goiter, asphyxiation, and death may occur;[163] lactation. Use iodides or iodine-containing drugs (eg, amiodarone) with caution in patients with untreated Hashimoto's thyroiditis, in iodide-deficient patients, in children with cystic fibrosis, and in euthyroid patients with a history of postpartum thyroiditis, subacute thyroiditis, amiodarone or lithium-induced thyroid disease, or Graves' disease previously treated with thioamides, radioactive iodine, or surgery because they may be particularly sensitive to iodide-induced hypothyroidism.[159–161,163] Patients with nontoxic multinodular goiters may be prone to development of hyperthyroidism.[164] Avoid iodides entirely in patients with toxic nodular goiter or toxic nodules, because thyrotoxicosis may be further aggravated.[164] Iodides are not recommended for use as expectorants because of their potential to induce acneiform eruptions, exacerbate existing lesions, and adversely affect the thyroid. Small-bowel lesions are associated with enteric-coated potassium-containing tablets, which can cause obstruction, hemorrhage, perforation, and possible death. This dosage form is not recommended.

Drug Interactions. Iodide prevents uptake of ^{131}I for several weeks and delays onset of thioamide action if given before the thioamide. Lithium may potentiate the antithyroid action of iodide. Serum iodine may be elevated if potassium-sparing diuretics are taken with potassium iodide.

Parameters to Monitor. Monitor for signs of iodism (*see* Adverse Reactions), hypothyroidism, hyperthyroidism, and parotitis occasionally during long-term use. Monitor thyroid function tests at least q 6–12 months during long-term use in patients with a family history of thyroid disease or goiter. Monitor serum potassium frequently in patients who are taking other drugs that may also affect serum potassium (eg, diuretics).

Notes. Iodide has the most rapid onset of any treatment for hyperthyroidism. In thyroid storm, iodide should theoretically be given 1 hr after the **thioamide** dose, but should not be withheld if oral thioamides cannot be given.[164] The therapeutic effects of iodide are variable and transient, with "escape" occurring after 10–14 days; do not use iodide alone in the therapy of hyperthyroidism.[165,166] Pharmacologic amounts of iodide can be present in serum from radiographic contrast agents and vaginal douches such as **povidone-iodine**.[164,167]

LEVOTHYROXINE SODIUM	Levothroid, Levoxyl, Synthroid, Various

Pharmacology. Levothyroxine is a synthetically prepared hormone identical to the thyroid hormone T_4. Thyroid hormones are responsible for normal growth, development, and energy metabolism.

Administration and Adult Dosage. **PO for replacement in hypothyroidism under 6 months in duration** full replacement dosage of 1.6–1.7 µg/kg/day initially, increasing if needed and tolerated in 25–50 µg/day increments at 6- to 8-

week intervals to a maintenance dosage that normalizes thyroid-stimulating hormone (TSH).[168–172] Usual maintenance dosages are 75–100 µg/day for women and 100–150 µg/day for men. Higher mean replacement dosages are required in patients with spontaneous hypothyroidism (1.7–1.8 µg/kg/day) than in those with iatrogenic hypothyroidism after radioiodine for Graves' disease (1.5–1.6 µg/kg/day).[168,171,172] **PO for suppression therapy of nodules** 100–150 µg/day initially, increasing, if necessary and tolerated, in 25–50 µg/day increments at 6- to 8-week intervals to suppress TSH to below normal, detectable limits to prevent further thyroid growth.[168,171,172] Dosages are usually higher than those required for replacement therapy. **PO for suppression therapy of thyroid cancer after thyroidectomy** 2.11 µg/kg/day initially, increasing, if needed and tolerated, in 25–50 µg/day increments at 6- to 8-week intervals to a dosage of 150–250 µg/day to suppress the TSH level to undetectable levels.[168,170–172] **IV for myxedema coma** 300–500 µg or 300 µg/m^2 to increase serum T_4 levels by 3–5 µg/dL (39–65 nmol/L), then 50–100 µg/day until oral administration is possible; use smaller dosages in cardiovascular disease.[168,170,172–174] **IM** indicated only for replacement therapy if patient cannot take oral medication; parenteral dosage is about 80% of oral dosage because of bioavailability difference.[168,170]

Special Populations. *Pediatric Dosage.* **PO for hypothyroidism** (preterm infants and fullterm neonates to 1 yr) 10–15 µg/kg/day to normalize T_4 to greater than 10 µg/dL (129 nmol/L) within 3–4 weeks; (>1 yr) 3–5 µg/kg/day (average 3.5).[170,172,175] Adjust maintenance dosage on the basis of growth, development, and T_4 and TSH values. Replacement by at least 24 months of age corrects short stature by age 5 yr.[176]

Geriatric Dosage. (>50 yr) **PO** start with 25–50 µg/day initially, then increase if tolerated in 6–8 weeks by 12.5–25 µg/day to a maintenance dosage necessary to normalize TSH; (>65 yr) less than 1 µg/kg/day may be required.[168–170,172] Poorly compliant elderly patients (mean age 86 yr) have been maintained on a twice-weekly dosing regimen; however, this regimen may be dangerous in cardiac patients.[177]

Other Conditions. In patients with cardiovascular disease or severe, long-standing (over 6 months) myxedema, PO 25–50 µg/day initially, increasing, if tolerated, at 6- to 8-week intervals by 12.5–25 µg/day to a maintenance dosage necessary to normalize TSH.[168–172] In patients with cardiovascular disease, particularly angina, increments should be balanced between exacerbation of angina and maintenance of euthyroidism. In some patients with severe coronary disease, incomplete control of hypothyroidism may be necessary to prevent further exacerbation of angina. During pregnancy, a 20–50% increase in dosage may be required to maintain a normal TSH level.[168–170,172]

Dosage Forms. **Tab** 25, 50, 75, 88, 100, 112, 125, 137, 150, 175, 200, 300 µg; **Inj** 200, 500 µg.

Patient Instructions. This medication must be taken regularly to maintain proper hormone levels in the body. Report immediately if chest pain (especially in elderly patients), palpitations, sweating, nervousness, or other signs of overactivity occur. Take any missed dose as soon as it is remembered, but if more than one dose is missed, do not double dosage.

Pharmacokinetics. *Onset and Duration.* PO onset 3–5 days; peak effect 3–4 weeks; duration after cessation of therapy 7–10 days. IV onset in myxedema coma 6–8 hr, maximum effect in 1 day.[168–173]

Serum Levels. (Physiologic and therapeutic during levothyroxine therapy) free T_4 6–21 ng/L (12–26 pmol/L); Total T_4 50–120 µg/L (65–155 nmol/L). Peak free T_4 levels can be 12.7 ± 2.6%, and total T_4 levels 8.1 ± 1.2% higher than trough levels or levels obtained 10 hr after a dose.[178] Many drugs, and pathologic and physiologic states affect binding and hence may affect results of some serum level determinations.[172,179–183]

Fate. Oral bioavailability ranges from 74 ± 11% to 93 ± 25% and is affected by many factors (eg, malabsorption, diet, cholesterol-binding resins, iron, aluminum-containing products).[168–170,172] A dose of 500 µg IV increases serum T_4 levels by 3–5 µg/dL (39–65 nmol/L)[168,173] Only 0.03% is unbound in plasma. V_d is (hypothyroid) 0.17 ± 0.22 L/kg; (euthyroid) 0.16 ± 0.09 L/kg; (hyperthyroid) 0.23 ± 0.44 L/kg. Turnover is (hypothyroid) 9.2 ± 1.7%/day; (euthyroid) 11.2 ± 1.7%/day; (hyperthyroid) 21 ± 4.9%/day. Cl is (hypothyroid) 0.0008 ± 0.0033 L/hr/kg; (euthyroid) 0.00074 ± 0.0017 L/hr/kg; (hyperthyroid) 0.002 ± 0.0007 L/hr/kg.[184] About 80% is deiodinated in the body; 35% is peripherally converted to the more active T_3 and 45% to inactive reverse T_3.[168,172] Another 15–20% is conjugated in the liver to form glucuronides and sulfates, which undergo an enterohepatic recirculation with reabsorption or excretion in the feces.[182,183]

$t_{1/2}$. (Hypothyroid) 7.5 ± 7.1 days; (euthyroid) 6.2 ± 4.7 days; (hyperthyroid) 3.2 ± 1.7 days.[184,185] Protein binding affects half-life (increased binding retards elimination and decreased binding increases elimination).[182]

Adverse Reactions. Most are dose related and can be avoided by increasing the initial dosage slowly to the minimum effective maintenance dosage. Signs of overdosage include headache, palpitations, chest pain, heat intolerance, sweating, leg cramps, weight loss, diarrhea, vomiting, nervousness, and other symptoms of hyperthyroidism. Long-term thyroid administration that results in TSH suppression may predispose to osteoporosis by increasing bone resorption; at greatest risk are postmenopausal women with a past history of hyperthyroidism.[168–170,172]

Contraindications. Thyrotoxicosis; uncorrected adrenal insufficiency.

Precautions. Initiate and increase dosage with caution in patients with cardiovascular disease, the elderly, and in long-standing hypothyroidism. In myxedema coma, give a corticosteroid concurrently.[173] The status of other metabolic diseases, including diabetes, adrenal insufficiency, hyperadrenalism, and panhypopituitarism may be affected by changes in thyroid status.

Drug Interactions. Phenytoin, carbamazepine, and other enzyme inducers; iron; aluminum-containing products; sodium polystyrene sulfonate; and cholesterol-binding resins can increase levothyroxine requirements. The action of some drugs (eg, digoxin, warfarin, insulin) may be altered by changing thyroid status.[170,172,179,181–183]

Parameters to Monitor. (Adults) TSH, free T_4 or free T_4 index, and clinical status of the patient q 6–8 weeks initially. Monitor trough levels or obtain levels at least 10 hr after tablet ingestion to avoid transient peak effects.[178] After stabilization, monitor free T_4 or free T_4 index, TSH, and clinical status at 6- to 12-month intervals. (Children) Monitor the parameters above q 4 weeks initially and q 3–4 months after stabilization. In congenital hypothyroidism, monitor T_4 because TSH may remain elevated despite adequate replacement doses.[172,175] (>50 yr) Evaluate the replacement dosage every year and adjust downward as necessary, because dosage requirements decrease with age.[168–172]

Notes. Levothyroxine is the drug of choice for thyroid replacement because of purity, standardization, long half-life, large body pool, and close simulation to normal physiologic hormone levels. Protect from light and moisture. Subpotent levothyroxine tablets are unlikely, because of USP requirements that all tablets be standardized by high-pressure liquid chromatography to be $\pm$ 10% of the labeled content.[168,172] Bioequivalence between Synthroid, Levothroid, and Levoxyl is likely.[168,170,187] Use of adjunctive thyroid hormones for depression and cardiopulmonary bypass is controversial.[172,189] Physiologic dosages of thyroid hormones in euthyroid patients are ineffective for weight reduction, obesity, and premenstrual tension; larger dosages may result in toxicity.[172] (*See* Thyroid Replacement Products Comparison Chart.)

LIOTHYRONINE SODIUM   Cytomel, Triostat, Various

Pharmacology. Liothyronine is a synthetic hormone identical to the thyroid hormone T_3, which is 4 times as potent by weight as T_4. (*See* Levothyroxine.)

Administration and Adult Dosage. **PO for replacement in hypothyroidism <6 months in duration** 25 µg/day initially, increasing, if needed and tolerated, in 12.5–25 µg/day increments at 1- to 2-week intervals to a maintenance dosage of 25–100 µg/day to normalize thyroid-stimulating hormone (TSH). **PO for severe hypothyroidism** 5 µg/day initially, increasing in 5–10 µg/day increments at 1- to 2-week intervals until 25 µg/day is reached, then increase in 12.5–25 µg/day increments at 1- to 2-week intervals until euthyroid. Dividing daily dosage into 2–3 doses may prevent wide serum level fluctuations.[181,188] **IV for myxedema coma** 25–50 µg initially, then 10–12.5 µg q 4–6 hr to a minimum of 10–15 µg q 12 hr until PO administration is possible; use smaller dosages of 10–20 µg IV initially in cardiovascular disease.[172,174] Limited experience with IV dosages over 100 µg/day. **PO for T_3 suppression test** 75–100 µg/day in 2–3 divided doses for 7 days, then repeat ^{131}I thyroid uptake test.

Special Populations. *Pediatric Dosage.* **PO for congenital hypothyroidism** 5 µg/day initially, increasing in 5 µg/day increments at 3- to 4-day intervals until desired effect is obtained. Usual maintenance dosage is (<1 yr) 20 µg/day; (1–3 yr) 50 µg/day; (>3 yr) 25–100 µg/day. Levothyroxine is the drug of choice in congenital hypothyroidism.[175]

Geriatric Dosage. Not recommended because of greater potential for cardiotoxicity.[172] If used, start at PO 5 µg/day and increase in 5 µg/day increments at 2-week intervals, if tolerated, until desired response is obtained (*see* Levothyroxine).

Other Conditions. Not recommended in those with cardiovascular disease but, if used, start at PO 5 µg/day and increase in 5 µg/day increments at 2-week intervals, if tolerated, until desired response is obtained (*see* Levothyroxine).

Dosage Forms. **Tab** 5, 25, 50 µg; **Inj** 10 µg/mL.

Patient Instructions. This medication must be taken regularly to maintain proper hormone levels in the body. Report immediately if chest pain (especially in elderly patients), palpitations, sweating, nervousness, or other signs of overactivity occur. Take any missed dose as soon as it is remembered, but if more than one dose is missed, do not double dosage.

Pharmacokinetics. *Onset and Duration.* PO onset 1–3 days; duration after cessation of therapy 3–5 days.

Serum Levels. During T_3 replacement, T_4 is maintained at ≤ 10 µg/L (13 nmol/L).[172,181,188]

Fate. Oral absorption is usually complete, but may be decreased in CHF.[181] With a typical replacement dose, T_3 has a peak of 4.5–7 µg/L (7–11 nmol/L) 1–2 hr postdose, returning to 0.88–1.6 µg/L (1.4–2.5 nmol/L) before the next dose 24 hr later.[172,181,188] V_d is: (hypothyroid) 0.53 ± 0.04 L/kg; (euthyroid) 0.52 ± 0.03 L/kg; (hyperthyroid) 0.94 ± 0.07 L/kg. Turnover is (hypothyroid) 50 ± 5%/day; (euthyroid) 68 ± 11%/day; (hyperthyroid) 110 ± 22%/day. Cl is (hypothyroid) 0.012 ± 0.002 L/hr/kg; (euthyroid) 0.020 ± 0.003 L/hr/kg; (hyperthyroid) 0.043 ± 0.013 L/hr/kg.[184,185] Excreted in urine as deiodinated metabolites and their conjugates.[189]

$t_{1/2}$. (Hypothyroid) 38 ± 6 hr; (euthyroid) 25 ± 3 hr; (hyperthyroid) 17 ± 4.7 hr.[184,185]

Adverse Reactions. *See* Levothyroxine. Dose-related adverse effects are more likely and appear more rapidly, because regulation of dosage is more difficult than with levothyroxine. Liothyronine and its mixtures (eg, desiccated thyroid, liotrix) cause "unphysiologic" toxic peaks in serum T_3 levels not found during levothyroxine replacement therapy.[181,188]

Contraindications. (*See* Levothyroxine.)

Precautions. (*See* Levothyroxine.)

Drug Interactions. Normal serum T_3 levels are age related and can be decreased by a wide variety of pharmacologic agents (eg, amiodarone, iodinated contrast dyes, corticosteroids, propylthiouracil) or clinical circumstances (eg, malnutrition, chronic renal, hepatic, pulmonary, or cardiac disease; or acute sepsis) which impair either peripheral or pituitary T_4 to T_3 conversion.[179,181,182] (*See also* Levothyroxine Drug Interactions.)

Parameters to Monitor. Serum TSH level and T_3 level (*see* Levothyroxine).

Notes. Liothyronine is not considered the drug of choice for replacement therapy in hypothyroidism because of its greater expense, shorter half-life (necessitating more frequent administration), and greater potential for cardiotoxicity, and the greater difficulty of monitoring.[168–170] Some claim liothyronine to be useful in patients with myxedema coma when impairment of T_4 to T_3 conversion is suspected[172–174] or in cardiac disease, because adverse effects will dissipate faster. Liothyronine is the preparation of choice when thyroid supplements must be stopped prior to isotope scanning. After scanning, maintenance therapy with levothyroxine is recommended. The use of T_3 for psychiatric disorders and cardiopulmonary bypass is controversial.[172,189] (*See* Thyroid Replacement Products Comparison Chart.)

THYROID REPLACEMENT PRODUCTS COMPARISON CHART

DRUG	DOSAGE FORMS	EQUIVALENT DOSAGE	CONTENTS	RELATIVE ONSET AND DURATION*	COMMENTS
Levothyroxine Levothroid Levoxyl Synthroid Various	Tab 25, 50, 75, 88, 100; 112, 125, 137, 150, 175, 200, 300 µg. Inj 200, 500 µg.	60 µg	T4	Long	Preparation of choice. T4 content is now standardized using HPLC and bioequivalence among products is likely.
Liothyronine Cytomel Triostat Various	Tab 5, 25, 50 µg Inj 10 µg/mL.	25 µg	T3	Short	Expensive; difficult to monitor. Preparation of choice if thyroid supplements are to be stopped for isotope scanning.
Liotrix Thyrolar	Tab ¼, ½, 1, 2, 3.†	#1 Tab‡	T4 and T3 in 4:1 ratio	Intermediate	No advantages; more costly and suffers from T3 content. (See Thyroid, Desiccated)
Thyroid, Desiccated Various	Tab 15, 30, 60, 90, 120, 180, 240, 300 mg.	60 mg	T4 and T3 in variable ratio	Intermediate	Inexpensive; allergy to animal protein rarely occurs; supraphysiologic elevations in T3 and T3-toxicosis may occur.

*With equivalent dosages.
†Numbers represent equivalent dosage of thyroid in grains (ie, 15, 30, 60, 120, 180 mg, respectively).
‡Thyrolar-1 contains T4 50 µg and T3 12.5 µg; other strengths are in the same proportion.
From references 172 and 187.

METHIMAZOLE
Tapazole

Pharmacology. Methimazole is a thioamide antithyroid drug that interferes with the synthesis of thyroid hormones by inhibiting iodide organification. Unlike propylthiouracil (PTU), methimazole does not block peripheral conversion of T_4 to T_3. Titers of thyroid receptor stimulating antibody (TRab) decline during therapy, suggesting an immunosuppressive effect. Methimazole is 10 times more potent than PTU on a weight basis.

Administration and Adult Dosage. PO for hyperthyroidism 30–40 mg/day as a single dose. If GI intolerance occurs, divide dosage q 8 hr initially until euthyroid (usually 6–8 weeks), then decrease by 33–50% over several weeks to a maintenance dosage of 5–15 mg/day in a single dose. Severe disease might require two divided doses. To prevent recurrence of hyperthyroidism, **levothyroxine** 75–100 µg/day may be added after 6 months once the patient is euthyroid; this may improve remission rates, but further study is warranted.[164,166,190–192] **PO for thyroid storm** 40–120 mg/day, divided q 8 hr until euthyroid. Traditional treatment duration for hyperthyroidism is 1–2 yr, although longer or shorter courses (eg, 6 months) might be effective.[164,166,169] Treatment may be continued indefinitely if necessary to control the disease and if no toxicity occurs. **PR** Methimazole can be formulated for rectal administration.[195]

Special Populations. *Pediatric Dosage.* **PO** 0.4 mg/kg/day or 15–20 mg/m^2/day given in 1–2 divided doses with a maintenance dosage of one-half the initial dosage.[170]

Geriatric Dosage. Same as adult dosage.

Other Conditions. In pregnancy, doses should be as low as possible to maintain maternal T_4 level in approximately the upper normal to mildly thyrotoxic range; initially give a maximum of 30 mg/day orally in single or 3 divided doses for 4–6 weeks, then decrease to 5–15 mg/day in a single dose.[164,166,169,194]

Dosage Forms. Tab 5, 10 mg.

Patient Instructions. Report sore throat, fever, or oral lesions immediately because they may be an early sign of a severe, but rare blood disorder. Also report any skin eruptions, itching, or yellowing of eyes and skin. Be sure to take at prescribed dosage intervals. If a dose is missed, take it as soon as possible. If it is time for the next dose, take both doses.

Pharmacokinetics. *Onset and Duration.* **PO** onset about 2–3 weeks, which is consistent with the elimination of existing T_4 stores. Duration intrathyroidally 40 hr.[196]

Serum Levels. <0.2 mg/L (1.8 µmol/L) inhibits iodide organification.[196]

Fate. Well absorbed orally. Considerable interindividual variation in pharmacokinetic parameters. Peak serum levels occur at 2.3 ± 0.8 hr; the peak after 30 mg orally is 0.8 ± 0.2 mg/L (6.8 ± 1.9 µmol/L); after 60 mg orally, 1.5 ± 0.5 mg/L (14 ± 4 µmol/L); after 60 mg rectally, 1.1 ± 0.5 mg/L (10 ± 5 µmol/L).[195–197] The drug is actively concentrated in thyroid gland with peak intrathyroidal levels of 0.11–1.1 mg/L (1–10 µmol/L) within 1 hr;[196] there is minimal plasma protein binding; it is distributed into breast milk 10 times greater than PTU.[194] V_d is 1.4 ± 0.6 L/kg; Cl is 0.072 ± 0.018 L/hr/kg. There are no active metabolites; 7–12% is excreted unchanged in urine, 6% excreted as inorganic sulfate, 1.5% as sulfur metabolites, and 50% as unknown metabolites.[196,197]

$t_{1/2}$. α phase 3 ± 1.4 hr; β phase 18.5 ± 13 hr in normal and hyperthyroid patients, increased to 21 hr in cirrhosis.[196] Intrathyroidal half-life is 20 hr.

Adverse Reactions. Maculopapular skin rashes and itching occur frequently and may disappear spontaneously with continued treatment; urticaria requires drug discontinuation.[164,166] Methimazole can be given to patients who develop only a nonurticarial maculopapular rash on PTU. Mild transient leukopenia occurs frequently in untreated Graves' disease, does not predispose to agranulocytosis, and is not an indication to discontinue the drug.[164,166,198,199] Agranulocytosis occurs occasionally, usually in the first 3 months of therapy. Risk increases with dosages over 40 mg/day in patients >40 yr; granulocyte colony-stimulating factors (eg, **filgrastim**) can hasten recovery.[198–201] Rarely, fever, arthralgias, cholestatic or hepatocellular toxicity, vasculitis, lupuslike syndrome, hypoprothrombinemia, aplastic anemia, thrombocytopenia, nephrotic syndrome, loss of taste, and spontaneous appearance of circulating antibodies to insulin or glucagon occur.[164,166,202–205]

Contraindications. Manufacturer states that breastfeeding is a contraindication, but some experts feel that breastfeeding may be performed with dosages of 10 mg/day or less and careful monitoring of infant thyroid function.[206]

Precautions. Although methimazole crosses the placenta at rates 4 times greater than **propylthiouracil** and has been associated with scalp defects (aplasia cutis), recent reports indicate methimazole can be given in pregnant patients intolerant to PTU.[164,194,207] Use with caution during lactation and in patients with severe allergic reactions to other thioamides. A low prevalence of cross-sensitivity occurs between thioamide compounds for nonurticarial skin rashes, so if these occur, another thioamide can be substituted. However, a 50% chance of cross-sensitivity exists for severe reactions (eg, agranulocytosis, hepatitis), so do not substitute another thioamide.[164,199]

Drug Interactions. Iodide given before a thioamide delays the response to the thioamide, especially in thyroid storm. Changes in thyroid status may alter pharmacodynamics and pharmacokinetics of digoxin, warfarin, theophylline, β-blockers, and insulin.

Parameters to Monitor. Monitor clinical status of patient; serum free T_4 or T_4 index, and TSH monthly initially until euthyroid, then q 3–6 months. Obtain occasional liver function tests and CBC with differential (but these are not recommended routinely, because they are not predictive of toxicity and transient leukopenia and elevations in liver function tests can occur); AST, ALT, total bilirubin, and alkaline phosphatase if patient reports signs of hepatitis; WBC and differential counts if patient reports signs of agranulocytosis such as fever, sore throat, or malaise.

Notes. Methimazole is the drug of choice for treatment of uncomplicated hyperthyroidism, because it is better tolerated and fewer tablets can be given once daily, improving patient compliance.[164,166,169] Remission rates of 20–40% are common after cessation of therapy. Favorable remission rates correlate with longer duration of therapy, higher dosages, mild disease, shrinkage of goiter size with therapy, disappearance of thyroid receptor stimulating antibodies, and initial presentation with T_3 toxicosis.[164,207] Concurrent administration of levothyroxine might also improve remission rates, but further study is required.[164,166,190–192] Most patients eventually require surgery or radioiodine; however, a trial of a thioamide is worthwhile in patients with minimal thyroid enlargement or very mild hyperthyroidism. In thyroid storm, pregnancy, and lactation, PTU is the drug of choice.

PROPYLTHIOURACIL   Various

Pharmacology. Propylthiouracil (PTU) is a thioamide antithyroid drug that blocks the synthesis of thyroid hormones and, at dosages over 450 mg/day, also decreases the peripheral conversion of T_4 to T_3. Titers of thyroid receptor stimulating antibody (TRab) decline during therapy, consistent with an immunosuppressive effect.

Administration and Adult Dosage. **PO for hyperthyroidism** 100–200 mg (depending on the severity of hyperthyroidism) q 6–8 hr initially until euthyroid (usually 6–8 weeks), then decrease by 33–50% over several weeks to a maintenance dosage of 50–150 mg/day in a single dose. Rarely, initial dosages of 1–1.2 g/day (maximum dosage) in 3–6 doses may be necessary.[164] **PO for thyroid storm** 200–250 mg q 6 hr until euthyroid; maintenance dosage is determined by patient response. Treatment duration for hyperthyroidism is 1–2 yr traditionally, although shorter courses of 6 months may also be effective in mild disease.[164,166,169] Treatment may be continued indefinitely if necessary to control the disease and if no toxicity occurs. To prevent recurrence of hyperthyroidism, **levothyroxine** 75–100 µg/day may be added after 6 months once the patient is euthyroid; this may improve remission rates, but further study is warranted.[164,166,190–192] **PR** PTU can be formulated for rectal administration.[208,209]

Special Populations. *Pediatric Dosage.* Give orally in 3 divided doses. **PO** 150–300 mg/m²/day. Alternatively, (6–10 yr) 5–10 mg/kg/day or 50–150 mg/day initially; (≥10 yr) 150–300 mg/day initially. Maintenance dosage is determined by patient response.

Geriatric Dosage. Same as adult dosage.

Other Conditions. In pregnancy, dosage should be as small as possible to maintain a mildly hyperthyroid maternal state; initially 300 mg/day orally in 3 divided doses for 4–6 weeks, then decrease to 50–150 mg/day in a single dose.[164,169,194]

Dosage Forms. **Tab** 50 mg.

Patient Instructions. Report sore throat, fever, or oral lesions immediately because they may be an early sign of a severe, but rare blood disorder. Also report any skin eruptions, itching, or yellowing of eyes and skin. Be sure to take at prescribed dosage intervals. If a dose is missed, take it as soon as possible. If it is time for the next dose, take both doses.

Pharmacokinetics. *Onset and Duration.* PO onset of therapeutic effect 2–3 weeks, consistent with the elimination of existing thyroxine stores.

Serum Levels. Peak PTU levels above 4 mg/L (24 µmol/L) produce antithyroid activity; 3 mg/L (18 µmol/L) reduces organification by 50%; 0.8 mg/L (5 µmol/L) reduces peripheral conversion activity by 50%.[197,210]

Fate. Oral bioavailability is 77 ± 13%. Peak levels occur 2 ± 0.3 hr after oral administration, and 4.7 ± 1 hr after rectal administration. Peak serum level after an oral dose of 50 mg is 1 ± 0.2 mg/L (6 ± 1.2 μmol/L); after 200 mg, 4.5 ± 0.7 mg/L (26 ± 4 μmol/L); after 300 mg, 7 ± 0.8 mg/L (42 ± 5 μmol/L); after 400 mg rectally, 3 ± 0.8 mg/L (18 ± 5 μmol/L).[196,208–210] Actively concentrated in the thyroid gland 40% as unknown metabolite, 32% as sulfate, and 20% as unchanged PTU; peak intrathyroidal levels of 0.17–1.7 mg/L (1–10 μmol/L) occur within 1 hr.[164,197] The drug is 80% plasma protein bound; it distributes poorly into breast milk. V_c is 0.21 ± 0.05 L/kg; $V_{dß}$ is 0.29 ± 0.06 L/kg; Cl is 0.23 ± 0.04 L/hr/kg. About 85% is excreted in 24 hr, 61% as glucuronides, 8–9% as inorganic sulfates, 8–10% as unknown sulfur metabolites, and <10% excreted unchanged in urine.[197]

$t_{1/2}$. α phase 7.5 ± 3.7 min; β phase 1.3 ± 0.6 hr.[164,197,210]

Adverse Reactions. *See* Methimazole; however, agranulocytosis is not more prevalent at higher dosages as it is with methimazole. Rarely, hepatitis occurs; hepatocellular toxicity is more frequent than cholestatic jaundice.[164,166,211] Transient transaminase elevations can occur in asymptomatic individuals which normalize within 3 months with continued drug administration.[190]

Contraindications. Manufacturer states that breastfeeding is a contraindication, but if necessary, it can be used with infant thyroid monitoring because of low milk levels and lack of effect on infants.[194,206]

Precautions. (*See* Methimazole.) Although it crosses the placenta poorly (one-fourth the rate of methimazole), it can cause fetal hypothyroidism and goiter.[164,166,194] Thyroid dysfunction may diminish as pregnancy progresses, allowing a reduction in dosage and, in some cases, a withdrawal of therapy 2–3 weeks before delivery. Adjunctive thyroid hormone therapy prevents maternal hypothyroidism, but because of minimal placental transfer, has little effect on the fetus.[194] Use with caution prior to surgery or during treatment with anticoagulants because of hypoprothrombinemic effect.

Drug Interactions. (*See* Methimazole.)

Parameters to Monitor. (*See* Methimazole.) Prothrombin time monitoring is advisable, particularly prior to surgery.

Notes. Because propylthiouracil decreases peripheral conversion of T_4 to T_3, it is considered the thioamide of choice in treating thyroid storm; it is also the drug of choice in pregnancy and breastfeeding.[164,194,205] PTU may decrease mortality because of alcoholic liver disease.[212]

■ REFERENCES

1. Kaye TB, Crapo L. The Cushing syndrome: an update on diagnostic tests. *Ann Intern Med* 1990;112:434–44.
2. Axelrod L. Corticosteroid therapy. In Becker KL, ed. *Principles and practice of endocrinology and metabolism.* Philadelphia: JB Lippincott; 1990:613–23.
3. Schimmer BP, Parker KL. Adrenocorticotropic hormone: adrenocortical steroids and their synthetic analogs; inhibitors of the synthesis and action of adrenal hormones. In Hardman JG et al., eds. *Goodman and Gilman's the pharmacological basis of therapeutics,* 9th ed. New York: McGraw-Hill; 1996:1459–85.
4. Clayton RN. Diagnosis of adrenal insufficiency. *Br Med J* 1989;298:271–2.
5. Cersosimo RJ, Karp DD. Adrenal corticosteroids as antiemetics during cancer chemotherapy. *Pharmacotherapy* 1986;6:118–27.
6. Anon. Ondansetron to prevent vomiting after cancer chemotherapy. *Med Lett Drugs Ther* 1991;33:63–4.

7. The Italian Group for Antiemetic Research. Dexamethasone, granisetron, or both for the prevention of nausea and vomiting during chemotherapy for cancer. *N Engl J Med* 1995;332:1–5.

8. Grunberg SM, Hesketh PJ. Control of chemotherapy-induced emesis. *N Engl J Med* 1993;329:1790–6.

9. Orth DN et al. The adrenal cortex. In Wilson JD, Foster DW, eds. *Williams textbook of endocrinology.* Philadelphia: WB Saunders; 1992:489–619.

10. Wildenradt SS, Hart LL. Antenatal dexamethasone as prophylaxis of respiratory distress syndrome. *Ann Pharmacother* 1994;28:475–7.

11. Bone RC et al. A controlled clinical trial of high-dose methylprednisolone in the treatment of severe sepsis and shock. *N Engl J Med* 1987;317:653–8.

12. McGowan JE et al. Guidelines for the use of systemic glucocorticoids in the management of selected infections. *J Infect Dis* 1992;165:1–13.

13. Benitz WE, Tatro DS. *The pediatric drug handbook,* 2nd ed. Chicago: Year Book; 1988.

14. Anon. Dexamethasone for bacterial meningitis in children. *Med Lett Drugs Ther* 1989;31:6–7.

15. Prober CG. The role of steroids in the management of children with bacterial meningitis. *Pediatrics* 1995;95:29–31.

16. Baxter JD. Minimizing the side effects of glucocorticoid therapy. *Adv Intern Med* 1990;35:173–94.

17. Tsuei SE et al. Disposition of synthetic glucocorticoids. I. Pharmacokinetics of dexamethasone in healthy adults. *J Pharmacokinet Biopharm* 1979;7:249–64.

18. Gustavson LE, Benet LZ. Pharmacokinetics of natural and synthetic glucocorticoids. In Anderson DC, Winter JSD, eds. *Butterworth's international medical reviews: clinical endocrinology.* Vol. 4, *Adrenal cortex.* London: Butterworth; 1985:235–81.

19. Baharav E et al. Dexamethasone-induced perineal irritation. *N Engl J Med* 1986;314:515–6. Letter.

20. Health and Public Policy Committee, American College of Physicians. The dexamethasone suppression test for the detection, diagnosis, and management of depression. *Ann Intern Med* 1984;100:307–8.

21. Nierenberg AA, Feinstein AR. How to evaluate a diagnostic marker test: lessons from the rise and fall of dexamethasone suppression test. *JAMA* 1988;259:1699–702.

22. Erstad BL. Severe cardiovascular adverse effects in association with acute, high-dose corticosteroid administration. *DICP* 1989;23:1019–23.

23. Kong AN et al. Pharmacokinetics and pharmacodynamic modeling of direct suppression effects of methylprednisolone on serum cortisol and blood histamine in human subjects. *Clin Pharmacol Ther* 1989;46:616–28.

24. Anon. Drugs for acute spinal cord injury. *Med Lett Drugs Ther* 1993;35:72–3.

25. Truhan AP, Ahmed AR. Corticosteroids: a review with emphasis on complications of prolonged systemic therapy. *Ann Allergy* 1989;62:375–90.

26. Breitenfield RV et al. Stability of renal transplant function with alternate-day corticosteroid therapy. *JAMA* 1980;244:151–6.

27. Bystryn J-C. Adjuvant therapy of pemphigus. *Arch Dermatol* 1984;120:941–51.

28. Siegel SC. Corticosteroid agents: overview of corticosteroid therapy. *J Allergy Clin Immunol* 1985;76:312–20.

29. Iafrate RP et al. Current concepts in clinical therapeutics: asthma. *Clin Pharm* 1986;5:206–27.

30. Haskell RJ et al. A double-blind, randomized clinical trial of methylprednisolone in status asthmaticus. *Arch Intern Med* 1983;143:1324–7.

31. Kelly HW, Murphy S. Corticosteroids for acute, severe asthma. *DICP* 1991;25:72–9.

32. The National Institutes of Health-University of California Expert Panel for Corticosteroids as Adjunctive Therapy for Pneumocystis Pneumonia. Consensus statement on the use of corticosteroids as adjunctive therapy for Pneumocystis pneumonia in the acquired immunodeficiency syndrome. *N Engl J Med* 1990;323:1500–4.

33. Groff GD et al. Systemic steroid therapy for acute gout: a clinical trial and review of the literature. *Semin Arthritis Rheum* 1990;19:329–36.

34. Hill MR et al. Monitoring glucocorticoid therapy: a pharmacokinetic approach. *Clin Pharmacol Ther* 1990;48:390–8.

35. Gambertoglio JG et al. Pharmacokinetics and bioavailability of prednisone and prednisolone in healthy volunteers and patients: a review. *J Pharmacokinet Biopharm* 1980;8:1–52.

36. Lewis GP et al. Prednisone side-effects and serum-protein levels. *Lancet* 1971;2:778–81.

37. Saag KG et al. Low dose long-term corticosteroid therapy in rheumatoid arthritis: an analysis of serious adverse events. *Am J Med* 1994;96:115–23.

38. Klein JF. Adverse psychiatric effects of systemic glucocorticoid therapy. *Am Fam Physician* 1992;46:1469–74.

39. Anon. Oral corticosteroids. *Med Lett Drugs Ther* 1975;17:99–100.

40. Callahan CM et al. Oral corticosteroid therapy for patients with stable chronic obstructive pulmonary disease: a meta-analysis. *Ann Intern Med* 1991;114:216–23.

41. Weinberger SE. Recent advances in pulmonary medicine. *N Engl J Med* 1993;328:1389–97.

42. Derendorf H et al. Pharmacokinetics of triamcinolone acetonide after intravenous, oral, and inhaled administration. *J Clin Pharmacol* 1995;35:302–5.

43. Mukwaya G. Immunosuppressive effects and infections associated with corticosteroid therapy. *Pediatr Infect Dis J* 1988;7:499–504.

44. Lebovitz HE. α-Glucosidase inhibitors in the treatment of hyperglycemia. In Lebovitz HE, ed. *Therapy for diabetes mellitus and related disorders,* 2nd ed. Alexandria, VA: American Diabetes Association; 1994.

45. Kirchain WR, Rendell MS. Aldose reductase inhibitors. *Pharmacotherapy* 1990;10:326–36

46. Zenon GJ III et al. Potential use of aldose reductase inhibitors to prevent diabetic complications. *Clin Pharm* 1990;47:446–57.

47. Giugliano D et al. Tolrestat for mild diabetic neuropathy. A 52-week, randomized, placebo-controlled trial. *Ann Intern Med* 1993;118:7–11.

48. White JR Jr, Campbell RK. Pharmacologic therapies. In Peragallo-Dittko V et al., eds. *A core curriculum for diabetes education,* 2nd ed. Chicago: American Association of Diabetes Educators; 1993:217–57.

49. Santiago JV, ed. *Medical management of insulin-dependent (type I) diabetes,* 2nd ed. Alexandria, VA: American Diabetes Association; 1993.

50. Adrogué HJ et al. Diabetic ketoacidosis: a practical approach. *Hosp Pract* 1989;(Feb. 15):83–112.

51. Sanson TH, Levine SN. Management of diabetic ketoacidosis. *Drugs* 1989;38:289–300.

52. Raskin P, ed. *Medical management of type II diabetes,* 3rd ed. Alexandria, VA: American Diabetes Association; 1994.

53. White JR Jr, Campbell RK. Guide to mixing insulins. *Hosp Pharm* 1991;26:1046–8.

54. Koda-Kimble MA. Diabetes mellitus. In Young LY, Koda-Kimble MA, eds. *Applied therapeutics,* 5th ed. Vancouver, WA: Applied Therapeutics; 1992:72-2–53.

55. Alberti KGMM, Nattrass M. Severe diabetic ketoacidosis. *Med Clin North Am* 1978;62:799–814.

56. The Diabetes Control and Complications Trial Research Group. The effect of intensive treatment of diabetes on the development and progression of long-term complications in insulin-dependent diabetes mellitus. *N Engl J Med* 1993;329:977–86.

57. White JR Jr, Campbell RK. Hypoglycemic drugs. *Clin Podiatr Med Surg* 1992;9;239–55.

58. White JR Jr, Campbell RK. Pharmacologic therapies in the management of diabetes mellitus. In Haire-Joshu D, ed. *Management of diabetes mellitus. Perspectives of care across the life span.* St. Louis: Mosby Year Book; 1994:119–48.

59. Peterson L et al. Insulin adsorbance to polyvinylchloride surfaces with implications for constant-infusion therapy. *Diabetes* 1976;25:72–4.

60. Brange J et al. Insulin analogues with improved absorption characteristics. *Horm Metab Res* 1992;26 (suppl):125–30.

61. Jørgensen S et al. NovoSol Basal: pharmacokinetics of a novel soluble long acting insulin analogue. *Br Med J* 1989;299:415–9.

62. Howley DC et al. [Lys (B28), Pro(B29)]-human insulin. A rapidly absorbed analogue of human insulin. *Diabetes* 1994;43:396–402.

63. DeFronzo RA et al. Mechanism of metformin action in obese and lean noninsulin-dependent diabetic subjects. *J Clin Endocrinol Metab* 1991;73:1294–301.

64. Bailey CJ. Biguanides and NIDDM. *Diabetes Care* 1992;15:755–72.

65. DeFronzo RA et al. Efficacy of metformin in patients with non-insulin-dependent diabetes mellitus. *N Engl J Med* 1995;333:541–9.

66. Somogyi A et al. Reduction of metformin tubular secretion by cimetidine in man. *Br J Clin Pharmacol* 1987;23:545–51.

67. Hermann LS et al. Therapeutic comparison of metformin and sulfonylurea, alone and in various combinations. *Diabetes Care* 1994;17:1100–8.

68. Gerich JE. Oral hypoglycemic agents. *N Engl J Med* 1989;321:1231–45.

69. Rydberg T et al. Hypoglycemic activity of glyburide (glibenclamide) metabolites in humans. *Diabetes Care* 1994;17:1026–30.

70. Davidson MB. Rational use of sulfonylureas. *Postgrad Med* 1992;92:69–85.

71. White JR Jr et al. Drug interactions and diabetes. The risk of losing glycemic control. *Postgrad Med* 1993;93:131–40.

72. Anon. The 1994 buyer's guide to diabetes supplies. *Diabetes Forecast* 1993;46(10):60–7.

73. Hatcher RA et al. *Contraceptive Technology,* 16th revised ed. New York: Irvington; 1994.

74. Van Look PFA, von Hertzen H. Emergency contraception. *Br Med Bull* 1993;49:158–70.

75. Weisberg E. Prescribing oral contraceptives. *Drugs* 1995;49:224–31.

76. Bayer SR, DeCherney AH. Clinical manifestations and treatment of dysfunctional uterine bleeding. *JAMA* 1993;269:1823–8.

77. Lu PY, Ory SJ. Endometriosis: current management. *Mayo Clin Proc* 1995;70:453–63.

78. Shenfield GM, Griffin JM. Clinical pharmacokinetics of contraceptive steroids. An update. *Clin Pharmacokinet* 1991;20:15–37.

79. Kuhl H. Pharmacokinetics of oestrogens and progestogens. *Maturitas* 1990;12:171–97.

80. Stanczyk FZ, Roy S. Metabolism of levonorgestrel, norethindrone, and structurally related contraceptive steroids. *Contraception* 1990;42:67–93.

81. Kuhnz W et al. Systemic availability of levonorgestrel after single oral administration of a norgestimate-containing combination oral contraceptive to 12 young women. *Contraception* 1994;49:255–63.

82. Fotherby K. Potency and pharmacokinetics of gestagens. *Contraception* 1990;41:533–50.

83. Back DJ et al. Comparative pharmacokinetics of levonorgestrel and ethinyloestradiol following intravenous, oral, and vaginal administration. *Contraception* 1987;36:471–9.

84. Goldzieher JW. Selected aspects of the pharmacokinetics and metabolism of ethinyl estrogens and their clinical implications. *Am J Obstet Gynecol* 1990;163:318–22.

85. Goldzieher JW. Pharmacokinetics and metabolism of ethinyl estrogens. In Goldzieher JW, Fotherby K, eds. *Pharmacology of the contraceptive steroids.* New York: Raven Press; 1994:140–51.

86. Kuhnz W et al. Pharmacokinetics of levonorgestrel and ethinylestradiol in 14 women during three months of treatment with a tri-step combination oral contraceptive: serum protein binding of levonorgestrel and influence of treatment on free and total testosterone levels in the serum. *Contraception* 1994;50:563–79.

87. Orme ML'E et al. Clinical pharmacokinetics of oral contraceptive steroids. *Clin Pharmacokinet* 1983;8:95–136.

88. Archer DF et al. Pharmacokinetics of a triphasic oral contraceptive containing desogestrel and ethinyl estradiol. *Fertil Steril* 1994;61:645–51.

89. McClamrock HD, Adashi EY. Pharmacokinetics of desogestrel. *Am J Obstet Gynecol* 1993;168:1021–8.

90. Orme M et al. The pharmacokinetics of ethinylestradiol in the presence and absence of gestodene and desogestrel. *Contraception* 1991;43:305–17.

91. Fotherby K. Pharmacokinetics and metabolism of progestins in humans. In Goldzieher JW, Fotherby K, eds. *Pharmacology of the contraceptive steroids.* New York: Raven Press; 1994:99–126.

92. Kubba A, Guillebaud J. Combined oral contraceptives: acceptability and effective use. *Br Med Bull* 1993;49:140–57.

93. McCann MF, Potter LS. Progestin-only oral contraception: a comprehensive review. *Contraception* 1994;50:S138–48.

94. Speroff L et al. Evaluation of a new generation of oral contraceptives. *Obstet Gynecol* 1993;81:1034–47.

95. Thorogood M, Villard-Mackintosh L. Combined oral contraceptives: risks and benefits. *Br Med Bull* 1993;49:124–39.

96. Upton GV, Corbin A. Contraception for the transitional years of women older than 40 years of age. *Clin Obstet Gynecol* 1992;35:855–64.

97. Schlesselman JJ. Net effect of oral contraceptive use on the risk of cancer in women in the United States. *Obstet Gynecol* 1995;85:793–801.

98. Shenfield GM. Oral contraceptives: are drug interactions of clinical significance? *Drug Saf* 1993;9:21–37.

99. Corson SL. A decade of experience with transdermal estrogen replacement therapy: overview of key pharmacologic and clinical findings. *Int J Fertil* 1993;38:79–91.

100. Kaunitz AM. Long-acting injectable contraception with depot medroxyprogesterone acetate. *Am J Obstet Gynecol* 1994;170:1543–9.

101. Kaunitz AM, Rosenfield A. Injectable contraception with depot medroxyprogesterone acetate. Current status. *Drugs* 1993;45:857–65.

102. Pardthaisong T et al. The long-term growth and development of children exposed to Depo-Provera during pregnancy or lactation. *Contraception* 1992;45:313–24.

103. World Health Organization Task Force for Epidemiological Research on Reproductive Health; Special Programme of Research, Development and Research Training in Human Reproduction. Progestogen-only contraceptives during lactation: I: infant growth. *Contraception* 1994;50:35–53.

104. World Health Organization Task Force for Epidemiological Research on Reproductive Health Special Programme of Research, Development and Research Training in Human Reproduction. Progestogen-only contraceptives during lactation: II: infant development. *Contraception* 1994;50:55–68.

105. Darney PD. Hormonal implants: contraception for a new century. *Am J Obstet Gynecol* 1994;170:1536–43.

106. Skegg DCG et al. Depot medroxyprogesterone acetate and breast cancer. A pooled analysis of the World Health Organization and New Zealand Studies. *JAMA* 1995;273:799–804.

107. Wysowski DK, Green L. Serious adverse events in Norplant users reported to the Food and Drug Administration's Med Watch spontaneous reporting system. *Obstet Gynecol* 1995;85:538–42.

108. Dunson TR et al. Complications and risk factors associated with the removal of Norplant implants. *Obstet Gynecol* 1995;85:543–48.

109. Bagshaw S. The combined oral contraceptive. Risks and adverse effects in perspective. *Drug Saf* 1995;12:91–6.

110. Anon. After the morning after and the morning after that. *Lancet* 1995;345:1381–2. Editorial.

111. Hannaford PC et al. Oral contraception and stroke. Evidence from the Royal College of General Practitioners' Oral Contraception Study. *Stroke* 1994;25:935–42.

112. Lidegaard O. Decline in cerebral thromboembolism among young women after introduction of low-dose oral contraceptives: an incidence study for the period 1980–1993. *Contraception* 1995;52:85–92.

113. Goldzieher JW, Zamah NM. Oral contraceptive side effects: where's the beef? *Contraception* 1995;52:327–35.

114. Anon. Oral contraceptive alert in UK sparks off controversy. *Lancet* 1995;346:1149–50. News.

115. Belchetz PE. Hormonal treatment of postmenopausal women. *N Engl J Med* 1994;330:1062–71.

116. Ettinger B et al. Cyclic hormone replacement therapy using quarterly progestin. *Obstet Gynecol* 1994;83:693–700.

117. The Postmenopausal Estrogen/Progestin Interventions (PEPI) Trial. Effects of estrogen or estrogen/progestin regimens on heart disease risk factors in postmenopausal women. *JAMA* 1995;273:199–208.

118. Lobo RA, Cassidenti DL. Pharmacokinetics of oral 17ß-estradiol. *J Reprod Med* 1992;37:77–84.

119. Anderson F. Kinetics and pharmacology of estrogens in pre- and postmenopausal women. *Int J Fertil* 1993;38(suppl 1):53–64.

120. Handa VL et al. Vaginal administration of low-dose conjugated estrogens: systemic absorption and effects on the endometrium. *Obstet Gynecol* 1994;84:215–8.

121. Pang SC et al. Long-term effects of transdermal estradiol with and without medroxyprogesterone acetate. *Fertil Steril* 1993;59:76–82.

122. Kuhnz W et al. Pharmacokinetics of estradiol free and total estrone, in young women following single intravenous and oral administration of 17 beta-estradiol. *Arzneimittelforschung* 1993;43:966–73.

123. Cobleigh MA et al. Estrogen replacement therapy in breast cancer survivors: a time for change. *JAMA* 1994;272:540–5.

124. Loprinzi CL et al. Megestrol acetate for the prevention of hot flashes. *N Engl J Med* 1994;331:347–52.

125. Campagnoli C et al. Long-term hormone replacement treatment in menopause: new choices, old apprehensions, recent findings. *Maturitas* 1993;18:21–46.

126. Lufkin EG et al. Treatment of postmenopausal osteoporosis with transdermal estrogen. *Ann Intern Med* 1992;117:1–9.

127. Walsh BW et al. Effects of postmenopausal estrogen replacement on the concentrations and metabolism of plasma lipoproteins. *N Engl J Med* 1991;325:1196–204.

128. Lindsay R. Prevention and treatment of osteoporosis. *Lancet* 1993;341:801–5.

129. Liberman UA et al. Effect of oral alendronate on bone mineral density and the incidence of fractures in postmenopausal osteoporosis. The Alendronate Phase III Osteoporosis Treatment Study Group. *N Engl J Med* 1995;333:1437–43.

130. Chesnut CH 3rd. Alendronate treatment of the postmenopausal osteoporotic woman: effect of multiple dosages on bone mass and bone remodeling. *Am J Med* 1995;99:144–52.

131. Overgaard K et al. Effect of salcatonin given intranasally on bone mass and fracture rates in established osteoporosis: a dose-response study. *Br Med J* 1992;305:556–61.

132. Wimalawansa SJ. Combined therapy with estrogen and etidronate has an additive effect on bone mineral density in the hip and vertebrae: four-year randomized study. *Am J Med* 1995;99:36–42.

133. Anon. New drugs for osteoporosis. *Med Lett Drugs Ther* 1996;38:1–3.

134. McCarthy ML, Stoukides CA. Estrogen therapy of uremic bleeding. *Ann Pharmacother* 1994;28:60–2.

135. Zachee P et al. Hematologic aspects of end-stage renal failure. *Ann Hematol* 1994;69:33–40.

136. Bhavnani BR, Cecutti A. Pharmacokinetics of 17ß-dihydroequilin sulfate and 17ß-dihydroequilin in normal postmenopausal women. *J Clin Endocrinol Metab* 1994;78:197–204.

137. Steinberg KK et al. A meta-analysis of the effect of estrogen replacement therapy on the risk of breast cancer. *JAMA* 1991;265:1985–90. {Erratum JAMA 1991;266:1362}.

138. Grady D et al. Hormone therapy to prevent disease and prolong life in postmenopausal women. *Ann Intern Med* 1992;117:1016–37.

139. American College of Physicians. Guidelines for counseling postmenopausal women about preventive hormone therapy. *Ann Intern Med* 1992;117:1038–41.

140. Lip GYH et al. Hormone replacement therapy and blood pressure in hypertensive women. *J Hum Hypertens* 1994;8:491–4.

141. Colditz GA et al. The use of estrogens and progestins and the risk of breast cancer in postmenopausal women. *N Engl J Med* 1995;332:1589–93.

142. Stanford JL et al. Combined estrogen and progestin hormone replacement therapy in relation to risk of breast cancer in middle-aged women. *JAMA* 1995;274:137–42.

143. Dupont WD, Page DL. Menopausal estrogen replacement therapy and breast cancer. *Arch Intern Med* 1991;151:67–72.

144. Ettinger B et al. Reduced mortality associated with long-term postmenopausal estrogen therapy. *Obstet Gynecol* 1996;87:6–12.

145. Udoff L et al. Combined continuous hormone replacement therapy: a critical review. *Obstet Gynecol* 1995;86:306–16.
146. Archer DF et al. Bleeding patterns in postmenopausal women taking continuous combined or sequential regimens of conjugated estrogens with medroxyprogesterone acetate. Menopause Study Group. *Obstet Gynecol* 1994;83:686–92.
147. Ravnikar V. Physiology and treatment of hot flushes. *Obstet Gynecol* 1995;75:3S–8.
148. Etienne MC et al. Improved bioavailability of a new oral preparation of medroxyprogesterone acetate. *J Pharm Sci* 1991;80:1130–2.
149. Wright CE et al. Effect of injection volume on the bioavailability of sterile medroxyprogesterone acetate suspension. *Clin Pharm* 1983;2:435–8.
150. Norman TR et al. Comparative bioavailability of orally and vaginally administered progesterone. *Fertil Steril* 1991;56:1034–9.
151. Munk-Jensen N et al. Continuous combined and sequential estradiol and norethindrone acetate treatment of postmenopausal women: effect of plasma lipoproteins in a two-year placebo-controlled trial. *Am J Obstet Gynecol* 1994;171:132–8.
152. Nahoul K et al. Profiles of plasma estrogens, progesterone and their metabolites after oral or vaginal administration of estradiol or progesterone. *Maturitas* 1993;16:185–202.
153. Padwick M et al. Absorption and metabolism of oral progesterone when administered twice daily. *Fertil Steril* 1986;46:402–7.
154. Ottoson UB et al. Serum levels of progesterone and some of its metabolites including deoxycorticosterone after oral and parenteral administration. *Br J Obstet Gynaecol* 1984;91:1111–9.
155. Freeman EW et al. A double-blind trial of oral progesterone, alprazolam, and placebo in treatment of severe premenstrual syndrome. *JAMA* 1995;274:51–7.
156. Freeman E et al. Ineffectiveness of progesterone suppository treatment for premenstrual syndrome. *JAMA* 1990;264:349–53.
157. Sternthal E et al. Suppression of thyroid radioiodine uptake by various doses of stable iodide. *N Engl J Med* 1980;303:1083–8.
158. Braverman LE, Utiger RD. *Werner & Ingbar's the thyroid*, 6th ed. Philadelphia: Lippincott; 1991.
159. Roti E et al. Effects of chronic iodine administration on thyroid status in euthyroid subjects previously treated with antithyroid drugs for Graves' hyperthyroidism. *J Clin Endocrinol Metab* 1993;76:928–32.
160. Roti E et al. Iodine-induced subclinical hypothyroidism in euthyroid subjects with a previous episode of amiodarone-induced thyrotoxicosis. *J Clin Endocrinol Metab* 1992;75:1273–7.
161. Roti E et al. Impaired intrathyroidal iodine organification and iodine-induced hypothyroidism in euthyroid women with a previous episode of postpartum thyroiditis. *J Clin Endocrinol Metab* 1991;73:958–63.
162. Mizukami Y et al. Iodine-induced hypothyroidism: a clinical and histological study of 29 patients. *J Clin Endocrinol Metab* 1993;76:466–71.
163. Delange F. The disorders induced by iodine deficiency. *Thyroid* 1994;4:107–28.
164. Klein I et al. Treatment of hyperthyroid disease. *Ann Intern Med* 1994;121:281–8.
165. Philippou G et al. The effect of iodide on serum thyroid hormone levels in normal persons, in hyperthyroid patients, and in hypothyroid patients on thyroxine replacement. *Clin Endocrinol (Oxf)* 1992;36:573–8.
166. Franklyn JA. The management of hyperthyroidism. *N Engl J Med* 1994;330:1731–8.
167. Mann K et al. Systemic iodine absorption during endoscopic application of radiographic contrast agents for endoscopic retrograde cholangiopancreaticography. *Eur J Endocrinol* 1994;130:498–501.
168. Mandel SJ et al. Levothyroxine therapy in patients with thyroid disease. *Ann Intern Med* 1993;119:492–502.
169. Singer PA et al. Treatment guidelines for patients with hyperthyroidism and hypothyroidism. *JAMA* 1995;273:808–12.
170. Toft AD. Thyroxine therapy. N Engl J Med 1994;331:174–81. [Erratum] *N Engl J Med* 1994;331:1035.
171. Burmeister LA et al. Levothyroxine dose requirements for thyrotropin suppression in the treatment of differentiated thyroid cancer. *J Clin Endocrinol Metab* 1992;75:344–50.
172. Roti E et al. The use and misuse of thyroid hormone. *Endocr Rev* 1993;14:401–23.
173. Nicoloff JT, LoPresti JS. Myxedema coma. A form of decompensated hypothyroidism. *Endocrinol Metab Clin North Am* 1993;22:279–90.
174. MacKerrow SD. Myxedema-associated cardiogenic shock treated with intravenous triiodothyronine. *Ann Intern Med* 1992;117:1014–5.
175. Fisher DA. Management of congenital hypothyroidism. *J Clin Endocrinol Metab* 1991;72:523–9.
176. Chiesa A et al. Growth follow-up in 100 children with congenital hypothyroidism before and during treatment. *J Pediatr Endocrinol* 1994;7:211–17.
177. Taylor J et al. Twice-weekly dosing for thyroxine replacement in elderly patients with primary hypothyroidism. *J Int Med Res* 1994;22:273–7.

178. Ain KA et al. Thyroid hormone levels affected by time of blood sampling in thyroxine-treated patients. *Thyroid* 1993;3:81–5.

179. Davies PH, Franklyn JA. The effects of drugs on tests of thyroid function. *Eur J Clin Pharmacol* 1991;40:439–51.

180. Bishnoi A et al. Effects of commonly prescribed nonsteroidal anti-inflammatory drugs on thyroid hormone measurements. *Am J Med* 1994;96:235–8.

181. Surks MI et al. American Thyroid Association guidelines for use of laboratory tests in thyroid disorders. *JAMA* 1990;263:1529–32.

182. Cavalieri RR, Pitt-Rivers R. The effects of drugs on the distribution and metabolism of thyroid hormones. *Pharmacol Rev* 1981;33:55–80.

183. Curran PG, DeGroot LJ. The effect of hepatic enzyme-inducing drugs on thyroid hormones and the thyroid gland. *Endocr Rev* 1991;12:135–50.

184. Nicoloff JT et al. Simultaneous measurement of thyroxine and triiodothyronine peripheral turnover kinetics in man. *J Clin Invest* 1972;51:473–83.

185. Inada M et al. Estimation of thyroxine and triiodothyronine distribution and of the conversion rate of thyroxine to triiodothyronine in man. *J Clin Invest* 1975;55:1337–48.

186. Faber J, Galloe AM. Changes in bone mass during prolonged subclinical hyperthyroidism due to L-thyroxine treatment: a meta-analysis. *Eur J Endocrinol* 1994;130:350–6.

187. Escalante DA et al. Assessment of interchangeability of two brands of levothyroxine preparations with a third-generation TSH assay. *Am J Med* 1995;98:374–8.

188. Salter DR et al. Triiodothyronine (T_3) and cardiovascular therapeutics: a review. *J Card Surg* 1992;7:363–74.

189. Pittman CS et al. Urinary metabolites of ^{14}C-labeled thyroxine in man. *J Clin Invest* 1972;51:1759–66.

190. Hashizume K et al. Administration of thyroxine in treated Graves' disease: effects on the level of antibodies to thyroid-stimulating hormone receptors and on the risk of recurrence of hyperthyroidism. *N Engl J Med* 1991;324:947–53.

191. McIver B et al. Lack of effect of thyroxine in patients with Graves' hyperthyroidism who are treated with an antithyroid drug. *N Engl J Med* 1996;334:220–4.

192. Tamai H et al. Lack of effect of thyroxine administration on elevated thyroid stimulating hormone receptor antibody levels in treated Graves' disease patients. *J Clin Endocrinol Metab* 1995;80:1481–4.

193. Perrild H et al. Diagnosis and treatment of thyrotoxicosis in childhood. A European questionnaire study. *Eur J Endocrinol* 1994;131:467–73.

194. Burrow GN. Thyroid function and hyperfunction during gestation. *Endocr Rev* 1993;14:194–202.

195. Nabil N et al. Methimazole: an alternative route of administration. *J Clin Endocrinol Metab* 1982;54:180–1.

196. Cooper DS et al. Methimazole pharmacology in man: studies using a newly developed radioimmunoassay for methimazole. *J Clin Endocrinol Metab* 1984;58:473–9.

197. Kampmann JP, Hansen JM. Clinical pharmacokinetics of antithyroid drugs. *Clin Pharmacokinet* 1981;6:401–28.

198. Meyer-Gessner H et al. Antithyroid drug-induced agranulocytosis: clinical experience with ten patients treated at one institution and review of the literature. *J Endocrinol Invest* 1994;17:29–36.

199. Tajiri J et al. Antithyroid drug-induced agranulocytosis: the usefulness of routine white blood cell count monitoring. *Arch Intern Med* 1990;150:621–4.

200. Tajiri J et al. Granulocyte colony-stimulating factor treatment of antithyroid drug-induced granulocytopenia. *Arch Intern Med* 1993;153:509–14.

201. Tamai H et al. Treatment of methimazole-induced agranulocytosis using recombinant human granulocyte-colony-stimulating factor (rhG-CSF). *J Clin Endocrinol Metab* 1993;77:1356–60.

202. Dolman KM et al. Vasculitis and antineutrophil cytoplasmic autoantibodies associated with propylthiouracil therapy. *Lancet* 1993;342:651–2.

203. Arab DM et al. Severe cholestatic jaundice in uncomplicated hyperthyroidism treated with methimazole. *J Clin Endocrinol Metab* 1995;80:1083–5.

204. Biswas N et al. Aplastic anemia associated with antithyroid drugs. *Am J Med Sci* 1991;301:190–4.

205. Liaw YF et al. Hepatic injury during propylthiouracil therapy in patients with hyperthyroidism. *Ann Intern Med* 1993;118:424–8.

206. Cooper DS. Antithyroid drugs: to breast-feed or not to breast-feed. *Am J Obstet Gynecol* 1987;157:234–5.

207. Wing DA et al. A comparison of propylthiouracil versus methimazole in the treatment of hyperthyroidism in pregnancy. *Am J Obstet Gynecol* 1994;170:90–5.

208. Walter RM, Bartle WR. Rectal administration of propylthiouracil in the treatment of Graves' disease. *Am J Med* 1990;88:69–70.

209. Bartle WR et al. Rectal absorption of propylthiouracil. *Int J Clin Pharmacol Ther Toxicol* 1988;26:285–7.

210. Cooper DS et al. Acute effects of propylthiouracil (PTU) on thyroidal iodide organification and peripheral iodothyronine deiodination: correlation with serum PTU levels measured by radioimmunoassay. *J Clin Endocrinol Metab* 1982;54:101–7.

211. Levy M. Propylthiouracil hepatotoxicity. A review and case presentation. *Clin Pediatr (Phila)* 1993;32:25–9.

212. Morgan TR. Treatment of alcoholic hepatitis. *Semin Liver Dis* 1993;13:384–94.

Renal and Electrolytes

DIURETICS

Class Instructions: Diuretics. If you are taking more than one dose a day, take the last dose in the afternoon or early evening to avoid having to void urine during the night. Avoid highly salted foods, but rigid salt restriction is not necessary. Avoid excessive water intake. Report any dizziness or lightheadedness (especially upon arising from sitting or lying), muscle cramps, weakness, lethargy, dry mouth, thirst, or low urine output.

AMILORIDE HYDROCHLORIDE   Midamor, Various

Amiloride is a potassium-sparing diuretic with a mechanism and site of action resembling triamterene. It has mild antihypertensive activity and a longer duration of action than triamterene. Adverse reactions are generally similar to triamterene; however, in contrast to triamterene, renal stone formation has not been reported with amiloride. Dosage is 10 mg/day in 1–2 doses, to a maximum of 20 mg/day. It is available as 5-mg tablets, and also in Moduretic 5–50 and generic products that contain hydrochlorothiazide 50 mg and amiloride 5 mg.[1–3]

FUROSEMIDE   Lasix, Various

Pharmacology. Furosemide is actively secreted via the nonspecific organic acid transport system into the lumen of the thick ascending limb of Henle's loop, where it decreases sodium reabsorption by competing for the chloride site on the Na^+-K^+-$2Cl^-$ cotransporter. Medullary hypertonicity is diminished, thereby decreasing the kidney's ability to reabsorb water. Excretion of sodium, chloride, potassium, hydrogen ion, calcium, magnesium, ammonium, bicarbonate, and possibly phosphate is enhanced. IV furosemide increases venous capacitance independent of diuretic effect, producing rapid improvement in pulmonary edema.[2,3]

Administration and Adult Dosage. PO for edema 20–80 mg as a single dose initially; double successive doses q 6–8 hr until response is obtained. The maximum single dose depends on the disease state: 160 mg for hepatic insufficiency; 240 mg for nephrotic syndrome; 80 mg for CHF (with normal kidney function);[4] however, dosages up to 2500 mg/day have been recommended in refractory CHF.[5] After response, effective dosage is given in 1–3 doses daily; usual daily maintenance dosage depends on the single dose to which the patient responded. **PO for chronic renal failure** 80 mg initially, increasing in 80 mg/day increments until response is obtained, to a maximum of 240 mg[4] (*see* Special Populations). **PO for hypertension** 40 mg bid. **IV** should be used only when oral administration is not feasible. IV doses can be given over 1–2 min, except the rate should not exceed 4 mg/min when large doses are given. **IM or IV for edema** use one-half the dose of PO furosemide (as outlined above);[4] may double the dose q 2 or more hr until desired response is obtained. This dosage is then given in 1–2 doses daily for maintenance. Dosages up to 4 g/day IV have been used in refractory CHF.[5] **IV for acute pulmonary edema** 40 mg initially, may repeat in 30–60 min with 80 mg, if necessary (assuming relatively normal kidney function). For patients with renal impairment, the initial and subsequent doses must be adjusted based on renal function. For example, if Cl_{cr} is 50 mL/min (about one-half normal), the dose must be doubled; if Cl_{cr} is 25 mL/min, the dose must be quadrupled. **Continuous IV infusion for edema or chronic renal failure** 40 mg loading dose followed by 20–40 mg/hr.

Special Populations. *Pediatric Dosage.* **PO for edema** 2 mg/kg in 1 dose initially, increasing by 1–2 mg/kg in 6–8 hr, if necessary, to a maximum of 6 mg/kg/day. **IM or IV** 1 mg/kg in 1 dose initially, increasing by 1 mg/kg q 2 or more hr until desired response is obtained or to a maximum of 6 mg/kg/day. Maximum single dose depends on renal function. *See* Notes.

Geriatric Dosage. Start with a low initial dose and titrate to response.

Other Conditions. For Cl_{cr} <15 mL/min, maximal response is attained with single IV doses of 200 mg (400 mg PO). Hence, there appears to be no need to administer larger single doses to such patients.[4] A diminished response may occur in severe decompensated CHF, caused in part by alterations in oral absorption[6] and decreased renal blood flow (despite relatively normal GFR), resulting in decreased delivery of furosemide to the renal tubule; IV administration circumvents absorption problems. However, decompensated CHF usually affects only the rate, rather than the extent of oral furosemide absorption.[7] Additionally, high-dose therapy may be of benefit in severe, refractory CHF[6] (*see* Administration and Adult Dosage). For patients with cirrhosis, dosage is based on renal function.

Dosage Forms. **Soln** 8, 10 mg/mL; **Tab** 20, 40, 80 mg; **Inj** 10 mg/mL.

Patient Instructions. (*See* Diuretics Class Instructions.)

Pharmacokinetics. *Onset and Duration.* (Venous capacitance) IV onset 5 min, duration >1 hr. (Diuresis) PO onset 30–60 min, peak 1–2 hr, duration <6 hr; IV onset 15 min, peak 30–60 min, duration 1–2 hr; duration may be prolonged in severe renal impairment. (Hypertension) Maximum effect on BP may not occur for several days.

Serum Levels. Site of action is within the renal tubules and not the serum; therefore, serum concentrations do not reflect diuretic activity. Serum levels >25 mg/L may be associated with ototoxicity.[8]

Fate. Pharmacokinetics are variable and absorption is erratic; 61 ± 17% (range 20–100) is bioavailable in normals, 30–100% in renal failure.[8,9] The rate, but not the extent, of absorption may be decreased in patients with edematous bowel caused by decompensated CHF;[7] 96–99% is plasma protein bound, reduced in CHF, renal disease or cirrhosis.[9] $V_{d\beta}$ is 0.11 L/kg; Cl is 0.12 ± 0.24 L/hr/kg; both V_d and Cl depend on protein binding.[8,9] Two possible inactive metabolites exist: a glucuronide, which is primarily excreted in urine (and to a lesser extent in the feces by passive diffusion into the GI lumen), and saluamine, which may be a true metabolite or an analytical artifact. Renal clearance is primarily by active secretion; 50–80% (IV) and 20–55% (PO) is excreted unchanged in urine. Renal clearance is decreased in renal failure consistent with decreased renal blood flow, a reduction of functioning nephrons, and the presence of competitive inhibitors for secretion.[9]

$t_{1/2}$. 92 ± 7 (range 30–120) min in normals, may be extended in cirrhosis to 81 ± 8 min or CHF to 122 min, and markedly prolonged in end-stage renal disease to 9.7 hr, and in multiorgan failure to 20–24 hr. Mean residence time has been proposed as a more appropriate estimate of duration: 51.4 min (IV); 135–195 min (PO).[8,9]

Adverse Reactions. Dehydration, hypotension, hypochloremic alkalosis, and hypokalemia are frequent. Hyperglycemia and glucose intolerance occur as with thiazides (*see* Hydrochlorothiazide). With high-dosage therapy (>250 mg/day), hyperuricemia occurs frequently. Tinnitus and hearing loss, occasionally permanent, occur, frequently in association with rapid IV injection of large doses in patients with renal impairment.[5,9,10] Rarely, thrombocytopenia, neutropenia, jaundice, pancreatitis, and a variety of skin reactions occur.

Contraindications. Pregnancy; anuria (except for single dose in acute anuria).

Precautions. Use with caution in patients with severe or progressive renal disease; discontinue if renal function worsens. Use with caution in liver disease (may precipitate hepatic encephalopathy), history of diabetes mellitus or gout, and in patients allergic to other sulfonamide derivatives. Use with caution in patients with hypokalemia, hypomagnesemia, or hypocalcemia.

Drug Interactions. Cholestyramine decreases furosemide absorption, and NSAIDs may decrease the diuretic effect of furosemide. Aminoglycoside toxicity may be enhanced in renally impaired patients. IV furosemide may produce flushing, sweating, and blood pressure variations in patients taking chloral hydrate.

Parameters to Monitor. Monitor serum potassium closely, other electrolytes periodically, and serum glucose, uric acid, BUN, and Cr_s occasionally. Observe for clinical signs of fluid or electrolyte depletion such as dry mouth, thirst, weakness, lethargy, muscle pains or cramps, hypotension, oliguria, tachycardia, and GI upset.

Notes. Furosemide is light-sensitive; oral solution must be refrigerated and protected from light. In severe proteinuria (>3.5 g/day), urinary albumin binds furosemide and reduces its effectiveness.[7] In general, clinical nonresponders tend to have a decreased fraction of loop diuretics excreted in the urine. For these patients, and for patients with CHF and renal impairment, larger doses may force more drug into the tubule; however, the risk of ototoxicity must be considered. Alternatively, combined use with a **thiazide** or **metolazone** orally may be effective by blocking sodium reabsorption at multiple tubule sites; however, these agents (especially metolazone) have a slow onset of action. If a rapid response is needed, IV **acetazolamide** or **chlorothiazide** can be given followed by the loop diuretic.[3,4,11,12] Combination with theophylline can also enhance diuresis.[12] (*See* Loop Diuretics Comparison Chart.)

LOOP DIURETICS COMPARISON CHART

DRUG	DOSAGE FORMS	ADULT DOSAGE*	PEDIATRIC DOSAGE*	DOSAGE IN RENAL IMPAIRMENT	COMMENTS
Bumetanide Bumex Various	Tab 0.5, 1, 2 mg. Inj 0.25 mg/mL.	PO for edema 0.5–2 mg/day, to a maximum of 10 mg/day IM or IV over 2–3 min 0.5–1 mg, to a maximum of 10 mg/day IV continuous infusion 1 mg, then 1–2 mg/hr.	PO, IM, or IV 0.01–0.02 mg/kg, to a maximum of 0.4 mg/kg or 10 mg total daily dosage.	For Cl_{cr} <15 mL/min, maximal response is attained with single PO or IV doses of 8–10 mg. IV infusion of 12 mg over 12 hr may be more effective and less toxic.	1 mg PO or IV = 40 mg IV furosemide.
Ethacrynic Acid Edecrin	Tab 25, 50 mg. Inj 50 mg.	PO minimal dose in the range of 50–200 mg/day initially, to a maximum of 200 mg bid IV 50 mg or 0.5–1 mg/kg, to maximum of 100 mg.	PO (infants) not established; (children) 25 mg or 1 mg/kg initially, increased in 25-mg increments to desired effect. IV not established. 1 mg/kg has been used.	Not recommended with Cl_{cr} <10 mL/min; for Cl_{cr} of 10–50 mL/min, increase interval to q 8–12 hr.	Nonsulfonamide. Reliable potency data not available; however, 50 mg IV is about equal to furosemide 35 mg IV.
Furosemide Lasix Various	Tab 20, 40, 80 mg. Soln 8, 10 mg/mL. Inj 10 mg/mL.	See monograph.	See monograph.	Maximal response occurs with 200 mg IV or an average of 400 mg PO, although quite variable.	IV dose averages 50% of PO dose, with great variability.
Torsemide Demadex	Tab 5, 10, 20, 100 mg. Inj 10 mg/mL.	See monograph.	See monograph.	Maximal response occurs with PO or IV dose of 50–100 mg.	5–10 mg PO or IV = 20 mg IV furosemide.

*Higher doses needed for patients with CHF, liver cirrhosis, and nephrotic syndrome.

From references 5–7, 31, 32, and product information.

HYDROCHLOROTHIAZIDE
Esidrix, Hydrodiuril, Oretic, Various

Pharmacology. Thiazides increase sodium and chloride excretion by interfering with their reabsorption in the cortical diluting segment of the nephron; a mild diuresis of slightly concentrated urine results. Potassium, bicarbonate, magnesium, phosphate, and iodide excretion are also increased; calcium excretion is decreased. Although thiazides decrease extracellular fluid volume, antihypertensive activity is primarily caused by direct vasodilation. Urine output is paradoxically decreased in diabetes insipidus.[2,3]

Administration and Adult Dosage. PO for edema 25–200 mg/day in 1–3 doses initially; 25–100 mg/day or intermittently for maintenance, to a maximum of 200 mg/day. **PO for hypertension** 12.5–50 mg/day. Maintenance dosages >50 mg/day provide little additional benefit in controlling essential hypertension and may increase the frequency of dose-related biochemical abnormalities.[13]

Special Populations. *Pediatric Dosage.* PO (<6 months) may require up to 3.3 mg/kg/day in 2 divided doses; (>6 months) 2–2.2 mg/kg/day in 2 divided doses.

Geriatric Dosage. Start with a low initial dose and titrate to response.

Other Conditions. At a Cl_{cr} <30 mL/min, usual dosages of thiazides and most related drugs are not very effective as diuretics.[4]

Dosage Forms. **Tab** 25, 50, 100 mg; **Soln** 10, 100 mg/mL.

Patient Instructions. (*See* Diuretics Class Instructions.) If stomach upset occurs, take drug with meals. Report persistent anorexia, nausea, or vomiting.

Pharmacokinetics. *Onset and Duration.* Onset of diuresis within 2 hr; peak in 4–6 hr; duration 6–12 hr. Onset of hypotensive effect in 3–4 days; duration 1 week or less after discontinuing therapy.

Serum Levels. The site of action is within the renal tubules and not the serum; therefore, serum concentrations do not reflect diuretic activity.

Fate. Oral bioavailability is 71 ± 15% in healthy individuals, increased when given with an anticholinergic, and decreased by one-half in CHF and after intestinal shunt surgery. There are no differences in absorption among single-entity formulations. The drug is 58 ± 17% plasma protein bound; V_d is 0.83 ± 0.31 L/kg; Cl is 0.29 ± 0.07 L/hr/kg. Over 95% is excreted unchanged in urine by filtration and secretion. In severe renal impairment, renal clearance is prolonged fivefold, with nonrenal clearance (mechanism as yet unidentified) playing an increased role in elimination.[8,14]

$t_{1/2}$. 2.5 ± 2 hr; prolonged in uncompensated CHF or renal impairment.[8,14,15]

Adverse Reactions. Hypokalemia is frequent; however, its treatment in otherwise healthy hypertensive patients is usually unnecessary. Potassium supplements or potassium-sparing diuretics (*see* Notes) may be indicated in patients with arrhythmias, MI, or severe ischemic heart disease; those with chronic liver disease; elderly eating a poor diet; patients taking digoxin, a corticosteroid, or drugs that interfere with ventricular repolarization such as phenothiazines and heterocyclic antidepressants; and those whose serum potassium falls below 3 mEq/L. Hyperuricemia occurs frequently but is reversible, and treatment is unnecessary unless the patient has renal impairment or a history of gout.[16] Hyperglycemia and alterations in glucose tolerance (usually reversible), loss of diabetic control, or precipitation of diabetes mellitus occur occasionally. Decreased glucose tolerance may increase in prevalence after several years of therapy.[17,18] Thrombocytopenia and pancreatitis occur rarely. Elevation of serum cholesterol and triglycerides occurs; the clinical importance is unknown, but it may increase the risk of coronary heart disease.

Contraindications. Anuria; pregnancy, unless accompanied by severe edema; allergy to sulfonamide derivatives.

Precautions. Use with caution in patients with renal function impairment, liver disease (may precipitate hepatic encephalopathy), history of diabetes mellitus, or gout. Use with caution in patients with diabetes mellitus, because thiazides may increase glucose intolerance.[17,18]

Drug Interactions. Cholestyramine decreases oral absorption of thiazides, and NSAIDs may decrease the diuretic effect of thiazides. Anticholinergics may increase oral bioavailability. Dosage of potent hypotensive agents may have to be reduced if a thiazide is added to the regimen. Concurrent calcium-containing antacids may cause hypercalcemia. Long-term thiazides may reduce lithium excretion.

Parameters to Monitor. Monitor serum potassium weekly to monthly initially; q 3–6 months when stable. Monitor other serum electrolytes periodically. Monitor all electrolytes more closely when other losses occur (eg, vomiting, diarrhea). Observe for clinical signs of fluid or electrolyte depletion such as dry mouth, thirst, weakness, lethargy, muscle pains or cramps, hypotension, oliguria, tachycardia, and GI upset. Monitor blood pressure periodically during antihypertensive therapy and serum glucose in patients with diabetes mellitus.

Notes. For the prevention of hypokalemia during thiazide therapy, a potassium-sparing diuretic may be preferred over potassium supplements in alkalotic patients, because these agents decrease hydrogen ion loss, which can correct alkalosis and drive more potassium extracellularly.[19] Potassium-sparing diuretics may also be preferred for patients predisposed to hypomagnesemia and for those with serum potassium <3 mEq/L, because potassium supplements rarely correct hypokalemia of this severity. (*See* Thiazides and Related Drugs Comparison Chart.)

THIAZIDES AND RELATED DIURETICS COMPARISON CHART[a]

DRUG	DOSAGE FORMS	ORAL DIURETIC DOSAGE RANGE (MG/DAY)	EQUIVALENT DIURETIC DOSAGE (MG)	PEAK EFFECT (HR)	DURATION OF DIURESIS (HR)
Bendroflumethiazide Naturetin	Tab 5, 10 mg.	2.5–15	5	4	6–12
Benzthiazide Exna Various	Tab 50 mg.	50–150	50	4–6	12–18
Chlorothiazide Diuril Various	Tab 250, 500 mg Susp 50 mg/mL Inj 500 mg.[b]	500–2000	500	2 (PO) 0.5 (IV)	6–12 (PO) 2 (IV)
Chlorthalidone[c] Hygroton Thalitone Various	Tab (Thalitone)[d] 15, 25 mg Tab 25, 50, 100 mg.	15–200	50	2	24–72
Hydrochlorothiazide Various	Tab 25, 50, 100 mg Soln 10, 100 mg/mL.	25–100	50	4–6	6–12
Hydroflumethiazide Diucardin Saluron Various	Tab 50 mg.	25–100	50	3–4	12–24
Indapamide[c] Lozol	Tab 1.25, 2.5 mg.	1.25–5	2.5	2	24–36

THIAZIDES AND RELATED DIURETICS COMPARISON CHART[a] (continued)

DRUG	DOSAGE FORMS	ORAL DIURETIC DOSAGE RANGE (MG/DAY)	EQUIVALENT DIURETIC DOSAGE (MG)	PEAK EFFECT (HR)	DURATION OF DIURESIS (HR)
Methyclothiazide Aquatensin Enduron Various	Tab 2.5, 5 mg.	2.5–10	5	6	24
Metolazone[c] Mykrox Zaroxolyn	Tab (Mykrox)[d] 0.5 mg. Tab 2.5, 5, 10 mg.	5–20 0.5–1 (Mykrox)	5 (Zaroxolyn)	2	12–24
Polythiazide Renese	Tab 1, 2, 4 mg.	1–4	2	6	24–48
Quinethazone[c] Hydromox	Tab 50 mg.	50–200	50	6	18–24
Trichlormethiazide Metahydrin Naqua	Tab 2, 4 mg.	2–4	2	6	24

[a]From USP-DI and product information; patients unresponsive to maximal dosage of one agent are unlikely to respond to another agent.
[b]There is no therapeutic advantage in giving the drug parenterally.
[c]Not a thiazide, but similar in structure and mechanism of action.
[d]Thalitone and Mykrox are more bioavailable than other formulations of the respective drugs.

MANNITOL
Osmitrol, Various

Pharmacology. Mannitol and other osmotic diuretics do not act on specific receptors, but rather on tubular fluid composition by distributing into extracellular fluid. Mannitol inhibits sodium and chloride reabsorption in the proximal tubule and ascending loop of Henle. Sodium, potassium, calcium, and phosphate excretion is increased. Renal blood flow is increased, the GFR of superficial nephrons is increased, and that of deep nephrons is decreased.[20] Mannitol increases serum osmolality, expanding intravascular volume and decreasing intraocular and intracranial pressures.[2,20]

Administration and Adult Dosage. *Never administer IM or SC, or add to whole blood for transfusion.* **IV as diagnostic evaluation of acute oliguria** (if blood pressure and CVP are normal and *after* cardiac output is maximized) give test dose of 12.5 g as a 15–20% solution over 3–5 min (often given with furosemide 80–120 mg IV), may repeat in 1 hr if urine output is less than 30–50 mL/hr. If no response after 2 doses, give no more mannitol and treat for acute tubular necrosis. If response occurs, look for underlying cause of oliguria (eg, hypovolemia). **IV for prevention of acute renal failure** give test dose as above to a total dose of 50 g or more in 1 hr as a loading dose, then maintain urine output at 50 mL/hr with continuous infusion of 5% solution, plus 20 mEq/L sodium chloride and 1 g/L calcium gluconate. **IV for reduction of intracranial or intraocular pressure** 1.5–2 g/kg over 30–60 min as a 15–25% solution. **IV to decrease nephrotoxicity of cisplatin** 12.5 g IV push just prior to cisplatin, then 10 g/hr for 6 hr as a 20% solution. Replace fluids with 0.45% sodium chloride with 20–30 mEq/L potassium chloride at 250 mL/hr for 6 hr. Maintain urine output >100 mL/hr with mannitol infusion.[21] (*See* Notes.)

Special Populations. *Pediatric Dosage.* **IV for oliguria or anuria** give test dose of 200 mg/kg as above; the therapeutic dose is 2 g/kg over 2–6 hr as a 15–20% solution. **IV for reduction of intracranial or intraocular pressure** 2 g/kg over 30–60 min as a 15–25% solution. **IV for intoxications** 2 g/kg as 5–10% solution as needed to maintain a high urinary output. (*See* Notes.)

Geriatric Dosage. Start with a low initial dose and titrate to response.

Dosage Forms. **Inj** 5, 10, 15, 20, 25%.

Pharmacokinetics. *Onset and Duration.* (Diuresis) onset 1–3 hr, duration depends on half-life. (Decrease in intraocular pressure) onset in 30–60 min duration 4–6 hr. (Decrease in intracranial pressure) onset within 15 min, peak 60–90 min duration 3–8 hr after stopping infusion.[22]

Serum Levels. The site of action is within the renal tubules and not the serum; therefore, serum concentrations do not reflect diuretic activity.

Fate. About 17% is absorbed orally. IV doses of 1 g/kg and 2 g/kg increase serum osmolality by 11 and 32 mOsm/kg, decrease serum sodium by 8.7 and 20.7 mEq/L, and decrease hemoglobin by 2.2 and 2.5 g/dL, respectively.[23] V_c is 0.074 L/kg; $V_{d\beta}$ is 0.23 L/kg; Cl is 0.086 L/hr/kg.[24] Mannitol is virtually completely eliminated unchanged in urine.

$t_{1/2}$. α phase 0.11 ± 0.12 hr; β phase 2.2 ± 1.3 hr.[24]

Adverse Reactions. Most serious and frequent are fluid and electrolyte imbalance, particularly symptoms of fluid overload such as pulmonary edema, hypertension, water intoxication, and CHF. Acute renal failure has been reported occasionally with high doses, especially in patients with renal impairment.[25,26] Dermal necrosis can occur if solution extravasates. Anaphylaxis has been reported rarely.

Contraindications. Patients with well-established anuria caused by severe renal disease or impaired renal function who do not respond to test dose; severe pulmonary congestion, frank pulmonary edema or severe CHF; severe dehydration; edema not caused by renal, cardiac, or hepatic disease that is associated with abnormal capillary fragility or membrane permeability; active intracranial bleeding, except during craniotomy.

Precautions. Pregnancy. Observe solution for crystals before administering (*see* Notes). Water intoxication may occur if fluid input exceeds urine output. Masking of inadequate hydration or hypovolemia may occur by drug-induced sustaining of diuresis. If extravasation occurs, aspirate any accessible extravasated solution, then remove the IV catheter and apply a cold compress to the area.

Drug Interactions. None known.

Parameters to Monitor. Monitor urine output closely and discontinue drug if output is low. Monitor serum electrolytes closely, taking care not to misinterpret low serum sodium as a sign of hypotonicity (*see* Fate). If serum sodium is low, measure serum osmolality. Observe for clinical signs of fluid or electrolyte depletion such as dry mouth, thirst, weakness, lethargy, muscle pains or cramps, hypotension, oliguria, tachycardia, and GI upset.

Notes. Mannitol may crystallize out of solution at concentrations above 15%. The crystals may be redissolved by warming in hot water and shaking or by autoclaving; cool to body temperature before administration. Administer solutions of 20% or greater through an inline filter. Addition of electrolytes to solutions of 20% or greater concentration may cause precipitation.

SPIRONOLACTONE   Aldactone, Various

Pharmacology. Spironolactone is a steroidal competitive aldosterone antagonist that acts from the interstitial side of the distal and collecting tubular epithelium to block sodium-potassium exchange, producing a delayed and mild diuresis. The diuretic effect is maximal in states of hyperaldosteronism. Sodium, chloride, and calcium excretion is increased; potassium and magnesium excretion is decreased. Spironolactone has mild antihypertensive activity and has a direct positive inotropic action on the heart.[27–29]

Administration and Adult Dosage. **PO for edema** 25–200 mg/day (usually 100 mg) in 2–4 divided doses initially, adjusting dosage after 5 days. If response is inadequate, add a thiazide or loop diuretic to the regimen. **PO for essential hypertension** 50–100 mg/day initially, adjusting dosage after 2 weeks. **PO for ascites** 100 mg/day initially, increasing to 200–400 mg/day in 2–4 divided doses. Restrict sodium to 2 g/day or less and, if necessary, fluid to 1 L/day. To eliminate delay in onset, a loading dose of 2–3 times the daily dosage may be given on the first day of therapy.[30]

Special Populations. *Pediatric Dosage.* **PO** 3.3 mg/kg/day, readjust dosage after 5 days; dosage may be increased up to triple this value. Restrict duration of therapy to 1 month.

Geriatric Dosage. Start with a low initial dose and titrate to response.

Dosage Forms. Tab 25, 50, 100 mg; **Tab** 25 mg with hydrochlorothiazide 25 mg (Aldactazide, various); **Tab** 50 mg with hydrochlorothiazide 50 mg (Aldactazide 50/50).

Patient Instructions. (*See* Diuretics Class Instructions.) Avoid excessive amounts of high-potassium foods or salt substitutes.

Pharmacokinetics. *Onset and Duration.* Onset gradual, peak 2–3 days with continued administration; onset can be hastened by giving loading dose; duration 2–3 days after cessation of therapy.

Serum Levels. Not established and not used clinically.

Fate. Bioavailability is about 90%;[27] food promotes absorption and possibly decreases first-pass effect.[31] Spironolactone undergoes rapid and extensive metabolism to canrenone (active metabolite), 7α-thiomethylspirolactone (major metabolite), and other sulfur-containing metabolites; together with the parent drug, these metabolites contribute to the overall antimineralocorticoid activity.[27,32] Metabolites are primarily eliminated renally, with minimal biliary excretion. Little or no parent drug is excreted unchanged in urine.[32,33]

$t_{1/2}$. (Spironolactone) 1.4 ± 0.5 hr; (7α-thiomethylspirolactone) 13.8 ± 6.4 hr; (canrenone) 16.5 ± 6.3 hr.[32]

Adverse Reactions. Hyperkalemia may occur, most frequently in patients with renal function impairment (especially those with diabetes mellitus) and those receiving potassium supplements or concomitant ACE inhibitors. Dehydration and hyponatremia occur occasionally, especially when the drug is combined with other diuretics. In patients receiving high dosages, frequent estrogenlike side effects including gynecomastia, decreased libido, and impotence in males occur; menstrual irregularities and breast tenderness occur in females. These effects are reversible after drug discontinuation.[34]

Contraindications. Anuria; acute renal insufficiency; rapidly deteriorating renal function; severe renal failure; serum potassium >5.5 mEq/L or development of hyperkalemia while taking the drug; hypermagnesemia.

Precautions. Pregnancy. Patients with renal impairment, especially those with diabetes mellitus and/or receiving an ACE inhibitor, are at risk for developing hyperkalemia. Use with caution in patients with hepatic disease. Do not use with triamterene or amiloride. Give potassium supplements only to patients with demonstrated hypokalemia who are taking a proximally acting diuretic and a corticosteroid concurrently with spironolactone or only for very short periods in treating cirrhosis and ascites.

Drug Interactions. Use with ACE inhibitors increases risk of hyperkalemia, especially in renal impairment. Spironolactone increases serum concentration of digoxin by reducing renal and possibly nonrenal clearance. Additionally, spironolactone and its metabolites may cross-react with digoxin-binding antibody in some digoxin immunoassays.

Parameters to Monitor. Monitor serum electrolytes, particularly potassium, periodically, especially early in the course of therapy. Monitor BUN and/or Cr_s periodically. In ascites, also obtain daily weight and urinary electrolytes, maintaining weight loss at no greater than 0.5–1 kg/day and urinary Na$^+$/K$^+$ ratio at greater than 1. Observe for clinical signs of fluid or electrolyte depletion such as dry mouth, thirst, weakness, lethargy, muscle pains or cramps, hypotension, oliguria, tachycardia, and GI upset.

Notes. Spironolactone is useful in patients with diabetes mellitus (with good renal function) or gout because it causes no impairment of glucose tolerance and minimal hyperuricemia. It is used in the diagnosis of primary aldosteronism and may be used in the management of the condition in patients unable to undergo surgery.

TORSEMIDE   Demadex

Torsemide is a loop diuretic similar to furosemide. Over the normal dosage range, its diuretic potency by weight is about 2–4 times that of furosemide. Onset of diuresis is similar; however, duration is longer (up to 8–12 hr orally). Oral bioavailability is 79–91% (median 80); V_d is 0.14–0.19 L/kg. In healthy individuals, the elimination half-life of torsemide is dose dependent, ranging from 2.2–3.8 hr. Nonrenal Cl remains essentially constant over a dosage range of 5–20 mg, but renal Cl and fraction excreted decrease, suggesting saturable renal clearance. Further studies are needed to clarify whether torsemide undergoes dose-dependent renal elimination. Renal impairment (Cl$_{cr}$ ≤60 mL/min) does not appreciably alter pharmacokinetic parameters; hemodialysis and hemofiltration do not markedly influence serum clearance. Although the potential for hypokalemia exists, torsemide's kaliuretic potency is less than that of furosemide, suggesting that it may be less potassium wasting during long-term therapy; however, the clinical relevance of this observation is unknown. Precautions and monitoring parameters are the same as for furosemide. Dosage for hypertension is 5–10 mg/day orally. Initial PO or IV dosage for edema or chronic renal failure is 20 mg/day; the dosage can be doubled until the desired response is obtained, to a usual maximum of 200 mg/day; or, IV by continuous infusion, give 20 mg loading dose, then 10–20 mg/hr. Initial PO or IV dosage for cirrhosis is 5–10 mg/day with a potassium-sparing diuretic, to a usual maximum of 40 mg/day.[35–38] Available as 5-, 10-, 20- and 100-mg tablets and 10 mg/mL injection. (*See* Furosemide Notes and Loop Diuretics Comparison Chart.)

TRIAMTERENE   Dyrenium

Pharmacology. Triamterene acts directly from the distal tubular lumen on active sodium exchange for potassium and hydrogen, producing a mild diuresis that is independent of aldosterone concentration. Sodium, chloride, calcium, and possibly bicarbonate excretion is increased; potassium and possibly magnesium excretion is decreased. Antihypertensive activity is inconsistent and less pronounced than with thiazides or spironolactone.[28,29]

Administration and Adult Dosage. PO initially 100 mg bid after meals if used alone; lower dosage if used with another diuretic. Adjust the maintenance dosage to the needs of the patient; it may range from 100 mg/day to 100 mg every other day, to a maximum of 300 mg/day.

Special Populations. *Pediatric Dosage.* **PO** 2–4 mg/kg/day initially, may increase to 6 mg/kg/day in 1–2 doses after meals, to a maximum of 300 mg/day. Decrease dosage if used with another diuretic.

Geriatric Dosage. Start with a low initial dose and titrate to response.

Dosage Forms. **Cap** 50, 100 mg; **Cap** 50 mg with hydrochlorothiazide 25 mg (Dyazide, various); **Tab** 75 mg with hydrochlorothiazide 50 mg (Maxzide, various); 37.5 mg with hydrochlorothiazide 25 mg (Maxzide-25, various).

Patient Instructions. (*See* Diuretics Class Instructions.) This drug may be taken with food or milk to minimize stomach upset. Report persistent loss of appetite, nausea, or vomiting. Avoid eating excessive amounts of high-potassium foods or salt substitutes.

Pharmacokinetics. *Onset and Duration.* Onset 2–4 hr; full therapeutic effect may not occur for several days; duration 7–9 hr.

Serum Levels. The site of action is within the renal tubules and not the serum; therefore, serum concentrations do not reflect diuretic activity.

Fate. Variable absorption, depending on formulation;[39,40] bioavailability is 52 ± 22%.[40] When the total urinary excretion of triamterene and its pharmacologically active metabolite is considered, the bioavailability value of triamterene reaches 83.2 ± 25.9%.[40] Triamterene undergoes marked first-pass metabolism with rapid hydroxylation followed by immediate conjugation to the sulfate ester, which is the predominant form in plasma and urine.[40] The sulfate conjugate is nearly equipotent with the parent in causing sodium excretion and sparing of potassium.[41,42] Triamterene is 50–55% plasma protein bound,[28,29] and its sulfate conjugate is 91% protein bound.[40] After oral administration, serum concentrations of both triamterene and its sulfate conjugate undergo a rapid decline over the first 6–8 hr after administration, followed by a slower terminal phase.[41] Both are eliminated renally by filtration and secretion. The fraction of a dose excreted as the parent is 3 ± 2%; that for the sulfate conjugate is 34 ± 8%.[41] The sulfate conjugate may accumulate in renal impairment.[42]

$t_{1/2}$. β phase (healthy adults) 4.3 ± 0.7 hr for triamterene and 3.1 ± 1.2 hr for sulfate;[40] up to 12 hr in cirrhosis.[43] Half-lives may also be prolonged in the elderly.[44]

Adverse Reactions. Nausea, vomiting, diarrhea, and dizziness occur occasionally. Dehydration and hyponatremia with an increase in BUN occur occasionally, especially when the drug is combined with other diuretics. Triamterene renal stones occur occasionally. Hyperkalemia occurs occasionally, especially in diabetics and in patients with renal impairment; metabolic acidosis has been reported. Megaloblastic anemia can occur in alcoholic cirrhosis.

Contraindications. Severe or progressive renal disease or dysfunction (except possibly nephrosis); severe renal failure; severe hepatic disease; serum potassium >5.5 mEq/L or development of hyperkalemia while taking the drug; hypermagnesemia.

Precautions. Pregnancy. Patients with renal impairment, especially those with diabetes mellitus and/or receiving an ACE inhibitor, are at risk for developing hyperkalemia. May cause elevation in serum uric acid in patients predisposed to gout. Do not use with spironolactone or amiloride.

Drug Interactions. Use with ACE inhibitors increases risk of hyperkalemia, especially in renal impairment. Indomethacin (and probably other NSAIDs) may reduce renal function when combined with triamterene.

Parameters to Monitor. Monitor serum electrolytes, particularly potassium, periodically, especially early in the course of therapy. Monitor BUN and/or Cr_s periodically. Observe for clinical signs of fluid or electrolyte depletion such as dry mouth, thirst, weakness, lethargy, muscle pains or cramps, hypotension, oliguria, tachycardia, and GI upset.

DIURETICS OF CHOICE COMPARISON CHART*

CONDITION	LOOP DIURETICS	OSMOTIC DIURETICS	THIAZIDES	POTASSIUM-SPARING AGENTS	COMMENTS
Relative Potency	>15%	10–15%	5–10%	<5%	Values refer to maximum fraction of filtered sodium excreted following maximally effective dose of drug.
Hypertension	A	—	A	D	Sustained antihypertensive effect of thiazides exhibits a flat dose-response curve and occurs at doses below the threshold for diuresis. Loop diuretics are diuretics of choice with Cl_{cr} <30 mL/min.
Congestive Heart Failure	A	—	A	D	Begin with thiazide with low dosage; if ineffective, substitute a loop diuretic. Loop diuretics are diuretics of choice with Cl_{cr} <30 mL/min. A loop diuretic plus a thiazide (in a high dose) can evoke a clinically useful diuresis even when Cl_{cr} <15 mL/min.
Pulmonary Edema	A (IV)	—	—	—	Prompt venodilation precedes diuretic effect.
Hepatic Ascites	B	—	—	A	Spironolactone is the agent of choice; urine Na:K ratio <1 indicates need for higher dosage (200–1000 mg/day). Rate of diuresis should not exceed 750 mL/day (no peripheral edema), or up to 2 L/day (if edema is present).

DIURETICS OF CHOICE COMPARISON CHART* (continued)

CONDITION	LOOP DIURETICS	OSMOTIC DIURETICS	THIAZIDES	POTASSIUM-SPARING AGENTS	COMMENTS
Renal Failure	A	C	—	—	A loop diuretic plus a thiazide (in a high dose) can evoke a clinically useful diuresis even when Cl_{cr} <15 mL/min; however, provocative diuretic challenges in oliguric patients can be potentially hazardous, especially if the cause of renal failure is uncertain.
Diabetes Insipidus	—	—	A	—	Thiazides are most useful in the nephrogenic form; a long-acting agent is preferred. In pituitary form, oral diuretics may be a useful alternative for patients who prefer oral therapy to the use of intranasal or IV desmopressin.
Hypercalcemia	A	—	—	—	High-dose furosemide (IV 80–100 mg q 1–2 hr) with IV saline for forced diuresis to promote calcium excretion.
Hypercalciuria	—	—	A	—	Thiazides cause marked reduction in urinary calcium excretion; they also appear effective in preventing calcium stone formation irrespective of whether urinary calcium is abnormally elevated.

A = Diuretic of choice; B = diuretic of second choice if patient unresponsive to first choice; C = useful in some circumstances; D = useful as an adjunct to a more potent diuretic to reduce potassium loss and possibly enhance therapeutic effect.

*This table is a guide to the selection of the most appropriate diuretic for the condition listed, but is not an all-inclusive guide to therapy.

From references 28, 29, and 45–47.

Electrolytes

Class Instructions: Oral Electrolytes. Take oral products (tablets) with or (liquids and powders) diluted in 6–8 fl oz of water or juice to avoid GI injury or laxative effect. This medication may be taken with food or after meals if upset stomach occurs.

CALCIUM SALTS   Various

Pharmacology. Calcium plays an important role in neuromuscular activity, pancreatic insulin release, gastric hydrogen secretion, blood coagulation, and platelet aggregation; as a cofactor for some enzyme reactions; and in bone and tooth metabolism.[48]

Administration and Adult Dosage. PO as dietary supplement (elemental calcium) 500–2000 mg bid–qid; RDA 800 mg/day;[49] for mature women, 1 g/day before menopause and 1.5 g/day thereafter has been recommended.[50] **PO to lower serum phosphate in ESRD** (calcium carbonate) 650 mg with each meal initially, adjust dosage to decrease serum phosphate to less than 6 mg/dL,[51] most patients require more than 1.3 g with each meal; (calcium acetate) 1334 mg with each meal initially, adjust dosage to decrease serum phosphate to less than 6 mg/dL (*see* Notes). **IV for emergency elevation of serum calcium** (calcium gluconate) 15 mg/kg in NS or D5W infused over 8–10 hr (typically raises serum calcium by 2–3 mg/dL),[52] may repeat q 1–3 days depending on response; (calcium gluceptate) 1.1–1.4 g infused at a rate not to exceed 36 mg/min of elemental calcium. **IV for hypocalcemic tetany** 10–20 mL calcium gluconate infused over 10 min, may repeat until tetany is controlled. *Faster IV infusion rates may result in cardiac dysfunction.*[52]

Special Populations. *Pediatric Dosage*. PO as dietary supplement (elemental calcium) RDA (<6 months) 400 mg/day; (6 months–1 yr) 600 mg/day; (1–10 yr) 800 mg/day; (11–18 yr) 1200 mg/day.[49] **PO for hypocalcemia** (elemental calcium) (neonates) 50–150 mg/kg/day in 4–6 divided doses, to a maximum of 1 g/day; (children) 20–65 mg/kg/day in 4 divided doses. **IV for emergency elevation of serum calcium** (infants) <1 mEq, may repeat q 1–3 days depending on response; (children) 1–7 mEq, may repeat q 1–3 days depending on response. **IV for hypocalcemic tetany** (infants) 2.4 mEq/day in divided doses; (children) 0.5–0.7 mEq/kg tid–qid, or more until tetany controlled.

Geriatric Dosage. Postmenopausal women may have a requirement of 1.5 g/day.[49] Lower dosage may be required in some patients because of the age-related decrease in renal function; however, requirements may increase with advanced renal insufficiency.

Other Conditions. Adolescence, renal impairment, and pregnancy may increase requirements; base maintenance dosage on serum calcium, serum phosphate, and diet.[49]

Dosage Forms. (*See* Oral Calcium Products Comparison Chart.) **Inj** (chloride) 1 g/10 mL (contains 273 mg or 13.6 mEq Ca); (gluconate) 1 g/10 mL (contains 93 mg or 4.65 mEq Ca); (gluceptate) 1.1 g/5 mL (contains 90 mg or 4.5 mEq Ca).

Patient Instructions. (*See* Oral Electrolytes Class Instructions.) Do not take within 2 hours of oral tetracycline or fluoroquinolone products. Take calcium tablets with food to maximize absorption. If used as a phosphate binder, calcium must be taken with food. Allow effervescent tablets to degas in a glass of water (about 4 minutes) before taking.

Pharmacokinetics. *Serum Levels.* Normal serum total calcium is 8.4–10.2 mg/dL (2.1–2.6 mmol/L) for an adult with a serum albumin of 4 g/dL. Because a lesser fraction of calcium is protein bound in hypoalbuminemia, the patient's value must be corrected based on serum albumin:

Corrected Serum Ca = Measured Serum Ca + 0.8 × (4 − Serum Albumin).

Fate. Oral calcium absorption is about 30% and depends on vitamin D and parathyroid hormone. Absorption decreases with age, high intake, achlorhydria, and estrogen loss at menopause;[49] absorption increases when taken with food[50,53] or in divided doses.[54] Bioavailability from various salt forms does not appear to differ substantially in normals;[55] however, differences in disintegration and dissolution among commercial formulations exist.[51,53] About 99% of total body calcium is found in bone; of the 1% in extracellular fluid, 40% is plasma protein bound (mostly to albumin); 9% is complexed to citrate, phosphate, and other anions; and 50% is diffusible and physiologically active. About 135–155 mg/day are secreted into the GI tract, with 85% reabsorbed. Fecal loss of unabsorbed dietary calcium and endogenous excretion is 100–130 mg/day, urine loss is 150 mg/day, and sweat loss is 15 mg/day.[54]

Adverse Reactions. IV calcium solutions, especially calcium chloride, are extremely irritating to the veins.[52] Constipation or flatulence occurs frequently, especially with high dosages; the frequency probably does not differ markedly among salt forms.[50] Calcium overload caused by oral calcium supplements is rare; immobilization, dosages in excess of 3–4 g/day, vitamin D therapy, and renal impairment may contribute to hypercalcemia, hypercalciuria, or nephrolithiasis during oral supplementation. Symptoms of hypercalcemia include nausea, vomiting, constipation, abdominal pain, dry mouth, and polyuria.

Contraindications. Hypercalcemia; sarcoidosis; severe cardiac disease; digitalis glycoside therapy; calcium nephrolithiasis; calcium-phosphate product greater than 70 (to determine calcium-phosphate product, multiply serum phosphate value [in mg/dL] by serum calcium value [in mg/dL]).

Precautions. Avoid extravasation of parenteral calcium products. If extravasation occurs, aspirate any accessible extravasated solution, then remove IV catheter and apply a cold compress to the area.

Drug Interactions. Concomitant thiazide diuretic therapy and sodium depletion or metabolic acidosis may increase tubular reabsorption of calcium. Calcium reduces oral absorption of fluoroquinolones, tetracyclines, and iron salts.

Parameters to Monitor. Serum calcium regularly, with frequency determined by patient's condition; BUN and/or Cr_s, serum phosphate, magnesium, and serum albumin (especially if low) periodically.

Notes. Calcium supplementation can also be achieved by dietary measures: skim milk provides 300 mg calcium/250 mL; cheese 300–400 mg calcium/28 g; and yogurt 43 mg calcium/28 g.[50] Calcium carbonate is inexpensive and a good first-line agent. However, dissolution of calcium from phosphate and carbonate salts is pH dependent. These salts may not be optimal calcium sources for patients with elevated GI pH, such as the elderly or those with achlorhydria. Calcium carbonate as a chewable tablet or nougat or the use of an alternative calcium salt have been recommended.[53] In ESRD, use calcium salts when serum phosphate is <8 mg/dL; when serum phosphate is >8 mg/dL, use aluminum hydroxide. Calcium acetate binds about twice the amount of phosphorus for the same quantity of calcium absorbed; however, the frequency of hypercalcemia does not seem to be diminished. (*See* Oral Calcium Products Comparison Chart.)

ORAL CALCIUM PRODUCTS COMPARISON CHART

PRODUCT	PERCENTAGE CALCIUM	ELEMENTAL CALCIUM CONTENT
Calcium Acetate	25	250 mg Tab = 62.5 mg
PhosEx		500 mg Tab = 125 mg
PhosLo		667 mg Tab = 169 mg
		1000 mg Tab = 250 mg
Calcium Carbonate	40	5 mL Susp = 500 mg
Calciday-667		650 mg Tab = 260 mg
Cal-Sup		667 mg Tab = 267 mg
Caltrate 600		750 mg Tab = 300 mg
Os-Cal		1250 mg Tab = 500 mg
Titralac		1500 mg Tab = 600 mg
Tums		
Calcium Citrate	21.1	950 mg Tab = 200 mg
Citracal		2376 mg Tab = 500 mg
Calcium Glubionate	6.5	5 mL Syrup = 115 mg
Neo-Calglucon		
Calcium Gluconate	9	500 mg Tab = 45 mg
Various		650 mg Tab = 58.5 mg
		975 mg Tab = 87.8 mg
		1000 mg Tab = 90 mg
Calcium Lactate	13	325 mg Tab = 42.3 mg
Various		650 mg Tab = 84.5 mg
Calcium Phosphate, Tribasic	39	1565 mg Tab = 600 mg
Posture		
Dairy Products	—	Cheese 28 g = 300–400 mg
		Skim Milk 250 mL = 300 mg
		Yogurt 28 g = 43 mg

From references 49–52 and product information.

MAGNESIUM SALTS   Various

Pharmacology. Magnesium is the second most abundant intracellular cation, with an essential role in neuromuscular function and protein and carbohydrate enzymatic systems; it functions as a cofactor for enzymes involved in transfer, storage, and utilization of intracellular energy. Magnesium is also an integral component of bone matrix.[56]

Administration and Adult Dosage. **PO as dietary supplement** (elemental magnesium) 20–130 mg daily–bid.[57] **PO for chronic deficiency** (elemental magnesium) 12–24 mg/kg in divided doses.[58] **IV for prevention of negative balance** (elemental magnesium) 100–200 mg/day in parenteral nutrition solution.[58] **IM for mild deficiency** 1 g $MgSO_4$ q 4–6 hr until serum magnesium is normalized or signs and symptoms abate;[58] **IM for severe hypomagnesemia** 2 g $MgSO_4$ as a 50% solution q 8 hr until serum magnesium is normalized or signs and symptoms abate; because IM injections are painful, continuous IV infusions may be preferred.[59] **IV infusion for severe hypomagnesemia** 48 mEq/day (6 g $MgSO_4$) for 3–7 days by continuous infusion.[59] **IV for life-threatening hypomagnesemia (acute arrhythmias and seizures)** 8–16 mEq (1–2 g $MgSO_4$) over 5–10 min, followed by continuous infusion of 48 mEq magnesium/day.[59] **IV for preeclampsia or eclampsia** 4-6 g $MgSO_4$, then 1–2 g/hr by continuous infusion to maintain target serum levels. (*See* Notes.)

Special Populations. *Pediatric Dosage.* **IV for hypomagnesemia** 25 mg/kg $MgSO_4$ as a 25% solution over 3–5 min q 6 hr for 3–4 doses. **IM for seizures** 20–40 mg/kg $MgSO_4$ as a 20% solution as needed. **IV for severe seizures** 100–200 mg/kg $MgSO_4$ as a 1–3% solution infused slowly with close monitoring of blood pressure. Administer one-half the dose during the initial 15–20 min and the total dose within 1 hr.

Geriatric Dosage. Lower dosage may be required in some patients because of the age-related decrease in renal function. Magnesium accumulates in advanced renal insufficiency.

Other Conditions. Base maintenance dosage on serum magnesium and diet. Renal impairment decreases requirement. In severe renal failure, reduce dosage by at least 50% of recommended amount and monitor serum magnesium after each dose.[60] Concomitant administration of potassium and calcium may be necessary, because many causes of hypomagnesemia also lead to hypocalcemia and hypokalemia.[58]

Dosage Forms. (*See* Magnesium Products Comparison Chart.)

Patient Instructions. (*See* Oral Electrolytes Class Instructions.)

Pharmacokinetics. *Onset and Duration.* Peak levels are achieved immediately after IV, 1 hr after IM. Duration (anticonvulsant) is 30 min with IV, 3–4 hr postonset with IM.

Serum Levels. (Normal) 1.3–2.1 mEq/L (0.65–1.1 mmol/L); (anticonvulsant) 4–7 mEq/L (2–3.5 mmol/L). Intracellular and extracellular concentrations can vary independently; hence, serum magnesium levels may not be indicative of total body stores.

Fate. Oral absorption varies inversely with intake; in general, 24–76% is absorbed,[61] principally in upper small intestine. Total body content is about 24 g,[57] of which 60% is in bone, 39% in tissues, and 1% in extracellular fluid; 30% is plasma protein bound. Elimination is primarily by the kidneys, with only 1–2% in feces. A renal threshold for magnesium excretion exists; therefore, replacement therapy must be continued slowly, usually over 5 days. Raising the serum concentration above normal exceeds the maximum tubular reabsorption capacity with subsequent excretion of excess.

Adverse Reactions. Serum concentration related: (3–5 mEq/L; 1.5–2.5 mmol/L) hypotension; (5–10 mEq/L; 2.5–5 mmol/L) PR interval changes, QRS prolongation, peaked T waves; (10 mEq/L; 5 mmol/L) areflexia; (15 mEq/L; 7.5 mmol/L) respiratory paralysis; (25 mEq/L; 12.5 mmol/L) cardiac arrest.[59] Pain on IM injection occurs very frequently.[60]

Contraindications. Hypermagnesemia; heart block; myocardial damage; severe renal failure.

Precautions. Use with caution in patients with renal impairment (Cl_{cr} <30 mL/min) and those concurrently taking a digitalis glycoside. With bolus $MgSO_4$ administration, 1 g of 10% calcium gluconate IV should be available in case apnea or heart block occurs.[61]

Drug Interactions. IV magnesium may potentiate neuromuscular blocking agents.

Parameters to Monitor. Serum magnesium regularly, frequency determined by condition of patient; BUN and/or Cr_s, serum potassium and calcium periodically. Deep tendon reflexes, respiratory rate, blood pressure, and ECG periodically.

Notes. For mild deficiencies, dietary supplementation may be sufficient to normalize magnesium stores; sources include cereals, nuts, green vegetables, meat, and fish.[61] Magnesium chloride is preferred for oral replacement and supplementation because it may be better absorbed and potentially causes less diarrhea.[62] Patients on long-term diuretic therapy who are prone to hypomagnesemia may benefit from using the minimally effective dose of diuretic and 20–30 mEq/day of magnesium orally or changing to a magnesium-sparing agent (eg, amiloride, spironolactone, triamterene).[63] Drugs known to produce hypomagnesemia include aminoglycoside antibiotics, amphotericin B, diuretics, alcohol, and cisplatin.[59,62] Coadministration of 3 g $MgSO_4$ IV with high-dose cisplatin chemotherapy has been recommended.[63] Although controversial, IV magnesium may reduce mortality post-MI.[64,65] Correction of refractory hypocalcemia and hypokalemia with concurrent hypomagnesemia requires magnesium replacement to restore mineral balance.[58] To avoid the precipitation reaction when $MgSO_4$ and calcium chloride are added to parenteral nutrition mixtures, use of calcium gluceptate has been recommended because it reacts more slowly than calcium chloride and a precipitate does not form.[66] (*See* Magnesium Products Comparison Chart.)

MAGNESIUM PRODUCTS COMPARISON CHART

PRODUCT	MAGNESIUM CONTENT* (MEQ/G)	DOSAGE FORMS†	COMMENTS
Magnesium, Chelated Chelated magnesium	8.3	Tab 500 mg = 100 mg Mg.	Amino acid chelate; sodium-free; oral use only.
Magnesium Chloride Slo-Mag Various	9.8 (PO) 20.8 (IV)	SR Tab 535 mg = 64 mg Mg. Inj 200 mg/mL = 23.6 mg/mL Mg.	Alternative to parenteral MgSO₄.
Magnesium Citrate Various	4.4	Soln 60 mg/mL = 3.2 mg/mL Mg.	Oral use only.
Magnesium Gluconate Almora Magatrate Magonate	4.5–4.8	Tab 500 mg = 27–29 mg Mg. Soln 11 mg/mL = 0.5 mg/mL Mg.	Very soluble; well absorbed; produces no diarrhea.
Magnesium Hydroxide Milk of magnesia	34	Susp 40 mg/mL = 13.6 mg/mL Mg. Susp 80 mg/mL = 27 mg/mL Mg. Tab 300 mg = 102 mg Mg. Tab 600 mg = 205 mg Mg.	Readily available in combination antacid formulations. Start with 5 mL susp or 1 tab, increase as tolerated to qid. Requires gastric acid for absorption. Inexpensive.
Magnesium Oxide	60.3	Cap 140 mg = 84 mg Mg. Tab 400 mg = 241 mg Mg.	Poorly soluble; net absorption low, especially in malabsorptive states.

(continued)

MAGNESIUM PRODUCTS COMPARISON CHART (continued)

PRODUCT	MAGNESIUM CONTENT* (MEQ/G)	DOSAGE FORMS†	COMMENTS
Magnesium Sulfate Epsom salt	8.1	Inj 10% = 9.6 mg/mL Mg. Inj 12.5% = 12 mg/mL Mg. Inj 20% = 23.6 mg/mL Mg. Inj 50% = 48 mg/mL Mg. Pwdr 1 g = 97.2 mg Mg.	Use IV, IM, or PO.

*1 mEq = 12 mg = 0.5 mmol Mg.
†Magnesium products exhibit variable oral absorption; increase dosage incrementally until no further rise in serum magnesium occurs or until diarrhea occurs.

PHOSPHATE SALTS

Various

Pharmacology. Phosphate is a structural element of bone and is involved in carbohydrate metabolism, energy transfer, and muscle contraction, and as a buffer in the renal excretion of hydrogen ion.[51] Many of the factors that influence serum calcium concentration also influence serum phosphate directly or indirectly.

Administration and Adult Dosage. **PO** 250–500 mg (8–16 mmol) of phosphorus qid initially, adjusted according to serum phosphate and calcium. **IV replacement** (recent and uncomplicated hypophosphatemia) 0.08 mmol/kg, to a maximum of 0.2 mmol/kg; (prolonged and multiple causes) 0.16 mmol/kg, to a maximum of 0.24 mmol/kg. Infuse doses over 6 hr and additional dosage guided by serum concentrations.[67] **IV for symptomatic hypophosphatemia** 1–3 g (31–94 mmol) of phosphate daily to maintain serum phosphate at 2–3 mg/dL.[68] When serum concentration reaches 2 mg/dL (0.67 mmol/L), and the patient is able to eat a normal diet, change to oral administration and phosphate-rich diet.[69]

Special Populations. *Pediatric Dosage.* **PO** (<4 yr) 250 mg (8 mmol) of phosphorus qid initially; (≥4 yr) same as adult dosage. **IV replacement** (for serum phosphate concentration 0.5–1 mg/dL) 0.05–0.08 mg/kg (0.15–0.25 mmol/kg) per dose over 4–6 hr; (for serum phosphate concentration <0.5 mg/dL) 0.08–0.12 mg/kg (0.25–0.35 mmol/kg) per dose over 6 hr.[55] Repeat doses as needed to achieve desired serum concentration. Actual dosage depends on signs, symptoms, and serum phosphate concentration.

Geriatric Dosage. Lower dosage may be required in some patients because of the age-related decrease in renal function.

Other Conditions. Renal impairment decreases requirement. Choose the appropriate salt form based on patient's sodium and potassium requirements. Requirement is increased during alcohol withdrawal, diabetic ketoacidosis, respiratory alkalosis, aluminum antacid therapy, burns, and anabolism.

Dosage Forms. (*See* Phosphate Products Comparison Chart.)

Patient Instructions. (*See* Oral Electrolytes Class Instructions.) Do not take capsules whole, but dissolve contents in 3/4 glass of water before taking. Powder in packets must be dissolved in one gallon of water before using. Chilling solution may improve palatability. Do not take with calcium-containing products.

Pharmacokinetics. *Serum Levels.* (As phosphorus) adults 2.7–4.5 mg/dL (0.9–1.5 mmol/L); children 4.5–5.5 mg/dL (1.5–1.8 mmol/L). Normal serum phosphorus concentrations may vary by as much as 2 mg/dL throughout the day, because of changes in transcellular distribution. Concentrations <1 mg/dL are dangerous and require replacement therapy.

Fate. Normal adult dietary intake is 1–1.5 g/day, of which 60–90% is absorbed, primarily in the jejunum. Most of the absorbed phosphorus is excreted in urine.[67]

Adverse Reactions. Frequently diarrhea and stomach upset occur with oral dosage forms.[67,70] Dose-related hyperphosphatemia, metastatic calcium deposition, dehydration, hypotension, hypomagnesemia, and hyperkalemia or hypernatremia (depending on salt used) can occur.

Contraindications. Hyperphosphatemia; hypocalcemia; hyperkalemia (potassium salt); hypernatremia (sodium salt); severe renal failure.

Precautions. Use cautiously in patients with renal impairment and in those with hypercalcemia. Dilute IV forms before use and administer slowly. Administer the potassium salt peripherally no faster than 10 mEq/hr to avoid vein irritation.[71]

Drug Interactions. None known.

Parameters to Monitor. Serum phosphorus regularly, frequency determined by condition of patient; BUN and/or Cr_s, serum calcium, and magnesium periodically.[72] Monitor serum sodium and/or potassium periodically, depending on salt form used.

Notes. Phosphate salts may precipitate in the presence of calcium salts in IV solutions; add no more than 40 mmol of phosphate and 5 mEq of calcium per liter. Calcium supplementation may be necessary to prevent hypocalcemic tetany during phosphate repletion. IV calcium gluconate or calcium chloride may be given until tetany subsides. Inorganic phosphorus exists in the body as the mono- and dibasic forms, the relative proportions of which are pH dependent. It is therefore preferable to report concentrations as mg/dL or mmol/L, rather than mEq/L.[67] (*See* Phosphate Products Comparison Chart.)

PHOSPHATE PRODUCTS COMPARISON CHART

PRODUCT	DOSAGE FORMS*	PHOSPHORUS CONTENT†		CATION CONTENT
		mg	mmol	
POTASSIUM SALTS				
K-Phos Original	Tab.	114	3.6	3.7 mEq K⁺/tablet.
Neutra-Phos K	Cap. Pwdr. Packet.	250 (per cap or packet)	8	14.3 mEq K⁺/cap or packet.
Potassium Phosphate	Inj.	94 (per mL)	3	4.4 mEq K⁺/mL.
SODIUM SALTS				
Fleet's Phospho-Soda	Soln.	128 (per mL)	4.1	111 mg (4.8 mEq) Na⁺/mL.
Sodium Phosphate	Inj.	94 (per mL)	3	93 mg (4 mEq) Na⁺/mL.
SODIUM-POTASSIUM SALTS				
K-Phos M.F.	Tab.	125 (per tablet)	4	67 mg (2.9 mEq) Na⁺ and 1.1 mEq K⁺/tablet.
K-Phos Neutral	Tab.	250 (per tablet)	8	298 mg (13 mEq) Na⁺ and 1.1 mEq K⁺/tablet.
K-Phos No. 2	Tab.	250 (per tablet)	8	134 mg (5.8 mEq) Na⁺ and 2.3 mEq K⁺/tablet.
Neutra-Phos Plain	Cap. Pwdr. Packet.	250 (per cap or packet)	8	164 mg (7.1 mEq) Na⁺ and 7.1 mEq K⁺/cap or packet.
Skim Milk	Liquid.	1000 (per quart)	32	552 mg (24 mEq) Na⁺ and 40 mEq K⁺/quart.

*Contents of capsules, tablets, and powders must be diluted in water before administration.
†31.25 mg = 1 mmol.
From references 67–69 and product information.

POTASSIUM SALTS   Various

Pharmacology. Potassium is the major cation of the intracellular space, where its major role is regulating muscle and nerve excitability. Other roles include control of intracellular volume (similar to sodium's control of extracellular volume), protein synthesis, enzymatic reaction, and carbohydrate metabolism.[73] The chloride salt is preferred for most uses, because concomitant chloride loss and metabolic alkalosis frequently accompany hypokalemia. Nonchloride salts are preferred in acidosis (eg, secondary to amphotericin B or carbonic anhydrase inhibitor therapy and in chronic diarrhea with bicarbonate loss).[74,75]

Administration and Adult Dosage. Variable, must be adjusted to needs of patient. **PO for prophylaxis with diuretic therapy** 40 mEq/day of potassium chloride prevents hypokalemia in most patients on long-term diuretic therapy.[74] For nonedematous, ambulatory patients with uncomplicated hypertension, generally no supplementation is needed; however, if serum potassium falls below 3 mEq/L, 50–60 mEq/day is recommended. For edematous patients (eg, CHF, cirrhosis with ascites) give 40–80 mEq/day (mild deficit) or 100–120 mEq/day (severe deficit), with careful monitoring of serum potassium.[76] **IV administration in peripheral vein** (serum potassium greater than 2.5 mEq/L) may be infused at 10–20 mEq/hr;[75] reserve rates faster than 20 mEq/hr for emergency situations; may repeat q 2–3 hr as needed; do not exceed a maximum concentration of 40 mEq/L; **IV administration in central vein** (serum potassium <2.5 mEq/L) up to 60 mEq/hr may be administered;[75] do not exceed a maximum concentration of 80 mEq/L. Infusion into a central vein requires use of a volume control device. Potassium concentration should not exceed 60 mEq/L unless the infusion site is via a large vein distal to the heart (eg, femoral vein) or more than one IV line is available; however, more concentrated solutions (200 mEq/L) infused at a slow rate (20 mEq/hr) have been used with relative safety.[77] (*See* Special Populations, Other Conditions.)

Special Populations. *Pediatric Dosage.* PO 1–2 mEq/kg/day during diuretic therapy.

Geriatric Dosage. Lower dosage may be required in some patients because of the age-related decrease in renal function.

Other Conditions. Base maintenance dosage on serum potassium; renal impairment decreases requirement. For patients with renal impairment or any form of heart block, decrease infusion rate by one-half and do not exceed 5–10 mEq/hr.[75]

Dosage Forms. **PO** (*see* Potassium Products Comparison Chart); **Inj** (potassium chloride) 2 mEq/mL; (potassium acetate) 2, 4 mEq/mL; (potassium phosphate) 4.4 mEq/mL of potassium and 3 mmol/mL of phosphate (*see* Phosphate Products Comparison Chart).

Patient Instructions. (*See* Oral Electrolytes Class Instructions.) Do not chew or crush tablets. The expanded wax matrix of sustained-release forms may be found in the stool, but this does not imply a lack of absorption.

Pharmacokinetics. *Onset and Duration.* Peak elevation of serum potassium concentrations following SR preparations is slightly delayed (2 hr) compared to the liquid form (1 hr). Effect on serum potassium is generally limited to the first 3 hr after administration.[78]

Serum Levels. May vary depending on laboratory. Normal serum levels are (newborn) 5–7.5 mEq/L; (adult and child) 3.5–5 mEq/L. Total body stores are about 50 mEq/kg or 3500 mEq. As a general rule, a decrease of 1 mEq/L in serum potassium reflects a 10–20% total body deficit; however, there is considerable variation;[76] signs of hypokalemia appear below 2.5 mEq/L; concentrations >7 mEq/L or <2.5 mEq/mL are dangerous. Clinical signs of hypokalemia or hyperkalemia are not reliable indicators of serum concentrations. Alkalosis decreases concentrations, and acidosis increases concentrations. Any hypokalemia-induced change in ECG must be treated as a medical emergency with IV potassium. Likewise, hyperkalemia-induced changes in ECG must also be treated as a medical emergency.

Fate. When initially administered, the rates of absorption and excretion are more rapid with the liquid than the SR forms; however, bioavailability is the same (78–90%) during long-term administration.[78,79] About 10 mEq/day are eliminated in feces; 60–90 mEq/day in urine, and 7.5 mEq/L in sweat.

Adverse Reactions. Bad taste, nausea, vomiting, diarrhea, and abdominal discomfort may occur frequently with oral liquids. Do not use enteric-coated tablets, because they may cause small-bowel and occasionally gastric ulceration.[76] Local tissue necrosis may occur if IV solution extravasates. Hyperkalemia may occur occasionally. Patients with diabetic nephropathy are at an increased risk for hyperkalemia.[80]

Contraindications. Severe renal impairment; untreated Addison's disease; adynamia episodica hereditaria; acute dehydration; heat cramps; hyperkalemia; concurrent ACE inhibitor or potassium-sparing diuretic in patients with renal impairment. Additionally, all solid dosage forms (including SR products) are contraindicated in patients in whom delay or arrest of the tablet through the GI tract may occur.

Precautions. Use with caution (if at all) in patients receiving potassium-sparing diuretics or ACE inhibitors, and in patients with digitalis-induced atrioventricular conduction disturbances or renal failure. Avoid extravasation of parenteral potassium products. If extravasation occurs, aspirate any accessible extravasated solution, then remove IV catheter and apply a cold compress to the area.

Drug Interactions. Use with an ACE inhibitor or potassium-sparing diuretic can result in hyperkalemia.

Parameters to Monitor. Serum potassium weekly to monthly initially, q 3–6 months when stable; BUN and/or Cr_s periodically. For supplementation in patients on long-term diuretic therapy, obtain a pretreatment serum potassium and magnesium, reassess after 2–3 weeks, and then monthly to determine pattern of potassium loss. Once steady state or normokalemia is achieved, assess quarterly or as condition requires.[76]

Notes. Place patient on a cardiac monitor before starting IV potassium.[75] A potassium-sparing diuretic may be preferable to potassium supplementation when large supplements are needed, aldosterone concentrations are elevated, enhanced diuretic response is desired, or magnesium loss is of concern. If large doses of potassium fail to correct hypokalemia, suspect hypomagnesemia, because potassium balance is strongly dependent on magnesium homeostasis.[74,81] If a hypokalemic patient is also hypomagnesemic, as occurs with **amphotericin B** therapy, the patient may not respond to potassium replacement therapy unless magnesium balance is restored. (*See* Oral Potassium Products Comparison Chart.)

POTASSIUM PRODUCTS COMPARISON CHART

PRODUCT	DOSAGE FORMS	COMMENTS
Potassium Acetate Various	Inj 2, 4 mEq/mL.	Useful in metabolic acidosis; avoid in metabolic alkalosis.
Potassium Acetate/ *Bicarbonate/Citrate* Trikates Tri-K	Soln 45 mEq/15 mL.[a]	Preferred form in patients with delayed GI transit time or metabolic acidosis; avoid nonchloride salts in metabolic alkalosis.
Potassium Chloride Kaochlor-Eff Klorvess K-Lyte/Cl Adolph's Morton No Salt NuSalt	Inj 2 mEq/mL; Soln 20, 30, 40, 45 　mEq/15 mL[a] Pwdr Packet 15, 20, 25 　mEq[b] SR Cap/Tab 6.7, 8, 10, 　20 mEq[c] Salt Substitutes 50–70 　mEq/tsp.[d]	Ideal for hypochloremic metabolic alkalosis.
Potassium Bicarbonate/ *Citrate* K-Lyte	Pwdr Packet 25, 50 mEq.[b]	Preferred form in patients with delayed GI transit time or metabolic acidosis; avoid nonchloride salts in metabolic alkalosis.
Potassium Gluconate Kaon	Soln 1.33 mEq/mL.[a]	Preferred form in patients with metabolic acidosis; avoid nonchloride salts in metabolic alkalosis.

[a]Liquids have rapid absorption, low frequency of GI ulceration, and unpleasant taste.
[b]Must be dissolved in water before use.
[c]Bioequivalent to liquid forms; avoid in patients with delayed GI transit time.
[d]Salt substitutes may also have large amounts of sodium.
From references 74–76 and product information.

ORAL REHYDRATION SOLUTIONS   Various

Pharmacology. Oral rehydration solutions supply sodium, chloride, potassium, and water to prevent or replace mild to moderate fluid loss (5–10% dehydration) in diarrhea or postoperative states, or when food and liquid intake are temporarily discontinued. A carbohydrate (usually glucose) is present to aid in sodium transport and subsequent water absorption.[82,83]

Administration and Adult Dosage. PO 1900–2850 mL (2–3 quarts)/day. Give only enough solution to supply the calculated water loss plus daily requirement.

Special Populations. *Pediatric Dosage.* Depends primarily on estimated fluid and electrolyte loss.[84] PO (infants) 150 mL/kg/day (one-half in the first 8 hr if possible, the remainder over the ensuing 16 hr) offered in frequent, small amounts (not to exceed 100 mL in a 20-min period).[85] Once the solution is well tolerated, it may be given less frequently (q 3–4 hr). For infants who finish the prescribed amount of solution in less than 24 hr, offer plain tap water to avoid hypernatremia.[86] PO (5–10 yr) 950–1900 mL (1–2 quarts)/day; (≥11 yr) same as adult dosage.

Geriatric Dosage. Lower dosage may be required in some patients because of the age-related decrease in renal function.

Other Conditions. Adjust intake based on fluid status and serum electrolytes. When electrolyte-containing foods are restarted, adjust solution intake accordingly.

Dosage Forms. *(See* Oral Rehydration Solutions Comparison Chart.)

Patient Instructions. These products are not for fluid replacement in prolonged or severe diarrhea. Reconstitute powdered products in tap water; do not mix with milk or fruit juices. If additional fluids are desired, drink water or other non-electrolyte-containing fluids to quench thirst.

Adverse Reactions. Hypernatremia, hyperkalemia, and acid-base disturbances may occur occasionally, especially in renal insufficiency or if errors occur in reconstituting bulk powders.

Contraindications. Intractable vomiting; adynamic ileus; intestinal obstruction; perforated bowel; shock; renal dysfunction (anuria, oliguria); monosaccharide malabsorption.[83]

Precautions. Use parenteral replacement to correct electrolyte imbalances caused by severe fluid loss (10–15% of body weight), inability to take oral fluids, severe gastric distention, or severe vomiting. Errors in reconstituting or diluting commercial powders may lead to severe consequences.

Drug Interactions. None known.

Parameters to Monitor. Serum sodium, potassium, chloride, and bicarbonate regularly, with frequency determined by condition of patient; BUN and/or Cr_s and urine specific gravity periodically; input and output, weight, and signs and symptoms of dehydration daily.

Notes. To prevent dehydration early in the course of diarrhea or to maintain hydration following parenteral replacement in adults and children, 90 mEq/L of sodium is acceptable. For infants, however, who have a higher insensible water loss, dilute solutions containing 50–60 mEq/L of sodium are suggested.[86] Alternatively, solutions of higher sodium concentration may be used in a ratio of 2:1 with additional free water.[82] Vomiting does not preclude use of oral replacement solutions; spooning small quantities into the mouth of the child who is experiencing some vomiting usually results in the administration of sufficient fluid to correct dehydration.[83]

ORAL REHYDRATION SOLUTIONS COMPARISON CHART

| SOLUTION | DOSAGE FORMS | ELECTROLYTES (MEQ/L)* | | | | OTHER | CARBOHYDRATE |
		Na+	K+	Cl⁻	BASE		
Infalyte	Soln 1000 mL.	50	25	45	34 Citrate	—	Rice syrup solids 3%.
Pedialyte	Soln 237, 946 mL.	45	20	35	30 Citrate	—	Dextrose 2.5%.
Rehydralyte	Soln 237 mL.	75	20	65	30 Citrate	—	Dextrose 2.5%.
Resol	Soln 960 mL.	50	20	50	34 Citrate	4 Ca++ 4 Mg++ 5 HPO₄=	Glucose 2%.
WHO Oral Rehydration Salts†	Powder.‡	90	20	80	30 Bicarbonate	—	Glucose 2%.

*Optimal solution (mEq/L): Na+ 75–100, K+ 20–30, Cl⁻ 65–100, base 20–30, carbohydrate 1.5–2%.
†WHO = World Health Organization Oral Rehydration Salts; available from Jianas Brothers Packaging, 2533 SW Boulevard, Kansas City, MO; tel (816) 421–2880.
‡Reconstitute powder in tap water; do not mix with milk or fruit juices.
From references 84–86 and product information.

SODIUM POLYSTYRENE SULFONATE
Kayexalate, Various

Pharmacology. A cation exchange resin that exchanges potassium for sodium. Each gram of resin binds up to 1 mEq of potassium and liberates 1–2 mEq of sodium.[87] Sorbitol is present in some products to induce diarrhea and to reduce the potential for fecal impaction. (*See* Notes.)

Administration and Adult Dosage. PO 15–20 g, may repeat as often as q 2 hr,[75] although doses up to 40 g have been recommended;[88] total dosage and duration of therapy depend on patient response. If suspension does not contain sorbitol, give powder with, or suspended in, a sorbitol solution (eg, 15 mL of 70% sorbitol). **PR as enema** 50 g retained for 30 min, if possible, may repeat as often as q 45 min.[75] Follow enema by an irrigation of up to 2 L of non-sodium-containing fluid to remove resin from bowel.

Special Populations. *Pediatric Dosage.* For small children and infants, calculate dosage on the basis of 1 g of resin binding 1 mEq of potassium.

Geriatric Dosage. Lower dosage may be required in some patients because of the age-related decrease in renal function.

Other Conditions. In severe situations, such as ongoing tissue damage or rapidly rising serum potassium in renal failure, a dosage of 80–100 g for every mEq/L of potassium above 5 mEq/L has been recommended.[88] However, under such circumstance, other forms of therapy may be considered.

Dosage Forms. Pwdr 454 g; **Susp** (containing sorbitol) 15 g/60 mL.

Pharmacokinetics. *Onset and Duration.* PO onset is 2–12 hr; PR onset is somewhat longer.

Fate. Not absorbed from GI tract; binds potassium and liberates sodium as it passes through intestine.

Adverse Reactions. Anorexia, nausea, and vomiting occur frequently with large doses; gastric irritation, constipation, and fecal impaction (especially in the elderly) occur occasionally. These effects may be avoided by using the enema. However, intestinal necrosis because of the enema has been reported. Use of **sorbitol** in the enema and failure to follow it with a cleansing enema may predispose uremic patients to potentially fatal intestinal necrosis.[87]

Precautions. Use with caution in patients who cannot tolerate any additional sodium load (eg, severe CHF, severe hypertension, marked edema). In addition to potassium, other cations (such as magnesium and calcium) may bind to the resin, causing electrolyte imbalances. If rapid potassium lowering is required, give insulin with or without glucose.

Drug Interactions. None known.

Parameters to Monitor. Serum potassium at least daily and more frequently if indicated; serum magnesium and calcium periodically; ECG and patient signs and symptoms may be useful in evaluating status.

Notes. On average, 50 g of resin will lower serum potassium by 0.5–1 mEq/L.[89] Rectal administration is less effective than oral use. Heating may alter the exchange properties of the resin. Sodium polystyrene sulfonate-induced constipation may be treated with 70% **sorbitol** in oral doses (ie, 10–20 mL/2 hr) sufficient to produce 1 or 2 watery stools/day.

Antigout Agents

ALLOPURINOL
Zyloprim, Various

Pharmacology. Allopurinol, a structural analogue of the purine base hypoxanthine, competitively inhibits xanthine oxidase. This reduces both serum and urinary uric acid levels by blocking the conversion of hypoxanthine and xanthine to uric acid and by decreasing purine synthesis.[90–92]

Administration and Adult Dosage. **PO for control of gout** 100 mg/day initially, increasing in 100 mg/day increments at weekly intervals until a serum uric acid level of 6 mg/dL or less is attained. **PO for maintenance of mild gout** 200–300 mg/day in single or divided doses; **PO for maintenance of moderately severe tophaceous gout** 400–600 mg/day, to a maximum of 800 mg/day for resistant cases. Give dosages that exceed 300 mg/day in divided doses. Give prophylactic colchicine 0.5–1.2 mg/day and/or an NSAID starting before allopurinol and continuing for 1 to several months after initiation of therapy because of an initial increased risk of gouty attacks.[90–93] A fluid intake sufficient to yield a daily urinary output of at least 2 L and the maintenance of a neutral or slightly alkaline urine are desirable. In transferring from a uricosuric agent to allopurinol, reduce the uricosuric dosage over a period of several weeks while gradually increasing the dosage of allopurinol. **PO or IV for secondary hyperuricemia associated with vigorous treatment of malignancies** 600–800 mg/day for 2–3 days is advisable with a high fluid intake, then reduce to 300 mg/day. Start at least 2–3 days (preferably 5 days) before initiation of cancer therapy. Discontinue when the potential for uric acid overproduction is no longer present.[94] IV should be used only in those who do not tolerate PO allopurinol. **PO for recurrent calcium oxalate stones in hyperuricosuria** 200–300 mg/day adjusted based on control of hyperuricosuria.

Special Populations. *Pediatric Dosage.* PO for secondary hyperuricemia associated with malignancies (<6 yr) 150 mg/day; (6–10 yr) 300 mg/day; alternatively, 2.5 mg/kg q 6 hr to a maximum of 600 mg/day. Start at least 2–3 days (preferably 5 days) before cancer therapy.[94] Evaluate response 48 hr after cancer therapy is started and adjust dosage as needed.

Geriatric Dosage. Lower dosage may be required in some patients because of the age-related decrease in renal function.

Other Conditions. In renal impairment, reduce initial dosage as follows: with Cl_{cr} of 80 mL/min, give 250 mg/day; with Cl_{cr} of 60 mL/min, give 200 mg/day; with Cl_{cr} of 40 mL/min, give 150 mg/day; with Cl_{cr} of 20 mL/min, give 100 mg/day; with Cl_{cr} of 10 mL/min, give 100 mg q 2 days; with Cl_{cr} <10 mL/min, give 100 mg q 3 days.[95] Base subsequent dosage adjustment on serum uric acid levels.

Dosage Forms. **Tab** 100, 300 mg; **Inj** 500 mg.

Patient Instructions. This drug may be taken with food, milk, or an antacid to minimize stomach upset. Adults should drink at least 10–12 full glasses (8 fl oz each) of fluid each day. Avoid large amounts of alcohol (may increase uric acid in blood) or vitamin C (may increase the possibility of kidney stones by making the urine more acidic). Report any skin rash, painful urination, blood in urine, eye irritation, swelling of lips or mouth, itching, chills, fever, sore throat, nausea, or vomiting while taking this drug. Allopurinol may cause drowsiness; use caution while driving or performing other tasks requiring alertness, coordination, or physical dexterity.

Pharmacokinetics. *Onset and Duration.* A measurable decrease in uric acid occurs in 2–3 days; normal serum uric acid is achieved in 1–3 weeks.

Fate. Well absorbed orally (67–81%), but rectal absorption is poor (0–6% of oral bioavailability). Rapidly oxidized to oxypurinol, an active, but less potent, inhibitor of xanthine oxidase. Protein binding of allopurinol or oxypurinol is negligible.[96] Allopurinol V_d is 1.5 ± 0.7 L/kg, Cl is 0.77 ± 0.22 L/hr/kg; oxypurinol V_d is about 1.6 L/kg.[96,97] Oxypurinol and allopurinol are excreted unchanged in urine in a ratio of about 10:1.[96]

$t_{1/2}$. (Allopurinol) 1.4 ± 0.4 hr; (oxypurinol) 19.7 ± 7.3 hr with normal renal function, 5–10 days in renal failure.[96]

Adverse Reactions. A mild maculopapular skin rash occurs in about 2% of patients, but the percentage increases to about 20% with concurrent ampicillin. These rashes may not recur if allopurinol is stopped and restarted at a lower dosage and oral desensitization to minor rashes from allopurinol in patients has been effective.[92,98] Exfoliative, urticarial, purpuric, and erythema multiforme lesions are also reported occasionally. These more severe reactions require drug discontinuation because severe hypersensitivity reactions such as vasculitis, toxic epidermal necrolysis, Stevens-Johnson syndrome, renal impairment, and hepatic damage can result. An occasional hypersensitivity syndrome (frequently marked by fever, rash, hepatitis, renal failure, and eosinophilia) has a mortality rate reportedly as high as 27%. It may begin 1 day to 2 yr (average 6 weeks) after start of therapy and appears related to preexisting renal dysfunction, elevated oxypurinol serum levels, or concurrent thiazide or other diuretic therapy.[95,99,100] Occasionally, nausea, vomiting, abdominal pain, and drowsiness occur. Rarely, alopecia, cataract formation, hepatotoxicity, bone marrow depression, leukopenia, leukocytosis, or renal xanthine stones occur.

Contraindications. Children (except for hyperuricemia secondary to malignancy). Do not restart the drug in patients who have developed a severe reaction (*see* Adverse Reactions).

Precautions. Pregnancy; lactation. Use with caution and in reduced dosage in renal impairment. Adjust dosage conservatively in patients with impaired renal function who are on a diuretic concomitantly.[95,100]

Drug Interactions. Diuretics may contribute to allopurinol toxicity, although a cause-and-effect relationship has not been established. Allopurinol markedly increases the toxicity of oral azathioprine and mercaptopurine. Allopurinol may increase the risk of hypersensitivity reactions to ampicillin and captopril, bone marrow suppression caused by cyclophosphamide, neurotoxicity of vidarabine, and nephrotoxicity of cyclosporine. Allopurinol may also increase the effect of oral anticoagulants. Concurrent use of salicylate for its antirheumatic effect does not compromise the action of allopurinol.

Parameters to Monitor. Monitor serum uric acid levels; pretreatment 24-hr urinary uric acid excretion.[90–92] Periodically determine liver function (particularly in patients with preexisting liver disease). Monitor renal function tests and CBC, especially during the first few months of therapy. Renal function is particularly important in patients on concurrent diuretic therapy.[95,100]

Notes. Allopurinol is the drug of choice for patients with impaired renal function who respond poorly to uricosuric agents; however, these patients should be monitored closely because of an increased frequency of adverse reactions.[90–93,95] Current data do not support the routine treatment of asymptomatic hyperuricemia in patients other than those receiving vigorous treatment of malignancies and in marked overexcreters.[90–92] Allopurinol has been used investigationally to reduce tissue damage during coronary artery bypass surgery, for organ transplantation storage solutions, and in the treatment of leishmaniasis.[101]

Because of limited studies showing very poor or no absorption of extemporaneously compounded allopurinol suppositories, this dosage form is not recommended.[96] Although preliminary reports indicated that extemporaneously prepared allopurinol mouthwash may be effective in protecting against **fluorouracil**-induced mucositis, one well-controlled clinical trial found it ineffective for this indication, and it is not recommended.[102]

COLCHICINE   Various

Pharmacology. Colchicine is an antiinflammatory agent relatively specific for gout, with activity probably because of the impairment of leukocyte chemotaxis, mobility, adhesion, and phagocytosis, and a reduction of the lactic acid production resulting from a decrease in urate crystal deposition.

Administration and Adult Dosage. **PO for acute gout** 1–1.2 mg initially, then 0.5–1.2 mg q 1–2 hr until pain is relieved or GI toxicity occurs (ie, nausea, vomiting, stomach pain, or diarrhea), to a maximum total dosage of 4–8 mg. Pain and swelling typically abate within 12 hr and usually are gone in 24–48 hr. An interval of 3 days is advised if a second course is required. **PO for prophylaxis in chronic gout** 0.5–1.8 mg/day or every other day depending on severity; divided doses are preferred with higher dosages. **PO for surgical prophylaxis in patients with gout** 0.5–0.6 mg tid, 3 days before and after surgery. **Slow IV for acute gout** (if patient cannot take oral preparation) 1–2 mg initially, diluted (if desired) in nonbacteriostatic NS, over 2–5 min, then 0.5 mg q 6–24 hr prn, to a maximum of 4 mg in 24 hr, or a maximum 4 mg for a single course of treatment.[103,104] Some clinicians recommend a single IV dose of 3 mg over 5 min; others recommend an initial dose of 1 mg or less, then 0.5 mg 1–2 times daily prn. If pain recurs, give IV 1–2 mg/day for several days; however, no more colchicine should be given by any route for at least 7 days after a full course (4 mg) of IV therapy.[103,104] IV colchicine is very irritating and extravasation must be avoided to prevent tissue and nerve damage; change to oral therapy as soon as possible. **Do not administer by SC or IM routes.** (*See* Notes.)

Special Populations. *Geriatric Dosage.* Reduce the maximum IV colchicine dosage to 2 mg with at least 3 weeks between courses, and lower the dosage further if previously maintained on oral colchicine.[103,104]

Other Conditions. Reduce the total IV and PO dosage of colchicine in renal impairment in proportion to the remaining renal function.[103–105] The dosage of prophylactic colchicine should not exceed 0.5 mg/day with a Cl_{cr} of ≤50 mL/min, because of an increased risk of peripheral neuritis and myopathy.[106] Not recommended in patients who require hemodialysis.[106]

Dosage Forms. **Tab** 500, 600 µg; **Inj** 500 µg/mL.

Patient Instructions. You should always have a supply of this drug at hand, and you should take it promptly at the earliest symptoms of a gouty attack. Relief of gout pain or occurrence of nausea, vomiting, stomach pain, or diarrhea indicate that the full therapeutic dosage has been attained and no more drug should be taken. After treatment of an attack, do not take any more colchicine for at least 3 days. Immediately report black tarry stools or bright red blood in the stools, which may indicate GI bleeding. Report any tiredness, weakness, numbness, or tingling. Also immediately report sore throat, fever, or oral lesions, which may be an early sign of a severe, but rare, blood disorder.

Pharmacokinetics. *Fate.* Rapidly but variably absorbed after oral administration (healthy young adults, 44 ± 17%; elderly, 45 ± 19%), with partial hepatic deacetylation. Plasma protein binding is approximately 50%; extensive leukocyte uptake occurs with levels found for up to 9 days. Distribution following IV administration is triphasic; V_d of the terminal phase for healthy young adults is 6.7 ± 1.4 L/kg, and for the elderly is 6.3 ± 2.3 L/kg. Cl for healthy young adults is 0.15 ± 0.02 L/hr/kg, and for the elderly 0.12 ± 0.01 L/hr/kg. Urinary (about 10% unchanged), biliary, and fecal elimination occur.[105,107,108]

$t_{1/2}$. (Healthy young adults) second phase 1.2 ± 0.2 hr; terminal phase 30 ± 6 hr; (elderly) second phase 1.2 ± 0.1 hr; terminal phase 34 ± 8 hr.[107]

Adverse Reactions. Nausea, vomiting, stomach pain, and diarrhea are frequent and may occur several hours after oral or IV drug administration; discontinue drug at first signs. Prolonged administration may occasionally cause bone marrow depression with agranulocytosis or thrombocytopenia, aplastic anemia, and purpura. Peripheral neuritis and myopathy with a characteristically elevated creatine kinase occur occasionally. This reaction usually resolves in 3–4 weeks after drug withdrawal and is associated with standard (unadjusted) dosage in renal insufficiency.[103–106,109] Alopecia, reversible malabsorption of vitamin B_{12}, and reversible azoospermia occur. Tissue and nerve damage may occur with IV extravasation. Overdosage can cause hemorrhagic gastroenteritis, vascular damage leading to shock, nephrotoxicity, and paralysis. As little as 7 mg has proved fatal, but much larger dosages have been survived.[104,105,110]

Contraindications. Serious GI, renal, hepatic, or cardiac disorders; combined hepatic, and renal dysfunction;[103–106] blood dyscrasias.

Precautions. Use with great caution in elderly or debilitated patients, especially those with early manifestations of hepatic, renal, GI, or heart disease. Reduce dosage if weakness, anorexia, nausea, vomiting, stomach pain, or diarrhea occurs.[105]

Drug Interactions. None known.

Notes. Colchicine is most effective when used early in the attack before most WBC chemotaxis takes place.[90,91,111] It may be an effective antiinflammatory agent in the therapy of the arthritis of pseudogout.[109] For acute gout, an **NSAID** or a corticosteroid may be preferred, but daily colchicine is often given for prophylaxis against recurrent gouty attacks before and during the first one to several months of allopurinol or uricosuric treatment.[90,91,111] Continuous prophylactic colchicine therapy can be effective in suppressing the acute attacks and renal dysfunction of familial Mediterranean fever.[105,109] Colchicine therapy may also be effective for primary biliary cirrhosis and certain inflammatory dermatoses.[105,109]

Pharmacology. Probenecid is an organic acid that inhibits renal tubular reabsorption of urate, thereby increasing the urinary excretion of uric acid and lowering serum urate. Probenecid also interferes with renal tubular secretion of many drugs, causing an increase or prolongation in their serum levels. (*See* Notes.)

Administration and Adult Dosage. PO for chronic gout 250 mg bid for 1 week, then 500 mg bid (not to be started during an acute attack). **Colchicine** 0.5–1.2 mg/day started before and continued for 1 to several months after initiation of uricosuric treatment diminishes exacerbation of uricosuric-induced gouty attacks.[90–92] To prevent hematuria, renal colic, costovertebral pain, and urate stone formation, liberal fluid intake and alkalinization of the urine with 3–7.5 g/day sodium bicarbonate or 7.5 g/day potassium citrate is recommended, at least until serum uric acid levels normalize and tophaceous deposits disappear. If an acute gouty attack is precipitated during therapy, increase the dosage of colchicine or add a corticosteroid or an NSAID to control the attack.[90–92] (*See* Precautions.) Decrease daily dosage by 500 mg q 6 months if no acute attacks occur, adjusted to maintain normal serum uric acid levels. **PO to prolong penicillin or cephalosporin action** 2 g/day in 4 divided doses. **PO with procaine penicillin G for neurosyphilis** 2 g/day in 4 divided doses for 10–14 days.[112]

Special Populations. *Pediatric Dosage* (<2 yr) contraindicated. **PO to prolong penicillin or cephalosporin action** (<50 kg) 25 mg/kg initially, then maintain at 40 mg/kg/day or 1.2 g/m^2/day in 4 divided doses; (>50 kg) same as adult dosage. **PO with amoxicillin for gonorrhea** (<45 kg) 25 mg/kg, to a maximum of 1 g.[112]

Geriatric Dosage. Same as adult dosage.

Other Conditions. For chronic gout in renal impairment (although probably ineffective when Cl_{cr} ≤ 30 mL/min), increase initial dosage of 500 mg bid in 500 mg/day increments monthly to the dosage that maintains normal serum uric acid levels, to a maximum of 2 g/day in divided doses.

Dosage Forms. **Tab** 500 mg; **Tab** 500 mg with colchicine 0.5 mg (ColBenemid, various).

Patient Instructions. This drug may be taken with food, milk, or an antacid to minimize stomach upset. Drink a large amount (10–12 full glasses) of fluids each day and avoid the use of aspirin- or salicylate-containing products unless directed otherwise.

Pharmacokinetics. *Fate.* Rapidly and completely absorbed from the GI tract; 74–99% plasma protein bound (decreasing with increasing dose), mostly to albumin.[113] V_d is 0.17 ± 0.03 L/kg.[8] Probenecid is extensively metabolized or conjugated, exhibiting Michaelis-Menten elimination; about 40% is excreted in urine as the monoacylglucuronide, less than 5% as unchanged drug, and the remainder as hydroxylated metabolites, which may have uricosuric activity.[114,115]

$t_{1/2}$. Dose dependent (increases with increasing dose): 4.5 ± 0.6 hr with 0.5 g; 12 hr with 2 g.[8,116]

Adverse Reactions. Headache, nausea, vomiting, urinary frequency, rash, and dizziness occur frequently. Exacerbation of gout and uric acid stones may occur. Nephrotic syndrome, hepatic necrosis, aplastic anemia, hemolytic anemia (possibly related to G-6-PD deficiency), and severe allergic reactions occur rarely.

Contraindications. Children <2 yr; known blood dyscrasias or uric acid kidney stones; initiation during an acute gouty attack.

Precautions. Hypersensitivity reactions require drug discontinuation. Use with caution in patients with a history of peptic ulcer or G-6-PD deficiency. (*See* Notes.)

Drug Interactions. Salicylates and pyrazinamide antagonize the uricosuric action of probenecid. Probenecid may increase the serum concentration of many drugs, including acyclovir, benzodiazepines, some β-lactams, clofibrate, dapsone, methotrexate, NSAIDs, penicillamine, sulfonylureas, thiopental, and zidovudine. NSAID clearance may be decreased by competitively inhibiting either formation or renal excretion of acylglucuronide metabolites.[117]

Parameters to Monitor. Serum uric acid weekly until stable when treating hyperuricemia; pretreatment 24-hr urinary uric acid excretion. If alkali is administered, periodically determine acid-base balance.

Notes. Current data do not support the treatment of patients with asymptomatic hyperuricemia caused by *undersecretion* of uric acid.[90,92,118] Most useful in symptomatic patients with reduced urinary excretion of urate: under 800 mg/day on an unrestricted diet; or under 600 mg/day on a purine-restricted diet.[90] Ineffective in prolonging the half-life of β-lactams that do not undergo renal tubular secretion (eg, ceftazidime, ceftriaxone, moxalactam).[119]

SULFINPYRAZONE Anturane, Various

Sulfinpyrazone is an analogue of phenylbutazone that lacks antiinflammatory and analgesic properties. It is a uricosuric agent with a mechanism and site of action resembling those of probenecid. It also has antiplatelet and antithrombotic activity. Oral absorption is rapid and complete, with peak serum levels occurring in 1–2 hr. V_d is 0.73 ± 0.23 L/kg; Cl of the parent compound is 0.14 ± 0.044 L/hr/kg; half-lives are 10 ± 1.3 hr (sulfinpyrazone) and 14.3 ± 4.5 hr (sulfide metabolite). Hepatic metabolism yields 4 metabolites. The parent compound is mainly responsible for uricosuric activity; the sulfide metabolite produces the antiplatelet effect. Adverse effects are similar to probenecid with occasional acute renal insufficiency, possibly caused by precipitation of uric acid in renal tubules or decrease in prostaglandin synthesis. Colchicine 0.5–1.2 mg/day started before and continued for 1 to several months after initiation of uricosuric treatment diminishes exacerbation of uricosuric-induced gouty attacks. Treat acute exacerbations of gout by increasing the colchicine dosage or by adding an NSAID or corticosteroid. Sulfinpyrazone is contraindicated in patients with peptic ulcers, symptoms of GI inflammation or ulceration, and blood dyscrasias. Avoid sulfinpyrazone in renal insufficiency because it may not be effective. Dosage as a uricosuric agent is 200–400 mg/day orally in 2 divided doses with meals or milk, increasing over 1 week to a maximum of 800 mg/day with an adequate fluid intake and alkalization of the urine. Reduce to the lowest dosage needed to control serum uric acid (as low as 200 mg/day). In elderly, azotemic cardiovascular patients, initiate therapy with 200 mg/day, and either increase in 200 mg/day increments q 4 days or keep constant for another 4 days depending upon Cr_s and serum uric acid, to a maximum maintenance dosage of 800 mg/day.[90–92,120–125] Available as 100-mg tablets and 200-mg capsules.

■ REFERENCES

1. Macfie HL et al. Amiloride. *Drug Intell Clin Pharm* 1981;15:94–8.
2. Rose BD. Diuretics. *Kidney Int* 1991;39:336–52.
3. Ellison DH. Diuretic drugs and the treatment of edema: from clinic to bench and back again. *Am J Kidney Dis* 1994;23:623–43.
4. Brater DC. Resistance to diuretics: mechanisms and clinical implications. *Adv Nephrol Necker Hosp* 1993;22:349–69.
5. Gerlag PG, van-Meijel JJ. High-dose furosemide in the treatment of refractory congestive heart failure. *Arch Intern Med* 1988;148:286–91.
6. Vasko MR et al. Furosemide absorption altered in decompensated congestive heart failure. *Ann Intern Med* 1985;102:314–8.
7. van Meyel JJ et al. Absorption of high dose furosemide (frusemide) in congestive heart failure. *Clin Pharmacokinet* 1992;22:308–18.
8. Benet LZ et al. Design and optimization of dosage regimens; pharmacokinetic data. In Hardman JG et al., eds. *Goodman and Gilman's the pharmacological basis of therapeutics*, 9th ed. New York: McGraw-Hill; 1996:1707–92.
9. Ponto LL, Schoenwald RD. Furosemide (frusemide): a pharmacokinetic/pharmacodynamic review (part I). *Clin Pharmacokinet* 1990;18:381–408.
10. Ponto LL, Schoenwald RD. Furosemide (frusemide): a pharmacokinetic/pharmacodynamic review (part II). *Clin Pharmacokinet* 1990;18:460–71.
11. Brater DC. Resistance to loop diuretics: why it happens and what to do about it. *Drugs* 1985;30:427–43.
12. Sica DA, Gehr TWB. Diuretic combinations in refractory oedema states. Pharmacokinetic-pharmacodynamic relationships. *Clin Pharmacokinet* 1996;30:229–49.
13. Myers MG. Hydrochlorothiazide with or without amiloride for hypertension in the elderly: a dose-titration study. *Arch Intern Med* 1987;147:1026–30.
14. Beermann B, Groschinsky-Grind M. Clinical pharmacokinetics of diuretics. *Clin Pharmacokinet* 1980;5:221–45.
15. Welling PG. Pharmacokinetics of the thiazide diuretics. *Biopharm Drug Dispos* 1986;7:501–35.
16. Langford HG et al. Is thiazide-produced uric acid elevation harmful? Analysis of data from the Hypertension Detection and Follow-up Program. *Arch Intern Med* 1987;147:645–9.
17. O'Bryne S, Feely J. Effects of drugs on glucose tolerance in non-insulin-dependent diabetes (part II). *Drugs* 1990;40:203–19.
18. O'Bryne S, Feely J. Effects of drugs on glucose tolerance in non-insulin-dependent diabetes (part I). *Drugs* 1990;40:6–18.
19. Womack PL, Hart LL. Potassium supplements vs. potassium-sparing diuretics. *DICP* 1990;24:710–1.
20. Lang F. Osmotic diuresis. *Renal Physiol* 1987;10:160–73.

21. Hoffman DM, Grossano D. Use of mannitol diuresis to reduce cis-platinum nephrotoxicity. *Drug Intell Clin Pharm* 1978;12:489–90. Letter.

22. Nissenson AR. Mannitol. *West J Med* 1979;131:277–84.

23. Manninen PH et al. The effect of high-dose mannitol on serum and urine electrolytes and osmolality in neuro-surgical patients. *Can J Anaesth* 1987;34:442–6.

24. Anderson P et al. Use of mannitol during neurosurgery: interpatient variability in the plasma and CSF levels. *Eur J Clin Pharmacol* 1988;35:643–9.

25. Dorman HR et al. Mannitol-induced acute renal failure. *Medicine* (Baltimore) 1990;69:153–9.

26. Horgan KJ et al. Acute renal failure due to mannitol intoxication. *Am J Nephrol* 1989;9:106–9.

27. Skluth HA, Gums JG. Spironolactone: a re-examination. *DICP* 1990;24:52–9.

28. Lant A. Diuretics: clinical pharmacology and therapeutic use (part II). *Drugs* 1985;29:162–88.

29. Lant A. Diuretics: clinical pharmacology and therapeutic use (part I). *Drugs* 1985;29:57–87.

30. Sadee W et al. Multiple dose kinetics of spironolactone and canrenoate-potassium in cardiac and hepatic failure. *Eur J Clin Pharmacol* 1974;7:195–200.

31. Overdiek JW, Merkus FW. Spironolactone metabolism and gynaecomastia. *Lancet* 1986;1:1103. Letter.

32. Gardiner P et al. Spironolactone metabolism: steady-state serum levels of the sulfur-containing metabolites. *J Clin Pharmacol* 1989;29:342–7.

33. Overdiek HW, Merkus FW. Influence of food on the bioavailability of spironolactone. *Clin Pharmacol Ther* 1986;40:531–6.

34. Jeunemaitre X et al. Efficacy and tolerance of spironolactone in essential hypertension. *Am J Cardiol* 1987;60:820–5.

35. Friedel HA, Buckley MM. Torasemide: a review of its pharmacological properties and therapeutic potential. *Drugs* 1991;41:81–103.

36. Brater DC et al. Clinical pharmacology of torasemide, a new loop diuretic. *Clin Pharmacol Ther* 1987;42:187–92.

37. Gehr TW et al. The pharmacokinetics of intravenous and oral torsemide in patients with chronic renal insufficiency. *Clin Pharmacol Ther* 1994;56:31–8.

38. Loute G et al. The influence of haemodialysis and haemofiltration on the clearance of torasemide in renal failure. *Eur J Clin Pharmacol* 1986;31(suppl):53–5.

39. Sharoky M et al. Comparative efficacy and bioequivalence of a brand-name and a generic triamterene-hydrochlorothiazide combination product. *Clin Pharm* 1989;8(7):496–500.

40. Gilfrich H et al. Pharmacokinetics of triamterene after i.v. administration to man: determination of bioavailability. *Eur J Clin Pharmacol* 1983;25:237–41.

41. Muirhead MR et al. Effect of cimetidine on renal and hepatic drug elimination: studies with triamterene. *Clin Pharmacol Ther* 1986;40:400–7.

42. Knauf H et al. Delayed elimination of triamterene and its active metabolite in chronic renal failure. *Eur J Clin Pharmacol* 1983;24:453–6.

43. Mutschler E et al. Pharmacokinetics of triamterene. *Clin Exp Hypertens [A]* 1983;5:249–69.

44. Sica DA, Gehr TW. Triamterene and the kidney. *Nephron* 1989;51:454–61.

45. Alaniz C. Management of cirrhotic ascites. *Clin Pharm* 1989;8:645–54.

46. Burns Schaiff R et al. Medical treatment of hypercalcemia. *Clin Pharm* 1989;8:108–21.

47. Sica DA, Gehr TWB. Diuretic combinations in refractory oedema states. Pharmacokinetic-pharmacodynamic relationships. *Clin Pharmacokinet* 1996;30:229–49.

48. Zaloga GP, Chernow B. Divalent ions: calcium, magnesium, and phosphorus. In Chernow B, ed.. *The pharmacologic approach to the critically ill patient,* 3rd ed. Baltimore: Williams & Wilkins; 1994:777–804.

49. Food and Nutrition Board, NRC. *Recommended dietary allowances,* 10th ed. Washington, DC: National Academy Press; 1989.

50. Anon. Calcium supplements. *Med Lett Drugs* Ther 1989;31:101–3.

51. Delmez JA, Slatopolsky E. Hyperphosphatemia: its consequences and treatment in patients with chronic renal disease. *Am J Kidney Dis* 1992;19:303–17.

52. Tohme JF, Bilezikian JP. Hypocalcemic emergencies. *Endocrinol Metab Clin North Am* 1993;22:363–75.

53. Carr CJ, Shangrew RF. Nutritional and pharmaceutical aspects of calcium supplementation. *Am Pharm* 1987;2:49–50, 54–7.

54. Blanchard J, Aeschlimann JM. Calcium absorption in man: some dosing recommendations. *J Pharmacokinet Biopharm* 1989;17:631–44.

55. Sheikh MS et al. Gastrointestinal absorption of calcium from milk and calcium salts. *N Engl J Med* 1987;317:532–6.

56. Altura BM. Basic biochemistry and physiology of magnesium: a brief review. *Magnes Trace Elem* 1991;10:167–71.

57. Gums JG. Clinical significance of magnesium: a review. *Drug Intell Clin Pharm* 1987;21:240–6.

58. Al-Ghamdi SMG et al. Magnesium deficiency: pathophysiologic and clinical overview. *Am J Kidney Dis* 1994;5:737–52.
59. Rude RK. Magnesium metabolism and deficiency. *Endocrinol Metab Clin North Am* 1993;22:377–95.
60. Montgomery P. Treatment of magnesium deficiency. *Clin Pharm* 1987;6:834–5.
61. Reinhart RA. Magnesium metabolism: a review with special reference to the relationship between intracellular content and serum levels. *Arch Intern Med* 1988;148:2415–20.
62. Kobrin SM, Goldfarb S. Magnesium deficiency. *Semin Nephrol* 1990;10:525–35.
63. Berkelhammer C, Bear RA. A clinical approach to common electrolyte problems: hypomagnesemia. *Can Med Assoc J* 1985;132:360–8.
64. Yusuf S et al. Intravenous magnesium in acute myocardial infarction: an effective, safe, simple, and inexpensive intervention. *Circulation* 1993;87:2043–6. Editorial.
65. Teo KK, Yusuf S. Role of magnesium in reducing mortality in acute myocardial infarction: a review of the evidence. *Drugs* 1993;46:347–59.
66. Chernow B et al. Hypomagnesemia: implications for the critical care specialist. *Crit Care Med* 1982;10:193–6.
67. Lloyd CW, Johnson CE. Management of hypophosphatemia. *Clin Pharm* 1988;7:123–8.
68. Rubin MF, Narins RG. Hypophosphatemia: pathophysiological and practical aspect of its therapy. *Semin Nephrol* 1990;10:536–45.
69. Hodgson SF, Hurley DL. Acquired hypophosphatemia. *Endocrinol Metab Clin North Am* 1993;22:397–409.
70. Peppers MP et al. Endocrine crises: hypophosphatemia and hyperphosphatemia. *Crit Care Clin* 1991;7:201–14.
71. Baker WL. Hypophosphatemia. *Am J Nurs* 1985;85:998–1003.
72. Kingston M, Al-Siba'i MB. Treatment of severe hypophosphatemia. *Crit Care Med* 1985;13:16–8.
73. Martin ML et al. Potassium. *Emerg Med Clin North Am* 1986;4:131–44.
74. Krishna GG. Hypokalemic states: current clinical issues. *Semin Nephrol* 1990;10:515–24.
75. Zull DN. Disorders of potassium metabolism. *Emerg Med Clin North Am* 1989;7:771–94.
76. Stanaszek WF, Romankiewicz JA. Current approaches to management of potassium deficiency. *Drug Intell Clin Pharm* 1985;19:176–84.
77. Kruse JA, Carlson RW. Rapid correction of hypokalemia using concentrated intravenous potassium chloride infusions. *Arch Intern Med* 1990;150:613–7.
78. Toner JM, Ramsay LE. Pharmacokinetics of potassium chloride in wax-based and syrup formulations. *Br J Clin Pharmacol* 1985;19:489–94.
79. Skoutakis VA et al. The comparative bioavailability of liquid, wax-matrix, and microencapsulated preparations of potassium chloride. *J Clin Pharmacol* 1985;25:619–21.
80. Breyer JA. Diabetic nephropathy in insulin-dependent patients. *Am J Kidney Dis* 1992;20:533–47.
81. Freedman BI, Burkart JM. Endocrine crises: hypokalemia. *Crit Care Clin* 1991;7:143–53.
82. Finch MH, Younoszai KM. Oral rehydration therapy. *South Med J* 1987;80:609–13.
83. Balistreri WF. Oral rehydration in acute infantile diarrhea. *Am J Med* 1990;88(6A):30S–3.
84. Grisanti KA, Jaffe DM. Dehydration syndromes: oral rehydration and fluid replacement. *Emerg Med Clin North Am* 1991;9:565–88.
85. Swedberg J, Steiner JF. Oral rehydration therapy in diarrhea: not just for Third World children. *Postgrad Med* 1983;74:335–41.
86. Anon. Oral rehydration solutions. *Med Lett Drugs Ther* 1983;25:19–20.
87. Lillemoe KD et al. Intestinal necrosis due to sodium polystyrene (Kayexalate) in sorbitol enemas: clinical and experimental support for the hypothesis. *Surgery* 1987;101:267–72.
88. Elms JJ. Potassium imbalance: causes and prevention. *Postgrad Med* 1982;72:165–71.
89. Alvo M, Warnock DG. Hyperkalemia. *West J Med* 1984;141:666–71.
90. Star VL, Hochberg MC. Prevention and management of gout. *Drugs* 1993;45:212–22.
91. Conaghan PG, Day RO. Risks and benefits of drugs used in the management and prevention of gout. *Drug Saf* 1994;11:252–8.
92. Emmerson BT. The management of gout. *N Engl J Med* 1996;334:445–51.
93. Campbell SM. Gout: how presentation, diagnosis, and treatment differ in the elderly. *Geriatrics* 1988;43(11):71–7.
94. Conger JD. Acute uric acid nephropathy. *Med Clin North Am* 1990;74:859–71.
95. Hande KR et al. Severe allopurinol toxicity: description and guidelines for prevention in patients with renal insufficiency. *Am J Med* 1984;76:47–56.
96. Murrell GAC, Rapeport WG. Clinical pharmacokinetics of allopurinol. *Clin Pharmacokinet* 1986;11:343–53.
97. Walter-Sack I et al. Disposition and uric acid lowering effect of oxipurinol: comparison of different oxipurinol formulations and allopurinol in healthy individuals. *Eur J Clin Pharmacol* 1995;49:215–20.
98. Fam AG et al. Desensitization to allopurinol in patients with gout and cutaneous reactions. *Am J Med* 1992;93:299–302.

99. Roujeau JC, Stern RS. Severe adverse cutaneous reactions to drugs. *N Engl J Med* 1994;331:1272–85.

100. Arellano F, Sacristán JA. Allopurinol hypersensitivity syndrome: a review. *Ann Pharmacother* 1993;27:337–43.

101. Day RO et al. New uses for allopurinol. *Drugs* 1994;48:339–44.

102. Loprinzi CL et al. A controlled evaluation of an allopurinol mouthwash as prophylaxis against 5-fluorouracil-induced stomatitis. *Cancer* 1990;65:1879–82.

103. Wallace SL, Singer JZ. Review: systemic toxicity associated with the intravenous administration of colchicine-guidelines for use. *J Rheumatol* 1988;15:495–9.

104. Roberts WN et al. Colchicine in acute gout: reassessment of risks and benefits. *JAMA* 1987;257:1920–2.

105. Levy M et al. Colchicine: a state-of-the-art review. *Pharmacotherapy* 1991;11:196–211.

106. Wallace SL et al. Renal function predicts colchicine toxicity: guidelines for the prophylactic use of colchicine in gout. *J Rheumatol* 1991;18:264–9.

107. Rochdi M et al. Pharmacokinetics and absolute bioavailability of colchicine after iv and oral administration in healthy human volunteers and elderly subjects. *Eur J Clin Pharmacol* 1994;46:351–4.

108. Jusko WJ, Gretch M. Plasma and tissue protein binding of drugs in pharmacokinetics. *Drug Metab Rev* 1976;5:43–140.

109. Famaey JP. Colchicine in therapy. State of the art and new perspectives for an old drug. *Clin Exp Rheumatol* 1988;6:305–17.

110. Hood RL. Colchicine poisoning. *J Emerg Med* 1994;12:171–7.

111. Wallace SL, Singer JZ. Therapy in gout. *Rheum Dis Clin North Am* 1988;14:441–57.

112. Anon. Drugs for sexually transmitted diseases. *Med Lett Drugs Ther* 1994;36:1–6.

113. Emanuelsson BM et al. Non-linear elimination and protein binding of probenecid. *Eur J Clin Pharmacol* 1987;32:395–401.

114. Israili ZH et al. Metabolites of probenecid. Chemical, physical, and pharmacological studies. *J Med Chem* 1972;15:709–13.

115. Perel JM et al. Identification and renal excretion of probenecid metabolites in man. *Life Sci* 1970;9:1337–43.

116. Dayton PG et al. The physiological disposition of probenecid, including renal clearance, in man, studied by an improved method for its estimation in biological material. *J Pharmacol Exp Ther* 1963;140:278–86.

117. Smith PC et al. Effect of probenecid on the formation and elimination of acyl glucuronides: studies with zomepirac. *Clin Pharmacol Ther* 1985;38:121–7.

118. Campbell SM. Gout: how presentation, diagnosis, and treatment differ in the elderly. *Geriatrics* 1988;43(11):71–7.

119. Brown GR. Cephalosporin-probenecid drug interactions. *Clin Pharmacokinet* 1993;24:289–300.

120. Hood WB. More on sulfinpyrazone after myocardial infarction. *N Engl J Med* 1982;306:988–9.

121. Palummeri E et al. Sulphinpyrazone in cardiovascular elderly azotemic patients: a proposal of a guided incremental dose schedule. *J Int Med Res* 1984;12:271–6.

122. Mahoney C et al. Kinetics and metabolism of sulfinpyrazone. *Clin Pharmacol Ther* 1983;33:491–7.

123. Schlicht F et al. Pharmacokinetics of sulfinpyrazone and its major metabolites after a single dose and during chronic treatment. *Eur J Clin Pharmacol* 1985;28:97–103.

124. Orlandini G, Brognoli M. Acute renal failure and treatment with sulfinpyrazone. *Clin Nephrol* 1983;20:161–2.

125. Rosenkranz B et al. Effects of sulfinpyrazone on renal function and prostaglandin formation in man. *Nephron* 1985;39:237–43.

Respiratory Drugs

ANTIHISTAMINES AND ANTIALLERGICS

Class Instructions: Antihistamines. This drug (with the exceptions of astemizole, fexofenadine, loratadine, and terfenadine) may cause drowsiness, dry mouth, or occasional dizziness. Until the extent of drowsiness is known, use caution when driving, operating machinery, or performing other tasks requiring mental alertness or motor coordination. Avoid excessive concurrent use of alcohol and other CNS depressants that cause drowsiness. This drug effectively suppresses seasonal allergic rhinitis only when taken continuously.

CETIRIZINE   Zyrtec

Cetirizine is a long-acting H_1-receptor antagonist that is a metabolite of hydroxyzine. Cetirizine is rapidly absorbed after oral administration; peak serum levels are reached within 1 hr. Food does not affect the amount absorbed, but may decrease the absorption rate. Protein binding averages 93%. Clearance in normal adults is 0.04–0.05 L/kg/hr. The elimination half-life is 7–10 hr in adults, 6–7 hr in children, and 18–21 hr in the elderly and patients with renal insufficiency. The alteration in half-life is caused by renal function changes rather than age per se. Cetirizine is not appreciably dialyzable. After oral administration of a 10-mg dose, 70% of the drug is excreted unchanged in the urine within 72 hr and 10% is excreted in feces. It is the only H_1-blocker not metabolized by the hepatic cytochrome P450 system. The most common side effects are sedation, headache, dry mouth, fatigue, and nausea. Early comparative trials suggested that sedation was similar to placebo and the nonsedating antihistamines; however, in some more recent comparisons, cetirizine 10 mg/day produced more sedation than loratadine 10 mg/day, terfenadine 120 mg/day, or placebo. The usual dosage in adults and children $\geq$12 yr is 10 mg given once daily. Cetirizine is not labeled for use in children <12 yr, but the following dosages have been reported: (2–6 yr) 5 mg/day; (6–11 yr) 10 mg/day. Reduce dosage to 5 mg/day in adults with moderate to severe renal impairment (Cl_{cr} <31 mL/min) or hepatic impairment.[1-3] Available as 5- and 10-mg tablets and 5 mg/mL syrup. (*See* Antihistamines Comparison Chart.)

CHLORPHENIRAMINE MALEATE   Chlor-Trimeton, Various

Pharmacology. Chlorpheniramine is a competitive antagonist of histamine at the H_1-histamine receptor. It also has anticholinergic and transient sedative effects when used intermittently.

Administration and Adult Dosage. PO for seasonal allergic rhinitis (effectiveness is maximized if given continuously, starting just prior to the pollen season) 4 mg hs initially, increasing gradually over 10 days as tolerated to 24 mg/day in 1–2 divided doses until the end of the season.[4] **PO for acute allergic reactions** 12 mg in 1–2 divided doses. **SC, IM, or IV for uncomplicated allergic reactions** 5–20 mg. **IV as adjunctive treatment in anaphylaxis** 10–20 mg. **SC, IM, or IV for allergic reactions to blood or plasma** 10–20 mg, to a maximum of 40 mg/day. **SR** (*see* Notes).

Special Populations. *Pediatric Dosage.* **PO for seasonal allergic rhinitis** (2–6 yr) 1 mg q 4–6 hr up to 4 mg/day; (6–12 yr) 2 mg hs initially, increasing gradually over 10 days as tolerated to 12 mg/day in 1–2 divided doses until the end of the season.[4] SR not recommended. (*See* Notes).

Geriatric Dosage. **PO** 4 mg daily–bid. Duration of action may be 36 hr or more, even when serum concentrations are low.[5]

Dosage Forms. **Cap** 12 mg; **Chew Tab** 2 mg; **Tab** 4, 8, 12 mg; **Syrup** 0.4 mg/mL; **SR Cap** 8, 12 mg (*see* Notes); **SR Tab** 8, 12 mg (*see* Notes); **Inj** 10 mg/mL (IM, IV, SC); 100 mg/mL (IM, SC only); **Tab** 4 mg with pseudoephedrine HCl 60 mg (Sudafed Plus, Isoclor, various); 4 mg with phenylpropanolamine HCl 25 mg (Allergy Relief Medicine, various); **Syrup** 0.4 mg/mL with phenylpropanolamine HCl 2.5 mg/mL (Triaminic, various).

Patient Instructions. (*See* Antihistamines Class Instructions.)

Pharmacokinetics. *Onset and Duration.* Onset is in 0.5–1 hr; duration of suppression of wheal and flare response (IgE-mediated) to skin tests with allergenic extract is 2 days.[6] Fast metabolizers have an earlier, greater, and more prolonged antihistaminic response than slow metabolizers because of rapid conversion to active metabolite.[7]

Serum Levels. Serum chlorpheniramine levels do not correlate with histamine antagonist activity because of an unidentified active metabolite.[7] (Children) 2.3–12 µg/L (6–31 nmol/L) suppress allergic rhinitis symptoms; (children) 4–10 µg/L (11–26 nmol/L) suppress histamine-induced wheal and flare.[4]

Fate. Oral bioavailability is about 34%; 72% is plasma protein bound.[5] V_d is (adults) 3.2 ± 0.3 L/kg; (children) 7 ± 2.8 L/kg; Cl is (adults) 0.1 ± 0.006 L/hr/kg; (children) 0.43 ± 0.19 L/hr/kg.[4,8] Rapidly and extensively metabolized by CYP2D6 to mono- and didesmethylchlorpheniramine and unidentified metabolites, one or more of which are active. Metabolites and a small amount of parent drug are excreted in urine.[7,9]

$t_{1/2}$. (Adults) 20 ± 5 hr;[8] (children) 13 ± 6 hr;[4] (chronic renal failure) 280–330 hr.[9]

Adverse Reactions. Frequent drowsiness, dry mouth, dizziness, and irritability occur with intermittent therapy; however, most patients develop tolerance to these side effects during continuous therapy, particularly if dosage is increased slowly.

Contraindications. Lactation; premature and newborn infants.

Precautions. Use chlorpheniramine with caution in the elderly (≥60 yr). It may cause paradoxical CNS stimulation in children. OTC labeling states to avoid in patients with narrow-angle glaucoma, symptomatic prostatic hypertrophy, asthma, emphysema, chronic pulmonary disease, shortness of breath, or breathing difficulties except under physician supervision; however, many studies have shown some bronchodilator effect of H_1-receptor antagonists.[6]

Drug Interactions. MAO inhibitors prolong and intensify the anticholinergic effects of antihistamines.[10] Alcohol or sedative-hypnotics may increase CNS depressant effects.

Parameters to Monitor. In seasonal allergic rhinitis, observe for sneezing, rhinorrhea, itchy nose, and conjunctivitis.

Notes. Not effective for nasal stuffiness. SR formulations offer no advantage over syrup or plain, uncoated tablets, because the drug has an inherently long duration of action. (*See* Antihistamines Comparison Chart.)

CROMOLYN SODIUM
Gastrocrom, Intal,
Nasalcrom, Opticrom, Various

Pharmacology. Cromolyn stabilizes the membrane of mast cells and other inflammatory cells (eg, eosinophils), inhibiting release and production of soluble mediators (eg, histamine, leukotrienes) that produce inflammation and bronchospasm. The mechanism appears to be the inhibition of calcium ion influx through the cell membrane. Cromolyn inhibits both the early and late responses to specific allergen and exercise challenges. It also prevents the increase in nonspecific bronchial hyperreactivity that occurs during a specific allergen season in atopic asthmatics.[11,12]

Administration and Adult Dosage. Inhal for asthma 20 mg qid at regular intervals via nebulizer (1 ampule inhalant solution) or 0.8–1.6 mg qid via a pressurized metered-dose inhaler. Initiate therapy in conjunction with an aerosolized β_2-agonist. (*See* Notes.) **Inhal for prevention of exercise-induced bronchospasm** single dose (as above) just prior to exercise. **Intranasal for prophylaxis of allergic rhinitis** 5.2 mg/nostril 3–6 times/day at regular intervals. **Ophth for allergic ocular disorders** 1–2 drops (1.6–3.2 mg) in each eye 4–6 times/day at regular intervals.[13] For chronic conditions the drug must be used continuously to be effective. **PO for mastocytosis** 200 mg qid, 30 min before meals and hs.

Special Populations. *Pediatric Dosage.* **Inhal** (<2 yr) dosage not established; (≥2 yr) same as adult dosage. **PO for mastocytosis** (term infants–2 yr) 20 mg/kg/day in 4 divided doses, to a maximum of 30 mg/kg/day; (2–12 yr) 100 mg qid, 30 min before meals and hs, increasing if necessary to a maximum of 40 mg/kg/day.

Geriatric Dosage. Same as adult dosage.

Other Conditions. The therapeutic effect is dose dependent, and patients with more severe disease may require more frequent administration initially. After a patient becomes symptom-free, the frequency of administration may be reduced to bid–tid.

Dosage Forms. **Inhal Soln** 10 mg/mL; **Inhal** 800 µg/puff (112, 200 doses/inhaler); **Nasal Inhal** 5.2 mg/spray (100 doses/inhaler)**; Ophth Drops** 40 mg/mL (250 drops/container); **PO Cap** 100 mg.

Patient Instructions. (Asthma) This medication must be used regularly and continuously to be effective. Do not stop therapy abruptly, except on medical advice. Carefully follow directions for inhaler use included with the device. Actuate (metered-dose device) during a *slow* deep inhalation, then hold breath for 5–10 seconds. Do not discontinue the use of the nebulizer solution during acute asthmatic attacks. You may mix the nebulizer solution with any bronchodilator inhalant solution. (Mastocytosis) Dissolve oral capsules in one-half glass (4 fl oz) of hot water, then add an equal amount of cold water and drink the entire amount. Do not mix with fruit juice, milk, or foods.

Pharmacokinetics. *Onset and Duration.* (Asthma) onset within 1 min for prevention of allergen-induced mast cell degranulation; duration dose dependent, 2–5 hr.[12] It may require 4–6 weeks to achieve maximal response, although most asthmatics have a response within 2 weeks.[14]

Fate. Oral bioavailability is 0.5–1%. Amount absorbed after inhalation is dependent on the delivery system; about 10% of the dosage for a Spinhaler and less than 2% with the nebulizer solution.[12] Peak serum levels occur 15–20 min after inhalation. V_d is 0.2 ± 0.04 L/kg; Cl is 0.35 ± 0.1 L/hr/kg. Rapidly excreted unchanged in equal portions in the bile and urine.[11,12]

$t_{1/2}$. 22.5 ± 1.6 min.[12]

Adverse Reactions. Mild burning or stinging may occur with ophthalmic solution.[13] Occasionally headache and diarrhea occur with oral capsules.

Precautions. Use with caution in patients with lactose sensitivity (capsules only). Watch for worsening of asthma in patients discontinuing the drug. Children <5 yr should receive cromolyn as the nebulizer solution. The ophthalmic solution contains 0.01% benzalkonium chloride; therefore, do not wear soft contact lenses during therapy.[13]

Drug Interactions. None known.

Parameters to Monitor. Monitor relief of asthmatic symptoms and the proper dosage and inhalation technique. Patient noncompliance or inappropriate inhalation technique often contribute to treatment failure. The measurement of peak expiratory flow rate with a peak flow meter is useful in severe chronic asthma. Periodic standard pulmonary function tests are indicated q 1–6 months in less severe asthma.

Notes. Comparative studies have shown cromolyn and **theophylline** to be equally effective for the prophylaxis of chronic asthma, although cromolyn produces fewer side effects.[11,12,14] The inhalant solution is stable with all β2-agonist and anticholinergic solutions for nebulization.[12] The nasal spray is most effective if started 1 week prior to the allergen season; however, patients receive benefit even if treatment is begun after symptoms occur.[14] Oral cromolyn has been used in the management of GI conditions such as food allergy and irritable bowel syndrome.[15]

CYPROHEPTADINE   Periactin, Various

Cyproheptadine is an H_1-receptor antagonist that is pharmacologically similar to chlorpheniramine. It also has antiserotonin activity. In addition to its antihistaminic properties, cyproheptadine is effective as an appetite stimulant and in treating cold urticaria, but it is relatively ineffective as an antipruritic. Cyproheptadine may be useful in treating patients with major depression who have a suppressible dexamethasone suppression test. Cyproheptadine is well absorbed after oral administration; peak action occurs in 6–9 hr. About 70% of a dose is excreted in feces as metabolites; unchanged drug is not detectable in urine. Cyproheptadine is contraindicated in premature and newborn infants, lactation, patients experiencing asthmatic attacks, and patients who have taken an MAO inhibitor within the preceding 2 weeks. Use with caution in patients who are at risk for complications from marked anticholinergic effects (eg, narrow angle glaucoma, symptomatic prostatic hypertrophy, pyloroduodenal or bladder neck obstruction, or stenosing peptic ulcer). The usual adult oral dosage is 4–20 mg/day (usually 4 mg tid–qid), to a maximum of 0.5 mg/kg/day; (<2 yr) safety and efficacy are not established; (2–6 yr) 2 mg bid–tid, to a maximum of 12 mg/day; (7–14 yr) 4 mg bid–tid, to a maximum of 16 mg/day. The initial dosage for geriatric patients is 4 mg bid. Reduce dosage in patients with marked hepatic dysfunction.[16–22] Available as 4 mg tablets and 0.4 mg/mL syrup. (*See* Antihistamines Comparison Chart.)

DIPHENHYDRAMINE HYDROCHLORIDE Benadryl, Various

Pharmacology. (*See* Chlorpheniramine.)

Administration and Adult Dosage. PO as an antihistamine or for parkinsonism 25–50 mg tid–qid. **PO for motion sickness** 50 mg 30 min before exposure, then ac and hs. **PO as a nighttime sleep aid** 25–50 mg hs. **PO as an antitussive** 25 mg q 4–6 hr. **Deep IM or IV as an antihistamine, or for allergic reactions to blood or plasma, motion sickness, adjunctive treatment of anaphylaxis, or parkinsonism** 10–50 mg/dose, 100 mg if required, to a maximum of 400 mg/day.

Special Populations. *Pediatric Dosage.* **PO as an antihistamine** 5 mg/kg/day, or (≤9 kg) 6.25–12.5 mg tid–qid. (>9 kg) 12.5–25 mg tid–qid, to a maximum of 300 mg/day. **PO as an antitussive** (2–6 yr) 6.25 mg q 4 hr, to a maximum of 25 mg/day; (6–12 yr) 12.5 mg q 4 hr, to a maximum of 75 mg/day. **Deep IM or IV** 5 mg/kg/day, in 4 divided doses, to a maximum of 300 mg/day.

Geriatric Dosage. **PO as an antihistamine** 25 mg bid–tid initially, then increase as needed.[23] (*See* Notes.)

Other Conditions. In renal impairment, increase dosage interval as follows: Cl_{cr} 10–50 mL/min, increase to 6–12 hr; Cl_{cr} <10 mL/min, increase to 12–18 hr.[23]

Dosage Forms. Cap 25, 50 mg; **Elxr** 2.5 mg/mL; **Syrup** 2.5 mg/mL; **Tab** 25, 50 mg; **Inj** 10, 50 mg/mL.

Patient Instructions. (*See* Antihistamines Class Instructions.)

Pharmacokinetics. *Onset and Duration.* Onset is 15 min after single oral dose; duration of suppression of wheal and flare is up to 2 days.[6,24] Duration of effect does not appear to be related to serum levels.

Serum Levels. (Antihistaminic effect) >25 µg/L (0.09 µmol/L); (sedation) 30–50 µg/L (0.1–0.17 µmol/L); (mental impairment) >60 µg/L (0.2 µmol/L).[8,24]

Fate. As a result of first-pass metabolism, oral bioavailability is variable, 61 ± 25%.[8,25] A single 50-mg oral dose in adults usually produces serum concentrations between 25–50 µg/L.[24] About 85% is plasma protein bound, lower in Asians and in cirrhosis.[26,27] V_d is 17.4 ± 4.8 L/kg in adults, larger in Asians and cirrhosis. Cl is 1.4 ± 0.6 L/hr/kg in adults, higher in Asians, and 0.7 ± 0.2 L/hr/kg in the elderly.[8,23,25,26] Metabolized to N-dealkylated and acidic metabolites.[25,2]

Less than 4% is excreted unchanged in urine.[29]

$t_{1/2}$. (Adults) 9.2 ± 2.5 hr; (elderly >65 yr) 13.5 ± 4.2 hr; (children 8–12 yr) 5.4 ± 1.8 hr;[8,25] (cirrhosis) 15 hr.[27]

Adverse Reactions. (*See* Chlorpheniramine.)

Contraindications. (*See* Chlorpheniramine.)

Precautions. (*See* Chlorpheniramine.)

Drug Interactions. MAO inhibitors prolong and intensify the anticholinergic effects of antihistamines.[10] Alcohol or sedative-hypnotics may increase CNS depressant effects.

Parameters to Monitor. In seasonal allergic rhinitis, observe for sneezing, rhinorrhea, itchy nose, and conjunctivitis.

Notes. Because of its low degree of efficacy for pruritus, weak suppression of IgE-mediated skin tests, and high sedative potential, diphenhydramine is not the antihistamine of choice for most conditions. In the elderly, diphenhydramine is discouraged as a nighttime sleep aid because of its high anticholinergic potential. **Dimenhydrinate** (Dramamine), used for motion sickness, is the 8-chlorotheophyllinate salt of diphenhydramine; 100 mg dimenhydrinate is about equal to 50 mg diphenhydramine.

HYDROXYZINE HYDROCHLORIDE	Atarax, Vistaril, Various
HYDROXYZINE PAMOATE	Vistaril, Various

Pharmacology. Hydroxyzine is a competitive antagonist of histamine at the H_1-histamine receptor. It also has antiemetic and sedative effects, thought to be a result of CNS subcortical suppression. Claims of long-term antianxiety properties have not been substantiated by well-designed studies.

Administration and Adult Dosage. **PO for pruritus** 25 mg tid–qid. **PO for seasonal allergic rhinitis** (effectiveness is maximized if given continuously just prior to the pollen season) 25 mg initially q hs until no sedation in morning, then increase dosage q 2–3 days to a maximum of 150 mg/day in 1–2 divided doses and maintain until end of season. Reduce dosage by one-third or more if sedation persists. Dosage may be increased, if tolerated, for symptoms during peak of pollen season.[30] **IM for sedation before and after general anesthesia** 50–100 mg. **IM for nausea and vomiting, and pre- and postoperative adjunctive medication** 25–100 mg. Preferred IM injection site is upper outer quadrant of gluteus maximus or midlateral thigh. **Not for SC or intra-arterial use.**

Special Populations. *Pediatric Dosage.* **PO for pruritus** (<6 yr) 50 mg/day in 2–3 divided doses; (≥6 yr) 50–100 mg/day in divided doses. **PO for seasonal allergic rhinitis** 10 mg initially q hs until no sedation in morning, then increase dosage q 2–3 days, to a maximum of 75 mg/day in 1–2 divided doses and maintain until end of season. Reduce dosage by one-third or more if sedation persists. Dosage may be increased, if tolerated, for symptoms during peak of pollen season.[30] **IM for pre- and postoperative sedation** 0.7 mg/kg.[31] **IM for nausea and vomiting**

and pre- and postoperative adjunctive medication 1.1 mg/kg. Preferred site in children is midlateral muscles of thigh.

Geriatric Dosage. **PO for pruritus** 10 mg tid–qid, increasing to 25 mg tid–qid if necessary.[32]

Dosage Forms. **Cap** (as pamoate equivalent of HCl salt) 25, 50, 100 mg; **Susp** (as pamoate equivalent of HCl salt) 5 mg/mL; **Syrup** (as HCl) 2 mg/mL; **Tab** (as HCl) 10, 25, 50, 100 mg; **Inj** (as HCl) 25, 50 mg/mL (IM only).

Patient Instructions. (*See* Antihistamines Class Instructions.)

Pharmacokinetics. *Onset and Duration.* Onset 15–30 min after oral administration. Duration of suppression of wheal and flare response to allergenic extract skin test is 4 days.[6,20]

Serum Levels. (Pruritus) 6–42 µg/L (14–102 nmol/L) suppress pruritus in children.[33]

Fate. Peak serum level of 73 ± 11 µg/L occurs 2 ± 0.4 hr after a 0.7 mg/kg dose in healthy adults, 117 ± 61 µg/L at 2.3 ± 0.7 hr in primary biliary cirrhosis (mean dose 44 mg).[34,35] V_d is (healthy adults) 16 ± 3 L/kg,[34] (elderly) 23 ± 6 L/kg, (children) 19 ± 9 L/kg,[33] and (primary biliary cirrhosis) 23 ± 13 L/kg.[32] Cl is (healthy young and elderly adults) 0.6 ± 0.2 L/hr/kg,[32,34] (children) 1.9 L/hr/kg,[33] (primary biliary cirrhosis) 0.5 ± 0.4 L/hr/kg.[35]

$t_{\frac{1}{2}}$. (Healthy adults) 20 ± 4 hr;[34] (elderly) 29 ± 10 hr;[32] (children) 7 hr, increasing with age;[34] (primary biliary cirrhosis) 37 ± 13 hr.[35]

Adverse Reactions. Transient drowsiness and dry mouth occur frequently when the drug is taken intermittently. Most patients develop tolerance to these effects when the drug is taken continuously, particularly if the dosage is slowly increased over 7–10 days. IM injection may be painful and has caused sterile abscess. Hemolysis has been associated with IV administration and tissue necrosis with SC or intra-arterial administration.

Contraindications. Early pregnancy; SC or intra-arterial use of injectable solution.

Precautions. Use with caution in the elderly.

Drug Interactions. MAO inhibitors prolong and intensify the anticholinergic effects of antihistamines.[10] Alcohol or sedative-hypnotics may increase CNS depressant effects.

Parameters to Monitor. In seasonal allergic rhinitis, observe for sneezing, rhinorrhea, itchy nose, and conjunctivitis.

Parameters to Monitor. In seasonal allergic rhinitis, observe for sneezing, rhinorrhea, itchy nose, and conjunctivitis.

Notes. Hydroxyzine suppresses wheal and flare response to the greatest degree and for the longest duration of all antihistamines,[6,20] including the newer nonsedating antihistamines.[31]

LORATADINE   Claritin

Loratadine is a long-acting antihistamine that is structurally similar to azatadine and pharmacologically similar to terfenadine, with little or no action at α-adrenergic or cholinergic receptors. The drug is rapidly absorbed; bioavailability and peak serum levels are increased by about 50% in geriatric subjects (66–78 yr). It is 97% bound to plasma proteins and extensively metabolized to an active metabolite, descarboethoxyloratadine. Approximately 80% of a dose is excreted equally in urine and feces as metabolites after 10 days. The mean elimination half-life in healthy adult patients is 8.4 hr (range 3–20) for loratadine and 24 hr (range 8.8–92) for descarboethoxyloratadine. Renal impairment does not seem to affect its elimination. Loratadine does not appear to be dialyzable. Coadminister drugs that inhibit hepatic metabolism with caution until definitive interaction studies are available. The usual dosage for children 2–9 yr is 5 mg/day; for adults and children >9 yr is 10 mg once a day on an empty stomach. In patients with hepatic impairment, begin with 10 mg every other day. The dosage of Claritin-D is 1 tablet bid on an empty stomach; Claritin-D 24-hr is given once daily.[36] Loratadine is available as 10-mg tablets, as 5-mg tablets with pseudoephedrine 120 mg (Claritin-D), and 10 mg tablets with pseudoephedrine 240 mg (Claritin-D 24-hr). (*See* Antihistamines Comparison Chart.)

NEDOCROMIL SODIUM Tilade

Nedocromil sodium is the disodium salt of a pyranoquinolone dicarboxylic acid that is chemically dissimilar but pharmacologically similar to cromolyn sodium. Like cromolyn, nedocromil inhibits the activation of and mediator release from inflammatory cells important in asthma and allergy. Nedocromil appears to have more potent in vitro activity against allergic response than cromolyn. Oral bioavailability is only 2–3%. Following inhalation, bioavailability is 5%, with peak serum concentrations occurring in 20–40 min; concentrations fall monoexponentially, with a half-life of 1.5–2.3 hr, reflecting absorption from lungs. Bronchospasm, headache, distinctive taste, nausea, and vomiting occur frequently. In a limited number of trials, nedocromil was effective for long-term prophylaxis of asthma. Like cromolyn, it can decrease bronchial hyperreactivity but is only partially effective in steroid-dependent asthmatics. Nedocromil sodium is intended for regular maintenance treatment and should not be used in acute asthma attacks. The recommended initial maintenance dosage for adults and children >12 yr is 2 actuations from a metered-dose inhaler qid. In patients under good control with qid administration (ie, patients requiring inhaled or oral β-agonists not more than twice a week), a lower dosage can be tried. First reduce to a tid regimen, then, after several weeks of continued good control, attempt to reduce to a bid regimen.[37–39] Available as 16.2-g inhalers, containing 112 2-mg doses (1.75 mg reaches the patient).

TERFENADINE Seldane

Pharmacology. A nonsedating competitive histamine H_1-receptor antagonist, terfenadine virtually lacks anticholinergic activity.

Administration and Adult Dosage. **PO for seasonal allergic rhinitis** 60 mg bid.

Special Populations. *Pediatric Dosage.* **PO for seasonal allergic rhinitis** (3–5 yr) 15 mg bid; (6–12 yr) 30–60 mg bid.[6]

Geriatric Dosage. **PO** 60 mg daily–bid.

Dosage Forms. **Tab** 60 mg; **SR Tab** 60 mg with pseudoephedrine 120 mg (Seldane-D).

Patient Instructions. (*See* Antihistamine Class Instructions.) Stop taking this medication immediately if you have a fainting spell.

Pharmacokinetics. *Onset and Duration.* Duration of suppression of histamine-induced wheal and flare response is 12 hr.[40]

Fate. Peak serum level of 1.5 ± 0.7 µg/L occurs 1–2 hr after a 60-mg oral dose.[41] The drug is rapidly and completely metabolized to two main metabolic products, an active carboxylic acid analogue (fexofenadine) and α,α-diphenyl-4-piperidinemethanol.[41] About 97% of terfenadine and 70% of fexofenadine are plasma protein bound.[8] About 40% is eliminated in urine and about 60% in feces in 12 days after a 60-mg oral dose;[41,42] 11–25% of a dose is eliminated in urine as fexofenadine after 24 hr.[8,42]

$t_{\frac{1}{2}}$. α phase 3.6 hr; ß phase 16–23 hr.[43]

Adverse Reactions. Frequency of sedation is comparable to placebo and about 50% less frequent than with chlorpheniramine or other antihistamines. Few anticholinergic side effects are reported.[46] Cardiotoxicity (eg, ventricular arrhythmias, prolonged QT interval, torsades de pointes) has been reported rarely,[47] sometimes preceded by syncope; the risk is markedly increased by drugs that inhibit CYP3A3/4, such as ketoconazole or erythromycin.

Contraindications. Patients taking ketoconazole, itraconazole, erythromycin, clarithromycin, or troleandomycin; significant hepatic dysfunction.

Precautions. Pregnancy. Discontinue if syncope occurs.

Drug Interactions. Inhibitors of CYP3A3/4 can markedly increase terfenadine cardiotoxicity. Avoid concurrent use with clarithromycin, erythromycin, fluoxetine, indinavir, itraconazole, ketoconazole, ritonavir, troleandomycin.

Parameters to Monitor. In seasonal allergic rhinitis, observe for sneezing, rhinorrhea, itchy nose, and conjunctivitis.

Notes. (*See* Antihistamines Comparison Chart.) **Fexofenadine** (Allegra) is a nonsedating antihistamine which is the active carboxylic acid metabolite of terfenadine. It has an elimination half-life of 14.4 hr (*see* Terfenadine Fate). Unlike terfenadine, fexofenadine does not prolong the QTc interval or predispose to torsades de pointes with high dosages or combined with CYP3A3/4 inhibitors such as erythromycin or ketoconazole. The oral dosage in adults and children >12 yr is 60 mg bid; in renal impairment, the dosage is 60 mg/day. It is available as 60 mg capsules.

ANTIHISTAMINES COMPARISON CHART

DRUG	DOSAGE FORMS	ADULT DOSAGE	PEDIATRIC DOSAGE	RELATIVE POTENCY	SIDE EFFECTS	
					Sedation*	Anticholinergic
Acrivastine	Tab 8 mg with pseudoephedrine 60 mg (Semprex-D).	8 mg qid.	PO (>12 yr) same as adult dosage	++	+	±
Astemizole Hismanal	Tab 10 mg.	PO 10 mg/day during allergy season—not for "prn" use.	PO (<6 yr) 0.2 mg/kg/day; (6–12 yr) 5 mg/day. Safety and efficacy not established.	+++	±	±
Azatadine Maleate Optimine	Tab 1 mg.	PO 1–2 mg bid.	Safety and efficacy not established <12 yr.	++	++	++
Brompheniramine Maleate Dimetane Various	Elxr 0.4 mg/mL Tab 4, 8, 12 mg SR Tab 8, 12 mg Inj 10 mg/mL.	PO 4 mg q 4–6 hr, to a maximum of 24 mg/day; SC, IM, or slow IV 5–20 mg q 12 hr, to a maximum of 40 mg/day.	PO (2–5 yr) 1 mg q 4–6 hr, to a maximum of 6 mg/day; (6–12 yr) 2 mg q 4–6 hr, to a maximum of 12 mg/day; SC, IM, or slow IV 0.5 mg/kg/day in 3–4 divided doses.	+++	+	++

(continued)

609

ANTIHISTAMINES COMPARISON CHART (continued)

DRUG	DOSAGE FORMS	ADULT DOSAGE	PEDIATRIC DOSAGE	RELATIVE POTENCY	SIDE EFFECTS	
					Sedation*	Anticholinergic
Carbinoxamine Maleate	Drp 2 mg with pseudoephedrine 25 mg and dextromethorphan 4 mg/mL. Syrup 0.8 mg with pseudoephedrine 12 mg and dextro-methorphan 13 mg/mL (Rondec).	PO 4–8 mg tid-qid.	PO 0.2–0.4 mg/kg/day; (1–3 yr) 2 mg tid-qid; (3–6 yr) 2–4 mg tid-qid; (>6 yr) 4–6 mg tid-qid.	+/++	++	+++
Cetirizine Zyrtec	Tab 5, 10 mg.	PO 10 mg/day.	PO (2–6 yr) 5 mg/day; (6–11 yr) 10 mg/day.	+++	+	±
Chlorpheniramine Maleate Chlor-Trimeton Various	Cap 12 mg SR Cap 8, 12 mg Syrup 0.4 mg/mL Chew Tab 2 mg Tab 4, 8, 12 mg SR Tab 8, 12 mg Inj 10, 100 mg/mL.	PO (acute allergic reactions) 12 mg/day in 1–2 divided doses PO (seasonal allergic rhinitis) 24 mg/day in 1–2 divided doses IV (acute allergic reactions) 5–40 mg/day.	PO (seasonal allergic rhinitis) (2–5 yr) 1 mg tid up to 4 mg/day, SR not recommended; (6–12 yr) 2 mg tid up to 12 mg/day.	++	+	++

(continued)

ANTIHISTAMINES COMPARISON CHART (continued)

DRUG	DOSAGE FORMS	ADULT DOSAGE	PEDIATRIC DOSAGE	RELATIVE POTENCY	SIDE EFFECTS Sedation*	SIDE EFFECTS Anticholinergic
Clemastine **Fumarate** Tavist Various	Syrup 0.13 mg (equivalent to 0.1 mg clemastine)/mL Tab 1.34, 2.68 mg (equivalent to 1 and 2 mg clemastine, respectively).	PO 1.34 mg bid–2.68 mg tid, to a maximum of 8.04 mg/day.	PO (6–12 yr) 0.67–1.34 mg bid, to a maximum of 4.02 mg/day.	++	++	+++
Cyproheptadine HCl Periactin Various	Tab 4 mg Syrup 0.4 mg/mL.	PO 4–20 mg/day, usually 4 mg tid–qid, to a maximum of 0.5 mg/kg/day.	PO (2–6 yr) 2 mg bid–tid, to a maximum of 12 mg/day; (7–14 yr) 4 mg bid–tid, to a maximum of 16 mg/day.	++	+	++
Dexchlorpheniramine **Maleate** Polaramine Various	Syrup 0.4 mg/mL Tab 2 mg SR Tab 4, 6 mg.	PO 2 mg q 4–6 hr, to a maximum of 12 mg/day or SR 4–6 mg hs or q 8–10 hr during the day.	PO (2–5 yr) 0.5 mg q 4–6 hr, to a maximum of 3 mg/day, SR not recommended; (6–11 yr) 1 mg q 4–6 hr or SR 4 mg at hs.	+++	+	++

(continued)

611

ANTIHISTAMINES COMPARISON CHART (continued)

| | | | RELATIVE POTENCY | | SIDE EFFECTS | |
DRUG	DOSAGE FORMS	ADULT DOSAGE	PEDIATRIC DOSAGE		Sedation*	Anticholinergic
Diphenhydramine HCl Benadryl Various	Cap 25, 50 mg Elxr 2.5 mg/mL Syrup 2.5 mg/mL Tab 25, 50 mg Inj 10, 50 mg/mL.	PO (antihistamine) 25–50 mg tid–qid PO (motion sickness) 50 mg 30 min before exposure, ac and hs PO (antitussive) 25 mg q 4 hr PO (nighttime sleep aid) 25–50 mg hs; IM, IV 10–50 mg, to a maximum o 400 mg/dayf	PO (>9 kg) 5 mg/kg/day, usually 12.5–25 mg tid–qid, to a maximum of 300 mg/day PO (antitussive) (6–12 yr) 12.5 mg q 4 hr, to a maximum of 75 mg/day. IM, IV 5 mg/kg, to a maximum of 300 mg/day.	+/++	+++	+++
Fexofenadine Allegra	Cap 60 mg.	PO 60 mg bid.	PO (>12 yr) same as adult dosage.	++	±|	±|

(continued)

ANTIHISTAMINES COMPARISON CHART (continued)

DRUG	DOSAGE FORMS	ADULT DOSAGE	PEDIATRIC DOSAGE	RELATIVE POTENCY	Sedation*	Anticholinergic
Hydroxyzine HCl **Pamoate** Atarax Vistaril Various	Cap (as pamoate equivalent of HCl salt) 25, 50, 100 mg Susp (as pamoate equivalent of HCl salt) 5 mg/mL Syrup (as HCl) 2 mg/mL Tab (as HCl) 10, 25, 50, 100 mg Inj (as HCl) 25, 50 mg/mL.	PO (pruritus) 25 mg tid–qid; (seasonal allergic rhinitis) titrate up to 150 mg/ day in 1–2 divided doses; IM 25–100 mg.	PO (pruritus) (<6 yr) 50 mg/day in 2–3 divided doses; (≥6 yr) 50–100 mg/day in divided doses; (seasonal allergic rhinitis) 25–75 mg/day in 1–2 divided doses IM (perioperative sedation) 0.7 mg/kg/dose; (nausea, vomiting, perioperative adjunctive medication) 1 mg/kg.	+++	++	++
Loratadine Claritin	Tab 10 mg.	PO 10 mg/day.	PO (2–9 yr) 5 mg/day; (>9 yr) 10 mg/day.	+++	±	±
Methdilazine HCl Tacaryl	Syrup 0.8 mg/mL Chew Tab 4 mg (equivalent to 3.6 mg methdilazine) Tab 8 mg.	PO 8 mg bid–qid.	PO (>3 yr) 4 mg bid–qid.	++/+++	+	+++

(continued)

613

ANTIHISTAMINES COMPARISON CHART (continued)

				RELATIVE	SIDE EFFECTS	
DRUG	DOSAGE FORMS	ADULT DOSAGE	PEDIATRIC DOSAGE	POTENCY	Sedation*	Anticholinergic
Promethazine HCl Phenergan Various	Syrup 1.25, 5 mg/mL Tab 12.5, 25, 50 mg Inj 25, 50 mg/mL Supp 12.5, 25, 50 mg	PO (allergy) 25 mg hs or 12.5 mg ac and hs; (nausea and vomiting) 25 mg initial dose, then 12.5–25 mg q 4–6 hr prn; (adjunctive preoperative use) 25–50 mg/dose IM, IV (IV maximum concentration 25 mg/mL, maximum rate 25 mg/min) or PR (allergy) 25 mg, may repeat in 2 hr; (nausea and vomiting) 12.5–25 mg q 4 hr prn; (adjunctive pre- and postoperative use) 25–50 mg/dose.	PO (allergy) 6.25–12.5 mg qid; (motion sickness or sedation) 12.5–25 mg bid IM, IV or PR (PR not recommended <2 yr); (allergy) 0.5 mg/kg/day in 4 divided doses; (adjunctive preoperative use) 1 mg/kg/dose, maximum dosage not to exceed one-half of adult dosage.	+++	++++	++++
Pyrilamine Maleate Various	Tab 25 mg.	PO (allergy) 25–50 mg tid–qid.	PO (<6 yr) safety and efficacy not established; (6–12 yr) 12.5–25 mg q 8 hr.	+/++	+	±1

(continued)

ANTIHISTAMINES COMPARISON CHART (continued)

DRUG	DOSAGE FORMS	ADULT DOSAGE	PEDIATRIC DOSAGE	RELATIVE POTENCY	SIDE EFFECTS Sedation*	SIDE EFFECTS Anticholinergic
Terfenadine Seldane	Tab 60 mg.	PO 60 mg bid.	PO (3–5 yr) 15 mg bid; (6–12 yr) 30–60 mg bid.	++	±	±
Trimeprazine Tartrate Temaril	SR Cap 5 mg Syrup 0.5 mg/mL Tab 2.5 mg.	PO 2.5 mg qid SR 5 mg q 12 hr.	PO (2–3 yr) 1.25 mg hs or tid prn; (>3 yr) 2.5 mg hs or tid prn SR not recommended <6 yr; (≥6 yr) 5 mg/day.	++/+++	++	+++
Tripelennamine HCl PBZ Various	Elxr 7.5 mg (citrate salt equivalent to 5 mg HCl)/mL Tab 25, 50 mg SR Tab 100 mg.	PO 25–50 mg q 4–6 hr, to a maximum of 600 mg/day.	PO 5 mg/kg/day in 4–6 divided doses, to a maximum of 300 mg/day SR not recommended.	+/++	++	±

(continued)

| | | | | | SIDE EFFECTS | |
| | | | | RELATIVE | | |
DRUG	DOSAGE FORMS	ADULT DOSAGE	PEDIATRIC DOSAGE	POTENCY	Sedation*	Anticholinergic
Triprolidine HCl Myidil	Syrup 1.25 mg/ 5 mL. Tab 2.5 mg with pseudoephedrine 60 mg (Actifed).	PO 2.5 mg q 4–6 hr, to a maximum of 10 mg/day.	PO (4 months–2 yr) 0.3 mg tid–qid; (2–5 yr) 0.625 mg tid–qid; (6–12 yr) 1.25 mg q 4–6 hr, to a maximum of 4 doses/day.	++/+++	++	++

+++++ = very high; +++ = high; ++ = moderate; + = low; ± = low to none
*Tolerance usually develops during long-term therapy.
From references 36, 50–54, and product information.

Bronchodilators

Class Instructions: Antiasthmatic Inhalers. Attach the mouthpiece to the spacer device (which slows the rate of inhalation and thereby increases penetration into airways). To use the inhaler, tilt head up and place mouthpiece of spacer device into mouth, making sure the teeth and tongue are not in the way. While inhaling slowly and deeply, release one dose of aerosolized medication, inhale, remove inhaler from mouth, and hold breath for 5–10 seconds. Wait at least 1 minute between puffs. Do not exceed prescribed dosage. Report if symptoms do not completely clear or the inhaler is required more than prescribed. Clean mouthpiece weekly with hot water and soap. Store away from heat and direct sunlight. Bronchodilators may cause nervousness, tremors (especially with terbutaline or albuterol), or rapid heart rate. Report if these effects continue after dosage reduction; if chest pain, dizziness, or headache occur; or if asthmatic symptoms are not relieved.

ALBUTEROL SULFATE
Epaq, Proventil, Ventolin, Volmax, Various

Pharmacology. Albuterol is a selective β_2-adrenergic agonist that produces bronchodilation, vasodilation, uterine relaxation, skeletal muscle stimulation, peripheral vasodilation, and tachycardia.[55,56]

Administration and Adult Dosage. **Inhal for asthma** (metered-dose inhaler) 90–180 µg (1–2 puffs), with 1–5 min between inhalations, q 4–6 hr prn and just before exercise;[56,57] (inhal soln) 2.5 mg by nebulization tid–qid; (inhal caps) 1–2 inhalation caps q 4–6 hr or 1 cap 15 min prior to exercise. **Inhal for severe bronchospasm** nebulized by compressed air or oxygen 2.5–5 mg (0.5–1 mL of 0.5% in 2–3 mL NS) q 4–6 hr prn (q 1–2 hr under medical supervision).[56,57] **PO for asthma** 2–4 mg q 6–8 hr, increase as tolerated to a maximum of 32 mg/day; **SR Tab** 4–8 mg q 12 hr to a maximum of 32 mg/day.

Special Populations. *Pediatric Dosage.* **Inhal for asthma** (metered-dose inhaler) (<12 yr) 90–180 µg (1–2 puffs) q 4–6 hr using spacer; (≥12 yr) same as adult dosage; (inhal soln) (<12 yr) 0.05–0.15 mg/kg q 4–6 hr prn, or (<20 kg) 0.25 mL of 0.5% solution; (>20 kg) 0.5 mL of 0.5% solution to a maximum of 1 mL diluted in 2–3 mL NS q 4–6 hr prn (q 1–2 hr for severe bronchospasm under medical supervision); (≥12 yr) same as adult dosage. **PO for asthma** (2–6 yr) 100–200 µg/kg/dose q 8 hr, to a maximum of 4 mg q 8 hr; (6–12 yr) 2 mg q 6–8 hr, to a maximum of 24 mg/day; (>12 yr) same as adult dosage. **SR Tab** (<12 yr) dosage not established; (>12 yr) same as adult dosage.

Geriatric Dosage. **Inhal for asthma** same as adult dosage. **PO** 2 mg tid–qid initially, increasing prn to a maximum of 8 mg tid–qid.

Dosage Forms. **Inhal** (metered-dose) 90 µg/puff (200 puffs/inhaler); **Inhal Soln** 0.5% (5 mg/mL), (unit dose soln, 3 mL) 0.083%; **Inhal Cap** (Rotacap) 200 µg for use with powder inhaler; **Tab** 2, 4 mg; **Syrup** 0.4 mg/mL; **SR Tab** 4, 8 mg. **Inhal** 90 µg plus ipratropium bromide 18 µg/puff (Combivent).

Patient Instructions. (*See* Antiasthmatic Inhalers Class Instructions.)

Pharmacokinetics. *Onset and Duration.* (Inhal) Onset within 15 min, peak 60–90 min or less; (PO) onset 30–60 min, peak 2–3 hr. Duration 4–6 hr, depending on the dose, dosage form, and clinical condition (*see* Sympathomimetic Bronchodilators Comparison Chart).

Fate. Peak serum level after 0.15 mg/kg by inhalation is 5.6 µg/L (23 nmol/L). Oral bioavailability is 50% because of hepatic first-pass metabolism; peak after 4-mg tab is 10 µg/L (42 nmol/L) in the liver; 50% is excreted in urine as an inactive sulfate conjugate. The drug does not appear to be metabolized in the lung.[58]

$t_{1/2}$. (IV) 2–3 hr; apparent half-life is 5–6 hr after oral and up to 7 hr after inhalation because of prolonged absorption.[59]

Adverse Reactions. Dose-related reflex tachycardia from peripheral vasodilation and from direct stimulation of cardiac β_2-receptors.[56,57] Tremor, palpitations, and nausea are other dose-related effects that are markedly reduced with aerosol administration. All β_2-agonists lower serum potassium concentrations.

Precautions. Pregnancy; cardiac disorders including coronary insufficiency and hypertension; diabetes. Excessive or prolonged use may lead to tolerance.

Drug Interactions. Concurrent β-blockers may antagonize effects.

Parameters to Monitor. Inhalation technique, asthma symptoms, frequency of use, pulmonary function, and heart rate.

Notes. A relationship between regular (ie, not prn) use of inhaled β_2-agonists and death from asthma has been a concern.[60,61] Regardless of whether β_2-agonists are directly responsible or are simply a marker for more severe asthma, heavy use (over 1 canister/month or 12 puffs/day) of these agents should alert clinicians that it is necessary to reevaluate the patient's condition. Epaq and Proventil HFA inhalers use a non-CFC propellant; drug delivery is similar, but not identical, to Ventolin and Proventil.

ATROPINE SULFATE   Various

Pharmacology. Atropine is a competitive antagonist of acetylcholine at peripheral muscarinic and central receptors, causing an increase in heart rate and decreased salivary secretion, GI motility, sweating, urinary bladder contractibility, and bronchodilation.

Administration and Adult Dosage. **PO, SC, IM, or IV for GI anticholinergic effect** 400–600 µg qid (with meals and hs); **SC, IM, or IV for preanesthetic medication** 300–600 µg about 1 hr before induction. **Inhal as a bronchodilator** 0.025–0.05 mg/kg q 4–6 hr diluted to 2–3 mL with NS and delivered by compressed air nebulizer.[62] **Ophthalmic for mydriasis or uveitis** 1–2 drops of 1% (10 mg/mL) soln (up to tid for uveitis).

Special Populations. *Pediatric Dosage.* **PO or SC for general use** 10 µg/kg q 4–6 hr; **Inhal as a bronchodilator** 0.05–0.075 mg/kg q 4–6 hr diluted to 2–3 mL with NS and delivered by compressed air nebulizer.[62]

Geriatric Dosage. Same as adult dosage, although the elderly may be more sensitive to adverse reactions.

Dosage Forms. **Inj** 0.1, 0.4, 0.5, 1 mg/mL; **Ophth Oint** 1%; **Ophth Soln** 1%.

Patient Instructions. This drug may cause dry mouth, constipation, urinary retention, blurring of vision, increased sensitivity to light, or drowsiness. Until the extent of these latter effects is known, use caution when driving, operating machinery, or performing other tasks requiring mental alertness. Avoid excessive concurrent use of alcohol and other drugs that cause drowsiness.

Pharmacokinetics. *Onset and Duration.* (Inhal) onset 3–5 min; peak 1–2 hr; duration 3–4 hr, dose dependent.[62]

Fate. Rapidly and completely absorbed from the GI tract, IM injection sites, and following inhalation.[63] Oral bioavailability is about 50%.[8] Only 10–15% of a nebulizer dose is effectively delivered to the lung. Plasma protein binding is 14–22%; V_d is 2 ± 1.1 L/kg; Cl is 0.48 ± 0.24 L/hr/kg.[8] Approximately 50% is excreted unchanged in urine; the remainder is metabolized.[64]

$t_{1/2}$. 3.5 ± 1.5 hr in healthy volunteers;[8,64] greater in infants, children, and the elderly.[65]

Adverse Reactions. Toxic effects are dose related and frequent, especially in children. Atropine may accumulate and produce systemic effects after multiple doses by inhalation in the elderly.[66] The following may occur in adults: at 0.5 mg, slight dryness of nose and mouth, bradycardia, and inhibition of sweating (may lead to fever); at 1 mg, definite dryness of nose and mouth, thirst, acceleration of heart rate (possibly preceded by slowing), and slight mydriasis; at 2 mg, marked dry mouth, tachycardia, palpitation, mydriasis, slight blurring of near vision, and flushed and dry skin; at 5 mg, increase in above symptoms, plus speech disturbance, swallowing difficulty, headache, hot and dry skin, and restlessness with asthenia; at >10 mg, above symptoms in the extreme, ataxia, excitement, disorientation, hallucinations, delirium, and coma.

Contraindications. Narrow-angle glaucoma; adhesions (synechiae) between the iris and lens of the eye; obstructive disease of GI tract; obstructive uropathy; intestinal atony; megacolon complicating ulcerative colitis; hiatal hernia with reflux esophagitis; unstable cardiovascular status in acute hemorrhage; tachycardia; myasthenia gravis.

Precautions. Pregnancy; patients >40 yr, particularly those with any severe heart disease, hypertension, ulcerative colitis, ileus, chronic lung disease, hyperthyroidism, autonomic neuropathy, hepatic or renal disease, or prostatic hypertrophy (these latter patients may experience urinary hesitancy, and should micturate at the time of administration). Overdosage may cause a curarelike action. The elderly may be at increased risk for confusion and hallucinations.

Drug Interactions. Anticholinergics may be potentiated by amantadine and may antagonize tacrine.

Parameters to Monitor. Monitor for anticholinergic symptoms.

Notes. As an inhaled bronchodilator, atropine is less effective than the β_2-adrenergic agents, but may produce additive bronchodilation with these drugs during acute asthma attacks. However, the quaternary compounds (eg, ipratropium) are preferred because of their decreased systemic absorption and longer duration of action.[62] Atropine may be combined directly with β_2-adrenergic agents in the nebulizer.

IPRATROPIUM BROMIDE   Atrovent

Pharmacology. Ipratropium is a competitive antagonist of acetylcholine at peripheral muscarinic receptors, but not centrally because of its quaternary structure.[67] It is used primarily as a bronchodilator in COPD, emphysema, and bronchitis.

Administration and Adult Dosage. Inhal for bronchospasm of COPD (including chronic bronchitis) 36–72 µg (2–4 puffs) qid by metered-dose inhaler, to a maximum of 288 µg (16 puffs)/day.[62,67] **Inhal for acute, severe asthma** 250–500 µg by nebulizer has been used.[68] **Nasal spray for rhinorrhea of perennial rhinitis** 2 sprays (84 µg)/nostril of 0.03% solution bid–tid; **Nasal spray for rhinorrhea of the common cold** 2 sprays (84 µg)/nostril tid–qid for up to 4 days.

Special Populations. *Pediatric Dosage.* (<12 yr.) safety and efficacy not established. **Inhal** (<2 yr) 125 µg/dose by nebulizer;[69] (>2 yr) 18–36 µg (1–2 puffs) q 6–8 hr by metered-dose inhaler or 250 µg q 6–8 hr by nebulizer has been used.[62,68,70]

Geriatric Dosage. Same as adult dosage.

Dosage Forms. **Inhal** 18 µg/puff (200 doses/inhaler); **Inhal Sol** 200 µg/mL (500 µg/vial). **Nasal Spray** 0.03, 0.06%. **Inhal** 18 µg plus 90 µg albuterol/puff (Combivent).

Patient Instructions. (*See* Antiasthmatic Inhalers Class Instructions.) Temporary blurring of vision may occur if the drug is sprayed into eyes.

Pharmacokinetics. *Onset and Duration.* Onset 3 min; peak 1–2 hr;[62] duration 4–6 hr, depending on intensity of response.[71]

Fate. Only 32% or less is orally absorbed and less than 1% of inhaled dose is absorbed.[62] Metabolized to 8 metabolites, which are excreted in the urine and bile.

$t_{1/2}$. 1.5–4 hr.[62]

Adverse Reactions. Dryness of the mouth. Because of quaternary nature of the molecule, typical systemic anticholinergic side effects are absent.[62,71] With the nasal spray, epistaxis, nasal dryness, dry mouth, or throat and nasal congestion occur in 1–10% of patients. During long-term use, headache, nausea, and upper respiratory tract infections also occur frequently.

Contraindications. (Aerosol inhaler) hypersensitivity to soy lecithin, soybeans, or related products.

Precautions. Use with caution in narrow-angle glaucoma, prostatic hypertrophy, or bladder neck obstruction.

Drug Interactions. None known.

Parameters to Monitor. Inhalation technique, asthma symptoms, frequency of use, pulmonary function, and anticholinergic symptoms.

Notes. Anticholinergics appear to be as potent bronchodilators as ß$_2$-adrenergic drugs in bronchitis and emphysema, but less potent in asthma.[62,67] Anticholinergics produce an additive bronchodilation with ß$_2$-adrenergic agents in severe asthma.[62,70]

SALMETEROL XINAFOATE   Serevent

Salmeterol is a β_2-agonist structurally and pharmacologically similar to albuterol. It produces bronchodilation for at least 12 hr following inhalation of a single 50-μg dose. After inhalation, salmeterol is extensively metabolized by hydroxylation, with the majority of a dose being eliminated within 72 hr. About 23% of administered radioactivity was recovered in the urine and 57% in the feces over a period of 168 hr. Onset of effective bronchodilation is achieved in 20–30 min; peak effect occurs within 3–4 hr. Salmeterol is intended for regular bid treatment of reversible airway obstruction and *not* for immediate symptomatic relief. The place of salmeterol in asthma therapy is being debated, in part because patients in need of regular β_2-agonist therapy should be regarded as candidates for an inhaled corticosteroid to treat underlying inflammation. Salmeterol dosages of 50 or 100 μg bid have been well tolerated in clinical trials. The usual dosage for adults and geriatric patients with mild to moderate asthma is 42 μg (2 puffs) bid by metered-dose inhaler. To prevent exercise-induced bronchospasm, inhale 2 puffs 30–60 min before exercise. Safety and efficacy in children <12 yr have not been established.[72] (*See* Sympathomimetic Bronchodilators Comparison Chart.) Available as metered-dose aerosol for inhalation 21 μg/puff in 6.5-g (60 actuations) and 13-g (120 actuations) canisters.

SYMPATHOMIMETIC BRONCHODILATORS COMPARISON CHART

		DOSAGE		RECEPTOR SELECTIVITY[b]		RELATIVE	DURATION OF ACTION
DRUG	DOSAGE FORMS	Adult	Pediatric[a]	β_1	β_2	β_2 POTENCY[c]	BY INHALATION (HR)
Albuterol Proventil Ventolin Volmax Various	Inhal (soln) 0.5%; (unit dose) 0.083%, (metered-dose) 0.09 mg/puff; (Rotacaps) 200 µg/cap SR Tab 4, 8 mg Syrup 0.4 mg/mL Tab 2, 4 mg.	Inhal (soln) 2.5–5 mg in 2–3 mL NS q 4–6 hr prn by nebulizer; may use q 1–2 hr prn status asthmaticus under medical supervision; (metered-dose) 1–2 puffs q 4–6 hr prn and prior to exercise; 1 Rotacap is equivalent to 2 metered-dose puffs PO 2–4 mg q 6–8 hr, to a maximum of 32 mg/day SR 4–8 mg q 12 hr to a maximum of 32 mg/day.	Inhal (soln) 0.05–0.15 mg/kg in 2–3 mL NS q 4–6 hr prn by nebulizer, may use q 1–2 hr prn or 0.5 mg/kg/hr continuously nebulized for status asthmaticus under medical supervision; (metered-dose) 1–2 puffs q 4–6 hr prn and prior to exercise PO 0.1–0.2 mg/kg q 6–8 hr to a maximum of 24 mg/day.	+	++++	5	4–6

(continued)

SYMPATHOMIMETIC BRONCHODILATORS COMPARISON CHART (continued)

DRUG	DOSAGE FORMS	DOSAGE Adult	DOSAGE Pediatric[a]	RECEPTOR SELECTIVITY[b] β_1	RECEPTOR SELECTIVITY[b] β_2	RELATIVE β_2 POTENCY[c]	DURATION OF ACTION BY INHALATION (HR)
Bitolterol[e] Tornalate Produral	Inhal (metered-dose) 0.37 mg/puff; (soln) 0.2%.	Inhal (metered-dose) 1–3 puffs q 4–6 hr prn.	Inhal (metered-dose) 1–2 puffs q 4–6 hr prn.	+	++++	2.5	4–8
Epinephrine Adrenalin Various	Inhal (soln) 1, 1.25, 2.25% (racemic) Inj 0.01, 0.1, 1 mg/mL.	See monograph.	See monograph.	+++	+++	5	0.5–2
Epinephrine Aq Suspension Sus-Phrine	Inj 500 μg/mL.	SC 0.5–1.5 mg q 6–10 hr.	SC 0.005 mL/kg q 6–10 hr.	+++	+++	5	0.5–2 (SC)
Isoetharine Bronkometer Bronkosol Various	Inhal (soln) 0.062, 0.08, 0.1, 0.125, 0.17, 0.2, 0.25, 0.5, 1%; (metered-dose) 340 μg/puff.	Inhal (soln) 2.5–10 mg diluted 1:3 in NS q 2–4 hr prn; (metered-dose) 1–2 puffs q 4–6 hr prn.	Inhal (soln) 0.1–0.2 mg/kg q 2–4 hr prn; (metered-dose) 1–2 puffs q 4–6 hr prn.	++	+++	1.7	0.5–2

(continued)

623

SYMPATHOMIMETIC BRONCHODILATORS COMPARISON CHART (continued)

DRUG	DOSAGE FORMS	DOSAGE Adult	DOSAGE Pediatric[a]	RECEPTOR SELECTIVITY[b] β_1	RECEPTOR SELECTIVITY[b] β_2	RELATIVE β_2 POTENCY[c]	DURATION OF ACTION BY INHALATION (HR)
Isoproterenol Isuprel Various	Inhal (soln) 0.25, 0.5, 1%; (metered-dose) 80, 131 µg/puff Inj 0.2 mg/mL SL Tab 10, 15 mg.	Not recommended because of short duration and lack of selectivity.		++++	++++	10	0.5–2
Metaproterenol Alupent Metaprel Various	Inhal (soln) 0.4% (unit dose 10 mg), 0.6% (unit dose 15 mg), 5%; (metered-dose) 0.65 mg/puff Syrup 2 mg/mL Tab 10, 20 mg.	Inhal (soln) 5–15 mg q 2–4 hr prn (q 1–2 hr under medical supervision); (metered-dose) 1–3 puffs q 4–6 hr prn and prior to exercise. PO 20 mg 3–4 times/day.	Inhal (soln) 0.25–0.5 mg/kg up to 15 mg q 2–4 hr prn; (metered-dose) 1–2 puffs prn and prior to exercise. PO 0.5 mg/kg q 4–6 hr, increase by 0.25 mg/kg as tolerated.	++	++	1	3–4

(continued)

SYMPATHOMIMETIC BRONCHODILATORS COMPARISON CHART (continued)

DRUG	DOSAGE FORMS	DOSAGE Adult	DOSAGE Pediatric[a]	RECEPTOR SELECTIVITY[b] β_1	RECEPTOR SELECTIVITY[b] β_2	RELATIVE β_2 POTENCY[c]	DURATION OF ACTION BY INHALATION (HR)
Pirbuterol Maxair	Inhal (metered-dose) 0.2 mg/puff.	Inhal 1–2 puffs q 4–6 hr and prior to exercise.	Inhal 1–2 puffs q 4–6 hr prm and prior to exercise.	+	++++	2.5	4–8
Salmeterol Serevent	Inhal (metered-dose) 21 µg/puff.	Inhal 2 puffs q 12 hr.[f]	(<12 yr) not established ; (≥12 yr) same as adult dosage.	+	++++	20	12
Terbutaline Brethaire Brethine	Inhal (metered-dose) 0.2 mg/puff Inj 1 mg/mL	Inhal 1–3 puffs q 4–6 hr prm; 5–7 mg undiluted by nebulizer q 4–6	Inhal 1–2 puffs q 4–6 hr prm; 0.1–0.3 mg/kg	+	++++	2.5	4–8

(continued)

SYMPATHOMIMETIC BRONCHODILATORS COMPARISON CHART (continued)

DRUG	DOSAGE FORMS	DOSAGE Adult[a]	DOSAGE Pediatric[a]	RECEPTOR SELECTIVITY[b] β₁	RECEPTOR SELECTIVITY[b] β₂	RELATIVE β₂ POTENCY[c]	DURATION OF ACTION BY INHALATION (HR)
Bricanyl	Tab 2.5, 5 mg.	hr prn[g] SC 0.25–0.5 mg q 2–6 hr prn PO 5 mg q 6–8 hr IV for preterm labor 10 μg/min, increased prn up to 80 μg/min for 4 hr, then PO for preterm labor (maintenance) 2.5 mg q 4–6 hr until term[h]	q 4–6 hr prn (q 1–2 hr under medical supervision)[e] SC 0.01 mg/kg up to 0.25 mg q 2–6 hr prn PO 0.075 mg/kg q 6–8 hr.				

[a]Isoproterenol and isoetharine are the only metered-dose aerosols labeled for use in children <12 yr.

[b]β₂-selectivity does not equate to bronchoselectivity; β₂-stimulation produces reflex tachycardia from vasodilation as well as stimulation of cardiac β₂-receptors.

[c]Molar potency relative to metaproterenol; large numbers indicate more potent compounds.

[d]Onset and duration data apply to aerosol therapy only. Duration of bronchodilation only applies to otherwise stable asthmatics and is not applicable to acute severe asthma or protection from severe provocation (eg, allergen, exercise, ozone). Duration may be shorter during acute exacerbation or with long-term therapy because of down-regulation of β-receptors (tolerance). Oral tablets (especially SR tablets) and syrups are slower in onset, but may be slightly longer acting than aerosols.

[e]Bitolterol is a prodrug converted in the body to **colterol**, the active drug, which is more potent than isoproterenol; the relative potency value because of incomplete conversion.

[f]For prophylaxis only; acute attacks must be treated with a short-acting agent.

[g]Use injectable solution; not a labeled indication.

[h]Preterm labor is not a labeled indication.

From references 56, 57, and 72.

THEOPHYLLINE

Theo-Dur, Slo-bid, Various

Pharmacology. Theophylline directly relaxes smooth muscle of bronchial airways and pulmonary blood vessels to act as a bronchodilator and pulmonary vasodilator. It is also a diuretic, coronary vasodilator, cardiac stimulant, and cerebral stimulant; it improves diaphragmatic contractility; and it lessens diaphragmatic fatigue. The exact cellular mechanism of smooth muscle relaxation is unknown, but intracellular calcium sequestration, inhibition of specific phosphodiesterase isozymes, adenosine receptor antagonism, and stimulation of endogenous catecholamine release have all been postulated to play a role.[73] **Aminophylline** is the ethylenediamine salt of theophylline.

Administration and Adult Dosage. **PO (theophylline) or IV (aminophylline) loading dose for acute asthma symptoms** 5 mg/kg (6 mg/kg aminophylline), if patient has taken no theophylline in previous 24 hr. In emergencies, 2.5 mg/kg (3 mg/kg aminophylline) may be given if an immediate serum level cannot be obtained. Each 1 mg/kg (1.25 mg/kg aminophylline) results in about a 2 mg/L increase in serum theophylline. Infuse IV aminophylline no faster than 25 mg/min. **Maintenance Dosage** (*see* Mean Clearances and Maintenance Dosages Comparison Chart). **PO for chronic asthma** (theophylline) initial dosage 400 mg/day in divided doses, then increase if tolerated in approximately 25% increments at 3-day intervals to 13 mg/kg/day or 900 mg/day, whichever is less. Use serum concentrations for subsequent dosage adjustment. For patients with CHF, liver dysfunction, or cor pulmonale, initial dosage must not exceed 400 mg/day unless serum levels are measured.[74,75] **IM PR suppositories not recommended.**

Special Populations. (*See* Mean Clearances and Maintenance Dosages Comparison Chart.) All dosage recommendations are based on the average theophylline clearance for a given population group. There is a wide interpatient variability (often greater than twofold) within all patient groups.[74–76] Therefore, it is essential that serum concentrations be monitored in all patients. If no doses have been missed or extra doses taken during the previous 48 hr, and if peak serum concentrations have been obtained (1–2 hr after liquid or plain uncoated tablet and 4–6 hr after most SR products), adjust dosage using Theophylline Dosage Adjustment Guide, which follows.

Pediatric Dosage. **PO or IV (infused over 20–30 min) for acute symptoms** same as adult dosage in mg/kg. **PO for chronic asthma** (theophylline) initial dosage (6–24 weeks) 8 mg/kg/day; (>24 weeks) 16 mg/kg/day or 400 mg/day (whichever is less) in divided doses; then increase, if tolerated, in approximately 25% increments at 3-day intervals to (6 weeks–1 yr) 0.2 × (age in weeks) + 5 mg/kg/day; (1–9 yr) 22 mg/kg/day; (9–12 yr) 20 mg/kg/day; (12–16 yr) 18 mg/kg/day; (>16 yr) 13 mg/kg/day.[74,76] **IM, PR suppositories not recommended.**

Geriatric Dosage. Not established; however, the elderly as a group have slower hepatic clearance. Therefore, use lower initial doses and monitor closely for response and adverse reactions.

Other Conditions. Many factors can alter theophylline dosage requirements (*see* Precautions). Use ideal body weight for dosage calculations in obese patients.[74]

THEOPHYLLINE DOSAGE ADJUSTMENT GUIDE	
SERUM CONCENTRATION (MG/L)*	ACTION†
Therapeutic	
10–20‡	Maintain dosage if tolerated; recheck serum level at 6- to 12-month intervals.
Too High	
20–25	Decrease dosage by 10%.
25–30	Skip next dose and decrease subsequent doses by 25%; recheck level.
Over 30	Skip next 2 doses and decrease subsequent doses by 50%; recheck level.
Too Low	
7.5–10	Increase dosage by 25%.
5–7.5	Increase dosage by 25%; recheck level.

*Appropriately measured peak (*see* Special Populations).
†Increase dosage only in patients whose condition is not well controlled.
‡Recent guidelines suggest that 5–15 mg/L may be a more appropriate range.[78]
From references 74, 76–78.

Dosage Forms. (*See* Theophylline Products Comparison Chart.)

Patient Instructions. Do not chew or crush sustained-release tablets or capsules. Take at equally spaced intervals around the clock. Report any nausea, vomiting, gastrointestinal pain, headache, or restlessness. Contents of sustained-release bead-filled capsules may be mixed with a vehicle (applesauce or jam) and swallowed without chewing for patients who have difficulty swallowing capsules. Take Theo-24 and Uniphyl products at least 1 hour before meals to avoid too rapid absorption of the drug.[79]

Pharmacokinetics. *Onset and Duration.* IV onset within 15 min with loading dose.[73]

Serum Levels. Well correlated with clinical effects: therapeutic is 10–20 mg/L (56–111 μmol/L);[73–75] however, improvement in respiratory function can be observed with serum concentrations of 5 mg/L (28 μmol/L).[78] A serum concentration of 5–10 mg/L is often adequate for treatment of neonatal apnea. Toxicity increases over 20 mg/L (*see* Adverse Reactions). Saliva concentration is an unreliable predictor of serum concentration.[74]

Fate. Plain uncoated tablets and solution are well absorbed orally; enteric-coated tablets and some SR dosage forms may be unreliably absorbed. Food may affect the rate and extent of absorption of some SR formulations, but has minimal effects on rapid-release forms. Food may either increase the rate of absorption (Theo-24, Uniphyl), producing dose dumping, or impair absorption (Theo-Dur Sprinkle).[75,79] Rectal suppository absorption is slow and erratic and suppositories (including aminophylline) are not recommended under any circumstances.[74,75] Rectal solutions may result in serum concentrations comparable to oral solution. About 60% is plasma protein bound (less in neonates); V_d is 0.5 ± 0.1 L/kg (greater in neonates). There may be marked intrapatient variability in clearance over time.[75] Cl is also affected by many factors (*see* Precautions). Smoking increases theophylline metabolism; this effect may last for 3 months to 2 yr after cessation of smoking.[74] Clearance progressively increases in infants during the first year of life.[75] Dose-dependent pharmacokinetics in therapeutic range occur often in children and rarely in adults.[75] In the elderly, clearance declines with age to about 35 mL/hr/kg.[80] Extensively metabolized in the liver to several inactive metabolites; 10% excreted unchanged in the urine.[75]

$t_{1/2}$. 8 ± 2 hr in adult nonsmokers, 4.4 ± 1 hr in adult smokers (1–2 packs per day); 3.7 ± 1.1 hr in children 1–9 yr. Newborn infants, older patients with COPD or cor pulmonale, and patients with CHF or liver disease may have a half-life >24 hr.

Adverse Reactions. Local GI irritation may occur. Reactions occur more frequently at serum concentrations >20 mg/L and include anorexia, nausea, vomiting, epigastric pain, diarrhea, restlessness, irritability, insomnia, and headache. Serious arrhythmias and convulsions (frequently leading to death or permanent brain damage) usually occur at levels >35 mg/L, but have occurred at lower concentrations and may *not* be preceded by less serious toxicity; cardiovascular reactions include sinus tachycardia and life-threatening ventricular arrhythmias with PVCs.[81] Rapid IV administration may be associated with hypotension, syncope, cardiac arrest (particularly if administered directly into central line), and death.[81] IM administration is painful and offers no advantage.

Contraindications. Active peptic ulcer disease; untreated seizure disorder. (Aminophylline) hypersensitivity to ethylenediamine.

Precautions. Use with caution in severe cardiac disease, hypoxemia, hepatic disease, acute myocardial injury, cor pulmonale, CHF, fever, viral illness, underlying seizure disorder, migraine, hepatic cirrhosis, and neonates. Do not give with other xanthine preparations. The alcohol in some oral liquid preparations may cause side effects in infants.

Drug Interactions. Numerous drugs and conditions can alter theophylline clearance and serum levels. Factors that can decrease serum levels include carbamazepine, charcoal-broiled beef, high-protein/low-carbohydrate diet, isoproterenol (IV), phenytoin, rifampin, and smoking. Factors that can increase serum levels include allopurinol (>600 mg/day), cimetidine, ciprofloxacin, cor pulmonale, macrolides (eg, erythromycin, troleandomycin), oral contraceptives, and propranolol.

Parameters to Monitor. (Inpatients) Obtain serum theophylline concentrations before starting therapy (if patient previously taking theophylline) and 1, 6, and 24 hr after start of infusion; Monitor daily during continuous infusion.[76] (Outpatients) Monitor serum concentrations q 6 months, 3–5 days after any dosage change, and whenever there are symptoms of toxicity.[74–76]

Notes. The oral theophylline preparations of choice for long-term use, to achieve both sustained therapeutic concentrations and improved compliance, are completely and slowly absorbed SR formulations that are minimally affected by food and pH[79] (*see* Theophylline Products Comparison Chart). Combination products containing **ephedrine** increase CNS toxicity and have no therapeutic advantage over adequate serum concentrations of theophylline alone.[74] **Dyphylline** is chemically related to, but not a salt of, theophylline; the amount of dyphylline equivalent to theophylline is unknown. Because its potency is less than theophylline and it has a short half-life (2 hr), its dosage is greater than theophylline and it must be given more frequently.[74]

MEAN CLEARANCES AND MAINTENANCE DOSAGES COMPARISON CHART

POPULATION GROUP	THEOPHYLLINE CLEARANCE (L/HR/KG)	ORAL THEOPHYLLINE* (MG/KG/DAY)	IV AMINOPHYLLINE[†] (MG/KG/HR)
Newborn up to 24 days (for apnea/bradycardia)	0.0174 ± 0.006	2	0.1
Newborn 24 days and older (for apnea/bradycardia)	0.0384 ± 0.018	3	0.15
Infants 6 weeks–1 yr	0.066 ± 0.028	0.2 x (age in weeks) + 5	0.05 x calculated daily theophylline
Children 1–9 yr	0.102 ± 0.036	22	1
Children 9–12 yr, adolescent daily smokers of cigarettes or marijuana, and otherwise healthy adult smokers <50 yr	0.093 ± 0.022	20	0.83
Adolescents 12–16 yr (nonsmokers)	0.077 ± 0.02	13	0.68
Otherwise healthy nonsmoking adults (including elderly patients)	0.052 ± 0.021	13	0.52
Cardiac decompensation, cor pulmonale, and/or liver dysfunction[‡]	0.026 ± 0.015	5	0.26

*To maintain a serum concentration of 10 mg/L (5 mg/L for newborn apnea/bradycardia). Dosage interval is dependent on preparation used.
[†]Aminophylline USP contains 80% anhydrous theophylline. Final infusion rate determined by serum concentration monitoring of theophylline.
[‡]Accumulation may occur over 5–7 days; do not exceed 400 mg/day unless serum concentrations are monitored.
From reference 74.

THEOPHYLLINE PRODUCTS COMPARISON CHART[a]

PRODUCT	ANHYDROUS THEOPHYLLINE CONTENT	MEASURABLE DOSE INCREMENT[b] (MG)	COMMENTS
RAPIDLY ABSORBED			
Plain Uncoated Tablets			
Various	Tab 100 mg scored.	50	Serum level fluctuations are 459%/117%.[c]
	Tab 125 mg scored.	62.5	
	Tab 200 mg scored.	100	
	Tab 250 mg scored.	125	
	Tab 300 mg scored.	150	
Oral Liquids (Alcohol-Free)			
Aerolate	10 mg/mL.	5	Sugar-free.
Somophyllin	18 mg/mL.	9	Contains aminophylline;[d] sugar-free.
Slo-Phyllin 80 Syrup	5.3 mg/mL.	5	Sugar-free.
Intravenous Solution			
Aminophylline[d]	20 mg/mL.	5	Use rubber stoppered vials to avoid glass particles from the breaking of ampules.
Theophylline	0.4, 0.8, 1.6, 2, 3.2, 4 mg/mL.	—	Available in large volume solutions only.
SLOW-RELEASE PRODUCTS[e]			
Somophyllin—CRT	Cap 100 mg.	50	Beads can be sprinkled on a small amount of food;
	Cap 200 mg.	100	serum level fluctuations are 130%/47%;[c] may require q 8 hr
	Cap 300 mg.	150	administration in children.

(continued)

THEOPHYLLINE PRODUCTS COMPARISON CHART[a] (continued)

PRODUCT	ANHYDROUS THEOPHYLLINE CONTENT	MEASURABLE DOSE INCREMENT[b] (MG)	COMMENTS
Slo-bid Gyrocaps	Cap 50 mg. Cap 75 mg. Cap 100 mg. Cap 125 mg. Cap 200 mg. Cap 300 mg.	25	Excellent bioavailability in young infants; beads can be sprinkled on small amount of food; serum level fluctuations are 43%/18%.[c]
Quibron-T/SR Dividose	Tab 300 mg multiscored (100, 150, 200, 300 mg).	100	Serum level fluctuations are 128%/46%;[c] may require q 8 hr administration in children.
Theo-Dur	Tab 100 mg scored. Tab 200 mg scored. Tab 300 mg scored. Tab 450 mg scored.	25 100 150 225	Serum level fluctuations are 38%/16% for 200-, 300- and 450-mg, and 87%/34% for 100-mg tablets;[c] some rapid metabolizers may require 8-hr dosage intervals to avoid breakthrough of symptoms.

[a]Only products with documented bioavailability that are minimally affected by food and with dosage forms that permit incremental changes in dose are listed.
[b]Accuracy of measurement decreases below 0.5 mL with suspensions and syrups, because of viscosity; smaller amounts cannot be accurately measured; measure all liquid dosage forms with a syringe.
[c]Predicted child/adult fluctuation between peak and trough (%) for 12-hr dosage interval; average child t ½ = 3.7 hr, average adult t ½ = 8.2 hr.[79]
[d]The ethylenediamine portion of aminophylline may cause urticaria or exfoliative dermatitis rarely.
[e]Only Slo-bid Gyrocaps and Theo-Dur tablets have sufficiently slow and complete absorption to allow 12-hr dosage intervals with minimal serum concentration fluctuations in most patients.[79] Many products advertised for bid dosage (eg, LaBID, Phyllocontin) do not maintain serum concentrations within the therapeutic range in many patients, especially children.[79] Some once-daily dosage products (eg, Theo-24, Uniphyl) are affected by food and may be unreliable.[75,80] The extent of absorption of Uni-Dur does not appear to be affected by food; however, large serum level fluctuations may render this agent unreliable for once-daily administration.[82,83]

ZAFIRLUKAST	Accolate
MONTELUKAST (Investigational, Merck)	Singulair
ZILEUTON	Zyflo

These drugs are potent, selective leukotriene antagonists. They have antiinflammatory activity and inhibit the antigen-induced contraction of the trachea and bronchospasm that occurs in asthma. Zafirlukast and montelukast are competitive leukotriene D_4 and E_4 receptor antagonists, whereas zileuton inhibits leukotriene synthesis. Monteleukast is orally absorbed; its oral absorption is increased by food and it has an elimination half-life of 4–5 hr. Single doses of 20 to 800 mg appear to be well tolerated. Zileuton is orally absorbed and eliminated by hepatic glucuronidation with a half-life of 1.5 hr. It is generally well tolerated, with headache reported in about 10% of patients in clinical trials; hepatic enzyme abnormalities have been reported. In trials of patient with mild to moderate asthma, oral zileuton dosages of 600 mg qid and 800 mg bid have been used. Dosage reduction may be necessary in hepatic dysfunction. Zafirlukast is well absorbed orally, although food reduces its bioavailability by 40%. It is metabolized by CYP2C9 and may inhibit CYP2C9 and CYP3A4; its half-life is 10 hr. The anticoagulant effect of warfarin is increased by zafirlukast; erythromycin, terfenadine, and theophylline decrease zafirlukast serum levels, whereas aspirin increases zafirlukast serum levels. Interactions with other drugs are not well studied. The dosage of zafirlukast in adults and children $\geq$12 yr is 20 mg bid on an empty stomach.[48,49] It is available as 20 mg tablets. The dosage of Zileuton is 600 mg qid. It is available as 600 mg tablets.

Inhaled Corticosteroids

| **BECLOMETHASONE DIPROPIONATE** | Beconase, Beclovent, Vancenase, Vanceril |

Pharmacology. Potent topical glucocorticoid with little systemic activity because of low systemic bioavailability.

Administration and Adult Dosage. Inhal for asthma 84 µg tid–qid, or 168 µg bid, to a maximum of 840 µg/day. (*See* Notes.) **Intranasal for nasal congestion** 42–84 µg/nostril bid–qid (168–336 µg/day total dosage) for several days, then decrease dosage (if symptoms do not recur) to minimum amount necessary to control stuffiness.

Special Populations. *Pediatric Dosage.* Inhal for asthma (6–12 yr) 42–84 µg (1–2 puffs) tid–qid or 168 µg bid, to a maximum of 420 µg/day; (>12 yr) same as adult dosage. **Intranasal for nasal congestion** (<6 yr) not recommended; (6–12 yr) 42 µg/nostril bid or tid.[84]

Geriatric Dosage. Same as adult dosage.

Other Conditions. During periods of a severe asthma attack, patients require supplementary treatment with systemic steroids.

Dosage Forms. Inhal (Beclovent, Vanceril) 42, 84 µg/inhalation (200 doses/inhaler); **Nasal Inhal** (Beconase, Vancenase) 42, 84 µg/spray (200 doses/inhaler); (Beconase AQ, Vancenase AQ); **Aq Susp** 42, 84 µg/spray (200 doses/bottle).

Patient Instructions. *Metered-dose oral inhaler.* Shake thoroughly; hold mouthpiece approximately two finger-spaces outside mouth with teeth and tongue out of the way. Tilt head back, actuate inhaler during slow deep breath, and hold breath for 5–10 seconds. Allow at least 1 minute between inhalations. Use any inhaled sympathomimetic bronchodilator (if prescribed) a few minutes prior to this drug to prevent bronchospasm and to enhance penetration of the corticosteroid into the bronchial tree. The use of "spacers" with corticosteroid inhalers decreases the frequency of local side effects, hoarseness, and oropharyngeal candidiasis. Rinsing your mouth and gargling with water or mouthwash following administration may also be beneficial. This medication is for preventive therapy and should not be used to treat acute asthma attacks. **Nasal Inhaler.** Blow your nose before use. Shake container well. Remove protective cap and hold inhaler between thumb and forefinger. Tilt head back slightly and insert the end of the inhaler into one nostril. While holding the other nostril closed with one finger, press down once to release one dose, and at the same time, inhale gently. Hold breath for a few seconds, then breathe out slowly through your mouth. Repeat the process in the other nostril. Avoid blowing your nose for the next 15 minutes.

Pharmacokinetics. *Onset and Duration.* Effect is usually evident within a few days, but it may take 2–4 weeks for maximum improvement.[85]

Fate. Only 10% or less of an inhaled dose is deposited in the lung; 80% is deposited in the mouth and swallowed. Oral absorption is slow and incomplete (61–90%), and undergoes extensive first-pass metabolism, resulting in oral bioavailability of less than 5%.[86] Well absorbed from the lung and extensively metabolized, with 65% excreted in the bile and less than 10% of unchanged drug and metabolites excreted in urine.[86]

$t_{1/2}$. 15 hr.

Adverse Reactions. After oral use, localized growth of *Candida* in the mouth occurs frequently, but clinically apparent infections occur only occasionally. Hoarseness and dry mouth occur occasionally; minimal to no suppression of the pituitary-adrenal axis occurs at the recommended dosage; however, dose-dependent suppression occurs at higher dosages.[85,87–90] After intranasal use, irritation and burning of the nasal mucosa and sneezing occur occasionally; intranasal and pharyngeal *Candida* infections, nasal ulceration, and epistaxis occur rarely.

Contraindications. Status asthmaticus or other acute episodes of asthma in which intensive measures are required; beclomethasone-exacerbated symptoms.

Precautions. During stress or severe asthmatic attacks, patients withdrawn from systemic corticosteroid should contact their physician immediately.

Drug Interactions. None known.

Parameters to Monitor. For treatment of asthma, frequency of daytime asthmatic symptoms; nocturnal use of prn sympathomimetic inhaler. For nasal congestion, relief of symptoms.

Notes. Patients needing a long-term, orally inhaled corticosteroid should be continued on therapeutic doses of a bronchodilator. Prior to use, a patient should be as free of symptoms as possible, which can be achieved with a 1-week course of oral prednisone. The nasal inhalation provides effective, prompt relief of nasal congestion when maximally tolerated dosage of oral sympathomimetics is inadequate. (*See also* Inhaled Corticosteroids Comparison Chart.)

INHALED CORTICOSTEROIDS COMPARISON CHART

DRUG	DOSAGE FORM	DOSE/PUFF (μG)	ADULT DOSAGE[a]	PEDIATRIC DOSAGE[b]	DOSAGE EQUIVALENCE (PUFFS/1000 μG)	SERUM HALF-LIFE (HR)
Beclomethasone Diproprionate	Inhal (metered-dose)	42, 84	Inhal 84 μg tid–qid or 168 μg bid, to a maximum of 840 μg/day	Inhal 42–84 μg tid–qid; 168 μg bid, to a maximum of 420 μg/day	12	15
Beclovent	Nasal Inhal (metered-dose)	42, 84				
Beconase Vancenase	(aqueous susp).	42, 84	Nasal Inhal 1–2 sprays into each nostril bid–qid.	Nasal Inhal 1 spray into each nostril bid–tid.		
Budesonide	Inhal (metered-dose)	50, 200	Inhal 400–1600 μg in divided doses bid–qid initially; adjust to 200–400 μg bid	Inhal (6–12 yr) 100–200 μg bid initially, decrease according to response; (>12 yr) same as adult dosage.	5	2–2.8
Pulmicort (Investigational, MSD)						
Rhinocort	Nasal Inhal (metered-dose).	32	Nasal Inhal 2 sprays into each nostril bid or 4 sprays into each nostril each morning, to a maximum of 800 μg/day.	Nasal Inhal (>6 yr) 2 sprays into each nostril bid or 4 sprays into each nostril each morning, to a maximum of 400 μg/day.		

(continued)

635

INHALED CORTICOSTEROIDS COMPARISON CHART (continued)

DRUG	DOSAGE FORM	DOSE/PUFF (µG)	ADULT DOSAGE[a]	PEDIATRIC DOSAGE[b]	DOSAGE EQUIVALENCE (PUFFS/1000 µG)	SERUM HALF-LIFE (HR)
Flunisolide AeroBid Nasalide Nasarel	Inhal (metered-dose) Nasal Inhal (aqueous soln; Nasarel).	250 25	Inhal 500 µg (2 puffs) bid to a maximum of 1 mg (4 puffs) bid Nasal Inhal 2 sprays into each nostril bid, to a maximum of 8 sprays into each nostril/day.	Inhal (<4 yr) not established; (4–12 yr) same as adult dosage. Dosages over 1 mg/day have not been studied Nasal Inhal 1 spray into each nostril tid–qid.	4	1.6
Fluticasone Propionate Flonase Flovent	Inhal (metered-dose) Inhal (dry pwdr) Nasal Inhal (aqueous susp).	44, 110, 220 50, 100, 250 50	Inhal 176–880 µg/day in 2 divided doses. Nasal Inhal 2 sprays into each nostril/day or 1 spray bid; maintenance 1 spray into each nostril/day, to a maximum of 200 µg/day.	Nasal Inhal (≥12 yr) 1 spray into each nostril/day, to a maximum of 200 µg/day.	4.5	7.8

(continued)

INHALED CORTICOSTEROIDS COMPARISON CHART (continued)

DRUG	DOSAGE FORM	DOSE/PUFF (µG)	ADULT DOSAGE[a]	PEDIATRIC DOSAGE[b]	DOSAGE EQUIVALENCE (PUFFS/1000 µG)	SERUM HALF-LIFE (HR)
Triamcinolone Acetonide						
Azmacort	Inhal (metered-dose)	100[e]	Inhal 200 µg (2 puffs) tid-qid; in severe asthma, 12–16 puffs/day. Adjust to bid for maintenance, to a maximum of 1600 µg (16 puffs)/day.	Inhal (6–12 yr) 100–200 µg (1–2 puffs) tid-qid, to a maximum of 1200 µg (12 puffs)/day.	5	0.5–1
Nasacort	Nasal Inhal. (aqueous soln; Nasacort Aq)	55	Nasal Inhal 2 sprays into each nostril once daily. Adjust to a maximum of 4 sprays/nostril/day in 1–4 divided doses; maintenance as low as 1 spray/day.	Nasal Inhal (>6 yr) Same as adult dosage.		

[a]Separate analyses of efficacy and safety in patients >60 yr are limited by small sample size.
[b]Unless stated otherwise, pediatric dosage is for patients 6–12 yr; dosages for patients <6 yr have generally not been established.
[c]There is little information on the relative antiasthmatic potencies between the inhaled corticosteroids. Assuming that the systemic activities are approximately equivalent µg for µg, this column provides a rough guide to the dosages likely to have equivalent efficacy and toxicity.
[e]200 µg/actuation, but 100 µg retained in the spacer.
From references 91–93.

637

Cough and Cold

DEXTROMETHORPHAN HYDROBROMIDE
Various

Pharmacology. Dextromethorphan is the nonanalgesic, nonaddictive d-isomer of the codeine analogue of levorphanol. With usual antitussive doses, the cough threshold is elevated centrally with little effect on the respiratory, cardiovascular, or GI systems.

Administration and Adult Dosage. PO as cough suppressant 10–30 mg q 4–8 hr, to a maximum of 120 mg/day; **SR** 60 mg q 12 hr.

Special Populations. *Pediatric Dosage.* **PO as cough suppressant** (<2 yr) not recommended; (2–6 yr) 2.5–7.5 mg q 4–8 hr, to a maximum of 30 mg/day (as syrup); (6–12 yr) 5–10 mg q 4 hr or 15 mg q 6–8 hr, to a maximum of 60 mg/day; (>12 yr) same as adult dosage. **SR** (2–5 yr) 15 mg q 12 hr; (6–12 yr) 30 mg q 12 hr. (*See* Notes.)

Geriatric Dosage. Same as adult dosage.

Dosage Forms. Cap 30 mg; **Lozenge** 2.5, 5, 7.5 mg; **Syrup** 0.7, 1, 1.5, 2, 3 mg/mL; **SR Susp** 6 mg/mL; (available in many combination products in variable concentrations).

Patient Instructions. Do not use this drug to suppress productive cough, or chronic cough that occurs with smoking, asthma, or emphysema. Report if your cough persists.

Pharmacokinetics. *Onset and Duration.* PO onset 1–2 hr; duration up to 6–8 hr with non-SR, 12 hr for SR suspension.[94]

Fate. Extensively metabolized, including appreciable first-pass effect, mainly to the active metabolite dextrorphan. Genetically determined polymorphic metabolism primarily by CYP2D6 with extensive (93%) and poor (7%) metabolizers.[95]

$t_{1/2}$. (Extensive metabolizers) <4 to about 9 hr; (poor metabolizers) 17–138 hr.[96]

Adverse Reactions. Occasional mild drowsiness and GI upset. Intoxication, bizarre behavior, CNS depression, and respiratory depression can occur with extremely high dosages. Naloxone may be effective in reversing these effects.[97–100] Reports of dextromethorphan abuse have increased, especially among teenagers.[101]

Contraindications. MAO inhibitor therapy.[102]

Precautions. Generally, do not use in patients with chronic cough or cough associated with excessive secretions.

Drug Interactions. Concurrent MAO inhibitors may cause hypotension, hyperpyrexia, nausea, and coma. Drugs that inhibit CYP2D6 may inhibit dextromethorphan metabolism, but serious effects are not reported.

Parameters to Monitor. Observe for relief of cough and CNS side effects.

Notes. Approximately equipotent with codeine in antitussive effectiveness in adults.[94,97] One trial of dextromethorphan and codeine for night cough in children found neither superior to placebo, and their efficacies have been questioned for this use.[103] (*See also* Codeine Salts.)

GUAIFENESIN   2/G, Robitussin, Organidin NR, Various

Pharmacology. Guaifenesin is proposed to have an expectorant action through an increased output of respiratory tract fluid, enhancing the flow of less viscid secretions, promoting ciliary action, and facilitating the removal of inspissated mucus. Evidence of the effectiveness of guaifenesin is largely subjective and not well established clinically.[97,104–108]

Administration and Adult Dosage. PO as an expectorant 100–400 mg q 4 hr; **SR** 600–1200 mg q 12 hr, to a maximum of 2.4 g/day.[107]

Special Populations. *Pediatric Dosage.* PO as an expectorant (2–6 yr) 50–100 mg q 4 hr, to a maximum of 600 mg/day; (6–12 yr) 100–200 mg q 4 hr, to a maximum of 1200 mg/day; (≥12 yr) same as adult dosage. **SR** (2–6 yr) 300 mg q 12 hr; (6–12 yr) 600 mg q 12 hr.

Geriatric Dosage. Same as adult dosage.

Dosage Forms. **Cap** 200 mg; **Syrup** 20, 40 mg/mL; **Tab** 100, 200 mg; **SR Cap** 300 mg; **SR Tab** 600 mg; **SR Tab** 400 mg with phenylpropanolamine 75 mg (Entex LA, various); 600 mg with pseudoephedrine 120 mg (Entex PSE).

Patient Instructions. Take this drug with a large quantity of fluid to ensure proper drug action. Report if your cough persists for more than one week, recurs, or is accompanied by a high fever, rash, or persistent headache.

Adverse Reactions. Occasional nausea and vomiting, especially with excessive dosage; dizziness, headache.

Precautions. Generally, do not use in patients with chronic cough or cough associated with excessive secretions.

Drug Interactions. None known.

Notes. May interfere with certain laboratory determinations of 5-hydroxyindoleacetic acid (5-HIAA) and vanilmandelic acid (VMA),[109] but does not cause a positive stool guaiac reaction in normal subjects.[108]

PSEUDOEPHEDRINE HYDROCHLORIDE   Efidac/24, Sudafed, Various

Pharmacology. Pseudoephedrine is an indirect-acting agent that stimulates α-, β_1- and β_2-adrenergic receptors via release of endogenous adrenergic amines. It is used primarily for decongestion of nasal mucosa.

Administration and Adult Dosage. PO as a decongestant 60 mg q 4–6 hr, to a maximum of 240 mg/day. PO SR Cap/Tab 120 mg q 12 hr; (Efidac/24) 240 mg once daily.

Special Populations. *Pediatric Dosage.* PO (3–12 months) 3 drops/kg q 4–6 hr, to a maximum of 4 doses/day; (1–2 yr) 7 drops (0.2 mL)/kg q 4–6 hr, to a maximum of 4 doses/day; (2–5 yr) 15 mg (as syrup) q 4–6 hr prn, to a maximum of 60 mg/day; (6–12 yr) 30 mg q 4–6 hr prn, to a maximum of 120 mg/day; (>12 yr) same as adult dosage. Do not give SR Cap/Tab 120 or 240 mg to patients <12 yr.

Geriatric Dosage. Demonstrate safe use of short-acting formulation before using an SR product.

Dosage Forms. **Cap** 60 mg; **SR Cap** 120 mg; **Drp** 9.4 mg/mL; **Syrup** 3, 6 mg/mL; **Tab** 30, 60 mg; **SR Tab** (12-hr) 120, 240 mg; (as sulfate) 120 mg (60 mg as immediate release, 60 mg as delayed release); (Efidac/24) 240 mg. **Tab** 60 mg with triprolidine HCl 2.5 mg (Actifed, various); **SR Cap** 120 mg with chlorpheniramine maleate 8 mg (Deconamine SR, Isoclor Timesules, various); **SR Tab** 120 mg with terfenadine 60 mg (Seldane-D).

Patient Instructions. Avoid taking the last dose of the day near bedtime if you have difficulty sleeping. Do not crush or chew SR preparations.

Pharmacokinetics. *Onset and Duration.* Onset within 30 min on an empty stomach, within 1 hr for SR forms; duration 3 hr or longer, 8–12 hr for most SR forms, 24 hr for Efidac/24.[110,111]

Fate. Solution and immediate-release tablets are rapidly and completely absorbed orally. SR dosage forms attain peak serum levels in (12-hr product) 4–6 hr or (24-hr product) 12 hr. Food appears to delay absorption of non-SR forms, but not the SR forms.[112,113] V_d is 2.7 ± 0.2 L/kg; Cl averages 0.44 L/hr/kg. Partially metabolized to inactive metabolite(s), and 6% metabolized to active metabolite, norpseudoephedrine; 45–90% excreted unchanged in urine depending on urinary pH and flow.[113,114]

$t_{1/2}$. Urinary flow and pH dependent: 13 ± 3 hr at pH 8; 6.9 ± 1.2 hr at pH 5.5–6; 4.7 ± 1.4 hr at pH 5.[114,115]

Adverse Reactions. Frequent mild transient nervousness, insomnia, irritability, or headache. Usually negligible pressor effect in normotensive patients.[116,117]

Contraindications. Severe hypertension; coronary artery disease; MAO inhibitor therapy.

Precautions. Use with caution in patients with renal failure,[118] hypertension, diabetes mellitus, ischemic heart disease, increased intraocular pressure, prostatic hypertrophy, urinary retention, or thyroid disease. Elderly patients may be particularly sensitive to CNS effects. If use is necessary in infants with phenylketonuria, reduce dosage to avoid possible increased agitation.[119]

Drug Interactions. Concurrent MAO inhibitors or furazolidone may increase pressor response. Urinary alkalinizers may decrease pseudoephedrine clearance.

Parameters to Monitor. Nasal stuffiness, CNS stimulation, blood pressure in hypertensive patients.

Notes. Combination with an antihistamine may provide additive benefit in seasonal allergic rhinitis, because antihistamines do not relieve nasal stuffiness.[120,121] Neither these combinations nor decongestants alone are of consistent long-term benefit for reduction of middle ear effusion in children with otitis media and are not recommended for this use.[122,123]

REFERENCES

1. Campoli-Richards DM et al. Cetirizine. A review of its pharmacological properties and clinical potential in allergic rhinitis, pollen-induced asthma, and chronic urticaria. *Drugs* 1990;40:762–81.

2. Mansmann HC et al. Efficacy and safety of cetirizine in perennial allergic rhinitis. *Ann Allergy* 1992;68:348–53.

3. Spencer CM et al. Cetirizine. A reappraisal of its pharmacological properties and therapeutic use in selected allergic disorders. *Drugs* 1993;46:1055–80.

4. Simons FER et al. Pharmacokinetics and efficacy of chlorpheniramine in children. *J Allergy Clin Immunol* 1982;69:376–81.

5. Huang SM et al. Pharmacokinetics of chlorpheniramine after intravenous and oral administration in normal adults. *Eur J Clin Pharmacol* 1982;22:359–65.

6. Cook TJ et al. Degree and duration of skin test suppression and side effects with antihistamines. *J Allergy Clin Immunol* 1973;51:71–7.

7. Usdin Yasuda S et al. Chlorpheniramine plasma concentration and histamine H_1-receptor occupancy. *Clin Pharmacol Ther* 1995;58:210–20.

8. Benet LZ et al. Design and optimization of dosage regimens; pharmacokinetic data. In Hardman JG et al., eds. *Goodman and Gilman's the pharmacological basis of therapeutics*, 9th ed. New York: McGraw-Hill; 1996:1707–92.

9. Paton DM, Webster DR. Clinical pharmacokinetics of H_1-receptor antagonists (the antihistamines). *Clin Pharmacokinet* 1985;10:477–97.

10. Simons FER. H_1-receptor antagonists: clinical pharmacology and therapeutics. *J Allergy Clin Immunol* 1989;84:845–61.

11. Shapiro GG, Konig P. Cromolyn sodium: a review. *Pharmacotherapy* 1985;5:156–70.

12. Murphy S, Kelly HW. Cromolyn sodium: a review of its mechanisms and clinical use in asthma. *Drug Intell Clin Pharm* 1987;21:22–35.

13. Sorkin EM, Ward A. Ocular sodium cromoglycate. An overview of its therapeutic efficacy in allergic eye disease. *Drugs* 1986;31:131–48.

14. Berman BA. Cromolyn: past, present, and future. *Pediatr Clin North Am* 1983;30:915–30.

15. Edwards AM. Oral sodium cromoglycate: its use in the management of food allergy. *Clin Exp Allergy* 1995;25(suppl 1):31–3.

16. Greenway SE et al. Treatment of depression with cyproheptadine. *Pharmacotherapy* 1995;15:357–60.

17. Krieger DT et al. Cyproheptadine-induced remission of Cushing's disease. *N Engl J Med* 1975;293:893–6.

18. Anon. Cyproheptadine as an appetite stimulant. *Drug Ther Bull* 1970;8:71–2.

19. Wanderer AA et al. Primary acquired cold urticaria. *Arch Dermatol* 1977;113:1375–7.

20. Rhoades RB et al. Suppression of histamine-induced pruritus by three antihistaminic drugs. *J Allergy Clin Immunol* 1975;55:180–5.

21. Baraf CS. Treatment of pruritus in allergic dermatoses: an evaluation of the relative efficacy of cyproheptadine and hydroxyzine. *Curr Ther Res* 1976;19:32–8.

22. Klein GL, Galant SP. A comparison of the antipruritic efficacy of hydroxyzine and cyproheptadine in children with atopic dermatitis. *Ann Allergy* 1980;44:142–5.

23. Simons KJ et al. Diphenhydramine: pharmacokinetics and pharmacodynamics in elderly adults, young adults, and children. *J Clin Pharmacol* 1990;30:665–71.

24. Carruthers SG et al. Correlation between plasma diphenhydramine level and sedative and antihistamine effects. *Clin Pharmacol Ther* 1978;23:375–82.

25. Blyden GT et al. Pharmacokinetics of diphenhydramine and a demethylated metabolite following intravenous and oral administration. *J Clin Pharmacol* 1986;26:529–33.

26. Spector R et al. Diphenhydramine in Orientals and Caucasians. *Clin Pharmacol Ther* 1980;28:229–34.

27. Meredith CG et al. Diphenhydramine disposition in chronic liver disease. *Clin Pharmacol Ther* 1984;35:474–9.

28. Glazko AJ et al. Metabolic disposition of diphenhydramine. *Clin Pharmacol Ther* 1974;16:1066–76.

29. Albert KS et al. Pharmacokinetics of diphenhydramine in man. *J Pharmacokinet Biopharm* 1975;3:159–70.

30. Schaaf L et al. Suppression of seasonal allergic rhinitis symptoms with daily hydroxyzine. *J Allergy Clin Immunol* 1979;63:129–33.

31. Gendreau-Reid L et al. Comparison of the suppressive effect of astemizole, terfenadine, and hydroxyzine on histamine-induced wheals and flares in humans. *J Allergy Clin Immunol* 1986;77:335–40.

32. Simons KJ et al. Pharmacokinetic and pharmacodynamic studies of the H_1-receptor antagonist hydroxyzine in the elderly. *Clin Pharmacol Ther* 1989;45:9–14.

33. Simons FER et al. Pharmacokinetics and antipruritic effects of hydroxyzine in children with atopic dermatitis. *J Pediatr* 1984;104:123–7.

34. Simons FE et al. The pharmacokinetics and antihistaminic of the H_1 receptor antagonist hydroxyzine. *J Allergy Clin Immunol* 1984;73(1 pt. 1):69–75.
35. Simons FER et al. The pharmacokinetics and pharmacodynamics of hydroxyzine in patients with primary biliary cirrhosis. *J Clin Pharmacol* 1989;29:809–15.
36. Simons FER, Simons KJ. Antihistamines. In Middleton E et al., eds. *Allergy. Principles and practice.* St. Louis: Mosby; 1993:856–79.
37. Wasserman SI. A review of some recent clinical studies with nedocromil sodium. *J Allergy Clin Immunol* 1993;92:210–5.
38. Kelly HW, Murphy S. Use of sodium cromoglycate and other anti-allergic drugs in asthma. In D'Arcy PF, McElnay JC, eds. *The pharmacy and pharmacotherapy of asthma.* Chichester: Ellis Horwood; 1989:86–103.
39. Brogden RN, Sorkin EM. Nedocromil sodium. An updated review of its pharmacological properties and therapeutic efficacy in asthma. *Drugs* 1993;45:693–715.
40. Simons FER, Simons KJ. Second-generation H_1-receptor antagonists. *Ann Allergy* 1991;66:5–19.
41. Okerholm RA et al. Bioavailability of terfenadine in man. *Biopharm Drug Dispos* 1981;2:185–90.
42. Garteiz DA et al. Pharmacokinetics and biotransformation studies of terfenadine in man. *Arzneimittelforschung* 1982;32:1185–90.
43. Woodward JK, Munro NL. Terfenadine, the first non-sedating antihistamine. *Arzneimittelforschung* 1982;32:1154–6.
44. Simons FER et al. Lack of subsensitivity to tefenadine during long-term terfenadine treatment. *J Allergy Clin Immunol* 1988;82:1068–75.
45. Simons KJ et al. Pharmacokinetics and pharmacodynamics of terfenadine and chlorpheniramine in the elderly. *J Allergy Clin Immunol* 1990;85:540–7.
46. McTavish D et al. Terfenadine. An updated review of its pharmacological properties and therapeutic efficacy. *Drugs* 1990;39:552–74.
47. Monahan BP et al. Torsades de pointes occurring in association with terfenadine use. *JAMA* 1990;264:2788–90.
48. Pauwels RA et al. Leukotrienes as therapeutic targets in asthma. *Allergy* 1995;50:615–22.
49. Schoors DF et al. Single dose pharmacokinetics, safety and tolerability of MK-0476, a new leukotriene D4-receptor antagonist, in healthy volunteers. *Br J Clin Pharmacol* 1995;40:277–80.
50. Olin BR, ed. *Facts and comparisons.* St. Louis: JB Lippincott; 1996.
51. Corey JP. Advances in the pharmacotherapy of allergic rhinitis: second-generation H_1-receptor antagonists. *Otolaryngol Head Neck Surg* 1993;109:584–92.
52. Krause HF. Antihistamines and decongestants. *Otolaryngol Head Neck Surg* 1992;107:835–40.
53. Korenblat PE, Wedner HJ. Allergy. *Theory and practice,* 2nd ed. Philadelphia: WB Saunders; 1992:300–3.
54. Desager J-P, Horsmans Y. Pharmacokinetic-pharmacodynamic relationships of H_1-antihistamines. *Clin Pharmacokinet* 1995;28:419–32.
55. Tashkin DP, Jenne JW. Beta adrenergic agonists. In Weiss EB et al., eds. *Bronchial asthma: mechanisms and therapeutics,* 3rd ed. Boston: Little, Brown; 1993:700–48.
56. Kelly HW. New β_2-adrenergic agonist aerosols. *Clin Pharm* 1985;4:393–403.
57. Hendeles L et al. Medical management of noninfectious rhinitis. *Am J Hosp Pharm* 1980;37:1496–504.
58. Hochhaus G, Möllmann H. Pharmacokinetic/pharmacodynamic characteristics of the β_2-agonists terbutaline, salbutamol and fenoterol. *Int J Clin Pharmacol Ther Toxicol* 1992;30:342–62.
59. Reynolds JEF, ed. *Salbutamol. Martindale the extra pharmacopoeia.* London: The Pharmaceutical Press; 1993:1255–7.
60. Spitzer OW et al. The use of β-agonists and the risk of death and near death from asthma. *N Engl J Med* 1992;326:501–6.
61. Mullen M et al. The association between β-agonist use and death from asthma. A meta-analytic integration of case-control studies. *JAMA* 1993;270:1842–5.
62. Gross NJ, Skorodin MS. Anticholinergic agents. In Jenne JW, Murphy S, eds. *Drug therapy for asthma: research and clinical practice.* New York: Marcel Dekker; 1987:615–68.
63. Harrison LI et al. Comparative absorption of inhaled and intramuscularly administered atropine. *Am Rev Respir Dis* 1986;134:254–7.
64. Hinderling PH et al. Integrated pharmacokinetics and pharmacodynamics of atropine in healthy humans. I: pharmacokinetics. *J Pharm Sci* 1985;74:703–10.
65. Pihlajamäki K et al. Pharmacokinetics of atropine in children. *Int J Clin Pharmacol Ther Toxicol* 1986;24:236–9.
66. Kradjan WA et al. Atropine serum concentrations after multiple inhaled doses of atropine sulfate. *Clin Pharmacol Ther* 1985;38:12–5.
67. Trujillo MH, Bellorin-Font E. Drugs commonly administered by intravenous infusion in intensive care units: a practical guide. *Crit Care Med* 1990;18:232–8.

68. Kelly HW, Murphy S. Should anticholinergics by used in acute severe asthma? *DICP* 1990;24:409–16.

69. Milner AD. Ipratropium bromide in airways obstruction in childhood. *Postgrad Med J* 1987;63(suppl 1):53–6.

70. Shuk S et al. Efficacy of frequent nebulized ipratropium bromide added to frequent high-dose albuterol therapy in severe childhood asthma. *J Pediatr* 1995;126:639–45.

71. Gross NJ. Ipratropium bromide. *N Engl J Med* 1988;319:486–94.

72. Brogden RN, Faulds D. Salmeterol xinafoate. A review of its pharmacological properties and therapeutic potential in reversible obstructive airway disease. *Drugs* 1991;42:895–912.

73. Jenne JW. Physiology and pharmacodynamics of the xanthines. In Jenne JW, Murphy S, eds. *Drug therapy for asthma: research and clinical practice*. New York: Marcel Dekker; 1987:297–334.

74. Hendeles L et al. Theophylline. In Evans WG et al., eds. *Applied pharmacokinetics: principles of therapeutic drug monitoring*, 2nd ed. Spokane, WA: Applied Therapeutics; 1986:1105–88.

75. Szefler SJ. Theophylline: pharmacokinetics and clinical applications. In Jenne JW, Murphy S, eds. *Drug therapy for asthma: research and clinical practice*. New York: Marcel Dekker; 1987:353–87.

76. Kelly HW et al. Appendix. In Jenne JW, Murphy S, eds. *Drug therapy for asthma: research and clinical practice*. New York: Marcel Dekker; 1987:1021–46.

77. International consensus report on diagnosis and treatment of asthma. Bethesda, MD: National Heart, Lung, and Blood Institute, National Asthma Education Program; U.S. Department of Health and Human Services publication 92–3091: 1992.

78. Self TH et al. Reassessing the therapeutic range for theophylline on laboratory report forms: the importance of 5–15 μg/ml. *Pharmacotherapy* 1993;13:590–4.

79. Hendeles L, Weinberger M. Selection of a slow-release theophylline product. *J Allergy Clin Immunol* 1986;78:743–51.

80. Morris JF. Geriatric considerations. In Weiss EB et al., eds. *Bronchial asthma: mechanisms and therapeutics*, 3rd ed. Boston: Little, Brown; 1993:1017–22.

81. Kelly HW. Theophylline toxicity. In Jenne JW, Murphy S, eds. *Drug therapy for asthma: research and clinical practice*. New York: Marcel Dekker; 1987:925–51.

82. González MA et al. Pharmacokinetic comparison of a once-daily and twice-daily theophylline delivery system. *Clin Ther* 1994;16:686–92.

83. González MA, Straughn AB. Effect of meals and dosage-form modification on theophylline bioavailability from a 24-hour sustained-release delivery system. *Clin Ther* 1994;16:804–14.

84. Kobayashi RH et al. Beclomethasone dipropionate aqueous nasal spray for seasonal allergic rhinitis in children. *Ann Allergy* 1989;62:205–8.

85. Fauci AS et al. Glucocorticoid therapy: mechanisms of action and clinical considerations. *Ann Intern Med* 1976;84:304–15.

86. Azarnoff DL ed. *Steroid therapy*. Philadelphia: WB Saunders, 1975.

87. Barnes PJ. Inhaled glucocorticoids for asthma. *N Engl J Med* 1995;332:868–75.

88. Barnes PJ, Pedersen S. Efficacy and safety of inhaled corticosteroid in asthma. *Am Rev Respir Dis* 1993;149:S1–26.

89. Szefler SJ. A comparison of aerosol glucocorticoids in the treatment of chronic bronchial asthma. *Pediatr Asthma Allergy Immunol* 1991;5:227–35.

90. Kamada AK. Therapeutic controversies in the treatment of asthma. *Ann Pharmacother* 1994;28:904–14.

91. Toogood JH et al. Aerosol corticosteroid. In Weiss EB et al., eds. *Bronchial asthma: mechanisms and therapeutics*, 2nd ed. Boston: Little, Brown; 1993:818–41.

92. McCubbin MM et al. A bioassay for topical and systemic effect of three inhaled steroids. *Clin Pharmacol Ther* 1995; 57:455–60.

93. Holliday SM et al. Inhaled fluticasone propionate. A review of its pharmacodynamic and pharmacokinetic properties, and therapeutic use in asthma. *Drugs* 1994;47:318–31.

94. Matthys H et al. Dextromethorphan and codeine: objective assessment of antitussive activity in patients with chronic cough. *J Int Med Res* 1983;11:92–100.

95. Jacqz-Aigrain E et al. CYP2D6- and CYP3A-dependent metabolism of dextromethorphan in humans. *Pharmacogenetics* 1993;3:197–204.

96. Woodworth JR et al. The polymorphic metabolism of dextromethorphan. *J Clin Pharmacol* 1987;27:139–43.

97. Bryant BG, Lombardi TP. Cold, cough, and allergy products. In Covington TR, ed. *Handbook of nonprescription drugs*, 10th ed. Washington, DC: American Pharmaceutical Association; 1993:89–115.

98. Committee on Drugs. Use of codeine- and dextromethorphan-containing cough syrups in pediatrics. *Pediatrics* 1978;62:118–22.

99. Shaul WL et al. Dextromethorphan toxicity: reversal by naloxone. *Pediatrics* 1977;59:117–9.

100. Katona B, Wason S. Dextromethorphan danger. *N Engl J Med* 1986;314:993. Letter.

101. Bem JL, Peck R. Dextromethorphan. An overview of safety issues. *Drug Saf* 1992;7:190–9.

102. Nierenberg DW, Semprebon M. The central nervous system serotonin syndrome. *Clin Pharmacol Ther* 1993;53:84–8.

103. Taylor JA et al. Efficacy of cough suppressants in children. *J Pediatr* 1993;122:799–802.

104. Hirsch SR et al. The expectorant effect of glyceryl guaiacolate in patients with chronic bronchitis. *Chest* 1973;63:9–14.

105. Heilborn H et al. Effect of bromhexine and guaiphenesine on clinical state, ventilatory capacity and sputum viscosity in chronic asthma. *Scand J Respir Dis* 1976;57:88–96.

106. Anon. Guaiphenesin and iodide. *Drug Ther Bull* 1985;23:62–4.

107. Anon. Cold, cough, allergy, bronchodilator, and antiasthmatic drug products for over-the-counter human use; expectorant drug products for over-the-counter human use; final monograph. *Fed Regist* 1989;54:8494–509.

108. Ziment I. Drugs modifying the sol-layer and the hydration of mucus. In Braga PC, Allegra L, eds. *Drugs in bronchial mucology.* New York: Raven Press; 1989:293–322.

109. Hansten PD. *Drug interactions,* 4th ed. Philadelphia: Lea & Febiger, 1979.

110. Roth RP et al. Nasal decongestant activity of pseudoephedrine. *Ann Otol Rhinol Laryngol* 1977;86:235–42.

111. Hamilton LH et al. A study of sustained action pseudoephedrine in allergic rhinitis. *Ann Allergy* 1982;48:87–92.

112. Hwang SS et al. In vitro and in vivo evaluation of a once-daily controlled-release pseudoephedrine product. *J Clin Pharmacol* 1995;35:259–67.

113. Kanfer I et al. Pharmacokinetics of oral decongestants. *Pharmacotherapy* 1993;13(6 pt 2):116S–28S.

114. Brater DC et al. Renal excretion of pseudoephedrine. *Clin Pharmacol Ther* 1980;28:690–4.

115. Kuntzman RG et al. The influence of urinary pH on the plasma half-life of pseudoephedrine in man and dog and a sensitive assay for its determination in human plasma. *Clin Pharmacol Ther* 1971;12:62–7.

116. Chua SS, Benrimoj SI. Non-prescription sympathomimetic agents and hypertension. *Med Toxicol* 1988;3:387–417.

117. Beck RA et al. Cardiovascular effects of pseudoephedrine in medically controlled hypertensive patients. *Arch Intern Med* 1992;152:1242–5.

118. Sica DA, Comstock TJ. Case report: pseudoephedrine accumulation in renal failure. *Am J Med Sci* 1989;298:261–3.

119. Spielberg SP, Schulman JD. A possible reaction to pseudoephedrine in a patient with phenylketonuria. *J Pediatr* 1977;90:1026.

120. Hendeles L. Selecting a decongestant. *Pharmacotherapy* 1993;13(6 pt 2):129S–34.

121. Bryant BG, Lombardi TP. Cold, cough, and allergy products. In Covington TR, ed. *Handbook of nonprescription drugs,* 10th ed. Washington, DC: American Pharmaceutical Association; 1993:89–115.

122. Thoene DE, Johnson CE. Pharmacotherapy of otitis media. *Pharmacotherapy* 1991;11:212–21.

123. Bahal N, Nahata MC. Recent advances in the treatment of otitis media. *J Clin Pharm Ther* 1992;17:201–15.

Part II

CLINICAL INFORMATION

- DRUG-INDUCED DISEASES
- DRUG INTERACTIONS AND INTERFERENCES
- DRUG USE IN SPECIAL POPULATIONS
- IMMUNIZATION
- MEDICAL EMERGENCIES
- NUTRITION SUPPORT

Drug-Induced Diseases

William G. Troutman

■ BLOOD DYSCRASIAS, HEPATOTOXICITY, NEPHROTOXICITY, OCULOTOXICITY, OTOTOXICITY, SEXUAL DYSFUNCTION, SKIN DISORDERS

The tables in the following sections provide information on specific drug-induced diseases. The tables identify drugs of major importance that are thought to be most frequently implicated in causing the disorder in question and thus do not include all drugs reported to cause the drug-induced disease.

When several members of a drug class are known to be similarly capable of producing a disorder, the class name (eg, phenothiazines, sulfonamides) is used, although individual agents may also be listed in boldface type for ease of location. Each entry briefly describes the clinical nature of the drug's toxicity and, when possible, gives its prevalence. Occasionally, the available literature reports that a drug is a possible cause of a disorder, but fails to adequately characterize the frequency and severity of the adverse reaction. In these cases, the phrase "scattered reports only" appears in the discussion section of the table. References are provided after each table for literature discussions and case reports of each particular drug-induced disorder.

Prior to using a table, it is important to read the introductory statement below to become familiar with any general information, inclusion criteria, and abbreviations which pertain to that table.

Drug-Induced Blood Dyscrasias, pages 649–658

This table does not include all drugs capable of causing the specified dyscrasias and excludes cancer chemotherapeutic agents, which are known for producing dose-related bone marrow suppression. Five major types of blood dyscrasias have been selected for inclusion in this table; the following abbreviations are used to indicate the specific blood dyscrasia:

A   – Aplastic Anemia
AGN – Agranulocytosis, Granulocytopenia, or Neutropenia
HA – Hemolytic Anemia
MA – Macrocytic Anemia
Th   – Thrombocytopenia

Drug-Induced Hepatotoxicity, pages 659–667

This table includes only those drugs with a well-established record of hepatotoxicity. Absence of a drug should not be interpreted to mean that a drug is incapable of producing liver damage, because virtually all drugs have been reported to produce elevations of serum liver enzymes. Combining drugs that have hepatotoxic potential commonly results in greater than additive liver damage. In general, drug-induced hepatotoxicity is most prevalent in older patients, women, and those with preexisting hepatic impairment.

Drug-Induced Nephrotoxicity, pages 668–675

This table includes agents that are associated with drug-induced nephrotoxicity, but excludes drugs that produce nephrotoxicity as a result of damage to tissues other than the kidney (eg, liver or skeletal muscle). The following abbreviations are used in the table:

Cl_{cr}	–	Creatinine Clearance
Cr_s	–	Serum Creatinine
GFR	–	Glomerular Filtration Rate
mOsm	–	Milliosmoles

Drug-Induced Oculotoxicity, pages 676–682

Occasionally, nonspecific blurred vision occurs with almost all drugs. The agents in this table are associated with a specific pattern of drug-induced oculotoxicity when administered *systemically*.

Drug-Induced Ototoxicity, pages 683–685

Drug-induced ototoxicity can affect hearing (auditory or cochlear function), balance (vestibular function), or both, depending upon the drug. Drugs of almost every class have been reported to produce tinnitus, as have placebos. The agents in this table are associated with a measurable change in hearing or vestibular defect when administered *systemically*.

Drug-Induced Sexual Dysfunction, pages 686–690

The large subjective component of human sexual response makes the evaluation of drug-induced sexual dysfunction difficult. Variations in study design have produced widely divergent reported rates of sexual dysfunction in the "normal" or control populations. Common drug-induced sexual dysfunctions include decreased libido or sexual drive, impotence (failure to achieve or maintain an erection in men), priapism (persistent and often painful erection), delayed ejaculation or failure of ejaculation, retrograde ejaculation (into the urinary bladder), and, in women, failure to achieve orgasm and decreased vaginal lubrication. Gynecomastia (enlargement of the male breast) has also been included in this table. Although it is not life-threatening, drug-induced sexual dysfunction has a negative impact on quality of life and is an important contributor to noncompliance with prescribed drug regimens.

Drug-Induced Skin Disorders, pages 691–693

Most drugs occasionally have been associated with rashes or other dermatologic reactions. The difficulty of determining a correct diagnosis of a skin disorder and the complexity of establishing a causal relationship with drug therapy make estimating of the frequency of occurrence of these reactions virtually impossible. Only skin disorders resulting from *systemic* administration of drugs are represented in this table. Drugs believed to be among the most common causes of a particular drug-induced skin disorder are designated by "XX" in the table. Stevens-Johnson syndrome, a potentially fatal form of erythema multiforme, is included in the table entries for erythema multiforme. The following abbreviations are used to indicate specific skin disorders:

AE – Acneiform Eruptions
Al   – Alopecia
ED – Exfoliative Dermatitis
EM – Erythema Multiforme
FE – Fixed Eruptions
LE – Lupus Erythematosus–Like Reactions
Ph – Photosensitivity and Phototoxicity Reactions
TN – Toxic Epidermal Necrolysis

Drug-Induced Blood Dyscrasias

See introductory information on page 647.

DRUG AND DYSCRASIA	NATURE OF DYSCRASIA
Acetaminophen	
Th	Scattered reports only; observed in 6 of 174 overdose patients in one report; may be an immune reaction.[1,2]
Alcohol	
HA	Most commonly encountered in chronic alcoholism.[3]
MA	Results from malnutrition and decreased folate absorption and/or utilization. Responds rapidly to folic acid administration.[3]
Th	Transient in many drinkers; persistent thrombocytopenia may accompany advanced alcoholic liver disease.[3]
Amphotericin B	
AGN	Scattered reports only.[3,4]
Th	Scattered reports only.[3–5]
Amrinone	
Th	18.6% prevalence in one study of oral therapy (oral form not marketed in the U.S.); the prevalence during parenteral therapy has been estimated at 2.4%, although 8 of 16 children receiving parenteral amrinone developed thrombocytopenia in one report. Thrombocytopenia may be caused by nonimmune peripheral platelet destruction.[6–8]
Antidepressants, Heterocyclic	
AGN	Idiosyncratic reaction, probably resulting from a direct toxic effect rather than allergy. Most commonly occurs between the second and eighth weeks of therapy.[3,9,10]
Ascorbic Acid	
HA	In G-6-PD deficiency with large doses.[3]

(continued)

DRUG AND DYSCRASIA	NATURE OF DYSCRASIA

Aspirin

HA   Almost always encountered in patients with G-6-PD deficiency, usually in conjunction with infection or other complicating factors.[3,11]

Th   May occur in addition to the drug's effects on platelet adhesiveness. Some evidence for an immune reaction.[1,3,12]

Azathioprine

AGN   Scattered reports only; leukopenia occurs frequently. May be influenced by genetically determined metabolic enzyme activity.[13]

Captopril

AGN   Prevalence estimated at 1/5000 patients. The prevalence increases greatly in patients with reduced renal function or collagen-vascular diseases and reaches 7% in patients with both renal impairment and a collagen-vascular disease. Most common during the first 3 weeks of therapy.[14]

Carbamazepine

AA   27 cases reported from 1964–1988; onset may be delayed until weeks or months after the initiation of therapy.[3,15]

AGN   Transient leukopenia occurs in about 10% of patients, usually during the first month of therapy. Recovery usually occurs within a week of drug withdrawal. Persistent leukopenia occurs in 2%.[15,16]

Th   Prevalence estimated at 2%.[15,17]

Cephalosporins

AGN   Rare; possibly the result of an immune reaction, but occurs most often with high dosages.[3,18]

HA   Positive direct Coombs' test occurs frequently and may persist for up to 2 months after discontinuation of therapy. Hemolysis is rare.[3,18]

Th   Rare; possibly the result of an immune reaction. Usually occurs late in the course of therapy.[3,18]

Chloramphenicol

AA   Prevalence estimated at 1/12,000 to 1/50,000 patients. Most cases develop with oral administration and after discontinuation of therapy, suggesting the development of a toxic metabolite. Blacks may be more susceptible than whites. It has occurred with parenteral and ophthalmic therapy. Aplastic anemia should not be confused with the dose-related anemia seen with chloramphenicol (Note: one case report suggests that a patient's dose-related anemia may have progressed to aplastic anemia, but most sources separate the two dyscrasias).[3,19–23]

AGN   Rare when compared with the prevalence of aplastic anemia.[3,19]

HA   In G-6-PD deficiency.[3]

Chloroquine

AGN   Scattered reports only; may be dose related.[3]

HA   Only a few cases have been reported; some association with G-6-PD deficiency is suspected.[3]

Cimetidine

AA   Scattered reports only; however, at least two fatalities reported (one fatality was also receiving chloramphenicol).[24]

AGN   Usually occurs in patients with systemic disease or other drug therapy which may have contributed to the dyscrasia.[24]

(continued)

DRUG AND DYSCRASIA	NATURE OF DYSCRASIA

Clozapine

AGN — Frequency of granulocytopenia is calculated to be as high as 1%, with mild to moderate neutropenia in up to 20%. Most cases occur in the first 4 months. Recovery usually occurs 2–3 weeks after drug withdrawal. Weekly WBC counts are mandated.[25,26]

Cocaine

Th — Reported with both IV and inhalational use.[27]

Contraceptives, Oral

MA — Results from impaired absorption and/or utilization of folate; of consequence only if the patient's folate status is markedly impaired.[3]

Dapsone

AGN — Many cases have occurred during combination therapy, so it is difficult to determine if dapsone alone is the causative agent.[3,28]

HA — In G-6-PD deficiency; may also have other mechanism(s). May be dose related; uncommon at 100 mg/day, but frequent at 200–300 mg/day.[3]

Digitoxin

Th — Scattered reports only; evidence of an immune mechanism.[1,29]

Digoxin

Th — Scattered reports only; evidence of an immune mechanism.[21,30]

Dimercaprol

HA — In G-6-PD deficiency.[3]

Dipyridamole

Th — Relative risk of thrombocytopenia calculated to be 14 times higher than in untreated individuals, but needs confirmation.[31]

Diuretics, Thiazide

HA — Exact mechanism is unclear; may be an immune reaction.[3,32]

Th — Mild thrombocytopenia occurs frequently, but severe cases are rare. May be caused by an immune reaction.[1,3,33]

Eflornithine

AA — Deaths caused by aplastic anemia have been reported.[34]

AGN — Leukopenia is reported in 18–37% of patients.[34]

MA — Megaloblastic anemia is frequently reported.[34]

Th — Thrombocytopenia is frequently reported.[34]

Felbamate

AA — More than 30 cases were reported shortly after the introduction of felbamate, resulting in the manufacturer and FDA urging withdrawal of patients from therapy. Most cases developed 2–6 months after initiation of therapy. Monitoring has not been effective for the early identification of cases.[35]

Fluconazole

Th — Scattered reports only.[36]

Flucytosine

AGN — Dose related; usually requires plasma level of 125 mg/L or greater.[37]

Th — Dose related; usually requires plasma level of 125 mg/L or greater.[37]

Foscarnet

AGN — Neutropenia occurs in 14% of patients treated for cytomegalovirus retinitis.[38]

Furosemide

Th — Uncommon, mild and asymptomatic.[3]

(continued)

DRUG AND DYSCRASIA	NATURE OF DYSCRASIA
Ganciclovir	
AGN	Granulocytopenia occurs in about 40% of patients; it is usually reversible upon drug discontinuation, but irreversible neutropenia and deaths have occurred.[38,39]
Th	Thrombocytopenia occurs in about 20% of patients.[39]
Gold Salts	
AA	Not dose dependent; while this reaction is not common, numerous fatalities have been reported.[13,40]
AGN	Often brief and self-limiting; usually responds to withdrawal of therapy.[41,42]
Th	Not dose or duration dependent; prevalence estimated at 1–3%; onset usually during the loading phase (first 1000 mg), but may be delayed until after the drug has been discontinued. Mechanism is unclear, but it often appears to be immunologically mediated.[1,3,43,44]
Heparin	
Th	Many patients demonstrate a mild, benign, transient decrease in platelets early in heparin therapy. Up to 3% experience immune-mediated, persistent thrombocytopenia, which is associated with increased development of life-threatening thrombosis. Intermittent, continuous infusion and "minidose" regimens have all been implicated; this is uncommon with SC administration. Prompt cessation of heparin minimizes serious complications; platelet count usually returns to normal within 48 hr. Lowest prevalence occurs with pork intestine-derived products. Low molecular weight heparins (eg, dalteparin, enoxaparin) are much less likely than unfractionated heparin to stimulate the formation of immune complexes leading to thrombocytopenia. Low molecular weight heparins offer no protection from thrombocytopenia in patients who have already formed heparin-associated antibodies.[45–48]
Immune Globulin	
AGN	Transient neutropenia frequently accompanies IV use.[49]
HA	Acute Coombs' positive hemolysis has been reported in patients receiving high-dose therapy.[49]
Indomethacin	
AA	Although rare, indomethacin has been associated with a risk 12.7 times higher than in untreated individuals, especially when used regularly and for a long duration.[50]
AGN	Although rare, risk may be 8.9 times higher than in untreated individuals.[50]
Interferon Alfa	
Th	Scattered reports only.[51]
Isoniazid	
AGN	Scattered reports only; some evidence of an immune reaction.[3,52]
Th	Scattered reports only; some evidence of an immune reaction.[1,3,52]
Lamotrigine	
AGN	Scattered reports only; too early to establish a pattern of risk.[53]
Levamisole	
AGN	May be the result of an autoimmune reaction with a prevalence of 4% or more in some series. Presence of the HLA-B27 phenotype in seropositive rheumatoid arthritis may be an important predisposing factor.[9,50,54]
Th	Scattered reports only.[1,55]

(continued)

DRUG AND DYSCRASIA	NATURE OF DYSCRASIA
Levodopa	
HA	Autoimmune reaction; positive direct and indirect Coombs' tests are frequent, but hemolysis is rare. **Carbidopa-levodopa** combinations have also produced hemolysis.[3]
Mefenamic Acid	
HA	Thought to be autoimmune.[3,11]
Mesalamine	
AA	Scattered reports only. One review of over 4000 cases found no adverse hematologic effects.[56,86]
Methimazole	
AA	Scattered reports only; however, some increased risk is present. Most cases occur during the first 3 months of therapy.[57,58]
AGN	Prevalence estimated at 0.31%. Encountered overwhelmingly in women and appears to increase with age. Most cases occur in the first 3 months of therapy, and monitoring during this time may detect agranulocytosis before it becomes clinically apparent.[3,57,59,60]
Methyldopa	
HA	Autoimmune reaction; positive direct Coombs' test occurs in 5–25% of patients, depending on dosage; hemolysis occurs in less than 1%, and its onset is gradual after 4 months or more of therapy. Recovery is rapid after discontinuation of the drug.[13,11,61]
Th	Rare; may be caused by an immune reaction.[1,3,62]
Methylene Blue	
HA	In G-6-PD deficiency.[3]
Nalidixic Acid	
HA	In G-6-PD deficiency; may also have other mechanisms.[3]
Th	Scattered reports only; possibly associated with renal impairment in one series.[63]
Nitrofurantoin	
HA	In G-6-PD deficiency; also encountered with enolase deficiency (mechanism unknown).[3]
Penicillamine	
AA	Rare; develops after several months of therapy; due to direct marrow toxicity.[64,65]
AGN	Rare; most cases occur during the first month of therapy.[3,65]
HA	Scattered reports only; may be caused by G-6-PD deficiency or fluctuations in copper levels during therapy of Wilson's disease.[65,66]
Th	Prevalence estimated at 10%; some decrease in platelet counts occurs in 75% of penicillamine-treated patients. May be the result of an immune reaction; most commonly occurs during the first 6 months of therapy.[3,65,67]
Penicillins	
AA	Prevalence very low when extent of use is considered.[3]
AGN	Uncommon with most penicillins, but frequent with **methicillin;** in one report, neutropenia developed in 23 of 68 methicillin-treated patients; resolution occurred within 3–7 days after drug withdrawal.[3,9,68]
HA	Positive direct Coombs' test occurs with large IV doses; hemolysis rare.[3,11]

(*continued*)

DRUG AND DYSCRASIA	NATURE OF DYSCRASIA
Phenazopyridine	
HA	Prevalence and mechanism unknown; renal insufficiency and overdose may be contributing factors. Often accompanied by methemoglobinemia.[3,69]
Phenobarbital	
MA	Over 100 cases reported; usually responds to folic acid.[3]
Phenothiazines	
AGN	Most common during the first 2 months of therapy and in older patients (>85% are >40 yr). Rapid onset and general lack of dose dependence suggest an idiosyncratic mechanism. Prevalence estimated as high as 1/1200.[13,9,70,71]
Phenytoin	
AA	Fewer than 25 reported cases, but the association with phenytoin is strong.[3]
AGN	Scattered reports only; onset after days to years of therapy.[3,9]
MA	Caused by impaired absorption and/or utilization of folate and responds to folic acid therapy (although folate replacement may lower phenytoin levels). Mild macrocytosis is very common (25% or more); onset is unpredictable, but usually appears after 6 months or more of therapy.[3]
Th	Scattered reports only; may be the result of an immune reaction.[1,3,72]
Primaquine	
HA	In G-6-PD deficiency.[3]
Primidone	
MA	Similar to phenobarbital, but prevalence may be lower; onset is unpredictable and may be delayed for several years during therapy. Some cases have responded to folic acid.[3]
Procainamide	
AGN	Prevalence usually estimated at less than 1%, but with a 25% fatal outcome. Occurs with both conventional and sustained-release products; usually occurs within the first 90 days of use. No relationship with daily or total dosage.[3,9,73–75]
Propylthiouracil	
AA	Scattered reports only; however, some increased risk is present. Most cases occur within the first 3 months of therapy.[57,58]
AGN	Prevalence estimated at 0.55%. Occurs overwhelmingly in women and appears to increase with age. Most cases occur in the first 3 months of therapy, and monitoring during this time may detect agranulocytosis before it becomes clinically apparent. Some evidence for an immune reaction.[3,9,57–60,76]
Quinacrine	
AA	About one-half of reported cases were preceded by a rash or lichenoid eruption; prevalence estimated at 3/100,000.[13,77]
HA	In G-6-PD deficiency; usually requires concurrent infection or other complicating factors.[3]
Quinidine	
AGN	Scattered reports only; an immune mechanism has been described.[9,78]
HA	In G-6-PD deficiency (but not in blacks). A rapid onset immune mechanism has also been described.[3,9,11,79]
Th	Caused by quinidine-specific antibodies; little or no cross-reactivity with quinine. Accounts for a large portion of drug-induced thrombocytopenia.[1,3,31,72,80]
Quinine	
AGN	Scattered reports only.[3]
HA	In G-6-PD deficiency (but not in blacks). An immune mechanism is also suspected.[3,81]

(continued)

DRUG AND DYSCRASIA	NATURE OF DYSCRASIA
Th	Caused by quinine-specific antibodies; little or no cross-reactivity with quinidine. Fatalities have been reported. It has occurred in people drinking quinine-containing tonic water.[1,3,31,82,83]
Rifampin	
HA	Rare, but many patients develop a positive Coombs' test; onset in hours in some sensitized patients.[3,52,84]
Th	Peripheral destruction of platelets appears to result from an immune reaction; difficult to separate rifampin contribution from that of other drugs, because it is usually used in combination therapy.[1,3,52]
Sulfasalazine	
AGN	Leukopenia reported in 5.6% of patients receiving the drug for rheumatoid arthritis and agranulocytosis/neutropenia in 4 of 1000 patients; prevalence of agranulocytosis/neutropenia among inflammatory bowel disease patients is considerably lower (0.3 of 1000 patients).[85,86]
HA	In G-6-PD deficiency, but also occurs in nondeficient patients. Hemolysis may be more common in slow acetylators.[3,86–88]
MA	One series of 130 arthritis patients reported macrocytosis in 21% and macrocytic anemia in 3%.[89]
Sulfonamides	
AA	Historically, an important cause of aplastic anemia, but most cases were reported following use of older sulfonamides; rarely occurs with products currently in use.[3]
AGN	Occurs mostly with older products; rarely occurs with products currently in use. Most current cases are in combined use with trimethoprim; also reported with **silver sulfadiazine**. Onset is usually rapid.[3,11,90,91]
HA	In G-6-PD deficiency; but also occurs in nondeficient patients.[3,92]
Th	Scattered reports only; probably an immune reaction. See also trimethoprim.[1,31,72]
Ticlopidine	
AGN	Neutropenia developed in 13 of 1518 patients in one study; onset was most common in the first 3 months of therapy. Neutropenia resolved within 3 weeks of drug discontinuation.[93]
Tocainide	
AGN	Prevalence estimated at 0.07–0.18% of patients.[94,95]
Triamterene	
MA	Few cases reported, but it is a potent inhibitor of dihydrofolate reductase; greatest risk in those with folate deficiency prior to therapy (eg, alcoholics).[3]
Trimethoprim	
AGN	Rare; occurs when used alone and in combination with sulfonamides, with the latter numerically more common.[3,91,96]
MA	Most cases occur after 1–2 weeks of therapy; this drug may have small antifolate action in humans, which becomes important only in those with folate deficiency prior to therapy (eg, alcoholics).[3]
Th	Thrombocytopenia is common, but severe cases are rare. Most commonly occured in combination therapy with sulfonamides. Relative risk calculated at 124 times that of untreated individuals.[1,3,31]
Valproic Acid	
MA	Macrocytosis occurs in 11 of 60 patients in one report.[97]
Th	Thrombocytopenia occurred in 12 of 60 patients in one report. Both immune and dose-dependent mechanisms have been suggested.[1,97]

(continued)

DRUG AND DYSCRASIA	NATURE OF DYSCRASIA
Vancomycin	
AGN	Scattered reports only; however, prevalence may be as high as 2%; mechanism unknown.[2,98,99]
Vitamin K	
HA	In G-6-PD deficiency; usually requires concurrent infection or other complicating factors. Hemolysis from high doses can contribute to jaundice in neonates; rarely toxic in older children and adults.[3]
Zidovudine	
AGN	Most patients experience at least a 25% reduction in neutrophil count; absolute neutrophil counts of less than 500/μL occur in 16% of patients. Usual onset is during the first 3 months of therapy.[100,101]
MA	Macrocytosis develops in most patients, usually beginning during the first few weeks of therapy. Zidovudine is now the leading cause of drug-induced macrocytosis.[100–102]

■ REFERENCES

1. Hackett T et al. Drug-induced platelet destruction. *Semin Thromb Hemost* 1982;8:116–37.
2. Fischereder M, Jaffe JP. Thrombocytopenia following acute acetaminophen overdose. *Am J Hematol* 1994;45:258–9.
3. Swanson M, Cook R. *Drugs chemicals and blood dyscrasias.* Hamilton, IL: Drug Intelligence Publications; 1977.
4. Wilson R, Feldman S. Toxicity of amphotericin B in children with cancer. *Am J Dis Child* 1979;133:731–4.
5. Chan CSP et al. Amphotericin-B-induced thrombocytopenia. *Ann Intern Med* 1982;96:332–3.
6. Ansell J et al. Amrinone-induced thrombocytopenia. *Arch Intern Med* 1984;144:949–52.
7. Treadway G. Clinical safety of intravenous amrinone—a review. *Am J Cardiol* 1985;56:39B-40.
8. Ross MP et al. Amrinone-associated thrombocytopenia: pharmacokinetic analysis. *Clin Pharmacol Ther* 1993;53:661–7.
9. Heimpel H. Drug-induced agranulocytosis. *Med Toxicol Adverse Drug Exp* 1988;3:449–62.
10. Levin GM, DeVane CL. A review of cyclic antidepressant-induced blood dyscrasias. *Ann Pharmacother* 1992;26:378–83.
11. Sanford-Driscoll M, Knodel LC. Induction of hemolytic anemia by nonsteroidal antiinflammatory drugs. *Drug Intell Clin Pharm* 1986;20:925–34.
12. Garg SK, Sarker CR. Aspirin-induced thrombocytopenia on an immune basis. *Am J Med Sci* 1974;267:129–32.
13. Anstey A et al. Pancytopenia related to azathioprine—an enzyme deficiency caused by a common genetic polymorphism: a review. *J R Soc Med* 1992;85:752–6.
14. Cooper RA. Captopril-associated neutropenia. Who is at risk? *Arch Intern Med* 1983;143:659–60. Editorial.
15. Sobotka JL et al. A review of carbamazepine's hematologic reactions and monitoring recommendations. *DICP* 1990;24:1214–9.
16. Tohen M et al. Blood dyscrasias with carbamazepine and valproate: a pharmacoepidemiological study of 2,228 patients at risk. *Am J Psychiatry* 1995;152:413–8.
17. Bradley JM et al. Carbamazepine-induced thrombocytopenia in a young child. *Clin Pharm* 1985;4:221–3.
18. Thompson JW, Jacobs RF. Adverse effects of newer cephalosporins. An update. *Drug Saf* 1993;9:132–42.
19. Chaplin S. Bone marrow depression due to mianserin, phenylbutazone, oxyphenbutazone, and chloramphenicol—part I. *Adverse Drug React Acute Poisoning Rev* 1986;2:97–136.
20. Chaplin S. Bone marrow depression due to mianserln phenylbutazone, oxyphenbutazone, and chloramphenicol—part II. *Adverse Drug React Acute Poisoning Rev* 1986;3:181–96.
21. Brodsky E et al. Topical application of chloramphenicol eye ointment followed by fatal bone marrow aplasia. *Isr J Med Sci* 1989;25:54.
22. Fraunfelder FT et al. Blood dyscrasias and topical ophthalmic chloramphenicol. *Am J Ophthalmol* 1993;115:812–3. Letter.
23. Flegg P et al. Chloramphenicol. Are concerns about aplastic anemia justified? *Drug Saf* 1992;7:167–9.
24. Aymard J-P et al. Haematological adverse effects of histamine H₂-receptor antagonists. *Med Toxicol Adverse Drug Exp* 1988;3:430–48.
25. Hummer M et al. Transient neutropenia induced by clozapine. *Psychopharmacol Bull* 1992;28:287–90.

26. Alvir JMJ et al. Clozapine-induced agranulocytosis. Incidence and risk factors in the United States. *N Engl J Med* 1993;329:162–7.

27. Leissinger CA. Severe thrombocytopenia associated with cocaine use. *Ann Intern Med* 1990;112:708–10.

28. Cockburn EM et al. Dapsone-induced agranulocytosis: spontaneous reporting data. *Br J Dermatol* 1993;128:702–3. Letter.

29. Young RC et al. Thrombocytopenia due to digitoxin. Demonstration of antibody and mechanisms of action. *Am J Med* 1966;41:605–14.

30. Pirovino M et al. Digoxin-associated thrombocytopaenia. *Eur J Clin Pharmacol* 1981;19:205–7.

31. Kaufman DW et al. Acute thrombocytopenic purpura in relation to the use of drugs. *Blood* 1993;82:2714–8.

32. Beck ML et al. Fatal intravascular immune hemolysis induced by hydrochlorothiazide. *Am J Clin Pathol* 1984;81:791–4.

33. Okafor KC et al. Hydrochlorothiazide-induced thrombocytopenic purpura. *Drug Intell Clin Pharm* 1986;20:60–1.

34. Sahai J, Berry AJ. Eflornithine for the treatment of *Pneumocystis carinii* pneumonia in patients with the acquired immunodeficiency syndrome: a preliminary review. *Pharmacotherapy* 1989;9:29–33.

35. Pennell PB et al. Aplastic anemia in a patient receiving felbamate for complex partial seizures. *Neurology* 1995;45:456–60.

36. Mercurio MG et al. Thrombocytopenia caused by fluconazole therapy. *J Am Acad Dermatol* 1995;32:525–6.

37. Kauffman CA, Frame PT. Bone marrow toxicity associated with 5-fluorocytosine therapy. *Antimicrob Agents Chemother* 1977;11:244–7.

38. Morbidity and toxic effects associated with ganciclovir or foscarnet therapy in a randomized cytomegalovirus retinitis trial. Studies of Ocular Complications of AIDS Research Group, in collaboration with the AIDS Clinical Trials Group. *Intern Med* 1995;155:65–74.

39. Cytovene product information. Palo Alto, CA: Syntex Laboratories; 1994.

40. Gibson J et al. Aplastic anemia in association with gold therapy for rheumatoid arthritis. *Aust N Z J Med* 1983;13:130–4.

41. Gibbons RB. Complications of chrysotherapy. A review of recent studies. *Arch Intern Med* 1979;139:343–6.

42. Gottlieb NL et al. The course of severe gold-associated granulocytopenia. *Clin Res* 1982;30:659A. Abstract.

43. Coblyn JS et al. Gold-induced thrombocytopenia. A clinical and immunogenetic study of twenty-three patients. *Ann Intern Med* 1981;95:178–81.

44. Adachi JD et al. Gold induced thrombocytopenia: platelet associated IgG and HLA typing in three patients. *J Rheumatol* 1984;11:355–7.

45. Warkentin TE et al. Heparin-induced thrombocytopenia in patients treated with low-molecular-weight heparin or unfractionated heparin. *N Engl J Med* 1995;332:1330–5.

46. Chong BH. Heparin-induced thrombocytopenia. *Aust N Z J Med* 1992;22:145–52.

47. Schmitt BP, Adelman B. Heparin-associated thrombocytopenia: a critical review and pooled analysis. *Am J Med Sci* 1993;305:208–15.

48. Phillips DE et al. Heparin-induced thrombotic thrombocytopenia. *Ann Pharmacother* 1994;28:43–6.

49. Misbah SA, Chapel HM. Adverse effects of intravenous immunoglobulin. *Drug Saf* 1993;9:254–62.

50. Risks of agranulocytosis and aplastic anemia. A first report of their relation to drug use with special reference to analgesics. The International Agranulocytosis and Aplastic Anemia Study. *JAMA* 1986;256:1749–57.

51. Murakami CS et al. Idiopathic thrombocytopenic purpura during interferon-α_{2B} treatment for chronic hepatitis. *Am J Gastroenterol* 1994;89:2244–5.

52. Holdiness MR. A review of blood dyscrasias induced by the antituberculosis drugs. *Tubercle* 1987;68:301–9.

53. Nicholson RJ et al. Leucopenia associated with lamotrigine. *BMJ* 1995;310:504.

54. Mielants H, Veys EM. A study of the hematological side effects of levamisole in rheumatoid arthritis with recommendations. *J Rheumatol* 1978;5(suppl 4):77–83.

55. El-Gobarey AF, Capell HA. Levamisole-induced thrombocytopenia. *Br Med J* 1977;2:555–6.

56. Abboudi ZH et al. Fatal aplastic anaemia after mesalazine. *Lancet* 1994;343:542. Letter.

57. Risk of agranulocytosis and aplastic anaemia in relation to use of antithyroid drugs. International Agranulocytosis and Aplastic Anaemia Study. *BMJ* 1988;297:262–5.

58. Biswas N et al. Case report: aplastic anemia associated with antithyroid drugs. *Am J Med Sci* 1991;301:190–4.

59. Tajiri J et al. Antithyroid drug-induced agranulocytosis. The usefulness of routine white blood cell count monitoring. *Arch Intern Med* 1990;150:621–4.

60. Meyer-Gebner M et al. Antithyroid drug-induced agranulocytosis: clinical experience with ten patients treated at one institution and review of the literature. *J Endocrinol Invest* 1994;17:29–36.

61. Kelton JG. Impaired reticuloendothelial function in patients treated with methyldopa. *N Engl J Med* 1985;313:596–600.

62. Manohitharajah SM et al. Methyldopa and associated thrombocytopenia. *Br Med J* 1971;1:494.

63. Meyboom RHB. Thrombocytopenia induced by nalidixic acid. *Br Med J* 1984;289:962.

64. Kay AGL. Myelotoxicity of D-penicillamine. *Ann Rheum Dis* 1979;38:232–6.

65. Camp AV. Hematologic toxicity from penicillamine in rheumatoid arthritis. *J Rheumatol* 1981;8(suppl 7):164–5.

66. Lyle WH. D-penicillamine and haemolytic anaemia. *Lancet* 1976;1:428. Letter.

67. Thomas D et al. A study of D-penicillamine induced thrombocytopenia in rheumatoid arthritis with Cr⁵¹-labelled autologous platelets. *Aust N Z J Med* 1981;11:722. Abstract.

68. Mallouh AA. Methicillin-induced neutropenia. *Pediatr Infect Dis J* 1985;4:262–4.

69. Jeffery WH et al. Acquired methemoglobinemia and hemolytic anemia after usual doses of phenazopyridine. *Drug Intell Clin Pharm* 1982;16:157–9.

70. Hollister LE. Allergic reactions to tranquilizing drugs. *Ann Intern Med* 1958;49:17–29.

71. Pisciotta AV et al. Agranulocytosis following administration of phenothiazine derivatives. *Am J Med* 1958;25:210–23.

72. Cimo PL et al. Detection of drug-dependent antibodies by the ⁵¹Cr platelet lysis test: documentation of immune thrombocytopenia induced by diphenylhydantoIn diazepam, and sulfisoxazole. *Am J Hematol* 1977;2:65–72.

73. Meyers DG et al. Severe neutropenia associated with procainamide: comparison of sustained release and conventional preparations. *Am Heart J* 1985;109:1393–5.

74. Thompson JF et al. Procainamide agranulocytosis: a case report and review of the literature. *Curr Ther Res* 1988;44:872–81.

75. Danielly J et al. Procainamide-associated blood dyscrasias. *Am J Cardiol* 1994;74:1179–80.

76. Fibbe WE et al. Agranulocytosis induced by propylthiouracil: evidence for a drug dependent antibody reacting with granulocytes, monocytes and haematopoietic progenitor cells. *Br J Haematol* 1986;64:363–73.

77. Custer RP. Aplastic anemia in soldiers treated with atabrine (quinacrine). *Am J Med Sci* 1946;212:211–24.

78. Ascensao JL et al. Quinidine-induced neutropenia: report of a case with drug-dependent inhibition of granulocyte colony generation. *Acta Haematol* 1984;72:349–54.

79. Geltner D et al. Quinidine hypersensitivity and liver involvement. A survey of 32 patients. *Gastroenterology* 1976;70:650–2.

80. Reid DM, Shulman NR. Drug purpura due to surreptitious quinidine intake. *Ann Intern Med* 1988;108:206–8.

81. Webb RF et al. Acute intravascular haemolysis due to quinine. *N Z Med J* 1980;91:14–6.

82. Murray JA et al. Bitter lemon purpura. *Br Med J* 1979;2:1551–2.

83. Freiman JP. Fatal quinine-induced thrombocytopenia. *Ann Intern Med* 1990;112:308–9. Letter.

84. Tahan SR et al. Acute hemolysis and renal failure with rifampicin-dependent antibodies after discontinuous administration. *Transfusion* 1985;25:124–7.

85. Marabani M et al. Leucopenia during sulfasalazine treatment for rheumatoid arthritis. *Ann Rheum Dis* 1989;48:505–7.

86. Jick H et al. The risk of sulfasalazine- and mesalazine-associated blood disorders. *Pharmacotherapy* 1995;15:176–81.

87. Cohen SM et al. Ulcerative colitis and erythrocyte G6PD deficiency. Salicylazosulfapyridine-provoked hemolysis. *JAMA* 1968;205:528–30.

88. Das KM et al. Adverse reactions during salicylazosulfapyridine therapy and the relation with drug metabolism and acetylator phenotype. *N Engl J Med* 1973;289:491–5.

89. Hopkinson ND et al. Haematological side-effects of sulphasalazine in inflammatory arthritis. *Br J Rheumatol* 1989;28:414–7.

90. Jarrett F et al. Acute leukopenia during topical burn therapy with silver sulfadiazine. *Am J Surg* 1978;135:818–9.

91. Anti-infective drug use in relation to the risk of agranulocytosis and aplastic anemia. The International Agranulocytosis and Aplastic Anemia Study. *Arch Intern Med* 1989;149:1036–40.

92. Zinkham WH. Unstable hemoglobins and the selective hemolytic action of sulfonamides. The International Agranulocytosis and Aplastic Anemia Study. *Arch Intern Med* 1977;137:1365–6. Editorial.

93. Hass WK et al. A randomized trial comparing ticlopidine hydrochloride with aspirin for the prevention of stroke in high-risk patients. *N Engl J Med* 1989;321:501–7.

94. Volosin K et al. Tocainide associated agranulocytosis. *Am Heart J* 1985;109:1392–3.

95. Roden DM, Woosley RL. Tocainide. *N Engl J Med* 1986;315:41–5.

96. Hawkins T et al. Severe trimethoprim induced neutropenia and thrombocytopenia. *N Z Med J* 1993;106:251–2.

97. May RB, Sunder TR. Hematologic manifestations of long-term valproate therapy. *Epilepsia* 1993; 34:1098–101.

98. Mackett RL, Guay DRP. Vancomycin-induced neutropenia. *Can Med Assoc J* 1985;132:39–40.

99. Sacho H, Moore PJ. Vancomycin-induced neutropenia. *S Afr Med J* 1989;76:701. Letter.

100. Richman DD et al. The toxicity of azidothymidine (AZT) in the treatment of patients with AIDS and AIDS-related complex. A double-blind, placebo-controlled trial. *N Engl J Med* 1987;317:192–7.

101. Rachlis A, Fanning MM. Zidovudine toxicity. Clinical features and management. *Drug Saf* 1993;8:312–20.

102. Snower DP, Weil SC. Changing etiology of macrocytosis. Zidovudine as a frequent causative factor. *Am J Clin Pathol* 1993;99:57–60.

Drug-Induced Hepatotoxicity

See introductory information on page 647.

DRUG	NATURE OF HEPATOTOXICITY
ACE Inhibitors	Hepatic injury occurs occasionally with angiotensin converting enzyme (ACE) inhibitors. **Captopril** and **enalapril** are implicated in most reported cases, but other ACE inhibitors likely have similar hepatotoxic potential. Most cases show cholestatic injury, but mixed and hepatocellular damage are also reported.[1–3]
Acetaminophen	Centrilobular hepatic necrosis may follow acute overdose with 140 mg/kg or more in children, or 6 g or more in adults. These doses saturate the normal metabolic pathways, producing large quantities of an hepatotoxic metabolite. Children appear to be have a lower risk than adults of developing acetaminophen-induced hepatitis. Laboratory evidence of hepatotoxicity peaks 3–4 days after the acute exposure. Therapy with **acetylcysteine** to bind the metabolite is indicated when the 4-hr postingestion serum acetaminophen level is over 150 mg/L. Even without acetylcysteine, fatalities are uncommon following acetaminophen overdose. Nonfatal cases usually recover fully in a few weeks. Chronic **alcohol** ingestion increases acetaminophen toxicity as does recent fasting. Acute alcohol ingestion is thought by some to have a protective action. Less destructive, but still detectable, hepatitis is reported in patients taking large doses for therapeutic purposes.[1,3,5,6]
Alcohol	Fatty infiltration of the liver occurs in 70–100% of alcoholics. Fatty liver is generally without clinical manifestation, but 30% of alcoholics progress to develop alcoholic hepatitis and about 10% develop cirrhosis. Malnutrition may potentiate alcoholic liver disease, and alcohol may enhance the hepatotoxicity of other drugs.[2]
Aldesleukin	Increases in serum bilirubin, alkaline phosphatase, and transaminases occur frequently. These primarily cholestatic changes are rapidly reversible after drug discontinuation.[7]
Allopurinol	Hepatitis and hepatic necrosis may accompany other symptoms (especially rash, fever, eosinophilia, and vasculitis) of allopurinol hypersensitivity. Damage is usually focal, but widespread damage is also reported. This reaction is rare, but serious when it occurs. Renal impairment may be a predisposing factor for allopurinol-induced hepatitis. Cholestasis has also been attributed to allopurinol.[1,2,8,9]
Aminoglutethimide	Laboratory evidence of hepatic dysfunction is common, but clinical evidence is rare.[1,8,10]
Aminosalicylic Acid	Up to 5% of patients develop a generalized hypersensitivity reaction. About 25% of these patients have evidence of mixed cholestatic and hepatocellular injury as part of their hypersensitivity reaction. Fatalities have been reported.[1,2,11]
Amiodarone	Mild increases in transaminases and LDH levels occur in up to one-half of patients, while phospholipidosis occurs in virtually all; normal values often return despite continued therapy. Symptoms of liver injury (eg, jaundice, nausea and vomiting, hepatomegaly, or weight loss) occur in 1–4% of patients. Onset is typically after 2–4 months of therapy, but may be delayed for 1 yr or more.

(continued)

DRUG	NATURE OF HEPATOTOXICITY
	Recovery after drug discontinuation may take from several months to 1 yr or more. The dose-related hepatotoxicity of amiodarone is reminiscent of alcoholic hepatitis. Cirrhosis and fatalities have also been reported.[1,2,4,12,13]
Amoxicillin and Clavulanic Acid	Fixed combinations of these drugs are occasionally associated with the development of relatively benign hepatocanalicular cholestasis. Jaundice usually resolves within 1–2 months of drug discontinuation, but laboratory test abnormalities may require up to 4 months for resolution. Since this reaction is rare with amoxicillin alone, it is assumed that clavulanic acid is primarily responsible.[2,14,15]
Androgens	*See* Steroids, C–17–α-Alkyl.
Antidepressants, Heterocyclic	The prevalence of hepatic injury is estimated at about 1%, with most of the cases presenting as cholestasis. This idiosyncratic reaction resembles the cholestasis associated with phenothiazines.[1,2,8]
Asparaginase	Slowly reversible steatosis occurs in 50–90% of patients, apparently as a result of the drug's influence on protein synthesis. Daily administration may be more hepatotoxic than weekly administration.[1,2,16–18]
Azathioprine	This drug is less hepatotoxic than its metabolite mercaptopurine. Azathioprine's hepatotoxicity is predominantly cholestatic rather than hepatocellular. Vascular lesions, including venous occlusion and peliosis hepatis, have been reported, but their prevalence is unknown. Nodular regenerative hyperplasia has followed use in kidney and liver transplantation.[2,8,16,19]
Busulfan	Use of this drug in bone marrow transplant patients is associated with apparently dose-related venoocclusive disease of the liver. Although the exact contribution of the drug is difficult to discern, this syndrome occurs in 20% of adults and in 5% of children treated with total doses of 16 mg/kg or more.[2,16,20,21]
Carbamazepine	Hepatic necrosis, granulomas, and cholestasis have all occurred, with some cases showing signs of hypersensitivity. Onset is most often in the first 4 weeks of therapy. Fatalities have been reported.[1,2,22]
Carmustine	Changes in liver function tests are found in 20–30% of patients, from a few days to several weeks after drug administration. These changes are usually mild and resolve quickly with drug discontinuation.[16]
Cephalosporins	Transient minor increases in AST, ALT, and alkaline phosphatase occur frequently. **Ceftriaxone** use is associated with development of "gallbladder sludge" in up to 25% of patients.[23]
Chenodiol.	Dose-related elevations in hepatic enzymes and a 0.4–3% prevalence of "clinically significant" hepatic injury occur.[1,24]
Chlorpropamide	Most reported hepatotoxic reactions are cholestatic, and are probably caused by an immune mechanism. Prevalence is estimated at 0.5–1.5%, with the onset usually within the first 2 months of therapy.[1,8]
Chlorzoxazone	Idiosyncratic hepatocellular damage occurs rarely, but fatalities have been reported. Discontinue the drug if elevated transaminases or bilirubin are detected.[25]
Cisplatin	Transient, dose-related elevations of hepatic enzymes occur frequently.[1,16]
Cocaine	Hepatic necrosis has been reported in cases of cocaine abuse, including at least one fatality. The prevalence of this reaction is not known.[2,4,26]
Contraceptives, Oral	Overt jaundice is estimated to occur in 1/4000–1/10,000 users, with most cases developing during the first 6 months of use. Patients who develop jaun- *(continued)*

DRUG	NATURE OF HEPATOTOXICITY
	dice during pregnancy have a greater chance of reacting similarly to oral contraceptives. The predominant lesion is cholestasis with little or no portal inflammation; pruritus is invariably present. Discontinuation of the drug is usually followed by resolution of the jaundice within a few weeks. Combination oral contraceptives are associated with an increase in the annual incidence of hepatic adenomas (3.4/100,000 vs. 1.3/100,000 in nonusers), especially after 5 or more years of use. These tumors may require resection. The frequency of gall bladder disease is also increased by oral contraceptives. An association between oral contraceptive use and any increased prevalence of hepatocellular carcinoma is unclear.[1,2,8,27]
Cyclosporine	Elevated serum levels of alkaline phosphatase and conjugated hyperbilirubin occur in 50–60% of patients. These changes are usually mild and pose little threat.[1,2,28,29]
Dantrolene	At least 1.8% of patients develop laboratory evidence of hepatic dysfunction, with symptomatic hepatitis in about 0.6%; the fatality rate among jaundiced patients is about 25%. Predisposing factors seem to include dosage (>300 mg/day), sex (women more than men), age (>30 yr), and duration of therapy (≥2 months).[1,30,31]
Dapsone	Hepatitis may occur as part of the "dapsone syndrome," which is a generalized hypersensitivity reaction including rash, fever, and lymphadenopathy. The true prevalence is unknown, but has been estimated to be as high as 5%. The onset is usually during the first 2 months of therapy. Although most dapsone-associated liver injury is hepatocellular, some cases of cholestasis have occurred.[1,2,8,32–34]
Disulfiram	This drug is occasionally associated with hepatitis, which may be caused by hypersensitivity. Most cases develop during the first few weeks of treatment. Deaths have been reported.[2,35,36]
Erythromycin	Erythromycin was thought to be a frequent cause of jaundice, but recent studies indicate that jaundice occurs only occasionally. Cholestasis apparently results from hypersensitivity (60% have eosinophilia and 50% have fever), which appears after 10–14 days of initial therapy or after 1–2 days in patients with a previous history of erythromycin exposure. Despite extensive use of the drug in children, most cases are reported in adults. Rapid reversal of symptoms follows drug discontinuation, but laboratory changes may persist for up to 6 months. Although most cases involve the **estolate** salt, hepatotoxicity has occurred with the **ethylsuccinate, stearate, and propionate** salts, and with erythromycin base.[1,2,8,37–39]
Ethionamide	Hepatitis may occur in 3–5% of patients, and serum enzyme elevations in 30% or more. Onset of hepatitis usually occurs after several months of therapy.[1,2,40]
Etretinate	Elevated hepatic enzymes occur in up to one-third of patients, but further evidence of hepatocellular damage is rare. Onset occurs most often 3–6 months after the start of therapy. Liver function tests should be monitored every 2–4 weeks for the first 4–6 months of therapy.[1,2,41]
Felbamate	Although the prevalence of hepatocellular destruction is unclear, it is of sufficient concern to limit the use of felbamate to carefully selected patients.[42]
Ferrous Salts	Hepatic necrosis may appear within 1–3 days of an acute overdose. The fatality rate is high if the patient is not treated promptly.[5]

(continued)

DRUG	NATURE OF HEPATOTOXICITY
Floxuridine	Hepatic arterial infusion of fludoxuridine results in 9% sclerosing cholangitis at 9 months and 26% after 1 yr. Elevations of liver enzyme levels are common, but are not predictive of greater hepatotoxicity.[2,16,43]
Flutamide	Elevated liver enzyme levels occur frequently, with clinically apparent hepatitis in 0.2% of patients.[2,44,45]
Gold Salts	Cholestasis occurs occasionally with normal doses of parenteral gold salts; hypersensitivity is the suspected mechanism. Onset is commonly within the first few weeks of therapy, and recovery usually occurs within 3 months after drug discontinuation. Lipogranulomas are frequently found in liver biopsies of parenteral gold-treated patients. These may persist long after drug withdrawal, but do not seem to impair liver function. Hepatic necrosis may result from overdose.[1,8,46,47]
Halothane	As many as 30% of patients may have increased serum transaminases or other evidence of mild hepatic impairment. Despite extensive publicity, the actual frequency of severe halothane hepatitis is low, ranging from 1/3500 to 1/35,000, with reported fatality rates of 17–96%. Susceptibility is greatest in adults, women, obese patients, and especially in patients with prior exposure to halothane. The mechanism of halothane hepatitis is poorly understood, but hypersensitivity is the most likely explanation. Fever precedes jaundice in most patients. The onset of jaundice is usually 5–8.5 days after exposure, but can occur between 1 and 26 days; shorter latent periods are associated with prior halothane exposure. **Methoxyflurane** and **enflurane** produce similar hepatotoxic reactions, although less frequently.[1,3,48,49]
Isoniazid	Elevated serum transaminase levels occur frequently, are presumed to be associated with subclinical hepatitis, resolve rapidly after drug discontinuation, and may resolve despite continued isoniazid therapy. A syndrome resembling viral hepatitis occurs in 1–2% of patients, with the onset usually during the first 3 months of therapy. The fatality rate from isoniazid hepatitis has fallen steadily over the past 2 decades, probably in response to more aggressive monitoring, and is now estimated to be as low as 0.001–0.005% of patients. **Alcohol** consumption increases the risk of hepatotoxicity, while the contribution of concomitant administration of **rifampin** is poorly defined. The role of acetylator phenotype remains unclear, with evidence for increased risk associated with both slow and fast acetylators.[1,2,4,50–52]
Ketoconazole	There is an 8–12% prevalence of mild elevation of hepatic enzymes. Hepatocellular necrosis with jaundice occurs in 0.03–0.1% of patients. There have been a few deaths attributed to ketoconazole hepatotoxicity.[1,2,8,53]
Mercaptopurine	Jaundice associated with cholestasis, hepatic necrosis, and mixed reactions occurs in 6–40% of patients, with the highest prevalence associated with doses of 2 mg/kg/day or more. Onset is usually during the first 2 months of therapy.[1,2,16,54]
Methotrexate	Hepatic injury (macrovesicular steatosis, necrosis, and bridging fibrosis) occurs frequently, depends on dose and duration of therapy, and may progress to cirrhosis if the drug is not stopped. Intermittent high doses pose less risk than daily low doses. Cirrhosis is reported in up to 24% of patients receiving long-term daily doses; other contributing factors include alcoholism and pre-existing liver or kidney disease. Hepatic fibrosis is not reflected by standard liver function tests and is best detected by biopsy. Biopsy has been recom- *(continued)*

DRUG	NATURE OF HEPATOTOXICITY
	mended at intervals of up to 36 months, after every 1.5 g of methotrexate, if 6 of 12 monthly transaminase levels are elevated, or if the serum albumin level drops below normal.[1-3,16,55,56]
Methyldopa	Mild changes in liver function tests occur in up to 35% of patients taking methyldopa, but the prevalence of clinical hepatitis is probably less than 1%. Most cases occur during the first 3 months of therapy. Hepatitis is more common in women, and most patients have rapid recovery after drug discontinuation. The fatality rate is less than 10% among patients who develop hepatitis. There is evidence to support a hypersensitivity mechanism in some patients.[1,57]
Niacin	Elevations of hepatic enzyme and bilirubin levels occur in 30–50% of patients taking sustained-release niacin in therapeutic doses. Symptomatic hepatic dysfunction occurs frequently and limits the use of the sustained-release product. Immediate-release niacin is also hepatotoxic, but to a lesser extent than sustained-release.[1,2,58]
Nitrofurantoin	Hepatic damage occurs occasionally, usually during the first month of therapy. Cholestasis is the most common presentation; hepatic necrosis is also reported. Hypersensitivity is the suspected mechanism, and the onset is frequently associated with fever, rash, and eosinophilia. Several late-developing cases of chronic active hepatitis have been reported; almost all are in women and after more than 6 months of therapy.[1,2,59]
Nonsteroidal Antiinflammatory Drugs	Most nonsalicylate NSAIDs do not seem to produce important hepatotoxicity. However, **diclofenac** is associated with predominantly hepatocellular damage and **sulindac** with cholestatic and mixed hepatocellular-cholestatic impairment. These reactions occur most commonly during the first 6 weeks of therapy and are often associated with fever, rash, or other signs of hypersensitivity.[1,2,4,60]
Papaverine	Numerous reports of hepatocellular injury and elevated liver enzymes in 27–43% of patients indicate a marked hepatotoxic potential.[1,2,61]
Penicillamine	Cholestasis occurs occasionally.[1,2,8,62]
Penicillins	**Cloxacillin** and **flucloxacillin** are rarely associated with cholestatic hepatitis. The effect is reversible, but it may persist for months after drug discontinuation.[1-3,50,65]
Phenothiazines	Most reports of liver damage involve **chlorpromazine**. The prevalence of hepatic enzyme elevation with this drug has been estimated to be as high as 42%, although 10% is probably more realistic. Similarly, cholestatic jaundice has been projected to occur in up to 5% of patients receiving chlorpromazine, but the actual prevalence is closer to 1%. The onset of cholestasis is generally in the first month of therapy and usually follows a prodrome of GI or influenzalike symptoms. About 70% of affected patients show signs of hypersensitivity, most frequently fever and eosinophilia, while only 5% have rash. Cholestasis usually follows a benign course, and most patients recover 1–2 months after drug discontinuation. A syndrome resembling primary biliary cirrhosis may occasionally occur. Despite the dominance of chlorpromazine in the reported cases, other phenothiazines are capable of producing similar hepatic damage.[1-3,50,65]
Phenytoin	Hepatocellular necrosis has been occasionally associated with phenytoin therapy. It is usually accompanied by other signs of hypersensitivity (eg, eosinophilia, fever, rash, lymphadenopathy). Onset usually occurs during the first 6 weeks of therapy. Reported fatality rates have been as high as 30%.[1,2,4,66,67]

(continued)

DRUG	NATURE OF HEPATOTOXICITY
Plicamycin	Dose-related laboratory evidence of hepatotoxicity occurs in virtually all patients. A common lesion is perivenous necrosis.[1–3,66,67]
Progestins	*See* Steroids, C–17–α–Alkyl.
Propoxyphene	A small number of cases of propoxyphene-induced cholestasis have been reported; these are thought to be the result of hypersensitivity.[1,2,8,69]
Propylthiouracil	Increases in ALT levels occur in up to 30% of patients. Onset is usually within the first 2 months of therapy, and ALT levels commonly return to normal with dosage reduction. Clinical hepatitis occurs rarely.[1,2,70]
Pyrazinamide	Pyrazinamide-induced hepatitis depends on dose and duration of therapy. Daily administration appears to present a greater risk than weekly administration.[1,71,72]
Quinidine	Hepatic damage is rare and usually accompanied by other signs of hypersensitivity, especially fever. Most reactions occur in the first month of therapy. The pathology is usually a mixture of hepatocellular necrosis and cholestasis; granulomas have also been reported.[1,73]
Salicylates	Up to 50% of patients taking antiarthritic dosages have laboratory evidence of liver damage. The risk of liver damage is greatest in patients with connective tissue disorders such as systemic lupus erythematosus (SLE) or juvenile rheumatoid arthritis. Clinically apparent salicylate-induced hepatitis is uncommon, usually mild, and readily reversible. Hepatotoxicity most often occurs at serum salicylate levels >250 mg/L, and only 7% of cases have serum salicylate levels <150 mg/L. Salicylates may cause microvesicular steatosis following intentional overdose.[1,2,60]
Steroids, C–17–α–Alkyl	Canalicular cholestasis occurs with a minimal amount of hepatic inflammation. The prevalence appears to be dose related; although laboratory changes are common (occurring in almost all patients taking anabolic steroids), jaundice is not. Jaundice may or may not be preceded by other clinical signs and usually follows 1–6 months of therapy. Peliosis hepatis has also been associated with these compounds, especially the anabolic steroids. Examples include **methyltestosterone, norethandrolone, methandrostenolone, fluoxymesterone, oxandrolone, oxymetholone and stanozolol.** C–17–α–ethinyl steroids such as **ethinyl estradiol, mestranol, norethindrone,** and **norethynodrel** may produce similar reactions. An association between C–17–α–alkyl steroids and an increase in the prevalence of hepatocellular carcinoma is unclear.[1,2,8,74]
Sulfasalazine	A small number of cases of sulfasalazine-associated hepatic damage, including fatalities, have been reported in both children and adults. Hepatic necrosis is apparently part of a generalized hypersensitivity reaction that includes rash, fever, and lymphadenopathy. Onset is usually within the first 4 weeks of therapy.[1,2,75]
Sulfonamides, Antibacterial	The sulfonamides currently in use appear to have a lower prevalence of hepatitis than their predecessors, with most reported cases appearing before 1947. Most cases of hepatotoxicity develop during the first 2 weeks of therapy and many are accompanied by other signs of hypersensitivity.[1,2,76] (*See also* Trimethoprim-Sulfamethoxazole.)
Tacrine	In a study of 2446 patients receiving tacrine, 25% had serum ALT levels at least 3 times greater than the upper limit of normal (ULN), 6% had levels at least 10 times greater than the ULN, and 2% had levels at least 25 times greater than the ULN. Most increases were detected in the first week of ther-

(*continued*)

DRUG	NATURE OF HEPATOTOXICITY
	apy. Most patients' ALT levels returned to no more than twice the ULN within 1 month after drug discontinuation, and no patients developed jaundice. Only 33% developed ALT levels more then 3 times the ULN on rechallenge.[77]
Tetracycline	Microvesicular steatosis may occur in patients receiving large doses of tetracycline IV, usually in excess of 1.5 g/day. Contributing factors include pregnancy, malnutrition, and impaired renal function, but hepatotoxicity has been reported in patients with none of these. Onset is most often during the first 10 days of therapy. Most cases of overt liver disease have resulted in death. Oral therapy may also produce signs of hepatotoxicity, although far less frequently.[1,2,39]
Trimethoprim-Sulfamethoxazole	"Clinically important" liver disease occurs in at least 5.2/100,000 patients (3.8/100,000 with trimethoprim alone). The available evidence supports hypersensitivity as the mechanism and cholestasis as the predominant form of injury. Fulminant hepatic failure has been reported.[2,39,78]
Troleandomycin	From 30–50% of patients receiving the drug show some laboratory evidence of abnormal liver function, and up to 4% develop jaundice.[1,2]
Valproic Acid	Hepatic enzyme elevations occur in 6–44% of patients, with clinically apparent liver disease in 0.05–1%. Fatal hepatotoxicity occurs most often in very young children (<2 yr old, 1/7000 on monotherapy and 1/500 on polydrug therapy; >2 yr old, 1/45,000 on monotherapy and 1/12,000 on polydrug therapy). The diffuse hepatocellular injury, microvesicular steatosis, and hepatic necrosis do not appear to be dose related and most commonly occur in the first 6 months of therapy. Serial liver function tests in asymptomatic patients do not predict patients at risk, but are commonly recommended because immediate discontinuation may reverse the condition.[1,2,67,79,80]
Vitamin A	Hepatomegaly, portal hypertension, and mild increases in liver enzyme levels are common features of chronic vitamin A toxicity. Central vein sclerosis and perisinusoidal fibrosis, which may progress to cirrhosis, have been reported in cases of chronic intoxication. These effects are associated with doses over 50,000 IU/day (sometimes with doses as low as 25,000 IU/day). Hepatotoxicity is also possible with acute doses over 600,000 IU.[1,2,81]

■ REFERENCES

1. Stricker BHCh, Spoelstra P. *Drug-induced hepatic injury.* Amsterdam: Elsevier; 1985.
2. Zimmerman HJ. Hepatotoxicity. *Dis Mon* 1993;39:675–787.
3. Hagley MT et al. Hepatotoxicity associated with angiotensin-converting enzyme inhibitors. *Ann Pharmacother* 1993;27:228–31.
4. Lee WM. Drug-induced hepatotoxicity. *N Engl J Med* 1995;333:1118–27.
5. Haddad LM, Winchester JF, eds. *Clinical management of poisoning and drug overdose,* 2nd ed. Philadelphia: WB Saunders; 1990.
6. Whitcomb DC, Block GD. Association of acetaminophen hepatotoxicity with fasting and ethanol use. *JAMA* 1994;272:1845–50.
7. Fisher B et al. Interleukin-2 induces profound reversible cholestasis: a detailed analysis in treated cancer patients. *J Clin Oncol* 1989;7:1852–62.
8. Zimmerman HJ, Lewis JH. Drug–induced cholestasis. *Med Toxicol* 1987;2:112–60.
9. Arellano F, Sacristán JA. Allopurinol hypersensitivity syndrome: a review. *Ann Pharmacother* 1993;27: 337–43.
10. Nagel GA et al. Phase II study of aminoglutethimide and medroxyprogesterone acetate in the treatment of patients with advanced breast cancer. *Cancer Res* 1982;42(suppl):3442S–4.
11. Simpson DG, Walker JH. Hypersensitivity to para-aminosalicylic acid. *Am J Med* 1960;29:297–306.

12. Guigui B et al. Amiodarone-induced hepatic phospholipidosis: a morphological alteration independent of pseudoalcoholic liver disease. *Hepatology* 1988;8:1063–8.

13. Richer M, Robert S. Fatal hepatotoxicity following oral administration of amiodarone. *Ann Pharmacother* 1995;29:582–6.

14. Reddy KR et al. Amoxicillin-clavulanate potassium-associated cholestasis. *Gastroenterology* 1989;96:1135–41.

15. Larrey D et al. Hepatitis associated with amoxycillin-clavulanic acid combination: report of 15 cases. *Gut* 1992;33:368–71.

16. Perry MC. Chemotherapeutic agents and hepatotoxicity. *Semin Oncol* 1992;19:551–65.

17. Pratt CB et al. Comparison of daily versus weekly L-asparaginase for the treatment of childhood acute leukemia. *J Pediatr* 1970;77:474–83.

18. Pratt CB, Johnson WW. Duration and severity of fatty metamorphosis of the liver following L-asparaginase therapy. *Cancer* 1971;28:361–4.

19. Gane E et al. Nodular regenerative hyperplasia of the liver graft after liver transplantation. *Hepatology* 1994;20:88–94.

20. Grochow LB et al. Pharmacokinetics of busulfan: correlation with veno-occlusive disease in patients undergoing bone marrow transplantation. *Cancer Chemother Pharmacol* 1989;25:55–61.

21. Vassal G et al. Busulfan and veno-occlusive disease of the liver. *Ann Intern Med* 1990;112:881. Letter.

22. Horowitz S et al. Hepatotoxic reactions associated with carbamazepine therapy. *Epilepsia* 1988;29:149–54.

23. Thompson JW, Jacobs RF. Adverse effects of newer cephalosporins. An update. *Drug Saf* 1993;9:132–42.

24. Schoenfield LJ et al. Chenodiol (chenodeoxycholic acid) for dissolution of gallstones: The National Cooperative Gallstone Study. A controlled trial of efficacy and safety. *Ann Intern Med* 1981;95:257–82.

25. Anon. Labeling change. *FDA Med Bull* 1996;26(1):3.

26. Wanless IR et al. Histopathology of cocaine hepatotoxicity. Report of four patients. *Gastroenterology* 1990;98:497–501.

27. Lindberg MC. Hepatobiliary complications of oral contraceptives. *J Gen Intern Med* 1992;7:199–209.

28. Atkinson K et al. Cyclosporine-associated hepatotoxicity after allogeneic marrow transplantation in man: differentiation from other causes of posttransplant liver disease. *Transplant Proc* 1983;15(suppl 1):2761–7.

29. Kassianides C et al. Liver injury from cyclosporine A. *Dig Dis Sci* 1990;35:693–7.

30. Utili R et al. Dantrolene-associated hepatic injury. Incidence and character. *Gastroenterology* 1977;72:610–6.

31. Ward A et al. Dantrolene. A review of its pharmacodynamic and pharmacokinetic properties and therapeutic use in malignant hyperthermia, the neuroleptic malignant syndrome and an update of its use in muscle spasticity. *Drugs* 1986;32:130–68.

32. Tomecki KJ, Catalano CJ. Dapsone hypersensitivity. The sulfone syndrome revisited. *Arch Dermatol* 1981;117:38–9.

33. Kromann NP et al. The dapsone syndrome. *Arch Dermatol* 1982;118:531–2.

34. Mohle-Boetani J et al. The sulfone syndrome in a patient receiving dapsone prophylaxis for *Pneumocystis carinii* pneumonia. *West J Med* 1992;156:303–6.

35. Wright C et al. Disulfiram-induced fulminating hepatitis: guidelines for liver-panel monitoring. *J Clin Psychiatry* 1988:49:430–4.

36. Mason NA. Disulfiram-induced hepatitis: case report and review of the literature. *DICP* 1989;23:872–5.

37. Inman WHW, Rawson NSB. Erythromycin estolate and jaundice. *Br Med J* 1983;286:1954–5.

38. Derby LE et al. Erythromycin-associated cholestatic hepatitis. *Med J Aust* 1993;158:600–2.

39. Carson JL et al. Acute liver disease associated with erythromycins, sulfonamides, and tetracyclines. *Ann Intern Med* 1993;119:576–83.

40. Conn HO et al. Ethionamide-induced hepatitis. A review with a report of an additional case. *Am Rev Resp Dis* 1964;90:542–52.

41. Sanchez MR et al. Retinoid hepatitis. *J Am Acad Dermatol* 1993;28:853–8.

42. Schmidt D, Krämer G. The new anticonvulsant drugs. Implications for avoidance of adverse effects. *Drug Saf* 1994;11:422–31.

43. Rougier P et al. Hepatic arterial infusion of floxuridine in patients with liver metastases from colorectal carcinoma: long-term results of a prospective randomized trial. *J Clin Oncol* 1992;10:1112–8.

44. Wysowski DK et al. Fatal and nonfatal hepatotoxicity associated with flutamide. *Ann Intern Med* 1993;118:860–4.

45. Gomez J-L et al. Incidence of liver toxicity associated with the use of flutamide in prostate cancer patients. *Am J Med* 1992;92:465–70.

46. Howrie DL, Gartner JC. Gold-induced hepatotoxicity: case report and review of the literature. *J Rheumatol* 1982;9:727–9.

47. Landas SK et al. Lipogranulomas and gold in the liver in rheumatoid arthritis. *Am J Surg Pathol* 1992;16:171–4.

48. Neuberger JM. Halothane and hepatitis. Incidence, predisposing factors and exposure guidelines. *Drug Saf* 1990;5:28–38.

49. Elliott RH, Strunin L. Hepatotoxicity of volatile anaesthetics. *Br J Anaesth* 1993;70:339–48.
50. Derby LE et al. Liver disorders in patients receiving chlorpromazine or isoniazid. *Pharmacotherapy* 1993;13:353–8.
51. Snider DE, Caras GJ. Isoniazid-associated hepatitis deaths: a review of available information. *Am Rev Resp Dis* 1992;145:494–7.
52. Salpeter SR. Fatal isoniazid-induced hepatitis—its risk during chemoprophylaxis. *West J Med* 1993;159:560–4.
53. Hay RJ. Risk/benefit ratio of modern antifungal therapy: focus on hepatic reactions. *J Am Acad Dermatol* 1993;29:S50–4.
54. Einhorn M, Davidsohn I. Hepatotoxicity of mercaptopurine. *JAMA* 1964;188:802–6.
55. Lewis JH, Schiff E. Methotrexate-induced chronic liver injury: guidelines for detection and prevention. *Am J Gastroenterol* 1988;88:1337–45.
56. Kremer JM et al. Methotrexate for rheumatoid arthritis. Suggested guidelines for monitoring liver toxicity. *Arthritis Rheum* 1994;37:316–28.
57. Rodman JS et al. Methyldopa hepatitis. A report of six cases and review of the literature. *Am J Med* 1976;60:941–8.
58. McKenney JM et al. A comparison of the efficacy and toxic effects of sustained- vs immediate-release niacin in hypercholesterolemic patients. *JAMA* 1994;271:672–7.
59. Stricker BH et al. Hepatic injury associated with the use of nitrofurans: a clinicopathological study of 52 reported cases. *Hepatology* 1988;8:599–606.
60. Rabinovitz M, Van Thiel DH. Hepatotoxicity of nonsteroidal anti-inflammatory drugs. *Am J Gastroenterol* 1992;87:1696–704.
61. Pathy MS, Reynolds AJ. Papaverine and hepatotoxicity. *Postgrad Med J* 1980;56:488–90.
62. Seibold JR et al. Cholestasis associated with D-penicillamine therapy: case report and review of the literature. *Arthritis Rheum* 1981;24:554–6.
63. Olsson R et al. Liver damage from flucloxacillIn cloxacillin and dicloxacillin. *J Hepatol* 1992;15:154–61.
64. Derby LE et al. Cholestatic hepatitis associated with flucloxacillin. *Med J Aust* 1993;158:596–600.
65. Regal RE et al. Phenothiazine-induced cholestatic jaundice. *Clin Pharm* 1987;6:787–94.
66. Smythe MA, Umstead GS. Phenytoin hepatotoxicity: a review of the literature. *DICP* 1989;23:13–8.
67. Wyllie E, Wyllie R. Routine laboratory monitoring for serious adverse effects of antiepileptic medications: the controversy. *Epilepsia* 1991;32(suppl 5):S74–9.
68. Green L, Donehower RC. Hepatic toxicity of low doses of mithramycin in hypercalcemia. *Cancer Treat Rep* 1984;68:1379–81.
69. Bassendine MF et al. Dextropropoxyphene induced hepatotoxicity mimicking biliary tract disease. *Gut* 1986;27:444–9.
70. Liaw Y-F et al. Hepatic injury during propylthiouracil therapy in patients with hyperthyroidism. A cohort study. *Ann Intern Med* 1993;118:424–8.
71. Hong Kong Chest Service/British Medical Research Council. Controlled trial of four thrice-weekly regimens and a daily regimen all given for 6 months for pulmonary tuberculosis. *Lancet* 1981;1:171–4.
72. Cohen CD et al. Hepatic complications of antituberculosis therapy revisited. *S Afr Med J* 1983;63:960–3.
73. Geltner D et al. Quinidine hypersensitivity and liver involvement. A survey of 32 patients. *Gastroenterology* 1976;70:650–2.
74. Haupt HA, Rovere GD. Anabolic steroids: a review of the literature. *Am J Sports Med* 1984;12:469–84.
75. Boyer DL et al. Sulfasalazine-induced hepatotoxicity in children with inflammatory bowel disease. *J Pediatr Gastroenterol Nutr* 1989;8:528–32.
76. Dujovne CA et al. Sulfonamide hepatic injury. Review of the literature and report of a case due to sulfamethoxazole. *N Engl J Med* 1967;277:785–8.
77. Watkins PB et al. Hepatotoxic effects of tacrine administration in patients with Alzheimer's disease. *JAMA* 1994;271:992–8.
78. Jick H, Derby LE. A large population-based follow-up study of trimethoprim-sulfamethoxazole, trimethoprim, and cephalexin for uncommon serious drug toxicity. *Pharmacotherapy* 1995;15:428–32.
79. Siemes H et al. Valproate (VPA) metabolites in various clinical conditions of probable VPA-associated hepatotoxicity. *Epilepsia* 1993;34:332–46.
80. Eadie MJ et al. Valproate-associated hepatotoxicity and its biochemical mechanisms. *Med Toxicol Adverse Drug Exp* 1988;3:85–106.
81. Kowalski TE et al. Vitamin A hepatotoxicity: a cautionary note regarding 25,000 IU supplements. *Am J Med* 1994;97:523–8.

Drug-Induced Nephrotoxicity

See introductory information on page 648.

DRUG	NATURE OF NEPHROTOXICITY
Acetaminophen	Tubular necrosis has been reported, usually in association with hepatotoxicity from acute overdose. Whether nephrotoxicity is a direct effect of acetaminophen or the result of the liver damage is the subject of controversy. It has been reported in cases without evidence of hepatotoxicity and with long-term use of therapeutic dosages. Acetaminophen is also implicated in some cases of analgesic nephropathy (see Analgesics) and with an increased risk of developing end-stage renal disease.[1,2,4–7]
ACE Inhibitors	Angiotensin-converting enzyme (ACE) inhibitors are frequently associated with the development of proteinuria and renal insufficiency. The prevalence of proteinuria in **captopril**-treated patients is estimated at 1%. The risks of renal insufficiency are greater with long-acting ACE inhibitors such as **enalapril** or **lisinopril** than with captopril. Immune complex glomerulopathy is a major contributor to ACE inhibitor nephrotoxicity. Hyponatremia, diuretic therapy (as well as other causes of hypovolemia), and diabetes mellitus contribute to an increased risk of nephrotoxicity. Recovery of renal function usually follows ACE inhibitor discontinuation, but complete renal artery occlusion has been reported.[1,2,8–13]
Acetazolamide	Glaucoma therapy with acetazolamide is associated with a tenfold increase in the risk of renal stone formation. Both calcium phosphate and calcium oxalate stones have been identified.[14,15]
Acyclovir	Acyclovir is concentrated in the urine and its precipitation in the collecting tubules with subsequent obstructive nephropathy may accompany high-dose (500 mg/m^2) IV use; oral therapy is apparently free from this problem. Adequate hydration should minimize the risk. Normal renal function usually returns within 6 weeks after drug withdrawal.[2,16]
Aldesleukin	Almost all patients receiving aldesleukin develop acute renal impairment marked by decreased Cl$_{cr}$, oliguria or anuria, and fluid retention. Most patients recover within 1 week after drug discontinuation, but some require 1 month or more.[52]
Allopurinol	Glomerulonephritis, interstitial nephritis and interstitial fibrosis occur rarely in allopurinol-treated patients. Most cases are associated with generalized hypersensitivity reactions to allopurinol (allopurinol hypersensitivity syndrome).[17,18]
Aminoglycosides	Proximal tubular necrosis occurs in up to 30% of patients treated with aminoglycosides for more than 7 days. Because of slow clearance of these drugs from renal tissue, they may still be present in high concentrations in the kidney after serum levels are undetectable, but there does not appear to be a good correlation between renal tissue concentrations of individual aminoglycosides and their nephrotoxic potential. Aminoglycoside-induced acute renal failure is usually nonoliguric, which may delay its recognition. It is often first detected as an asymptomatic increase in Cr$_s$. Detectable changes in GFR usually occur at least 5 days after initiation of therapy and may progress after drug discontinuation. Aminoglycoside-induced renal damage is related to total dosage and duration of treatment. Elevated steady-state trough concentrations may increase the risk

(continued)

DRUG	NATURE OF NEPHROTOXICITY
	of nephrotoxicity, while single daily doses may reduce it. Recovery of some to all lost renal function may occur over several weeks after drug discontinuation. Monitoring of aminoglycoside plasma levels and serial renal function tests may be of value in recognizing nephrotoxicity. **Neomycin** has the greatest and **streptomycin** the least nephrotoxic potential of the aminoglycosides. All other currently marketed aminoglycosides have intermediate nephrotoxic potentials. Concomitant therapy with other nephrotoxic drugs should be avoided.[1,2,8–10,19–22]
Amphotericin B	Some degree of nephrotoxicity occurs in almost all patients treated with amphotericin B. The drug causes a reduction in renal plasma flow as well as glomerular and tubular damage. Most patients experience a rapid decline in GFR, which often stabilizes at 20–60% of normal, and may not return to normal until several months after drug discontinuation. Distal tubular damage may lead to loss of concentrating ability, renal tubular acidosis, and electrolyte disturbances (most commonly hypokalemia, but also hyponatremia and hypomagnesemia). These effects appear to be dosage related, and many patients respond favorably to temporary drug discontinuation or a reduction in dosage. Sodium supplementation (eg, 1 L normal saline IV daily) or coadministration with fat emulsion may have prophylactic effects, although the latter is an unstable mixture. Some authors suggest that the total dosage of amphotericin B should be kept below 3–5 g to minimize permanent nephrotoxicity.[1,8–10,23–25]
Analgesics	Analgesic nephropathy is a syndrome of papillary necrosis and progressive renal medullary impairment that occurs in persons with long-term consumption of large quantities of oral analgesic products, especially combination products. Most reported patients are 30–70 yr old, and women usually outnumber men. The syndrome is characterized by proteinuria, reduced renal concentrating ability, and the presence of RBCs and WBCs in the urine. Analgesic nephropathy has been historically attributed to **phenacetin**, but the removal of phenacetin from nonprescription analgesic products has not been consistently associated with a decline in analgesic nephropathy mortality. **Acetaminophen** (a metabolite of phenacetin) and **salicylates** are also likely contributors, especially in combination, but salicylates taken alone do not seem to be associated with renal damage or any increase in risk for end-stage renal disease. Historically, this syndrome has been responsible for a large percentage of chronic renal failure deaths, with a considerable variation in prevalence among nations (high in Australia and Germany, low in the U.S.), apparently reflecting analgesic abuse patterns. Mild cases are reversible, but severe cases may continue to deteriorate after the discontinuation of analgesics. The prevalence of urinary tract cancer appears higher than normal among chronic analgesic abusers.[1,2,5–7,26]
Azacitidine	Proximal and distal tubular dysfunction, polyuria, glucosuria, and decreases in serum bicarbonate occur occasionally during azacitidine therapy.[27]
Carboplatin	Although apparently less nephrotoxic than cisplatin, carboplatin therapy is frequently associated with reductions in GFR and increased electrolyte losses (especially calcium and magnesium). Patients with preexisting renal impairment and those who receive inadequate hydration during drug administration are at greatest risk.[28]
Cephalosporins	The cephalosporin (and cephamycin) antibiotics are capable of producing rare interstitial nephritis similar to the penicillins. Increases in BUN and Cr$_s$ occur oc-

(*continued*)

DRUG	NATURE OF NEPHROTOXICITY
	casionally. The nephrotoxicity of the newer cephalosporins is minimal compared to older drugs such as **cephalothin**.[8,9,29–31]
Cidofovir	Proteinuria occurs frequently during cidofovir therapy. **Probenecid** decreases the prevalence and magnitude of proteinuria.[32]
Cisplatin	Dosage-related proximal tubular impairment is the major limiting factor in cisplatin therapy, and may occur in 50–75% of patients. Cl_{cr} is typically reduced to 60–80% of baseline with repeated courses of therapy. The greatest damage occurs in the first month of therapy, and it appears to be more likely when the drug is administered repetitively at close time intervals. Forced hydration and mannitol diuresis may reduce renal toxicity, at least for the first cycle of therapy. Magnesium and calcium loss are common manifestations of cisplatin-induced nephrotoxicity. Cisplatin-induced renal effects may be detected as long as 6 months after the end of therapy.[1,18,28,33]
Contrast Media	Increased Cr_s occurs frequently in patients receiving contrast media. In unselected patients, the prevalence of Cr_s >0.5 mg/dL or greater than 50% above pretreatment is 2–7%. A variety of renal lesions are described including medullary necrosis and proximal tubular vacuolation and necrosis as well as the deposition of urate and oxalate crystals. The most common pattern is acute oliguric renal failure developing within 24 hr after the administration of the contrast agent and lasting 2–5 days; nonoliguric renal failure has also been reported. Most patients recover fully, but permanent renal impairment has been reported. Patients with preexisting renal impairment are at much greater risk and constitute 60% of patients experiencing nephrotoxicity. Vigorous hydration before, during, and after drug administration reduces the risk of nephrotoxicity. High-osmolality ionic contrast media are worse than low-osmolality ionic contrast media. Newer, nonionic contrast agents have yet to demonstrate any advantage.[1,2,10,34–36]
Cyclosporine	Dose-related nephrotoxicity, usually accompanied by increased cyclosporine trough concentrations, frequently limits the usefulness of cyclosporine. Reduction in dosage usually reduces the renal toxicity. The drug produces a decrease in GFR, impaired tubular function, interstitial nephritis, hypertension, fluid retention, and hyperkalemia. Cyclosporine causes vasoconstriction in preglomerular arterioles, which may lead to chronic arteriopathy and tubular atrophy if the dosage is not reduced. Cyclosporine nephrotoxicity is usually reversible during the first 6 months of therapy, but the risk of permanent renal impairment increases with time. Calcium-channel blockers appear to reduce the prevalence of cyclosporine-induced nephrotoxicity in renal transplant patients.[1,2,8–10,20,37–40]
Demeclocycline	This drug is capable of producing nephrogenic diabetes insipidus, which is usually, but not always, dosage-related. For this reason, it has been used in the management of the syndrome of inappropriate antidiuretic hormone secretion.[20,41] (*See also* Tetracyclines.)
Diuretics, Thiazide	Occasional cases of interstitial nephritis have been reported, which may be the result of hypersensitivity reactions.[2,8]
Foscarnet	Acute tubular necrosis occurs frequently with foscarnet. Cr_s increased during 35 of 56 courses of therapy in one retrospective study. Hydration with normal saline appears to markedly decrease the severity and frequency of nephrotoxicity.[42]

(*continued*)

DRUG	NATURE OF NEPHROTOXICITY
Furosemide	Nephrocalcinosis and nephrolithiasis are encountered in up to 64% of low-birthweight infants treated with furosemide. These effects usually resolve following drug discontinuation.[43]
Gallium Nitrate	Nephrotoxicity is the most frequent adverse effect of gallium and elevations in BUN and Cr_s may occur after only one dose. At least one death has been associated with gallium-induced nephrotoxicity.[44,45]
Gold Salts	A lesion resembling membranous glomerulonephritis with proteinuria may occur in 3–10% of patients receiving parenteral gold therapy. Microhematuria and nephrotic syndrome are less frequent. One-half of the cases of proteinuria develop in the first 6 months of therapy. Occasionally, acute tubular necrosis and interstitial nephritis are reported. Although recovery may take up to 18 months, permanent renal impairment after drug withdrawal is uncommon. There is evidence for both immune and direct toxic mechanisms for gold nephrotoxicity. Oral **auranofin** appears to be less nephrotoxic than parenteral gold products.[1,2,10,46,47]
Ifosamide	Nephrotoxicity occurred in most patients in some reports, with both proximal and distal tubular damage encountered. Some patients demonstrate Fanconi syndrome–like symptoms including renal loss of glucose, electrolytes, and small proteins, and occasionally acute renal failure.[28,48,49]
Immune Globulin	Intravenous administration of immune globulin can produce rare acute renal failure after the first or repeated exposures. Prompt discontinuation results in rapid recovery of renal function.[50,51]
Lithium	Lithium frequently produces nephrogenic diabetes insipidus, which is at least in part dosage related. This typically mild effect is usually reversible upon drug withdrawal. It appears that long-term therapy (10–15 yr) is associated with an increased prevalence of reduced Cl_{cr} and renal concentrating ability beyond what would be explained by aging alone. Interstitial nephritis and nephrotic syndrome have also been reported.[1,2,9,10,20,41,53–56]
Mannitol	High doses (>200 g/day or >400 g/2 days) are associated with the development of acute oliguric renal failure. Although low doses act as renal vasodilators, high doses produce renal vasoconstriction. Keeping the osmolal gap to no more than 55 mOsm/kg should minimize the risk. Acute renal failure may require 7–10 days for recovery; dialysis shortens the recovery period to 1–2 days.[57,58]
Methotrexate	This drug is directly toxic to the kidney in large doses, producing acute tubular necrosis. Methotrexate is primarily eliminated through the kidney, and its nephrotoxicity compounds itself by causing the serum level of the drug to rise. About 20% of deaths associated with methotrexate therapy are caused by acute renal failure. The drug and its metabolites may precipitate in the distal tubule. Close monitoring of methotrexate serum levels and adjustment of dosage may help to minimize the risk of nephrotoxicity, as do vigorous hydration and alkalinization during drug administration.[2,47,59,60]
Methoxyflurane	Nephrogenic diabetes insipidus, proximal tubular damage, and interstitial nephritis are reported. The nephrotoxicity of methoxyflurane appears to be dose related and may be caused by increased circulating fluoride ion concentrations. Fluoride causes distal tubular dysfunction by inhibiting sodium and chloride transport in the ascending loop of Henle, and reducing the response to antidiuretic hormone. Urinary oxalate crystallization has also been reported following methoxyflurane anesthesia.[20,61,62]

(*continued*)

DRUG	NATURE OF NEPHROTOXICITY
Mitomycin	Tubular necrosis occurs most frequently with daily therapy, but is also reported with the intermittent therapy now recommended. Nephrotoxicity appears to be related to the total dosage administered, with the risk of renal impairment rising when the total dosage exceeds 30 mg/m^2. Onset may be delayed for many months.[47,63,64]
Nitrosoureas	The nitrosoureas can produce insidious nephrotoxicity in patients on long-term therapy. **Lomustine** seems to have the greatest nephrotoxic potential. Some cases of permanent renal function impairment have been reported.[65]
Nonsteroidal Antiinflammatory Drugs	NSAIDs can reduce Cl$_{cr}$ and produce nonoliguric renal insufficiency as a result of renal circulatory changes caused by inhibition of prostaglandin synthesis. These effects tend to be relatively minor and usually reversible. The prevalence is usually low (0.5–1% of patients), but some patients are at increased risk; predisposing factors include advanced age, preexisting renal impairment, and states of renal hypoperfusion (eg, sodium depletion, hypotension, diuretic use, hepatic cirrhosis, and CHF). Reversible acute interstitial nephritis and necrosis occur occasionally. Long-term NSAID use (>5000 tablets) increases the risk of developing end-stage renal disease by a factor of 8.8. It is not possible at this time to accurately categorize the prevalence associated with each NSAID, although **sulindac** is thought to pose the least risk; **fenoprofen** is the NSAID most commonly associated with interstitial nephritis and nephrotic syndrome.[1,2,6,7,10,20,66–68]
Penicillamine	Slight to moderate proteinuria occurs in 7–30% of patients on long-term (>6 months) therapy with penicillamine for rheumatoid arthritis. Most cases develop in the first year. Proteinuria is usually benign and slowly reversible over 6–12 months, but nephrotic syndrome is occasionally encountered. The lesions appear to be perimembranous glomerulonephritis resulting from the deposition of antigen-antibody complexes on the renal basement membrane.[1,2,10,20,69]
Penicillins	Interstitial nephritis has been reported with most penicillins. **Methicillin** is by far the most frequently implicated penicillin (frequency 10–16%); the reason for its dominance in unknown. Penicillin-induced interstitial nephritis is an immune reaction that most commonly occurs during a long course of therapy. The reaction is usually accompanied by other signs of hypersensitivity such as fever, rash, and eosinophilia; hematuria may also occur. The reduction of renal function may not be oliguric, so urine volume is not a reliable parameter to monitor. Recovery usually occurs within weeks to months after drug discontinuation.[1,2,20,70]
Pentamidine	Reversible acute renal failure (indicated by increased Cr$_s$, BUN, and potassium) is regularly encountered in IV pentamidine-treated patients (73–95%). Pentamidine-induced nephrotoxicity depends on total dosage and duration of therapy.[71,72]
Plicamycin	High doses (50 µg/kg/day) produced renal impairment in 40% of patients, including some who die of acute renal failure. Nephrotoxicity is far less likely at the 25–30 µg/kg/day (or lower) dosage used most often.[73]
Polymyxins	Adverse reactions involving the kidney occur in about 20% of patients receiving **colistimethate** parenterally. Tubular necrosis is the most frequently described lesion, but interstitial nephritis is also reported. High dosage, long duration of therapy, and renal impairment are predisposing factors. Polymyxin-induced renal damage is usually reversible, but some patients continue to deteriorate after drug withdrawal.[74]

(continued)

DRUG	NATURE OF NEPHROTOXICITY
Rifampin	There are scattered reports of rifampin-induced acute renal failure resulting from tubulointerstitial nephritis. This appears to be a hypersensitivity reaction and most commonly occurs with intermittent dosage regimens, but has also been accompanied continuous therapy.[75]
Streptozocin	Nephrotoxicity is the most common dosage-limiting side effect. The prevalence increases with prolonged administration until virtually all patients demonstrate renal impairment. Dosages below 1.5 g/m^2/week are less toxic. The damage is both glomerular and tubular. The drug should be discontinued as soon as renal damage is detected.[28,73]
Sulfonamides, Antibacterial	Early sulfonamides were poorly soluble, and urinary crystallization was a common problem. Today crystallization occurs in fewer than 0.3% of patients receiving the more soluble sulfonamides and adequate hydration. Interstitial nephritis, glomerulonephritis, and tubular necrosis are reported rarely. These reactions are probably allergic in origin.[2,8,76]
Tacrolimus	Acute nephrotoxicity occurs with a prevalence similar to that of cyclosporine. Progressive nephrotoxicity is reported with long-term (>1 yr) therapy.[39,49,77]
Tetracyclines	Fanconi syndrome, characterized by tubular damage with proteinuria, glycosuria, aminoaciduria, and electrolyte disturbances, was associated with the use of outdated tetracycline products. Because of changes in the manufacturing process, this syndrome is now unlikely to occur. The antianabolic effects of tetracyclines can contribute to azotemia in patients with preexisting renal impairment.[78] (*See also* Demeclocycline.)
Triamterene	Triamterene therapy is associated with an increase in urinary sediment, and the drug may be incorporated into existing renal calculi. One report suggests that one in 1500 users of the drug will develop triamterene-associated calculi during the course of 1 yr. As a precaution, the drug should probably not be used in patients with a history of renal calculi. Triamterene may also be associated with the development of interstitial nephritis.[79,80]
Vancomycin	Nephrotoxicity from vancomycin was commonly reported early in its history. Currently, the prevalence of vancomycin-induced renal impairment (usually mild) is 5–17%. It is usually reversible after discontinuation of the drug. Concomitant administration of **aminoglycosides** results in at least additive nephrotoxicity.[2,81–84]

■ REFERENCES

1. Koren G. The nephrotoxic potential of drugs and chemicals. Pharmacological basis and clinical relevance. *Med Toxicol Adverse Drug Exp* 1989;4:59–72.
2. Wang AYM, Lai KN. Drug-induced renal diseases. *Adverse Drug React Bull* 1994;Oct(168):635–8.
3. Cobden I et al. Paracetamol-induced acute renal failure in the absence of fulminant liver damage. *Br Med J* 1982;284:21–2.
4. Segasothy M et al. Paracetamol: a cause for analgesic nephropathy and end-stage renal disease. *Nephron* 1988;50:50–4.
5. Sandler DP et al. Analgesic use and chronic renal disease. *N Engl J Med* 1989;320:1238–43.
6. Perneger TV et al. Risk of kidney failure associated with the use of acetaminophen, aspirin, and nonsteroidal antiinflammatory drugs. *N Engl J Med* 1994;331:1675–9.
7. Whelton A. Renal effects of over-the-counter analgesics. *J Clin Pharmacol* 1995;35:454–63.
8. Paller MS. Drug-induced nephropathies. *Med Clin North Am* 1990;74:909–17.
9. Walker RJ, Duggin GG. Drug nephrotoxicity. *Ann Rev Pharmacol Toxicol* 1988;28:331–45.
10. Hoitsma AJ et al. Drug-induced nephrotoxicity. Aetiology, clinical features and management. *Drug Saf* 1991;6:131–47.

11. Packer M. Identification of risk factors predisposing to the development of functional renal insufficiency during treatment with converting-enzyme inhibitors in chronic heart failure. *Cardiology* 1989;76(suppl 2):50–5.

12. Mandal AK et al. Diuretics potentiate angiotensin converting enzyme inhibitor-induced acute renal failure. *Clin Nephrol* 1994;42:170–4.

13. Parish RC, Miller LJ. Adverse effects of angiotensin converting enzyme (ACE) inhibitors. An update. *Drug Saf* 1992;7:14–31.

14. Kass MA et al. Acetazolamide and urolithiasis. *Ophthalmology* 1981;88:261–5.

15. Tawil R et al. Acetazolamide-induced nephrolithiasis: implications for treatment of neuromuscular disorders. *Neurology* 1993;43:1105–6.

16. Sawyer MH et al. Acyclovir-induced renal failure. Clinical course and histology. *Am J Med* 1988;84:1067–71.

17. Elasy T et al. Allopurinol hypersensitivity syndrome revisited. *West J Med* 1995;162:360–1.

18. Arellano F, Sacristán JA. Allopurinol hypersensitivity syndrome: a review. *Ann Pharmacother* 1993;27:337–43.

19. Appel GB. Aminoglycoside nephrotoxicity. *Am J Med* 1990;88(suppl 3C):16S–20.

20. Werner M, Costa MJ. Nephrotoxicity of xenobiotics. *Clin Chim Acta* 1995;237:107–54.

21. Barclay ML, Begg EJ. Aminoglycoside toxicity and relation to dose regimen. *Adverse Drug React Toxicol Rev* 1994;13:207–34.

22. Bertino JS et al. Incidence of and significant risk factors for aminoglycoside-associated nephrotoxicity in patients dosed by using individualized pharmacokinetic monitoring. *J Infect Dis* 1993;167:173–9.

23. Sabra R, Branch RA. Amphotericin B nephrotoxicity. *Drug Saf* 1990;5:94–108.

24. Anderson CM. Sodium chloride treatment of amphotericin B nephrotoxicity—standard of care? *West J Med* 1995;162:313–7.

25. Vita E, Schroeder DJ. Intralipid in prophylaxis of amphotericin B nephrotoxicity. *Ann Pharmacother* 1994;28:1182–3.

26. Bennett WM, DeBroe ME. Analgesic nephropathy—a preventable renal disease. *N Engl J Med* 1989;320:1269–71.

27. Kintzel PE, Dorr RT. Anticancer drug renal toxicity and elimination: dosing guidelines for altered renal function. *Cancer Treat Rev* 1995;21:33–64.

28. Cornelison TL, Reed E. Nephrotoxicity and hydration management for cisplatin, carboplatin, and ormaplatin. *Gynecol Oncol* 1993;50:147–58.

29. Quin JD. The nephrotoxicity of cephalosporins. *Adverse Drug React Acute Poisoning Rev* 1989;8:63–72.

30. Zhanel GG. Cephalosporin-induced nephrotoxicity: does it exist? *DICP* 1990;24:262–5.

31. Thompson JW, Jacobs RF. Adverse effects of newer cephalosporins. An update. *Drug Saf* 1993;9:132–42.

32. Polis MA et al. Anticytomegaloviral activity and safety of cidofovir in patients with human immunodeficiency virus infection and cytomegalovirus viuria. *Antimicrob Agents Chemother* 1995;39:882–6.

33. Anand AJ, Bashey B. Newer insights into cisplatin nephrotoxicity. *Ann Pharmacother* 1993;27:1519–25.

34. Cronin RE. Southwestern Internal Medicine Conference: renal failure following radiologic procedures. *Am J Med Sci* 1989;298:342–56.

35. Spinler SA, Goldfarb S. Nephrotoxicity of contrast media following cardiac angiography: pathogenesis, clinical course, and preventive measures, including the role of low-osmolality contrast media. *Ann Pharmacother* 1992;26:56–64.

36. Porter GA. Contrast medium-associated nephrotoxicity. Recognition and management. *Invest Radiol* 1993;28(suppl 4):S11-8.

37. Bennett WM et al. Nephrotoxicity of immunosuppressive drugs. *Nephrol Dial Transplant* 1994;9(suppl 4):141–5.

38. Rossi SJ et al. Prevention and management of the adverse effects associated with immunosuppressive therapy. *Drug Saf* 1993;9:104–31.

39. Bennett WM. The nephrotoxicity of immunosuppressive drugs. *Clin Nephrol* 1995;43(suppl 1):S3–7.

40. Platz K-P et al. Nephrotoxicity following orthotopic liver transplantation. *Transplantation* 1994;58:170–8.

41. Forrest JN et al. Superiority of demeclocycline over lithium in the treatment of chronic syndrome of inappropriate secretion of antidiuretic hormone. *N Engl J Med* 1978;298:173–7.

42. Deray G et al. Foscarnet nephrotoxicity: mechanism, incidence and prevention. *Am J Nephrol* 1989;9:316–21.

43. Alon US et al. Nephrocalcinosis and nephrolithiasis in infants with congestive heart failure treated with furosemide. *J Pediatr* 1994;125:149–51.

44. Samson MK et al. Phase I-II clinical trial of gallium nitrate (NSC–15200). *Cancer Clin Trials* 1980;3:131–6.

45. Warrell RP et al. Treatment of patients with advanced malignant lymphoma using gallium nitrate administered as a seven-day continuous infusion. *Cancer* 1983;51:1982–7.

46. Hall CL. Gold nephropathy. *Nephron* 1988;50:265–72.

47. Newton P et al. Proteinuria with gold therapy: when should gold be permanently stopped? *Br J Rheumatol* 1983;22:11–7.

48. Berns JS et al. Severe, irreversible renal failure after ifosamide treatment. A clinicopathologic report of two patients. *Cancer* 1995;76:497–500.
49. Ashraf MS et al. Ifosamide nephrotoxicity in paediatric cancer patients. *Eur J Pediatr* 1994;153:90–4.
50. Cantú TG et al. Acute renal failure associated with immunoglobulin therapy. *Am J Kidney Dis* 1995;25:228–34.
51. Misbah SA, Chapel HM. Adverse effects of intravenous immunoglobulin. *Drug Saf* 1993;9:254–62.
52. Vial T, Descotes J. Clinical toxicity of interleukin-2. *Drug Saf* 1992;7:417–33.
53. Jorkasky DK et al. Lithium-induced renal disease: a prospective study. *Clin Nephrol* 1988;30:293–302.
54. Schou M. Effects of long-term lithium treatment on kidney function: an overview. *J Psychiatr Res* 1988;22:287–96.
55. Bendz H et al. Kidney damage in long-term lithium patients: a cross-sectional study of patients with 15 years or more on lithium. *Nephrol Dial Transplant* 1994;9:1250–4.
56. Walker RG. Lithium nephrotoxicity. *Kidney Int* 1993;44(suppl 42):S93–8.
57. Dorman HR et al. Mannitol-induced acute renal failure. *Medicine* 1990;69:153–9.
58. Gadallah MF et al. Case report: mannitol nephrotoxicity syndrome: role of hemodialysis and postulate of mechanisms. *Am J Med Sci* 1995;309:219–22.
59. Condit PT et al. Renal toxicity of methotrexate. *Cancer* 1969;23:126–31.
60. Stoller RG et al. Use of plasma pharmacokinetics to predict and prevent methotrexate toxicity. *N Engl J Med* 1977;297:630–4.
61. Cousins MJ, Mazze RI. Methoxyflurane nephrotoxicity. A study of dose response in man. *JAMA* 1973;225:1611–6.
62. Desmond JW. Methoxyflurane nephrotoxicity. *Can Anaesth Soc J* 1974;21:294–307.
63. Valavaara R, Nordman E. Renal complications of mitomycin C therapy with special reference to the total dose. *Cancer* 1985;55:47–50.
64. Verwey J et al. Mitomycin C–induced renal toxicity, a dose-dependent side effect? *Eur J Cancer Clin Oncol* 1987;23:195–9.
65. Weiss RB et al. Nephrotoxicity of semustine. *Cancer Treat Rep* 1983;67:1105–12.
66. Stillman MT, Schlesinger PA. Nonsteroidal anti-inflammatory drug nephrotoxicity. Should we be concerned? *Arch Intern Med* 1990:150:268–70.
67. Porile JL et al. Acute interstitial nephritis with glomerulopathy due to nonsteroidal anti-inflammatory agents: a review of its clinical spectrum and effects of steroid therapy. *J Clin Pharmacol* 1990;30:468–75.
68. Murray MD, Brater DC. Renal toxicity of the nonsteroidal anti-inflammatory drugs. *Ann Rev Pharmacol Toxicol* 1993;32:435–65.
69. Hall CL et al. Natural course of penicillamine nephropathy: a long term study of 33 patients. *Br Med J* 1988:296:1083–6.
70. Appel GB. A decade of penicillin related acute interstitial nephritis—more questions than answers. *Clin Nephrol* 1980;13:151–4.
71. Lachaal M, Venuto RC. Nephrotoxicity and hyperkalemia in patients with acquired immunodeficiency syndrome treated with pentamidine. *Am J Med* 1989;87:260–3.
72. Briceland LL, Bailie GR. Pentamidine-associated nephrotoxicity and hyperkalemia in patients with AIDS. *DICP* 1991;25:1171–4.
73. Ries F. Nephrotoxicity of chemotherapy. *Eur J Cancer Clin Oncol* 1988;24:951–3.
74. Koch-Weser J et al. Adverse effects of sodium colistimethate. Manifestations and specific reaction rates during 317 courses of therapy. *Ann Intern Med* 1970;72:857–68.
75. Utas C et al. Acute renal failure due to rifampicin therapy. *Nephron* 1994;67:367–8. Letter.
76. Appel GB, Neu HC. The nephrotoxicity of antimicrobial agents (third of three parts). *N Engl J Med* 1977;296:784–7.
77. Porayko MK et al. Nephrotoxicity of FK 506 and cyclosporine when used as primary immunosuppression in liver transplant recipients. *Transplant Proc* 1993;25:665–8.
78. Appel GB, Neu HC. The nephrotoxicity of antimicrobial agents (second of three parts). *N Engl J Med* 1977;296:722–8.
79. Ettinger B et al. Triamterene nephrolithiasis. *JAMA* 1980;244:2443–5.
80. Sica DA, Gehr TWB. Triamterene and the kidney. *Nephron* 1989;51:454–61.
81. Bailie GR, Neal D. Vancomycin ototoxicity and nephrotoxicity. A review. *Med Toxicol Adverse Drug Exp* 1988;3:376–86.
82. Eng RHK et al. Effect of intravenous vancomycin on renal function. *Chemotherapy* 1989;35:320–5.
83. Rybak MJ et al. Nephrotoxicity of vancomycin, alone and with an aminoglycoside. *J Antimicrob Chemother* 1990;25:679–87.
84. Duffull SB, Begg EJ. Vancomycin toxicity. What is the evidence for dose dependency? *Adverse Drug React Toxicol Rev* 1994;13:103–14

Drug-Induced Oculotoxicity

See introductory information on page 648.

DRUG	NATURE OF OCULOTOXICITY
Allopurinol	Despite the discovery of allopurinol in cataractous lenses taken from patients on long-term (>2 yr) therapy, there is no clinical evidence for an increased risk of cataracts in allopurinol-treated patients.[1–3]
Amantadine	At least 9 cases of diffuse, white, subendothelial corneal opacities have been reported. These opacities usually resolved within a few weeks after amantadine discontinuation.[4]
Amiodarone	Most patients treated with amiodarone develop bilateral corneal microdeposits (75% after 1 yr of therapy). Visual symptoms occur in 6–14%. Halo vision at night is most commonly reported, but patients may also complain of photophobia and blurred vision. The deposits are apparently dose related and reversible, disappearing 3–7 months after drug discontinuation. Minute lens opacities occurred in 7 of 14 amiodarone-treated patients in one study.[5–7]
Anticholinergic Agents	Blurring of vision can result from paralysis of accommodation (cycloplegia). These drugs also dilate the pupil (mydriasis), which may produce photophobia and precipitate narrow-angle glaucoma. With systemic administration, large doses are usually required to produce mydriasis, which is most commonly associated with potent anticholinergics such as **atropine**, **scopolamine**, or **benztropine**. Patients being treated for narrow-angle glaucoma can usually tolerate systemic anticholinergic therapy, but should nevertheless avoid these drugs unless absolutely necessary. Patients with open-angle glaucoma, particularly if treated, can receive anticholinergic medications without much risk. Patients receiving nebulized **ipratropium** by face mask are at risk for developing increased intraocular pressure and precipitation of narrow-angle glaucoma, probably from the drug escaping from beneath ill-fitting masks and directly affecting the eyes. All of the ocular effects of anticholinergics are dose related and reversible.[5,8–10]
Anticonvulsants	Diplopia and nystagmus occur frequently. Blurred vision may be caused by mydriasis (**phenytoin**) or cycloplegia (**carbamazepine**). All of these effects are dose related.[11]
Antidepressants, Heterocyclic	These drugs have anticholinergic properties and are capable of precipitating narrow-angle glaucoma and cycloplegia at usual doses (*see* Anticholinergic Agents). There is a 10–30% prevalence of blurred vision resulting from cycloplegia, but it is rarely troublesome and is reversible upon drug discontinuation. Blurred vision usually resolves despite continued antidepressant use as the eye becomes tolerant to the drug's effects. **Selective serotonin reuptake inhibitors** (SSRIs) do not seem to produce any important ocular effects.[5,12,13]
Antihistamine Drugs (H$_1$-Blockers)	With the exception of **astemizole**, **loratadine**, and **terfenadine**, these drugs have some anticholinergic properties and are capable of precipitating narrow-angle glaucoma and cycloplegia (*see* Anticholinergic Agents). These effects are minor and are reversible upon drug discontinuation. Antihistamines (most notably **diphenhydramine**) may reduce night vision.[5,9,14]
β-Adrenergic Blocking Agents	A reduction in tear production occurs, which can produce a hot, dry, gritty sensation in the eyes. This is rapidly reversible upon drug discontinuation.

(continued)

DRUG	NATURE OF OCULOTOXICITY
Bromocriptine	Myopia is a frequent complication of long-term bromocriptine therapy and often goes unappreciated until the patient complains of blurred vision. The cause is not fully determined, but it may be due to lens swelling. Myopia is reversible within 1–2 weeks after drug discontinuation.[5,15,16]
Busulfan	Long-term therapy (usually ≥1 yr) with busulfan is associated with the development of posterior subcapsular cataracts in about 10% of patients.[3,17,18]
Chloramphenicol	Optic neuritis, papilledema, and visual field defects are occasionally reported. These effects can occur after weeks or years of therapy, but are most common after several months of chloramphenicol use. Most cases are reported in children with cystic fibrosis, but the association with this disorder is unclear and may only reflect the types of patients who receive long-term chloramphenicol therapy. Both permanent visual impairment and recovery are reported after drug discontinuation. There are anecdotal reports that large doses of vitamins B_6 and B_{12} may have a beneficial impact on these adverse effects.[5,19–22]
Chloroquine	The oculotoxicity of chloroquine limits its usefulness; two general types of ocular change occur: corneal deposits and retinopathy. About 50% of patients demonstrate corneal deposits, less than one-half of whom have visual impairment resulting from these deposits. Opacities present as punctate or whirling patterns. They may appear after as little as 2 months and usually do not interfere with vision. They are usually reversible in 6–8 weeks after drug discontinuation. Early changes in the retina (deposition of pigment in the macula) are usually asymptomatic and reversible. More advanced damage includes hyperpigmentation of the macula surrounded by a depigmented ring and hyperpigmented retina ("bull's-eye" retinopathy). Patients complain of reading difficulty, blurred vision, visual field defects, and photophobia; some may also report defective color vision and light flashes. The prevalence ranges from 3–45% in various reports. The drug should be discontinued if these symptoms develop. Patients receiving long-term therapy with chloroquine should have ophthalmologic examinations at least every 6 months initially and then annually if their vision remains stable. Daily dosage seems to be more important than the total dosage or duration of therapy for the development of retinopathy; limiting the daily dosage to 4 mg/kg up to a maximum of 250 mg in adults minimizes the risk. The prognosis of chloroquine-induced retinopathy is uncertain. Weekly use of chloroquine for malarial prophylaxis does not seem to cause retinopathy.[15,23–26]
Cisplatin	Blurred vision and altered color perception are frequently associated with high-dose cisplatin. Blurred vision gradually improves after drug discontinuation, while altered color vision may persist. Pigmentary retinopathy is also reported.[3,18]
Clomiphene	Visual disturbances, most commonly blurred vision, occur frequently with clomiphene. These disturbances usually disappear after the drug is withdrawn, but one report of three patients describes prolonged afterimages, shimmering of the peripheral visual field, and photophobia.[27]
Contraceptives, Oral	A variety of retinal vascular disorders have been attributed to oral contraceptives, but the association remains unproved. It is purported that some oral contraceptive users cannot tolerate contact lenses, possibly because of ocular edema or dryness; however, a prospective study failed to show any differences in lens tolerance between oral contraceptive users and nonusers.[28,29]
Corticosteroids	These drugs can produce a variety of ocular disorders, most notably glaucoma and cataracts. Corticosteroid-induced increases in intraocular pressure appear to be

(continued)

DRUG	NATURE OF OCULOTOXICITY
	dose related and may persist for several months after drug discontinuation. Corticosteroid-induced cataracts (usually posterior subcapsular) are found frequently in patients on long-term, systemic therapy and are correlated with total dosage and duration of therapy. Outcome is variable, ranging from improvement despite continued therapy to rare loss of sight. Most patients have no vision impairment. Although they most commonly occur with large oral doses, increased intraocular pressure and cataracts are reported in patients receiving corticosteroids by the topical ophthalmic, inhalation, and intranasal routes. Children develop cataracts more frequently than adults.[2,3,5,18,30–32]
Cyclophosphamide	One report showed a 17% prevalence of transient reversible blurred vision during high-dose cyclophosphamide therapy. Recovery took from 1 hr to 14 days. Keratoconjunctivitis is also common.[3,18,33]
Cyclosporine	Severe visual disturbances, including cortical blindness, occur occasionally with cyclosporine. Oculotoxicity appears to be dose related and resolves after drug discontinuation.[34]
Cytarabine	Keratoconjunctivitis, corneal damage, and photophobia are frequent, dose-related side effects of cytarabine. These symptoms usually resolve 1–2 weeks after drug discontinuation. Corticosteroid eye drops may have a beneficial effect, but should be used with caution in patients with corneal damage.[3,18,35,36]
Deferoxamine	Oculotoxicity, including blurred vision, impaired color vision, night blindness, and retinal deposits, occurs in 4–11% of patients receiving deferoxamine for chronic iron overload. These effects appear to be dose related and may be because of the chelation of trace minerals.[37–40]
Digitalis Glycosides	The most unique ocular effect is the frosted or snowy appearance of objects or colored halos around them. These effects are most noticeable in bright light. Color vision may be affected such that objects appear yellow (green or other colors are reported, but far less frequently). With **digoxin**, color changes usually occur when the plasma level exceeds 1.5 µg/L. Digitalis glycosides are also reported to produce photophobia, blurred vision, central scotomas, and flickering or light flashes before the eyes. Reversible ocular side effects occur in up to 25% of patients with digitalis intoxication.[5,41,42]
Disulfiram	A few cases of retrobulbar neuritis have occurred, manifested by a dramatic decline in visual acuity and impairment of color vision. In most patients, vision returns to normal after drug discontinuation.[5,43]
Doxorubicin	This drug stimulates excessive lacrimation shortly after administration in about 25% of patients. Conjunctivitis has also been reported.[18,44]
Ethambutol	Retrobulbar neuritis is the primary ocular complication. Symptoms include blurred vision, scotoma, and reduction of the visual field. Color vision defects also occur, usually presenting as a reduction in green perception. Retrobulbar neuritis is dose related, occurring most frequently with dosages of 25 mg/kg/day or more. Its onset is usually after 3–6 months of therapy and it is slowly reversible after drug discontinuation. Dosages up to 15 mg/kg/day appear relatively free of ocular side effects.[5]
Fluorouracil	Ocular irritation and reversible excessive lacrimation occur in about 50% of patients treated with systemic fluorouracil. Some patients may develop eversion of the eyelid margin (cicatricial ectropion) or potentially irreversible fibrosis of the tear duct (dacryostenosis) with prolonged therapy.[3,5,18,45–47]

(continued)

DRUG	NATURE OF OCULOTOXICITY
Gold Salts	Parenteral gold can produce microscopic crystalline deposits in the cornea, most commonly in the superficial layers. These deposits are dose related and rarely occur until the total dosage of parenteral gold exceeds 1 g. The deposits slowly resolve after drug discontinuation, do not appear to affect vision, and are not a reason to stop gold therapy. **Auranofin** does not seem to produce these ocular effects.[5,48,49]
Hydroxychloroquine	This drug can produce the same spectrum of ocular toxicity as **chloroquine** (*see* Chloroquine). Although it is often said that hydroxychloroquine produces less oculotoxicity than chloroquine, there are no substantial data to support this. Limiting the daily dosage to 6.5 mg/kg up to a maximum of 400 mg in adults minimizes the risk of retinopathy.[5,23–25,50,51]
Interferon Alfa	Although the prevalence cannot be accurately determined, retinal vascular complications have been reported. These effects appear to be reversible after drug discontinuation.[52]
Isoniazid	Optic neuritis occurs occasionally, most commonly in malnourished or alcoholic patients, and often manifests itself as impaired red-green perception. It responds to **pyridoxine** therapy.[5]
Methotrexate	Adverse ocular effects frequently associated with systemic methotrexate include conjunctivitis, increased or decreased lacrimation, photophobia, and eye pain. Onset is during the first week of therapy, and resolution usually occurs within one week after drug discontinuation.[13,18]
Muromonab-CD3	Conjunctivitis and photophobia occur frequently.[53]
Oxygen	Retrolental fibroplasia is an important complication of oxygen therapy in neonates, particularly premature or other low-birthweight neonates. The risk of retrolental fibroplasia in these patients increases whenever the concentration of inspired oxygen exceeds normal.[54–56]
Paclitaxel	Scintillating scotomas or photopsia occur frequently during paclitaxel infusions. The onset of these short-lived effects is usually during the last hour of the infusion. They do not always recur during subsequent infusions.[57,58]
Pamidronate	Reversible anterior uveitis and conjunctivitis are occasional complications of pamidronate therapy.[59]
Pentostatin	Conjunctivitis and keratitis frequently occur during pentostatin therapy. Although conjunctivitis is usually mild, keratitis can be severe.[3]
Phenothiazines	Lesions of the lens, cornea, and retina are the most important features of phenothiazine-induced oculotoxicity. White to yellow-brown deposits in the lens most frequently occur with long-term, high-total-dosage (over 600 g) **chlorpromazine** therapy. Similar deposits are also found in the corneas of chlorpromazine-treated patients. Epithelial keratopathy, possibly resulting from a photosensitivity reaction, can occur after only a few months of high-dosage therapy. It is characterized by a diffuse opacification of the corneal epithelium. The consistent use of sunglasses may reduce the risk of keratopathy. Lens and corneal deposits usually do not interfere with vision, and all of these effects may be slowly reversible. **Thioridazine** is most noted for producing pigmentary retinopathy. As with most phenothiazine-induced ocular effects, pigmentary retinopathy is dose related. Patients may complain of blurred vision, decreased night vision, brown discoloration of vision, and central scotoma. Vision may improve if the drug is withdrawn soon enough; however, some cases continue to deteriorate despite drug discontinuation. Other phe- *(continued)*

DRUG	NATURE OF OCULOTOXICITY
	nothiazines may cause pigmentary retinopathy, but the supporting data are limited to case reports. Phenothiazines (especially thioridazine) have anticholinergic effects and may precipitate narrow-angle glaucoma. Corneal edema is a rare, but dangerous, complication of phenothiazine use requiring immediate discontinuation of therapy.[12,60,61]
Psoralens	The combination of psoralens and long-wave ultraviolet light (PUVA therapy) radiation is associated with the development of conjunctivitis, photophobia, and other signs of ocular irritation. The use of UVA protective lenses greatly reduces the prevalence. An experimentally demonstrated connection between PUVA therapy and cataracts has not been confirmed clinically.[5,62,63]
Quinine	Loss of visual acuity and reduction of the visual field to the point of blindness can occur with quinine therapy or (especially) overdose. Other reported ocular effects include impaired color vision and night blindness. These effects are usually reversible, but permanent constriction of the visual field and blindness are reported. The ocular effects of quinine may be the result of changes in the retinal vasculature.[5,64,65]
Retinoids	Blepharoconjunctivitis occurs in >50% of patients receiving **isotretinoin**. This painful condition appears to be dose related, and its onset is usually during the first 2 months of therapy. Dry eyes may occur with or without blepharoconjunctivitis. Corneal opacities, which clear in 6–7 weeks after drug discontinuation, are also reported. Similar effects are reported with **etretinate**.[5,66–69]
Rifabutin	Although the prevalence is unclear, uveitis is associated with prophylactic rifabutin therapy in AIDS patients.[70,71]
Rifampin	Exudative conjunctivitis, ocular pain, and orange staining of tears (and consequent staining of soft contact lenses) are occasionally reported with rifampin. These effects are rapidly reversible when the drug is withdrawn.[72–74]
Sympathomimetic Agents	These drugs are capable of dilating the pupil and precipitating narrow-angle glaucoma. Sympathomimetics with marked α-adrenergic activity (eg, **ephedrine, phenylpropanolamine, tetrahydrozoline**) should be avoided. The risk of this reaction is slight unless large doses are taken orally or the drugs are applied topically.[9]
Tamoxifen	Fine, refractile retinal opacities and retinal edema may occur; some corneal opacities are also reported. These lesions are associated with both high- and low-dose therapy. They may result in reduced visual acuity and are slowly reversible after drug discontinuation.[3,5,18,75,76]
Vinca Alkaloids	Various ocular disorders occur. Most (ptosis, blurred vision, night blindness) are thought to be the result of cranial nerve impairment. Some evidence of cranial nerve impairment occurs in up to 50% of vincristine-treated patients. **Vincristine** may be more oculotoxic than **vinblastine**.[3,5,18,77]

■ REFERENCES

1. Lerman S et al. Further studies on allopurinol therapy and human cataractogenesis. *Am J Ophthalmol* 1984;97:205–9.
2. Clair WK et al. Allopurinol use and the risk of cataract formation. *Br J Ophthalmol* 1989;73:173–6.
3. Burns LJ. Ocular toxicities of chemotherapy. *Semin Oncol* 1992;19:492–500.
4. Fraunfelder FT, Meyer SM. Amantadine and corneal deposits. *Am J Ophthalmol* 1990;110:96–7. Letter.
5. Davidson SI, Rennie IG. Ocular toxicity from systemic drug therapy. An overview of clinically important adverse reactions. *Med Toxicol* 1986;1:217–24.

6. Flach AJ et al. Amiodarone-induced lens opacities. *Arch Ophthalmol* 1983;101:1554–6.

7. Naccarelli GV et al. Adverse effects of amiodarone. Pathogenesis, incidence and management. *Med Toxicol Adverse Drug Exp* 1989;4:246–53.

8. Hiatt RL et al. Systemically administered anticholinergic drugs and intraocular pressure. *Arch Ophthalmol* 1970;84:735–40.

9. Durkee DP, Bryant BG. Drug therapy reviews: drug therapy of glaucoma. *Am J Hosp Pharm* 1978;35:682–90.

10. Singh J et al. Nebulized bronchodilator therapy causes acute angle closure glaucoma in predisposed individuals. *Respir Med* 1993;87:559–61. Letter.

11. Goldman MJ, Schultz-Ross RA. Adverse ocular effects of anticonvulsants. *Psychosomatics* 1993;34:154–8.

12. Oshika T. Ocular adverse effects of neuropsychiatric agents. Incidence and management. *Drug Saf* 1995;12:256–63.

13. Ritch R et al. Oral imipramine and acute angle closure glaucoma. *Arch Ophthalmol* 1994;112:67–8.

14. Luria SM et al. Effects of aspirin and dimenhydrinate (Dramamine) on visual processes. *Br J Clin Pharmacol* 1979;7:585–93.

15. Calne DB et al. Long-term treatment of parkinsonism with bromocriptine. *Lancet* 1978;1:735–8.

16. Manor RS et al. Myopia during bromocriptine treatment. *Lancet* 1981;1:102. Letter.

17. Podos SM, Canellos GP. Lens changes in chronic granulocytic leukemia. Possible relationship to chemotherapy. *Am J Ophthalmol* 1969;68:500–4.

18. Imperia PS et al. Ocular complications of systemic cancer chemotherapy. *Surv Ophthalmol* 1989;34:209–30.

19. Cocke JG et al. Optic neuritis with prolonged use of chloramphenicol. Case report and relationship to fundus changes in cystic fibrosis. *J Pediatr* 1966;68:27–31.

20. Huang NN et al. Visual disturbances in cystic fibrosis following chloramphenicol administration. *J Pediatr* 1966;68:32–44.

21. Cocke JG. Chloramphenicol optic neuritis. Apparent protective effects of very high daily doses of pyridoxine and cyanocobalamin. *Am J Dis Child* 1967;114:424–6.

22. Harley RD et al. Optic neuritis and optic atrophy following chloramphenicol in cystic fibrosis patients. *Trans Am Acad Ophthalmol Otolaryngol* 1970;74:1011–31.

23. Mackenzie AH. Dose refinements in long-term therapy of rheumatoid arthritis with antimalarials. *Am J Med* 1983;75(July 18, suppl):40–5.

24. Easterbrook M. Ocular effects and safety of antimalarial agents. *Am J Med* 1988;85(suppl 4A):23–9.

25. Kerdel F et al. Antimalarial agents and the eye. *Dermatol Clin* 1992;10:513–9.

26. Lange WR et al. No evidence for chloroquine-associated retinopathy among missionaries on long-term malaria chemoprophylaxis. *Am J Trop Med Hyg* 1994;51:389–92.

27. Purvin VA. Visual disturbance secondary to clomiphene citrate. *Arch Ophthalmol* 1995;113:482–4.

28. De Vries Reilingh A et al. Contact lens tolerance and oral contraceptives. *Ann Ophthalmol* 1978;10:947–52.

29. Petursson GJ. Oral contraceptives. *Ophthalmology* 1981;88:368–71.

30. Renfro L, Snow JS. Ocular effects of topical and systemic steroids. *Dermatol Clin* 1992;10:505–12.

31. Toogood JH et al. Association of ocular cataracts with inhaled and oral steroid therapy during long-term treatment of asthma. *J Allergy Clin Immunol* 1993;91:571–9.

32. Opatowsky I et al. Intraocular pressure elevation associated with inhalation and nasal corticosteroids. *Ophthalmology* 1995;102:177–9.

33. Kende G et al. Blurring of vision. A previously undescribed complication of cyclophosphamide therapy. *Cancer* 1979;44:69–71.

34. Memon M et al. Reversible cyclosporine-induced cortical blindness in allogenic bone marrow transplant recipients. *Bone Marrow Transplant* 1995;15:283–6.

35. Lass JH et al. Topical corticosteroid therapy for corneal toxicity from systemically administered cytarabine. *Am J Ophthalmol* 1982;94:617–21.

36. Herzig RH et al. High-dose cytosine arabinoside therapy for refractory leukemia. *Blood* 1983;62:361–9.

37. Olivieri NF et al. Visual and auditory neurotoxicity in patients receiving subcutaneous deferoxamine infusions. *N Engl J Med* 1986;314:869–73.

38. De Virgiliis S et al. Depletion of trace elements and acute ocular toxicity induced by desferrioxamine in patients with thalassaemia. *Arch Dis Child* 1988;63:250–5.

39. Cases A et al. Acute visual and auditory neurotoxicity in patients with end-stage renal disease receiving desferrioxamine. *Clin Nephrol* 1988;29:176–8.

40. Cases A et al. Ocular and auditory toxicity in hemodialyzed patients receiving desferrioxamine. *Nephron* 1990;56:19–23.

41. Robertson DM et al. Ocular manifestations of digitalis toxicity. Discussion and report of three cases of central scotomas. *Arch Ophthalmol* 1966;76:640–5.

42. Aronson JK, Ford AR. The use of colour vision measurement in the diagnosis of digoxin toxicity. *Q J Med* 1980;49:273–82.

43. Norton AL, Walsh FB. Disulfiram-induced optic neuritis. *Trans Am Acad Ophthalmol Otolaryngol* 1972;76:1263–5.

44. Curran CF, Luce JK. Ocular adverse reactions associated with Adriamycin (doxorubicin). *Am J Ophthalmol* 1989;108:709–11.

45. Straus DJ et al. Cicatricial ectropion secondary to 5-fluorouracil therapy. *Med Pediatr Oncol* 1977;3:15–9.

46. Haidak DJ et al. Tear-duct fibrosis (dacryostenosis) due to 5-fluorouracil. *Ann Intern Med* 1978;88:657.

47. Christophidis N et al. Ocular side effects with 5-fluorouracil. *Aust N Z J Med* 1979;9:143–4.

48. Bron AJ et al. Epithelial deposition of gold in the cornea in patients receiving systemic therapy. *Am J Ophthalmol* 1979;88:354–60.

49. Kincaid MC et al. Ocular chrysiasis. *Arch Ophthalmol* 1982;100:1791–4.

50. Easterbrook M. The ocular safety of hydroxychloroquine. *Semin Arthritis Rheum* 1993;23(suppl 1):62–7.

51. Bernstein HN. Ocular safety of hydroxychloroquine sulfate (Plaquenil). *South Med J* 1992;85:274–9.

52. Guyer DR et al. Interferon-associated retinopathy. *Arch Ophthalmol* 1993;111:350–6.

53. Dukar O, Barr CC. Visual loss complicating OKT3 monoclonal antibody therapy. *Am J Ophthalmol* 1993;115:781–5.

54. Committee on Fetus and Newborn, American Academy of Pediatrics. History of oxygen therapy and retrolental fibroplasia. *Pediatrics* 1976;57(suppl):591–642.

55. Betts EK et al. Retrolental fibroplasia and oxygen administration during general anesthesia. *Anesthesiology* 1977;47:518–20.

56. Naiman J et al. Retrolental fibroplasia in hypoxic newborn. *Am J Ophthalmol* 1979;88:55–8.

57. Capri G et al. Optic nerve disturbances: a new form of paclitaxel neurotoxicity. *J Natl Cancer Inst* 1994;86:1099–101.

58. Seidman AD, Barrett S. Photopsia during 3-hour paclitaxel administration at doses ≥250 mg/m². *J Clin Oncol* 1994;12:1741–2. Letter.

59. Macarol V, Fraunfelder FT. Pamidronate disodium and possible ocular adverse drug reactions. *Am J Ophthalmol* 1994;118:220–4.

60. Bond WS, Yee GC. Ocular and cutaneous effects of chronic phenothiazine therapy. *Am J Hosp Pharm* 1980;37:74–8.

61. Ngen CC, Singh P. Long-term phenothiazine administration and the eye in 100 Malaysians. *Br J Psychiatry* 1988;152:278–80.

62. Farber EM et al. Current status of oral PUVA therapy for psoriasis. Eye protection revisions. *J Am Acad Dermatol* 1982;6:851–5.

63. Stern RS. Ocular lens findings in patients treated with PUVA. Photochemotherapy follow-up-study. *J Invest Dermatol* 1994;103:534–8.

64. Gangitano JL, Keltner JL. Abnormalities of the pupil and visual-evoked potential in quinine amblyopia. *Am J Ophthalmol* 1980;89:425–30.

65. Dyson EH et al. Death and blindness due to overdose of quinine. *Br Med J* 1985;291:31–3.

66. Fraunfelder FT et al. Adverse ocular reactions possibly associated with isotretinoin. *Am J Ophthalmol* 1985;100:534–7.

67. Lebowitz MA, Berson DS. Ocular effects of oral retinoids. *J Am Acad Dermatol* 1988;19:209–11.

68. Gold JA et al. Ocular side effects of the retinoids. *Int J Dermatol* 1989;28:218–25.

69. Gross EG, Helfgott MA. Retinoids and the eye. *Dermatol Clin* 1992;10:521–31.

70. Saran BR et al. Hypopyon uveitis in patients with acquired immunodeficiency syndrome treated for systemic *Mycobacterium avium* complex infection with rifabutin. *Arch Ophthalmol* 1994;112:1159–65.

71. Karbassi M, Nikou S. Acute uveitis in patients with acquired immunodeficiency syndrome receiving prophylactic rifabutin. *Arch Ophthalmol* 1995;113:699–701.

72. Cayley FE, Majumdar SK. Ocular toxicity due to rifampicin. *Br Med J* 1976;1:199–200.

73. Lyons RW. Orange contact lenses from rifampin. *N Engl J Med* 1979;300:372–3. Letter.

74. Harris J, Jenkins P. Discoloration of soft contact lenses by rifampicin. *Lancet* 1985;2:1133. Letter.

75. Mihm LM, Barton TL. Tamoxifen-induced ocular toxicity. *Ann Pharmacother* 1994;28:740–2.

76. Pavlidis NA et al. Clear evidence that long-term, low-dose tamoxifen treatment can induce ocular toxicity. A prospective study of 63 patients. *Cancer* 1992;69:2961–4.

77. Albert DM et al. Ocular complications of vincristine therapy. *Arch Ophthalmol* 1967;78:709–13.

Drug-Induced Ototoxicity

See introductory information on page 648.

DRUG	NATURE OF OTOTOXICITY
Aminoglycosides	Aminoglycoside antibiotics can cause both cochlear and vestibular toxicity. Cochlear toxicity presents as progressive hearing loss starting with the highest tones and advancing to lower tones. Thus, considerable damage may occur before the patient is cognizant of it. Vestibular damage presents as dizziness, vertigo, or ataxia. Both forms of ototoxicity are usually bilateral and potentially reversible, but permanent damage is common and may progress after aminoglycoside discontinuation. Estimates of the prevalence of aminoglycoside-induced ototoxicity vary widely depending on the criteria applied. Clinically detectable ototoxicity probably occurs in as many as 5% of patients, with a much higher percentage demonstrating audiometrically detectable damage. Most aminoglycoside-induced ototoxicity is associated with parenteral therapy, but it has followed topical, oral, and irrigation use of these drugs, especially **neomycin**. A patient should receive dosages by these routes that are no greater than the dosages given by injection. Possible predisposing factors for ototoxicity include decreased renal function, duration of therapy, total dosage, plasma levels exceeding the therapeutic range, previous aminoglycoside use, concurrent use of other ototoxic drugs, dehydration, and old age. There is some evidence of an inherited susceptibility to aminoglycoside-induced ototoxicity. Hearing impairment is less common in neonates and children. Once-daily administration may produce less hearing loss than multiple daily doses. Serial audiometry may be useful in early detection of ototoxicity. Each aminoglycoside has a slightly different spectrum of ototoxicity; the table below serves as a general guide to their relative ototoxic potential.[1–7]

RELATIVE OTOTOXIC POTENTIAL

DRUG	COCHLEAR	VESTIBULAR
Amikacin	++	+
Gentamicin	++	++
Kanamycin	+++	+
Neomycin	+++	+
Netilmicin	+	+
Streptomycin	++	+++
Tobramycin	++	++

DRUG	NATURE OF OTOTOXICITY
Antidepressants, Heterocyclic	The prevalence of **tricyclic antidepressant** (TCA)-associated tinnitus is estimated to be 1%. Tinnitus may subside despite continued therapy.[2,8]
Carboplatin	(*See* Cisplatin.)
Chloroquine	Nerve deafness is a rare but consistent feature of chloroquine therapy. Its onset is usually delayed and is usually thought of as irreversible and accompanying long-term therapy. A partially reversible case and a case resulting from only 1 g of chloroquine have been reported.[2,3,9,10]

(*continued*)

DRUG	NATURE OF OTOTOXICITY
Cisplatin	Tinnitus occurs frequently and usually subsides within 1 week of drug discontinuation. It cannot be relied upon to predict further ototoxicity. Hearing loss occurs frequently in patients receiving cisplatin and may be dose limiting. Audiometric abnormalities can be detected in most patients and may appear within a few days after the drug is started. High frequencies are lost first, and hearing loss occurs early or not at all. If therapy continues despite early hearing loss, the majority of patients experience hearing loss in the speech frequencies. Effects are cumulative, dose related, and probably irreversible. Prolonged, low-dose therapy may produce less ototoxicity than short-term, high-dose treatment. Ototoxicity may occur more frequently in children and the elderly, and those with preexisting hearing loss appear to be at increased risk. **Carboplatin** seems to produce far less ototoxicity.[1–3,11–15]
Deferoxamine	Dosage-related hearing impairment occurs during chronic deferoxamine therapy. The prevalence is difficult to estimate, but it occurs frequently. High-frequency hearing is affected first, and both reversible and irreversible hearing loss have been reported.[16–18]
Diuretics, Loop	Rapid-onset hearing loss is a frequent feature of high-dose, rapid IV administration of **furosemide**. The onset may be more gradual with **ethacrynic acid**. Renal failure is usually listed as a predisposing factor, but only renal failure patients are likely to receive large IV doses. Coadministration with **aminoglycoside antibiotics** is often said to result in increased ototoxicity, but one study failed to confirm this. The hearing loss is usually transient, but permanent loss has been reported, more often with ethacrynic acid than with furosemide. Hearing loss and vestibular toxicity after oral therapy have been reported. **Bumetanide** or **torsemide** produce less ototoxicity than ethacrynic acid or furosemide.[1–3,19,20]
Eflornithine	High- and low-frequency hearing impairment is reported frequently and dizziness occurs occasionally.[14]
Erythromycin	Hearing loss has occasionally followed high-dosage (>4 g/day) parenteral or oral therapy, and does not seem to be caused by any particular salt form. Impaired hepatic or renal function and advanced age may increase the risk. The loss occurs at speech frequencies and is usually reversible, but irreversible hearing loss has been reported. Recovery usually begins within 24 hr of drug discontinuation.[1,3,21,22]
Minocycline	Reversible vestibular toxicity, manifested primarily by dizziness, loss of balance, and lightheadedness, is a frequent occurrence. This adverse effect was noted in an average of 76% of patients in 6 studies and required 12–52% of affected patients to either discontinue the drug or to stop working. Other studies have found lower, but still large, percentages of patients with vestibular toxicity. Women may be more susceptible than men. Onset is often during the first 2 days of therapy, and recovery begins soon after minocycline discontinuation.[1,23–25]
Nonsteroidal Anti-inflammatory Drugs	Although not as common as with salicylates, NSAIDs have been associated with hearing impairment and deafness. Tinnitus and vestibular dysfunction have also been reported.[1–3,26]
Quinine	Tinnitus and high-frequency hearing impairment occur frequently. Although these effects are usually reversible, permanent hearing impairment has occurred with long-term therapy. Vestibular effects have also been described.[1–3,26]
Salicylates	Tinnitus, high-frequency hearing loss, and occasional vertigo are common features of salicylate intoxication. Hearing loss appears to be related to the unbound plasma salicylate level, explaining the marked interpatient variability in the total salicylate serum

(continued)

DRUG	NATURE OF OTOTOXICITY
	level at which it is first detected. Most patients demonstrating ototoxicity from salicylates are receiving long-term, high-dose therapy, such as for rheumatoid arthritis. Salicylate ototoxicity, even if severe, is almost always reversible in 48–72 hr, but permanent hearing loss has been reported.[1-3,26,27]
Vancomycin.	Transient and permanent hearing loss, tinnitus, and dizziness have occurred. Hearing impairment is rare with plasma levels <30 mg/L (21 µmol/L). In many of the reported cases, the patient had also been exposed to other ototoxic drugs, especially **aminoglycoside antibiotics**. The prevalence of purely vancomycin-induced ototoxicity is unknown, but it is probably low.[1,28,29]

■ REFERENCES

1. Huang MY, Schacht J. Drug-induced ototoxicity. Pathogenesis and prevention. *Med Toxicol Adverse Drug Exp* 1989;4:452–67.
2. Griffin JP. Drug-induced ototoxicity. *Br J Audiol* 1988;22:195–210.
3. Norris CH. Drugs affecting the inner ear. A review of their clinical efficacy, mechanisms of action, toxicity, and place in therapy. *Drugs* 1988;36:754–72.
4. Brummett RE, Fox KE. Aminoglycoside-induced hearing loss in humans. *Antimicrob Agents Chemother* 1989;33:797–800.
5. Garrison MW et al. Aminoglycosides: another perspective. *DICP* 1990;24:267–72.
6. Matz GJ. Aminoglycoside cochlear ototoxicity. *Otolaryngol Clin North Am* 1993;26:705–12.
7. Barclay ML, Begg EJ. Aminoglycoside toxicity and relation to dose regimen. *Adverse Drug React Toxicol Rev* 1994;13:207–34.
8. Tandon R et al. Imipramine and tinnitus. *J Clin Psychiatry* 1987;48:109–11.
9. Dwivedi GS, Mehra YN. Ototoxicity of chloroquine phosphate. A case report. *J Laryngol Otol* 1978;92:701–3.
10. Mukherjee DK. Chloroquine ototoxicity—a reversible phenomenon? *J Laryngol Otol* 1979;93:809–15.
11. van der Hulst RJAM et al. High frequency audiometry in prospective clinical research of ototoxicity due to platinum derivatives. *Ann Otol Rhinol Laryngol* 1988;97:133–7.
12. Skinner R et al. Ototoxicity of cisplatinum in children and adolescents. *Br J Cancer* 1990;61:927–31.
13. Blakley BW, Myers SF. Patterns of hearing loss resulting from *cis*-platinum therapy. *Otolaryngol Head Neck Surg* 1993;109:385–91.
14. Schweitzer VG. Ototoxicity of chemotherapeutic agents. *Otolaryngol Clin North Am* 1993;26:759–89.
15. Kennedy ICS et al. Carboplatin is ototoxic. *Cancer Chemother Pharmacol* 1990;26:232–4.
16. Olivieri NF et al. Visual and auditory neurotoxicity in patients receiving subcutaneous deferoxamine infusions. *N Engl J Med* 1986;314:869–73.
17. Gallant T et al. Serial studies of auditory neurotoxicity in patients receiving deferoxamine therapy. *Am J Med* 1987;83:1085–90.
18. Cases A et al. Ocular and auditory toxicity in hemodialyzed patients receiving desferrioxamine. *Nephron* 1990;56:19–23.
19. Rybak LP. Ototoxicity of loop diuretics. *Otolaryngol Clin North Am* 1993;26:829–44.
20. Smith CR, Lietman PS. Effect of furosemide on aminoglycoside-induced nephrotoxicity and auditory toxicity in humans. *Antimicrob Agents Chemother* 1983;23:133–7.
21. Brummett RE. Ototoxic liability of erythromycin and analogues. *Otolaryngol Clin North Am* 1993;26:811–9.
22. Sacristán JA et al. Erythromycin-induced hypoacusis: 11 new cases and literature review. *Ann Pharmacother* 1993;27:950–5.
23. Schofield CBS, Masterton G. Vestibular reactions to minocycline. *MMWR* 1976;25:31.
24. Gump DW et al. Side effects of minocycline: different dosage regimens. *Antimicrob Agents Chemother* 1977;12:642–6.
25. Greco TP et al. Minocycline toxicity: experience with an altered dosage regimen. *Curr Ther Res* 1979;25:193–201.
26. Jung TTK et al. Ototoxicity of salicylate, nonsteroidal anti-inflammatory drugs, and quinine. *Otolaryngol Clin North Am* 1993;26:791–810.
27. Brien J. Ototoxicity associated with salicylates. A brief review. *Drug Saf* 1993;9:143–8.
28. Brummett RE. Ototoxicity of vancomycin and analogues. *Otolaryngol Clin North Am* 1993;26:821–8.
29. Duffull SB, Begg EJ. Vancomycin toxicity. What is the evidence for dose dependency? *Adverse Drug React Toxicol Rev* 1994;13:103–14.

Drug-Induced Sexual Dysfunction

See introductory information on page 648.

DRUG	NATURE OF DYSFUNCTION
Alcohol	Low doses result in behavioral disinhibition. With higher doses, sexual response is impaired, frequently resulting in failure of erection in men and reduced vaginal vasodilation and delayed orgasm in women. In chronic alcoholics, sexual dysfunction frequently persists long after alcohol withdrawal and is permanent in some. The long-term effects are probably both neurologic and endocrine in origin; alcohol reduces testosterone levels and increases luteinizing hormone levels. Long-term effects are independent of liver disease.[1–7]
Alprostadil	Penile pain was reported at least once in 37% of patients in early clinical trials of intracavernous alprostadil. Similarly, 4% of patients reported prolonged (4–6 hr) erection and 0.4% reported priapism (erection >6 hr).[8]
Aminocaproic Acid	This drug may inhibit ejaculation without affecting libido and has produced "dry" ejaculation. Effects are rapidly reversible upon drug discontinuation.[1,9,10]
Amphetamines	Low doses may increase libido and produce a delay in male orgasm. High doses have been associated with failure to achieve an erection in men and loss of orgasm in both sexes.[1,11–13]
Anabolic Steroids	Impotence and gynecomastia occur frequently in men and may be the result of reduction in the circulating levels of natural testosterone.[2,14]
Anticonvulsants	Both female and male libido may be reduced. Self-reported sexual dysfunction has been described in a widely varying percentage of patients. Social and psychological aspects of epilepsy probably play an important role in these findings. Some effects may be caused by a reduction in the level of free testosterone, resulting from hepatic enzyme induction and higher concentrations of sex hormone binding globulins.[3,15–17]
Antidepressants, Heterocyclic	Impotence, delayed ejaculation, and painful ejaculation have been reported in men. Women have reported delayed orgasm and anorgasmia. Both increased and, more commonly, decreased libido have been reported in men and women. The frequency of these effects varies considerably among published reports, perhaps reflecting the influence of the underlying depressive illness. One recent report found some type of sexual dysfunction in 20 of 41 patients receiving heterocyclic antidepressants.[1–3,9,13,18–23] *See also* Selective Serotonin Reuptake Inhibitors, and Trazodone.
β-Adrenergic Blocking Agents	These drugs are associated with a variety of sexual problems, most commonly impotence. In a study of 46 men taking **propranolol**, 7 experienced "complete" impotence, 13 noted reduced potency, and 2 complained of reduced libido. In a larger trial, the frequencies of impotence during propranolol therapy were 13.8% and 13.2% after 12 weeks and 2 years, respectively. However, these figures did not differ significantly from placebo. Most of the published reports implicate propranolol, and it appears that other more cardioselective β-blockers are less frequently associated with complaints of adverse sexual effects. There have been at least 25 reported patients who complained of sexual dysfunction (18 impotence, 9 decreased libido) while receiving topical ophthalmic treatment with **timolol**. Some of these patients were rechallenged with positive results.[1–3,9,21,24–29]
Calcium- Channel Blockers	Although these drugs are generally thought to be free of adverse effects on sexual function, they are associated with gynecomastia. **Verapamil** is the most commonly implicated calcium-channel blocker, but **nifedipine** and **diltiazem** can also produce gy-

(continued)

DRUG	NATURE OF DYSFUNCTION
	necomastia. Other calcium channel blockers seem to be less likely to cause gynecomastia.[30]
Carbonic Anhydrase Inhibitors	Many patients receiving carbonic anhydrase inhibitors (eg, **acetazolamide**, **methazolamide**) develop a syndrome of malaise, fatigue, weight loss, and depression that often includes loss of libido. These patients appear to be more acidotic than those without the syndrome and some respond to therapy with sodium bicarbonate. Decreased libido has occurred in both men and women and usually requires 2 weeks of carbonic anhydrase inhibitor therapy to develop.[1,31,32]
Cimetidine	In a group of 22 men treated with high dosages of cimetidine for hypersecretory states, 11 developed gynecomastia and 9 experienced impotence. These effects appear to be dose related and readily reversible, and are not an important problem at dosages used for peptic ulcers. Cimetidine has some antiandrogenic effects, possibly the result of hyperprolactinemia, which are thought to be responsible for sexual dysfunction. Displacement of androgens from breast androgen receptors may contribute to the development of gynecomastia. **Ranitidine** does not appear to be associated with as high a prevalence of sexual dysfunction, and **famotidine** is not antiandrogenic.[1–3,9,14,30,33]
Clofibrate	In large multicenter trials, impotence has been reported more frequently than with placebo.[1–3,9,34,35]
Clonidine	Although some reports have indicated no sexual problems, others have indicated problems in up to 24% of patients. Impotence is the most frequently noted effect, but delayed or retrograde ejaculation in men and failure of orgasm in women have also been described.[1–3,9,21,27,36]
Cocaine	Although cocaine is often perceived as a sexual stimulant, its use is associated with difficulty in establishing an erection and delayed ejaculation.[1,13,37,38]
Cyproterone	Gynecomastia may result from the antiandrogen effects of cyproterone.[14]
Digoxin	Digitalis glycosides have some estrogenlike activity, and digoxin has been associated with decreased libido, impotence, and gynecomastia in men. In one study, digoxin use was associated with a 60% decrease in testosterone and a similar increase in estrogen in men.[1–3,9,39]
Diuretics, Thiazide	Thiazide diuretics and **chlorthalidone** are thought to produce adverse sexual effects, but the prevalence remains difficult to quantify. In one large study, the prevalence of impotence was reported to be significantly higher with **bendroflumethiazide** than with placebo (23% after 2 years compared with 10% for placebo), and in another **hydrochlorothiazide** was reported to produce more impotence and loss of libido than **propranolol**. In a well-designed study, 14% of men taking **chlorothiazide** complained of impotence as did 14% of placebo-treated men. In a third study, 6 months of chlorthalidone therapy increased erectile difficulty in 23% of men.[1–3,9,26–28,36,40–42]
Estrogens	Impotence and gynecomastia occur frequently in men taking estrogens for prostate cancer. Estrogens have been used to reduce libido and sexual activity of male sex offenders.[1–3,43]
Finasteride	Gynecomastia has been reported with finasteride.[62]
Flutamide	Gynecomastia may result from the antiandrogen effects of flutamide.[14]
Guanadrel	Poorly characterized "sexual dysfunction" and "ejaculatory disturbances" have been reported.[9,21]
Guanethidine	Up to 54% of men have reported impotence and up to 71% have reported ejaculatory impairment. Guanethidine does not affect parasympathetic function and would not be expected to produce impotence, leading some to suggest that the impotence is secondary to the inhibition of ejaculation. Retrograde ejaculation occurs as a result of the *(continued)*

DRUG	NATURE OF DYSFUNCTION
	failure of the internal urethral sphincter to close; this action is sympathetically mediated. Although it is not well characterized, decreased libido in women taking guanethidine has been reported. Guanethidine effects are reversible upon drug discontinuation and may be alleviated by a reduction in dosage.[1–3,9,36,40,44,45]
Ketoconazole	Gynecomastia has been reported, apparently the result of the inhibition of testosterone synthesis.[14,30]
Marijuana	Both positive and negative effects on sexual function are possible. Low doses may have a disinhibiting effect, while large doses have been associated with decreased libido and impotence. Long-term use may also result in gynecomastia.[1,30,46]
Methyldopa	Impotence and ejaculatory failure in men, and reduced libido in both sexes have been described. The frequency of sexual dysfunction varies from quite low in some reports to greater than 50% in response to direct questioning. These effects are dose related and reversible. They may be the result of drug-induced sympathetic inhibition and mild CNS depression. Gynecomastia in men and painful breast enlargement in women have occurred.[1–3,9,21,28,36,40]
Monoamine Oxidase Inhibitors	Reported adverse sexual effects of MAOIs are highly variable. Impotence, spontaneous erections, and ejaculatory delay, as well as orgasmic failure in both men and women, have been described. The true prevalence of these effects cannot be determined from available data, but MAOIs may be associated with more sexual dysfunction than heterocyclic antidepressants.[1,3,13,18–21,23]
Narcotics	Long-term narcotic use (especially abuse) is frequently associated with decreased libido and orgasmic failure in both sexes, and impotence in men. These effects are dose related, with the highest frequency of impotence reported in narcotic addicts (80–90% in some series), and are reversible upon drug discontinuation.[1,47–49]
Nitrates and Nitrites	These vasodilators have been used (primarily by inhalation) to enhance the perception of orgasm. When they are used too soon before orgasm, however, the vasodilation rapidly produces loss of erection. This effect has been used therapeutically to reduce spontaneous erections in men undergoing urologic procedures.[1,50,51]
Omeprazole	Although the prevalence is unclear, impotence and gynecomastia in men and breast enlargement in women have been described.[52]
Papaverine	Intracavernous injection of papaverine resulted in priapism (defined as an erection lasting longer than 3 hr) in 17% of 400 patients. Those with psychogenic or neurogenic impotence were more likely to experience priapism than those with vasculogenic impotence.[53]
Phenothiazines	These drugs have been implicated in producing a wide variety of adverse sexual effects including impotence and priapism, absent and spontaneous ejaculation, painful ejaculation, retrograde ejaculation, menstrual irregularities, and decreased libido. These effects result from the complex actions of the drugs on the patient's hormonal balance and central sympathetic and parasympathetic pathways. With the exception of priapism, these effects are usually benign and respond to drug discontinuation. **Thioridazine** is the most commonly implicated drug. The possible contribution of the underlying disease state cannot be overlooked.[1–3,13,23,54]
Phenoxybenzamine	This α-adrenergic blocker is associated with dosage-related failure of ejaculation, but not interference with orgasm. This effect was present in all 19 patients in one study and reversed 24–48 hr after drug discontinuation.[1,2,55]
Progestins	Impotence has been reported in 25–70% of men receiving progestins for prostatic hypertrophy. Progestins have been used to reduce libido and sexual activity of male sex offenders.[1,43,56]
Reserpine.	Impotence and failure of ejaculation in men and reduced libido in both sexes may occur.[1,3,9,36]

(continued)

DRUG	NATURE OF DYSFUNCTION
Sedative-Hypnotics	In a manner similar to alcohol, low doses may produce some disinhibition, whereas large doses may reduce sexual performance.[1-3,20]
Selective Serotonin Reuptake Inhibitors	Anorgasmia and inhibition of orgasm are frequent adverse effects. Although most of the reports describe problems with **fluoxetine**, most SSRIs have been implicated. **Sertraline** appears to be the SSRI with the greatest prevalence of sexual dysfunction.[2,21,57-59]
Spironolactone	Gynecomastia in men and painful breast enlargement or menstrual irregularities in women are frequent with large dosages. Less frequently reported effects are impotence, inhibition of vaginal lubrication, and loss of libido. The structural similarity of the drug to estrogens and progestins is thought to be a key factor in the genesis of adverse sexual effects. Spironolactone may inhibit the formation of testosterone and breast receptor binding. It may also increase the metabolic clearance of testosterone and its rate of peripheral conversion to estradiol. These effects appear to be dosage related.[1,3,9,14,30,36,60]
Trazodone	Numerous cases of priapism have been reported, usually during the first month of therapy.[3,9,21,23,54,61]

■ REFERENCES

1. Buffum J. Pharmacosexology: the effects of drugs on sexual function. A review. *J Psychoact Drugs* 1982;14:5–44.
2. Brock GB, Lue TF. Drug-induced male sexual dysfunction. An update. *Drug Saf* 1993;8:414–26.
3. McWaine DE, Procci WR. Drug-induced sexual dysfunction. *Med Toxicol Adverse Drug Exp* 1988;3:289–306.
4. Lemere F, Smith JW. Alcohol-induced sexual impotence. *Am J Psychiatry* 1973;130:212–3.
5. Wilson GT, Lawson DM. Effects of alcohol on sexual arousal in women. *J Abnorm Psychol* 1976;85:489–97.
6. Gordon GG et al. Effect of alcohol (ethanol) administration on sex-hormone metabolism in normal men. *N Engl J Med* 1976;295:793–7.
7. Dudek FA, Turner DS. Alcoholism and sexual functioning. *J Psychoact Drugs* 1982;14:47–54.
8. Caverject prescribing information. Upjohn; 1995.
9. Buffum J. Pharmacosexology update: prescription drugs and sexual function. *J Psychoact Drugs* 1986;18:97–106.
10. Evans BE, Aledort LM. Inhibition of ejaculation due to epsilon aminocaproic acid. *N Engl J Med* 1978;298:166–7. Letter.
11. Greaves G. Sexual disturbances among chronic amphetamine users. *J Nerv Ment Dis* 1972;155:363–5.
12. Smith DE et al. *Amphetamine abuse and sexual dysfunction: clinical and research considerations.* In Smith DE et al., eds. Amphetamine use, misuse, and abuse: proceedings of the National Amphetamine Conference, 1978. Boston: GK Hall; 1979:228–48.
13. Sagraves RT. Effects of psychotropic drugs on human erection and ejaculation. *Arch Gen Psychiatry* 1989;46:275–84.
14. Braunstein GD. Gynecomastia. *N Engl J Med* 1993;328:490–5.
15. Toone BK et al. Sex hormone changes in male epileptics. *Clin Endocrinol* 1980;12:391–5.
16. Dana-Haeri J et al. Reduction of free testosterone by antiepileptic drugs. *Br Med J* 1982;284:85–6.
17. Morrell MJ. Sexual dysfunction in epilepsy. *Epilepsia* 1991;32(suppl 6):S38–45.
18. Mitchell JE, Popkin MK. Antidepressant drug therapy and sexual dysfunction in men: a review. *J Clin Psychopharmacol* 1983;3:76–9.
19. Harrison WM et al. Effects of antidepressant medication on sexual function: a controlled study. *J Clin Psychopharmacol* 1986;6:144–9.
20. Shen WW, Sata LS. Inhibited female orgasm resulting from psychotropic drugs. A five-year, updated, clinical review. *J Reprod Med* 1990;35:11–4.
21. Anon. Drugs that cause sexual dysfunction: an update. *Med Lett Drugs Ther* 1992;34:73–8.
22. Balon R et al. Sexual dysfunction during antidepressant treatment. *J Clin Psychiatry* 1993;54:209–12.
23. Pollack MH et al. Genitourinary and sexual adverse effects of psychotropic medication. *Int J Psychiatry Med* 1992;22:305–27.
24. Burnett WC, Chahine RA. Sexual dysfunction as a complication of propranolol therapy in men. *Cardiovasc Med* 1979;4:811–5.

690   DRUG-INDUCED DISEASES

25. Fraunfelder FT, Meyer SM. Sexual dysfunction secondary to topical ophthalmic timolol. *JAMA* 1985;253:3092–3. Letter.
26. Medical Research Council Working Party on Mild to Moderate Hypertension. Adverse reactions to bendrofluazide and propranolol for the treatment of mild hypertension. *Lancet* 1981;2:539–42.
27. Veterans Administration Cooperative Study Group on Antihypertensive Agents. Comparison of propranolol and hydrochlorothiazide for the initial treatment of hypertension. II. Results of long-term therapy. *JAMA* 1982;248:2004–11.
28. Bansal S. Sexual dysfunction in hypertensive men. A critical review of the literature. *Hypertension* 1988;12:1–10.
29. Prisant LM et al. Sexual dysfunction with antihypertensive drugs. *Arch Intern Med* 1994;154:730–6.
30. Thompson DF, Carter JR. Drug-induced gynecomastia. *Pharmacotherapy* 1993;13:37–45.
31. Epstein DL, Grant WM. Carbonic anhydrase inhibitor side effects. Serum chemical analysis. *Arch Ophthalmol* 1977;95:1378–82.
32. Wallace TR et al. Decreased libido—a side effect of carbonic anhydrase inhibitor. *Ann Ophthalmol* 1979;11:1563–6.
33. Jensen RT et al. Cimetidine-induced impotence and breast changes in patients with gastric hypersecretory states. *N Engl J Med* 1983;308:883–7.
34. The Coronary Drug Project Research Group. Clofibrate and niacin in coronary heart disease. *JAMA* 1975;231:360–81.
35. Oliver MF et al. A co-operative trial in the primary prevention of ischaemic heart disease using clofibrate. Report from the Committee of Principal Investigators. *Br Heart J* 1978;40:1069–118.
36. Duncan L, Bateman DN. Sexual function in women. Do antihypertensive drugs have an impact? *Drug Saf* 1993;8:225–34.
37. Siegel RK. Cocaine and sexual dysfunction: the curse of mama coca. *J Psychoact Drugs* 1982;14:71–4.
38. Wesson DR. Cocaine use by masseuses. *J Psychoact Drugs* 1982;14:75–6.
39. Neri A et al. Subjective assessment of sexual dysfunction of patients on long-term administration of digoxin. *Arch Sex Behav* 1980;9:343–7.
40. Bulpitt CJ, Dollery CT. Side effects of hypotensive agents evaluated by a self-administered questionnaire. *Br Med J* 1973;3:485–90.
41. Wassertheil-Smoller S et al. Effect of antihypertensives on sexual function and quality of life: the TAIM study. *Ann Intern Med* 1991;114:613–20.
42. Chang SW et al. The impact of diuretic therapy on reported sexual function. *Arch Intern Med* 1991;151:2402–8.
43. Bancroft J et al. The control of deviant sexual behaviour by drugs: I. Behavioural changes following oestrogens and anti-androgens. *Br J Psychiatry* 1974;125:310–5.
44. Bauer GE et al. The reversibility of side effects of guanethidine therapy. *Med J Aust* 1973;1:930–3.
45. Veterans Administration Cooperative Study Group on Antihypertensive Agents. Multiclinic controlled trial of bethanidine and guanethidine in severe hypertension. *Circulation* 1977;55:519–25.
46. Halikas J et al. Effects of regular marijuana use on sexual performance. *J Psychoact Drugs* 1982;14:59–70.
47. Cushman P. Sexual behavior in heroin addiction and methadone maintenance. Correlation with plasma luteinizing hormone. *N Y State J Med* 1972;72:1261–5.
48. Langrod J et al. Methadone treatment and physical complaints: a clinical analysis. *Int J Addict* 1981;16:947–52.
49. Rosenbaum M. When drugs come into the picture, love flies out the window: women addicts' love relationships. *Int J Addict* 1981;16:1197–206.
50. Sigell LT et al. Popping and snorting volatile nitrites: a current fad for getting high. *Am J Psychiatry* 1978;135:1216–8.
51. Welti RS, Brodsky JB. Treatment of intraoperative penile tumescence. *J Urol* 1980;124:925–6.
52. Lindquist M, Edwards IR. Endocrine adverse effects of omeprazole. *BMJ* 1992;305:451–2.
53. Lomas GM, Jarow JP. Risk factors for papaverine-induced priapism. *J Urol* 1992;147:1280–1.
54. Thompson JW et al. Psychotropic medication and priapism: a comprehensive review. *J Clin Psychiatry* 1990;51:430–3.
55. Kedia KR, Persky L. Effect of phenoxybenzamine (dibenzyline) on sexual function in man. *Urology* 1981;18:620–2.
56. Meiraz D et al. Treatment of benign prostatic hyperplasia with hydroxyprogesterone-caproate: placebo-controlled study. *Urology* 1977;9:144–8.
57. Herman JB et al. Fluoxetine-induced sexual dysfunction. *J Clin Psychiatry* 1990;51:25–7.
58. Musher JS. Anorgasmia with the use of fluoxetine. *Am J Psychiatry* 1990;147:948. Letter.
59. Zajecka J et al. The role of serotonin in sexual dysfunction: fluoxetine-associated orgasm dysfunction. *J Clin Psychiatry* 1991;52:66–8.
60. Rose LI et al. Pathophysiology of spironolactone-induced gynecomastia. *Ann Intern Med* 1977;87:398–403.
61. Warner MD et al. Trazodone and priapism. *J Clin Psychiatry* 1987;48:244–5.
62. Green L et al. Gynecomastia and breast cancer during finasteride therapy. *N Engl J Med* 1996;335:823. Letter.

Drug-Induced Skin Disorders

See introductory information on page 648.

DRUG	AE	AI	ED	EM	FE	LE	Ph	TN	REFERENCES
Acetaminophen		X			X			X	1–3
Allopurinol				X	X			XX	1–6
Amantadine		X					X		1
Aminosalicylic Acid			X						5
Amiodarone		X					X		1,4,7
Amphetamines		X							2
Androgens	XX	X							1,2,4,5
Antidepressants, Heterocyclic	X						X		1,4,7
Auranofin		X							1
Azathioprine		X							1
Barbiturates	X			XX	X			XX	1–6,8
Bleomycin		XX							1,2
Bromocriptine		X							1,2,4
Captopril		X	X						1
Carbamazepine			X	X	X			X	1–3,5,8
Carboplatin		X							1
Chloral Hydrate	X			X	X				1,2
Chlordiazepoxide					X				1
Chloroquine				X	X		X	X	2,4,7
Cimetidine				X				X	2,4
Clofibrate		X							2,5
Colchicine		XX		X				X	1–3,5
Contraceptives, Oral	X	X			X	X	X		1,2,4,5,7
Corticosteroids	XX								1,2,4,5
Cyclophosphamide		XX						X	1,2
Cyclosporine	X	X							1
Cytarabine		XX							1
Dacarbazine							X		1,2,7
Dactinomycin	XX							X	1,2,5
Danazol	XX								1,2
Dapsone				X	X		X	X	1,2,7
Daunorubicin		X							1,2
Disulfiram	X								1
Diuretics, Thiazide				X				XX	1,2,4,5,7

(continued)

DRUG	AE	AI	ED	EM	FE	LE	Ph	TN	REFERENCES
Doxorubicin		XX							1
Ethionamide	X								1
Etoposide		XX							1
Etretinate		XX					X		1,2,4,7
Fluoroquinolones							XX		1,7
Fluorouracil		XX					X		1,2,4,7
Furosemide				X					2,4
Gold Salts		X	XX	X	X		X	X	1,2,5,7
Griseofulvin				X	X		X		2,4,7
Heparin		X							1,2
Hydralazine						XX			1,2,5,9
Ifosfamide		XX							1
Interferon Alfa (2a, 2b)		XX							1,2
Isoniazid	X	X	X		X	X	X	X	1,2,4,5,9
Isotretinoin		XX					X		1,2,4,7
Ketoconazole		X							1
Levodopa		X							2,5
Lithium	XX	X	X						1,2,4,5
Meprobamate				X					1
Methotrexate		XX		X			X	X	1,2,4,7
Methyldopa					X				1,5,9
Methysergide		X							1
Metronidazole				X					1,2
Mitomycin		X							1
Nalidixic Acid							X		2,7
Nitrofurantoin		X		X	X			X	2,4
NSAIDs		X		X	X		X	X	1–4,7
Paclitaxel		XX							1
Penicillamine		X		XX	X	X			1,2,4,9
Penicillins			XX	XX	X			X	1–6,8
Phenolphthalein				X	X			X	1,2,4,5
Phenothiazines			X	X	X	X	XX		1,2,4,5,7,9
Phenytoin	X		X	X	X	X		X	1,2,4,5,8,9
Plicamycin								X	2,4
Procainamide						XX			1,5,9
Propranolol		X			X				4,5
Propylthiouracil		X					X		1,2,5
Psoralens	X					X	XX		1,2
Quinacrine		X		X					2,5

(*continued*)

DRUG	AE	AI	ED	EM	FE	LE	Ph	TN	REFERENCES
Quinidine	X		X		X	X	X		2,5,7,9
Quinine	X			X	X		X		1,2
Rifampin	X								1
Salicylates				XX	X			X	1–4
Streptomycin			XX	X	X			X	1,2,4
Sulfonamides			XX	XX	X	X	XX	XX	1–9
Sulfonylureas				X			X	X	1,2,4–7
Tamoxifen		X							1
Tetracyclines				X	X		XX		1,2,4–7
Tretinoin							X		1,7
Trimethadione	X	X		X		X			1,2,5
Valproic Acid		X		X					1,2,5,6
Vinblastine		XX					X		1,2,4,7
Vincristine		XX							1
Vitamin A		X		X					1,2,4,5
Warfarin		X							1,2,4,5

■ REFERENCES

1. Zürcher K, Krebs A. *Cutaneous drug reactions*, 2nd ed. Basel: S Karger; 1992.
2. Bork K. *Cutaneous side effects of drugs*. Philadelphia: WB Saunders; 1988.
3. Roujeau J-C et al. Toxic epidermal necrolysis (Lyell syndrome). Incidence and drug etiology in France, 1981–1985. *Arch Dermatol* 1990;126:37–42.
4. Blacker KL et al. Cutaneous reactions to drugs. In Fitzpatrick TB et al., eds. *Dermatology in general medicine*, 4th ed. New York: McGraw-Hill; 1993:1783–1806.
5. Millikan LE. Drug eruptions (dermatitis medicamentosa). In Moschella SL, Hurley HJ, eds. *Dermatology*, 3rd ed. Philadelphia: WB Saunders; 1992:535–73.
6. Chan H-L et al. The incidence of erythema multiforme, Stevens-Johnson syndrome, and toxic epidermal necrolysis. A population-based study with particular reference to reactions caused by drugs among outpatients. *Arch Dermatol* 1990;126:43–7.
7. Drugs that cause photosensitivity. *Med Lett Drugs Ther* 1995;37:35–6.
8. Roujeau JC, Stern RS. Severe adverse cutaneous reactions to drugs. *N Engl J Med* 1994;331:1272–85.
9. Price EJ, Venables PJW. Drug-induced lupus. *Drug Saf* 1995;12:283–90.

Drug Interactions and Interferences

Cytochrome P450 Enzyme Interactions

Philip O. Anderson

Cytochrome P450 enzymes are found throughout the body and are important role in the metabolism of many drugs, catalyzing a hydroxylation, N-demethylation, ring oxidation, and more.[1,2] Most substrates are metabolized by a specific enzyme, whereas each cytochrome P450 enzyme is generally capable of metabolizing many different compounds.[2,3] Induction or inhibition of these enzymes can drastically affect the outcome of drug therapy.

Cytochrome P450 enzymes are identified by the prefix "CYP" followed by an Arabic number identifying the family, although Roman numerals are still sometimes used. The three important enzyme families in humans are CYP1, CYP2, and CYP3. Subfamilies are given letters (eg, CYP2B, CYP2C). This is followed by a number identifying the specific enzyme.

Although most concentrated in the liver, cytochrome P450 enzymes exist in all tissues of the human body.[2,3] Intestinal mucosal cytochrome P450 enzymes appear to be primarily from the P450IIIA family, probably CYP3A4 in humans.[3] These enzymes affect the bioavailability of some drugs.

INDUCTION AND INHIBITION

When the amount of enzyme present in the body is increased by a drug or chemical, the enzyme is said to be "induced." Although most inducers are P450 substrates, this is not always the case. Induction can increase the rate of clearance of a drug, decreasing its efficacy. It can also increase the rate of formation of an active or toxic metabolite, resulting in exaggeration of therapeutic effect or increased toxicity.

Theoretically, all substrates metabolized by the same enzyme can compete for the same binding site, causing competitive inhibition. However, the clinical relevance depends on the concentration, relative affinities, and other elimination pathways of each substrate. Like inducers, not all inhibitors are enzyme substrates. Some drugs or their metabolites can form an inactive complex with a cytochrome P450 enzyme or its heme group. Inhibition may lead to increased toxic effects by causing drug accumulation, or it can lower toxic or therapeutic effects by decreasing the amount of toxic or active metabolite(s).

DRUG INTERACTIONS

Knowing which drugs are metabolized by each cytochrome P450 enzyme and the drugs that influence those enzymes can help in predicting drug-drug interactions. However, there are additional points to consider when predicting drug interactions.

The effect of inhibition on drug elimination depends on whether a substrate has alternate elimination pathways. Inhibition of an enzyme may not be clinically important if there are alternative metabolic pathways.

Therapeutic range is also important. If a drug has a wide therapeutic range, factors such as induction or inhibition become clinically unimportant. The opposite is true for drugs with a narrow therapeutic range, such as tricyclic antidepressants (TCAs) and antiarrhythmics.[4,5]

Last, consider metabolites. Not only does inhibition and induction of cytochrome P450 enzymes influence the formation of active metabolites, the formation of active metabolites may enhance inhibition or induction. Fluoxetine, an inhibitor of CYP2D6, has an active metabolite norfluoxetine, which also inhibits CYP2D6.[6,7]

The table following is meant to serve as an aid in the prediction of drug-drug interactions. However, it is also important to consider many other parameters: whether the patient is a poor or extensive metabolizer, the affinity of the drug for the binding site, the concentration of drug in the liver, the presence of alternate elimination pathways, and the therapeutic range. Because research on P450 metabolism is currently being published at a rapid rate, the table is not complete. The absence of a drug from the table does not necessarily imply that it is not metabolized by one of the P450 enzymes.

COMMON DRUGS THAT INTERACT WITH P450 ENZYMES

	SUBFAMILY SUBSTRATES	INDUCERS	INHIBITORS
1A2	acetaminophen, amitriptyline, antipyrine, caffeine, clomipramine, clozapine, imipramine, propranolol, tacrine, theophylline, (R)-warfarin	charcoal-broiled food, omeprazole, smoking	ciprofloxacin, fluvoxamine, grapefruit juice, macrolides*
2B6	cyclophosphamide, ifosfamide	phenobarbital, phenytoin	
2C8	benzphetamine, diazepam, diclofenac, (R)-mephenytoin, paclitaxel, tolbutamide		
2C9/10	diclofenac, hexobarbital, ibuprofen, (R)-mephenytoin, naproxen, phenytoin, piroxicam, tolbutamide, (S)-warfarin		fluconazole, fluoxetine, fluvastatin, ritonavir, sulfaphenazole
2C18	cimetidine, (S)-mephenytoin, propranolol, retinoic acid	omeprazole, piroxicam	
2C19	amitriptyline, clomipramine, diazepam, hexobarbital, imipramine, mephenytoin, mephobarbital, omeprazole, propranolol		fluoxetine, fluvoxamine, omeprazole, ritonavir
2D6	chlorpheniramine, clozapine, codeine, debrisoquine, dextromethorphan, flecainide, fluoxetine, haloperidol, loratadine, metoprolol, mexiletine, paroxetine, perphenazine, propafenone, propranolol, risperidone, thioridazine, timolol, tricyclic antidepressants, venlafaxine		cimetidine, haloperidol, perphenazine, propoxyphene, quinidine, ritonavir, SSRIs,† thioridazine
2E1	acetaminophen, alcohol, chlorzoxazone,	alcohol (chronic),	disulfiram

(continued)

	SUBFAMILY SUBSTRATES	INDUCERS	INHIBITORS
	dapsone, halothane, isoflurane, methoxyflurane, sevoflurane	isoniazid	
3A3/4	alfentanil, alprazolam, amiodarone, amitriptyline, androgens, astemizole, benzphetamine, bromocriptine, carbamazepine, cisapride, clomipramine, clonazepam, clozapine, cocaine, corticosteroids, cyclosporine, dapsone, dexamethasone, diazepam, diltiazem, disopyramide, erythromycin, ethinylestradiol, ethosuximide, etoposide, felodipine, ifosfamide, imipramine, isradipine, ketoconazole, lidocaine, oratadine, lovastatin, miconazole (IV), midazolam, nifedipine, nimodipine, omeprazole, paclitaxel, progesterone, propafenone, quinidine, quinine, saquinavir, sertraline, tacrolimus, tamoxifen, teniposide, terfenadine, testosterone, theophylline, triazolam, troleandomycin, verapamil, vinca alkaloids, (R)-warfarin	aminoglutethimide, carbamazepine, glucocorticoids, phenobarbital, phenytoin, rifampin, sulfinpyrazone	cimetidine, cyclophosphamide, cyclosporine, diltiazem, fluvoxamine, grapefruit juice, ifosfamide, itraconazole, ketoconazole, macrolides,* metronidazole, miconazole (IV), nefazodone, nifedipine, ritonavir, verapamil

SSRIs, selective serotonin reuptake inhibitors.
*CYP3A4 enzyme inhibition by macrolide antibiotics varies by drug: troleandomycin > erythromycin > clarithromycin > azithromycin = dirithromycin = 0.
[†]CYP2D6 enzyme inhibition by SSRI varies by drug: paroxetine > fluoxetine > sertraline > fluvoxamine.
Compiled from references 3, 8–24.

■ REFERENCES

1. Almira M. Drug biotransformation. In Katzung BG, ed. *Basic and clinical pharmacology.* Norwalk, CT: Appleton & Lange; 1992:49–59.

2. Watkins PB. Role of cytochromes P450 in drug metabolism and hepatotoxicity. *Semin Liver Dis* 1990;10:235–50.

3. Watkins PB. Drug metabolism by cytochromes P450 in the liver and small bowel. *Gastroenterol Clin North Am* 1992;21:511–26.

4. DeVane CL. Pharmacogenetics and drug metabolism of newer antidepressant agents. *J Clin Psychiatry* 1994;55(suppl):38-4–5.

5. Lennard M. Genetically determined adverse drug reactions involving metabolism. *Drug Saf* 1993;9:60–77.

6. Crewe HK et al. The effect of selective serotonin reuptake inhibitors on cytochrome P4502D6 (CYP2D6) activity in human liver microsomes. *Br J Clin Pharmacol* 1992;34:262–5.

7. Otton SV et al. Inhibition by fluoxetine of cytochrome P450 2D6 activity. *Clin Pharmacol Ther* 1993;53:401–9.

8. Spinler SA et al. Possible inhibition of hepatic metabolism of quinidine by erythromycin. *Clin Pharmacol Ther* 1995;57:89–94.

9. Ereshefsky L et al. Antidepressant drug interactions and the cytochrome P450 system. the role of cytochrome P4502D6. *Clin Pharmacokinet* 1995;29(suppl):10–9.

10. von Moltke LL et al. Metabolism of drugs by cytochrome P450 3A isoforms. *Clin Pharmacokinet* 1995;29(suppl):33–44.

11. Flockhart DA. Drug interactions and the cytochrome P450 system. *Clin Pharmacokinet* 1995;29(suppl):45–52.

12. Slaughter RL, Edwards DJ. Recent advances: the cytochrome P450 enzymes. *Ann Pharmacother* 1995;29:619–24.

13. Pollock BG. Recent developments in drug metabolism of relevance to psychiatrists. *Harvard Rev Psychiatr* 1994;2:204–13.

14. Gonzalez FJ. Human cytochromes P450: problems and prospects. *Trends Pharmacol Sci* 1992;13:346–52.

15. Tatro DS, ed. *Drug interactions facts.* St. Louis: Facts and Comparisons; 1995.

16. Riesenman C. Antidepressant drug interactions and the cytochrome P450 system: a critical appraisal. *Pharmacotherapy* 1995;6(pt 2):84S–99.

17. Kivisto KT et al. The role of human cytochrome P450 enzymes in the metabolism of anticancer agents: implications for drug interactions. *Br J Clin Pharmacol* 1995;40:523–30.

18. Schein JR. Cigarette smoking and clinically significant drug interactions. *Ann Pharmacother* 1995;29:1139–48.

19. Mitra AK et al. Metabolism of dapsone to its hydroxylamine by CYP2E1 in vitro and in vivo. *Clin Pharmacol Ther* 1995;58:556–66.

20. Transon C et al. In vivo inhibition profile of cytochrome P450TB (CYP2C9) by (+/−)-fluvastatin. *Clin Pharmacol Ther* 1995;58:412–7.

21. Periti P et al. Pharmacokinetic drug interactions of macrolides. *Clin Pharmacokinet* 1992;23:106–31.

22. Crewe HK et al. The effect of selective serotonin re-uptake inhibitors on cytochrome P4502D6 (CYP2D6) activity in human liver microsomes. *Br J Clin Pharmacol* 1992;34:262–5.

23. Manufacturer's Product Information.

24. Ketter TA et al. The emerging role of cytochrome P4503A in psychopharmacology. *J Clin Psychopharmacol* 1995;15:387–98.

Drug-Drug Interactions

Philip D. Hansten

This section is a list of drug-drug interactions which are most likely to be important in clinical practice. In the drug interactions list, minor or poorly documented interactions have been omitted, as have obvious interactions such as drugs with pharmacologic actions which are clearly similar (barbiturates-benzodiazepines) or opposite (isoproterenol-propranolol). For a more comprehensive review, the reader is directed to references 1 and 2 at the end of this section. It is important to remember that the presence of a drug interaction in this list does not necessarily imply that the two drugs should not be used together. In the majority of cases, the drugs may be used concomitantly as long as appropriate measures are taken.

In preparing this section, collective drug group or drug class names have been used whenever possible; drugs that are members of one of these groups are not listed individually. The following drug group names are used:

Aminoglycosides
Amphetamines
Angiotensin-Converting
    Enzyme (ACE) Inhibitors
Antacids, Oral
Anticholinergic Agents
Anticoagulants, Oral
Antidepressants, Heterocyclic*
Antidiabetic Agents
Barbiturates
Benzodiazepines
β-Adrenergic Blocking Agents
Calcium-Channel Blocking
    Agents
Calcium Salts
Cephalosporins
Contraceptives, Oral
Corticosteroids
Digitalis Glycosides
Diuretics, Potassium-Sparing

Diuretics, Thiazide
Iron Preparations
Monoamine Oxidase Inhibitors (MAOIs)
Nitrates
Nonsteroidal Antiinflammatory
    Drugs (NSAIDs)
Penicillins
Phenothiazines
Potassium Salts
Quinolones
Salicylates
Selective Serotonin Reuptake
    Inhibitors (SSRIs)
Skeletal Muscle Relaxants
    (Surgical)
Sulfonamides, Antibacterial
Sympathomimetic Agents
Tetracyclines
Thyroid Hormones
Zinc Salts

*Tricyclic Antidepressants, Maprotiline, Amoxapine.

Acetaminophen

- *Alcohol:* chronic alcohol abuse may increase the likelihood of acetaminophen hepatotoxicity, probably because of increased production of hepatotoxic acetaminophen metabolites; hepatotoxicity may occur with high therapeutic acetaminophen doses; alcoholics should limit their use of acetaminophen.[1-3]

Acetazolamide

- *Quinidine:* alkalinization of the urine may decrease quinidine elimination, increasing the risk of quinidine toxicity.[1,2]
- (*See also* Salicylates; Sympathomimetic Agents.)

Alcohol

- *Chloral Hydrate:* these drugs may inhibit each other's metabolism and prolong CNS depression; may produce vasodilation and hypotension.[1,2]
- *Disulfiram:* ingestion of even small amounts of alcohol may produce the disulfiram reaction, consisting of vasodilation, hypotension, nausea, vomiting, chest pain, weakness, and confusion; patients should also be warned about products whose alcohol content may not be obvious (eg, pharmaceuticals, topical preparations).[1]
- *Guanadrel:* response same as Alcohol–Guanethidine.
- *Guanethidine:* alcohol-induced vasodilation may accentuate guanethidine's orthostatic hypotension.[1,2]
- *Methotrexate:* chronic coadministration may increase the risk of methotrexate-induced liver damage; patients receiving methotrexate should minimize their consumption of alcohol.[1,2]
- *Metronidazole:* disulfiramlike reactions are reported, but are uncommon; patients should be warned about the possibility of their occurrence.[1,2]
- *Nitrates:* the vasodilation produced by both drugs may combine to produce marked hypotension.[1,2]
- *Phenytoin:* chronic use of large quantities of alcohol may stimulate metabolism of phenytoin; monitor phenytoin levels in alcoholics.[1,2]
- (*See also* Acetaminophen; Anticoagulants, Oral; Antidiabetic Agents; Salicylates.)

Allopurinol

- *Ampicillin:* Allopurinol appears to increase the risk of ampicillin rash; mechanism is unknown.[4]
- *Angiotensin-Converting Enzyme Inhibitors:* increased risk of hypersensitivity reactions (eg, skin eruptions, fever, arthralgias) with concurrent **captopril** and allopurinol.[1,2]
- *Azathioprine:* allopurinol inhibits first-pass metabolism of **mercaptopurine** (active metabolite of azathioprine) to inactive products, resulting in

increased mercaptopurine toxicity; when coadministration cannot be avoided, oral azathioprine dosage should be reduced by 75%.[1,2]

- *Cyclophosphamide:* cyclophosphamide-induced bone marrow suppression may be enhanced by allopurinol administration; mechanism is unknown.[1,2]
- *Mercaptopurine:* (*See* Allopurinol–Azathioprine [*Note:* the interaction described probably does not occur with IV mercaptopurine].)[2]
- (*See also* Anticoagulants, Oral.)

Amantadine: (*See* Anticholinergic Agents.)

Aminoglycosides

- *Amphotericin B:* possible additive nephrotoxicity; monitor renal function.[1,2]
- *Cephalosporins:* additive nephrotoxicity is possible, primarily with cephalothin; prolonged therapy merits repeated renal function tests.[1,2]
- *Cisplatin:* possible additive nephrotoxic effect; if combination cannot be avoided, monitor renal function closely.[5]
- *Digitalis Glycosides:* oral **neomycin** may impair digoxin absorption; monitor digitalis glycoside levels if long-term oral neomycin therapy is begun.[1,2]
- *Ethacrynic Acid:* additive ototoxicity has been reported; impaired renal function is an important predisposing factor.[1,2]
- *Methoxyflurane:* additive nephrotoxicity is possible; less nephrotoxic antibiotics should be used whenever possible.[1,2]
- *Penicillins:* the absorption of oral **penicillin V** is impaired by as much as 50% by oral **neomycin;** use parenteral penicillin until neomycin therapy is completed; also, **ticarcillin** and other penicillins appear to inactivate aminoglycosides when mixed in vitro, and possibly also in patients with severe renal impairment.[1,2]
- *Skeletal Muscle Relaxants (Surgical):* aminoglycoside antibiotics can produce neuromuscular blockade, which can enhance that of the muscle relaxant, prolonging recovery time and sometimes causing respiratory paralysis; avoid coadministration when ventilatory assistance equipment is not available.[1,2]

Aminophylline: (*See* Theophylline.)

Amiodarone

- *Anticoagulants, Oral:* enhanced anticoagulant response; if combination cannot be avoided, monitor prothrombin time carefully and reduce anticoagulant dosage accordingly.[1,2]
- *Cyclosporine:* increased cyclosporine serum concentrations; monitor closely for excessive cyclosporine levels and effect, and reduce cyclosporine dosage if needed.[1,2]
- *Digitalis Glycosides:* increased serum **digoxin** levels; monitor for evidence of increased digoxin effect, using serum digoxin determinations if possible.[1,2]
- *Phenytoin:* increased serum phenytoin levels; monitor phenytoin serum levels, and reduce phenytoin dosage if needed.[1,2]
- *Quinidine:* possible reduction in quinidine clearance; monitor quinidine levels and effect, and reduce quinidine dosage if needed.[6]

Amphetamines: (*See* Sympathomimetic Agents.)

Amphotericin B

- *Cyclosporine:* possible additive nephrotoxicity; if combination cannot be avoided, monitor renal function closely.[7]
- (*See also* Aminoglycosides; Corticosteroids; Digitalis Glycosides.)

Angiotensin-Converting Enzyme (ACE) Inhibitors

- *Diuretics, Potassium-Sparing:* ACE inhibitors and potassium-sparing diuretics may produce additive hyperkalemia, especially with marked renal impairment; monitor potassium status closely.[8]
- *Furosemide:* starting an ACE inhibitor in the presence of sodium depletion and hypovolemia caused by loop diuretics may result in a precipitous fall in blood pressure and consequent renal insufficiency.[1,2]
- *Lithium:* ACE inhibitors may increase serum lithium concentrations, probably by reducing renal lithium elimination.[9,10]
- *Nonsteroidal Antiinflammatory Drugs (NSAIDs):* NSAIDs may inhibit the antihypertensive response to ACE inhibitors; effect may be less likely with **sulindac** and possibly **nabumetone;** monitor blood pressure closely.[11,12]
- *Potassium Salts:* ACE inhibitors and potassium supplements may produce additive hyperkalemia, especially with marked renal impairment; monitor potassium status closely.[1,2]
- (*See also* Allopurinol.)

Antacids, Oral

- *Digitalis Glycosides:* antacids may modestly reduce the extent of **digoxin** absorption; give digoxin 2 hr before antacids.[1]
- *Diuretics, Thiazide:* large doses of calcium antacids may produce hypercalcemia in the presence of thiazides in predisposed patients (eg, high vitamin D intake, hyperparathyroidism); mechanism is thiazide-induced reduction of urinary calcium excretion.[13]
- *Iron Preparations:* calcium carbonate, sodium bicarbonate, and possibly magnesium trisilicate reduce absorption of oral iron, but aluminum and magnesium hydroxides apparently do not; separate doses by 2 hr or more.[1,2,14]
- *Isoniazid:* aluminum-containing antacids may interfere with isoniazid absorption; separate doses by 2 hr or select another antacid.[1,2]
- *Quinidine:* antacid-induced increases in urinary pH can decrease the amount of quinidine excreted by the kidney; watch for evidence of increased quinidine effect.[1,2]
- *Quinolones:* antacids may reduce extent of absorption of **ciprofloxacin, enoxacin, norfloxacin,** and **ofloxacin;** give quinolone 2 hr before or 6 hr after antacid.[15,16]
- *Salicylates:* appreciably reduced salicylate levels, caused by enhanced renal elimination in patients receiving large doses of a salicylate; serum salicylate levels should be monitored in patients requiring long-term salicylate therapy.[17]

- *Sodium Polystyrene Sulfonate:* this resin can bind magnesium and calcium ions from the antacid in the gut, resulting in systemic alkalosis; rectal use of the resin may avoid this problem.[1,2]
- *Tetracyclines:* antacids containing di- or trivalent ions interfere with absorption of oral tetracyclines; separate doses by 2 hr.[1,2]
- (*See also* Cimetidine–Ketoconazole.)

Anticholinergic Agents

- *Amantadine:* amantadine potentiates the effects of high dosages of anticholinergics, especially the CNS activity.[1,2]
- *Tacrine:* tacrine is a cholinergic agent, and combined use with anticholinergic agents may result in inhibition of the effect of one or both drugs.[18,19]

Anticoagulants, Oral

- *Alcohol:* increased anticoagulant activity occurs with large amounts of alcohol, but the mechanism has not been clearly defined; 1 or 2 drinks per day is not likely to have any effect.[1,2]
- *Allopurinol:* increased anticoagulant activity in some patients; monitor prothrombin time carefully.[1,2]
- *Aminoglutethimide:* decreased anticoagulant effect, probably caused by enhanced anticoagulant metabolism.[1,2]
- *Anabolic Steroids:* although mechanism is unknown, increased anticoagulant activity commonly occurs; monitor prothrombin time closely.[1,2]
- *Antidiabetic Agents:* **dicumarol** may inhibit sulfonylurea metabolism; **warfarin** appears to be less likely to interact.[1,2]
- *Barbiturates:* decreased anticoagulant effect, mostly caused by stimulation of hepatic metabolism of the anticoagulant; monitor prothrombin time carefully if the barbiturate is being used as an anticonvulsant; **benzodiazepines** are more suitable if only sedative or hypnotic effects are desired.[1,2]
- *Carbamazepine:* decreased anticoagulant effect, most likely caused by stimulation of hepatic metabolism of anticoagulant; monitor prothrombin time carefully.[1,2]
- *Chloral Hydrate:* chloral hydrate may temporarily increase hypoprothrombinemic effect of **warfarin** because of serum protein binding displacement; long-term therapy with both drugs is unlikely to cause problems.[1,2]
- *Chloramphenicol:* marked increase in **dicumarol** activity is well documented, probably caused by inhibition of dicumarol metabolism; although less evidence is available for **warfarin,** caution is advised.[1,2]
- *Cholestyramine:* decreased absorption of **warfarin;** separate administration by 6 hr; some interaction occurs even if doses are separated, because of enterohepatic circulation of warfarin.[1,2]
- *Cimetidine:* enhanced hypoprothrombinemic response to **warfarin** because of inhibition of warfarin metabolism; may necessitate reduction in warfarin dosage; **famotidine, nizatidine,** and **ranitidine** are less likely to interact with warfarin.[1,2]

- *Clofibrate:* well-documented increase in anticoagulant activity; monitor prothrombin time carefully.[1,2]
- *Colestipol:* response same as Anticoagulants, Oral–Cholestyramine.
- *Danazol:* increased anticoagulant activity; monitor prothrombin time carefully.[1,2]
- *Dextrothyroxine:* well-documented increase in anticoagulant effect; monitor prothrombin time carefully.[1,2]
- *Disulfiram:* increased anticoagulant activity because of inhibition of anticoagulant metabolism; monitor prothrombin time carefully.[1,2]
- *Erythromycin:* increased anticoagulant activity because of inhibition of **warfarin** metabolism; monitor prothrombin time carefully.[20]
- *Fluconazole:* increased **warfarin** activity in some patients; monitor prothrombin time carefully.[21]
- *Gemfibrozil:* response same as Anticoagulants, Oral–Clofibrate.
- *Glutethimide:* decreased anticoagulant effect, probably caused by stimulation of hepatic metabolism of anticoagulant; **benzodiazepines** are preferred in patients taking oral anticoagulants.[1,2]
- *Griseofulvin:* decreased anticoagulant effect reported; monitor prothrombin time carefully.[1,2]
- *Itraconazole:* possible increase in **warfarin** anticoagulant effect; monitor prothrombin time carefully.[22]
- *Ketoconazole:* possible increase in **warfarin** anticoagulant effect; monitor prothrombin time carefully.[23]
- *Lovastatin:* increased **warfarin** activity in some patients; monitor prothrombin time carefully.[1,2]
- *Meclofenamate:* enhanced hypoprothrombinemic response to **warfarin;** avoid concurrent use or monitor prothrombin time carefully.[1,2]
- *Metronidazole:* enhanced hypoprothrombinemic response to **warfarin** because of inhibition of metabolism; monitor prothrombin time carefully.[1,2]
- *Miconazole:* possible increase in anticoagulant activity with either systemic or topical miconazole; monitor prothrombin time carefully.[1,2]
- *Nonsteroidal Antiinflammatory Drugs (NSAIDs):* most NSAIDs do not regularly affect hypoprothrombinemic response to oral anticoagulants; use caution because of possible GI bleeding and antiplatelet effect of NSAIDs.[1,2]
- *Phenytoin:* **dicumarol** may inhibit phenytoin metabolism, whereas phenytoin may stimulate dicumarol metabolism; the use of **warfarin** may reduce the importance of this interaction, but watch for evidence of reduced (may be preceded by transient increase) warfarin effect caused by phenytoin-induced enzyme stimulation.[1,2]
- *Propafenone:* increased **warfarin** activity, probably caused by inhibition of warfarin metabolism; monitor prothrombin time carefully.[1]
- *Quinidine:* may enhance hypoprothrombinemic response to **warfarin** occasionally; monitor prothrombin time carefully.[1,2]

- *Quinolones:* increased **warfarin** activity with **ciprofloxacin,** probably caused by inhibition of warfarin metabolism; monitor prothrombin time carefully.[1]
- *Rifampin:* decreases anticoagulant activity by stimulating **warfarin** metabolism; monitor prothrombin time carefully.[1,2]
- *Salicylates:* large doses of salicylates increase anticoagulant effect; monitor prothrombin time carefully; smaller doses may cause problems because of possible GI bleeding and antiplatelet effect (with aspirin only).[1,2]
- *Selective Serotonin Reuptake Inhibitors (SSRIs):* **fluvoxamine** may substantially increase the hypoprothrombinemic response to **warfarin,** whereas **fluoxetine, paroxetine,** and **sertraline** appear to have little or no effect on warfarin response; some evidence suggests that SSRIs increase the risk of bleeding even in the absence of hypoprothrombinemia.[24–28]
- *Sulfinpyrazone:* increased anticoagulant activity, primarily caused by inhibition of **warfarin** metabolism; monitor prothrombin time carefully.[1,2]
- *Sulfonamides, Antibacterial:* some sulfonamides may enhance hypoprothrombinemic response to oral anticoagulants; monitor prothrombin time carefully.[1,2]
- *Thyroid Hormones:* increased anticoagulant effect, probably because of increased catabolism of clotting factors; monitor prothrombin time carefully.[1,2]
- *Trimethoprim/Sulfamethoxazole:* well-documented increase in **warfarin** response; does not occur in all patients; probably caused by sulfamethoxazole; monitor prothrombin time carefully.[1,2]
- (*See also* Amiodarone.)

Antidepressants, Heterocyclic

- *Barbiturates:* may stimulate antidepressant metabolism; watch for reduced antidepressant effect.[1,2]
- *Carbamazepine:* may stimulate antidepressant metabolism; watch for reduced antidepressant effect.[1]
- *Cimetidine:* inhibition of tricyclic antidepressant (TCA) metabolism; monitor for excessive tricyclic effect (eg, severe anticholinergic effects) and reduce tricyclic dosage if needed; **famotidine, nizatidine,** and **ranitidine** may be less likely than cimetidine to interact with tricyclics.[1,2]
- *Clonidine:* reduced antihypertensive response to clonidine; use another antihypertensive (but not guanadrel or guanethidine).[1,2]
- *Guanadrel:* response same as Antidepressants, Heterocyclic–Guanethidine.
- *Guanethidine:* antidepressants inhibit the uptake (and therefore action) of guanethidine by the adrenergic neurons; effects noted after 2 days of antidepressant therapy; use another antihypertensive agent (but not guanadrel or clonidine).[1,2]
- *Monoamine Oxidase Inhibitors (MAOIs):* symptoms of CNS stimulation with convulsions and death have been reported; combination can be used if large dosages are avoided and patient closely monitored.[1,2]

- **Propoxyphene:** possible inhibition of **doxepin** metabolism; monitor for excessive doxepin response and reduce doxepin dosage if needed.[1,2]
- **Quinidine:** possible increase in serum levels of TCAs; watch for tricyclic toxicity.[1,2]
- **Selective Serotonin Reuptake Inhibitors (SSRIs):** increased serum levels of TCAs; watch for tricyclic toxicity.[1,2]
- **Sympathomimetic Agents:** TCAs may increase pressor response to parenteral **epinephrine, norepinephrine, phenylephrine,** and possibly other sympathomimetics; effect of oral or nasal sympathomimetics not established, but caution is warranted; monitor blood pressure when sympathomimetics are given to patients receiving heterocyclic antidepressants.[1,2]

Antidiabetic Agents

- **Alcohol:** alcohol may produce hypoglycemia, especially in fasting patients; moderate increases in blood glucose may occur in nonfasting patients. Disulfiramlike reactions have occurred with **sulfonylureas,** and patients should be warned about that possibility.[1,2]
- **Anabolic Steroids:** enhanced hypoglycemic effect; antidiabetic agent dosage reduction may be required.[1,2]
- **β-Adrenergic Blocking Agents:** β-blockers prolong hypoglycemic episodes and inhibit tachycardia and tremors that are signs of hypoglycemia (sweating is not inhibited); hypertension may occur during hypoglycemia; cardioselective β-blockers (eg, **atenolol, metoprolol**) are less likely to cause problems than nonselective types (eg, **nadolol, propranolol**).[29]
- **Chloramphenicol:** prolonged half-lives have been reported for **tolbutamide** and **chlorpropamide,** probably resulting from inhibition of metabolism; reduction of **sulfonylurea** dosage may be necessary with prolonged chloramphenicol use.[1,2]
- **Cimetidine:** may increase the hypoglycemic effect of **glipizide;** other H_2-receptor antagonists may also interact, since mechanism appears to be increased gastric pH. **Tolbutamide** effect may also be increased by cimetidine dosage of 1 g/day or more. Reduction of glipizide or tolbutamide dosage may be required.[30,31]
- **Clofibrate:** enhanced hypoglycemic effect of **sulfonylureas** may occur; may require decrease of sulfonylurea dosage.[1,2]
- **Corticosteroids:** corticosteroids may increase serum glucose levels; increase of antidiabetic dosage may be required.[1,2]
- **Diuretics, Thiazide:** thiazides may aggravate diabetes; increased dosage of antidiabetic agent may be needed to maintain control; patients stabilized on both drugs are not likely to have problems.[1,2]
- **Fluconazole:** may increase serum levels of **tolbutamide, glipizide,** and **glyburide,** probably because of inhibition of metabolism; other **sulfonylureas** may also be affected; may need to decrease sulfonylurea dosage.[2]
- **Methyldopa:** reduced **tolbutamide** metabolism; possible enhanced tolbutamide hypoglycemia; effect on other sulfonylureas not known.[32]

- *Monoamine Oxidase Inhibitors (MAOIs):* MAOIs may interfere with normal adrenergic response to hypoglycemia, prolonging the action of antidiabetic agents; MAOIs should be avoided in diabetics.[1,2]
- *Rifampin:* stimulates metabolism of **tolbutamide** and possibly other **sulfonylureas;** may require increased sulfonylurea dosage.[1,2]
- *Salicylates:* enhanced response to **sulfonylureas** (especially **chlorpropamide**) is possible; several possible mechanisms; reduction of antidiabetic dosage may be necessary if prolonged high-dose salicylate is planned.[1,2]
- *Sulfonamides, Antibacterial:* several sulfonamides reported to increase the activity of **sulfonylureas** by inhibition of metabolism or displacement from serum protein binding sites; use another antiinfective whenever possible.[1,2]
- *Thyroid Hormones:* may increase antidiabetic drug requirements; mechanism unknown.[1,2]
- (*See also* Anticoagulants, Oral.)

Astemizole Interactions similar to Terfenadine.

Azathioprine (*See* Allopurinol.)

Barbiturates

- *β-Adrenergic Blocking Agents:* enhanced metabolism of β-blockers that are primarily metabolized by the liver (eg, **propranolol, metoprolol**); monitor for reduced β-blocker effect and increase β-blocker dosage if needed.[1,2]
- *Calcium-Channel Blocking Agents:* barbiturates may enhance metabolism of oral **verapamil, nifedipine,** and possibly other calcium-channel blockers; watch for reduced effect of calcium-channel blocker.[1,2]
- *Contraceptives, Oral:* barbiturates may stimulate metabolism of contraceptives; menstrual irregularities and unplanned pregnancies may occur; more likely with low-dose oral contraceptives.[1,33]
- *Corticosteroids:* **phenobarbital** increases the metabolism of corticosteroids (other barbiturates probably produce a similar effect); patients may require increased corticosteroid dosage.[1,2]
- *Cyclosporine:* barbiturates enhance cyclosporine metabolism; monitor for reduced cyclosporine levels and effect, and increase cyclosporine dosage if needed.[1,2]
- *Griseofulvin:* impaired griseofulvin absorption; numerous small doses of griseofulvin may provide greater absorption in the presence of barbiturates than single large doses.[1,2]
- *Phenothiazines:* barbiturates may enhance phenothiazine metabolism; possible decrease in antipsychotic effect.[1,2]
- *Quinidine:* barbiturates may enhance quinidine metabolism; monitor for reduced quinidine levels and effect.[1,2]
- *Tetracyclines:* barbiturates may enhance **doxycycline** metabolism; possible decrease in antimicrobial effect.[1,2]

- *Theophylline:* barbiturates enhance theophylline metabolism; monitor theophylline serum levels and increase theophylline dosage if needed.[1,2]
- *Valproic Acid:* valproic acid inhibits phenobarbital metabolism; reduced phenobarbital dosage may be necessary.[34]
- *(See also* Anticoagulants, Oral; Antidepressants, Heterocyclic.)

Benzodiazepines

- *Calcium-Channel Blocking Agents:* **diltiazem** and **verapamil** can markedly increase oral **midazolam** serum concentrations, leading to increased sedative effects; parenteral midazolam probably interacts to a lesser extent.[35]
- *Cimetidine:* cimetidine may inhibit the elimination of **chlordiazepoxide** and **diazepam,** but not **lorazepam** or **oxazepam**—reduction in diazepam or chlordiazepoxide dosage may be needed;[36,37] cimetidine (or other drugs that increase gastric pH) may modestly increase the bioavailability of **triazolam.**[1,2]
- *Disulfiram:* disulfiram may inhibit the elimination of **chlordiazepoxide** and **diazepam,** but not **lorazepam** or **oxazepam;** reduction in diazepam or chlordiazepoxide dosage may be necessary.[38,39]
- *Itraconazole:* marked increase in oral **midazolam** serum concentrations, leading to increased sedative effects; parenteral midazolam probably interacts to a lesser extent; avoid combination.[40]
- *Ketoconazole:* marked increase in oral **midazolam** serum concentrations, leading to increased sedative effects; parenteral midazolam probably interacts to a lesser extent; avoid combination.[40]
- *Nefazodone:* inhibition of **alprazolam** and **triazolam** metabolism; avoid combinations or monitor for excessive benzodiazepine effect and decrease benzodiazepine dosage if needed.
- *Selective Serotonin Reuptake Inhibitors (SSRIs):* **fluoxetine** and **fluvoxamine** increase levels of **alprazolam** and **diazepam;** reduction in benzodiazepine dosage may be necessary.[41-44]
- *Theophylline:* inhibition of benzodiazepine sedation; watch for altered benzodiazepine response if theophylline is initiated or discontinued.[45]
- *(See also* Omeprazole.)

β-Adrenergic Blocking Agents

- *Cimetidine:* enhanced **propranolol** effect; may require reduction of propranolol dosage.[46]
- *Clonidine:* combined use with **propranolol** may result in *hyper*tensive reactions, especially if clonidine is abruptly discontinued.[1,2]
- *Digitalis Glycosides:* β-blockers may worsen CHF or digitalis-induced bradycardia.[1,2]
- *Nonsteroidal Antiinflammatory Drugs:* antihypertensive effect of β-blockers may be inhibited; mechanism may be prostaglandin inhibition. **Sulindac** and possibly **nabumetone** may be less likely to interact.[1,2]

- **Prazosin:** enhanced hypotensive reaction to first dose of prazosin; anticipate hypotensive episode and take appropriate precautions (eg, take first prazosin dose at bedtime).[1,2] A similar effect may be seen with **doxazosin** or **terazosin.**
- **Rifampin:** enhanced metabolism of β-blockers primarily metabolized by the liver (eg, **propranolol, metoprolol**); monitor for reduced β-blocker effect and increase β-blocker dosage if necessary.[1,2]
- **Sympathomimetic Agents: epinephrine** may produce hypertensive reactions in patients on **propranolol** (and probably other nonselective blockers such as **nadolol**); may also occur with other sympathomimetics such as **phenylephrine** and **phenylpropanolamine;** avoid such combinations if possible; if used, monitor closely for hypertensive response.[1,2]
- **Theophylline:** mutual inhibition of effect may occur; β-blockers (especially nonselective) may worsen asthma.[1,2]
- (*See also* Antidiabetic Agents; Barbiturates; Digitalis Glycosides.)

Bismuth Subsalicylate

- **Tetracycline:** bismuth subsalicylate may reduce GI absorption of tetracycline; separate doses by 2 hr, with tetracycline given first.[2]

Calcium-Channel Blocking Agents

- **Carbamazepine: verapamil** and **diltiazem** inhibit carbamazepine metabolism; monitor for increased carbamazepine levels and effect, and decrease carbamazepine dosage if needed.[1,2]
- **Cyclosporine: verapamil, diltiazem,** and **nicardipine** inhibit cyclosporine metabolism; monitor for increased cyclosporine levels and effect, and reduce cyclosporine dosage if needed.[1,2]
- **Digitalis Glycosides:** increased serum digoxin levels with **verapamil,** and to a lesser extent with **bepridil, diltiazem,** and **nitrendipine** (minimal effects with **felodipine, nicardipine,** or **nifedipine**); monitor for excessive digoxin effect and decrease digoxin dosage if needed.[1,2]
- **Rifampin:** enhanced metabolism of oral **verapamil,** and probably also other calcium-channel blockers; monitor for reduced calcium-channel blocker effect.[1,2]
- **Theophylline: verapamil** and **diltiazem** may inhibit theophylline metabolism; monitor for excessive theophylline levels and decrease theophylline dosage if needed.[1,2]
- (*See also* Barbiturates; Benzodiazepines.)

Calcium Salts: (*See* Digitalis Glycosides.)

Carbamazepine

- **Cimetidine:** inhibition of carbamazepine metabolism; monitor for excessive carbamazepine levels and effect, and decrease carbamazepine dosage if needed.[1,2]
- **Clarithromycin:** inhibition of carbamazepine metabolism; monitor for excessive carbamazepine levels and effect, and decrease carbamazepine dosage if needed.[1,2]

- *Contraceptives, Oral:* oral contraceptive metabolism may be increased; menstrual irregularities and unplanned pregnancies may occur; may be more likely with low-dose oral contraceptives. [1,2]
- *Corticosteroids:* increase in corticosteroid metabolism; may require increased corticosteroid dosage.[1,2]
- *Cyclosporine:* enhanced cyclosporine metabolism; monitor for reduced cyclosporine levels and effect, and increase cyclosporine dosage if needed.[1,2]
- *Danazol:* inhibition of carbamazepine metabolism; monitor for excessive carbamazepine levels and effect, and decrease carbamazepine dosage if needed.[1,2]
- *Erythromycin:* inhibition of carbamazepine metabolism; monitor for excessive carbamazepine levels and effect, and decrease carbamazepine dosage if needed.[1,2]
- *Haloperidol:* enhanced haloperidol metabolism; monitor for reduced haloperidol response and increase haloperidol dosage if needed.[47]
- *Isoniazid:* inhibition of carbamazepine metabolism; monitor for excessive carbamazepine levels and effect, and decrease carbamazepine dosage if needed.[1,2]
- *Propoxyphene:* inhibition of carbamazepine metabolism; monitor for excessive carbamazepine levels and effect, and decrease carbamazepine dosage if needed.[1,2]
- *Quinine:* inhibition of carbamazepine metabolism; monitor for excessive carbamazepine levels and effect, and decrease carbamazepine dosage if needed.[48]
- *Selective Serotonin Reuptake Inhibitors (SSRIs):* **fluoxetine** inhibits carbamazepine metabolism; monitor for excessive carbamazepine levels and effect, and decrease carbamazepine dosage if needed.[1,2]
- *Theophylline:* enhanced theophylline metabolism; monitor theophylline serum levels and increase theophylline dosage if needed.[49]
- *Troleandomycin:* inhibition of carbamazepine metabolism; monitor for excessive carbamazepine levels and effect, and decrease carbamazepine dosage if needed.[1,2]
- (*See also* Anticoagulants, Oral; Antidepressants, Heterocyclic; Calcium-Channel Blocking Agents; Tetracyclines.)

Cephalosporins

- *Probenecid:* renal elimination of cephalosporins that undergo tubular secretion is reduced.[1,2]
- (*See also* Aminoglycosides.)

Chloral Hydrate

- *Furosemide:* IV furosemide may produce flushing, sweating, and blood pressure variations in patients taking chloral hydrate.[1,2]
- (*See also* Alcohol; Anticoagulants, Oral.)

Chloramphenicol

- *Phenytoin:* concomitant therapy may cause enhanced phenytoin levels through inhibition of phenytoin metabolism; use another antiinfective whenever possible.[1,2]

- (*See also* Anticoagulants, Oral; Antidiabetic Agents.)

Chloroquine

- *Cyclosporine:* chloroquine may increase cyclosporine levels and lead to cyclosporine toxicity; monitor for excessive cyclosporine effect and decrease cyclosporine dosage if needed.[50,51]

Cholestyramine

- *Diuretics, Thiazide:* reduced thiazide absorption; administer thiazide at least 2 hr before cholestyramine and monitor for reduced thiazide response.[1,2]

- *Furosemide:* markedly reduced furosemide absorption; administer furosemide at least 2 hr before or 6 hr after cholestyramine.[52]

- *Methotrexate:* reduced methotrexate absorption; separate doses as much as possible and monitor for reduced methotrexate effect.[53]

- (*See also* Anticoagulants, Oral; Digitalis Glycosides; Thyroid Hormones.)

Cimetidine

- *Clozapine:* increased clozapine serum concentrations, probably through inhibition of CYP1A2; monitor for excessive clozapine effect and decrease clozapine dosage if needed.[54]

- *Ketoconazole:* increased gastric pH may reduce GI absorption of ketoconazole; same effect with other H_2-receptor antagonists, **antacids,** and probably **omeprazole** and **lansoprazole.**[1,2]

- *Lidocaine:* inhibition of lidocaine elimination; monitor for excessive lidocaine levels and effect, and decrease lidocaine dosage if needed; **famotidine, nizatidine,** and **ranitidine** are less likely to interact with lidocaine.[1,2]

- *Phenytoin:* inhibition of phenytoin metabolism; monitor for increased phenytoin levels and effect, and decrease phenytoin dosage if needed; **famotidine, nizatidine,** and **ranitidine** are less likely to interact with phenytoin.[55]

- *Procainamide:* inhibition of renal excretion of both procainamide and N-acetylprocainamide; monitor for excessive procainamide levels and effect, and decrease procainamide dosage if needed; **ranitidine** may also increase procainamide levels, although probably not to the same extent as cimetidine; **famotidine** does not appear to affect procainamide elimination.[1,2]

- *Quinidine:* inhibition of quinidine metabolism; monitor for excessive quinidine levels and effect, and decrease quinidine dosage if needed; **famotidine, nizatidine,** and **ranitidine** are less likely to interact with quinidine.[1,2]

- *Tacrine:* increased tacrine serum concentrations, possibly increasing tacrine cholinergic effects (eg, nausea, vomiting, anorexia, diarrhea).[56]

- *Theophylline:* cimetidine may reduce elimination of theophylline; watch for theophylline toxicity and monitor theophylline serum levels; reduced theophylline dosage may be required.[57] **Famotidine, nizatidine,** and **ranitidine** are less likely to interact with theophylline.
- (*See also* Anticoagulants, Oral; Antidepressants, Heterocyclic; Antidiabetic Agents; Benzodiazepines; β-Adrenergic Blocking Agents; Carbamazepine.)

Cisapride

- *Itraconazole:* cisapride metabolism by CYP3A4 may be reduced, possibly resulting in serious ventricular arrhythmias; avoid combination.[58]
- *Ketoconazole:* cisapride metabolism by CYP3A4 may be reduced, possibly resulting in serious ventricular arrhythmias; avoid combination.[58]
- *Miconazole:* cisapride metabolism by CYP3A4 may be reduced by IV miconazole, possibly resulting in serious ventricular arrhythmias; avoid combination.[58]
- *Troleandomycin:* cisapride metabolism by CYP3A4 may be reduced, possibly resulting in serious ventricular arrhythmias; avoid combination.[58]

Cisplatin

- *Methotrexate:* reduced methotrexate elimination; monitor for increased methotrexate response.[5]
- (*See also* Aminoglycosides.)

Clarithromycin

- *Terfenadine:* reduced terfenadine metabolism; possible increased risk of cardiac arrhythmias; avoid combination; **astemizole** may interact with clarithromycin similarly.[59]
- (*See also* Carbamazepine.)

Clofibrate

- *Furosemide:* clofibrate-induced myopathy (eg, muscle pain, stiffness) may be more likely in presence of furosemide; hypoalbuminemia is also a predisposing factor.[1,2]
- (*See also* Anticoagulants, Oral; Antidiabetic Agents.)

Clonidine

- *Levodopa:* antiparkinson effect of levodopa may be inhibited; avoid combined use or monitor closely for impaired levodopa effect.[1]
- (*See also* Antidepressants, Heterocyclic; β-Adrenergic Blocking Agents.)

Clozapine

- *Selective Serotonin Reuptake Inhibitors (SSRIs):* **Fluvoxamine** appears to increase clozapine serum concentrations, probably through inhibition of CYP1A2; monitor for excessive clozapine effect and decrease clozapine dosage if needed.[60]
- (*See also* Cimetidine.)

Colestipol: Interactions same as Cholestyramine.

Contraceptives, Oral

- *Griseofulvin:* possible reduction of oral contraceptive efficacy; if combination cannot be avoided, monitor for menstrual irregularities and consider adding another form of contraception during griseofulvin use.[61]

- *Penicillins:* data are inconclusive; **ampicillin** may interfere with enterohepatic circulation of contraceptive hormones; menstrual irregularities and unplanned pregnancies may occur; more likely with low-dose oral contraceptives; use alternative contraception instead of, or in addition to, oral contraceptives while on ampicillin.[1,33]

- *Phenytoin:* oral contraceptive metabolism may be increased; menstrual irregularities and unplanned pregnancies may occur; more likely with low-dose oral contraceptives.[33]

- *Rifampin:* rifampin may interfere with the action of oral contraceptives, increasing the risk of unplanned pregnancy; another method of birth control should be used.[1,33]

- *Tetracyclines:* possibly same effect as penicillins, but documentation is poor.

- (*See also* Barbiturates; Carbamazepine.)

Corticosteroids

- *Aminoglutethimide:* decreased **dexamethasone** effect, probably because of enhanced dexamethasone metabolism; other corticosteroids might be similarly affected.[1,2]

- *Amphotericin B:* enhancement of amphotericin B-induced potassium depletion; monitor serum potassium levels regularly and supplement with potassium salts if needed.[1,2]

- *Diuretics, Thiazide:* enhancement of potassium depletion; monitor serum potassium levels regularly and supplement with potassium chloride if needed.[1,2]

- *Furosemide:* loop diuretics may enhance corticosteroid-induced potassium depletion; monitor serum potassium levels regularly and supplement with potassium chloride if needed.[1,2]

- *Ketoconazole:* reduced **methylprednisolone** elimination; monitor for excessive methylprednisolone response; effect on other corticosteroids is not well established.[1,2]

- *Phenytoin:* increased **dexamethasone** metabolism; other corticosteroids may be similarly affected.[1,2]

- *Rifampin:* increased in corticosteroid metabolism; may require increased corticosteroid dosage.[1,2]

- *Salicylates:* decreased salicylate levels, possibly because of corticosteroid effects on salicylate elimination; salicylate intoxication possible if patient is on large doses of salicylate and corticosteroid dosage is reduced.[1,2]

- (*See also* Aminoglutethimide; Antidiabetic Agents; Barbiturates; Carbamazepine.)

Cyclophosphamide: (*See* Allopurinol.)

Cyclosporine

- *Anabolic Steroids:* increased serum cyclosporine levels; monitor cyclosporine levels and effect, and renal function carefully.[1,2]

- *Erythromycin:* inhibition of cyclosporine metabolism; monitor for increased cyclosporine levels and effect, and reduce cyclosporine dosage if needed.[62,63]

- *Fluconazole:* possible inhibition of cyclosporine metabolism, especially with higher fluconazole dosages; monitor for increased cyclosporine levels and effect, and reduce cyclosporine dosage if needed.[64]

- *Itraconazole:* possible inhibition of cyclosporine metabolism; monitor for increased cyclosporine levels and effect, and reduce cyclosporine dosage if needed.[1,2]

- *Ketoconazole:* possible inhibition of cyclosporine metabolism; monitor for increased cyclosporine levels and effect, and reduce cyclosporine dosage if needed.[1,2]

- *Lovastatin:* increased risk of myopathy (eg, muscle pain, weakness); rhabdomyolysis has been reported.[1,2]

- *Miconazole:* inhibition of cyclosporine metabolism likely; monitor for increased cyclosporine levels and effect, and reduce cyclosporine dosage if needed.[65]

- *Phenytoin:* enhanced cyclosporine metabolism; monitor for reduced cyclosporine levels and effect, and increase cyclosporine dosage if needed.[66]

- *Rifampin:* enhanced cyclosporine metabolism; monitor for reduced cyclosporine levels and effect, and increase cyclosporine dosage if needed.[67]

- *Sulfonamides, Antibacterial:* reduced serum cyclosporine levels and possible enhanced nephrotoxicity; monitor cyclosporine levels and effect, and renal function.[68,69]

- (*See also* Amiodarone; Amphotericin B; Barbiturates; Calcium-Channel Blocking Agents; Carbamazepine; Chloroquine.)

Danazol: (*See* Anticoagulants, Oral; Carbamazepine.)

Dapsone

- *Probenecid:* probenecid may reduce the renal elimination of dapsone; reduction of dapsone dosage may be required.[1,2]

Dextrothyroxine: (*See* Anticoagulants, Oral.)

Didanosine: (*See* Quinolones.)

Digitalis Glycosides

- *Amphotericin B:* amphotericin B–induced potassium loss may contribute to digitalis toxicity; monitor serum potassium levels regularly, and supplement with a potassium salt if needed.[1,2]

- *Calcium Salts:* both have similar myocardial actions; use parenteral calcium salts with caution.[1,2]
- *Cholestyramine:* may bind **digitoxin** (and possibly **digoxin**) in the gut; separate doses and monitor for reduced digitalis effect.[1,2]
- *Colestipol:* interaction same as Digitalis Glycosides–Cholestyramine.
- *Diuretics, Thiazide:* long-term diuretic-induced potassium loss may contribute to digitalis intoxication; monitor serum potassium levels and supplement with potassium chloride or give a potassium-sparing diuretic if needed.[1,2]
- *Ethacrynic Acid* (*See* Digitalis Glycosides–Diuretics, Thiazide.)
- *Furosemide* (*See* Digitalis Glycosides–Diuretics, Thiazide.)
- *Kaolin-Pectin:* reduced GI absorption of digoxin; give **digoxin** 2 or more hr before kaolin-pectin.[1,2]
- *Penicillamine:* reduced serum **digoxin** levels may occur; assess need for increase in digoxin dosage.[70]
- *Quinidine:* reduced renal clearance and tissue binding of **digoxin** resulting in average twofold increase in serum digoxin; **digitoxin** may also be affected, probably by different mechanisms; monitor for increased digitalis effect, serum **digoxin** levels useful; may necessitate reduction in digitalis dosage.[71]
- *Rifampin:* enhanced hepatic metabolism of **digitoxin;** monitor for reduced digitoxin effect; **digoxin** probably less likely to interact with rifampin.[1,2]
- *Spironolactone:* reduced elimination of **digitoxin** and **digoxin** reported, but spironolactone metabolites may also produce false increases in serum levels of digitalis glycosides by some methods; watch for clinical evidence of excessive digitalis effect.[1,72]
- *Sulfasalazine:* reduced GI absorption of **digoxin;** spacing doses may not avoid interaction; monitor for reduced digoxin effect.[1,2]
- (*See also* Aminoglycosides; Amiodarone; Antacids, Oral; β-Adrenergic Blocking Agents; Calcium-Channel Blocking Agents.)

Disulfiram

- *Isoniazid:* mental changes may result from effects of both drugs on metabolism of adrenergic neurotransmitters; avoid the use of disulfiram in patients who must take isoniazid.[1,2]
- *Metronidazole:* confusion and psychotic episodes have been reported; avoid combination or monitor for psychiatric reactions.[1,2]
- *Phenytoin:* disulfiram inhibits the hepatic metabolism of phenytoin; phenytoin dosage reduction may be necessary.[1,2]
- *Theophylline:* inhibition of theophylline metabolism; monitor for excessive theophylline response and decrease theophylline dosage if needed.[73]
- (*See also* Alcohol; Anticoagulants, Oral; Benzodiazepines.)

Diuretics, Potassium-Sparing: (*See* Angiotensin-Converting Enzyme Inhibitors; Nonsteroidal Antiinflammatory Drugs; Potassium Salts.)

Diuretics, Thiazide

- *Lithium Carbonate:* long-term diuretic use may result in decreased lithium elimination; monitor serum lithium levels until the patient is stabilized in the therapeutic range.[1,2]
- *Nonsteroidal Antiinflammatory Drugs (NSAIDs):* NSAIDs may slightly inhibit the natriuretic and antihypertensive effects of thiazides; increased thiazide dosage may be needed in some patients.[74,75]
- (*See also* Antacids, Oral; Antidiabetic Agents; Cholestyramine; Colestipol; Corticosteroids; Digitalis Glycosides.)

Dopamine

- *Phenytoin:* IV phenytoin may produce hypotension in severely ill patients receiving IV dopamine; monitor blood pressure closely if combination used.[76]

Erythromycin

- *Lovastatin:* increased risk of myopathy (eg, muscle pain, weakness); rhabdomyolysis has been reported.[1,2]
- *Tacrolimus:* reduced tacrolimus metabolism; possible increase in tacrolimus toxicity.[77]
- *Terfenadine:* reduced terfenadine metabolism; possible increased risk of cardiac arrhythmias; avoid combination; **astemizole** appears to interact with erythromycin in a similar way.[78,79]
- *Theophylline:* erythromycin may reduce theophylline elimination in some patients; risk of theophylline toxicity is greatest in patients on relatively large dosages of theophylline.[80]
- (*See also* Anticoagulants, Oral; Carbamazepine; Cyclosporine.)

Estrogens: (*See* Contraceptives, Oral.)

Ethacrynic Acid: (*See* Aminoglycosides; Digitalis Glycosides.)

Fluconazole

- *Phenytoin:* increased serum phenytoin levels, probably caused by inhibition of metabolism; monitor for excessive phenytoin levels and effect, and reduce phenytoin dosage if needed.[1,2]
- (*See also* Anticoagulants, Oral; Antidiabetic Agents; Cyclosporine.)

Furosemide

- *Nonsteroidal Antiinflammatory Drugs (NSAIDs):* the hypotensive and natriuretic effects of furosemide may be inhibited by NSAIDs; possible need for increased furosemide dosage.[74]
- (*See also* Angiotensin-Converting Enzyme Inhibitors; Chloral Hydrate; Cholestyramine; Clofibrate; Colestipol; Corticosteroids; Digitalis Glycosides.)

Gemfibrozil

- *Lovastatin:* increased risk of myopathy (eg, muscle pain, weakness); rhabdomyolysis has been reported.[1,2]

- (*See also* Anticoagulants, Oral.)

Glutethimide: (*See* Anticoagulants, Oral.)

Griseofulvin: (*See* Anticoagulants, Oral; Barbiturates; Contraceptives, Oral.)

Guanadrel: (*See* Alcohol; Antidepressants, Heterocyclic; Phenothiazines; Sympathomimetic Agents.)

Guanethidine: (*See* Alcohol; Antidepressants, Heterocyclic; Phenothiazines; Sympathomimetic Agents.)

Haloperidol

- *Lithium:* CNS toxicity (eg, lethargy, confusion, extrapyramidal symptoms, fever) occasionally with this combination; avoid combination in acute mania if possible; if combination is used, adjust dosages carefully and monitor for neurotoxicity.[1,2]
- *Methyldopa:* combined use may cause dementia (eg, confusion, disorientation); avoid combination or monitor for adverse psychiatric effects.[1,2]
- (*See also* Carbamazepine.)

Heparin: (*See* Salicylates.)

Hydralazine

- *Nonsteroidal Antiinflammatory Drugs (NSAIDs):* reduced antihypertensive response to hydralazine; monitor blood pressure.[81]

Iron Preparations

- *Methyldopa:* reduced methyldopa absorption; monitor for reduced antihypertensive response.[1,2]
- *Quinolones:* decreased extent of absorption of **ciprofloxacin, norfloxacin, lomefloxacin,** and **ofloxacin** (latter two less affected); give quinolone at least 2 hr before or 6 hr after iron.[1,2]
- *Tetracyclines:* decreased tetracycline absorption, probably due to chelation in gut; give tetracycline at least 2 hr before or 4 hr after iron preparations.[1,2]
- *Thyroid Hormones:* decreased thyroid hormone absorption; give thyroid at least 2 hr before or 4 hr after iron.[1,2]
- *Vitamin E:* large doses of vitamin E impair utilization of iron in patients with iron deficiency anemia; avoid vitamin E in such patients.[1,2]
- (*See also* Antacids, Oral.)

Isoniazid

- *Phenytoin:* isoniazid inhibits the hepatic metabolism of phenytoin, increasing the risk of toxicity, particularly in slow acetylators; reduction of phenytoin dosage may be required.[1,2]
- *Rifampin:* metabolism of isoniazid to hepatotoxic metabolites may be enhanced by rifampin; monitor for hepatotoxicity.[1,2]
- (*See also* Antacids, Oral; Carbamazepine; Disulfiram.)

Itraconazole

- *Terfenadine:* reduced terfenadine metabolism; possible increased risk of cardiac arrhythmias; avoid combination; **astemizole** may interact with itraconazole in a similar way.[82,83]
- (*See also* Anticoagulants, Oral; Benzodiazepines; Cisapride; Cyclosporine.)

Kaolin-Pectin (*See* Digitalis Glycosides.)

Ketoconazole

- *Terfenadine:* reduced terfenadine metabolism; possible increased risk of cardiac arrhythmias; avoid combination; **astemizole** appears to interact with ketoconazole in a similar way.[79,84-86]
- (*See also* Anticoagulants, Oral; Benzodiazepines; Cimetidine; Cisapride; Corticosteroids; Cyclosporine.)

Levodopa

- *Papaverine:* antiparkinson effect of levodopa may be inhibited; avoid papaverine in such patients.[1,2]
- *Phenytoin:* antiparkinson effect of levodopa may be inhibited; if phenytoin must be used with levodopa, monitor for reduced levodopa response; theoretically, increasing levodopa dosage might restore antiparkinson response.[1,2]
- *Pyridoxine:* pyridoxine increases levodopa metabolism, markedly decreasing its effectiveness; this interaction does not occur if a peripheral decarboxylase inhibitor (eg, **carbidopa**) is used in conjunction with levodopa.[1,2]
- (*See also* Clonidine; Monoamine Oxidase Inhibitors; Phenothiazines.)

Lidocaine: (*See* Cimetidine.)

Lithium

- *Methyldopa:* signs of lithium toxicity may occur in the absence of increased serum lithium; if interaction occurs, select another antihypertensive.[87]
- *Nonsteroidal Antiinflammatory Drugs (NSAIDs):* reduced renal clearance of lithium; monitor for excessive lithium effect and decrease lithium dosage if needed; **sulindac** (and possibly **ibuprofen** and **nabumetone**) may be less likely to increase lithium than other NSAIDs.[88-90]
- *Phenytoin:* signs of lithium toxicity may occur in the absence of increased serum lithium; monitor for clinical evidence of lithium toxicity if combined use cannot be avoided.[91]
- *Sodium Chloride:* excess sodium increases lithium excretion; sodium deficiency may promote lithium retention and increase risk of toxicity; patients taking lithium should not be on low-salt diets.[1]
- *Theophylline:* enhanced renal lithium clearance; monitor lithium levels and increase lithium dosage if needed.[92,93]
- (*See also* Angiotensin-Converting Enzyme Inhibitors; Diuretics, Thiazide; Haloperidol.)

Lovastatin: (*See* Anticoagulants, Oral; Cyclosporine; Erythromycin; Gemfibrozil.)

Meclofenamate: (*See* Anticoagulants, Oral.)

Mercaptopurine: (*See* Allopurinol.)

Methotrexate

- *Nonsteroidal Antiinflammatory Drugs (NSAIDs):* NSAIDs such as **ketoprofen** and **indomethacin** (and probably others) may reduce renal methotrexate excretion; avoid combination in patients receiving antineoplastic dosages of methotrexate until risks are better described.[94,95]

- *Omeprazole:* omeprazole may inhibit the renal elimination of methotrexate, increasing methotrexate serum concentrations; monitor for excessive methotrexate effect and decrease methotrexate dosage if needed.[96]

- *Para-Aminobenzoic Acid (PABA):* PABA may displace methotrexate from serum protein binding sites; do not give PABA-containing products systemically during methotrexate therapy.[1,2]

- *Probenecid:* reduced renal excretion of methotrexate; may necessitate decreases in methotrexate dosage.[1,2]

- (*See also* Alcohol; Cholestyramine; Cisplatin; Colestipol; Salicylates.)

Methoxyflurane: (*See* Aminoglycosides; Tetracyclines.)

Methyldopa: (*See* Antidiabetic Agents; Haloperidol; Iron Preparations; Lithium; Sympathomimetic Agents.)

Metronidazole: (*See* Alcohol; Anticoagulants, Oral; Disulfiram.)

Mexiletine

- *Phenytoin:* enhanced mexiletine metabolism; monitor for reduced mexiletine response and increase mexiletine dosage if needed.[97]

- *Rifampin:* enhanced mexiletine metabolism; monitor for reduced mexiletine response and increase mexiletine dosage if needed.[98]

Miconazole: (*See* Anticoagulants, Oral; Cisapride; Cyclosporine.)

Monoamine Oxidase Inhibitors (MAOIs)

- *Levodopa:* increased levels of dopamine and norepinephrine, and hypertensive reaction may occur; **carbidopa** seems to protect against this interaction.[1,2]

- *Meperidine:* a variety of reactions may occur, including hypertension, excitement, rigidity and, occasionally, hypotension and coma; avoid meperidine in patients on MAOIs; other narcotics are apparently safer.[1,2]

- *Nefazodone:* nefazodone inhibits the neuronal uptake of serotonin. Since fatal reactions have occurred with combined use of SSRIs and MAOIs, nefazodone should also be considered contraindicated with MAOIs.[1]

- *Selective Serotonin Reuptake Inhibitors (SSRIs):* severe or fatal reactions have been reported when **tranylcypromine** was given to patients receiving **fluoxetine.** Avoid fluoxetine (and other SSRIs) within 2 weeks of stopping tranylcypromine (or other nonselective MAOIs); avoid starting a nonselective MAOI within 5 weeks of stopping fluoxetine or within 2 weeks of stopping other SSRIs (**fluvoxamine, paroxetine, sertraline**).[1,2]

- *Sympathomimetic Agents:* indirect-acting agents such as **amphetamines, ephedrine, metaraminol, phenylpropanolamine, pseudoephedrine,** and possibly **methylphenidate** may cause a hypertensive crisis in patients on MAOIs; of the direct-acting agents, **phenylephrine** may also produce hypertension in patients on MAOIs, whereas the response to **epinephrine** and **norepinephrine** is minimally affected.[1,2]

- (*See also* Antidepressants, Heterocyclic; Antidiabetic Agents.)

Nefazodone

- *Terfenadine:* nefazodone inhibits CYP3A4 and may inhibit terfenadine metabolism; possible increased risk of cardiac arrhythmias; avoid combination; **astemizole** may interact with nefazodone in a similar way.

- (*See also* Benzodiazepines; Monoamine Oxidase Inhibitors.)

Nitrates: (*See* Alcohol.)

Nonsteroidal Antiinflammatory Drugs (NSAIDs)

- *Diuretics, Potassium-Sparing:* indomethacin (and probably other NSAIDs) may reduce renal function when combined with **triamterene;** preliminary evidence indicates that **spironolactone** does not produce the same effect.[99]

- (*See also* Angiotensin-Converting Enzyme Inhibitors; Anticoagulants, Oral; β-Adrenergic Blocking Agents; Diuretics, Thiazide; Furosemide; Hydralazine; Lithium; Methotrexate; Sympathomimetic Agents.)

Omeprazole

- *Benzodiazepines:* increased serum **diazepam** levels, probably because of inhibition of metabolism; monitor for excessive diazepam effect.[100]

- *Phenytoin:* modest increase in serum phenytoin levels; monitor for excessive phenytoin levels and effect.[100,101]

- (*See also* Cimetidine–Ketoconazole; Methotrexate.)

Papaverine: (*See* Levodopa.)

Para-Aminobenzoic Acid: (*See* Methotrexate; Sulfonamides, Antibacterial.)

Penicillamine: (*See* Digitalis Glycosides.)

Penicillins

- *Probenecid:* renal elimination of penicillins is reduced; this may be used to therapeutic advantage when high levels of penicillin are desired.[2]

- *Tetracyclines:* bacteriostatic agents, such as tetracyclines, inhibit bacterial growth, whereas penicillins require actively growing bacteria to exert their effect; coadministration could nullify the action of the penicillins; however, clinical problems are infrequent in patients receiving adequate dosages of both drugs.[1,2]

- (*See also* Aminoglycosides; Contraceptives, Oral.)

Phenothiazines

- *Guanethidine:* phenothiazines may inhibit the uptake of guanethidine (and perhaps **guanadrel**) by the adrenergic neurons, thereby reducing its hypotensive effects; at the same time, phenothiazines have hypotensive effects of their own, so use of both drugs requires close monitoring of blood pressure.[1,2]

- *Levodopa:* levodopa does not block phenothiazine-induced extrapyramidal symptoms, but phenothiazines may inhibit the antiparkinson activity of levodopa.[1,2]

- (*See also* Barbiturates.)

Phenytoin

- *Quinidine:* enhanced quinidine metabolism; monitor for reduced quinidine levels and effect, and increase quinidine dosage if needed.[1,2]

- *Rifampin:* enhanced phenytoin metabolism; monitor for reduced phenytoin levels and increase phenytoin dosage if needed.[102,103]

- *Selective Serotonin Reuptake Inhibitors (SSRIs):* **fluoxetine** appears to inhibit phenytoin metabolism, and may produce phenytoin toxicity in some patients.[104]

- *Theophylline:* enhanced theophylline metabolism; monitor theophylline serum levels and increase theophylline dosage if needed.[49]

- *Valproic Acid:* valproic acid displaces phenytoin from serum protein binding sites; total serum phenytoin levels are reduced; free phenytoin is increased only temporarily, so a change in phenytoin dosage is usually not necessary.[105,106]

- (*See also* Alcohol; Amiodarone; Anticoagulants, Oral; Chloramphenicol; Cimetidine; Contraceptives, Oral; Corticosteroids; Cyclosporine; Disulfiram; Dopamine; Fluconazole; Isoniazid; Levodopa; Lithium; Mexiletine; Omeprazole; Sulfonamides, Antibacterial; Tetracyclines.)

Potassium Salts

- **Diuretics, Potassium-Sparing:** serious hyperkalemia may result if a potassium salt and a potassium-sparing compound such as **amiloride, spironolactone,** or **triamterene** are given to the same patient; monitor serum potassium levels very closely.[1,2]

- (*See* also Angiotensin-Converting Enzyme Inhibitors.)

Prazosin: (*See* β-Adrenergic Blocking Agents.)

Probenecid: (*See* Cephalosporins; Dapsone; Methotrexate; Penicillins; Salicylates.)

Procainamide: (*See* Cimetidine.)

Propafenone: (*See* Anticoagulants, Oral.)

Propoxyphene: (*See* Antidepressants, Heterocyclic; Carbamazepine.)

Pyridoxine: (*See* Levodopa.)

Quinidine

- **Rifampin:** rifampin stimulates quinidine metabolism; quinidine dosage may need to be increased if the combination cannot be avoided.[107]
- **Sodium Bicarbonate:** alkalinization of the urine may decrease quinidine elimination, thereby increasing the risk of quinidine toxicity.[1]
- (*See also* Acetazolamide; Amiodarone; Antacids, Oral; Anticoagulants, Oral; Antidepressants, Heterocyclic; Barbiturates; Cimetidine; Digitalis Glycosides; Phenytoin.)

Quinine: (*See* Carbamazepine.)

Quinolones

- **Didanosine:** the buffers in didanosine contain aluminum and magnesium ions that can markedly reduce the oral absorption and serum levels of **ciprofloxacin;** other quinolones may be similarly affected. Avoid combination or give quinolone at least 2 hr before didanosine.[108]
- **Sucralfate:** sucralfate markedly reduces the oral absorption and serum levels of **ciprofloxacin, norfloxacin,** and **ofloxacin;** avoid sucralfate or give quinolone at least 2 hr before sucralfate.[1,2,109]
- **Theophylline: ciprofloxacin** and **enoxacin** reduce theophylline clearance; monitor for excessive theophylline levels and effect, and reduce theophylline dosage if needed.[110,111]
- *See also* Antacids, Oral; Anticoagulants, Oral; Iron Preparations.

Rifampin

- **Methadone:** rifampin may stimulate metabolism of methadone; withdrawal symptoms are possible in patients on methadone maintenance.[1]
- **Theophylline:** enhanced theophylline metabolism; monitor theophylline serum levels and increase theophylline dosage if needed.[112]
- **Zidovudine:** reduced zidovudine serum levels; monitor for reduced zidovudine effect and increase zidovudine dosage if needed.[113]
- (*See also* Anticoagulants, Oral; Antidiabetic Agents; β-Adrenergic Blocking Agents; Calcium-Channel Blocking Agents; Contraceptives, Oral; Corticosteroids; Cyclosporine; Digitalis Glycosides; Isoniazid; Mexiletine; Phenytoin; Quinidine.)

Salicylates

- **Acetazolamide:** acetazolamide may enhance renal salicylate excretion and increase salicylate penetration into the brain; the latter effect may produce CNS salicylate toxicity if patient is on a large salicylate dosage.[1,114]
- **Alcohol:** enhanced risk of GI blood loss.[1,2]
- **Heparin:** aspirin effects on platelet adhesiveness might leave the heparin-treated patient more prone to hemorrhage; some patients are given the combination intentionally for the combined anticoagulant effects.[1,2]
- **Methotrexate:** salicylate displaces methotrexate from serum protein binding sites and also inhibits its renal elimination; may increase the risk of

methotrexate toxicity; do not give a salicylate to patients taking antineoplastic dosages of methotrexate; warn patient about the use of OTC products that contain salicylate.[1,2]

- *Probenecid:* salicylate inhibits the uricosuric effect of probenecid, particularly with large doses of salicylate; occasional small doses present no problem.[1,2]
- *Sulfinpyrazone:* salicylate inhibits the uricosuric effect of sulfinpyrazone;
occasional small doses present no problem.[1,2]
- (*See also* Antacids, Oral; Anticoagulants, Oral; Antidiabetic Agents; Corticosteroids.)

Selective Serotonin Reuptake Inhibitors (SSRIs)

- *Theophylline:* Fluvoxamine can increase theophylline levels, probably by
inhibiting theophylline hepatic metabolism; monitor for excessive theophylline effect and decrease theophylline dosage if needed.[115,116]
- (*See also* Anticoagulants, Oral; Antidepressants, Heterocyclic; Benzodiazepines; Carbamazepine; Clozapine; Monoamine Oxidase Inhibitors;
Phenytoin.)

Simvastatin: Interactions same as Lovastatin.

Skeletal Muscle Relaxants (Surgical): (*See* Aminoglycosides.)

Sodium Bicarbonate: (*See* Quinidine; Sympathomimetic Agents; Tetracyclines.)

Sodium Chloride: (*See* Lithium.)

Sodium Polystyrene Sulfonate: (*See* Antacids, Oral.)

Spironolactone: (*See* Digitalis Glycosides; Potassium Salts.)

Sucralfate: (*See* Quinolones.)

Trimethoprim/Sulfamethoxazole: (*See* Anticoagulants, Oral.)

Sulfasalazine: (*See* Digitalis Glycosides.)

Sulfinpyrazone: (*See* Anticoagulants, Oral; Salicylates.)

Sulfonamides, Antibacterial

- *Para-Aminobenzoic Acid (PABA):* systemically administered PABA antagonizes the antibacterial effects of the sulfonamides, which work by competing with PABA in bacteria.[1]
- *Phenytoin:* sulfonamides may inhibit the metabolism of phenytoin and displace it from serum protein binding sites; monitor serum phenytoin levels
if more than a few days of sulfonamide therapy are planned.[1,2]
- (*See also* Anticoagulants, Oral; Antidiabetic Agents; Cyclosporine; Digitalis Glycosides.)

Sympathomimetic Agents

- *Acetazolamide:* alkalinization of the urine decreases elimination of **amphetamines, pseudoephedrine,** and possibly other sympathomimetics.[1]
- *Guanethidine:* sympathomimetics with indirect activity, such as **amphetamines** and **ephedrine,** may inhibit the antihypertensive effect of guanethi-

dine (and perhaps **guanadrel**); direct-acting sympathomimetics, such as **norepinephrine** and **phenylephrine,** may produce an exaggerated response in patients on guanethidine (and perhaps **guanadrel**); avoid sympathomimetics in patients on guanethidine.[1,2]

- *Methyldopa:* possible increase in pressor response to **norepinephrine;** mechanism not established.[1]
- *Sodium Bicarbonate:* alkalinization of the urine decreases elimination of **amphetamines, pseudoephedrine,** and possibly other sympathomimetics.[1]
- (*See also* Antidepressants, Heterocyclic; β-Adrenergic Blocking Agents; Monoamine Oxidase Inhibitors.)

Tacrine

- *Theophylline:* increased theophylline serum concentrations; possible increase in risk of theophylline toxicity.[117]
- (*See also* Anticholinergic Agents; Cimetidine.)

Tacrolimus: (*See* Erythromycin.)

Terfenadine

- *Troleandomycin:* reduced terfenadine metabolism; possible increased risk of cardiac arrhythmias; avoid combination; **astemizole** may interact with troleandomycin in a similar way.[118]
- (*See also* Clarithromycin; Erythromycin; Itraconazole; Ketoconazole; Nefazodone.)

Tetracyclines

- *Carbamazepine:* carbamazepine may stimulate **doxycycline** metabolism; possible decrease in antimicrobial effect.[1,2]
- *Methoxyflurane:* additive nephrotoxicity has been reported.[1,2]
- *Phenytoin:* phenytoin may stimulate **doxycycline** metabolism, possibly decreasing antimicrobial effect.[1,2]
- *Zinc Salts:* large doses of zinc salts (eg, 200 mg) may reduce tetracycline absorption; space doses by 2 hr or more and give tetracycline first.[1,2]
- (*See also* Antacids, Oral; Barbiturates; Bismuth Subsalicylate; Contraceptives, Oral; Iron Preparations; Penicillins.)

Theophylline

- *Troleandomycin:* elevated serum theophylline levels may occur; mechanism is probably inhibition of theophylline metabolism; monitor theophylline serum levels; may need to reduce theophylline dosage.[1,2]
- *Vaccination, Influenza:* theophylline elimination may be reduced following influenza vaccination, but this may not occur with purified subviron (split) influenza vaccines; monitor theophylline serum levels if patient receives whole viron influenza vaccine.[119,120]
- (*See also* Barbiturates; Benzodiazepines; β-Adrenergic Blocking Agents; Calcium-Channel Blocking Agents; Carbamazepine; Cimetidine; Disulfiram; Erythromycin; Lithium; Phenytoin; Quinolones; Rifampin; Selective Serotonin Reuptake Inhibitors; Tacrine.)

Thyroid Hormones

- *Cholestyramine:* cholestyramine binds both T3 and T4 in the gut, preventing their absorption; separate doses by at least 4 hr.[1,2]
- *Colestipol:* interactions same as Thyroid Hormones–Cholestyramine.
- (*See also* Anticoagulants, Oral; Antidiabetic Agents; Iron Preparations.)

Triamterene: (*See* Potassium Salts.)

Troleandomycin: (*See* Carbamazepine; Cisapride; Terfenadine; Theophylline.)

Vaccination, Influenza: (*See* Theophylline.)

Valproic Acid: (*See* Barbiturates; Phenytoin.)

Vitamin E: (*See* Iron Preparations.)

Zidovudine: (*See* Rifampin.)

Zinc Salts: (*See* Tetracyclines.)

■ REFERENCES

1. Hansten PD, Horn JR. *Drug interactions and updates quarterly.* Vancouver: Applied Therapeutics; 1996 (updated quarterly).
2. Tatro DS, ed. *Drug interaction facts.* St. Louis: JB Lippincott; 1996 (updated quarterly).
3. Hansten PD, Horn JR. Acetaminophen and alcohol—a potentially toxic combination. *Drug Interact Newsl* 1986;6:31–4.
4. Boston Collaborative Drug Surveillance Program. Excess of ampicillin rashes associated with allopurinol or hyperuricemia. *N Engl J Med* 1972;286:505–7.
5. Hansten PD, Horn JR. Cisplatin drug interactions. *Drug Interact Newsl* 1985;5:49–50.
6. Saal AK et al. Effect of amiodarone on serum quinidine and procainamide levels. *Am J Cardiol* 1984;53:1264–7.
7. Hansten PD, Horn JR. Amphotericin B interaction. *Drug Interact Newsl* 1985;5:U-7.
8. Hansten PD, Horn JR. Captopril (Capoten) interactions. *Drug Interact Newsl* 1985;5:U-10–1.
9. Navis GJ et al. Volume homeostasis, angiotensin converting enzyme inhibition, and lithium therapy. *Am J Med* 1989;86:621.
10. Baldwin CM, Safferman AZ. A case of lisinopril-induced lithium toxicity. *DICP* 1990;24:946–7.
11. Fujita T et al. Effect of indomethacin on antihypertensive action of captopril in hypertensive patients. *Clin Exp Hypertens [A]* 1981;3:939–52.
12. Silberbauer K et al. Acute hypotensive effect of captopril in man modified by prostaglandin synthesis inhibition. *Br J Clin Pharmacol* 1982;14(suppl):87S–93S.
13. Hakim R et al. Severe hypercalcemia associated with hydrochlorothiazide and calcium carbonate therapy. *Can Med Assoc J* 1979;121:591–4.
14. O'Neil-Cutting MA, Crosby WH. The effect of antacids on the absorption of simultaneously ingested iron. *JAMA* 1986;255:1468–70.
15. Nix DE et al. Effects of aluminum and magnesium antacids and ranitidine on the absorption of ciprofloxacin. *Clin Pharmacol Ther* 1989;46:700–5.
16. Gugler R, Allgayer H. Effect of antacids on the clinical pharmacokinetics of drugs. An update. *Clin Pharmacokinet* 1990;18:210–9.
17. Hansten PD, Hayton WL. Effect of antacid and ascorbic acid on serum salicylate concentration. *J Clin Pharmacol* 1980;20:326–31.
18. Ott BR, Lannon MC. Exacerbation of parkinsonism by tacrine. *Clin Neuropharmacol* 1992;15:322–5.
19. Summers WK et al. Use of THA in treatment of Alzheimer-like dementia: pilot study in twelve patients. *Biol Psychiatry* 1981;16:145–53.
20. Hansten PD, Horn JR. Erythromycin and warfarin. *Drug Interact Newsl* 1985;5:37–40.
21. Seaton TL et al. Possible potentiation of warfarin by fluconazole. *DICP* 1990;24:1177–8.
22. Yeh J et al. Potentiation of action of warfarin by itraconazole. *BMJ* 1990;301:669.
23. Smith AG. Potentiation of oral anticoagulants by ketoconazole. *Br Med J* 1984;288:188–9.

24. Benfield P, Ward A. Fluvoxamine. A review of its pharmacodynamic and pharmacokinetic properties, and therapeutic efficacy in depressive illness. *Drugs* 1986;32:313–34.

25. Claire RJ et al. Potential interaction between warfarin sodium and fluoxetine. *Am J Psychiatry* 1991;148:1604. Letter.

26. Aranth J, Lindberg C. Bleeding, a side effect of fluoxetine. *Am J Psychiatry* 1992;149:412. Letter.

27. Bannister SJ et al. Evaluation of the potential for interactions of paroxetine with diazepam, cimetidine, warfarin, and digoxin. *Acta Psychiatr Scand* 1989;80(suppl 350):102–6.

28. Wilner KD et al. The effects of sertraline on the pharmacodynamics of warfarin in healthy volunteers. *Biol Psychiatry* 1991;29:354S–5S.

29. Hansten PD. Beta-blocking agents and antidiabetic drugs. *Drug Intell Clin Pharm* 1980;14:46–50.

30. Feely J, Peden N. Enhanced sulfonylurea-induced hypoglycaemia with cimetidine. *Br J Clin Pharmacol* 1983;15:607P.

31. Cate EW et al. Inhibition of tolbutamide elimination by cimetidine but not ranitidine. *J Clin Pharmacol* 1986;26:372–7.

32. Gachalyi B et al. Effect of alphamethyldopa on the half-lives of antipyrine, tolbutamide and D-glucaric acid excretion in man. *Int J Clin Pharmacol Ther Toxicol* 1980;18:133–5.

33. Hansten PD. Drug interactions that inhibit oral contraceptive efficacy. *Drug Interact Newsl* 1981;1:9–11.

34. Patel IH et al. Phenobarbital-valproic acid interaction. *Clin Pharmacol Ther* 1980;27:515–21.

35. Backman JT et al. Dose of midazolam should be reduced during diltiazem and verapamil treatments. *Br J Clin Pharmacol* 1994;37:221–5.

36. Klotz U, Reimann I. Delayed clearance of diazepam due to cimetidine. *N Engl J Med* 1980;302:1012–4.

37. Patwardhan RV et al. Cimetidine spares the glucuronidation of lorazepam and oxazepam. *Gastroenterology* 1980;79:912–6.

38. MacLeod SM et al. Interaction of disulfiram with benzodiazepines. *Clin Pharmacol Ther* 1978;24:583–9.

39. Sellers EM et al. Differential effects on benzodiazepine disposition by disulfiram and ethanol. *Arzneimittelforschung* 1980;30:882–6.

40. Olkkola KT et al. Midazolam should be avoided in patients receiving the systemic antimycotics ketoconazole or itraconazole. *Clin Pharmacol Ther* 1994;55:481–5.

41. Lasher TA et al. Pharmacokinetic pharmacodynamic evaluation of the combined administration of alprazolam and fluoxetine. *Psychopharmacology* 1991;104:323–7.

42. Greenblatt DJ et al. Fluoxetine impairs clearance of alprazolam but not of clonazepam. *Clin Pharmacol Ther* 1992;52:479–86.

43. Lemberger L et al. The effect of fluoxetine on the pharmacokinetics and psychomotor responses of diazepam. *Clin Pharmacol Ther* 1988;43:412–9.

44. Fleishaker JC, Hulst LK. A pharmacokinetic and pharmacodynamic evaluation of the combined administration of alprazolam and fluvoxamine. *Eur J Clin Pharmacol* 1994;46:35-91991;11:85–7.

45. Bonfiglio MF, Dasta JF. Clinical significance of the benzodiazepine-theophylline interaction. *Pharmacotherapy* 1991;11:85–87.

46. Feely J et al. Reduction of liver blood flow and propranolol metabolism by cimetidine. *N Engl J Med* 1981;304:692–5.

47. Hansten PD, Horn JR. Carbamazepine (Tegretol) interactions. *Drug Interact Newsl* 1986;6:U-13.

48. Amabeoku GJ et al. Pharmacokinetic interaction of single doses of quinine and carbamazepine, phenobarbitone and phenytoin in healthy volunteers. *East Afr Med J* 1993;70:90–3.

49. Hansten PD, Horn JR. Enzyme inducers and theophylline. *Drug Interact Newsl* 1985;5:41–3.

50. Finielz P et al. Interaction between cyclosporin and chloroquine. *Nephron* 1993;65:333. Letter.

51. Nampoory MRN et al. Drug interaction of chloroquine with cyclosporin. *Nephron* 1992;62:108-9. Letter.

52. Neuvonen PJ et al. Effects of resins and activated charcoal on the absorption of digoxin, carbamazepine and frusemide. *Br J Clin Pharmacol* 1988;25:229–33.

53. Ertmann R, Landbeck G. Effect of oral cholestyramine on the elimination of high-dose methotrexate. *J Cancer Res Clin Oncol* 1985;110:48–50.

54. Szymanski S et al. A case report of cimetidine-induced clozapine toxicity. *J Clin Psychiatry* 1991;52:21–2.

55. Hansten PD, Horn JR. Phenytoin interaction. *Drug Interact Newsl* 1985;5:U-1.

56. deVries TM et al. Effect of cimetidine and low-dose quinidine on tacrine pharmacokinetics in humans. *Pharm Res* 1993;10:S337. Abstract.

57. Jackson JE et al. Cimetidine-theophylline interaction. *Pharmacologist* 1980;22:231. Abstract.

58. Ahmad SR, Wolfe SM. Cisapride and torsades de pointes. *Lancet* 1995;345:508.

59. Honig P et al. Effect of erythromycin, clarithromycin and azithromycin on the pharmacokinetics of terfenadine. *Clin Pharmacol Ther* 1993;53:161. Abstract.

60. Hiemke C et al. Elevated levels of clozapine in serum after addition of fluvoxamine. *J Clin Psychopharmacol* 1994;14:279–81. Letter.

61. van Dijke CPH, Weber JCP. Interaction between oral contraceptives and griseofulvin. *Br Med J* 1984;288:1125–6.

62. Freeman DJ et al. The effect of erythromycin on the pharmacokinetics of cyclosporine. *Clin Pharmacol Ther* 1986;39:193. Abstract.

63. Kohan DE. Possible interaction between cyclosporine and erythromycin. *N Engl J Med* 1986;314:448. Letter.

64. Yee GC, McGuire TR. Pharmacokinetic drug interactions with cyclosporin (part I). *Clin Pharmacokinet* 1990;19:319–32.

65. Horton CM et al. Cyclosporine interactions with miconazole and other azole-antimycotics: a case report and review of the literature. *J Heart Lung Transplant* 1992;11:1127–32.

66. Hansten PD, Horn JR. Phenytoin interactions. *Drug Interact Newsl* 1985;5:U-3.

67. Hansten PD, Horn JR. Rifampin interactions. *Drug Interact Newsl* 1985;5:U-8.

68. Ringden O et al. Nephrotoxicity by co-trimoxazole and cyclosporine in transplanted patients. *Lancet* 1984;1:1016–7.

69. Jones DK et al. Serious interaction between cyclosporin A and sulphadimidine. *Br Med J* 1986;292:728–9.

70. Moezzi B et al. The effect of penicillamine on serum digoxin levels. *Jpn Heart J* 1978;19:366–70.

71. Hansten PD. Quinidine and digoxin. *Drug Interact Newsl* 1981;1:13–5.

72. Carruthers SG, Dujovne CA. Cholestyramine and spironolactone and their combination in digitoxin elimination. *Clin Pharmacol Ther* 1980;27:184–7.

73. Loi C-M et al. Dose-dependent inhibition of theophylline metabolism by disulfiram in recovering alcoholics. *Clin Pharmacol Ther* 1989;45:476–86.

74. Hansten PD, Horn JR. Diuretics and nonsteroidal anti-inflammatory drugs. *Drug Interact Newsl* 1986;6:27–9.

75. Watkins J et al. Attenuation of hypotensive effect of propranolol and thiazide diuretics by indomethacin. *Br Med J* 1980;281:702–5.

76. Bivins BA et al. Dopamine-phenytoin interaction. *Arch Surg* 1978;113:245–9.

77. Shaeffer MS et al. Interaction between FK506 and erythromycin. *Ann Pharmacother* 1994;28:280–1. Letter.

78. Honig PK et al. Changes in the pharmacokinetics and electrocardiographic pharmacodynamics of terfenadine with concomitant administration of erythromycin. *Clin Pharmacol Ther* 1992;52:231–8.

79. Honig PK et al. Comparison of the effect of the macrolide antibiotics erythromycin, clarithromycin and azithromycin on terfenadine steady-state pharmacokinetics and electrocardiographic parameters. *Drug Invest* 1994;7:148–56.

80. Hansten PD. Erythromycin and theophylline. *Drug Interact Newsl* 1981;1:5–6.

81. Cinquegrani MP, Liang CS. Indomethacin attenuates the hypotensive action of hydralazine. *Clin Pharmacol Ther* 1986;39:564–70.

82. Crane JK, Shih HT. Syncope and cardiac arrhythmia due to an interaction between itraconazole and terfenadine. *Am J Med* 1993;95:445–6.

83. Pohjola-Sintonen S et al. Itraconazole prevents terfenadine metabolism and increases risk of torsades de pointes ventricular tachycardia. *Eur J Clin Pharmacol* 1993;45:191–3.

84. Eller MG et al. Pharmacokinetic interaction between terfenadine and ketoconazole. *Clin Pharmacol Ther* 1991;49:130. Abstract.

85. Honig PK et al. Terfenadine-ketoconazole interaction. Pharmacokinetic and electrocardiographic consequences. *JAMA* 1993;269:1513–8.

86. Lavrijsen K et al. The interaction of ketoconazole, itraconazole and erythromycin with the in vitro metabolism of antihistamines in human liver microsomes. *Allergy* 1993;48(suppl):34.

87. Hansten PD. Lithium and methyldopa. *Drug Interact Newsl* 1981;1:11.

88. Ragheb MA, Powell AL. Failure of sulindac to increase serum lithium levels. *J Clin Psychiatry* 1986;47:33–4.

89. Frolich JC et al. Indomethacin increases plasma lithium. *Br Med J* 1979;1:1115–6.

90. Furnell MM, Davies J. The effect of sulindac on lithium therapy. *Drug Intell Clin Pharm* 1985;19:374–6.

91. MacCallum WAG. Interaction of lithium and phenytoin. *Br Med J* 1980;280:610–1.

92. Cook BL et al. Theophylline-lithium interaction. *J Clin Psychiatry* 1985;46:278–9.

93. Sieries FS, Ossowski MG. Concurrent use of theophylline and lithium in a patient with chronic obstructive lung disease and bipolar disorder. *Am J Psychiatry* 1982;139:117–8.

94. Thyss A et al. Clinical and pharmacokinetic evidence of a life-threatening interaction between methotrexate and ketoprofen. *Lancet* 1986;1:256–8.

95. Ellison NM, Servi RJ. Acute renal failure and death following sequential intermediate-dose methotrexate and 5-FU. A possible adverse effect due to concomitant indomethacin administration. *Cancer Treat Rep* 1985;69:342–3.

96. Reid T et al. Impact of omeprazole on the plasma clearance of methotrexate. *Cancer Chemother Pharmacol* 1993;33:82–4.

97. Hansten PD, Horn JR. Mexiletine (Mexitil) interactions. *Drug Interact Newsl* 1985;5:U-9.

98. Pentikainen PJ et al. Effect of rifampicin treatment on the kinetics of mexiletine. *Eur J Clin Pharmacol* 1982;23:261–6.

99. Hansten PD, Horn JR. Indomethacin and triamterene. *Drug Interact Newsl* 1985;5:43.

100. Gugler R, Jensen JC. Omeprazole inhibits oxidative drug metabolism. Studies with diazepam and phenytoin in vivo and 7-ethoxycoumarin in vitro. *Gastroenterology* 1985;89:1235–41.

101. Prichard PJ et al. Oral phenytoin pharmacokinetics during omeprazole therapy. *Br J Clin Pharmacol* 1987;24:543–5.

102. Kay L et al. Influence of rifampicin and isoniazid on the kinetics of phenytoin. *Br J Clin Pharmacol* 1985;20:323–6.

103. Wagner JC, Slama TG. Rifampin-phenytoin drug interaction. *Drug Intell Clin Pharm* 1984;18:497. Abstract.

104. Nightingale SL. Fluoxetine labeling revised to identify phenytoin interaction and to recommend against use in nursing mothers. *JAMA* 1994;271:1067.

105. Bruni J et al. Valproic acid and plasma levels of phenytoin. *Neurology* 1979;29:904–5.

106. Monks A, Richens A. Effect of single doses of sodium valproate on serum phenytoin levels and protein binding in epileptic patients. *Clin Pharmacol Ther* 1980;27:89–95.

107. Twum-Barima Y, Carruthers SG. Evaluation of rifampin-quinidine interaction. *Clin Pharmacol Ther* 1980;27:290. Abstract.

108. Sahai J et al. Cations in the didanosine tablet reduce ciprofloxacin bioavailability. *Clin Pharmacol Ther* 1993;53:292–7.

109. Lehto P, Kivisto KT. Effect of sucralfate on absorption of norfloxacin and ofloxacin. *Antimicrob Agents Chemother* 1994;38:248–51.

110. Karki SD et al. Seizure with ciprofloxacin and theophylline combined therapy. *DICP* 1990;24:595–6.

111. Parent M, LeBel M. Meta-analysis of quinolone-theophylline interactions. *DICP* 1991;25:191–4.

112. Hansten PD, Horn JR. Rifampin interactions. *Drug Interact Newsl* 1985;5:U-1.

113. Burger DM et al. Pharmacokinetic interaction between rifampin and zidovudine. *Antimicrob Agents Chemother* 1993;37:1426–31.

114. Anderson CJ et al. Toxicity of combined therapy with carbonic anhydrase inhibitors and aspirin. *Am J Ophthalmol* 1978;86:516–9.

115. Sperber AD. Toxic interaction between fluvoxamine and sustained release theophylline in an 11-year-old boy. *Drug Saf* 1991;6:460–2.

116. Rasmussen BB et al. Selective serotonin reuptake inhibitors and theophylline metabolism in human liver microsomes: potent inhibition by fluvoxamine. *Br J Clin Pharmacol* 1995;39:151–9.

117. deVries TM et al. Effect of multiple-dose tacrine administration on single-dose pharmacokinetics of digoxin, diazepam, and theophylline. *Pharm Res* 1993;10:S333. Abstract.

118. Fournier P et al. Une nouvelle cause de torsades de pointes: association terfenadine et troleandomycine. *Ann Cardiol Angeiol (Paris)* 1993;42:249–52.

119. Renton KW et al. Decreased elimination of theophylline after influenza vaccination. *Can Med Assoc J* 1980;123:288–90.

120. Hansten PD, Horn JR. Theophylline interactions. *Drug Interact Newsl* 1986;6:U-4.

Drug-Laboratory Test Interferences: Blood, Serum, Plasma Chemistry; Urine Tests; Hematology

David G. Dunlop

The following table lists common clinical laboratory tests and drugs that may interfere with those tests. Drugs may interfere with laboratory tests through a pharmacologic or toxic effect, or through actual chemical interference with the testing process. Either effect may lead to an altered value of the laboratory test, resulting in an inappropriate diagnosis or treatment. It is essential that the clinician recognize possible drug–laboratory test interferences and use this information in the overall assessment of a patient's clinical status.

For the purposes of this section, a pharmacologic or toxic effect refers to change in a laboratory test that occurs because of the action of the drug in vivo. The alteration in laboratory value is often expected and reflects a true measure of what is taking place in the body. With a change of this type, the test is interpreted as being accurate even if it falls outside the normal range. Examples are hyperglycemia following corticosteroid administration or electrolyte disturbances after diuretic use. An illustration of a toxic effect is elevated transaminase levels subsequent to an acetaminophen overdose.

An analytical interference differs from a pharmacologic effect, in that the true laboratory value is not measured accurately. The result is inaccurate because of a problem with in vitro laboratory test procedures. The chemical and physical characteristics of a drug may account for the interference. Examples of an analytical interference include cefoxitin mimicking creatinine in a colorimetric assay or fluoride being misread as chloride due to chemical similarities.

This table lists drug interferences with the most common laboratory tests. For detailed information on laboratory tests not covered here, refer to references 1–3 at the end of this section. A drug may interfere with various laboratory tests by different mechanisms. Also, a drug may cause more than one type of interference (eg, a physiologic increase and an analytical decrease). New laboratory procedures and improved assays are being developed at a rapid pace and this information is constantly changing. Therefore, it may be necessary to compare the original citation against the procedures carried out at your laboratory. Refer to the references cited in the table, as well as other relevant sources, to obtain further information about a specific test.

The following abbreviations are used in the table:

(B)	– Blood
(CSF)	– Cerebrospinal Fluid
(S)	– Serum
(I)	– Analytical Interference of Drug
(P)	– Pharmacologic/Toxic Effect of Drug

DRUG–LABORATORY TEST INTERFERENCES

TEST	DRUGS THAT MAY AFFECT RESULTS AND CAUSE OF INTERFERENCE

BLOOD, SERUM, PLASMA CHEMISTRY

Alkaline Phosphatase (S)

Elevated by albumin (I), anticonvulsants (P), hepatotoxins (P), ticlopidine (P).[1,3,4]

Decreased by citrate salts (I), diphosphonates (eg, etidronate) (P), EDTA (I), estrogens (P), fluoride salts (I), vitamin D (P), zinc salts (I).[1,3]

Aminotransferases (ALT [SGPT]/AST [SGOT]) (S)

Elevated by acarbose (P), acetaminophen (I,P), ascorbic acid (I), cholinergic drugs (P), danazol (P), dexrazoxane (P), erythromycin (I,P), hepatotoxins (P), HMG-CoA reductase inhibitors (P), IM injections (P), isotretinoin (P), methyldopa (I), narcotics (P), parenteral nutrition (P), salicylate (P), tacrine (P), ticlopidine (P).[1–5]

Decreased by interferon alfa (P), interferon beta (P), naltrexone (P).[1]

Ammonia (B)

Elevated by acetazolamide (P), alcohol (P), ammonium chloride (P), asparaginase (P), barbiturates (P), carbamazepine (P), diuretics (loop, thiazide) (P), divalproex (P), isoniazid (P), parenteral nutrition (P), valproic acid (P).[1,3,6]

Decreased by cefotaxime (I), kanamycin (oral) (P), lactulose (P), neomycin (oral) (P), potassium salts (P), tetracyclines (P).[1,2,4]

Amylase (S)

Elevated by asparaginase (P), chloride salts (I), cholinergic drugs (P), contraceptives (oral, combination) (P), dexrazoxane (P), fluoride salts (I), narcotics (P), pancreatotoxins (P), potassium iodide (P).[1,3,6]

Decreased by somatostatin (P).[1]

Bilirubin, Total (S)

Elevated by ascorbic acid (I), dexrazoxane (P), dextran (I), epinephrine (I), hemolytic agents (P), hepatotoxins (P), isoproterenol (I), levodopa (I), methyldopa (I,P), narcotics (I), nitrofurantoin (I,P), phenazopyridine (diazo reaction) (I), phenelzine (I), propranolol (I), rifampin (I,P), sulfonamides (I), theophylline (I).[1–3,6]

Decreased by barbiturates (especially in newborns) (P), corticosteroids (P), phenazopyridine (colorimetric) (I), pindolol (P), sulfonamides (P).[3,4]

Calcium (S)

Elevated by anabolic steroids (P), androgens (P), calcium salts (P), cefotaxime (I), chlorpropamide (I), contraceptives (oral, combination) (P), diuretics (thiazide) (P), estrogens (P), ferrous salts (I), hydralazine (I), interferons (I), lithium salts (P), magnesium salts (I), progestins (P), tamoxifen (P), thyroid (P), vitamin A (P), vitamin D (P).[1–4,6]

Decreased by acetazolamide (P), albuterol (P), alcohol (P), aldesleukin (P), amifostine (P), asparaginase (P), aspirin (P), calcitonin (P), carbamazepine (P), cisplatin (P), corticosteroids (P), diphosphonates (eg, etidronate) (P), diuretics (loop) (P), EDTA (I), fluoride salts (I,P), foscarnet (P), heparin (I), laxatives (P), magnesium salts (P), phenobarbital (P), phenytoin (P), phosphate salts (P), plicamycin (P), saquinavir (P), sulfisoxazole (I), zalcitabine (P).[1–4,6]

Carbon Dioxide (B)

Elevated by bicarbonate salts (P), diuretics (loop, thiazide) (P), respiratory depressants (P).[1,3]

Decreased by aldesleukin (P), aspirin overdose (P), nephrotoxins (P), theophylline (P).[1,3]

Chloride (S)

Elevated by androgens (P), carbamazepine (P), cefotaxime (I), cholestyramine (P), corticosteroids (by salt retention) (P), cyclosporine (P), diuretics (carbonic

(continued)

TEST	DRUGS THAT MAY AFFECT RESULTS AND CAUSE OF INTERFERENCE

BLOOD, SERUM, PLASMA CHEMISTRY

anhydrase inhibitor, thiazide—chronically by alkalosis) (P), estrogens (P), guanethidine (P), halides (eg, fluoride salts) (I), lithium salts (P), methyldopa (P), NSAIDs (P), propantheline (I), pyridostigmine (I).[1,3]

Decreased by bicarbonate salts (P), cefotaxime (metabolite) (P), chlorpropamide (P), corticosteroids (by alkalosis) (P), diuretics (loop, thiazide—by acute diuresis) (P), fludrocortisone (by alkalosis) (P), laxatives (long-term use) (P).[1,3]

Cholesterol (S)
[Does not include antilipemics]. *Elevated* by alcohol (P), anabolic steroids (by cholestasis) (P), ascorbic acid (I), aspirin (I), β-adrenergic blockers (P), cefotaxime (I), contraceptives (oral, combination) (P), corticosteroids (I,P), cyclosporine (P), diuretics (thiazide) (P), hepatotoxins (cholestatic effect) (P), isotretinoin (I), mycophenolate (P), phenothiazines (I,P), smoking (P), ticlopidine (I), vitamin A (I), vitamin D (I).[1–4,6]

Decreased by aldesleukin (P), anabolic steroids (by inhibiting synthesis) (P), ascorbic acid (I,P), chlorpropamide (P), estrogens (P), haloperidol (P), heparin (I), hepatotoxins (decreased synthesis) (P), kanamycin (oral) (P), metformin (P), metronidazole (P), neomycin (oral) (P), niacin (P), nitrates (I), penicillamine (I).[1–4,6]

Coombs' [Direct]
Positive by cephalosporins (P), chlorpromazine (P), chlorpropamide (P), ethosuximide (P), hemolytic agents (P), hydralazine (P), indomethacin (P), isoniazid (P), levodopa (P), mefenamic acid (P), methyldopa (P), penicillins (P), rifampin (P), quinidine (P), quinine (P), sulfonamides (P), tetracyclines (P).[1,3–5]

Creatine Kinase (S)
Elevated by alcohol (chronic) (P), aminocaproic acid (P), cefotaxime (I), clofibrate (P), danazol (P), gemfibrozil (P), HMG-CoA reductase inhibitors (P), IM injections (P), niacin (P), probucol (P), succimer (I).[1,2,4]

Creatinine (S)
Elevated by acetohexamide (I), aldesleukin (P), ascorbic acid (I), cephalosporins (Jaffe method) (I,P), cimetidine (P), cyclosporine (P), flucytosine (I), furosemide (I), lactulose (I), levodopa (I), lidocaine (I), lithium salts (P), methyldopa (I), nephrotoxins (P), nitrofurantoin (I), penicillin (I), pentamidine (P), salicylates (P), trimethoprim/sulfamethoxazole (P).[1–4,7]

Glucose (S)
Elevated by acetaminophen (SMA 12/60 method) (I), albuterol (P), antidepressants (heterocyclic) (P), ascorbic acid (neocuproin method) (I), asparaginase (P), β-adrenergic blockers (type I diabetes) (P), cefotaxime (I), clonidine (P), corticosteroids (P), cyclosporine (P), dextran (I), dextrothyroxine (P), diazoxide (P), diuretics (loop, thiazide) (P), epinephrine (I,P), estrogens (P), glucagon (P), isoniazid (P), levodopa (SMA 12/60 method) (I), lithium salts (P), methyldopa (I), metronidazole (I), mycophenolate (P), niacin (I,P), pentamidine (IV) (P), phenothiazines (P), phenytoin (P), progestins (P), salicylates (acute toxicity) (I,P), somatostatin (P), tacrolimus (P), thiabendazole (P), thyroid (P), zalcitabine (P).[1–4,6]

Decreased by acetaminophen (GOD-Perid method) (I,P), alcohol (P), anabolic steroids (P), ascorbic acid (GOD-Perid method) (I), β-adrenergic blockers (in type II diabetes) (P), clofibrate (P), disopyramide (P), gemfibrozil (P), isoniazid (I), levodopa (glucose oxidase) (I), MAOIs (P), metformin (P), pentamidine (IV) (P), salicylates (acute and long-term toxicity) (P), sulfonamides (P).[1–3,5]

(*continued*)

TEST	DRUGS THAT MAY AFFECT RESULTS AND CAUSE OF INTERFERENCE

BLOOD, SERUM, PLASMA CHEMISTRY

Iron (S)
Elevated by cefotaxime (I), chloramphenicol (P), cisplatin (P), citrate salts (I), contraceptives (oral, combination) (P), dexrazoxane (P), estrogens (P), ferrous salts (I), iron dextran (I,P), methyldopa (P), rifampin (I).[1,3,6]
Decreased by acarbose (P), cholestyramine (P), colchicine (P), deferoxamine (I), heparin (I).[1,3,6]

Iron-Binding Capacity, Total (S)
Elevated by estrogen (P).[1,3,6]
Decreased by chloramphenicol (P), corticotropin (P).[1,3,6]

Magnesium (S)
Elevated by amiloride (P), calcium salts (I), cefotaxime (I), lithium salts (P), magnesium salts (P).[1,3–5]
Decreased by albuterol (P), alcohol (P), aldesleukin (P), amifostine (P), amino-glycosides (P), amphotericin B (P), calcium salts (I), cefotaxime (I), cisplatin (P), cyclosporine (P), digitalis glycosides (toxic concentrations) (P), diphosphonates (eg, etidronate) (P), diuretics (loop, thiazide) (P), foscarnet (P), insulin (P), phosphate salts (I), tacrolimus (P).[1,3–5]

Osmolality (S)
Elevated by alcohol (ADH suppression) (P), corticosteroids (P), demeclocycline (ADH inhibition) (P), glucose (I), lithium salts (ADH inhibition) (P), mannitol (I,P).[1,4]
Decreased by carbamazepine (P), chlorpropamide (P), vasopressin (P).[1,4]

Phosphorus, Inorganic (S)
Elevated by foscarnet (P), vitamin D (excessive) (P).[1,4]
Decreased by aldesleukin (P), anabolic steroids (P), androgens (P), antacids (phosphate binders) (P), anticonvulsants (P), diphosphonates (eg, etidronate) (P), foscarnet (P), lithium salts (P), mycophenolate (P), parenteral nutrition (P), sucralfate (P).[1,4–6]

Potassium (S)
Elevated by aminocaproic acid (P), ACE inhibitors (P), antineoplastics (cytotoxic effect) (P), β-adrenergic blockers (P), cyclosporine (P), diuretics (potassium-sparing) (P), iodine salts (I), isoniazid (P), lithium salts (P), mannitol (P), my-cophenolate (P), nephrotoxins (P), NSAIDs (especially indomethacin) (P), pentamidine (P), potassium penicillin (P), propranolol (P), salt substitutes (P), succinylcholine (P), tacrolimus (P).[1–6]
Decreased by acetazolamide (P), aminoglycosides (P), ammonium chloride (P), amphotericin B (P), bicarbonate salts (P), β-adrenergic agonists (P), corticosteroids (P), diphosphonates (eg, etidronate) (P), diuretics (loop, thiazide) (P), fludrocortisone (P), foscarnet (P), glucose (P), insulin (P), laxatives (P), mycophenolate (P), ondansetron (P), penicillins (extended-spectrum) (P), salicylates (P), saquinavir (P).[1–6]

Protein, Total (S)
Elevated by anabolic steroids (P), corticosteroids (P), heparin (I), phenazopyridine (I).[1–3]
Decreased by estrogens (P), hepatotoxins (P).[1–3]

Protein, Total (CSF)
Elevated by methotrexate (I), penicillins (I), phenothiazines (I), sulfonamides (I), tetracyclines (I).[1–3]
Decreased by cytarabine (P).[1–3]

Sodium (S)
Elevated by anabolic steroids (P), carbamazepine (P), clonidine (P), contraceptives (oral, combination) (P), corticosteroids (P), diazoxide (P), estrogens (P), fludrocortisone (P), methyldopa (P), NSAIDs (P), tetracycline (P).[1,3,6]

(continued)

TEST	DRUGS THAT MAY AFFECT RESULTS AND CAUSE OF INTERFERENCE

BLOOD, SERUM, PLASMA CHEMISTRY

Thyroxine (S)

Decreased by ammonium chloride (P), amphotericin B (P), carbamazepine (P), chlorpropamide (P), diuretics (P), interferons (P), lithium salts (P), sulfonylureas (P), vasopressin and analogues (P), vincristine (P).[1,3,4,6]

Elevated by amiodarone (P), clofibrate (P), contraceptives (oral, combination) (P), estrogens (P), heparin (I), insulin (P), levodopa (P), propranolol (P), radiographic agents (I,P), tamoxifen (P).[1-6]

Decreased by anabolic steroids (P), androgens (P), asparaginase (P), carbamazepine (P), cholestyramine (P), clofibrate (P), corticosteroids (P), danazol (I), heparin (I), iodide (P), lithium salts (P), phenytoin (P), salicylates (P), sulfonamides (P), sulfonylureas (P).[1-4,6]

Triglycerides (S)

Elevated by alcohol (P), β-adrenergic blockers (P), cholestyramine (P), colestipol (P), contraceptives (oral, combination) (P), dexrazoxane (P), diuretics (loop, thiazide) (P), estrogens (P), isotretinoin (P).[2-4,6]

Decreased by ascorbic acid (I,P), asparaginase (P), clofibrate (P), danazol (P), gemfibrozil (P), metformin (P), niacin (P), sulfonylureas (P).[1-4]

Urea Nitrogen (S)

Elevated by acetohexamide (I), aldesleukin (P), anabolic steroids (P), chloral hydrate (I), chloramphenicol (Nesslerization method) (I), dextran (I), diuretics (loop, thiazide) (P), nephrotoxins (P), pentamidine (P), sulfonamides (I), tetracyclines (P).[1,3,4,6]

Decreased by ascorbic acid (I), chloramphenicol (Berthelot method) (I), fluoride salts (I), streptomycin (I).[1,3,4,6]

Uric Acid (S)

Elevated by acetaminophen (I), acetazolamide (P), anabolic steroids (P), androgens (P), antineoplastics (P), ascorbic acid (I), caffeine (Bittner method) (I), cyclosporine (P), diazoxide (P), diuretics (carbonic anhydrase inhibitor, loop, thiazide) (P), epinephrine (I), ethambutol (I), hydralazine (I), isoniazid (I), levodopa (I,P), methyldopa (I), niacin (P), phenytoin (P), propranolol (P), pyrazinamide (P), rifampin (I), salicylates (low doses) (I,P), spironolactone (P), tacrolimus (P), theophylline (I,P).[2-4,6]

Decreased by acetohexamide (P), allopurinol (P), ascorbic acid (by seralyzer) (I), clofibrate (P), contrast media (iodinated) (P), corticosteroids (P), diflunisal (P), glucose infusions (P), guaifenesin (I), indomethacin (P), levodopa (I), lithium salts (P), methyldopa (I), phenothiazines (P), probenecid (P), salicylates (large doses) (P), sulfinpyrazone (P).[2-4,6]

URINE TESTS

Bilirubin

Elevated by hepatotoxins (P), mefenamic acid (I), phenazopyridine (I), phenothiazines (I,P).[1,6]

Catecholamines

Elevated by acetaminophen (I), alcohol (P), α_1-adrenergic blockers (P), aspirin (I), caffeine (P), chloral hydrate (I), chlorpromazine (I), epinephrine (I), erythromycin (I), hydralazine (I), insulin (P), labetalol (I), levodopa (I), methenamine (I), methyldopa (I), niacin (I), nitroglycerin (P), quinidine (I), reserpine (P), tetracyclines (I,P).[1,2,4,6]

Decreased by α_2-adrenergic blockers (P), bromocriptine (P), clonidine (P), contrast media (iodinated) (I), disulfiram (P), guanethidine (P), methenamine (destroys catecholamines in bladder urine) (P), reserpine (P).[1,2,4]

(continued)

TEST	DRUGS THAT MAY AFFECT RESULTS AND CAUSE OF INTERFERENCE
URINE TESTS	
Creatinine	*Elevated* by ascorbic acid (I), cephalosporins (except cefotaxime, ceftazidime; Jaffe method) (I), corticosteroids (P), levodopa (I), methyldopa (I), nephrotoxins (P), nitrofurantoin (I).[1,4,6]
	Decreased by anabolic steroids (P), androgens (P), cimetidine (P), diuretics (thiazide) (P).[1,4,6]
Glucose	*False positive* by aminosalicylic acid (copper reduction) (I), ascorbic acid (copper reduction) (I), aspirin (copper reduction) (I,P), cephalosporins (except cefotaxime; copper reduction) (I), chloral hydrate (copper reduction) (I), corticosteroids (P), diuretics (loop, thiazide) (P), ifosfamide (P), levodopa (copper reduction) (I), niacin (P), penicillins (P), phenazopyridine (Tes-Tape) (I), phenothiazines (P).[1–6]
	False negative by ascorbic acid (glucose oxidase) (I), bisacodyl (I), chloral hydrate (glucose oxidase) (I), diazepam (I), digoxin (I), ferrous salts (I), levodopa (glucose oxidase) (I), phenazopyridine (glucose oxidase) (I), tetracyclines (I).[1–6]
Gonadotropins (Pregnancy Test)	*False positive* by phenothiazines (I).[1,6]
Ketones	*Elevated* by albuterol (P), ifosfamide (I), isoniazid (P), levodopa (Labstix) (I), mesna (I), phenazopyridine (I), phenothiazines (I), salicylates (I), succimer (I).[1,2,4,6]
Protein	*Elevated* by acetazolamide (I), bicarbonate salts (I), captopril (I), cephalosporins (I), chlorpromazine (I), contrast media (iodinated) (I), diuretics (carbonic anhydrase inhibitor) (I or P), ifosfamide (P), nephrotoxins (P), phenazopyridine (I), salicylates (I), sulfonamides (I), tolbutamide (I).[1,6]
Specific Gravity	*Elevated* by contrast media (iodinated) (P), dextran (P), sucrose (P).[1,4,6]
	Decreased by lithium salts. (P).[1]
HEMATOLOGY	
Erythrocyte Sedimentation Rate (B)	*Elevated* by dextran (P), methyldopa (P), methysergide (P), penicillamine (P), theophylline (P), vitamin A (P).[1,6]
	Decreased by corticosteroids (P), gold salts (P), penicillamine (P), quinine (P), salicylates (P), drugs that cause hyperglycemia (P).[1,6]
Prothrombin Time (B)	[Does not include anticoagulants or drugs that potentiate or antagonize them]. *Elevated* by antibiotics (gut sterilizing) (P), aspirin (P), cephalosporins (P), chloral hydrate (P), chloramphenicol (P), cholestyramine (P), colestipol (P), cyclophosphamide (P), dexrazoxane (P), hepatotoxins (P), laxatives (P), mercaptopurine (P), propylthiouracil (P), quinidine (P), quinine (P), sulfonamides (P).[1,4,6]
	Decreased by anabolic steroids (P), azathioprine (P), contraceptives (oral, combination) (P), estrogens (P), vitamin K (P).[1,3,6]

◼ REFERENCES

1. Young DS. *Effects of drugs on clinical laboratory tests,* 3rd ed. Washington, DC: AACC Press; 1990, and Supplement, 1991.
2. Salway JG ed. *Drug-test interaction handbook,* 1st ed. New York: Raven Press; 1990.
3. Sher PP. *Drug interferences with clinical laboratory tests.* Drugs 1982;24:24–63.
4. McEvoy GK, ed. *AHFS drug information 96.* Bethesda, MD: American Society of Health-System Pharmacists; 1996.
5. Dukes MNG, ed. *Meyler's side effects of drugs,* 12th ed. Amsterdam: Elsevier; 1992.
6. Wallach J. *Interpretation of diagnostic tests: a synopsis of laboratory medicine,* 5th ed. Boston: Little, Brown; 1992.
7. Ducharme MP et al. Drug-induced alterations in serum creatinine concentrations. *Ann Pharmacother* 1993;27:622–33.

Drug-Induced Discoloration of Feces and Urine

The drugs and drug classes in the following tables have been associated with the discoloration of feces or urine. Drugs and drug classes are listed generically.

DRUGS THAT MAY DISCOLOR FECES	
DRUG/DRUG CLASS	COLOR PRODUCED
Antacids, Aluminum Hydroxide Types	Whitish or speckling
Anthraquinones	Brownish staining of rectal mucosa
Antibiotics, Oral	Greenish gray
Anticoagulants	Pink to red or black*
Bismuth Salts	Greenish black
Charcoal	Black
Clofazimine	Red to brownish black
Ferrous Salts	Black
Heparin	Pink to red or black*
Indocyanine Green	Green
Indomethacin	Green because of biliverdinemia
Nonsteroidal Antiinflammatory Drugs	Pink to red or black*
Omeprazole	Discoloration
Phenazopyridine	Orange-red
Pyrvinium Pamoate	Red
Rifampin	Red-orange
Risperidone	Discoloration
Salicylates (especially Aspirin)	Pink to red or black*

*These colors may indicate intestinal bleeding.

DRUGS THAT MAY DISCOLOR URINE

DRUG/DRUG CLASS	COLOR PRODUCED
Aminopyrine	Red
Aminosalicylic Acid	Discoloration; red in hypochlorite solution*
Amitriptyline	Blue-green
Anthraquinones	Yellow-brown in acid urine; yellow-pink-red in alkaline urine
Antipyrine	Red-brown
Azuresin	Blue or green
Chloroquine	Rust yellow to brown
Chlorzoxazone	Orange or purplish red
Cimetidine (injection)	Green[†]
Clofazimine	Red to brownish black
Daunorubicin	Red
Deferoxamine	Reddish
Doxorubicin	Red
Ethoxazene	Orange to orange-brown
Ferrous Salts	Black
Flutamide	Amber or yellow-green
Furazolidone	Brown
Idarubicin	Red
Indandiones	Orange-red in alkaline urine
Indomethacin	Green because of biliverdinemia
Iron Sorbitex	Brown-black
Levodopa	Red-brown; dark on standing in hypochlorite solution*
Loratadine	Discoloration
Methocarbamol	Dark to brown, black or green on standing
Methyldopa	Dark on standing in hypochlorite solution*
Methylene Blue	Blue or green
Metronidazole	Dark, brown
Mitoxantrone	Blue-green
Niacin	Dark
Nitrofurantoin	Rust yellow to brown
Pamaquine	Rust yellow to brown
Phenacetin	Dark brown to black on standing
Phenazopyridine	Orange to red
Phenolphthalein	Pink to purplish red in alkaline urine
Phenothiazines	Pink to red or red-brown
Phensuximide	Pink to red or red-brown
Phenytoin	Pink to red or red-brown
Primaquine	Rust yellow to brown

(continued)

DRUG/DRUG CLASS	COLOR PRODUCED
Promethazine (injection)	Green[†]
Propofol (injection)	Green,[†] white
Quinacrine	Deep yellow in acidic urine
Quinine	Brown to black
Resorcinol	Dark green
Riboflavin	Yellow fluorescence
Rifabutin	Discoloration
Rifampin	Red-orange
Sulfasalazine	Orange-yellow in alkaline urine
Sulfonamides, Antibacterial	Rust yellow to brown
Sulindac	Discoloration
Tolonium	Blue-green
Triamterene	Pale blue fluorescence
Warfarin	Orange

[*]Hypochlorite solution in toilet bowl from prior use of chlorine bleach.
[†]Caused by phenol as a preservative in the injectable formulation.

■ REFERENCES

1. Anon. *Physicians' desk reference,* 49th ed. Montvale, NJ: Medical Economics Data Production; 1995.
2. Baran RB, Rowles B. Factors affecting coloration of urine and feces. *J Am Pharm Assoc* 1973;NS13:139–42.
3. Bodenham A et al. Propofol infusion and green urine. *Lancet* 1987;2:740. Letter.
4. Bowling P et al. Intravenous medications and green urine. *JAMA* 1981;246:216. Letter.
5. Devereaux MW, Mancall EL. Brown urine, bleach, and L-DOPA. *N Engl J Med* 1974;291:1142. Letter.
6. Michaels RM, ed. Discolored urine. *Physicians' Drug Alert* 1981;2(9):71.
7. Nates J et al. Appearance of white urine during propofol anesthesia. *Anesth Analg* 1995;81:204–13. Letter.
8. Raymond JR, Yarger WE. Abnormal urine color: differential diagnosis. *South Med J* 1988;81:837–41.
9. Wallach J. *Interpretation of diagnostic tests,* 5th ed. Boston: Little, Brown; 1992:737–8, 747.

Drug Use in Special Populations

Drugs and Pregnancy

Andrea J. Anderson

In the United States, fetal malformations occur in 3–6% of pregnancies. These include major and minor malformations from any cause, be it drug, infection, maternal disease state, genetic, or pollutant.[1,2] Drug use during pregnancy may be associated with risk to the developing fetus as well as to the pregnant woman. Drugs are probably responsible for only about 1–5% of fetal malformations; 60–70% of malformations have unknown causes.[2–4]

The genetic makeup of both the fetus and the mother influences the extent to which an agent may affect the developing fetus. For example, the rates of absorption, metabolism, and elimination of an agent by the mother, its rate of placental transfer, or the way it interacts with cells and tissues of the embryo are all genetically determined factors. Thus, human teratogenicity cannot be predicted based only on animal data or extrapolated from one pregnancy to another.

■ PHYSIOLOGIC AND DEVELOPMENTAL FACTORS

Teratogenic substances rarely cause a single defect. Most often, a spectrum of defects occurs that corresponds with the systems undergoing major development at the time of exposure. Major malformations are usually the result of first trimester exposure during critical periods of organogenesis. Exposures during the second and third trimesters may result in alterations or damage in fine structure and function. Intrauterine growth retardation (IUGR) is perhaps the most reliable indicator that a teratogen was present during the second and third trimesters of fetal development. Several organs and systems continue to develop after birth. Therefore, exposure to agents later in pregnancy carries some risk and may result in debilitating alterations in development such as mental retardation. Figure 3–1 depicts the stages of human structural development in relation to teratogenic potential.[5]

■ DRUG FACTORS

Most chemicals in the maternal bloodstream cross the placenta. Movement of compounds across the placenta is generally bidirectional, although the net transfer occurs from mother to fetus in most instances.[6,7] Although active and facilitated transport of some substances across the placenta have been demonstrated, the transplacental passage of most agents occurs primarily by simple diffusion.[6,8,9]

737

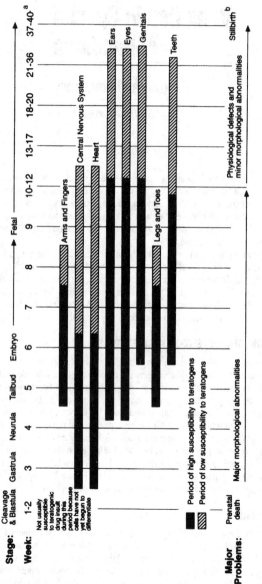

Figure 3–1. Variation in Teratogenic Susceptibility of Organ Systems during Stages of Human Intrauterine Development.

[a]Average time from fertilization to parturition is 38 weeks

[b]Drugs administered during this period may cause neonatal depression at birth (or other effects directly related to the pharmacological effect of the administered drug)

From Pagliaro LA, Pagliaro AM. Problems in pediatric drug therapy, 3rd ed. Hamilton, IL: Drug Intelligence Publications; 1995, reproduced with permission.

Only the unbound (free) fraction of a drug is subject to placental transfer; there-fore, the greater degree of protein binding exhibited by a drug, the less that is likely to be transferred to the fetus.[6,8,9] Early in pregnancy the placental membrane is relatively thick, and this characteristic tends to reduce permeability.[6] The thick-ness of the trophoblastic epithelium decreases and surface area increases in the last trimester. The passage of drugs is increased during this stage of pregnancy.[6,10]

The rate-limiting factors in placental transfer of drugs are the same as those that govern membrane diffusion by molecules in general. Thus, the rate of diffu-sion across the placental barrier is directly proportional to the maternal-fetal con-centration gradient and the surface area of the placenta.[6,8,9] Higher concentrations are generally attained in fetal serum and amniotic fluid after bolus than after con-tinuous infusion of drug into the mother, and by multiple-dose rather than sin-gle-dose therapy.[6] Certain physicochemical properties of drugs or chemicals favor transport to the fetus, including low molecular weight, lipid solubility, and non-ionization at pH 7.4.[7,9,10]

Each drug has a threshold above which fetal defects can occur and below which no effects are discernible. Whether an agent reaches a "threshold concen-tration" in the fetus depends on maternal factors (eg, rates of absorption and clear-ance) as well as the chemical nature of the agent.

Administration of drugs near term poses another potential threat to the fetus. Before birth, the fetus relies on maternal systems for drug elimination. After birth, the infant must rely on its own metabolic and excretory capabilities, which have not yet fully developed. Drugs given near term or during birth, especially those with long half-lives, may have an even more prolonged action in the neonate. Drugs that cause maternal addiction are also known to cause fetal addiction. Neonatal withdrawal symptoms may occur when mothers have been addicted to drugs during pregnancy or when they have taken addicting drugs near term, even though the mothers themselves are not addicted.

■ EFFECTS OF PREGNANCY ON THE MOTHER

Maternal physiology changes as pregnancy progresses and may have an effect on drug disposition and clearance. Maternal plasma volume increases by about 20% at midgestation and 50% at term,[9] and then falls toward prepregnancy levels post-partum. The apparent volume of distribution for many drugs increases as the fetal compartment enlarges, causing changes in maternal serum drug concentrations. Drugs with a narrow therapeutic range require careful monitoring during preg-nancy, and possibly dosage increases. As maternal plasma volume returns to nor-mal, dosages of many drugs require reduction. Changes in plasma protein concen-trations during pregnancy may affect the degree of binding and thus the amount of unbound drug.[8,9] Despite an increase in production of serum albumin, the in-creased intracellular and intravascular volumes cause the serum albumin concen-trations to decline.[11] A decrease in total plasma protein concentrations of about 10 g/L occurs during pregnancy.[8] Body fat increases by 3–4 kg during pregnancy and may act as a depot for fat-soluble drugs, thereby increasing their apparent volume of distribution (V_d).[9] Renal blood flow and glomerular filtration rate increase by almost 50% during pregnancy due to increased cardiac output. Renally excreted drugs may therefore have increased rates of clearance.[9]

■ INTERPRETATION OF STUDIES

There are few controlled, prospective studies of drug use in pregnancy. Most of the available information comes from case reports or case control studies. Cause-and-effect relationships between drugs and teratogenicity are difficult to establish retrospectively because of the numerous variables associated with each report. These include maternal drug dosage, time of ingestion relative to the date of conception, duration of therapy, concomitant exposures to other potential teratogens, and questionable study design or methodology. Because studies cannot disprove that a slight teratogenic risk may be associated with in utero exposure to drugs, drugs should be used during pregnancy only when absolutely necessary. The following table provides information concerning the effects of drugs used during pregnancy on the pregnant woman and on pregnancy outcome. For a more thorough discussion of the principles of teratology, the reader should consult reference 1.

The following abbreviation is used in the table:

- IUGR—intrauterine growth retardation, less than the tenth percentile (of an appropriate standard) birth weight for gestational age.[12]

DRUGS AND PREGNANCY

DRUG	NATURE OF EFFECT

ANALGESICS AND ANTIINFLAMMATORY DRUGS

Acetaminophen

Acetaminophen does not appear to be associated with congenital malformations. Acetaminophen is the analgesic-antipyretic of choice for use near term, because it does not affect platelet function or peripheral prostaglandin synthesis.[13,14] In maternal acetaminophen overdose, most infants are normal at birth,[15-18] but there have been a few cases of neonatal liver toxicity.[15,19] Acetaminophen may prevent fetal distress in laboring women with chorioamnionitis and fever.[20]

Narcotics

Narcotic analgesics are not associated with any fetal malformations, but narcotic abuse during pregnancy or use near term may lead to fetal addiction and neonatal withdrawal. Meconium may be present in the amniotic fluid, caused most likely by increased bowel activity during periods of fetal withdrawal and/or hypoxia, putting the fetus at risk for meconium aspiration.[21] See Heroin. Withdrawal symptoms, including irritability, increased muscle tone, sleep disturbances, vague autonomic nervous system symptoms, tremulousness, high-pitched crying, frantic and uncoordinated sucking, and seizures may occur in neonates born to narcotic-addicted women and nonaddicted women using narcotics near term. Neonatal respiratory depression may occur when narcotic analgesics are given during labor and is dependent on the drug, dose, interval, and route of administration (IV > IM).[22-25] There is conflicting information on the effects of narcotics on subsequent mental and motor development during the first year of life.[23,24]

Butorphanol[26] and, to a lesser degree, **meperidine**, when used during labor, frequently cause a sinusoidal fetal heart rate pattern. Meperidine crosses the placenta rapidly and is eliminated by the fetus at a rate much slower than that of the mother.[27] Furthermore, its metabolite, **normeperidine**, is very long-acting. Meperidine given during delivery interferes with the early establishment of breastfeeding because of infant sedation.[28] Epidural **alfentanil** does not provide good analgesia and is associated with neonatal hypotonus.[29] **Nalbuphine** is more rapidly transferred to the placenta and causes more abnormal Apgar scores (<7) at 1 min than meperidine.[30]

Infants born to narcotic-dependent women maintained on **methadone** during pregnancy may have smaller birth weights, lengths, and head circumferences than nonexposed infants, but they are usually not growth retarded.[22,23] A crossover study in seven women in a methadone maintenance program showed that divided doses of methadone stabilized the fetal activity pattern (which may indicate fetal withdrawal) before and after drug administration compared with single daily doses.[31] Women can be offered bid drug administration when single-dose treatment produces maternal withdrawal symptoms or abnormal fetal activity patterns. Prolonged thrombocytosis has been observed in infants born to women taking methadone alone or with other addictive drugs.[24] Anecdotal case reports of **pentazocine** use alone or with **tripelennamine** ("T's and Blues") throughout pregnancy have described infants who demonstrate withdrawal symptoms similar to those reported in offspring of heroin and methadone addicts.[24] Small-for-gestational-age infants, prematurity, and fetal distress have also been observed.[32] Maternal **propoxyphene** use may also lead to neonatal withdrawal symptoms.[24]

(continued)

DRUGS AND PREGNANCY (continued)

DRUG	NATURE OF EFFECT
Nonsteroidal Antiinflammatory Drugs	
	The early case reports that implicate **indomethacin** as etiologic in prenatal closure of the ductus arteriosus are inconclusive.[33–38] Indomethacin may cause oligohydramnios because of decreased fetal urine output, thereby placing the fetus at potential risk for pulmonary hypoplasia and umbilical cord compromise.[37–40] Two studies have shown transient decreases in amniotic fluid volumes with maternal indomethacin use,[37,40] but another demonstrated no change in volume even though fetal urine output decreased.[35] However, no effect on neonatal renal function was noted in one study.[39]
	First trimester use of **aspirin** did not increase the risk of congenital heart defects in relation to that of other structural malformations.[41] Repeated third trimester administration of aspirin 325 mg may result in prolonged constriction of the ductus arteriosus and pulmonary hypertension.[42] Maternal ingestion of aspirin 325 mg during the third trimester may interfere with uterine contractility and prolong gestation and labor.[42,43] Maternal and neonatal platelet function may be affected, resulting in increased maternal blood loss at delivery and abnormal platelet function tests and clinical bleeding in newborns, including intracranial hemorrhage.[33,43] Second or third trimester use of low-dose (20–100 mg/day) aspirin in mothers at risk of developing pregnancy-related hypertension decreased the frequency of this disorder and its complications.[43–45] A follow-up 18 months postdelivery of infants exposed in utero to aspirin 50 mg/day showed no increase in malformations or abnormalities in height, weight, or physical problems. Fine motor and language development were also normal.[46]
	Systematic evaluation of other commonly used NSAIDs have not been conducted in humans, but no substantive reports of NSAID teratogenicity exist.[33,34,47] Out of 50 spontaneous reports to one **ibuprofen** manufacturer of exposure during pregnancy, there appeared to be no drug-induced abnormalities.[47] However, caution is warranted because of the similarity to indomethacin and aspirin. **Naproxen** has been associated with persistent pulmonary hypertension in a neonate whose mother had ingested 5 g naproxen 8 hr before delivery.[33]

ANTICOAGULANTS

Heparin	Heparin has not been associated with an increased risk for structural or functional defects or with IUGR. Maternal thrombocytopenia and hemorrhage may occur.[48–51]
Warfarin	Warfarin and related anticoagulants may produce the "fetal warfarin syndrome" or "warfarin embryopathy." The critical period of risk appears to be between 6 and 12 weeks of gestation. Features include nasal hypoplasia, neonatal respiratory distress secondary to upper airway obstruction, stippled epiphyses, IUGR, and varying degrees of hypoplasia of the extremities. Eye abnormalities, including blindness, have also been reported. About one-third of exposed cases resulted in adverse pregnancy outcomes.[2,48–56] A few cases of diaphragmatic malformation have been reported when warfarin was used early in pregnancy.[57] CNS defects occur in about 3% of those exposed and appear to occur independent of the fetal warfarin syndrome. Critical periods of risk for CNS effects appear to be during the second and third trimesters.[56] Warfarin also increases the risk for fetal as well as maternal hemorrhage, especially when used near term.[48,52]

(continued)

DRUGS AND PREGNANCY (continued)

DRUG	NATURE OF EFFECT

ANTICONVULSANTS

Many congenital malformations have been reported in children of epileptic mothers, and all anticonvulsants (except felbamate, lamotrigine, and gabapentin, for which human data are inadequate) have been implicated as possible causes of malformations. Epileptic mothers have a two- to fourfold increased frequency of fetal malformation compared with nonepileptic mothers, although it is difficult to separate the effects of the disease from possible drug effects.[58-63] Major malformations seem to be more common following combination therapy than with monotherapy, particularly with triple combinations that include valproic acid.[59,64-67] Some evidence suggests that fetal deficiency of epoxide hydrolase, a major enzyme in the metabolic pathway of many anticonvulsants (eg, phenytoin, carbamazepine, valproic acid) that helps eliminate toxic intermediates, mediates teratogenic effects. Deficient function of this enzyme may be inherited as an autosomal recessive trait.[58,68-71] Total concentrations of carbamazepine, phenytoin, phenobarbital, and valproic acid decline as pregnancy progresses, caused mainly by changes in plasma protein binding.[72,73] However, free or unbound drug concentrations fall appreciably only for phenobarbital. Free concentrations of valproic acid increase. Measurement of free anticonvulsant drug concentrations allows for appropriate dosage adjustment.[72]

Carbamazepine	Evidence showing that women taking carbamazepine are at no increased risk beyond that of other epileptic mothers has been questioned.[23,60,74-78] Recent evidence suggests that carbamazepine might increase the risk for certain abnormalities, including spina bifida, when taken during pregnancy.[79-86] The malformations are similar to those ascribed to other anticonvulsants: specific facial features, nail hypoplasia, smaller head circumference, and developmental delay. Data concerning developmental delay or impairment, as well as those concerning cardiac defects, require substantiation. Some evidence suggests there may be increased teratogenicity when carbamazepine is combined with valproic acid and phenytoin with or without other anticonvulsants.[66,82,83] Higher serum concentrations of carbamazepine were found in mothers of abnormal offspring than in mothers of normal offspring.[66]
Oxazolidinediones	Long-term use of **trimethadione** or **paramethadione** during pregnancy has resulted in children with abnormalities, including varying features of the following: mental deficiency, speech disorders, IUGR, mild midfacial hypoplasia, short upturned nose with uroad and low nasal bridge, prominent forehead with V-shaped eyebrows, epicanthal folds, high arched palate, ventricular septal defects, micrognathia, microcephaly, strabismus, low-set ears with anteriorly folded helix, short stature, ambiguous genitalia, hypospadias, and clitoral hypertrophy. The frequency of spontaneous abortion may also be increased.[2,24,53,87]
Phenobarbital	Abnormalities have been reported with phenobarbital alone and in combination, but causality has not been convincingly established. Malformations similar to those occurring with phenytoin have been reported when phenobarbital was used alone or in combination with primidone. These include craniofacial anomalies (eg, short noses with low nasal bridges, hypertelorism, low-set ears, wide mouth, prominent lips, cleft soft palate), cardiac defects, and digital hypoplasia.[59] These effects may be more likely when maternal serum concentrations exceed usual therapeutic concentrations. Barbiturates can cause a decrease in vitamin K–dependent clotting factors, leading to bleeding in the newborn.[24,64] Decreased fetal folic acid concentrations have been reported; some suggest folic acid supplementation during pregnancy may decrease the risk of abnormal offspring.[65,88-90] Neonatal withdrawal may occur after phenobarbital use during pregnancy. Data concerning developmental delay or impairment require substantiation.[74] Anecdotal reports of tumors in 10 children prenatally exposed to phenytoin and a barbiturate have caused concern that in utero exposure may potentiate cancer.[91]

(continued)

743

DRUGS AND PREGNANCY (continued)

DRUG	NATURE OF EFFECT
Phenytoin	Phenytoin serum concentrations may decrease during pregnancy as a result of increased plasma clearance. Adjustment of phenytoin dosage to maintain serum free drug concentrations seems to improve seizure control.[92] The risk of developing the full-blown fetal hydantoin syndrome (FHS) is about 5–10% when phenytoin is taken throughout pregnancy; the risk of a less serious effect is 30%.[53] Serum anticonvulsant concentrations were higher in mothers of malformed infants than in mothers of normal infants in some studies.[93] The principal features of FHS are craniofacial anomalies (eg, bowed upper lip, ocular hypertelorism, broad nasal bridge, short nose, microcephaly, cleft lip and/or palate), epicanthal folds, digital hypoplasia with small or absent nails, cardiac defects, and pre- and postnatal growth deficiency. Umbilical and inguinal hernias, hypospadias, and brain malformations have also been reported.[2,59,85,94–98] Phenytoin can cause a decrease in vitamin K–dependent clotting factors, leading to bleeding in the newborn.[24,64,85] Decreased fetal folic acid concentrations have been reported; folic acid supplementation may decrease the risk of abnormal offspring.[65,88–90] Maternal phenytoin use has also been associated with developmental delay and intellectual impairment.[93,95] Anecdotal reports of tumors in ten children prenatally exposed to phenytoin and a barbiturate have caused concern that in utero exposure may potentiate carcinogenicity.[91]
Primidone	The teratogenicity of primidone is difficult to assess, because of few reported cases and primidone being taken with other anticonvulsants, primarily phenytoin. Anecdotal reports and one small prospective study have reported abnormalities in offspring of women taking primidone alone. Although no specific pattern has been established, reported malformations include craniofacial alterations; cardiac defects, pre- and postnatal growth retardation, digital hypoplasia with small or flat nails, inguinal hernias, and hypospadias.[24] Some developmental delay has also been reported. These effects may be more likely when maternal serum concentrations exceed usual therapeutic concentrations. Phenobarbital is one metabolite of primidone (see Phenobarbital).
Valproic Acid	Neural tube defects (eg, spina bifida) occurred in 1.4% of valproic acid-exposed fetuses compared with 0.4% in fetuses exposed to other anticonvulsants.[53,65,94] The risk for neural tube defects may be five- to tenfold higher with valproic acid compared with the background frequency.[58] The neural tube closes between 22 and 29 days after conception; disruption of programmed events during this period of development results in an open defect of the cranium (if disruption occurs early) or spine (if disruption occurs later).[98] External ear anomalies, congenital heart defects, hypospadias, craniofacial anomalies, low birthweight, and small head circumference have been reported.[53,62,65,66,94,99–103] Cases of limb reduction defects, radial ray aplasia, talipes equinovarus, developmental delay, neurologic abnormality, and brain atrophy have also been reported.[53,101] The risk for adverse pregnancy outcome is higher when valproic acid is taken with other anticonvulsant drugs, particularly carbamazepine.[66,82,83] Serum concentrations of valproic acid tend to be higher in pregnancies with abnormal outcome than in those with normal outcome.[66] Decreased fetal folic acid concentrations or altered folate metabolism have been reported; folic acid supplementation during pregnancy may decrease the risk of neural tube defects.[58,88,104]

(continued)

DRUGS AND PREGNANCY (continued)

DRUG	NATURE OF EFFECT

ANTIHISTAMINES

Despite reports implicating both **meclizine** and **Bendectin (doxylamine and pyridoxine** with or without **dicyclomine)** as teratogens, large-scale studies have shown no association between these agents and fetal malformation.[3,24,105–107] **Brompheniramine** or **chlorpheniramine** use during pregnancy has not been associated with an increased risk of fetal malformations.[24,106,108–110] **Diphenhydramine and dimenhydrinate** have been suggested by one retrospective study to be the causes of cleft lip and/or palate in the neonate, but this is unconfirmed.[23,106] Dimenhydrinate may have an oxytocic effect on the term uterus, causing shortened labor. The same concerns associated with oxytocin (hyperstimulation and the possibility of uterine rupture) apply.[106,111]

ANTIMICROBIAL DRUGS

Aminoglycosides

Streptomycin has been reported to cause congenital hearing loss, ranging from minor high-frequency loss to total deafness, when given to pregnant women for the treatment of tuberculosis. Prevalence is low, especially with careful dosage calculation and limited duration of therapy.[6,24,112,113] Other aminoglycosides (eg, **gentamicin, tobramycin)** may pose a similar risk.[6,24,114]

Antimalarials

Chloroquine malaria prophylaxis has not been associated with adverse fetal effects. Larger antiinflammatory doses, however, have resulted in spontaneous abortion and fetal retinal and vestibular damage.[6,112,115–117] **Hydroxychloroquine** may increase the risk for intravascular hemolysis and methemoglobinemia because the fetus has relative deficiencies of glutathione and G-6-PD.[6,112] There are no reports of **primaquine** teratogenicity, but it may induce hemolysis in neonates because of their relative deficiencies of G-6-PD and glutathione.[22,115,116] **Pyrimethamine** is a microbial folate antagonist and should be used cautiously because the mammalian folate antagonist methotrexate is teratogenic, and folic acid supplementation may be warranted during treatment.[6,24,112,115,116,118] **Quinine** has been used as a folk remedy for inducing abortion, despite its relatively poor efficacy. When abortion attempts fail, quinine produces more maternal deaths than abortions performed by a licensed practitioner. Fetal anomalies include blindness, optic nerve hypoplasia, deafness, and hearing impairment.[6,24,112,116]

Antituberculars

Ethambutol does not appear to cause malformations. Several anomalies involving the CNS occurred in 655 reported exposures.[6,24,112,113] Of the reported **isoniazid** exposures during pregnancy, only 1% demonstrated any malformations. No pattern of malformation was revealed, but several abnormalities involved the CNS.[6,24,112,113] Exposures were confounded by concomitant ethambutol therapy. Isoniazid appears to be the safest and most effective antitubercular during pregnancy,[6] although there may be an increased risk of hepatotoxicity in pregnant women. **Rifampin** safety during pregnancy is less well established than isoniazid. However, it has not been associated with an increased risk of fetal malformations. In most reports, rifampin was taken with either isoniazid or ethambutol. Neonatal hypoprothrombinemia has been reported and raises some concern about the use of this drug, especially near term.[6,24,112,113] If rifampin is given during pregnancy, maternal oral prophylaxis with vitamin K 20 mg/day for 2 weeks prior to delivery is recommended.[6,24,112] Infants should receive 0.5–1 mg of vitamin K IM or SC immediately after delivery and 6–8 hr later.[22]

(continued)

DRUGS AND PREGNANCY (continued)

DRUG	NATURE OF EFFECT
Cephalosporins	Cephalosporins are thought to be without teratogenic risk.[6,8,112,114,119]
Chloramphenicol	Although reports of fetal abnormality or toxicity associated with maternal chloramphenicol are lacking, there is a theoretical risk for development of blood dyscrasias and aplastic anemia. Particular caution should be exercised near term because the "gray baby" syndrome is a result of toxic accumulation of chloramphenicol in neonates caused by their relative inability to eliminate the drug.[6,112,114]
Erythromycins	Pregnant women are at increased risk for hepatotoxicity caused by erythromycin estolate. About 10–15% of women treated with the estolate in the second trimester had abnormally elevated AST (SGOT) concentrations, which normalized when therapy was discontinued.[22] There is no evidence that erythromycin is harmful to the fetus.[6,24,112,119]
Penicillins	Penicillins are without teratogenic risk.[6,112,114,119,120] Treatment of early syphilis with penicillin (or other drugs) during pregnancy may produce the Jarisch-Herxheimer reaction, resulting in uterine cramping, decreased fetal movement, and in some cases fetal death.[121]
Quinolones	**Nalidixic acid** use during pregnancy has been reported to cause increased intracranial pressure, papilledema, and bulging fontanelles in the newborn. Avoid first trimester use.[6,112,114] **Fluoroquinolones** (eg, **ciprofloxacin, norfloxacin, ofloxacin**) cause arthropathy in immature animals and therefore should not be used in pregnancy.[112]
Sulfonamides	There are occasional reports of abnormalities, but no distinct malformation pattern has emerged. Evidence associating sulfonamide use near term with neonatal kernicterus is lacking, despite sulfonamide displacement of bilirubin from albumin binding sites.[6,111,112,114,118,119,122,123] There is a theoretical risk for hemolysis in the fetus or neonate because of their relative deficiencies of G-6-PD and glutathione.[6,112] Because **trimethoprim** is a folate antagonist, caution is advised in pregnancy (*see* Methotrexate and Pyrimethamine).[6,12] However, data suggest a lack of teratogenicity.[6,114,119,120,122,123,125,126] In one prospective, randomized study, single-dose trimethoprim 600 mg was compared with the usual five–day course (300 mg/day) for asymptomatic bacteriuria in 60 pregnant women between the 16th and 30th weeks of gestation. There were no detrimental effects on pregnancy outcome.[126]
Sulfones	**Dapsone** use does not appear to increase the risk of fetal abnormalities.[127] A woman on dapsone throughout her first pregnancy had a male infant who developed hyperbilirubinemia necessitating phototherapy. In a subsequent pregnancy, dapsone was discontinued 1 month prior to delivery and the infant did not develop hyperbilirubinemia. The authors postulated that because dapsone is similar to sulfonamides, it could displace bilirubin from albumin binding sites.[6,112,128] *See* Sulfonamides.
Tetracyclines	Fetal effects of tetracyclines are caused by interference with protein synthesis and chelation with calcium and other di- and trivalent cations. Tetracyclines can cause hypoplasia and permanent staining of the teeth when taken after the 12th week of pregnancy. The risk of discoloration increases with dose, duration of therapy, and advancing pregnancy; one-third to one-half of third trimester exposures may be affected. Tetracyclines are also incorporated into calcifying bone, and inhibition of bone growth has been reported. As bone is resorbed, the tetracycline is released.[6,112,114,119] Pregnant women with pyelonephritis or underlying renal disease, or following an overdose, appear at risk for developing acute fatty necrosis of the liver and azotemia.[6,112,114,119] *(continued)*

DRUGS AND PREGNANCY (continued)

DRUG	NATURE OF EFFECT
Urinary Germicides	No fetal abnormalities or neonatal hemolytic anemia have been observed with **nitrofurantoin** use during pregnancy.[6,114,129–131] A theoretical risk for the development of hemolysis in neonates exists if the drug is taken by the mother near term due to infants' relative G-6-PD and glutathione deficiencies.[131]
Miscellaneous Antiinfectives	Maternal **acyclovir** use during the second and third trimesters does not appear to be associated with fetal toxicity.[112,124,132–138] Acyclovir may mediate a delay in maternal humoral antibody response that could result in delayed transfer of IgG to the fetus, thereby increasing the risk of neonatal HSV infection.[132]
	Twenty years' experience and several studies demonstrate no association of **metronidazole** with congenital malformations, abortions, or stillbirths.[139–142] However, a few cases of facial clefting have been reported.[143]
	There are few data concerning the teratogenic effects of **vancomycin**. There is a theoretical risk for auditory and renal toxicity in the fetus.[6,112] However, in one small prospective trial, IV administration of vancomycin to ten women during the second or third trimesters produced no cases of fetal renal toxicity or hearing impairment.[144]
	Zidovudine therapy has not been associated with an increase in birth defects greater than normal.[145–147] Concentrations of zidovudine are 2.5–7 times higher in amniotic fluid than in cord blood; concentrations in cord blood were higher (113–140%) than those in maternal blood.[148,149] In a case report, neonatal elimination of zidovudine or its metabolite was minimal during the first 24–36 hr of life.[148] In another report, the elimination half-life in infants was 9–18 times that seen in their mothers (*n* = 3).[149] Transmission of HIV from mother to fetus is substantially reduced with zidovudine treatment.[146]

ANTINEOPLASTICS AND IMMUNOSUPPRESSANTS

Antineoplastic agents have both teratogenic and mutagenic potential, and reports of infertility and congenital defects exist. Nevertheless, several studies indicate that fertility is preserved, with normal pregnancy outcome, among both women and men treated for cancer prior to conception. Although aggressive treatment of malignancy is necessary on occasion, avoidance or minimum use of these drugs, especially during the first trimester, is recommended. Chemotherapy generally produces a decrease in birthweight, but not IUGR.[150] The occupational risk for hospital personnel exposed through inhalation or skin absorption has not been fully determined, although there are retrospective studies that suggest occupational exposure during the first trimester results in increased fetal loss.[2,151] Use of antineoplastics near delivery may cause neonatal bone marrow suppression.[152] However, normal pregnancy outcome has been reported, particularly if exposure is very early in gestation (first week after conception).[153] **Busulfan** has been associated with IUGR and multiple malformations, although no specific pattern is evident. **Chlorambucil** use during the first and second trimesters may cause spontaneous abortion and urogenital malformation. **Cyclophosphamide** use during the first trimester has resulted in fetal malformations, particularly of the toes, syndactyly, and cleft palate.[154] No malformations have been reported with second or third trimester use. A report of malignancies in a child that occurred 10 and 14 yr after exposure in utero raises the question whether intrauterine exposure to cyclophosphamide can cause iatrogenic or second cancers. Adults and children exposed to alkylating agents such as cyclophosphamide have developed second malignancies years after their exposure.[155] Experience with **fluorouracil** is limited, but it has been reported to cause malformations consistent with inhibition of cell division and cell growth.[24] Inadvertent first trimester topical administration of 5% fluorouracil to the lower genital tract did not result in abnormal appearing infants in ten pregnancies.[156,157] First trimester use of the folate antagonist **methotrexate** is known to cause spontaneous abortion and congenital abnormalities, including cranial anomalies, cleft palate, syndactyly, growth retardation,

(continued)

DRUGS AND PREGNANCY (continued)

DRUG	NATURE OF EFFECT

and developmental abnormalities.[2,158] One study of ten pregnancies in eight women taking methotrexate 7.5–10 mg/week during the first trimester for arthritis resulted in three spontaneous abortions, two elective abortions, and the birth of five full-term normal infants. The infants had no medical illnesses or learning disabilities.[158] Normal pregnancy outcome has been reported after use in the second and third trimesters.[2,158,159] **Procarbazine** use in pregnancy is limited, but has been associated with several fetal abnormalities, all occurring with first trimester exposure.[24] **Thioguanine** has been associated with abnormalities following its use in both the first and second trimesters.

Normal pregnancy outcome has been reported with **azathioprine** taken for renal transplantation, SLE, or acute or chronic leukemias.[34,161] However, there have been reports of IUGR, neonatal lymphopenia, hypogammaglobulinemia, thymic hypoplasia, fetal bone marrow suppression, leukopenia, and thrombocytopenia.[34,162] A retrospective review examined the outcome of 16 pregnancies in 14 women who took azathioprine for inflammatory bowel disease up until 16 weeks' gestation or throughout gestation. Most women were taking either prednisone or prednisolone plus sulfasalazine in addition to azathioprine. There were no congenital anomalies or developmental problems.[162] Previous studies showed some abnormal chromosomal aberrations; however, there is no evidence of permanent genomal or gonadal damage. **Cyclosporine**, used throughout pregnancy following renal or hepatic transplant, does not appear to be associated with malformations, although experience is limited. IUGR occurred in 11 of 20 infants, and six of these cases had severe IUGR (below the third percentile); however, normal size for gestational age infants are often delivered. No neonatal distress or increased mortality has been reported.[163–166]

CARDIOVASCULAR DRUGS

Antiarrhythmics.

Neonatal hypothyroidism with and without goiter, as well as hyperthyroidism, has occurred with **amiodarone** use.[167] A child with transient congenital hypothyroidism showed some delay in motor development and impaired speech performance at age 5.[167] **Digoxin** is not a teratogen. It may be given to pregnant women to treat fetal CHF and supraventricular tachycardia (SVT). Maternal digitalis toxicity has been associated with fetal toxicity and miscarriage in one case and neonatal ECG changes with subsequent infant death in another. Maternal concentrations should be monitored closely because, as pregnancy progresses, renal clearance of digoxin increases. However, digoxin bioavailability may also increase. Therefore, serum concentrations may decrease or increase.[168,169] **Disopyramide** use during pregnancy has not been well studied, but in one report it was associated with the initiation of uterine contractions that subsided when the drug was discontinued.[168] **Procainamide** use during pregnancy is probably safe. However, because of its association with systemic lupus erythematosus (SLE), caution is advised.[168] **Quinidine** use during pregnancy appears to be without teratogenic effect.[24,168] Neonatal thrombocytopenia has been reported after maternal use of quinidine.[24]

(continued)

DRUGS AND PREGNANCY (continued)

DRUG	NATURE OF EFFECT
β-Adrenergic Blocking Agents	**Atenolol, pindolol, metoprolol,** or **propranolol** are thought to be generally safe in pregnancy. Maternal hypertension has been shown to cause IUGR, decreased placental size, neonatal respiratory depression, and hypoglycemia. These agents have also been associated with IUGR and neonatal hypoglycemia and hypotension. Whether these effects are caused by the drugs or by maternal disease has not been established. Mild neonatal bradycardia may be caused by these agents. One author suggests that β-blockers may adversely affect fetal adaptation to intrauterine hypoxia, such as that associated with umbilical cord compression.[168,170–176] An **esmolol** bolus and infusion administered to a mother near term in an attempt to treat SVT was associated with severe fetal bradycardia that required emergency cesarean section.[177] Although generally regarded as safe during pregnancy, **labetalol** given IV to control severe hypertension has caused neonatal bradycardia, weak femoral pulses, inadequate breathing, hypotonia, hypotension, and hypoglycemia.[174,176,178,179]
Hypotensive Agents	Although normal fetal outcome has been reported with maternal use of **angiotensin-converting enzyme (ACE) inhibitors,**[180] several cases of IUGR and prolonged neonatal anuria and hypotension with resultant renal failure have been associated with maternal ingestion of **captopril** or **enalapril**.[170,180–182] Oligohydramnios or anhydramnios was present in seven of nine cases (not recorded in the other two cases) and led to pulmonary hypoplasia and death in some. Respiratory problems occurred in several neonates. Some infants had altered or absent skull formation with dysmorphic facial features; others had persistent ductus arteriosus (this may have been caused by low birthweight).[181,182] Nineteen women who had filled an ACE inhibitor prescription during pregnancy gave birth to 19 live infants, two of which were preterm. One infant exposed during the first and second trimesters had microcephaly and occipital encephalocele; one infant exposed during the second and third trimesters had prolonged anuria and hypotension requiring dialysis; and one infant exposed all through pregnancy had hypoglycemia.[183] The FDA warns against their use in the second and third trimesters. There may be an increased frequency of fetal loss associated with ACE inhibitors.
Calcium-Channel Blocking Agents	No malformations have been associated with use of calcium-channel blocking agents during pregnancy.[184–186] Bolus doses of IV **isradipine** during labor effectively reduce maternal blood pressure while causing a concomitant increase in heart rate.[184] Fetal heart rate increased 3, 8, and 10% after maternal IV bolus doses of 0.5, 1, and 1.5 mg, respectively. One woman developed hypotension for 7 min following the 1.5-mg dose with concomitant fetal bradycardia for 5 min, which returned to normal with no sequelae. A small, transient decrease in uterine activity occurred with all doses.[184] **Nifedipine** does not appear to alter uterine arterial resistance when given at 17–22 weeks,[185] or 26–35 weeks gestational age.[186]

Diazoxide administered by rapid IV bolus has been associated with excessive maternal hypotension and fetal distress. Slow IV infusion or minibolus administration may prevent this occurrence. Other reported effects include inhibition of labor, neonatal hyperglycemia when exposure preceded delivery, alopecia, hypertrichosis languinosa, and decreased bone age after exposure in the last 19–70 days of gestation. Other investigators report no problems after long-term oral administration of diazoxide.[168,174,178]

(continued) |

DRUGS AND PREGNANCY (continued)

DRUG	NATURE OF EFFECT
	Hydralazine use in pregnancy may cause reduced uteroplacental blood flow, fetal heart rate changes after acute administration, and neonatal hypothermia and thrombocytopenia.[168,174,178] There is little information concerning first trimester use.
	Methyldopa use during pregnancy has been studied more extensively than any other antihypertensive. Available data show teratogenicity. Transient reduction in neonatal blood pressure has been noted after maternal methyldopa ingestion. There is a questionable association of IUGR after maternal treatment with methyldopa. One study suggested IUGR was caused by chronic hypertension rather than by methyldopa.[168,174,178]
	Reserpine, when given to mothers within 24 hr of delivery, produces edema of the nasal mucosa in the neonate. This effect is especially important because newborns are obligate nose breathers. Lethargy, hypothermia, and bradycardia have also been reported in infants whose mothers received antenatal reserpine.[174,187]
DIURETICS	Diuretics should be used with great caution during pregnancy because they can cause a decrease in maternal intravascular volume and consequently diminish uteroplacental perfusion, thereby compromising fetal oxygenation. This effect is most rapid and severe with **loop diuretics** (eg, **bumetanide, furosemide, torsemide**). IV furosemide administration to the pregnant woman has enabled ultrasonic imaging of the fetal bladder because of increased fetal urine output. **Thiazide** use in pregnancy may produce neonatal hypoglycemia, hyponatremia, hypokalemia, and thrombocytopenia.[168,174,178,188]
ERGOT ALKALOIDS	The use of **ergonovine, ergotamine**, or **methylergonovine** before delivery carries the same risk of uterine stimulation as oxytocin.[189] (See Hormones and Synthetic Substitutes, Oxytocin.)
GASTROINTESTINAL DRUGS	
Antacids	The safety of antacid use during the first trimester of pregnancy has not been established.[105,111] Second and third trimester use appears to be without adverse effects.
Histamine H₂-Receptor Antagonists	No reports link **cimetidine** or **ranitidine** to adverse pregnancy outcome.[190] Manufacturer data on cimetidine in 50 pregnant women reveal no increased risk to the developing fetus, although time of exposure was not noted. The use of H₂-antagonists as preanesthetic agents to prevent aspiration of acidic stomach contents has no reported adverse effects on the course of delivery or on the neonate.[105,111,191,192]
Mesalamine Derivatives	**Sulfasalazine** has been associated with IUGR. However, one large survey found the prevalence of IUGR, prematurity, pregnancy loss, and developmental defects to be lower in women taking sulfasalazine for Crohn's disease than in the general population.[111,193,194] (See also Antimicrobial Drugs, Sulfonamides.)

(continued)

750

DRUGS AND PREGNANCY (continued)

DRUG	NATURE OF EFFECT
Metoclopramide	There are no reports of adverse fetal outcome associated with use of metoclopramide during pregnancy; however, the drug has not been used widely in this setting.[105,106,111] One study of 120 women with hyperemesis gravidarum treated with metoclopramide, prochlorperazine, or placebo found no malformations or neonatal problems. The use of metoclopramide during labor, anesthesia, or cesarean section to prevent acid aspiration has not been associated with adverse maternal, fetal, or neonatal outcome.[105,106,111]
Sucralfate	There have been no adequate studies on sucralfate in pregnant women. Because little of the drug is absorbed, little risk is expected.[105,111]
HORMONAL DRUGS	
Androgens	Androgen (eg, **testosterone, methyltestosterone, danazol**) exposure during the first week of gestation has been associated with masculinization of the female embryo. Clitoromegaly, with or without fusion of the labia minora, may occur. In some cases a urogenital sinus opening at the base of the clitoris has been observed. The extent of the defect is correlated with the time of exposure, and the effects are more apparent with higher dosages.[2,195,196] Although danazol dosages under 400 mg/day may carry a lower risk, virilization was observed with 200 mg/day in one case.[196] Because differentiation of external genitalia occurs 8–12 weeks postconception, exposure beyond the 12th week of gestation is expected to produce only clitoral hypertrophy. If danazol is discontinued by the 8th week of gestation, the risk is substantially lower. Internal genitalia are unaffected because they are not androgen responsive. The male fetus does not appear to be adversely affected.
Clomiphene	Clomiphene-induced ovulation results in an increased frequency of multiple ovulations (primarily twinning), delayed follicular rupture, ectopic pregnancy, and female fetuses. There is also an increase in abnormal karyotypes in oocytes and abortuses. The high proportion of abnormal karyotypes could be related to the increase in spontaneous abortions and low pregnancy rate noted after ovulation induction and in vitro fertilization.[197,198] The rate of birth defects reported after ovulation induction in most studies has been within the expected range.[197,199,200]
Corticosteroids	Although teratogenic in animals, corticosteroids have not been demonstrated to be teratogenic in humans. Large prospective investigations, together with cases of pregnant women with inflammatory bowel disease, asthma, or rheumatoid arthritis, do not show an increase in spontaneous abortions or congenital defects in infants exposed prenatally. Some studies show decreased birth weight and increased rates of prematurity, although these effects may have been due to the underlying maternal disease.[34,108,201–203] Women who had status asthmaticus during pregnancy were more likely to have infants with low birthweight or IUGR.[203] A placental enzyme (11-β-OH-dehydrogenase) inactivates certain corticosteroids, leading to low fetal concentrations. This inactivation is most prominent with **hydrocortisone, prednisone,** or **prednisolone** compared with **betamethasone** or **beclomethasone**.[34,108] The fetal liver is relatively ineffective in converting prednisone into the active prednisolone, even at term.[108] Therefore, prednisone or hydrocortisone may be preferred during pregnancy. When appropriate, corticosteroids can be administered by aerosol inhalation or intrasynovial injection to minimize systemic availability.[33,34,108,109,194,201–203] Neonates born to women taking long-term corticosteroids should be monitored for adrenal insufficiency, although this rarely occurs. Maternal **betametha-**

(continued)

DRUGS AND PREGNANCY (continued)

DRUG	NATURE OF EFFECT
	sone therapy has been used to prevent respiratory distress in infants born between 28 and 34 weeks of gestation with no apparent adverse effects.[108,204,205] No differences in psychologic or physical development, pulmonary function, ophthalmologic findings, or neurologic function were noted between exposed and nonexposed children between 10 and 12 years of age.[206] However, there was a significantly increased frequency of hospitalizations for infections during early childhood in the exposed group. Corticosteroid use during pregnancy may cause an increased risk for maternal gestational diabetes, hypertension, and excessive weight gain.[109,201,202]
Diethylstilbestrol (DES)	Daughters of DES-exposed mothers have an increased frequency of vaginal adenosis; structural defects of the cervix, vagina, uterus, and fallopian tubes; and reproductive complications. Adverse reproductive effects include infertility, spontaneous abortion, ectopic pregnancy, premature deliveries, and perinatal deaths.[2,207–210] Two large cohort studies do not confirm the relation of DES to clear cell carcinoma. Early studies showing such an association were retrospective and had serious methodologic flaws.[211] If an association exists, the risk of developing this cancer in exposed females is very low. Data on DES-exposed males are suggestive of an increased risk for infertility, various urogenital abnormalities, and testicular cancer.[212]
Oxytocin	Oxytocin given for induction of labor may cause tetanic uterine contractions, causing decreased uterine blood flow and fetal distress. The risk of neonatal hyperbilirubinemia appears to be increased 1.6-fold following oxytocin-induced labor compared with spontaneous labor, and neonatal jaundice has occurred.[213]
Progestins	High doses of progestins (eg, **medroxyprogesterone, norethindrone, norethynodrel**) during pregnancy may cause masculinization of female external genitalia (clitoral hypertrophy or labioscrotal fusion). Hypospadias has been reported in males.[214,215] This most likely occurs during the period of external genitalia development (8–12 weeks postconception).[2,24,216–218] Doses used in oral or implantable contraceptives do not appear to carry these risks.[219]
Prostaglandins	**Misoprostol** has uterotonic effects and should not be used during pregnancy. In 56 pregnant women who requested first trimester abortions, 1 or 2 oral doses of misoprostol 400 μg resulted in spontaneous fetal expulsions.[220] Twenty-five women had uterine bleeding. High doses of misoprostol in early pregnancy, such as those used to induce abortion, might be associated with defects resulting from vascular disruption.[221,222] Anomalies reported include limb deficiency/reduction defects, mobius sequence, convergent strabismus, and defects of the cranium and overlying scalp.[221–223] Further substantiation of the association between high-dose misoprostol exposure and these defects is required. Misoprostol has been used with methotrexate for first trimester pregnancy termination (see the Methotrexate monograph). **Dinoprostone**, when administered as vaginal tablets to mildly hypertensive women at term to induce labor, produced significant decreases in the percentage of time occupied by fetal body and breathing movements 3–4 hr later.[224] Fetal outcome was normal. Dinoprostone may shorten labor more than oxytocin.[225,226]

(continued)

DRUGS AND PREGNANCY (continued)

DRUG	NATURE OF EFFECT
Sulfonylureas	Maternal diabetes is known to increase the rate of malformations and perinatal mortality.[227,228] Pregnancy in 20 women exposed to an oral hypoglycemic (16 to a sulfonylurea, 3 to a biguanide, 1 unknown) during organogenesis resulted in a higher proportion of major and minor malformations than a similar unexposed control group.[228] A retrospective case review did not find a similar increase in malformations.[229] Malformations reported include auricular, vertebral, cardiac, neural tube, and limb defects.[228–230] Complicating the issue is a study that shows glyburide does not cross the human placenta ex vivo in appreciable amounts.[231] Sulfonylureas (eg, **chlorpropamide, glyburide, glipizide**) and biguanides (eg, **metformin**) may cause prolonged hypoglycemia or hyperinsulinism in the newborn.[2,24,53,228,232] Pregnant diabetics should be treated with **insulin**.
Thyroid and Antithyroid Agents	**Propylthiouracil** and **methimazole** were associated with neonatal goiter in early reports, possibly because of the use of iodine in addition to unnecessarily high dosages of antithyroid medication. However, even conservative management does not completely eliminate the risk of congenital goiter. Transient neonatal hypothyroidism and neonatal thyrotoxicosis may occur. Monitor infants for thyrotoxicosis, because it may be masked by the antithyroid agent. Hypothyroidism may be prevented by discontinuing the drug, if the mother has remained euthyroid, 4–6 weeks before delivery. Case reports of four infants with ulcerlike midline scalp defects have been associated with maternal methimazole. Mothers with moderate to severe hyperthyroidism not receiving treatment have an increased risk of complications including toxemia, small-for-gestational-age babies, and neonatal morbidity.[233–235] Excessive **iodine** use during pregnancy is associated with congenital goiter and hypothyroidism. Goiters may be large enough to cause tracheal compression and interfere with delivery. Severe maternal iodine deficiency produces hypothyroidism and cretinism.[233,234]

No adverse effects have been reported after inadvertent exposure to **131I** prior to 10 weeks' gestation. After 10 weeks' gestation, the fetal thyroid actively concentrates iodine; any radioactive iodine ingested by the mother will cross the placenta and destroy fetal thyroid tissue.[2,233] |

PSYCHOTHERAPEUTIC AGENTS

Antidepressants	Although there are several case reports of maternal use of **tricyclic antidepressants** (TCAs) during pregnancy associated with varied fetal anomalies, no consistent pattern of malformation has been confirmed.[78] An early association with limb reductions has not been confirmed. Maternal use of TCAs (eg, **clomipramine, desipramine, imipramine**) during pregnancy has occasionally produced neonatal symptoms of breathlessness, respiratory distress, hypertonia with tremor, clonus, spasm, cyanosis, tachypnea, irritability, and feeding difficulties. In one case, maternal **nortriptyline** use was associated with neonatal urinary retention.[78,236] Prospective follow-up of exposed pregnancies, including first trimester exposure, and spontaneous reports to the manufacturer of adverse fetal outcome following use, do not implicate **fluoxetine** as a teratogen.[237–238] However, a prospective study found increased risks of multiple minor malformations, prematurity, admission to a special care nursery, and poor neonatal adaptation.[239]

(continued)

DRUG	NATURE OF EFFECT
Lithium	Lithium use during the first trimester of pregnancy, particularly from the third to eighth weeks, may be associated with an increased risk of cardiovascular abnormalities, including Ebstein's anomaly.[78,240-244] Anomalies of the external ear, ureters, CNS, and endocrine system, as well as macrosomia, have also been reported.[242,243] A case of polyhydramnios possibly caused by lithium-induced fetal polyuria has been reported.[245] Of lithium-exposed pregnancies followed by the Lithium Registry, 39% delivered prematurely, 36% had macrosomia (>90th percentile body weight for gestational age), and there was an 8.3% perinatal mortality rate.[78] Symptoms of lithium toxicity, including lethargy, hypotonia, poor sucking reflex, respiratory distress, cyanosis, arrhythmias, and hypothermia have been reported in newborns of women on long-term lithium therapy. Newborn blood concentrations were 0.6–1 mEq/L. Monitor maternal serum concentrations frequently during pregnancy, because lithium clearance varies as pregnancy progresses.[78,238,240-242]
Phenothiazines	Most data do not implicate phenothiazines as teratogens.[78,106,246] However, a reanalysis of some early data questions initial negative findings and suggests an increased risk of malformations in association with first trimester antinauseant phenothiazine use during the fourth to tenth weeks of gestation.[78,246] Phenothiazine use near term has resulted in some cases of extrapyramidal effects in the neonate, which have persisted up to 9 months.[78,111,246] Leukemia, hyperbilirubinemia, and jaundice (primarily in premature neonates), decreased gastric motility, poor sucking, and respiratory depression have also been reported.[78]

SEDATIVES AND HYPNOTICS

High dosages of any sedative-hypnotic close to or during delivery may result in neonatal CNS and respiratory depression.

Anesthetics, General	There is a possible association between general anesthesia for surgery performed between gestational weeks four and five and neural tube defects,[247] and first trimester exposure to general anesthesia is associated with hydrocephalus and eye defects.[248] However, not all patients in these studies received the same preoperative medications or inhalation anesthetics, although **nitrous oxide** was received by over 98% in one study.[247] Definitive conclusions await further study. **Halothane**, teratogenic in rats, has questionable effects on the developing human embryo.[249] Although a two- to fourfold increase in the rate of spontaneous abortion in pregnant women with long-term exposure to inhalation anesthetics (eg, operating room and dental personnel) has been suggested, poor study design makes conclusions very suspect.[249,250] Inhalation anesthetic use during labor is associated with CNS and respiratory depression in the neonate. When given intermittently during labor, equilibrium between mother and fetus is usually not reached. This and the comparatively large minute volume of the newborn favor the rapid elimination of inhalational agents. However, when inhaled continuously, high fetal tissue concentrations may occur causing neonatal depression, especially in the premature or poor-risk infant.[251] During labor, halothane is not recommended due to its low analgesic activity. Nitrous oxide, **methoxyflurane**, and **enflurane** are commonly used.[251] Neonatal EEG recordings have documented that **thiopental** general anesthesia has more depressant effects than 0.5% **bupivacaine** epidural anesthesia when used for cesarean section.[252]
Barbiturates	Barbiturate addiction during pregnancy can result in neonatal withdrawal. Symptoms include tremors, irritability, restlessness, high-pitched crying, increased tone, hyperphagia, and overreaction to stimuli, which may persist for up to 6 months.[24] (*See* Anticonvulsants, Phenobarbital.)

(continued)

DRUGS AND PREGNANCY (continued)

DRUG	NATURE OF EFFECT
Benzodiazepines	Recent data do not support an association between **diazepam** or **chlordiazepoxide** and oral clefting.[24,78,236,253-256] However, there is a case report describing an acentric cranio-facial cleft in a child whose mother took 580 mg diazepam as a single dose about 43 days after her last menstrual period.[257] Infants of mothers using benzodiazepines near term may exhibit withdrawal symptoms (including tremors, irritability, and hypertonicity) and cardiovascular, respiratory, and CNS effects consistent with benzodiazepine pharmacology. Many exhibit the "floppy baby syndrome" characterized by muscular relaxation, poor sucking, disturbances in thermoregulation and regurgitation.[24,78,251,253,254,258-262] **Oxazepam**, **lorazepam**, and **temazepam** are short-acting and predominately metabolized into inactive glucuronides and subsequently excreted via the kidneys; they therefore may be preferred over diazepam, although irritability, feeding difficulties, and muscle tone disorders lasting 2 months were reported in two infants of mothers who used lorazepam 2–3 mg/day throughout pregnancy.[251,263]
Meprobamate	In one study, meprobamate ingestion during the first 42 days of pregnancy resulted in eight children with abnormalities (12.1% of those exposed, five of whom had cardiovascular malformations). Other large-scale investigations have not confirmed these findings.[24] Alternative agents are advised, especially during the first trimester.
VACCINES	
See Immunization, page 851, for information regarding vaccination during pregnancy.	
MISCELLANEOUS AGENTS	
Anesthetics, Local	There is no association between maternal exposure to local anesthetics during the first 4 months of pregnancy and fetal malformations.[162,251,252,264] However, local anesthetics have been associated with fetal and neonatal CNS and myocardial depression following maternal use during labor. Fetal bradycardia may occur after paracervical blocks. Epidural administration of **bupivacaine** or **lidocaine** appear to be the safest method for obstetric analgesia. Epidural lidocaine was shown to decrease neonatal neurobehavioral performance, but the effect was short-lived and of minimal clinical consequence.[251] High-concentration (0.75%) bupivacaine is not recommended for use in obstetrics because of the profound neonatal myocardial depression and prolonged difficult resuscitation associated with accidental intravascular injection.[251,264] Lower concentrations are popular because of the high quality of analgesia with minimal degree of motor block.[251] The bisulfite-free preparation of **chloroprocaine** had no adverse effects on mother, fetus, or neonate.[252] **Mepivacaine** should not be used in obstetric anesthesia because the neonate is unable to metabolize it.[251,252]
Antiallergics	**Cromolyn** sodium use during pregnancy is not known to have any teratogenic effects.[108,109,201,202] A prescription event monitoring study of **nedocromil** in the United Kingdom identified 79 pregnancies exposed.[265] Routine follow-up showed no abnormalities among the 33 infants with first trimester exposure to nedocromil.
Gold Salts	Although teratogenic in animals, gold salts have not been demonstrated to be harmful to the human fetus. Several anecdotal reports have described normal children born to women using gold salts during pregnancy. Definitive conclusions await further study.[33,34]

(continued)

755

DRUGS AND PREGNANCY (continued)

DRUG	NATURE OF EFFECT
Magnesium Sulfate	Long-term infusion of magnesium sulfate during the second trimester occasionally causes bone abnormalities and dental enamel hypoplasia.[266,267] However, infusions between 24 and 34 weeks' gestation in women with preterm labor generally does not cause adverse neonatal outcomes.[268] Use of magnesium sulfate as a tocolytic agent near term has been associated with neonatal hypotonia, hyporeflexia, respiratory distress, hypocalcemia, and hypermagnesemia.[189,266]
Penicillamine	Data on the teratogenicity of penicillamine are contradictory. The majority of pregnant women taking penicillamine deliver normal healthy babies, even at the high dosages used in treatment of Wilson's disease.[33,34,269,270] No abnormalities were found in 50 children of 27 patients with Wilson's disease and seven with cystinuria treated with 0.5–2 g/day during early pregnancy or throughout gestation.[271] In another study of 19 patients with rheumatoid arthritis taking penicillamine, the only congenital defect noted was a ventricular septal defect.[271] However, penicillamine may increase the solubility of dermal collagen and decrease molecular cross-linking. There have been cases of fetal connective tissue disease as well as cutis laxa in children born to mothers who ingested penicillamine during pregnancy.[33,34]
Podophyllin	Podophyllotoxins are antimitotic agents, and their use during pregnancy is contraindicated. Maternal oral use during the fifth through ninth weeks of gestation was associated with congenital malformation. High doses used topically at the 34th week resulted in severe maternal toxicity and a stillborn fetus. There are several cases in which topical podophyllin use during pregnancy produced no adverse outcome.[272–275]
Retinoids	**Etretinate** is a known teratogen in humans. Fetal abnormalities include facial dysmorphia, syndactyies; absence of terminal phalanges; neural tube closure defects, malformations of hip, ankle, and forearm, low-set ears, high palate, decreased cranial volume, and alterations of the skull and cervical vertebrae.[276] Etretinate accumulates in adipose tissue with repeated administration and has been detected in the serum of some patients up to 3 yr after discontinuing therapy. The importance of this, relative to the risk of teratogenicity, is unknown. An effective form of contraception must be used for at least 1 month before etretinate therapy, during therapy, and for an indefinite time following therapy, some say for at least 2 yr.[276–281] Unpublished data from the manufacturer indicate suspected teratogenicity in 8 out of 95 fetuses reportedly exposed 1–24 months following drug discontinuation.[278] **Isotretinoin** use during pregnancy is associated with defects of the CNS, heart, external ear, and thymus.[53,282–290] Other reported malformations include cleft palate, microphthalmia, micrognathia, facial dysmorphia, and limb reduction defects. Infants may exhibit hearing and visual impairment and mental retardation.[288] One report estimated the relative risk for major birth defects from isotretinoin to be 25.6.[282] Data suggest that the risk is substantial even when exposure to isotretinoin is brief or dosage is low.[289] In an analysis of cases reported to the manufacturer, 28% of exposed fetuses were malformed.[289] Exposures before day 14 of gestation resulted in the same rates of malformation and spontaneous/missed abortion as exposures between day 14 and 83 of gestation.[289] The risk for spontaneous abortion is also increased.[283,284,289] Topical application of 1 g of a 0.1% **tretinoin** preparation daily, assuming a maximum penetration of 33%, would result in absorption equivalent to approximately 12 IU/kg/day of vitamin A. Most prenatal vitamins contain 5000 IU of vitamin A and result in absorption of about 80 IU/kg/day.[291] Therefore, teratogenicity of this retinoid, although theoretically possible, is unlikely when used topically as directed.[292,293] Retrospective review of women receiving topical retinoids during the first trimester and review of cases of malformations typical of those observed with *(continued)*

DRUGS AND PREGNANCY (continued)

DRUG	NATURE OF EFFECT
	exposure to retinoids showed no association between topical retinoids and malformations.[292,293] However, two case reports of malformations similar to those associated with isotretinoin after first trimester tretinoin exposure have been published.[294,295]
	Vitamin A (retinol or retinyl esters, but not beta-carotene) in toxic doses is teratogenic in experimental animals, producing defects in almost all organ systems. Such research and the discovery of the teratogenicity of isotretinoin and etretinate has raised concern about the effects of excess vitamin A on the human fetus. Daily ingestion of 833 IU/kg of vitamin A produced a 600% and 400% increase in serum concentrations of the two main retinoids present in serum during isotretinoin therapy.[296] Human data on vitamin A teratogenicity consist of only a few anecdotal reports and epidemiologic studies, and the range of malformations associated with maternal use of high-dose vitamin A has not been well defined. Epidemiologic studies show that doses of vitamin A contained in prenatal vitamin supplements (ie. ≤10,000 IU) are not associated with an increased risk of fetal malformation.[297-300] However, because of methodologic flaws and incomplete data, the degree of risk associated with higher daily dosages of vitamin A is unclear. Further research is warranted. Defects observed when mothers ingested ≥25,000 IU/day vitamin A during pregnancy include craniofacial, CNS, cardiac, urinary, vertebral, and other skeletal malformations.[2,301,302]
Sympathomimetic Agents	The treatment of hypotension during pregnancy with sympathomimetic agents is complicated by the fact that the uterine vasculature is supplied solely with α-adrenergic receptors and is maximally dilated under basal conditions. Pure α-adrenergic agents markedly constrict uterine vessels and decrease blood flow, thereby compromising the fetus. β-adrenergic agents cause peripheral vasodilation and tend to shunt blood away from the uterus and also may cause fetal compromise. Volume-expanding agents seem to be the most prudent treatment for sudden hypotension in pregnancy. Use of sympathomimetics for treatment of nasal congestion may be associated with an increase in fetal activity and fetal tachycardia. Systemically administered sympathomimetics should be avoided in patients with hypertension or eclampsia, or situations in which there is poor fetal cardiac reserve.[24,303] Aerosol inhalation of **metaproterenol, albuterol, isoetharine,** or **terbutaline** is probably safe during pregnancy.[108,109,201,202] Less is known about the oral use of these products, but experience suggests no adverse outcome. **Salmeterol** was taken during the first trimester during 64 pregnancies and only during the second and third trimesters in three pregnancies.[304] The 67 pregnancies resulted in live births in 50, spontaneous abortion in 6, ectopic termination in 2, elective termination in 4, and unknown outcomes in 5 of these pregnancies. The small number of fetuses exposed to salmeterol during this study precludes any definitive conclusions about the safety of salmeterol during pregnancy. Albuterol, terbutaline, and **ritodrine** have been given in large IV or PO doses for their tocolytic effects in the third trimester without permanent harm to the fetus, although hypertension, hypoglycemia, hypokalemia, and hypocalcemia have been reported.[252] **Ephedrine** use during labor may cause altered neonatal sleep patterns.[252]
Thalidomide	Thalidomide, the first drug established as a human teratogen, causes bilateral limb reduction defects, facial hemangioma, esophageal or duodenal atresia, and anomalies of the external ears, kidneys, and heart. The time of greatest risk is between gestational days 22 and 32. If exposure occurs between days 27 and 30, the arms are most often affected; with exposure between days 30 and 33, the legs and arms are all affected.[2]

(continued)

DRUGS AND PREGNANCY (continued)

DRUG	NATURE OF EFFECT
Theophylline	No adverse fetal effects from long-term theophylline use during pregnancy are known.[108,109,201,202,305] Theophylline toxicity has been reported in three newborns whose mothers received theophylline or **aminophylline** in late pregnancy and during labor. Symptoms included jitteriness, vomiting, tachycardia, and irritability, all of which resolved in all cases.[24,108] Maternal theophylline pharmacokinetics may change during the second and third trimesters, with decreased theophylline protein binding, decreased nonrenal clearance, and increased renal clearance.[306] Both V_d and half-life increase during the third trimester.[306] Pregnant women should have theophylline concentrations monitored frequently for dosage adjustments.
Vaginal Spermicides	Vaginal spermicide use was associated with major congenital anomalies in two retrospective analyses, casting doubt on the results.[307,308] Subsequent studies, including a meta-analysis of nine studies, indicate a lack of association between these agents and congenital malformations.[219,309–312]
Vitamins	For **vitamin A**, *see* Retinoids. **Vitamin D** excess has been associated with an idiopathic hypercalcemic syndrome including cardiovascular malformation, abnormal bone mineralization, elfin facies, mental retardation, hypercalcemia, and nephrocalcinosis. Definitive conclusions await further investigation.[2,313,314]

DRUGS FOR NONMEDICAL USE

Alcohol	Animal studies show that alcohol and acetaldehyde exposure in utero results in morphologic changes in the structure as well as in protein and endocrine content of the CNS.[315–317] As many as 5% of human congenital anomalies may be due to maternal alcohol consumption,[318] and it may be responsible for 10% of all cases of mental retardation (alcohol is the most frequent recognizable cause of mental retardation).[318,319] A twofold increase in spontaneous abortion was noted among women who drank one to two drinks daily for the first 2 months of pregnancy; the rate was higher in those who drank more than two drinks daily. Moderate drinking (1–13 fl oz of absolute alcohol per week) is associated with an increase in some of the features of the fetal alcohol syndrome (FAS), including IUGR.[319,320] Alcohol-related birth defects may occur at rates higher than that of FAS, and CNS dysfunction may occur with lower alcohol exposure than that required to produce the FAS.[319] Chronic heavy alcohol consumption is associated with the full-blown FAS in 10–50% of children exposed in utero. Features of FAS include IUGR, microcephaly, postnatal growth deficiency, developmental delay, mental retardation, and craniofacial anomalies. Joint, limb, cardiac, ocular, brain, and urogenital defects along with eustachian tube dysfunction also occur as well as neonatal withdrawal symptoms similar to those in adults.[53,315–329] Alcohol consumption during pregnancy should be avoided, because the minimal dosage that may produce adverse fetal effects has not been established. One author proposed that the threshold dosage for alcohol teratogenesis may be 1 fl oz of absolute alcohol per day.[319] Eliminating or even reducing alcohol consumption at any time during pregnancy may improve fetal outcome and should be encouraged.

(continued)

DRUGS AND PREGNANCY (continued)

DRUG	NATURE OF EFFECT
Amphetamines	Data on the effect of prenatal amphetamines, both prescribed and abused, are conflicting; however, no consistent pattern of abnormalities has emerged.[24,330] Most studies found no increase in severe congenital malformations, but others report biliary atresia, congenital heart disease, and eye and CNS defects.[24,330] Reports of decreased birth weight and length, head circumference, and IUGR may be caused by poor maternal nutrition, but use of other drugs and alcohol may have confounded these findings. Investigations with term neonates exposed antenatally to **methamphetamine**, with or without cocaine, document an increased prevalence of prematurity, IUGR, altered behavioral patterns (abnormal sleep patterns, poor feeding, tremors, and hypertonia).[331,332] One case of labor onset 8 hr after ingestion of amphetamines resulted in emergency cesarean section for fetal distress.[333] The placenta appeared to be vasoconstricted and the infant died 4 days postpartum from respiratory arrest and intracranial bleeding. (See also Cocaine.)
Caffeine	Caffeine is not suspected of causing fetal malformations. Data suggest that caffeine use before and during pregnancy may increase the rate of spontaneous abortion, although substantiation of these data is required.[334,335] A small reduction in birthweight has been observed when caffeine consumption during pregnancy exceeded 300 mg/day; cigarette smoking may have contributed to these findings. There are conflicting data about whether 400–600 mg/day of caffeine increases the risk of miscarriage, stillbirth, or prematurity.[335–340] One study showed increased rates of infant central and obstructive apnea positively associated with increasing maternal caffeine consumption.[341]
Cocaine	Maternal cocaine use during pregnancy has been associated with adverse fetal and maternal outcomes. Although most data relate to use near term, preliminary findings suggest some risks from exposure early in pregnancy. Poor health care and nutrition, a high infection rate, and frequent concomitant drug (eg, narcotics, nicotine, marijuana) and alcohol use complicate risk evaluation. Maternal cocaine use is associated with an increase in the frequency of spontaneous abortion, placental hemorrhage, abruptio placentae, and still-births. There is also an increase in frequency of prematurity as well as premature rupture of the membranes. A few cases of precipitate delivery have been reported, as well as two cases of precipitate rupture of ectopic pregnancy. Fetal genitourinary malformations and intrauterine death in mothers who used cocaine have been reported.[342–347] Because of the very small number of studies, the association of other adverse effects with cocaine use are questionable. Reports published include small-for-gestational-age infants, micro-cephaly, CNS abnormalities, limb defects, abnormal facies, cardiovascular abnormalities, necrotizing enterocolitis and intestinal atresia, cranial-spinal abnormalities, and ophthal-mologic abnormalities (eg, optic nerve abnormalities, delayed visual maturation, prolonged eyelid edema).[329,343,346–361] Infants may experience a "withdrawal" syndrome consisting of jitteriness, tremor, hyperreflexia, hypertonia, irritability, high-pitched crying, frantic sucking, poor feeding, tachypnea, abnormal sleep patterns, vomiting, or loose stools. Neurologic signs of toxicity, including seizures, have also been reported. Exposed infants have an increased frequency of abnormal pneumograms, respiratory distress, or other cardiorespiratory abnormalities. Some authors feel these abnormalities may predispose infants to sudden infant death syndrome (SIDS). Retrospective population-based stud-ies found that the risk of SIDS in cocaine-exposed infants was higher than that of infants whose mothers did not abuse any drugs; however, several confounding risks *(continued)*

DRUGS AND PREGNANCY (continued)

DRUG	NATURE OF EFFECT
	for SIDS could not be controlled.[362,363] Several reports of neonatal or fetal cerebral infarction or intracranial hemorrhage exist.[342,343,360,364–394] A case of hydranencephaly in an infant exposed during the first few months of pregnancy might be explained by vasospasm in the internal carotid artery secondary to cocaine.[342,343,357,364–390,393,394]
Heroin	Determining adverse fetal effects related to heroin use is difficult. Poor health care and nutrition, lack of prenatal care, a high infection rate, and frequent concomitant nicotine, nonmedical drug, or alcohol use complicate risk assessment. No specific pattern of fetal malformation has been noted. Some studies have associated maternal heroin use with a decrease in birthweight and length, head circumference, small-for-gestational-age-infants, low Apgar scores, meconium staining, neonatal respiratory distress, jaundice, and increased neonatal mortality. A narcotic withdrawal syndrome occurs frequently, usually within the first 24–48 hr after birth, although it can be delayed for as long as 6 days. The symptoms, which have persisted for as long as 20 days, include irritability, feeding and sleeping problems, hyperactivity, excessive sneezing, yawning, vomiting, mucous secretion, sweating, and face scratching. Other withdrawal symptoms (including increased muscle tone, vague autonomic nervous system symptoms; tremulousness, high-pitched crying, frantic and uncoordinated sucking, and seizures) may occur in neonates born to narcotic-addicted women and nonaddicted women using narcotics near term. The frequency of withdrawal is directly related to the daily dosage and duration of maternal addiction. The results of studies evaluating development show conflicting results ranging from no effect to problems with behavior, perceptual, and organizational abilities.[22,24,391] One retrospective population-based study found that the relative risk of SIDS was 15.5 in infants of mothers who abused illicit opiates during all or part of pregnancy.[362]
Marijuana	Marijuana smoke contains carbon monoxide and may cause constriction of uterine and placental vessels resulting in fetal hypoxia and decreased nutrient supply.[392,395] Marijuana use during pregnancy has not been associated with any specific pattern of malformation, but exposures were confounded by nicotine and other nonmedical drug and alcohol use.[392,393,395–397]
Phencyclidine	Long-term phencyclidine use during pregnancy, especially near term, may produce neonatal withdrawal symptoms of hypertonicity, occasional darting eye movements, and lethargy, contrasted with coarse flappy tremors after stimulation. These infants have a marked increase in lability of behavioral states and poor consolability.[398,399] Some children at 9 and 18 months of age exhibited fine motor, adaptive, and language scores in the low-normal range. Motor movements in the lower extremities were also awkward.[392,398]

(continued)

DRUGS AND PREGNANCY (continued)

DRUG	NATURE OF EFFECT
Tobacco	Cigarette smoke contains numerous toxins, including carbon monoxide and **nicotine**, which are probably responsible for reported fetal hypoxia because of decreased oxygen exchange and by placental vasoconstriction.[400,401] Smoking during pregnancy is associated with increased rates of IUGR or low birth weight (5% decrease per pack smoked daily), prematurity, spontaneous abortion, neonatal and postnatal deaths, abruptio placentae, premature rupture of membranes, and placenta previa.[2,232,401–405] Such conditions occur particularly in women who are regular smokers of 10 or more cigarettes daily. Cigarette smoking has been shown to alter the placental arterial linings as well as to accelerate placental senescence, which may explain the placental complications associated with smoking.[401,404–406] One study involving 17,152 infants (15.7% of the mothers were smokers) found an increased frequency of minor malformations in infants of mothers aged 35 yr or older who smoked.[407] Some data suggest infants of smokers have increased nervous system excitation, hypertonicity, and altered breathing patterns with an increased rate of central apnea.[341,393,408] These children have also been shown to have altered language, auditory, and lower cognitive functions. Women exposed to second-hand or side-stream smoke may also be at risk for delivering a growth-retarded or preterm infant.[402] If a woman stops smoking by the 20th week of pregnancy, the risk of a low-birthweight infant is similar to that of the general population.[400] Tobacco chewing during pregnancy is also associated with a greatly increased rate of stillbirth, IUGR, and prematurity.[402] Some studies suggest an increased risk of childhood acute lymphocytic and lymphoblastic leukemias and lymphoma in those whose fathers and/or mothers smoked before or during pregnancy.[409,410]

■ REFERENCES

1. Wilson JG, Fraser RC, eds. *Handbook of teratology.* Vol I. General principles and etiology. New York: Plenum Press; 1977.
2. Beckman DA, Brent RL. Mechanism of known environmental teratogens: drugs and chemicals. *Clin Perinatol* 1986;13:649–87.
3. Brent RL. The complexities of solving the problem of human malformations. *Clin Perinatol* 1986;13:491–503.
4. Friedman JM et al. Potential human teratogenicity of frequently prescribed drugs. *Obstet Gynecol* 1990;75:594–9.
5. Pagliaro LA, Pagliaro AM, eds. *Problems in pediatric drug therapy,* 3rd ed. Hamilton, IL: Drug Intelligence Publications; 1995.
6. Chow AW, Jewesson PJ. Pharmacokinetics and safety of antimicrobial agents during pregnancy. *Rev Infect Dis* 1985;7:287–313.
7. Berlin CM. Effects of drugs on the fetus. *Pediatr Rev* 1991;12:282–7.
8. Landers DV et al. Antibiotic use during pregnancy and the postpartum period. *Clin Obstet Gynecol* 1983;26:391–406.
9. Murray L, Seger D. Drug therapy during pregnancy and lactation. *Emerg Med Clin North Am* 1994;12:129–49.
10. Pacifici GM, Nottoli R. Placental transfer of drugs administered to the mother. *Clin Pharmacokinet* 1995;28:235–69.
11. Frey BM, O'Donnell J. Drug therapy in pregnancy and lactation. *J Pharm Pract* 1989;2:2–12.
12. Kramer MS. Intrauterine growth and gestational duration determinants. *Pediatrics* 1987;80:502–11.
13. Streissguth AP et al. Aspirin and acetaminophen use by pregnant women and subsequent child IQ and attention decrements. *Teratology* 1987;35:211–9.
14. Heymann MA. Non-narcotic analgesics: use in pregnancy and fetal and perinatal effects. *Drugs* 1986;32(suppl 4):164–76.
15. Ludmir J et al. Maternal acetaminophen overdose at 15 weeks of gestation. *Obstet Gynecol* 1986;67:750–1.
16. McElhatton PR et al. Paracetamol poisoning in pregnancy: an analysis of the outcomes of cases referred to the teratology information service of the national poisons information service. *Hum Exp Toxicol* 1990;9:147–53.
17. Rosevear SK, Hope PL. Favourable neonatal outcome following maternal paracetamol overdose and severe fetal distress: case report. *Br J Obstet Gynaecol* 1989;96:491–3.
18. Robertson RG et al. Acetaminophen overdose in the second trimester of pregnancy. *J Fam Pract* 1986;23:267–8.
19. Kurzel RB. Can acetaminophen excess result in maternal and fetal toxicity? *South Med J* 1990;83:953–5.
20. Kirshon B et al. Effect of acetaminophen on fetal acid-base balance in chorioamnionitis. *J Reprod Med* 1989;34:955–9.
21. Edelin KC et al. Methadone maintenance in pregnancy: consequences to care and outcome. *Obstet Gynecol* 1988;71:399–404.
22. Lifschitz MH et al. Factors affecting head growth and intellectual function in children of drug addicts. *Pediatrics* 1985;75:269–74.
23. Kaltenbach KA, Finnegan LP. Prenatal narcotic exposure: perinatal and developmental effects. *Neurotoxicology* 1989;10:597–604.
24. Briggs GG et al. *Drugs in pregnancy and lactation,* 3rd ed. Baltimore: Williams & Wilkins; 1990.
25. Roy S, Basu RK. Role of sublingual administration of tablet buprenorphine hydrochloride on relief of labour pain. *J Indian Med Assoc* 1992;90:151–3.
26. Hatjis CG, Meis PJ. Sinusoidal fetal heart rate pattern associated with butorphanol administration. *Obstet Gynecol* 1986;67:377–80.
27. Savona-Ventura C et al. Pethidine blood concentrations at time of birth. *Int J Gynecol Obstet* 1991;36:103–7.
28. Righard L, Alade M-O. Effect of delivery room routines on success of first breast feed. *Lancet* 1990;336:1105–7.
29. Curran MJA. Options for labor analgesia: techniques of epidural and spinal analgesia. *Semin Perinatol* 1991;15:348–57.
30. Dan U et al. Intravenous pethidine and nalbuphine during labor: a prospective double-blind comparative study. *Gynecol Obstet Invest* 1991;32:39–43.
31. Wittmann BK, Segal S. Comparison of the effects of single- and split-dose methadone administration on the fetus: ultrasound evaluation. *Int J Addiction* 1991;26:213–8.
32. Little BB et al. Effects of T's and blues abuse on pregnancy outcome and infant health status. *Am J Perinatol* 1990;7:359–62.
33. Brooks PM, Needs CJ. The use of antirheumatic medication during pregnancy and in the puerperium. *Rheum Dis Clin North Am* 1989;15:789–806.
34. Klipple GL, Cecere FA. Rheumatoid arthritis and pregnancy. *Rheum Dis Clin North Am* 1989;15:213–39.

35. Kirshon B et al. Influence of short-term indomethacin therapy on fetal urine output. *Obstet Gynecol* 1988;72:51–3.

36. Moise KJ et al. Indomethacin in the treatment of premature labor: effects on the fetal ductus arteriosus. *N Engl J Med* 1988;319:327–31.

37. Morales WJ et al. Efficacy and safety of indomethacin versus ritodrine in the management of preterm labor: a randomized study. *Obstet Gynecol* 1989;74:567–72.

38. Hallak M et al. Indomethacin for preterm labor: fetal toxicity in a dizygotic twin gestation. *Obstet Gynecol* 1991;78:911–3.

39. Wurtzel D. Prenatal administration of indomethacin as a tocolytic agent: effect on neonatal renal function. *Obstet Gynecol* 1990;76:689–92.

40. Hickok DE et al. The association between decreased amniotic fluid volume and treatment with nonsteroidal anti-inflammatory agents for preterm labor. *Am J Obstet Gynecol* 1989;160:1525–31.

41. Werler MM et al. The relation of aspirin use during the first trimester of pregnancy to congenital cardiac defects. *N Engl J Med* 1989;321:1639–42.

42. Rudolph AM. Effects of aspirin and acetaminophen in pregnancy and in the newborn. *Arch Intern Med* 1981;141:358–63.

43. Benigni A et al. Effect of low-dose aspirin on fetal and maternal generation of thromboxane by platelets in women at risk for pregnancy-induced hypertension. *N Engl J Med* 1989;321:357–62.

44. Sibai BM et al. Low-dose aspirin in pregnancy. *Obstet Gynecol* 1989;74:551–7.

45. Schiff E et al. The use of aspirin to prevent pregnancy-induced hypertension and lower the ratio of thromboxane A2 to prostacyclin in relatively high risk pregnancies. *N Engl J Med* 1989;321:351–6.

46. Parazzini F et al. Follow-up of children in the Italian Study of Aspirin in Pregnancy. *Lancet* 1994;343:1235. Letter.

47. Barry WS et al. Ibuprofen overdose and exposure in utero: results from a postmarketing voluntary reporting system. *Am J Med* 1984;77(suppl 1a):35–9.

48. Hall JG et al. Maternal and fetal sequelae of anticoagulation during pregnancy. *Am J Med* 1980;68:122–40.

49. Ginsberg JS et al. Risks to the fetus of anticoagulant therapy during pregnancy. *Thromb Haemost* 1989;61:197–203.

50. Ginsberg JS, Hirsh J. Use of anticoagulants during pregnancy. *Chest* 1989;95(suppl):156S–60.

51. Nageotte MP et al. Anticoagulation in pregnancy. *Am J Obstet Gynecol* 1981;141:472–3.

52. Iturbe-Alessio I et al. Risks of anticoagulant therapy in pregnant women with artificial heart valves. *N Engl J Med* 1986;315:1390–3.

53. Cohen MM. Syndromology: an updated conceptual overview. VII. Aspects of teratogenesis. *Int J Oral Maxillofac Surg* 1990;19:26–32.

54. Born D et al. Pregnancy in patients with prosthetic heart valves: the effects of anticoagulation on mother, fetus, and neonate. *Am Heart J* 1992;124:413–7.

55. Gärtner BC et al. Phenprocoumon therapy during pregnancy: case report and comparison of the teratogenic risk of different coumarin derivatives. *Z Geburtshilfe Perinatol* 1993;197:262–5.

56. Pati S, Helmbrecht GD. Congenital schizencephaly associated with in utero warfarin exposure. *Reprod Toxicol* 1994;8:115–20.

57. Normann EK, Stray-Pedersen B. Warfarin-induced fetal diaphragmatic hernia: case report. *Br J Obstet Gynaecol* 1989;96:729–30.

58. Kaneko S. Antiepileptic drug therapy and reproductive consequences: functional and morphologic effects. *Reprod Toxicol* 1991;5:179–98.

59. Dravet C et al. Epilepsy, antiepileptic drugs, and malformations in children of women with epilepsy: a French prospective cohort study. *Neurology* 1992;42(suppl 5):75–82.

60. Waters CH et al. Outcomes of pregnancy associated with antiepileptic drugs. *Arch Neurol* 1994;51:250–3.

61. Gaily E, Granström M-L. Minor anomalies in children of mothers with epilepsy. *Neurology* 1992;42(suppl 5):128–31.

62. Koch S et al. Major and minor birth malformations and antiepileptic drugs. *Neurology* 1992;42(suppl 5):83–8.

63. Yerby MS et al. Antiepileptics and the development of congenital anomalies. *Neurology* 1992;42(suppl 5):132–40.

64. Yerby MS. Problems and management of the pregnant woman with epilepsy. *Epilepsia* 1987;28(suppl 3):S29–36.

65. Froscher W. Teratogenic effects of anti-epileptic drugs. *Drugs Today* 1989;25:563–7.

66. Lindhout D et al. Antiepileptic drugs and teratogenesis in two consecutive cohorts: changes in prescription policy paralleled by changes in pattern of malformations. *Neurology* 1992;42(suppl 5):94–110.

67. Lander CM, Eadie MJ. Antiepileptic drug intake during pregnancy and malformed offspring. *Epilepsy Res* 1990;7:77–82.

68. Sharony R, Graham JM. Identification of fetal problems associated with anticonvulsant usage and maternal epilepsy. *Obstet Gynecol Clin North Am* 1991;18:933–51.

69. Finnell RH et al. Clinical and experimental studies linking oxidative metabolism to phenytoin-induced teratogenesis. *Neurology* 1992;42(suppl 5):25–31.

70. Omtzigt JGC et al. The 10,11-epoxide-10,11-diol pathway of carbamazepine in early pregnancy in maternal serum, urine, and amniotic fluid: effect of dose, comedication, and relation to outcome of pregnancy. *Ther Drug Monit* 1993;15:1–10.

71. Van Dyke DC et al. Differences in phenytoin biotransformation and susceptibility to congenital malformations: a review. *DICP* 1991;25:987–92.

72. Yerby MS et al. Antiepileptic drug disposition during pregnancy. *Neurology* 1992;42(suppl 5):12–6.

73. Luef G et al. Management of epilepsy. *Lancet* 1990;336:1126–7. Letter.

74. van der Pol MC et al. Antiepileptic medication in pregnancy: late effects on the children's central nervous system development. *Am J Obstet Gynecol* 1991;164:121–8.

75. Saunders M. Epilepsy in women of childbearing age. *Br Med J* 1989;299:581.

76. Jones KL et al. Teratogenic effects of carbamazepine. *N Engl J Med* 1989;321:1481. Letter.

77. Scialli AR, Lione A. Teratogenic effects of carbamazepine. *N Engl J Med* 1989;321:1480. Letter.

78. Elia J et al. Teratogenicity of psychotherapeutic medications. *Psychopharmacol Bull* 1987;23:531–86.

79. Rosa FW. Spina bifida in infants of women treated with carbamazepine during pregnancy. *N Engl J Med* 1991;324:674–7.

80. Källén AJB. Maternal carbamazepine and infant spina bifida. *Reprod Toxicol* 1994;8:203–5.

81. Oakeshott P, Hunt GM. Carbamazepine and spina bifida. *BMJ* 1991;303:651.

82. Lindhout D et al. Teratogenicity of antiepileptic drug combinations with special emphasis on epoxidation (of carbamazepine). *Epilepsia* 1984;25:77–83.

83. Kaneko S et al. Teratogenicity of antiepileptic drugs: analysis of possible risk factors. *Epilepsia* 1988;29:459–67.

84. Jones KL et al. Pattern of malformations in the children of women treated with carbamazepine during pregnancy. *N Engl J Med* 1989;320:1661–6.

85. Gladstone DJ et al. Course of pregnancy and fetal outcome following maternal exposure to carbamazepine and phenytoin: a prospective study. *Reprod Toxicol* 1992;6:257–61.

86. Vestermark V, Vestermark S. Teratogenic effect of carbamazepine. *Arch Dis Child* 1991;66:641–2.

87. Smith DW. *Recognizable patterns of human malformation*, 3rd ed. Philadelphia: WB Saunders; 1982.

88. Biale Y, Lewenthal H. Effect of folic acid supplementation on congenital malformations due to anticonvulsive drugs. *Eur J Obstet Gynecol Reprod Biol* 1984;18:211–6.

89. Finnell RH. Genetic differences in susceptibility to anticonvulsant drug-induced developmental defects. *Pharmacol Toxicol* 1991;69:223–7.

90. Hopkins A. Epilepsy and anticonvulsant drugs. *Br Med J* 1987;294:497–501.

91. Lipson A, Bale P. Ependymoblastoma associated with prenatal exposure to diphenylhydantoin and methylphenobarbitone. *Cancer* 1985;55:1859–62.

92. Dickinson RG et al. The effect of pregnancy in humans on the pharmacokinetics of stable isotope labelled phenytoin. *Br J Clin Pharmacol* 1989;28:17–27.

93. Scolnik D et al. Neurodevelopment of children exposed in utero to phenytoin and carbamazepine monotherapy. *JAMA* 1994;271:767–70.

94. Adams J et al. Developmental neurotoxicity of anticonvulsants: human and animal evidence on phenytoin. *Neurotoxicol Teratol* 1990;12:203–14.

95. Kotzot D et al. Hydantoin syndrome with holoprosencephaly: a possible rare teratogenic effect. *Teratology* 1993;48:15–9.

96. Squier W et al. Neocerebellar hypoplasia in a neonate following intra-uterine exposure to anticonvulsants. *Dev Med Child Neurol* 1990;32:737–42.

97. Nanda A et al. Fetal hydantoin syndrome: a case report. *Pediatr Dermatol* 1989;6:130–3.

98. Hobbins JC. Diagnosis and management of neural-tube defects today. *N Engl J Med* 1991;324:690–1.

99. Garden AS et al. Valproic acid therapy and neural tube defects. *Arch Neurol* 1985;132:933–6.

100. Tein I, MacGregor DL. Possible valproate teratogenicity. *Arch Neurol* 1985;42:291–3.

101. Verloes A et al. Proximal phocomelia and radial ray aplasia in fetal valproic syndrome. *Eur J Pediatr* 1990;149:266–7.

102. Hubert A et al. Aplasia cutis congenita of the scalp in an infant exposed to valproic acid in utero. *Acta Paediatr* 1994;83:789–90.

103. Sharony R et al. Preaxial ray reduction defects as part of valproic acid embryofetopathy. *Prenatal Diag* 1993;13:909–18.

104. Nau H et al. Valproic acid-induced neural tube defects in mouse and human: aspects of chirality, alternative drug development, pharmacokinetics, and possible mechanisms. *Pharmacol Toxicol* 1991;69:310–21.

105. Howden CW. Treatment of common minor ailments. *Br Med J* 1986;293:1549–50.

106. Leathem AM. Safety and efficacy of antiemetics used to treat nausea and vomiting in pregnancy. *Clin Pharm* 1986;5:660–8.

107. McKeigue PM et al. Bendectin and birth defects: I. a meta-analysis of the epidemiologic studies. *Teratology* 1994;50:27–37.

108. Ziment I, Au JP. Managing asthma in the pregnant patient. *J Respir Dis* 1988;9:66–74.

109. Mawhinney H, Spector SL. Optimum management of asthma in pregnancy. *Drugs* 1986:32;178–87.

110. Seto A et al.Evaluation of brompheniramine safety in pregnancy. *Reprod Toxicol* 1993;7:393–5. Letter.

111. Lewis JH et al. The use of gastrointestinal drugs during pregnancy and lactation. *Am J Gastroenterol* 1985;80:912–23.

112. Anon. Safety of antimicrobial drugs in pregnancy. *Med Lett Drugs Ther* 1987;29:61–3.

113. Holdiness MR. Teratology of the antituberculosis drugs. *Early Hum Dev* 1987;15:61–74.

114. Pedler SJ, Bint AJ. Management of bacteriuria in pregnancy. *Drugs* 1987;33:413–21.

115. Wolfe MS, Cordero JF. Safety of chloroquine in chemosuppression of malaria during pregnancy. *Br Med J* 1985;290:1466–7.

116. Ellis CJ. Antiparasitic agents in pregnancy. *Clin Obstet Gynecol* 1986;13:269–74.

117. Levy M et al. Pregnancy outcome following first trimester exposure to chloroquine. *Am J Perinatol* 1991;8:174–8.

118. Pajor A. Pancytopenia in a patient given pyrimethamine and sulphamethoxidiazine during pregnancy. *Arch Gynecol Obstet* 1990;247:215–7.

119. Chapman ST. Bacterial infections in pregnancy. *Clin Obstet Gynecol* 1986;13:397–417.

120. Cruikshank DP, Warenski JC. First-trimester maternal *Listeria* monocytogenes sepsis and chorioamnionitis with normal neonatal outcome. *Obstet Gynecol* 1989;73:469–71.

121. Klein VR et al. The Jarisch-Herxheimer reaction complicating syphilotherapy in pregnancy. *Obstet Gynecol* 1990;75:375–80.

122. Soper DE, Merrill-Nach S. Successful therapy of penicillinase-producing *Neisseria gonorrhoeae* pharyngeal infection during pregnancy. *Obstet Gynecol* 1986;68:290–1.

123. Czeizel A. A case-control analysis of the teratogenic effects of co-trimoxazole. *Reprod Toxicol* 1990;4:305–13.

124. Landsberger EJ et al. Successful management of varicella pneumonia complicating pregnancy: a report of three cases. *J Reprod Med* 1986;31:311–4.

125. Kelly RT, Bibbins B. Pregnancy and brucellosis. *Tex Med* 1987;83:39–41.

126. Bailey RR et al. Comparison of single dose with a five-day course of trimethoprim for asymptomatic (covert) bacteriuria of pregnancy. *N Z Med J* 1986;99:501–3.

127. Anon. Dapsone. In Barnhart ER, ed. *Physicians' desk reference*, 44th ed. Oradell, NJ: Medical Economics; 1990:1079–80.

128. Thornton YS, Bowe ET. Neonatal hyperbilirubinemia after treatment of maternal leprosy. *South Med J* 1989;82:668.

129. Hailey FJ et al. Foetal safety of nitrofurantoin macrocrystals therapy during pregnancy: a retrospective analysis. *J Int Med Res* 1983;11:364–9.

130. D'Arcy PF. Nitrofurantoin. *Drug Intell Clin Pharm* 1985;19:540–7.

131. Personal communication, Carol A. Bixler, Norwich Eaton Pharmaceuticals, February 12, 1991.

132. Brown ZA, Baker DA. Acyclovir therapy during pregnancy. *Obstet Gynecol* 1989;73:526–31.

133. Leen CLS et al. Acyclovir and pregnancy. *Br Med J* 1987;294:308. Letter.

134. Hankins GDV et al. Acyclovir treatment of varicella pneumonia in pregnancy. *Crit Care Med* 1987;15:336–7.

135. Boyd K, Walker E. Use of acyclovir to treat chickenpox in pregnancy. *Br Med J* 1988;296:393–4.

136. Eder SE et al. *Varicella* pneumonia during pregnancy: treatment of two cases with acyclovir. *Am J Perinatol* 1988;5:16–8.

137. Klein NA et al. Herpes simplex virus hepatitis in pregnancy. Two patients successfully treated with acyclovir. *Gastroenterology* 1991;100:239–44.

138. Anon. Pregnancy outcomes following systemic prenatal acyclovir exposure—June 1, 1984–June 30, 1993. *MMWR* 1993;42:806–9.

139. Amon I. Placental transfer of metronidazole. *J Perinat Med* 1985;13:97–8. Letter.

140. Drinkwater P. Metronidazole. *Aust N Z J Obstet Gynaecol* 1987;27:228–30.

141. Roe FJC. Safety of nitroimidazoles. *Scand J Infect Dis* 1985;46(suppl):72–81.

142. Piper JM et al. Prenatal use of metronidazole and birth defects: no association. *Obstet Gynecol* 1993;82:348–52.

143. Greenberg F. Possible metronidazole teratogenicity and clefting. *Am J Med Genetics* 1985;22:825. Letter.

144. Reyes MP et al. Vancomycin during pregnancy: does it cause hearing loss or nephrotoxicity in the infant? *Am J Obstet Gynecol* 1989;161:977–81.

145. Sperling RS et al. A survey of zidovudine use in pregnant women with human immunodeficiency virus infection. *N Engl J Med* 1992;326:857–61.

146. Anon. Birth outcomes following zidovudine therapy in pregnant women. *MMWR* 1994;43:409,415–6.

147. Kumar RM et al. Zidovudine use in pregnancy: a report on 104 cases and the occurrence of birth defects. *J Acquir Immune Defic Syndr* 1994;7:1034–9.

148. Chavanet P et al. Perinatal pharmacokinetics of zidovudine. *N Engl J Med* 1989;321:1548–9. Letter.

149. Watts DH et al. Pharmacokinetic disposition of zidovudine during pregnancy. *J Infect Dis* 1991;163:226–32.

150. Kim DS, Park MI. Maternal and fetal survival following surgery and chemotherapy of endodermal sinus tumor of the ovary during pregnancy: a case report. *Obstet Gynecol* 1989;73:503–7.

151. Selevan SG et al. A study of occupational exposure to antineoplastic drugs and fetal loss in nurses. *N Engl J Med* 1985;313:1173–8.

152. Raffles A et al. Transplacental effects of maternal cancer chemotherapy. Case report. *Br J Obstet Gynaecol* 1989;96:1099–100.

153. Odom LD et al. 5-fluorouracil exposure during the period of conception: report on two cases. *Am J Obstet Gynecol* 1990;163:76–7.

154. Kirshon B et al. Teratogenic effects of first-trimester cyclophosphamide therapy. *Obstet Gynecol* 1988;72:462–4.

155. Zemlickis D et al. Teratogenicity and carcinogenicity in a twin exposed in utero to cyclophosphamide. *Teratogenesis Carcinog Mutagen* 1993;13:139–43.

156. Kopelman JN, Miyazawa K. Inadvertent 5-fluorouracil treatment in early pregnancy: a report of three cases. *Reprod Toxicol* 1990;4:233–5.

157. Van Le L et al. Accidental use of low-dose 5-fluorouracil in pregnancy. *J Reprod Med* 1991;36:872–4.

158. Kozlowski RD et al. Outcome of first-trimester exposure to low-dose methotrexate in eight patients with rheumatic disease. *Am J Med* 1990;88:589–92.

159. Blatt J et al. Pregnancy outcome following cancer chemotherapy. *Am J Med* 1980;69:828–32.

160. Artlich A et al. Teratogenic effects in a case of maternal treatment for acute myelocytic leukaemia—neonatal and infantile course. *Eur J Pediatr* 1994;153:488–91.

161. Korelitz BI. Pregnancy, fertility, and inflammatory bowel disease. *Am J Gastroenterol* 1985;80:365–70.

162. Alstead EM et al. Safety of azathioprine in pregnancy in inflammatory bowel disease. *Gastroenterology* 1990;99:443–6.

163. Pickrell MD et al. Pregnancy after renal transplantation: severe intrauterine growth retardation during treatment with cyclosporin A. *Br Med J* 1988;296:825.

164. Pujals JM et al. Osseous malformation in baby born to woman on cyclosporin. *Lancet* 1989;1:667. Letter.

165. Haagsma EB et al. Successful pregnancy after orthotopic liver transplantation. *Obstet Gynecol* 1989;74:442–3.

166. Burrows DA et al. Successful twin pregnancy after renal transplant maintained on cyclosporine A immunosuppression. *Obstet Gynecol* 1988;72:459–61.

167. Plomp TA et al. Use of amiodarone during pregnancy. *Eur J Obstet Gynecol Reprod Biol* 1992;43:201–7.

168. Lees KR, Rubin PC. Treatment of cardiovascular diseases. *Br Med J* 1987;294:358–60.

169. Moriguchi Mitani G et al. The pharmacokinetics of antiarrhythmic agents in pregnancy and lactation. *Clin Pharmacokinet* 1987;12:253–91.

170. Kaler SG et al. Hypertrichosis and congenital anomalies associated with maternal use of minoxidil. *Pediatrics* 1987;79:434–6.

171. Al Kasab SM et al. β-Adrenergic receptor blockade in the management of pregnant women with mitral stenosis. *Am J Obstet Gynecol* 1990;163:37–40.

172. Ellenbogen A et al. Metabolic effects of pindolol on both mother and fetus. *Curr Ther Res* 1988;43:1038–41.

173. Lyons CW, Colmorgen GHC. Medical management of pheochromocytoma in pregnancy. *Obstet Gynecol* 1988;72:450–1.

174. Lubbe WF. Hypertension in pregnancy: pathophysiology and management. *Drugs* 1984;28:170–88.

175. Devoe LD et al. Metastatic pheochromocytoma in pregnancy and fetal biophysical assessment after maternal administration of alpha-adrenergic, beta-adrenergic, and dopamine antagonists. *Obstet Gynecol* 1986;68 (suppl):15S–8.

176. Haraldsson A, Geven W. Severe adverse effects of maternal labetalol in a premature infant. *Acta Paediatr Scand* 1989;78:956–8.

177. Ducey JP, Knape KG. Maternal esmolol administration resulting in fetal distress and cesarean section in a term pregnancy. *Anesthesiology* 1992;77:829–32.

178. Naden RP, Redman CWG. Antihypertensive drugs in pregnancy. *Clin Perinatol* 1985;12:521–38.

179. Haraldsson A, Geven W. Half-life of maternal labetalol in a premature infant. *Pharm Weekbl Sci* 1989;11:229–31.

180. Rosa FW et al. Neonatal anuria with maternal angiotensin-converting enzyme inhibition. *Obstet Gynecol* 1989;74:371–4.

181. Mehta N, Modi N. ACE inhibitors in pregnancy. *Lancet* 1989;2:96. Letter.

182. Cunniff C et al. Oligohydramnios sequence and renal tubular malformation associated with maternal enalapril use. *Am J Obstet Gynecol* 1990;162:187–9.

183. Piper JM et al. Pregnancy outcome following exposure to angiotensin-converting enzyme inhibitors. *Obstet Gynecol* 1992;80:429–32.

184. Wide-Swensson D et al. Effects of isradipine, a new calcium antagonist, on maternal cardiovascular system and uterine activity in labour. *Br J Obstet Gynaecol* 1990;97:945–9.

185. Thaler I et al. Effect of calcium channel blocker nifedipine on uterine artery flow velocity waveforms. *J Ultrasound Med* 1991;10:301–4.

186. Moretti MM et al. The effect of nifedipine therapy on fetal and placental Doppler waveforms in preeclampsia remote from term. *Am J Obstet Gynecol* 1990;163:1844–8.

187. Mabie WC et al. Chronic hypertension in pregnancy. *Obstet Gynecol* 1986;67:197–205.

188. Sibai BM et al. Effects of diuretics on plasma volume in pregnancies with long-term hypertension. *Am J Obstet Gynecol* 1984;150:831–5.

189. Doan-Wiggins L. Drug therapy for obstetric emergencies. *Emerg Med Clin North Am* 1994;12:257–3.

190. Koren G, Zemlickis DM. Outcome of pregnancy after first trimester exposure to H₂ receptor antagonists. *Am J Perinatol* 1991;8:37–8.

191. Qvist N et al. Cimetidine as pre-anesthetic agent for cesarean section: perinatal effects on the infant, the placental transfer of cimetidine and its elimination in the infants. *J Perinat Med* 1985;13:179–83.

192. Ikenoue T et al. Effects of ranitidine on maternal gastric juice and neonates when administered prior to caesarean section. *Aliment Pharmacol Ther* 1991;5:315–8.

193. Baiocco PJ, Korelitz BI. The influence of inflammatory bowel disease and its treatment on pregnancy and fetal outcome. *J Clin Gastroenterol* 1984;6:211–6.

194. Meyers S, Sachar DB. Medical management of Crohn's disease. *Hepatogastroenterology* 1990;37:42–55.

195. Saenger P. Abnormal sex differentiation. *J Pediatr* 1984;104:1–17.

196. Brunskill PJ. The effect of fetal exposure to danazol. *Br J Obstet Gynaecol* 1992;99:212–5.

197. Fischer K. A rapid evolution mechanism may contribute to changes in sex ratio, multiple birth incidence, frequency of autoimmune disease and frequency of birth defects in Clomid conceptions. *Med Hypotheses* 1990;31:59–65.

198. Wramsby H et al. Chromosome analysis of human oocytes recovered from preovulatory follicles in stimulated cycles. *N Engl J Med* 1987;316:121–4.

199. Shoham Z et al. Early miscarriage and fetal malformations after induction of ovulation (by clomiphene citrate and/or human menotropins), in vitro fertilization, and gamete intrafallopian transfer. *Fertil Steril* 1991;55:1–11.

200. Mills JL et al. Risk of neural tube defects in relation to maternal fertility and fertility drug use. *Lancet* 1990;336:103–4.

201. Noble PW et al. Respiratory diseases in pregnancy. *Obstet Gynecol Clin North Am* 1988;15:391–428.

202. Greenberger PA, Patterson R. Management of asthma during pregnancy. *N Engl J Med* 1985;312:897–902.

203. Fitzsimons R et al. Outcome of pregnancy in women requiring corticosteroids for severe asthma. *J Allergy Clin Immunol* 1986;78:349–53.

204. Avery ME et al. Update on prenatal steroid for prevention of respiratory distress. *Am J Obstet Gynecol* 1986;155:2–5.

205. Van Marter LJ et al. Maternal glucocorticoid therapy and reduced risk of bronchopulmonary dysplasia. *Pediatrics* 1990;86:331–6.

206. Smolder-de Haas H et al. Physical development and medical history of children who were treated antenatally with corticosteroids to prevent respiratory distress syndrome: a 10- to 12-year follow-up. *Pediatrics* 1990;85:65–70.

207. Melnick S et al. Rates and risks of diethylstilbestrol-related clear-cell adenocarcinoma of the vagina and cervix. An update. *N Engl J Med* 1987;316:514–6.

208. Anon. Infertility among daughters exposed to diethylstilbestrol. *Drug Newsl* 1988;7:59. Abstract.

209. Adams DM et al. Intrapartum uterine rupture. *Obstet Gynecol* 1989;73:471–3.

210. Claman P, Berger MJ. Phenotypic differences in upper genital tract abnormalities and reproductive history in dizygotic twins exposed to diethylstilbestrol. *J Reprod Med* 1990;35:431–3.

211. McFarlane MJ et al. Diethylstilbestrol and clear cell vaginal carcinoma: reappraisal of the epidemiologic evidence. *Am J Med* 1986;81:855–63.

212. Leary FJ et al. Males exposed in utero to diethylstilbestrol. *JAMA* 1984;252:2984–9.

213. Singhi S et al. Iatrogenic neonatal and maternal hyponatraemia following oxytocin and aqueous glucose infusion during labour. *Br J Obstet Gynaecol* 1985;92:356–63.

214. Harris EL. Genetic epidemiology of hypospadias. *Epidemiol Rev* 1990;12:29–40.

215. Blickstein I, Katz Z. Possible relationship of bladder exstrophy and epispadias with progestins taken during early pregnancy. *Br J Urol* 1991;68:105–6.

216. Stoll C et al. Genetic and environmental factors in hypospadias. *J Med Genet* 1990;27:559–63.

217. Anon. Progestational drug birth defects warning statement. *FDC Rep* 1987;49(2):T&G1–2.

218. Lammer EJ, Cordero JF. Exogenous sex hormone exposure and the risk for major malformations. *JAMA* 1986;255:3128–32.

219. Simpson JL, Phillips OP. Spermicides, hormonal contraception and congenital malformations. *Adv Contraception* 1990;6:141–67.

220. Schönhöfer PS. Brazil: misuse of misoprostol as an abortifacient may induce malformations. *Lancet* 1991;337:1534–5.

221. Gonzalez CH et al. Limb deficiency with or without Möbius sequence in seven Brazilian children associated with misoprostol use in the first trimester of pregnancy. *Am J Med Genet* 1993;47:59–64.

222. Castilla EE, Orioli IM. Teratogenicity of misoprostol: data from the Latin-American Collaborative Study of Congenital Malformations (ECLAMC). *Am J Med Genet* 1994;51:161–2. Letter.

223. Fonseca W et al. Misoprostol and congenital malformations. *Lancet* 1991;338:56. Letter.

224. Sorokin Y et al. Effects of induction of labor with prostaglandin E_2 on fetal breathing and body movements: controlled, randomized, double-blind study. *Obstet Gynecol* 1992;80:788–91.

225. Papageorgiou I et al. Labor characteristics of uncomplicated prolonged pregnancies after induction with intracervical prostaglandin E_2 gel versus intravenous oxytocin. *Gynecol Obstet Invest* 1992;34:92–6.

226. Ray DA, Garite TJ. Prostaglandin E_2 for induction of labor in patients with premature rupture of membranes at term. *Am J Obstet Gynecol* 1992;166:836–43.

227. Rosenn B et al. Minor congenital malformations in infants of insulin-dependent diabetic women: association with poor glycemic control. *Obstet Gynecol* 1990;70:745–9.

228. Piacquadio K et al. Effects of in-utero exposure to oral hypoglycaemic drugs. *Lancet* 1991;338:866–9.

229. Hellmuth E et al. Congenital malformations in offspring of diabetic women treated with oral hypoglycaemic agents during embryogenesis. *Diabetic Med* 1994;11:471–4.

230. Saili A, Sarna MS. Tolbutamide: teratogenic effects. *Indian Pediatr* 1991;28:936–40.

231. Elliott BD et al. Insignificant transfer of glyburide occurs across the human placenta. *Am J Obstet Gynecol* 1991;165:807–12.

232. Kramer MS et al. Determinants of fetal growth and body proportionality. *Pediatrics* 1990;86:18–26.

233. Mestman JH. Thyroid disease in pregnancy. *Clin Perinatol* 1985;12:651–7.

234. Momotani N et al. Antithyroid drug therapy for Graves' disease during pregnancy. *N Engl J Med* 1986;315:24–8.

235. Martinez-Frias ML et al. Methimazole in animal feed and congenital aplasia cutis. *Lancet* 1992;339:742–3. Letter.

236. Calabrese JR, Gulledge AD. Psychotropics during pregnancy and lactation: a review. *Psychosomatics* 1985;26:413–29.

237. Pastuszak A et al. Pregnancy outcome following first-trimester exposure to fluoxetine (Prozac). *JAMA* 1993;269:2246–8.

238. Goldstein DJ, Marvel DE. Psychotropic medications during pregnancy: risk to the fetus. *JAMA* 1993;270:2177. Letter.

239. Chambers CD et al. Birth outcomes in pregnant women taking fluoxetine. *N Engl J Med* 1996;335:1010–5.

240. Zalzstein E et al. A case-control study on the association between first trimester exposure to lithium and Ebstein's anomaly. *Am J Cardiol* 1990;65:817–8.

241. Warkany J. Teratogen update: lithium. *Teratology* 1988;38:593–6.

242. Chapman WS. Lithium use during pregnancy. *J Fla Med Assoc* 1989;76:454–8.

243. Jacobson SJ et al. Prospective multicentre study of pregnancy outcome after lithium exposure during first trimester. *Lancet* 1992;339:530–3.

244. Cohen LS et al. A reevaluation of risk of in utero exposure to lithium. *JAMA* 1994;271:146–50.

245. Ang MS et al. Maternal lithium therapy and polyhydramnios. *Obstet Gynecol* 1990;76:517–9.

246. Marken PA et al. Treatment of psychosis in pregnancy. *DICP* 1989;23:598–9.

247. Kallen B, Mazze RI. Neural tube defects and first trimester operations. *Teratology* 1990;41:717–20.

248. Sylvester GC et al. First-trimester anesthesia exposure and the risk of central nervous system defects: a population-based case-control study. *Am J Public Health* 1994;84:1757–60.

249. Baeder Ch, Albrecht M. Embryotoxic/teratogenic potential of halothane. *Int Arch Occup Environ Health* 1990;62:263–71.

250. Tannenbaum TN, Goldberg RJ. Exposure to anesthetic gases and reproductive outcome. A review of the epidemiologic literature. *J Occup Med* 1985;27:659–68.

251. Kanto J. Obstetric analgesia: clinical pharmacokientic considerations. *Clin Pharmacokinet* 1986;11:283–98.

252. Janowsky EC. Pharmacologic aspects of local anesthetic use. *Anesthesiol Clin North Am* 1990;8:1–25.

253. Rosenberg L et al. Lack of relation of oral clefts to diazepam use during pregnancy. *N Engl J Med* 1983;309:1282–5.

254. Shiono PH, Mills JL. Oral clefts and diazepam use during pregnancy. *N Engl J Med* 1984;311:919–20. Letter.

255. Bergman U et al. Teratogenic effects of benzodiazepine use during pregnancy. *J Pediatr* 1990;116:490–1. Letter.

256. Czeizel A. Lack of evidence of teratogenicity of benzodiazepine drugs in Hungary. *Reprod Toxicol* 1988:1:183–8.

257. Rivas F et al. Acentric craniofacial cleft in a newborn female prenatally exposed to a high dose of diazepam. *Teratology* 1984;30:179–80.

258. Laegreid L et al. Teratogenic effects of benzodiazepine use during pregnancy. *J Pediatr* 1989;114:126–31.

259. Laegreid L et al. Congenital malformations and maternal consumption of benzodiazepines: a case-control study. *Dev Med Child Neurol* 1990;32:432–41.

260. Fisher JB et al. Neonatal apnea associated with maternal clonazepam therapy: a case report. *Obstet Gynecol* 1985;66(suppl):34S–5.

261. St Clair SM, Schirmer RG. First-trimester exposure to alprazolam. *Obstet Gynecol* 1992;80:843–6.

262. Laegreid L et al. The effect of benzodiazepines on the fetus and the newborn. *Neuropediatrics* 1992;23:18–23.

263. Sanchis A et al. Adverse effects of maternal lorazepam on neonates. *DICP* 1991;25:1137–8.

264. Gormley DE. Cutaneous surgery and the pregnant patient. *J Am Acad Dermatol* 1990;23:269–79.

265. Anon. *Asthma.* PEM News No. 7. Drug Safety Research Unit, Southampton, England. August 1990.

266. Lamm CI et al. Congenital rickets associated with magnesium sulfate infusion for tocolysis. *J Pediatr* 1988;113:1078–82.

267. Holcomb WL et al. Magnesium tocolysis and neonatal bone abnormalities: a controlled study. *Obstet Gynecol* 1991;78:611–4.

268. Cox SM et al. Randomized investigation of magnesium sulfate for prevention of preterm birth. *Am J Obstet Gynecol* 1990;163:767–72.

269. Dupont P et al. Pregnancy in a patient with treated Wilson's disease: a case report. *Am J Obstet Gynecol* 1990;163:1527–8.

270. Soong Y-K et al. Successful pregnancy after D-penicillamine therapy in a patient with Wilson's disease. *J Formosan Med Assoc* 1991;90:693–6.

271. Ostensen M, Husby G. Antirheumatic drug treatment during pregnancy and lactation. *Scand J Rheumatol* 1985;14:1–7.

272. Chamberlain MJ et al. Toxic effect of podophyllum application in pregnancy. *Br Med J* 1972;3:391–2.

273. Ridley CM. Toxicity of podophyllum. *Br Med J* 1972;3:698. Letter.

274. Karol MD et al. Podophyllum: suspected teratogenicity from topical application. *Clin Toxicol* 1980;16:283–6.

275. Sundharam JA. Is podophyllin safe for use in pregnancy? *Arch Dermatol* 1989;125:1000–1.

276. Stamatos MN. The most important step forward in years (etretinate). Nutley, NJ: Roche Laboratories; 1986. Promotional letter.

277. Anon. Etretinate approved. *FDA Drug Bull* 1986;16(2):16–7.

278. Vahlquist A, Rollman O. Etretinate and the risk for teratogenicity: drug monitoring in a pregnant woman for 9 months after stopping treatment. *Br J Dermatol* 1990;123:131. Letter.

279. Personal communication. Joseph B Laudano, Roche Laboratories, January 29, 1987.

280. Anon. Etretinate for psoriasis. *Med Lett Drugs Ther* 1987;29:9–10.

281. Geiger J-M et al. Teratogenic risk with etretinate and acitretin treatment. *Dermatology* 1994;189:109–16.

282. Lammer EJ et al. Retinoic acid embryopathy. *N Engl J Med* 1985;313:837–41.

283. Holmes A, Wolfe S. When a uniquely effective drug is teratogenic: the case of isotretinoin. *N Engl J Med* 1989;321:756. Letter.

284. Faich G, Rosa F. When a uniquely effective drug is teratogenic: the case of isotretinoin. *N Engl J Med* 1989;321:756–7. Letter.

285. Rappaport EB, Knapp M. Isotretinoin embryopathy—a continuing problem. *J Clin Pharmacol* 1989;29:463–5.

286. Hansen LA, Pearl GS. Isotretinoin teratogenicity. Case report with neuropathologic findings. *Acta Neuropathol* 1985;65:335–7.

287. McBride WG. Limb reduction deformities in child exposed to isotretinoin in utero on gestation days 26–40 only. *Lancet* 1985;1:1276. Letter.

288. Anon. Birth defects caused by isotretinoin-New Jersey. *MMWR* 1988;37:171–2, 177.

289. Dai WS et al. Epidemiology of isotretinoin exposure during pregnancy. *J Am Acad Dermatol* 1992;26:599–606.

290. Rizzo R et al. Limb reduction defects in humans associated with prenatal isotretinoin exposure. *Teratology* 1991;44:599–604.

291. Zbinden G. Investigations on the toxicity of tretinoin administered systemically to animals. *Acta Derm Venereol Stockh Suppl* 1975;74:36–40.

292. deWals P et al. Association between holoprosencephaly and exposure to topical retinoids: results of the EUROCAT survey. *Paediatr Perinat Epidemiol* 1991;5:445–7.

293. Jick SS et al. First trimester topical tretinoin and congenital disorders. *Lancet* 1993;341:1181–2.

294. Camera G, Pregliasco P. Ear malformation in baby born to mother using tretinoin cream. *Lancet* 1992;339:687. Letter.

295. Lipson AH et al. Multiple congenital defects associated with maternal use of topical tretinoin. *Lancet* 1993;341:1352–3. Letter.

296. Eckhoff Ch, Nau H. Vitamin A supplementation increases levels of retinoic acid compounds in human plasma: possible implications for teratogenesis. *Arch Toxicol* 1990;64:502–3.

297. Martínez-Frías ML, Salvador J. Epidemiological aspects of prenatal exposure to high doses of vitamin A in Spain. *Eur J Epidemiol* 1990;6:118–23.

298. Werler MM et al. Maternal vitamin A supplementation in relation to selected birth defects. *Teratology* 1990;42:497–503.

299. Rothman KJ et al. Teratogenicity of high vitamin A intake. *N Engl J Med* 1995;333:1369–73.

300. Oakley GP, Erickson JD. Vitamin A and birth defects. Continuing caution is needed. *N Engl J Med* 1995;333:1414–5. Editorial.

301. Anon. Use of supplements containing high-dose vitamin A—New York State, 1983–1984. *MMWR* 1987;36:80–2.

302. Committee on Safety of Medicines. Vitamin A and teratogenesis. *Lancet* 1985;1:319–20.

303. Wright JW et al. Effect of tocolytic agents on fetal umbilical velocimetry. *Am J Obstet Gynecol* 1990;163:748–50.

304. Mann RD et al. *Salmeterol*. PEM Report No. 25. Drug Safety Research Unit, Southampton, England; July, 1994.

305. Stenius-Aarniala B et al. Slow-release theophylline in pregnant asthmatics. *Chest* 1995;107:642–7.

306. Frederiksen MC et al. Theophylline pharmacokinetics in pregnancy. *Clin Pharmacol Ther* 1986;40:321–8.

307. Shapiro S et al. Birth defects and vaginal spermicides. *JAMA* 1982;247:2381–4.

308. Jick H et al. Vaginal spermicides and congenital disorders. *JAMA* 1981;245:1329–32.

309. Louik C et al. Maternal exposure to spermicides in relation to certain birth defects. *N Engl J Med* 1987;317:474–8.

310. Warburton D et al. Lack of association between spermicide use and trisomy. *N Engl J Med* 1987;317:478–82.

311. Einarson TR et al. Maternal spermicide use and adverse reproductive outcome: a meta-analysis. *Am J Obstet Gynecol* 1990;162:655–60.

312. Anon. Data do not support association between spermicides, birth defects. *FDA Drug Bull* 1986;16:21.

313. Martin NDT et al. Increased plasma 1,25-dihydroxyvitamin D in infants with hypercalcemia and elfin facies. *N Engl J Med* 1985;313:888–9. Letter.

314. Chesney RW et al. Increased plasma 1,25-dihydroxyvitamin D in infants with hypercalcemia and elfin facies. *N Engl J Med* 1985;313:889–90. Letter.

315. Rudeen PK, Creighton JA. Mechanisms of central nervous system alcohol-related birth defects. In *Molecular mechanisms of alcohol teratogenesis*. Clifton, NJ: Humana Press; 1989:147–165.

316. Goodwin FK. Acetaldehyde produced and transferred by human placenta. *JAMA* 1988;260:3563.

317. Blakley PM, Scott WJ. Determination of the proximate teratogen of the mouse fetal alcohol syndrome. 1. Teratogenicity of ethanol and acetaldehyde. *Toxicol Applied Pharmacol* 1984;72:355–63.

318. Little BB et al. Alcohol abuse during pregnancy: changes in frequency in a large urban hospital. *Obstet Gynecol* 1989;74:547–50.

319. Clarren SK. Fetal alcohol syndrome: diagnosis, treatment, and mechanisms of teratogenesis. In *Transplacental disorders: perinatal detection, treatment, and management (including pediatric AIDS)*. Proceedings of the 1988 Albany Birth Defects Symposium XIX. New York: Alan R. Liss, Inc.; 1990:37–55.

320. Virji SK. The relationship between alcohol consumption during pregnancy and infant birthweight. An epidemiologic study. *Acta Obstet Gynecol Scand* 1991;70:303–8.

321. Kline J et al. Drinking during pregnancy and spontaneous abortion. *Lancet* 1980;2:176–80.

322. Harlap S, Shiono PH. Alcohol, smoking, and incidence of spontaneous abortions in the first and second trimester. *Lancet* 1980;2:173–6.

323. Streissguth AP et al. Natural history of the fetal alcohol syndrome: a 10-year follow-up of eleven patients. *Lancet* 1985;2:85–91.

324. Halmesmaki E et al. Low somatomedin C and high growth hormone levels in newborns damaged by maternal alcohol abuse. *Obstet Gynecol* 1989;74:366–70.

325. Strömland K. Contribution of ocular examination to the diagnosis of foetal alcohol syndrome in mentally retarded children. *J Mental Defic Res* 1990;34:429–35.

326. Froster UG, Baird PA. Congenital defects of the limbs and alcohol exposure in pregnancy: data from a population based study. *Am J Med Genet* 1992;44:782–5.

327. Ronen GM, Andrews WL. Holoprosencephaly as a possible embryonic alcohol effect. *Am J Med Genet* 1991;40:151–4.

328. Bonnemann C, Meinecke P. Holoprosencephaly as a possible embryonic alcohol effect: another observation. *Am J Med Genet* 1990;37:431–2.

329. Astley SJ et al. Analysis of facial shape in children gestationally exposed to marijuana, alcohol, and/or cocaine. *Pediatrics* 1992;89:67–77.

330. Little BB et al. Methamphetamine abuse during pregnancy: outcome and fetal effects. *Obstet Gynecol* 1988;72:541–4.

331. Oro AS, Dixon SD. Perinatal cocaine and methamphetamine exposure: maternal and neonatal correlates. *J Pediatr* 1987;111:571–8.

332. Dixon SD, Bejar R. Echoencephalographic findings in neonates associated with maternal cocaine and methamphetamine use: incidence and clinical correlates. *J Pediatr* 1989;115:770–8.

333. Smith DS, Gutsche BB. Amphetamine abuse and obstetrical anesthesia. *Anesth Analg* 1980;59:710–1. Letter.

334. Infante-Rivard C et al. Fetal loss associated with caffeine intake before and during pregnancy. *JAMA* 1993;270:2940–3.

335. Dlugosz L, Bracken MB. Reproductive effects of caffeine: a review and theoretical analysis. *Epidemiol Rev* 1992;14:83–100.

336. Watkinson B, Fried PA. Maternal caffeine use before, during and after pregnancy and effects upon offspring. *Neurobehav Toxicol Teratol* 1985;7:9–17.

337. Cerrato PL. Caffeine: how much is too much? *RN* 1990;53:77–80.

338. Szucs Myers VA, Miwa LJ. Caffeine consumption during pregnancy. *Drug Intell Clin Pharm* 1988;22:614–6

339. Olsen J et al. Coffee consumption, birthweight, and reproductive failures. *Epidemiology* 1991;2:370–4.

340. Narod SA et al. Coffee during pregnancy: a reproductive hazard? *Am J Obstet Gynecol* 1991;164:1109–14.

341. Toubas PL et al. Effects of maternal smoking and caffeine habits on infantile apnea: a retrospective study. *Pediatrics* 1986;78:159–63.

342. Lutiger B et al. Relationship between gestational cocaine use and pregnancy outcome: a meta-analysis. *Teratology* 1991;44:405–14.

343. Chen C et al. Respiratory instability in neonates with in utero exposure to cocaine. *J Pediatr* 1991;119:111–3.

344. Ho J et al. Renal vascular abnormalities associated with prenatal cocaine exposure. *Clin Pediatr* 1994;33:155–6.

345. Lezcano L et al. Crossed renal ectopia associated with maternal alkaloid cocaine abuse: a case report. *J Perinatol* 1994;14:230–3.

346. Viscarello RR et al. Limb–body wall complex associated with cocaine abuse: further evidence of cocaine's teratogenicity. *Obstet Gynecol* 1992;80:523–6.

347. Hume RF Jr et al. Ultrasound diagnosis of fetal anomalies associated with in utero cocaine exposure: further support for cocaine-induced vascular disruption teratogenesis. *Fetal Diagn Ther* 1994;9:239–45.

348. Teske MP, Trese MT. Retinopathy of prematurity-like fundus and persistent hyperplastic primary vitreous associated with maternal cocaine use. *Am J Ophthalmol* 1987;103:719–20.

349. Good WV et al. Abnormalities of the visual system in infants exposed to cocaine. *Ophthalmology* 1992;99:341–6.

350. Downing GJ et al. Characteristics of perinatal cocaine-exposed infants with necrotizing enterocolitis. *Am J Dis Child* 1991;145:26–7. Letter.

351. Lipshultz SE et al. Cardiovascular abnormalities in infants prenatally exposed to cocaine. *J Pediatr* 1991;118:44–51.

352. van den Anker JN et al. Prenatal diagnosis of limb-reduction defects due to maternal cocaine use. *Lancet* 1991;338:1332. Letter.

353. McCalla S et al. The biologic and social consequences of perinatal cocaine use in an inner-city population: results of an anonymous cross-sectional study. *Am J Obstet Gynecol* 1991;164:625–30.

354. Little BB, Snell LM. Brain growth among fetuses exposed to cocaine in utero: asymmetrical growth retardation. *Obstet Gynecol* 1991;77:361–4.

355. Sheinbaum KA, Badell A. Physiatric management of two neonates with limb deficiencies and prenatal cocaine exposure. *Arch Phys Med Rehabil* 1992;73:385–8.

356. Gieron-Korthals MA et al. Expanding spectrum of cocaine induced central nervous system malformations. *Brain Develop* 1994;16:253–6.

357. Rais-Bahrami K, Naqvi M. Hydranencephaly and maternal cocaine use: a case report. *Clin Pediatr* 1990;29:729–30.

358. Hannig VL, Phillips JA. Maternal cocaine abuse and fetal anomalies: evidence for teratogenic effects of cocaine. *South Med J* 1991;84:498–9.

359. Spinazzola R et al. Neonatal gastrointestinal complications of maternal cocaine abuse. *N Y State J Med* 1992;92:22–3.

360. Hoyme HE et al. Prenatal cocaine exposure and fetal vascular disruption. *Pediatrics* 1990;85:743–7.

361. Greenfield SP et al. Genitourinary tract malformations and maternal cocaine abuse. *Urology* 1991;37:455–9.

362. Davidson Ward SL et al. Sudden infant death syndrome in infants of substance-abusing mothers. *J Pediatr* 1990;117:876–81.

363. Durand DJ et al. Association between prenatal cocaine exposure and sudden infant death syndrome. *J Pediatr* 1990;117:909–11.

364. Lowenstein DH et al. Acute neurologic and psychiatric complications associated with cociane abuse. *Am J Med* 1987;83:841–6.

365. Chasnoff IJ et al. Perinatal cerebral infarction and maternal cocaine use. *J Pediatr* 1986;108:456–9.

366. Chasnoff IJ et al. Cocaine use in pregnancy. *N Engl J Med* 1985;313:666–9.

367. Oro AS, Dixon SD. Perinatal cocaine and methamphetamine exposure: maternal and neonatal correlates. *J Pediatr* 1987;111:571–8.

368. Anon. Cocaine. In Briggs GG et al., eds. *Update: drugs in pregnancy and lactation.* Baltimore: Williams & Wilkins; 1989;2:31–8.

369. Burkett G et al. Perinatal implications of cocaine exposure. *J Reprod Med* 1990;35:35–42.

370. Collins E et al. Perinatal cocaine intoxication. *Med J Aust* 1989;150:331–4.

371. Cherukuri R et al. A cohort study of alkaloidal cocaine ("crack") in pregnancy. *Obstet Gynecol* 1988;72:147–51.

372. Kaye K et al. Birth outcomes for infants of drug abusing mothers. *N Y State J Med* 1989;89:256–61.

373. Bingol N et al. Teratogenicity of cocaine in humans. *J Pediatr* 1987;110:93–6.

374. Keith LG et al. Substance abuse in pregnant women: recent experience at the Perinatal Center for Chemical Dependence of Northwestern Memorial Hospital. *Obstet Gynecol* 1989;73:715–20.

375. Roland EH, Volpe JJ. Effect of maternal cocaine use on the fetus and newborn: review of the literature. *Pediatr Neurosci* 1989;15:88–94.

376. Doering PL et al. Effects of cocaine on the human fetus: a review of clinical studies. *DICP* 1989;23:639–45.

377. Mastrogiannis DS et al. Perinatal outcome after recent cocaine usage. *Obstet Gynecol* 1990;76:8–11.

378. Cravey RH. Cocaine deaths in infants. *J Anal Toxicol* 1988;12:354–5.

379. Chouteau M et al. The effect of cocaine abuse on birth weight and gestational age. *Obstet Gynecol* 1988;72:351–4.

380. Little BB et al. Cocaine abuse during pregnancy: maternal and fetal implications. *Obstet Gynecol* 1989;73:157–60.

381. Mercado A et al. Cocaine, pregnancy, and postpartum intracerebral hemorrhage. *Obstet Gynecol* 1989;73:467–8.

382. Ney JA et al. The prevalence of substance abuse in patients with suspected preterm labor. *Am J Obstet Gynecol* 1990;162:1562–7.

383. Thatcher SS et al. Cocaine use and acute rupture of ectopic pregnancies. *Obstet Gynecol* 1989;74:478–9.

384. Gonsoulin W et al. Rupture of unscarred uterus in primigravid woman in association with cocaine abuse. *Am J Obstet Gynecol* 1990;163:526–7.

385. Madden JD et al. Maternal cocaine abuse and effect on the newborn. *Pediatrics* 1986;77:209–11.

386. Rosenstein BJ et al. Congenital renal abnormalities in infants with in utero cocaine exposure. *J Urol* 1990;144:110–2.

387. Chavez GF et al. Maternal cocaine use during early pregnancy as a risk factor for congenital urogenital anomalies. *JAMA* 1989;262:795–8.

388. Ward SLD et al. Abnormal sleeping ventilatory pattern in infants of substance-abusing mothers. *Am J Dis Child* 1986;140:1015–20.

389. Chasnoff IJ et al. Prenatal cocaine exposure is associated with respiratory pattern abnormalities. *Am J Dis Child* 1989;143:583–7.

390. Cregler LL, Mark H. Medical complications of cocaine abuse. *N Engl Med J* 1986;315:1495–500.

391. Klenka HM. Babies born in a district general hospital to mothers taking heroin. *Br Med J* 1986;293:745–6.

392. Braude MC et al. Perinatal effects of drugs of abuse. *Fed Proc* 1987;46:2446–53.

393. Zuckerman B et al. Effects of maternal marijuana and cocaine use on fetal growth. *N Engl J Med* 1989;320:762–8.

394. Feldman JG et al. A cohort study of the impact of perinatal drug use on prematurity in an inner-city population. *Am J Public Health* 1992;82:726–8.

395. Fried PA. Cigarettes and marijuana: are there measurable long-term neurobehavioral teratogenic effects? *Neurotoxicology* 1989;10:577–84.

396. Hatch EE, Bracken MB. Effect of marijuana use in pregnancy on fetal growth. *Am J Epidemiol* 1986;124:986–93.

397. Tansley BW et al. Visual processing in children exposed prenatally to marihuana and nicotine: a preliminary report. *Can J Public Health* 1986;77(suppl 1):72–8.

398. Chasnoff IJ et al. Phencyclidine: effects on the fetus and neonate. *Dev Pharmacol Ther* 1983;6:404–8.

399. Golden NL et al. Phencyclidine use during pregnancy. *Am J Obstet Gynecol* 1984;148:254–9.

400. Lindblad A et al. Effect of nicotine on human fetal blood flow. Obstet Gynecol 1988;72:371–82.
401. Pinette MG et al. Maternal smoking and accelerated placental maturation. *Obstet Gynecol* 1989;73:379–82.
402. Cole H. Studying reproductive risks, smoking. *JAMA* 1986;255:22–3.
403. Shiono PH et al. Smoking and drinking during pregnancy: their effects on preterm birth. *JAMA* 1986;255:82–4.
404. Brown HL et al. Premature placental calcification in maternal cigarette smokers. *Obstet Gynecol* 1988;71:914–7.
405. Newnham JP et al. Effects of maternal cigarette smoking on ultrasonic measurements of fetal growth and on Doppler flow velocity waveforms. *Early Hum Dev* 1990;24:23–6.
406. Jauniaux E, Burton GJ. The effect of smoking in pregnancy on early placental morphology. *Obstet Gynecol* 1992;79:645–8.
407. Seidman DS et al. Effect of maternal smoking and age on congenital anomalies. *Obstet Gynecol* 1990;76:1046–50.
408. Brown RW et al. Effect of maternal smoking during pregnancy on passive respiratory mechanics in early infancy. *Pediatr Pulmonol* 1995;19:23–8.
409. John EM et al. Prenatal exposure to parents' smoking and childhood cancer. *Am J Epidemiol* 1991;133:123–32.
410. Stjernfeldt M et al. Maternal smoking and irradiation during pregnancy as risk factors for child leukemia. *Cancer Detect Prev* 1992;16:129–35.

Drugs and Breastfeeding

Philip O. Anderson

With the increasing recognition of the benefits of breastfeeding, the clinician must often weigh the benefits versus risks of drug therapy in lactating women. The physicochemical, pharmacokinetic, and clinical factors involved with drug use in nursing women have been described.[1-7] These factors are summarized below.

■ PHYSICOCHEMICAL FACTORS

Small water-soluble nonelectrolytes pass into milk by simple diffusion through pores in the mammary epithelial membrane that separates plasma from milk. Equilibration between the two fluids is rapid, and milk levels of drugs approximate plasma levels. For larger molecules, only the lipid-soluble, nonionized forms pass through the membrane by dissolving in the cell wall and diffusing across the interior of the cell to reach the milk. Because the pH of milk is generally lower than that of plasma, milk can act as an "ion trap" for basic drugs. At equilibrium, these compounds may be concentrated in milk relative to plasma. Conversely, acidic drugs are inhibited from entering milk. The pKa of weak electrolytes is an important determinant of their equilibrium concentration in milk.

Protein binding is also an important determinant because plasma proteins bind drugs much more avidly than do milk proteins. Highly protein-bound drugs do not pass into milk in high concentrations. Lipid solubility favors passage of drugs into milk, because the fat component of milk can concentrate lipid-soluble drugs. However, because milk contains only 3–5% fat, its capacity for concentrating drugs is limited. Active transport of drugs into breastmilk may occur, but it is rare.[8]

■ PHARMACOKINETIC FACTORS

Because the breast is periodically emptied and replaced with newly formed milk, equilibrium between plasma and milk is rarely reached. The rate of passage from plasma into milk is therefore important in determining the concentration of a drug in milk. Factors favoring rapid passage into milk are high lipid solubility and low molecular weight.

Passage of drugs between plasma and milk occurs in two directions. When the concentration of nonionized free drug in milk is higher than is in plasma, net transfer of drug from milk to plasma occurs. Thus, pumping and discarding milk does not appreciably hasten the elimination of most drugs from milk, nor does it have a marked effect on overall clearance of the drug from the mother's body.

■ METHODS OF EXPRESSING THE EXTENT OF PASSAGE

The ratio of concentrations of a drug in milk and plasma (the milk/plasma or M/P ratio) has often been used as a measure of a drug's passage into breastmilk. However, the M/P ratio has shortcomings that make it meaningless as a measure of drug safety during nursing: There is no standard method of calculating the value, and the value is not constant, as often calculated, but varies with the time after the dose and with the number of doses given.

The percentage of the maternal dose that is excreted into milk is also used to express the extent of passage. This value alone is not predictive of safety in a nursing infant, but can be used to calculate the actual dosage received by the infant.

Drug clearance can be a useful factor for identifying drugs that may accumulate in infants and have a pharmacologic effect.[9] Drugs with a total body clearance of 0.6 L/hr/kg or greater and that have no active metabolites are unlikely to cause a pharmacologic effect in a nursing infant.

Knowledge of the actual dosage received by an infant via milk, either from the literature or by calculation, and comparison of this dosage with the therapeutic infant dosage is the most reliable way to measure drug safety in the nursing infant.

All of the above methods fall short of providing a complete assessment of the safety of a drug during breastfeeding in a specific mother-infant pair, however. Several other drug and clinical factors must be considered in addition.

■ CLINICAL CONSIDERATIONS

Factors that should be considered when determining the advisability of using a particular drug in a nursing mother include the potential acute toxicity of the drug, dosage and duration of therapy, age of the infant, quantity of milk consumed, experience with the drug in infants, oral absorption of the drug by the infant, potential long-term effects, possible interference with lactation, and non-dose-related toxicities.[1,7]

A stepwise approach to using medications in breastfeeding women can be followed in order to minimize infant exposure to medications in milk.[1] Starting from the strategies that are least disruptive to nursing and progressing to those that are most disruptive, the prescriber can consider the following steps: withhold the drug, delay drug therapy temporarily, choose drugs that pass poorly into milk, use alternative routes of administration (eg, topical, inhalation), avoid nursing at peak times, administer the drug before the infant's longest sleep period, and withhold breastfeeding temporarily.

Another consideration is non-dose-related adverse effects, such as allergic reactions, and some hemolytic anemias; however, these are relatively uncommon. GI intolerance caused by antiinfective agents in breastmilk can occur whether or not the drugs are absorbed by the infant. Antiinfective agents are among the most commonly used maternal medications during nursing. Although serious side effects are rare, diarrhea is not infrequent, occurring in about 12% of infants.[10] Disruption of the infant's GI flora is uncommon, but it can lead to pseudomembranous colitis rarely.[11] Severe diarrhea or blood in the infant's stool during maternal antimicrobial use is an indication to stop nursing and seek medical attention.

Although the above considerations are important, follow-up of mothers who took medications while breastfeeding their infants has shown that serious side effects are rare.[10] Only infrequently must nursing be discontinued completely because of concern of acute toxicity from maternal drug therapy.

The following table contains information on the use of specific drugs during nursing. The risks are assessed and alternatives are presented based on the above principles. Information in the table is from reference 1 unless noted otherwise.

DRUGS EXCRETED INTO BREASTMILK

DRUG	NATURE OF EFFECT

ANALGESICS AND ANTIINFLAMMATORIES

Acetaminophen

The amount of acetaminophen excreted into milk is small. Acetaminophen is a good analgesic choice during nursing.

Narcotics

Neonates are particularly susceptible to narcotics in breastmilk.[7] Postpartum maternal opiates (oral **codeine** or **propoxyphene** with or without prior IM **meperidine**) may be a causative factor in episodes of apnea, bradycardia, and cyanosis during the first week of life. Avoid maternal narcotics when the breast-fed neonate has experienced such an episode.[7] Although single analgesic doses of most narcotics are excreted into milk in small amounts, infant drowsiness caused by repeated administration of postpartum oral narcotics in milk is more prevalent than commonly thought — about 20% in one study.[10] Drowsiness is dose related and can be severe with the maximum dosage. Limiting oral dosage to one tablet (eg, **codeine** 30 mg, **hydrocodone** 5 mg, or **oxycodone** 5 mg) q 4 hr is advisable; analgesia can be supplemented with additional acetaminophen or ibuprofen.[7]

Intravenous narcotics and narcotic agonist/antagonists (eg, **butorphanol, nalbuphine**) given during labor can interfere with establishment of lactation.[12–14] **Meperidine** is particularly likely to interfere with lactation when given during labor.[12,13,15] Furthermore, repeated postpartum meperidine doses result in high concentrations of meperidine and **normeperidine** in milk, causing more neurobehavioral depression in breast-fed neonates than equivalent doses of morphine. Meperidine is best avoided during labor and nursing. **Morphine** 10–15 mg in single parenteral doses produces only low concentrations in milk, but repeated doses may result in drug accumulation in infant plasma to near therapeutic concentrations. Morphine glucuronides in milk contribute an additional 50–100% to the infant dose via deconjugation in the infant's gut to the active drug. Epidural administration and patient-controlled analgesia cause fewer infant effects than IV and are preferred.[7,16] Butorphanol and nalbuphine levels in milk are low, and oral bioavailability in the infant should be low.[17,18] IV or epidural **fentanyl** and epidural **sufentanil** produce low milk levels.[19–21] Additionally, these drugs have poor oral bioavailability, so they are good choices for maternal analgesia during nursing.

Nonsteroidal Antiinflammatory Drugs (NSAIDs)

Amounts of most NSAIDs in milk are low because they are weak acids that are extensively plasma protein bound. However, short-acting agents are preferred, particularly in the case of neonates. Some agents have active metabolites (eg, **sulindac**) or glucuronide metabolites (eg, **salicylate, fenoprofen, ketoprofen**) that can add to infant intake. Because of the increased likelihood of accumulation, long-acting agents such as **diflunisal, naproxen, piroxicam,** and **sulindac** should be avoided in mothers of neonates, although amounts of piroxicam in milk are low.[1,7] The more toxic NSAIDs such as **mefenamic acid** and **indomethacin** should probably be avoided, although recent studies on indomethacin indicate that it may not be contraindicated.[22,23] **Ketorolac** is contraindicated during nursing.

Ibuprofen and **flurbiprofen** have the best documentation of safety during breastfeeding; amounts of ibuprofen in milk are unmeasurable after dosages of up to 1.6 g/day, and flurbiprofen levels are low to undetectable after dosages

(continued)

DRUG	NATURE OF EFFECT
	up to 50 mg tid. **Diclofenac** was not detected in milk after a single dose of 50 mg IM, or 100 mg/day for 1 week, and the amount of **tolmetin** in one woman's milk was low.
Salicylate	Salicylate enters milk in a low concentration relative to that in plasma, although its glucuronide metabolite increases the overall amount. Doses over 1 g yield markedly higher salicylate concentrations in milk and may result in high infant plasma concentrations. The risk of Reye's syndrome caused by salicylate in milk is unknown. NSAIDs such as ibuprofen are preferred over aspirin for long-term therapy. However, when a salicylate is used for long-term maternal therapy, infant salicylate plasma concentrations should be monitored, particularly in neonates. Although acetaminophen or ibuprofen is preferred, occasional **aspirin** in analgesic dosages should pose a minimal risk to the infant except for the potential antiplatelet effect. Avoidance of breastfeeding for 1–2 hr after a dose should avoid this effect.

ANTICHOLINERGIC AGENTS

Excretion of anticholinergic agents into milk has not been well studied. Theoretical hazards include anticholinergic effects such as drying of secretions, temperature elevations, and CNS disturbances in the infant. Infants should be carefully observed when anticholinergics are given to the mother. Centrally acting anticholinergics may also inhibit milk ejection (ie. oxytocin secretion).

ANTICOAGULANTS

Indandiones (eg, **anisindione, phenindione**) are contraindicated because infant hemorrhage has occurred. Although minimal documentation exists, it is unlikely that **heparin** or **low molecular weight heparins** (eg, **enoxaparin, dalteparin**) pass into milk or are absorbed orally by the infant. Amounts of **warfarin** in milk are of no clinical consequence with maternal dosage of 12 mg/day or less, probably because of extensive protein binding;[1,9] higher dosages have not been studied. Other coumarin derivatives (eg, **acenocoumarol, dicumarol, phenprocoumon**) also appear to be safe.[1,24]

ANTICONVULSANTS

Infants of mothers taking anticonvulsants may have more difficulty nursing and may breast feed for a shorter duration.[25,26] Breast-fed infants may achieve plasma drug concentrations that produce pharmacologic effects; mild drowsiness is common in the infants of mothers taking anticonvulsants, especially in the early neonatal period. Breastfeeding can mitigate withdrawal symptoms in infants whose mothers took anticonvulsants during pregnancy, and withdrawal symptoms have been observed after abrupt weaning. Long-term effects of exposure are not well studied. Plasma concentration monitoring in breast-fed infants may be indicated, particularly in infants who are excessively drowsy, feed poorly, or gain weight inadequately. Strategies suggested to minimize sedation include alternating breastfeeding and bottle feeding, providing most or all of the day's dosage at once and providing bottle feeding(s) for 1 or 2 feedings afterward, and withholding breastfeeding during the early neonatal period.

Carbamazepine	Carbamazepine and its major metabolite are excreted into milk and can be detected in nursing infants' plasma; concentrations are usually low, but near the therapeutic range in some infants. Two cases of hepatic dysfunction in breast-fed neonates have been reported.[27,28] Carbamazepine can be used during lactation, but occasional measurements of infant plasma concentration may be indicated, as well as close observations of the infant for jaundice and other signs of possible adverse idiosyncratic effects.
Clonazepam	Plasma concentrations were low in two nursing infants, and no effects were noted.[1] Breastfeeding increased another infant's plasma levels over those transmitted transplacentally.[29] Observation of the infant for drowsiness and monitoring of the infant's plasma concentration may be indicated. *(continued)*

DRUG	NATURE OF EFFECT
Ethosuximide	Breast-fed infants may attain ethosuximide plasma concentrations near the therapeutic range, and some infants may show signs of drowsiness or fussiness. Breastfeeding should be undertaken with caution, and the mother's plasma concentrations should be kept as low as possible while remaining in the therapeutic range. Infant plasma drug concentration monitoring is indicated.
Phenobarbital	The effect of phenobarbital is unpredictable: drowsiness leading to feeding difficulties can occur; breastfeeding can prevent withdrawal symptoms in infants whose mothers took phenobarbital during pregnancy; and withdrawal symptoms have been observed after abrupt weaning. Phenobarbital can be used in low to moderate dosages, but infant behavior, weight gain, and plasma concentrations should be monitored if there is concern. Sometimes breastfeeding will have to be discontinued because of excessive drowsiness and poor weight gain.
Phenytoin	Phenytoin is excreted into milk in small amounts. Rarely infants may experience idiosyncratic reactions such as cyanosis and methemoglobinemia, but infants generally tolerate phenytoin in milk well.
Primidone	Primidone and its metabolites (**phenylethylmalonamide**, **phenobarbital**, and **parahydroxyphenobarbital**) appear in milk in relatively large amounts. Considerations are the same as for phenobarbital (above).
Valproic Acid	Valproic acid passes into milk in low concentrations, and no effects have been noted in infants. Infants should be observed for rare idiosyncratic effects such as hepatotoxicity.

ANTIHISTAMINES

There are few studies on antihistamine use during lactation. One study found drowsiness or irritability occurred in 12% of breast-fed infants.[10] Older sedating (and more anticholinergic) antihistamines appear to be more problematic. **Cyproheptadine** lowers maternal serum prolactin and should be avoided. **Triprolidine** and **loratadine** are excreted in seemingly unimportant amounts. **Terfenadine** levels in milk are low, and the drug is well tolerated, with irritability reported in some infants.[10,30] Single bedtime doses of antihistamines (preferably short-acting and/or nonsedating drugs) after the last feeding of the day may be adequate for many women and minimize the amount the infant receives. High dosages or sustained-release formulations of sedating antihistamines or combinations containing a sympathomimetic agent should be avoided.

ANTIMICROBIAL DRUGS

Aminoglycosides	Systemic effects in infants are unlikely because of the small amounts in milk and poor oral absorption; however, infants should be observed for disruptions of the GI flora, such as diarrhea and thrush.
Antifungals	**Amphotericin B** and **nystatin** are virtually unabsorbed orally, and the latter is frequently used orally for thrush in infants; therefore, both are safe for use in nursing mothers, including topical application to the nipples. Likewise, **clotrimazole** has poor oral bioavailability and has also been used orally in infants with thrush, sometimes successfully after nystatin has failed.[31] **Miconazole** appears to have efficacy and safety similar to clotrimazole.[32] When vaginal administration is used, these agents are preferred. **Fluconazole** amounts in milk are much less than the dosage prescribed for infants and can be used for recalcitrant *Candida* infections.[33,34] **Ketoconazole** levels in milk are low,[35] but it should probably be avoided in nursing mothers either orally or topically to the nipples because of its occasional hepatotoxicity and the availability of safer alternatives. Other imidazole antifungals have not been studied. **Gentian violet** is potentially toxic (toxic to mucous membranes, carcinogenic and

(continued)

DRUG	NATURE OF EFFECT
	mutagenic in rodents, potential tattooing of the skin) and is best avoided topically on the nipples or in the infant's mouth.[36,37]
Antimalarials	Breastfeeding should be undertaken cautiously during daily therapy with **chloroquine** or **hydroxychloroquine**, because the importance of the small amounts of drug and metabolites in mile is unclear and accumulation may occur. Weekly prophylactic doses are probably safe, because the amount of drug in milk is less than the infant prophylactic dose. Small amounts of **quinine** in milk are unlikely to harm the infant, although allergic reactions may occur. **Pyrimethamine** appears to be safe and may be excreted into milk in quantities sufficient to treat or protect infants less than 6 months of age against malaria; however, breastfeeding is not a reliable method of drug administration. **Mefloquine** appears in milk in small amounts after a single dose, but has not been studied after repeated weekly administration for malaria prophylaxis.
Antiparasitics	**Mebendazole** was undetectable in milk in one woman and is poorly absorbed orally; therefore, it is unlikely to cause adverse effects in a breast-fed infant. Contrary to an earlier report, it does not appear to inhibit lactation.[38] Only a small amount of **praziquantel** reaches the infant, and the drug appears safe during nursing.
Antituberculars	Antituberculars appear to pass into milk in small quantities. Use caution in nursing mothers because many of these drugs can cause hepatic damage. However, inadequate maternal therapy probably poses a much greater risk to the infant than the drugs in milk. The mother may take single daily doses of many of these drugs at bedtime and substitute a bottle for a nighttime feeding to minimize infant exposure. **Isoniazid** is excreted into milk in amounts that are less than those given to treat an infant. **Pyrazinamide** concentrations in milk in one woman were low and would give the baby less than a therapeutic dosage. **Rifampin** has not been well studied, but amounts in milk appear to be small. **Cycloserine** is excreted in small amounts, and no adverse reactions have been reported in infants. **Ethambutol** has not been adequately studied.
Cephalosporins	Cephalosporins appear in trace amounts in milk and can lead to disruption of the GI flora or, rarely, allergic sensitization. Breastfeeding is safe with first- and second-generation agents. The risk may be greater with the third-generation cephalosporins and similar agents (eg, **moxalactam**, **aztreonam**) that are more active against GI flora. Infants exposed to cephalosporins in milk should be observed for diarrhea, thrush, and rashes.
Macrolides	**Erythromycin**, **clarithromycin**, and **azithromycin** are excreted into the milk in amounts much smaller than a typical infant dosage and are usually safe.[1,39,40]
Penicillins	Penicillins appear in trace amounts in milk that can occasionally lead to allergic sensitization, allergic reactions in previously sensitized infants, or disruption of the GI flora, especially with the broader-spectrum agents. Unless the infant is allergic to penicillin, breastfeeding is generally safe with penicillins. Infants exposed to penicillins in milk should be observed for diarrhea, rash or thrush.
Quinolones	**Ciprofloxacin**, **ofloxacin**, and **pefloxacin** are concentrated in milk; **nalidixic acid**, **fleroxacin**, and **temafloxacin** have also been detected.[41,42] Ciprofloxacin appears to have caused pseudomembranous colitis in a breast-fed infant via breastmilk,[11] and nalidixic acid caused hemolytic anemia in a breast-fed neonate. Most fluoroquinolones are probably best avoided during nursing. **Norfloxacin** was undetectable in milk after a 200-mg dose,

(continued)

DRUG	NATURE OF EFFECT
	and may be acceptable for maternal UTI treatment because of its low milk excretion and poor oral bioavailability.
Sulfonamides	Some sulfonamides may cause hemolysis in G-6-PD-deficient infants; theoretically, sulfonamides may increase the risk of kernicterus in neonates. **Sulfamethoxazole**, with or without trimethoprim, and **sulfisoxazole** can be used by mothers of healthy, full-term infants over 2 months of age.
Sulfones	Newborns and G-6-PD-deficient infants are particularly susceptible to **dapsone** hemolysis. Older infants may be able to tolerate the amounts of sulfones excreted into milk.
Tetracyclines	Milk calcium apparently inhibits absorption of the small amounts of **tetracycline** in milk. Infant absorption and plasma concentrations have not been reported with other tetracyclines, but infants would only receive a few milligrams per day of **demeclocycline, doxycycline,** or **minocycline** with usual maternal dosages. Doxycycline concentrations in milk progressively increased with duration of therapy in one study. Although other drugs are preferred for most infections, tetracyclines can be used for a short time (7–10 days); prolonged or repeat courses should be avoided during nursing. **Minocycline** has caused black milk.[43]
Urinary Germicides	**Methenamine hippurate** and **methenamine mandelate** pass into milk in small quantities and seem safe to use. **Nitrofurantoin** is excreted into milk in pharmacologically unimportant amounts, but it should be avoided with infants under 1 month of age and those with G-6-PD deficiency.

MISCELLANEOUS ANTIMICROBIALS

Acyclovir	Acyclovir has not been well studied, but a breast-fed infant would receive about 1% of the mother's weight-adjusted oral dosage. Some controversy exists, but the low dosage in milk and its poor oral bioavailability indicate that it may be well tolerated by the nursing infant, even with large IV doses.[44,45] Topical acyclovir applied to small areas of the mother's body away from the breast should pose no risk to the infant.
Amantadine	Amantadine is a dopamine agonist that decreases serum prolactin and may decrease lactation. The drug is probably best avoided during nursing. It is not known if **rimantadine** has the same effect, so it should be used cautiously during nursing.
Chloramphenicol	Chloramphenicol milk concentrations are not sufficient to induce "gray baby" syndrome, but theoretically may be enough to cause the rare, idiosyncratic aplastic anemia. Adverse reactions in infants, including refusal of the breast, falling asleep during feeding, and vomiting after feeding, have occurred. Breastfeeding is contraindicated during maternal chloramphenicol treatment.
Clindamycin	Clindamycin is excreted variably in small amounts into milk. It is not certain what effects these amounts may have on infants' GI flora (eg, induction of pseudomembranous colitis), but a single case of bloody stools in an infant with normal stool flora was reported during maternal clindamycin use. Clindamycin is best avoided if possible, but a few days of therapy with close monitoring of the infant is probably acceptable. Vaginal clindamycin presents less infant risk than oral or IV use.
Clofazimine	Maternal clofazimine use resulted in a breast-fed infant developing the typical skin discoloration and becoming hypermelanotic. The skin color returned to normal 5 months after the end of therapy.
Metronidazole	Metronidazole and its hydroxy metabolite are found in the plasma of nursing infants in concentrations that are 10–20% of maternal plasma concentrations.

(*continued*)

DRUG	NATURE OF EFFECT
	Anecdotal cases of diarrhea and isolation of *Candida* species from breast-fed infants have been reported, but most infants do not have immediate reactions. Because of the carcinogenicity in animals and possible mutagenicity and the relatively high infant plasma concentrations achieved, metronidazole should be avoided in nursing mothers.[1,46] When essential to treat trichomoniasis, metronidazole may be given as a single 2-g dose, and an alternative feeding method used for the next 24 hr. After longer courses for anaerobic infections, nursing can resume 12–24 hr after the final dose. **Furazolidone,** which is poorly absorbed orally, can be used to treat maternal giardiasis if the infant is over 1 month of age.
Trimethoprim	Trimethoprim is excreted into milk in amounts that are probably not harmful.
Vancomycin`	Vancomycin is excreted into milk in only small amounts,[47] and because it is not orally absorbed, its use during nursing is safe.

ANTINEOPLASTICS AND IMMUNOSUPPRESSANTS

Antineoplastics
    Breastfeeding is generally considered to be contraindicated in women receiving antineoplastic drugs. **Busulfan** in a dosage of 4 mg/day for 5 weeks was taken by one woman while breastfeeding with no apparent adverse effects on her infant's leukocytes or hemoglobin. This case is by no means conclusive, however, and breastfeeding is not recommended. In one patient, platinum was not detected in milk at any time after an IV infusion of 100 mg/m^2 of **cisplatin.** In another patient, milk platinum was 0.9 mg/L 19.5 hr after her third daily dose of 20 mg/m^2. Because the platinum may be in a reactive form, nursing is not recommended during cisplatin therapy. **Cyclophosphamide** is detectable in milk, and has caused bone marrow depression in infants of women who nursed while receiving the drug. **Doxorubicin** and its primary active metabolite, doxorubicinol, appear in rather large amounts in milk, with their highest milk concentrations occurring 24 hr after a dose. **Etoposide** milk levels are undetectable 24 hr after a dose.[48] **Hydroxyurea** is excreted in small amounts into milk, but breastfeeding is not advised. **Methotrexate** was found in low amounts in milk in one patient; however, this case is not conclusive. Low weekly doses for arthritis probably pose only a slight risk to the infant. **Mitoxantrone** was measurable in milk for at least 28 days after a 6 mg/kg dosage was given daily for 3 days.[48]

Immunosuppressants
    Three infants were reportedly breast-fed safely during maternal **azathioprine** use (75–100 mg/day) after renal transplantation. Low concentrations of the azathioprine metabolite **mercaptopurine** were found in milk. Breastfeeding can be undertaken with close infant monitoring during azathioprine immunosuppressive therapy. There is no information on the safety of **cyclosporine** therapy during breastfeeding, and breastfeeding should be avoided until further data are available.

CARDIOVASCULAR DRUGS

Antiarrhythmics
    Some antiarrhythmics reach near-therapeutic concentrations in breast-fed infants. **Amiodarone** is excreted in amounts that may pose a hazard to the infant and it should not be used during nursing.[1,49] Data on **disopyramide** indicate that infants may receive relatively large amounts of the drug and its metabolite, with plasma concentrations below (but near) the therapeutic range. Disopyramide may be used cautiously during lactation when other alternatives

(continued)

DRUG	NATURE OF EFFECT
	are unacceptable., The infant should be observed for anticholinergic symptoms, and plasma concentrations should be monitored if there is a concern. Sparse data from one patient indicate that **tocainide** may be concentrated in milk and should be used with caution during nursing.
	Because of its low oral bioavailability, maternal **bretylium** is unlikely to produce effects in nursing infants; 400 mg q 8 hr was taken orally by one mother while nursing with no apparent effects on her infant. Infants receive trivial doses of **digoxin** via breastmilk. Amounts of **flecainide** in milk are small and unlikely to affect the infant. **Lidocaine** concentrations in milk during continuous IV infusion and as a local anesthetic are low and poorly absorbed by the infant, so it poses no hazard to the infant.[50,51] Concentrations of **mexiletine** in milk are low and cannot be detected in the plasma of breast-fed infants, but poor feeding may have occurred in one infant. **Procainamide** and its active metabolite, **N-acetylprocainamide**, are more concentrated in milk than in plasma, but absolute amounts are small; procainamide may be used with caution in nursing mothers. **Propafenone** milk levels are very low, but no clinical experience has been reported.[52] **Quinidine** excretion appears to be inconsequential.
β-Adrenergic Blocking Agents	The excretion of β-blockers into breastmilk has been extensively studied. The infant's dosage varies greatly among the different compounds, allowing a range of choices. The most water-soluble drugs reach the infant in the greatest amounts because plasma protein binding, which is directly related to lipid solubility, is the primary determinant of the extent of passage. Additionally, the water-soluble agents have the longest half-lives, are renally eliminated, and therefore are more likely to accumulate in infants. Maternal therapy with **atenolol** and **acebutolol** have resulted in adverse effects (eg, bradycardia, hypotension, tachypnea, cyanosis) in breast-fed infants. These two drugs, as well as **betaxolol**, **nadolol**, **sotalol**, and **timolol**, should be avoided in mothers of newborn infants and when high dosage is required. **Oxprenolol** and **mepindolol** excretion is intermediate and they should probably be avoided during the early neonatal period. **Propranolol**, **metoprolol**, and **labetalol** (and its isomer, **dilevalol**) are excreted in low enough quantities to allow nursing even in the neonatal period.
Calcium-Channel Blocking Agents	Single case reports indicate that only small amounts of **diltiazem** and **nimodipine** are excreted into milk. More data are needed to judge the safety of these drugs during nursing.[1,53] Two case reports indicate that only small amounts of **nifedipine** enter milk. A study of three mothers likewise found only small amounts of **nitrendipine** in milk. Although these drugs appear safe in nursing mothers, caution should be used until more data are available. Several case reports indicate that the amounts of **verapamil** and **norverapamil** in milk and infant plasma are low. Verapamil appears to be safe during nursing.
Hypotensive Agents	Certain antihypertensives are less desirable than others during nursing. Milk concentrations of **clonidine** are much higher than maternal plasma concentrations, and breast-fed infants have plasma concentrations approaching those of the mother.[1,54] Clonidine and **guanfacine** may also decrease prolactin secretion. These drugs must be used with caution during breastfeeding, and avoided if possible. **Reserpine** should be avoided because it may cause nasal stuffiness and increased tracheobronchial secretions.
	The **angiotensin-converting enzyme (ACE) inhibitors**, benazepril, captopril, and enalapril, are found in small amounts and no adverse effects have occurred in breast-fed infants.[1,55] Additionally, milk ACE activity was in the nor

(continued)

DRUG	NATURE OF EFFECT

mal range after a dose of enalapril. These ACE inhibitors appear to be good choices during lactation. Limited data indicate that low-dose, short-term use of **hydralazine** (ie, a few days postpartum) is probably safe. There is limited information on **minoxidil** in milk, but amounts appear to be low. However, minoxidil should be used with caution, particularly when therapy involves large dosages and long-term use. Several studies indicate that **methyldopa** is excreted in unimportant amounts.

DIURETICS

Large dosages of short-acting thiazide-type or usual dosages of loop diuretics (eg, **furosemide**) or long-acting **thiazide**-type diuretics (eg, **chlorthalidone**, **bendroflumethiazide**) can suppress lactation and should be avoided. Long-acting agents may also accumulate in infants' plasma. Low dosages of short-acting thiazide-type diuretics should pose no problems to the infant or suppress lactation, although theoretically, thrombocytopenia or allergic reactions to sulfonamide diuretics might occur. **Acetazolamide** appears in milk in small amounts that are unlikely to harm the infant. The amounts of **spironolactone** and its metabolites in milk appear to be inconsequential.

ERGOT ALKALOIDS

Some ergot alkaloids have dopaminergic activity that can suppress prolactin release and lactation. **Bromocriptine** was used therapeutically for this purpose, but has lost this indication in the United States because of potentially serious toxicity. Although **ergonovine** can lower postpartum serum prolactin concentrations, **methylergonovine** apparently does not, nor is methylergonovine found in milk in important quantities. Short-term, low-dose regimens of these agents immediately postpartum pose no hazard to the infant, but methylergonovine is preferred because it does not inhibit lactation. Courses of these drugs given several days postpartum may expose the infant to greater risk because of the larger amount of milk consumed at this age. **Ergotamine** daily for 6 days postpartum did not affect lactation or infant weight in one study; however, the excretion of ergotamine into milk during lactation has not been studied. Its use probably should be avoided during lactation, because older ergot preparations have produced toxic effects in infants.

GASTROINTESTINAL DRUGS

Antacids	Although **aluminum**, **calcium**, and **magnesium** antacids are partially absorbed, they are unlikely to appreciably increase concentrations of these ions in milk and are safe to use.
Antidiarrheals	Nonabsorbable products such as **kaolin-pectin** are preferred in nursing mothers. The **loperamide** prodrug loperamide oxide results in only small amounts of loperamide in breastmilk.[56] **Diphenoxylate** excretion into milk has not been studied. One or two small doses of loperamide or diphenoxylate daily should pose little risk to the nursing infant. **Bismuth subsalicylate** should be avoided because of systemic salicylate absorption.
Antiulcer Drugs	**Cimetidine** is concentrated in milk because of ion trapping and possibly active secretion;[8] **ranitidine** is also concentrated, but to a lesser extent. Cimetidine and ranitidine are best taken as a single dose at bedtime with avoidance of night feedings. **Famotidine** and **nizatidine** are less concentrated in milk and may be preferable during nursing. However, **sucralfate**, which is virtually nonabsorbable, may be preferable to all H_2-receptor antagonists. Proton pump inhibitors (**omeprazole**, **lansoprazole**) have not been studied, but are considered too potent to use during nursing.
Cathartics and Laxatives	Some **anthraquinone** derivatives, such as **aloe** and **cascara**, and other stimulant cathartics (eg, **phenolphthalein**) should be avoided during nursing because of a laxative effect in breast-fed infants. Laxatives that are nonabsorbable or poorly absorbed, such as bulk-forming (eg, **psyllium**), osmotic (eg,

(continued)

DRUG	NATURE OF EFFECT
	magnesium or phosphate salts) or stool-softening (eg, **docusate**) types, are preferred during lactation. **Senna** in moderate dosages appears to be acceptable if other measures fail. **Bisacodyl** is virtually unabsorbed from the GI tract and should be safe.
Gastrokinetic Agents	**Metoclopramide** elevates serum prolactin via central dopaminergic antagonism and results in increased milk production and a more rapid transition from colostrum to mature milk. It may be used therapeutically in mothers who are producing insufficient quantities of milk, such as the mothers of premature or sick infants, or adoptive mothers. Metoclopramide may induce or worsen depression in some women, so caution is warranted. Although infant dosages of metoclopramide from milk are low, the infant's serum prolactin concentrations may sometimes be elevated. Concern has been raised because of possible defects in neural development in newborn animals exposed to dopamine receptor antagonists. Avoiding breastfeeding for 3–4 hr after the dose and limiting the duration of therapy to 14 days should minimize infant exposure when metoclopramide use is essential. Milk **cisapride** concentrations are low, but its effects on maternal prolactin or infants are not known.
Mesalamine Derivatives	Small amounts of **sulfasalazine** and **sulfapyridine** have been found in milk and infant's plasma after oral sulfasalazine use. The small amount of sulfapyridine released should cause no bilirubin displacement. Following **olsalazine**, the drug is not detectable in milk, but its metabolite acetyl-5-ASA is found in small amounts.[57] Small amounts of **mesalamine** and larger amounts of its metabolite were found in milk after oral administration of mesalamine.[1,58] Diarrhea (bloody in once case) has occurred in infants of mothers using mesalamine derivatives. Sulfasalazine, mesalamine, and its derivatives may be used cautiously during nursing with close infant observation.

HORMONAL DRUGS

Contraceptives, Combined Estrogen-Progestin	Although present in milk in small amounts, estrogens and progestins are readily metabolized by nursing infants. Rare case reports of breast enlargement in infants and proliferation of the vaginal epithelium in female infants have been attributed to combination oral contraceptives. One case of megaloblastic anemia in an infant, possibly caused by contraceptive steroids in milk, was reported. These effects occur primarily with products containing >50 μg of estrogen. These high-estrogen contraceptives also markedly suppress lactation, especially when administered immediately postpartum. When currently available low-dose **estrogen** plus **progestin** combination contraceptives are begun 6 or more weeks postpartum, a dramatic effect is usually not seen, but long-term negative effects on milk yield lead to early feeding supplementation and discontinuation of breastfeeding, and perhaps to decreased infant growth. An 8-year follow-up of breast-fed infants of mothers taking contraceptives containing 50 μg **ethinyl estradiol** found no adverse effects on the infants' development or behavior. Progestin-only contraceptives are preferred during lactation.
Contraceptives, Progestin-Only	No immediate effects have been reported with progestin-only contraceptives, such as **levonorgestrel** implants, **depot medroxyprogesterone acetate**, or oral **norethindrone** or **norgestrel**. Progestin-only contraceptives generally enhance or have no effect on milk supply and may extend the duration of lactation. Although infant growth may undergo a slight, transient depression after insertion of **levonorgestrel** implants, large, multicenter studies have found no

(continued)

DRUG	NATURE OF EFFECT
	effect of progestin-only contraceptives on growth and development of infants and children up to puberty.[59–62] Progestin-only contraceptives started at least 6 weeks postpartum are the preferred hormonal contraceptives during lactation.[63,64] (*See also* Progesterone.)
Corticosteriods	**Prednisone** and **prednisolone** excretion into milk is minimal even with large oral doses.[65] The infant dosage can be reduced even further by using prednisolone rather than prednisone and avoiding nursing for 3–4 hr after a dose. Three infants have been breast-fed during long-term maternal use of **methylprednisolone** 6–8 mg/day with apparent safety. Large IV doses of corticosteroids or use of long-acting agents such as **dexamethasone** have not been studied, and caution is warranted during these uses in nursing mothers. Depot injections, inhaled corticosteroids (eg, **beclomethasone**), or topical corticosteriods should present little or no risk to the infant because of low maternal plasma concentrations.
Desmopressin	Desmopressin is excreted in negligible amounts into milk and is poorly absorbed orally by the infant, so it appears safe to use.
Insulin	Diabetic mothers using insulin may nurse their infants. However, it has been empirically found that the mother may need to reduce her insulin dosage to about 75% of her prepregnancy dosage.
Progesterone	Progesterone used as a contraceptive via implants (investigationally) or intrauterine devices transfers little drug to the breast-fed infant, and any drug in milk is minimally absorbed by the infant.[1,63,64] Milk progesterone concentrations have not been measured after higher doses used to treat premenstrual syndrome.
Thyroid and Antithyroid Agents	Thyroid hormones are necessary for normal lactation. It appears that **levothyroxine** (T_4) passes into milk poorly, although **liothyronine** (T_3) may pass in more physiologically relevant amounts. Milk concentrations of thyroid hormones have not been measured after exogenous administration, but a physiologic replacement dosage of levothyroxine to a breastfeeding mother is not expected to result in excessive thyroid administration to the infant. Replacement therapy with liothyronine or supraphysiologic maternal levothyroxine dosage may transfer larger amounts of liothyronine to the infant. **Protirelin (thyrotropin-releasing hormone, TRH)** causes an increase in prolactin secretion and may enhance milk yield.[66]
	Propylthiouracil in dosages of 300 mg/day or less is the antithyroid drug of choice during lactation. **Methimazole** 20 mg/day or less or **carbimazole** (a methimazole prodrug) 15 mg/day or less may also be used, but these drugs pass into milk better and have a longer half-life than propylthiouracil; thus, they are less desirable alternatives.[67] A potential for idiosyncratic reactions and hypothyroidism exists, and measurement of the infant's serum thyroxine and TSH concentrations at 2–4 week intervals is prudent with all antithyroid drugs.

PSYCHOTHERAPEUTIC AGENTS

Antidepressants	**Heterocyclic antidepressants** have not been well studied during lactation, and no agreement exists on the advisability of therapy during lactation. Some authors have recommended against use of antidepressants because of potential (but undemonstrated) long-term effects on infants' neurologic development. Others consider tricyclic antidepressants (TCAs) to be acceptable; follow-up for 1–3 yr in a small group of breast-fed infants indicates no adverse effects on growth and development. Sedating TCAs with active metabolites

(continued)

DRUG	NATURE OF EFFECT

areless desirable than other TCAs, though. Respiratory depression was reported in one breast-fed infant whose mother was taking **doxepin** 25 mg tid, but an infant whose mother was taking 150 mg at night had no problems. Maternal dosages of **amitriptyline** up to 150 mg/day, **desipramine** 300 mg/day, **imipramine** 200 mg/day, **nortriptyline** 125 mg/day, or **clomipramine** 150 mg/day have not caused observable effects in the few infants studied, and in several infants, nortriptyline plasma levels were undetectable with maternal nortriptyline dosages of up to 125 mg/day or amitriptyline 175 mg/day. [1,68–70] Infant exposure to the tricyclic antidepressants can be minimized by using a secondary amine (eg, nortriptyline, desipramine) and giving the drug as a single dose at bedtime, skipping nighttime feeding(s), if necessary; these drugs have low milk levels and no active metabolites, and are eliminated from the milk relatively rapidly. Avoidance of nursing may be indicated with preterm infants and when unusually high maternal dosages are prescribed. A single 50-mg dose of **trazodone**, 250 mg/day of **amoxapine**, or 100–150 mg/day of **maprotiline** produce low drug concentrations in milk, but effects of these drugs on infants have not been well studied. **Bupropion** and its metabolite were concentrated in milk, but were undetectable in the plasma of one 14-month-old infant whose mother was taking 300 mg/day and nursing twice daily. [71] Its safety in younger infants is not known.

Selective Serotonin Reuptake Inhibitors (SSRIs) **Fluoxetine** use during nursing is considered inadvisable. Although daily dosage of the drug and metabolite in milk are less than 10% of the mother's weight-adjusted dosage, [72] their half-lives are very long. One case of colic symptoms and unexplained high serum levels was reported in a breast-fed 6-week-old. [73] Several infants have reportedly been safely breast-fed during maternal fluoxetine use. [72,74,75] Older infants may be less likely to be affected than newborns who eliminate the drug more slowly. **Sertraline** concentrations were undetectable in the plasma of a breast-fed infant whose mother was taking a dosage of 100 mg/day, [69] but little other information is available. **Paroxetine** and **fluvoxamine** appear in milk in amounts similar to or less than fluoxetine, [76,77] but there is much less experience with them. No long-term follow-up has been performed on infants who were nursed during maternal therapy with any SSRI.

Monoamine Oxidase Inhibitors (MAOIs) There are no data on the amounts of MAOIs excreted into milk. Because of their potential toxicity, MAOIs should be avoided during nursing. These drugs also reportedly inhibit lactation.

Antipsychotics Data on the use of antipsychotics during lactation are sparse. [70,78,79] **Haloperidol** has been studied in only two patients; small quantities were found in milk. Infants were not affected, but long-term effects are not known. **Phenothiazines** and **thioxanthenes** pass into milk somewhat unpredictably, but usually in small amounts. Drowsiness can occur with the more sedating agents, such as **chlorpromazine**. Other effects, such as extrapyramidal symptoms, may be possible, but have not been reported. Limited follow-up, ranging from 15 months to 6 yr, indicates no long-term effects on infant development. Breastfeeding during **clozapine** use is not recommended. [80] Outside the United States, **sulpiride** is used to stimulate prolactin secretion and enhance milk supply in a dosage of 50 mg PO bid or tid for up to 14 days.

Lithium Lithium in milk can adversely affect the infant when lithium elimination is impaired, as in dehydration or in neonates and premature infants. Neonates may also have transplacentally acquired plasma lithium levels. The long-term ef-

(continued)

DRUG	NATURE OF EFFECT
	fects of lithium on infants are not known; many authors consider lithium therapy a contraindication to breastfeeding, but others do not. Lithium can probably be used cautiously in mothers who are carefully selected for their ability to monitor their full-term infants. Breastfeeding should be discontinued immediately if the infant appears restless or looks ill. Measurement of plasma lithium concentrations in the infant can help rule out lithium toxicity.[1,70]

SEDATIVES AND HYPNOTICS

Many sedatives and hypnotics pass into breastmilk in measurable and potentially important amounts. Sedative and hypnotic intake should be minimized during lactation.

General Anesthetics	Compared with epidural anesthesia, general anesthesia used during cesarean delivery can decrease both the frequency and duration of breastfeeding.[81] Excretion of most inhalation anesthetics into breastmilk has not been well studied. Blood levels of anesthetic gases such as **desflurane, enflurane, halothane, isoflurane, nitrous oxide,** and **sevoflurane** drop rapidly following anesthesia, are predicted to pass poorly into milk, and are probably poorly absorbed by the infant.[82,83] **Etomidate** milk levels in milk drop rapidly after a dose and should pose little risk to the infant.[84] Amounts of **propofol** in milk are small and probably do not have good oral bioavailability in the infant. Typical IV doses of **thiopental** for induction of anesthesia produce low concentrations in milk that do not appear to cause effects in the infant.[1,84] Recent opinion suggests that breastfeeding can be resumed as soon as the mother has recovered from general anesthesia sufficiently to nurse.[82,83]
Barbiturates	Barbiturates may stimulate metabolism of endogenous compounds in the infant when small amounts pass into milk. Short-acting agents appear to be preferable to long-acting agents, because smaller amounts are excreted into milk. Large single doses may have more potential for causing infant drowsiness than multiple small doses. *See also* Anesthetics and Anticonvulsants.
Benzodiazepines	Long-acting benzodiazepines and those with active metabolites (eg, diazepam) can accumulate and cause adverse effects in infants, especially neonates, because of their immature excretory mechanisms. Milk **alprazolam** levels are relatively low,[85] but infant drowsiness and withdrawal symptoms have been reported with alprazolam use during nursing.[1,10] Long-term benzodiazepine therapy should be avoided during breastfeeding, particularly in the neonatal period. When oral therapy is essential, the short-acting agents, **oxazepam** or **lorazepam**, appear to be preferable; **temazepam** may also be acceptable.[86] Breastmilk should be withheld for 6–8 hr after a single dose of **diazepam** for short dental, surgical, or diagnostic procedures. **Midazolam** concentrations in milk are low and unlikely to affect the infant after a single dose or short course of therapy.[82,83]
Miscellaneous Sedative-Hypnotics	**Chloral hydrate** and its active metabolite, **trichloroethanol,** appear in milk in dosages that approximate an infant sedative dosage and are detectable for up to 24 hr after a single dose. **Meprobamate** concentrations peak in milk at 4 hr, which is 2 hr after peak maternal plasma concentrations. **Zolpidem** milk levels are low for 3 hr after a dose and undetectable thereafter.[87]

MISCELLANEOUS AGENTS

Allopurinol	**Allopurinol** and its active metabolite **oxypurinol** are excreted into milk in nearly therapeutic amounts and oxypurinol is detectable in the nursing infant's plasma in near-therapeutic levels.[88] Although one infant breast-fed without

(continued)

DRUG	NATURE OF EFFECT
	harm, infants should be observed for side effects, especially hypersensitivity reactions. If possible, give allopurinol to the mother in a single dose after the last nursing of the evening.
Baclofen	Baclofen appears in milk in small amounts, and it may be used in nursing mothers with caution.
Bupivacaine	Bupivacaine is undetectable in milk when administered to the mother by the intrapleural or epidural routes.
Colchicine	Several infants have been breast-fed safely during long-term, low-dose administration of colchicine for familial Mediterranean fever.[89,90] The amounts excreted in milk indicate that toxicity might occur with higher dosages.[90] Colchicine is known to decrease milk production and alter milk composition in animals when infused into the udder. It should only be used with great caution and in low dosages when breastfeeding.
Fluorescein	Fluorescein is detectable in milk after IV or topical administration. After IV administration, it had a milk half-life of 62 hr in one mother. The drug may present a risk to neonates who are undergoing phototherapy. Temporarily withholding nursing after fluorescein use (especially IV) appears to be appropriate in this situation.
Fluoride	Fluoride concentrations in milk are low and virtually unrelated to maternal intake. Although there are no definitive studies, most authors recommend fluoride supplementation in breast-fed infants.
Gadodiamide and Gadopentetate	These noniodine, **gadolinium**-containing contrast media used in magnetic resonance imaging are detectable in milk, but have poor oral absorption and are rapidly excreted renally. Withholding of nursing for 6–12 hr should provide adequate safety.
Gold	During maternal administration of **aurothioglucose** and **gold sodium thiomalate**, gold was detected in the blood and urine of some nursing infants. The weight-adjusted infant dosage may be greater than the maternal dosage, but the amount of gold that infants absorb is not clear. Sufficient amounts are absorbed, however, to potentially cause adverse effects. Opinions vary, but gold therapy is a reason to very carefully monitor the breast-fed infant, and may be a reason for withholding breastfeeding.
Iodides	Inorganic iodide is contraindicated during breastfeeding, because of possible thyroid suppression and rash. Topical and vaginal **povidone-iodine** in nursing mothers results in elevated milk iodine concentrations and occasional thyroid suppression in nursing infants. Povidone iodine preparations should not be used while nursing. **Iopanoic acid** contains free iodide that can be detected in milk. **Diatrizoate**, **iodamide**, **iohexol**, **metrizoate**, and **metrizamide** are detectable in milk after IV administration. Although no adverse effects have been reported in infants, breastfeeding should probably be withheld for 24 hr after administration of most iodinated contrast media. Large amounts of iodine are excreted in milk into milk for weeks after lymphangiography with **ethiodized oil**, and nursing should be discontinued after this procedure.
Levodopa	Levodopa decreases serum prolactin in nonnursing women with hyperprolactinemia and galactorrhea. It decreases serum prolactin in a dose-dependent fashion and inhibits lactation in animals at high dosages. It is likely that levodopa would interfere with lactation in nursing mothers. Effects in breast-fed infants have not been studied.

(continued)

DRUG	NATURE OF EFFECT
Lindane	Lindane was excreted into milk at up to 30 times the typical background concentration (from environmental pollution) after maternal topical application of a 0.3% emulsion daily for 3 days. Milk concentrations remained elevated over background concentrations for at least 7 days. Although they have not been studied, alternative drugs (eg, **permethrin, pyrethrins**) are preferred for nursing mothers because of their low order of toxicity.
Magnesium	Therapy with IV magnesium increases milk magnesium concentrations only slightly. Oral absorption of magnesium is poor, so maternal magnesium therapy is not a contraindication to breastfeeding. Difficulty in establishing a milk supply by the mother and difficulty in nursing by the infant are sometimes observed after mothers have received magnesium sulfate infusions for the treatment of eclampsia.
Neostigmine	Six infants of mothers treated with neostigmine for myasthenia gravis were reportedly breast-fed successfully. Neostigmine was not found in milk, but one infant appeared to have abdominal cramps after each breastfeeding.
Pyridostigmine	Pyridostigmine has been used safely during breastfeeding in three patients with myasthenia gravis.
Pyridoxine	High-dose pyridoxine (600 mg/day in three doses) has been used therapeutically to suppress lactation, although it is often not effective. With usual dosages found in foods and low-dose vitamin supplements, pyridoxine has no effect on prolactin or lactation.
Retinoids	The primary active metabolite of **etretinate, acitretin,** passes into breastmilk in a quantity sufficient to recommend avoidance of nursing while taking either of these drugs. Although there is no information on use during lactation, the manufacturers of topical **tretinoin** and oral **isotretinoin** state that they are not compatible with nursing. Based on the systemic bioavailability of tretinoin applied topically to a small area such as the face, it seems unlikely that harmful amounts reach the infant via breastmilk. Caution should be used to avoid contact of the infant's skin with treated areas of the mother's skin, regardless of whether she is nursing.
Sulfonylureas	**Tolbutamide** is excreted in milk in small amounts that should cause no harm. The manufacturer reports that **chlorpropamide** levels in milk are low, but no published clinical data are available. No information is available on the other oral sulfonylurea agents.
Sympathomimetic Agents	Sympathomimetics decrease milk flow in animals by central inhibition of secretion and release of oxytocin, and by peripheral vasoconstriction, which limits the access of oxytocin to myoepithelial cells in the breast. **Norepinephrine** may also decrease prolactin release. Although these effects are not well documented in humans, lactation inhibition seems to occur occasionally with oral decongestants (eg, **pseudoephedrine**); therefore, sympathomimetic nasal sprays (eg, **oxymetazoline**) are recommended over oral decongestant products. **Pseudoephedrine** may also cause irritability in some infants.[10] Use of oral **terbutaline** results in low milk terbutaline concentrations, causes no symptoms in breast-fed infants, and is not expected to decrease milk supply. β_2-receptor agonists are probably safe to use orally, but inhaler products should transfer less drug to the infant and are preferred.
Sumatriptan	Sumatriptan poses little risk during breastfeeding.[91]
Theophyllines	Maternal theophylline use may occasionally cause irritability and fretful sleep in (*continued*)

DRUG	NATURE OF EFFECT
	infants. Newborn infants are most likely to be affected because of their slow elimination and low plasma protein binding of theophylline. There is no need to avoid theophylline products; however, maternal plasma concentrations should be kept in the lower part of the therapeutical range and infant plasma concentrations may be measured if side effects appear to occur. The related drug **dyphylline** is excreted into milk in greater amounts and is best avoided.
Vaccines	Breastfeeding is not a contraindication to the use of *any* vaccine in the mother.[92]

DRUGS FOR NONMEDICAL USE

Alcohol	Alcohol equilibrates rapidly between blood and milk, resulting in milk concentrations equivalent to simultaneous blood concentrations. Peak maternal plasma alcohol levels occur later in nursing mothers than in nonnursing women;[93] alteration in milk odor parallels milk alcohol levels.[93,94] Potential effects on infants vary, depending on the pattern of use. Drunkenness (deep, unarousable sleep with snoring, deep respiration, no reaction to pain, inability to suck, excessive perspiration, and a feeble pulse) was reported after maternal binge drinking.
	Pseudo-Cushing's syndrome was reported in the infant of a chronic alcoholic mother. One prospective study suggests that as little as 1 drink daily can cause slight impairment of the infant's motor development that increases in a dose-dependent fashion.[1] Infants suck more, but consume less milk after maternal alcohol ingestion.[94] Alcohol also affects lactation; it inhibits the milk ejection reflex in a dose-dependent fashion, with single doses over 2 g/kg completely blocking suckling-induced oxytocin release. Animal studies show that alcohol consumption results in a reduced suckling-induced prolactin release and reduced milk yield. An unknown substance in beer increases maternal serum prolactin, but this effect also occurs with nonalcoholic beer.[1,95] Alcohol should be used in moderation during lactation. Nursing should probably be withheld temporarily after alcohol consumption, with the duration dependent on the amount consumed — at least 2 hr per drink is suggested.[96]
Amphetamines	In a mother taking amphetamine 20 mg/day therapeutically, amphetamine concentrations in milk were less than those in plasma and no adverse effects on the infant were noted. However, there is likely to be substantial intersubject variation in excretion, and concentrations in milk during high-dose abuse of amphetamines have not been measured. Anecdotally, infants seem to experience drug-induced behavioral abnormalities, such as agitation and crying. Amphetamine also inhibits prolactin release and, in high dosages, may interfere with lactation.
Caffeine	Anecdotal reports of infant jitteriness and difficulty sleeping have been reported with very high maternal intake of caffeine, but infant serum caffeine concentrations were not measured. Systematic studies have indicated that caffeine and its metabolites are excreted into milk in relatively small amounts with usual maternal intake and infants are usually not affected, even with rather high maternal intake.[1,97,98] Effects are more likely in premature and newborn infants, because of their greatly diminished ability to metabolize caffeine.
Cocaine	Although not well studied in humans, the chemical nature of cocaine and results from animal studies indicate that it would be expected to appear in milk in amounts that would affect the infant.[1,99] In addition, plasma cholinesterase, which is needed to metabolize the drug, is low in newborns. Cocaine and its toxic metabolite can be detected in milk and cause adverse effects (consisting of vomiting, diarrhea, irritability, and dilated pupils) in breast-fed infants.[1,99]

(continued)

DRUG	NATURE OF EFFECT
	Cocaine was detectable in milk for 24–36 hr after use. Convulsions occurred in an infant whose mother used topical cocaine to treat sore nipples. Breast-feeding is not recommended when the mother is a chronic cocaine user, and even occasional use of cocaine is discouraged during breastfeeding. Breast-feeding should be withheld for at least 24 hr after occasional cocaine use.
Heroin	Heroin abuse can result in high enough concentrations in milk to cause addiction or alleviate withdrawal symptoms in infants; however, breastfeeding is not a reliable method of preventing withdrawal. Although most authorities do not consider **methadone** maintenance a contraindication to breastfeeding, it is best to avoid breastfeeding for 2–6 hr after the dose, when peak milk concentrations occur.
Marijuana	Marijuana excretion into milk has not been well studied, but **dronabinol** (**tetrahydrocannabinol**) may reach high concentrations in milk and may be detected in the infant, particularly with heavy maternal use. Short-term effects in infants have not been reported, but a decrement in motor development at 1 yr in the infants of marijuana-smoking mothers was reported in one study. Marijuana lowers serum prolactin slightly in nonlactating women and oxytocin release in rodents; however, the effect of marijuana on lactation in nursing mothers is not known. Breastfeeding should be avoided when the mother is a heavy marijuana user and during therapeutic dronabinol use. Breastfeeding should be withheld for several hours after occasional marijuana use and caution should be used to avoid exposing the infant to marijuana smoke.
Phencyclidine	Phencyclidine is concentrated in milk and remains detectable for weeks after heavy use. Breastfeeding should be avoided after phencyclidine use, but a sufficient duration of abstinence is undefined.
Tobacco	**Nicotine** and its metabolite, **cotinine**, are excreted into breastmilk in amounts proportional to the number of cigarettes smoked by the mother.[1,100] The milk of smokers contains higher concentrations of **cadmium** than the milk of nonsmokers, but other toxins in smoke have not been measured. Smokers also produce lower milk volumes, have lower milkfat content, use formula supplements more often, and wean their infants from breastfeeding earlier than non-smokers, in part because nicotine lowers maternal basal prolactin concentrations.[1,101,102] fants of smoking mothers have an increased frequency of infantile colic, large postnursing decreases in respiratory rate and oxygen saturation, and more respiratory infections.[1,100] However, among infants of smokers, those who are *not* breast-fed have almost the double the risk of respiratory illness of breast-fed infants.[103] In nonsmokers, breastfeeding reduces the risk of sudden infant death syndrome (SIDS) compared to bottle feeding, but smoking negates this advantage.[104] Nursing mothers should be advised to (1) stop or decrease smoking to the greatest degree possible, (2) not breastfeed right after smoking, and (3) not smoke in the same room with the infant.[1,105] The use of nicotine chewing gum or topical patches has not been studied during lactation. Although they are not recommended by the manufacturer during nursing, these products are likely to be less hazardous to the nursing infant than maternal smoking.

RADIOPHARMACEUTICALS

Exposure of the infant to excessive amounts of radioactivity is usually the primary concern raised by administration of radiopharmaceuticals to nursing mothers, rather than any inherent pharmacologic toxicity of the agent. Breastfeeding should be discontinued, at least temporarily, after administration of a radiopharmaceutical to a nursing mother. The length of time needed for milk radioactivity to decline (by means of both radioactive decay

(continued)

DRUG	NATURE OF EFFECT

and maternal excretion) to a safe exposure level depends on several factors: dosage, biological half-life, radionuclide half-life, "contamination" with other isotopes, age of the infant, potential for oral absorption of the radionuclide from the infant's GI tract, and threshold level that is considered safe. Two reviews deal comprehensively with the topic of radiopharmaceutical use in nursing mothers and provide more detailed information.[106,107]

■ REFERENCES

1. Anderson PO. Drug use during breast feeding. *Clin Pharm* 1991;10:594–624.

2. Rasmussen F. The mechanisms of drug secretion into milk. In Galli C et al., eds. *Dietary lipids and postnatal development*. New York: Raven Press; 1973;231:45

3. Richter O, Reinhardt D. The transference of drugs from breast-feeding mothers to their infants: a pharmacokinetic model. *Biol Res Preg* 1980;1:112–7.

4. Wilson JT et al. Pharmacokinetic pitfalls in the estimation of the breast milk/plasma ratio for drugs. *Annu Rev Pharmacol Toxicol* 1985;25:667–89.

5. Fleishaker JC et al. Factors affecting the milk-to-plasma drug concentration ratio in lactating women: physical interactions with protein and fat. *J Pharm Sci* 1987;76:189–93.

6. Atkinson HC, Begg EJ. Prediction of drug distribution into human milk from physicochemical characteristics. *Clin Pharmacokinet* 1990;18:151–67.

7. Anderson PO. Medication use while breast feeding a neonate. *Neonatal Pharmacol Q* 1993; 2:3–14.

8. Oo CY et al. Active transport of cimetidine into human milk. *Clin Pharmacol Ther* 1995;58:548–55.

9. Ito S, Koren G. A novel index for expressing exposure of the infant to drugs in breast milk. *Br J Clin Pharmacol* 1994;38:99–102.

10. Ito S et al. Prospective follow-up of adverse reactions in breast-fed infants exposed to maternal medication. *Am J Obstet Gynecol* 1993;168:1393–9.

11. Harmon T et al. Perforated pseudomembranous colitis in the breast-fed infant. *J Pediatr Surg* 1992;27:744–46.

12. Righard L, Alade MO. Effect of delivery room routines on success of first breast-feed. *Lancet* 1990;336:1105–7.

13. Rajan L. The impact of obstetric procedures and analgesia/anesthesia during labour and delivery on breast feeding. *Midwifery* 1994;10:87–103.

14. Crowell MK et al. Relationship between obstetric analgesia and time of effective breast feeding. *J Nurse Midwifery* 1994;39:150–5.

15. Nissen E et al. Effects of maternal pethidine on infants' developing breast feeding behavior. *Acta Paediatr* 1995;84:140–5.

16. Zakowski MI et al. A two-dose epidural morphine regimen in cesarean section patients: pharmacokinetic profile. *Acta Anaesthesiol Scand* 1993;37:584–9.

17. Pittman KA et al. Human perinatal distribution of butorphanol. *Am J Obstet Gynecol* 1980;138:797–800.

18. Wischnik A et al. Elimination von nalbuphin in die muttermilch. *Arzneimittelforschung* 1988;38:1496–8.

19. Madej TH, Strunin L. Comparison of epidural fentanyl with sufentanil. *Anesthesia* 1987;42:1156–61.

20. Leuschen MP et al. Fentanyl excretion in breast milk. *Clin Pharm* 1990;9:336–7. Letter.

21. Steer PL et al. Concentration of fentanyl in colostrum after an analgesic dose. *Can J Anaesth* 1992;39:231–5.

22. Lebedevs TH et al. Excretion of indomethacin in breast milk. *Br J Clin Pharmacol* 1991;32:751–4.

23. Beaulac-Baillargeon L, Allard G. Distribution of indomethacin in human milk and estimation of its milk to plasma ratio in vitro. *Br J Clin Pharmacol* 1993;36:413–6.

24. von Kries R et al. Transfer von phenprocoumon in die muttermilch. *Monatsschr Kinderheilkd* 1993;141:505–7.

25. Ito S et al. Initiation and duration of breast-feeding in women receiving antiepileptics. *Am J Obstet Gynecol* 1995;172:881–6.

26. Hartmann AM et al. Stillen, gewichtszunanme und verhalten bei neugeborenen epileptischer frauen. *Monatsschr Kinderheilkd* 1994;142:505–12.

27. Frey B et al. Transient cholestatic hepatitis in a neonate associated with carbamazepine exposure during pregnancy and breast-feeding. *Eur J Pediatr* 1990;150:136–8.

28. Merlob P et al. Transient hepatic dysfunction in an infant of an epileptic mother treated with carbamazepine during pregnancy and breastfeeding. *Ann Pharmacother* 1992;26:1563–5.

29. Bossi L et al. Pharmacokinetics and clinical effects of antiepileptic drugs in newborns of chronically treated epileptic mothers. In Janz D et al., eds. *Epilepsy, pregnancy and the child*. New York: Raven Press; 1982:373–81.

30. Lucas BD Jr. et al. Terfenadine breast milk excretion and pharmacokinetic in lactating women. *Pharmacotherapy* 1992;12:506. Abstract.

31. Johnstone HA, Marcinak JF. Candidiasis in the breastfeeding mother and infant. *J Obstet Gynecol Neonatal Nurs* 1990;19:171–3.

32. Amir LH, Pakula S. Nipple pain, mastalgia and candidiasis in the lactating breast. *Aust N Z J Obstet Gynecol* 1991;31:378–80.

33. Schilling CG et al. Excretion of fluconazole in human breast milk. *Pharmacotherapy* 1993;13:387. Abstract.

34. Force RW. Fluconazole concentrations in breast milk. *Pediatr Infect Dis J* 1995;14:235–6.

35. Moretti ME et al. Disposition of maternal ketoconazole in breast milk. *Am J Obstet Gynecol* 1995;173:1625–6.

36. Utter AR. Gentian violet treatment for thrush: can its use cause breastfeeding problems? *J Human Lact* 1990;6:178–80.

37. *USP-DI*, 16th ed. Volume I. Drug Information for the health care professional. Rockville, MD: US Pharmacopoeial Convention; 1996:1539–60.

38. Kurzel RB et al. Mebendazole and postpartum lactation. *N Z J Med* 1994;107:439. Letter.

39. Sedlmayr T et al. Clarithromycin, ein neues makrolid-antibiotikum. *Geburtshilfe Frauenheilkd* 1993;53:488–91.

40. Kelsey JJ et al. Presence of azithromycin breast milk concentrations: a case report. *Am J Obstet Gynecol* 1994;170:1375–6.

41. Dan M et al. Penetration of fleroxacin into breast milk and pharmacokinetic in lactating women. *Antimicrob Agents Chemother* 1993;37:293–6.

42. Giamarellou H et al. Temafloxacin pharmacokinetics in the breast milk of lactating women. Presented at the 32nd Interscience Conference on Antimicrobial Agents and Chemotherapy. Anaheim, CA; 1992. Abstract 428.

43. Hunt MJ. Black breast milk due to minocycline therapy. *Br J Dermatol* 1996;134:943–4.

44. Taddio A et al. Acyclovir excretion in human breast milk. *Ann Pharmacother* 1994;28:585–7.

45. Bork K, Benes P. Concentration and kinetic studies of intravenous acyclovir in serum and breast milk of a patient with eczema herpeticum. *J Am Acad Dermatol* 1995;32:1053–5.

46. Dobias L et al. Genotoxicity and carcinogenicity of metronidazole. *Mutation Res* 1994;317:177–94.

47. Reyes MP et al. Vancomycin during pregnancy: does it cause hearing loss or nephrotoxicity in the infant? *Am J Obstet Gynecol* 1989;161:977–81.

48. Azuno Y et al. Mitoxantrone and etoposide in breast milk. *Am J Hematol* 1995;48:131–2.

49. Plomp TA et al. Use of amiodarone during pregnancy. *Eur J Obstet Gynecol Reprod Biol* 1992;43:201–7.

50. Zeisler JA et al. Lidocaine excretion in breast milk. *Drug Intell Clin Pharm* 1981;57:691–3.

51. Lebedevs TH et al. Excretion of lignocaine and its metobolite monoethylglycinexylidide in breast milk following its use in a dental procedure. *J Clin Periodontol* 1993;20:606–8.

52. Libardoni M et al. Transfer of propafenone and 5-OH-propafenone to foetal plasma and maternal milk. *Br J Clin Pharmacol* 1991;32:527–8. Letter.

53. Carcas AJ et al. Nimodipine transfer into human breast milk and cerebrospinal fluid. *Ann Pharmacother* 1996;30:148–50.

54. Bunjes R et al. Clonidine and breast feeding. *Clin Pharm* 1993;12:178–9. Letter.

55. Kaiser G et al. Benazepril and benazeprilat in human plasma and breast milk. *Eur J Clin Pharmacol* 1989;36(suppl):A303. Abstract.

56. Nikodem VC, Hofmeyr GJ. Secretion of the antidiarrhoeal agent loperamide oxide in breast milk. *Eur J Clin Pharmacol* 1992;42:695–6. Letter.

57. Miller LG et al. Disposition of olsalazine and metabolites in breast milk. *J Clin Pharmacol* 1993;33:703–6.

58. Klotz U, Harings-Kaim A. Negligible amounts of 5-aminosalicylic acid in breast milk. *Lancet* 1993;342:618–9. Letter.

59. Pardthaisong T et al. The long-term growth and development of children exposed to Depo-Provera during pregnancy or lactation. *Contraception* 1992;45:313–24.

60. Dunson TR et al. A multicenter clinical trial of a progestin-only oral contraceptive in lactating women. *Contraception* 1993;47:23–35.

61. Progestogen-only contraceptives during lactation: I. Infant growth. World Health Organization Task force for Epidemiological Research on Reproductive Health; Special Programme of Research, Development and Research Training in Human Reproduction. *Contraception* 1994;50:35–53.

62. Progestogen-only contraceptives during lactation: II. Infant development. World Health Organization Task Force for Epidemiological Research on Reproductive Health; Special Programme of Research, Development and Research Training in Human Reproduction. *Contraception* 1994;50:55–68.

63. Chi I-C et al. The progestin-only oral contraceptive-its place in postpartum contraception. *Adv Contraception* 1992;8:93–103.

64. Díaz S, Croxatto HB. Contraception in lactating women. *Curr Opin Obstet Gynecol* 1993;5:815–22.

65. Greenberger PA et al. Pharmacokinetics of prednisolone transfer to breast milk. *Clin Pharmacol Ther* 1993;53:324–8.

66. Hanew K et al. Simultaneous administration of TRH and sulpiride caused additive but not synergistic PRL responses in normal subjects. *Endocrinol Jpn* 1992;39:465–8.

67. Aziz F. Effect of methimazole treatment of maternal thyrotoxicosis on thyroid function in breast-feeding infants. *J Pediatr* 1996;128:855–8.

68. Wisner KL et al. Antidepressant treatment during breast-feeding. *Am J Psychiatr* 1996;153:1132–7.

69. Altshuler LL et al. Breastfeeding and sertraline: a 24-hour analysis. *J Clin Psychiatr* 1995;56:243–5.

70. Yoshida K, Kumar R. Breast feeding and psychotropic drugs. *Int Rev Psychiatr* 1996;8:117–24.

71. Briggs GG et al. Excretion of bupropion in breast milk. *Ann Pharmaco Ther* 1993;27:431–3.

72. Taddio A et al. Excretion of fluoxetine and its metabolite, norfluoxetine, in human breast milk. *J Clin Pharmacol* 1996;36:42–7.

73. Lester BM et al. Possible association between fluoxetine hydrochloride and colic in an infant. *J Am Acad Child Adolesc Psychiatry* 1993;32:1253–5.

74. Isenberg KE. Excretion of fluoxetine in human breast milk. *J Clin Psychiatry* 1990;51:169. Letter.

75. Burch KJ, Wells, BG. Fluoxetine/norfluoxetine concentrations in human milk. *Pediatrics* 1992;89:676–7.

76. Spigset O et al. Paroxetine levels in breast milk. *J Clin Psychiatr* 1996;57:29. Letter.

77. Wright S et al. Excretion of fluvoxamine in breast milk. *Br J Clin Pharmacol* 1991;31:209. Letter.

78. McElhatton PR. The use of phenothiazines during pregnancy and lactation. *Reprod Toxicol* 1992;6:475–90.

79. Pons G et al. Excretion of psychoactive drugs into breast milk. *Clin Pharmacokinet* 1994;27:270–89.

80. Barnas C et al. Clozapine concentrations in maternal and fetal plasma, amniotic fluid, and breast milk. *Am J Psychiatr* 1994;151:945. Letter.

81. Lie B, Juul J. Effect of epidural vs. general anesthesia on breastfeeding. *Acta Obstet Gynecol Scand* 1988;67:207–9.

82. Lee JJ, Rubin AP. Breast feeding and anaesthesia. *Anesthesia* 1993;48:616:25.

83. Spigset O. Anaesthetic agents and excretion in breast milk. *Acta Anaesthesiol Scand* 1994;38:94–103.

84. Esener Z et al. Thiopentone and etomidate concentrations in maternal and umbilical plasma, and in colostrum. *Br J Anaesthesia* 1992;69:586–8.

85. Oo Cy et al. Pharmacokinetics in lactating women; prediction of alprazolam transfer into milk. *Br J Clin Pharmacol* 1995;40:231–6.

86. Lebedevs TH et al. Excretion of temazepam in breast milk. *Br J Clin Pharmacol* 1992;33:204–6. Letter.

87. Pons G et al. Zolpidem excretion in breast milk. *Eur J Clin Pharmacol* 1989;37:245–8.

88. Kamilli I, Gresser U. Allopurinol and oxypurinol in human breast milk. *Clin Invest* 1993;71:161–4.

89. Ben-Chetrit E et al. Colchicine in breast milk of patients with familial Mediterranean fever. *Arth Rheum* 1996;39:1213–7.

90. Guillonneau M. et al. Colchicine is excreted at high concentrations in human breast milk. *Eur J Obstet Gynecol* 1995;61:177–8.

91. Wonjar-Horton RE et al. Distribution and excretion of sumatriptan in human milk. *Br J Clin Pharmacol* 1996;41:217–21

92. Gizurarson S. Optimal delivery of vaccines. Clinical pharmacokinetic considerations. *Clin Pharmacokinet* 1996;30:1–15.

93. da-Silva VA et al. Ethanol pharmacokinetics in lactating women. *Braz J Med Biol Res* 1993;26:1097–103.

94. Mennella JA, Beauchamp GK. The transfer of alcohol in human milk. Effects on flavor and the infant's behavior. *N Engl J Med* 1991;325:981–5.

95. Menella JA, Beauchamp GK. Beer, breastfeeding, and folklore. *Dev Psychobiol* 1993;16:459–66.

96. Anderson PO. Alcohol and breast feeding. *J Hum Lact* 1995;11:321–3.

97. Blanchard J et al. Methylxanthine levels in breast milk of lactating women in different ethnic and socioeconomic classes. *Biopharm Drug Dispos* 1992;13:187–96.

98. Oo CY et al. Pharmacokinetics of caffeine and its demethylated metabolites in lactation: predictions of milk to serum concentration ratios. *Pharm Res* 1995;12:313–6.

99. Dickson PH et al. The routine analysis of breast milk for drugs of abuse in a clinical toxicology laboratory. *J Forensic Sci* 1994;39:207–14.

100. Stephans MBF, Wilkerson N. Physiologic effects of maternal smoking on breast-feeding infants. *J Acad Nurse Pract* 1993;5:105–13.

101. Mansbach IK et al. Onset and duration of breast feeding among Israeli mothers: relationships with smoking and types of delivery. *Soc Sci Med* 1991;33:1391–7.

102. Hopkinson LM et al. Milk production by mothers of premature infants: influence of cigarette smoking. *Pediatrics* 1992;90:934–8.

103. Jin C, Rossignol AM. Effects of passive smoking on respiratory illness from birth to eighteen months, in Shanghai, People Republic of China. *J Pediatr* 1993;123:553–8.

104. Klonoff-Cohen HS et al. The effect of passive smoking and tobacco exposure through breast milk on sudden infant death syndrome. *JAMA* 1995;273:795–8.

105. Hakansson A, Cars H. Maternal cigarette smoking; breast-feeding, and respiratory tract infections in infancy; a matched-pairs study. *Scand J Primary Health Care* 1991;9:115–9.

106. Romney BM et al. Radionuclide administration to nursing mothers; mathematically derived guidelines. *Radiology* 1986;160:549–54.

107. Mountford PJ, Coakley AJ. A review of the secretion of radioactivity in human breast milk: data, quantitative analysis and recommendations. *Nucl Med Commun* 1989;10:15–27.

Pediatric Drug Therapy

William E. Murray

Pediatric drug therapy presents a challenge to the practitioner in many respects. The pediatric population is comprised of a range of patient weights and organ maturity. There is often a lack of pediatric-specific data in the literature from which to derive appropriate dosage regimens. At times, medications must be used for which data are extrapolated on the basis of limited pharmacokinetic knowledge about the pediatric population. It must be remembered that children should not be treated as "little adults" when designing dosage regimens. Dosage administration nomograms derived from adult data should not be used in the pediatric population. Pharmacodynamic responses for the majority of medications used in children are even less well known. Children often react much differently from adults to certain medications. Examples are the use of stimulants such as methylphenidate to control hyperactivity common with attention deficit disorders and paradoxical hyperactivity, which may be observed in children when taking phenobarbital. With therapeutically monitored medications, the standard adult therapeutic range is typically used, because age-specific, concentration-effect information is scarce. Due to protein binding differences, infants may respond to lower total drug concentrations than adults for certain medications (eg, phenytoin, theophylline).

One of the problems facing the clinician and caregiver of small children is the administration of medications. Dosage forms are usually designed with the adult population in mind, and the dosage cannot easily be individualized in small patients. This is especially true for most sustained-release products. Most young children cannot swallow tablets and capsules; thus, liquid preparations are generally preferred in this age group. For many drugs, liquid forms are not commercially available and must be extemporaneously compounded. Stability of these preparations is often unknown or of limited duration. Even when appropriate dosage forms suitable for young children are available, palatability, resistance to taking medications, and compliance issues may hinder optimal therapy.

■ PHARMACOKINETICS

Absorption

At birth, gastric pH is neutral but falls to values of 1–3 in the first day of life. Subsequently, gastric pH returns toward neutrality, because gastric acid secretion is low in the first several weeks to months. Adult values are usually achieved after the age of 2 yr.[1,2] Medications that require gastric acidity for absorption may have poor bioavailability in this age group, rendering them ineffective or requiring much higher doses than normal in order for therapeutic serum concentrations to be reached. Examples of medications in this group include phenytoin, ketoconazole, and itraconazole.[1,3] Alternative agents may have to be used if adequate serum levels cannot be documented when these drugs are administered orally. Certain medications that are acid-labile may actually have increased bioavailability in infants. These include antibiotics such as penicillin G and ampicillin.[4]

Gastric emptying time can be delayed in infants, especially premature infants.[1,3,5] Peak drug concentrations may occur much later during infancy than in older children and adults. Other factors that may influence overall bioavailability of a particular medication in infants include the relatively high frequencies of gastroesophageal reflux, which may cause the dose to be spit up or vomited, and acute gastroenteritis (diarrhea), which may considerably shorten intestinal transit time. The oral route must be used with caution in these instances, especially in critically ill patients.

Other routes of administration can also pose difficulties in the pediatric population. Overall muscle mass is decreased, and intramuscular administration may not be practical and is certainly not appreciated by most children. Most adults still remember their first injections in the doctor's office when they were children. Also, the dose of drug to be administered may require multiple injections.

Rectal administration may be used in situations where the oral route is not practical or available; however, absorption may be incomplete and/or erratic. Topical administration of medications can lead to undesired systemic absorption, especially in infancy when the skin thickness is less and the total skin surface area is proportionally greater than in adults.[1,2,4]

Distribution

Rapid changes in body composition can dramatically alter the volume of distribution (V_d) for many medications during the first several months of life. Newborns have a higher percentage of total body water and extracellular fluid than older children and adults.[1,3,6] Hydrophilic drugs such as the aminoglycosides have a much larger V_d in newborns; this gradually decreases over the first year of life to approach adult values.

Total body fat in newborns (especially premature infants) is much lower than in older children and adults.[6] Medications that are lipophilic may have a lower weight-adjusted V_d in the very young.

Protein binding is an important determinant of the V_d for drugs that are bound by albumin and other plasma proteins. In the neonatal period, the binding affinity of albumin is decreased compared with older children and adults (because of the persistence of fetal albumin).[1–3] Highly protein-bound drugs such as phenytoin have a higher free fraction in neonates, and there may be an increased pharmacodynamic response at lower concentrations of total drug. The V_d of these drugs is inversely related to the degree of protein binding.

Additionally, the clinician must be aware of the potential for highly protein-bound substances to displace bilirubin from binding sites on albumin, particularly in the newborn.[1–3,7] The blood-brain barrier in newborns is more permeable than in older patients, and free bilirubin can readily cross into the CNS and cause kernicterus.

Tissue-binding characteristics for many medications are unknown, but can vary dramatically from that in adults. One example is digoxin, which binds to erythrocytes in pediatric patients to a much greater extent than in adult patients.[2,4] Digoxin has a much larger V_d in pediatric patients, and recommended loading dose regimens in this age group are much larger on a mg/kg basis than in adult patients. Generally, drug distribution volumes are larger in neonates and gradually approach adult values (in L/kg) by the first year of life.

Metabolism

Metabolic processes show dramatic changes in the first weeks to months of life. At birth, most hepatic enzymes are immature and drug metabolizing capacity is greatly reduced. Phase I reactions (ie, oxidation) are largely controlled by the mixed-function oxidase system, of which the cytochrome P450 enzymes are the major determinant. These enzymes are largely undeveloped in newborns, especially premature infants, but maturation may take place quickly in the first weeks to months of life. Phase II reactions (ie, conjugation) include glucuronidation, sulfation, and acetylation. These reactions are also immature at birth, and drug toxicity has resulted (eg, with chloramphenicol) because of the absence of knowledge about dosage requirements in newborns.[1–3,6]

The liver size relative to body weight in newborns is much larger than in adults.[1] Rapid weight gain, with subsequent increases in liver size and metabolic capacity, may require many dosage adjustments to prevent newborns from growing out of their dosages for many medications. When full metabolic capacity is reached in the pediatric patient, the hepatic clearance may greatly exceed that observed in adult patients on a weight-adjusted basis. Pediatric dosages of many medications on a mg/kg basis are often much greater than in adults. Figure 3–2 illustrates the change in clearance with age for theophylline.[6] Most medications have similar curves, but may be shifted to the left or have different relative peaks compared with adult values. A decrease in hepatic clearance relative to body weight typically begins after a child weighs approximately 30 kg.[8] Thereafter, the increase in total body weight in proportion to liver size becomes greater. Thus in adolescence, drug dosages typically begin to approach adult values. Drug toxicity can be observed in the adolescent patient if drug dosages on a mg/kg basis (designed for younger patients) are used.

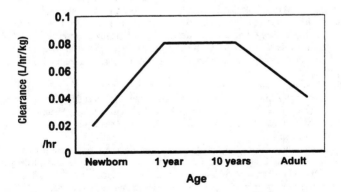

Figure 3–2. Maturation of Theophylline Metabolism

Renal Elimination

The kidneys are the major route of drug elimination for many drugs. The kidneys are functionally immature at birth with regard to both glomerular filtration and tubular secretion. Glomerular filtration at birth adjusted for body surface area is only 30–40% of values in older infants and healthy young adults.[1-3] Premature infants often have even lower values during the first few weeks of life. Dosages of many medications (eg, aminoglycosides, vancomycin) that are eliminated largely by glomerular filtration must be decreased on the basis of the relative immaturity of the kidneys at birth. Maturation of glomerular filtration occurs over the first several weeks to months of life. The dosages of most medications are similar to those in older children by 4–6 months of age. Although the frequency of renal disease in children is much lower than in the adult population, factors that may alter renal function, such as shock, nonsteroidal antiinflammatory drugs, or hypoxia, must be considered when evaluating dosage regimens. Serum creatinine, the usual marker for renal function, is usually lower in young children compared with adults. This is because of children's lower muscle mass. Thus, a serum creatinine that indicates normal renal function in an adult may indicate renal impairment in a young child.

Tubular secretion is also diminished in the newborn. Drugs that have a component of tubular secretion (eg, penicillin) are typically administered at reduced dosages in the newborn. Maturation of tubular secretion occurs somewhat more slowly than glomerular filtration, but approaches adult values by 8–12 months of age.[1-3]

Evaluating Drug Data in Children

With the numerous maturational changes observed in children from birth through adolescence, results of pediatric drug studies must be used with caution in children whose age differs from that in the study. Dosages extrapolated only on a weight basis have the potential to underdose or overdose other age groups, depending on the population studied. Body surface area may correlate better with total body water and extracellular water than body weight, and may be useful in certain instances in calculating dosage regimens. With the exception of cancer chemotherapeutic agents, information on drug dosage is more widely available in mg/kg than by body surface area.[5] Medications with narrow therapeutic ranges should have serum concentrations measured to aid in individualizing drug therapy, especially in critically ill children or those with known decreased renal or hepatic function.

Pharmacodynamic changes are poorly studied in the pediatric population, and responses to specific drug concentrations may be much different than in the adult population. Diseases of childhood often differ from those in adults. Medications that may be tolerated by adult patients may be inappropriate for the pediatric population (eg, aspirin for fever).

Caution must be used in the interpretation of drug levels, as there may be much greater fluctuation in serum concentrations because of shorter drug half-lives in children than in adults. Additionally, the total volume of blood needed for drug level monitoring in small children may limit serum level monitoring.

Detailed information on specific drugs can be found in the Pediatric Dosage sections of the individual drug monographs.

REFERENCES

1. Stewart CF, Hampton EM. Effect of maturation on drug disposition in pediatric patients. *Clin Pharm* 1987;6:548–64.

2. Besunder JB et al. Principles of drug biodisposition in the neonate. A critical evaluation of the pharmacokinetic-pharmacodynamic interface (part I). *Clin Pharmacokinet* 1988;14:189–216.

3. Milsap RL et al. Special pharmacokinetic considerations in children. In Evans WE et al., eds. *Applied pharmacokinetics. Principles of therapeutic drug monitoring,* 3rd ed. Vancouver, WA: Applied Therapeutics; 1992:10-1–32.

4. Morselli PL et al. Clinical pharmacokinetics in newborns and infants. Age-related differences and therapeutic implications. In Gibaldi M, Prescott LF, eds. *Handbook of clinical pharmacokinetics,* Section II. Balgowlah, NSW, Australia: ADIS Health Science Press; 1983:98–141.

5. Maxwell GM. Paediatric drug dosing. Bodyweight versus surface area. *Drugs* 1989;37:113–5.

6. McLeod HL, Evans WE. Pediatric pharmacokinetics and therapeutic drug monitoring. *Pediatr Rev* 1992;13:413–21.

7. Morselli PL. Clinical pharmacokinetics in neonates. In Gibaldi M, Prescott LF, eds. *Handbook of clinical pharmacokinetics,* Section II. Balgowlah, NSW, Australia: ADIS Health Science Press; 1983:79–97.

8. Rane A, Wilson JT. Clinical pharmacokinetics in infants and children. In Gibaldi M, Prescott LF, eds. *Handbook of clinical pharmacokinetics,* Section II. Balgowlah, NSW, Australia: ADIS Health Science Press; 1983:142–68.

Geriatric Drug Therapy

Dianne E. Tobias

Geriatric drug therapy is an important area of therapeutics and research, because of the growing elderly population, their disproportionately high use of medications, and their increased risk of drug misadventures. Although they represent approximately 12% of the U.S. population, the elderly consume more than 30% of all medications.[1] Trends include increasing numbers of the extreme elderly (over age 80) and elderly with functional disabilities. It is estimated that the number of elderly who are dependent in their activities of daily living will triple from 1985 to 2060. Ethical considerations, such as a patient's right to exercise decisions regarding treatment, are particularly relevant to the elderly population.[2,3] As the number of elderly increases and health care resources diminish, cost-benefit considerations will become increasingly important.[4]

The elderly are the most physiologically heterogenous category of the adult population. The rate of normal aging varies considerably, and comparing data from persons of chronologically similar age can be misleading; health status is probably as important as age. Optimization of drug therapy in the elderly requires an understanding of how aging and concomitant pathology affect the pharmacokinetics and pharmacodynamics of drugs, the need to assess elderly patients individually, and of the elderly patients' expectations of therapy.[5]

Compliance issues leading to misuse and medication errors can be important in the elderly.[6] The cost of medications, physical difficulty in opening medication containers, swallowing large tablets, reading the prescription label, and the presence of depression or cognitive impairment can contribute to compliance problems.[7–9]

Adverse drug reactions are more common in the elderly,[10–13] although the correlation with age alone is debatable.[1,14] Increased medication use, especially medications with greater potential for toxicity, and chronic pathology with intermittent acute exacerbations are thought to contribute to the higher frequency and severity of adverse drug reactions. Most reactions in the elderly are dose-related rather than idiosyncratic as a result of changes in pharmacokinetics and/or pharmacodynamics. Given the wide physiologic variability in the elderly population, the contribution of pharmacokinetic and pharmacodynamic changes can vary considerably. Additionally, the elderly are more sensitive to specific adverse reactions. For example, they have an increased sensitivity to anticholinergic side effects, especially central effects such as disorientation and memory impairment. These effects can be additive because many drugs commonly taken by the elderly are centrally active.[15–17] Varying degrees of cognitive impairment or even delirium can be induced by drugs in several classes including benzodiazepines, centrally acting antihypertensive agents, and antidepressants.[15,18] The onset can be insidious and mistakenly attributed solely to the aging process.

■ PHARMACOKINETICS

Absorption

With aging there is some decrease in gastric secretions, acidity, gastric emptying, peristalsis, absorptive surface area, and splanchnic blood flow,[9,19] although the effect on gastric pH may not be as pronounced as previously believed.[20,21] Taken together, the changes predict an altered extent or rate of absorption of orally administered drugs, yet most formal studies show no difference in oral bioavailability. Some factors might counterbalance each other (eg, acidity and gastric emptying; decreased absorptive surface and longer transit time). Some drugs (eg, digoxin) have shown a clinically unimportant slowed rate of absorption with equivalent quantities absorbed. Drugs with high extraction ratios may have increased bioavailability in the elderly compared with young patients, because of a decreased first-pass effect secondary to reduced hepatic blood flow. Impaired first-pass metabolism in the elderly has been shown for labetalol, propranolol, lidocaine, and verapamil.[22] It is known that the elderly have drier skin with lower lipid content, which is expected to be less permeable to hydrophilic compounds. Although neither conclusively nor well studied, percutaneous drug absorption appears to decrease with age.[23]

Distribution

Body weight generally decreases, but more important, body composition changes with age. Total body water and lean body mass decrease, while body fat increases in proportion to total body weight. The percentage of body weight contributed by fat changes from 18% and 33% in young men and women, respectively, to 36% and 45% in their elderly counterparts.[24] These factors can alter the apparent volume of distribution (V_d) of drugs in the elderly, although other aspects of drug disposition (binding, metabolism, elimination) can be additive or negate the effect. The V_d changes are most marked for highly lipophilic and hydrophilic drugs, and elderly patients are particularly susceptible to overdosage from drugs that should be dosed on ideal body weight or lean body weight.[25] Theoretically, highly lipid-soluble drugs (eg, long-acting benzodiazepines, lidocaine) may have an increased V_d and a prolonged effect if drug clearance remains constant. Conversely, water-soluble drugs (eg, digoxin) may have a decreased V_d, and at least transiently increased serum levels, leading to possible toxicity if initial doses are not conservative.[9] Although cardiac output does not appear to decrease with age,[26] some chronic diseases affecting the elderly do contribute to a decrease in cardiac output and regional blood flow. There is some evidence that blood is preferentially shunted away from the liver and kidneys to the brain, heart, and muscles.[27] These changes could explain the slowed elimination of some drugs and the heightened sensitivity to others.

Protein Binding

The proportion of albumin among total plasma proteins decreases with frailty, catabolic disease states, and immobility seen in many elderly,[28] but it is no longer believed that serum albumin decreases with age alone.[23] Serum albumin determinations should be performed to aid monitoring and dosage adjustment of drugs that are highly protein bound in the chronically immobile or ill elderly. A decrease in serum albumin can increase the percentage of free drug available for pharmacologic effect and elimination. Changes in albumin binding are more important with highly bound (greater than 90%) acidic drugs such as salicylates, phenytoin, and warfarin.[9] Conversely, basic drugs, including lidocaine, propranolol, and meperidine, have affinity for α_1-acid-glycoprotein, which may increase with age, especially when associated with conditions such as inflammatory diseases and malignancies.[9] Protein binding theoretically may be increased and result in less free drug available, although clinical relevance of this is unclear.[23] With both types of binding, the net effect on clearance varies, depending on metabolism and elimination. Although not always clinically available, free drug concentration measurements are often desirable in the elderly. There is also some evidence that the elderly may have a greater potential for protein displacement drug interactions.[29,30]

Metabolism

Liver size and hepatic blood flow decrease with age and especially with disease. Studies show hepatic blood flow decreases by 35%, and liver volume by 44% and 28% in elderly women and men, respectively, when compared to younger counterparts.[13] Such a decrease in hepatic blood flow can limit the first-pass effect of drugs with high extraction ratios and markedly reduce their systemic clearance. Studies on phase I drug metabolism (ie, oxidation) do not consistently show a correlation with age,[23] although most show that the elderly, especially men, have prolonged elimination. Differences may be explained by environmental factors such as smoking habits and genetics. Phase II metabolism (ie, conjugation) does not appear to be influenced as much by age, although there has been less study in this area.[9,13,23] The effect of aging on drug acetylation is inconsistent and the importance unclear.[9,23] There does not appear to be any age difference in the degree of inhibition or induction of cytochrome P450 isoenzymes.[13,31] Monitoring and management of interactions with drugs such as cimetidine should be handled in the same manner as in younger patients. The changes described in liver size and metabolic function help to explain why certain drugs may have prolonged elimination; however, the variability of data cautions against generalizing about the effect of age alone. The initial dosage of metabolized drugs should be conservative and subsequent dosage adjustments based on careful monitoring of therapeutic and toxic parameters.

Renal Elimination

The effect of aging on the renal elimination of drugs is probably the most completely understood and important aspect affecting geriatric drug therapy. Glomerular filtration, tubular secretion, and renal blood flow all decrease with age. Creatinine clearance (Cl_{cr}) decreases approximately 1% per year after age 40;[32] the effect is variable, and volume depletion, congestive heart failure, and renal disease can further decrease organ function. Because creatinine production also decreases with age, serum creatinine may be normal despite a substantial decrease in renal function. It is therefore recommended that Cl_{cr} be measured or estimated using a method that incorporates age and weight.[33,34] The dosage of renally excreted drugs with low therapeutic indices should be conservative initially, with subsequent dosage titrated by close clinical and serum drug level monitoring, if applicable.

■ PHARMACODYNAMICS

Heightened drug effects that cannot be explained by altered pharmacokinetic variables alone have been hypothesized to be caused by changes in compensatory homeostasis, drug receptor sensitivity, or complications of chronic diseases that occur in the elderly. There is a gradual decrease in homeostatic reserve with aging. Postural control and orthostatic circulatory response are examples of compensatory mechanisms that are slowed in aging. Adequate postural blood pressure control relies on several factors, including central coordination, muscle tone, and proprioception, all of which can be blunted in the elderly.[15] As a result, side effects that are minimal or absent in a young patient with normal compensatory response, can be marked in the elderly. The administration of long-acting anxiolytics, hypnotics, or antipsychotics can further alter these mechanisms and lead to an increased risk of falls in the elderly.[9,35] Similarly, symptomatic postural hypotension can result from the administration of a variety of antihypertensive agents (especially calcium-channel blockers and ACE inhibitors) and other drugs (eg, antipsychotics, antidepressants) that affect vasomotor tone. Physiologic mechanisms such as vasoconstriction and tachycardia are unable to fully compensate for the postural hypotension in the elderly.[15] Temperature regulation and intestinal motility are other homeostatic mechanisms that change with aging and can explain heightened effects of certain drugs.

The number and characteristics of drug receptors can change with aging and produce altered, often heightened, drug response. Research has shown age-related decreases in several autonomic receptors. There is some evidence of increased sensitivity to oral anticoagulants and digoxin, apart from the alterations in pharmacokinetics, which might contribute to the higher frequency of adverse reactions to these two agents in the elderly.[15]

Preliminary data indicate a possible increase in brain sensitivity to certain drugs with aging. It is unknown whether this effect is caused by changes in blood-brain permeability or tissue receptor sensitivity.[9] More research into drug pharmacodynamics in the elderly is needed, especially the interrelationship with pharmacokinetic alterations. The presence and impact of multiple concurrent pathologies and their treatments cannot be overemphasized in their contribution to the various drug effects seen in the elderly.

■ OTHER FACTORS

Cigarette smoking can cause clinically important induction of the metabolism of some drugs to a similar degree in both the elderly and the young.[23,36] This, and the fact that many published studies do not indicate smoking history, could explain some interpatient variability of pharmacokinetic data.

Nutritional intake is sometimes diminished in the elderly and can lead to nutritional and vitamin deficiencies. Nutritional status of the elderly can impact the outcome of drug therapy and, conversely, drug therapy can affect nutritional status.[19,36,37]

■ EVALUATING DRUG DATA FOR THE ELDERLY

Because of age-related changes that may impact the outcome of drug therapy as outlined in this chapter, the results of drug studies using young subjects cannot always be extrapolated accurately to the elderly. Studies on diseases and drugs in the elderly do not always include sufficient numbers of elderly, especially extremely aged subjects, to draw appropriate conclusions.[38] Studies that include the elderly do not always separate results by decade of age and health status, two criteria that are helpful in assessing applicability of data in this heterogeneous population. Many studies also do not mention data on nutrition, alcohol, and smoking, which might explain some variability of results.[19] Although single-dose studies in healthy volunteers can be useful, long-term studies in afflicted elderly patients often yield data more applicable to therapeutics. Drugs are often not studied over a wide dosage range, so a minimal effective dosage in the elderly cannot be determined.[39]

When reviewing studies that include the elderly, one should consider the following potential problems: numbers of subjects must be sufficient to allow for high attrition rates and the typically wide variation in this population; study length must be sufficient for a chronic disease; concomitant diseases and medications must be acknowledged and their impact assessed; and "normal" values can be different from those of a younger population.[40–42]

■ CONCLUSION

The effects of aging as related to drug therapy illustrate the challenges in caring for the elderly. Clinical practice guidelines that have been developed for conditions commonly afflicting the elderly, such as those published by the Agency for Health Care Policy and Research, can be a helpful guide.[43] Conservative dosage, especially initially, with close clinical monitoring for dose-dependent effects is critical and should be emphasized by all health care practitioners caring for the elderly. For detailed information on specific drugs in the elderly, refer to the Geriatric Dosage section of the individual drug monographs.

■ REFERENCES

 1. Gerety MB et al. Adverse events related to drugs and drug withdrawal in nursing home residents. *J Am Geriatr Soc* 1993;41:1326–32.
 2. Faden R, German PS. Quality of life. Considerations in geriatrics. *Clin Geriatr Med* 1994;10:541–55.
 3. Goldstein MK. Ethical considerations in pharmacotherapy of the aged. *Drugs Aging* 1991;1:91–7.
 4. Livesley B. Cost-benefit considerations in the treatment of elderly people. *Drugs Aging* 1991;1:249–53.
 5. Tobias DE. Ensuring and documenting the quality of drug therapy in the elderly. *Generations* 1994;18:40–2.
 6. Burns JMA et al. Elderly patients and their medication: a post-discharge follow-up study. *Age Ageing* 1992;21:178–81.
 7. Honig PK, Cantilena LR. Polypharmacy. Pharmacokinetic perspectives. *Clin Pharmacokinet* 1994;26:85–90.
 8. Botelho RJ, Dudrak R. Home assessment of adherence to long-term medication in the elderly. *J Fam Pract* 1992;35:61–5.
 9. Tregaskis BF, Stevenson IH. Pharmacokinetics in old age. *Br Med Bull* 1990;46:9–21.
10. Denham MJ. Adverse drug reactions. *Br Med Bull* 1990;46:53–62.

11. Beard K. Adverse reactions as a cause of hospital admission in the aged. *Drugs Aging* 1992;2:356–67.

12. Owens NJ et al. Distinguishing between the fit and frail elderly, and optimising pharmacotherapy. *Drugs Aging* 1994;4:47–55.

13. Woodhouse KW, James OFW. Hepatic drug metabolism and ageing. *Br Med Bull* 1990;46:22–35.

14. Walker J, Wynne H. Review: the frequency and severity of adverse drug reactions in elderly people. *Age Ageing* 1994;23:255–9.

15. Swift CG. Pharmacodynamics: changes in homeostatic mechanisms, receptor and target organ sensitivity in the elderly. *Br Med Bull* 1990;46:36–52.

16. Feinberg M. The problems of anticholinergic adverse effects in older patients. *Drugs Aging* 1993;3:335–48.

17. Nolan L, O'Malley K. Adverse effects of antidepressants in the elderly. *Drugs Aging* 1992;2:450–8.

18. Bowen JD, Larson EB. Drug-induced cognitive impairment. Defining the problem and finding solutions. *Drugs Aging* 1993;3:349–57.

19. Iber FL et al. Age-related changes in the gastrointestinal system. Effects on drug therapy. *Drugs Aging* 1994;5:34–48.

20. Gainsborough N et al. The association of age with gastric emptying. *Age Ageing* 1993;22:37–40.

21. Russell TL et al. Upper gastrointestinal pH in seventy-nine healthy, elderly, North American men and women. *Pharm Res* 1993;10:187–96.

22. Durnas C et al. Hepatic drug metabolism and aging. *Clin Pharmacokinet* 1990;19:359–89.

23. Roskos KV, Maibach HI. Percutaneous absorption and age. Implications for therapy. *Drugs Aging* 1992;2:432–49.

24. Novak LP. Aging, total body potassium, fat-free mass, and cell mass in males and females between ages 18 and 85 years. *J Gerontol* 1972;27:438–43.

25. Morgan DJ, Bray KM. Lean body mass as a predictor of drug dosage. Implications for drug therapy. *Clin Pharmacokinet* 1994;26:292–307.

26. Rodeheffer RJ et al. Exercise cardiac output is maintained with advancing age in healthy human subjects: cardiac dilatation and increased stroke volume compensate for a diminished heart rate. *Circulation* 1984;69:208–13.

27. Schumacher GE. Using pharmacokinetics in drug therapy. VII: pharmacokinetic factors influencing drug therapy in the aged. *Am J Hosp Pharm* 1980;37:559–62.

28. Woo J et al. Effect of age and disease on two drug binding proteins: albumin and α-1-acid glycoprotein. *Clin Biochem* 1994;27:289–92.

29. Wallace S et al. Factors affecting drug binding in plasma of elderly patients. *Br J Clin Pharmacol* 1976;3:327–30.

30. Ritschel WA. Drug disposition in the elderly: gerontokinetics. *Methods Find Exp Clin Pharmacol* 1992;14:555–72.

31. Vestal RE et al. Aging and the response to inhibition and induction of theophylline metabolism. *Exp Gerontol* 1993;28:421–33.

32. Lindeman RD. Changes in renal function with aging. Implications for treatment. *Drugs Aging* 1992;2:423–31.

33. Siersbaek-Nielsen K et al. Rapid evaluation of creatinine clearance. *Lancet* 1971;1:1133–4.

34. Cockcroft DW, Gault MH. Prediction of creatinine clearance from serum creatinine. *Nephron* 1976;16:31–41.

35. Campbell AJ. Drug treatment as a cause of falls in old age. A review of the offending agents. *Drugs Aging* 1991;1:289–302.

36. O'Mahony MS, Woodhouse KW. Age, environmental factors and drug metabolism. *Pharmacol Ther* 1994;61:279–87.

37. Roe DA. Medications and nutrition in the elderly. *Prim Care* 1994;21:135–47.

38. Gurwitz JH et al. The exclusion of the elderly and women from clinical trials in acute myocardial infarction. *JAMA* 1992;268:1417–22.

39. Kitler ME. Clinical trials and clinical practice in the elderly. A focus on hypertension. *Drugs Aging* 1992;2:86–94.

40. Zimmer AW et al. Conducting clinical research in geriatric populations. *Ann Intern Med* 1985;103:276–83.

41. Butler RN. The importance of basic research in gerontology. *Age Ageing* 1993;22:S53–4.

42. Fraser CG. Age-related changes in laboratory test results. Clinical implications. *Drugs Aging* 1993;3:246–57.

43. Agency for Health Care Policy and Research. Guidelines for pressure ulcer prevention: improving practice and a stimulus for research. *J Gerontol* 1993;48:M3–5.

Renal Disease

John G. Gambertoglio

■ DOSAGE MODIFICATION IN RENAL IMPAIRMENT

The number of individuals with impaired kidney function is increasing steadily. In the United States, over 100,000 patients with end-stage renal disease are undergoing either hemodialysis or continuous ambulatory peritoneal dialysis, and over 1000 patients each year undergo kidney transplantation. Therapeutic advances in immunosuppressive drugs and dialysis techniques have made increased survival and quality of life possible for patients with kidney diseases.

Invariably, these patients have multiple medical problems that either contributed to the development of their renal dysfunction or are sequelae of having chronic renal disease. Hypertension, diabetes, infection, bone disease, neurologic dysfunction, GI disturbances, and bleeding abnormalities are but a few of the frequently encountered medical conditions in renal failure patients. These patients are prescribed a number of medications; in one survey of dialysis patients, it was determined that they received an average of over eight drugs per patient.[1] Thus, renal patients are at increased risk for adverse reactions to drugs because of the number of drugs received, concurrent medical problems, and the impaired drug excretory pathway.[2,3] Complications resulting from drug administration can be minimized by the rational use of drugs and knowledge of their pharmacokinetic and pharmacodynamic characteristics in renal failure patients.

Since the advent of specific and sensitive methods for measuring drug concentrations in biological fluids, a voluminous literature has evolved concerning drug disposition in renal disease and the effects of dialysis.[4–6] This section provides a conceptual discussion of how renal disease alters drug disposition. It also describes an approach for determining the appropriate dosage adjustment necessary in the presence of renal disease to achieve the optimal therapeutic effect with minimal toxicity. The next section, Dialysis of Drugs, discusses the concepts of drug removal by dialysis and provides specific data on the amount removed by dialysis and dosage modification for a number of drugs during dialysis.

Four Basic Questions

A practical approach to drug therapy in patients with renal insufficiency is to answer the following questions:

1. What is the patient's renal function status?
2. What alterations exist in the pharmacokinetics or pharmacodynamics of the specific drug in renal failure?
3. What approaches to dosage modification are useful for a specific drug?
4. What is the dialysis removal of the drug and is dosage supplementation necessary?

Determining Renal Function

The usual tests to measure a patient's renal function include blood urea nitrogen (BUN), serum creatinine (Cr_s), and creatinine clearance (Cl_{cr}).[7]

The BUN is useful as a correlate of uremic symptoms and helps the clinician determine the adequacy of treatment modalities such as dialysis. However, the level of BUN can change because of many factors in addition to changes in renal function. Urea is both filtered and reabsorbed by the nephron, and its renal excretion is a function of urine flow. For example, excessive diuretic use, dehydration, or bleeding can all increase the BUN without there being a decline in renal function.[7]

For adults, creatinine production and elimination are constant at approximately 20 mg/kg/day under steady-state conditions.[8] Creatinine is filtered by the glomerulus with little renal tubular secretion; however, secretion becomes important at low levels of renal function. Decreases in renal function are reflected by increases in Cr_s and corresponding decreases in Cl_{cr}. Nonrenal factors that can affect the BUN do not alter Cr_s, so Cr_s and Cl_{cr} serve as better markers of changing renal function. The relationship between Cr_s and Cl_{cr} is a hyperbolic one, as is shown in Figure 3–3. Initial small increases in Cr_s represent larger decreases in renal function (flatter part of the curve) than do similar increases in Cr_s at higher levels of Cr_s. Furthermore, for every doubling in Cr_s there is a halving in Cl_{cr} (ie, as Cr_s changes from 1 to 2 mg/dL, the Cl_{cr} declines from 120 to 60 mL/min; 2 to 4

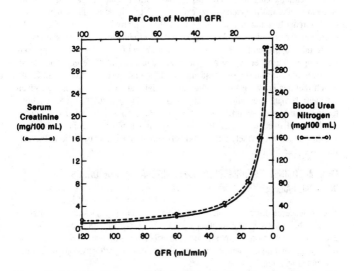

Figure 3–3. The Relationship Between Steady-State Values for Serum Creatinine, Blood Urea Nitrogen, and Glomerular Filtration Rate (GFR). It is assumed that creatinine clearance is equal to GFR and that creatinine production is constant, even under conditions of severe impairment of glomerular function.

From Kassirer JP. Clinical evaluation of kidney function-glomerular function. N Engl J Med 1971;285:385–9. Reproduced with permission.

mg/dL represents a decrease in Cl_{cr} from 60 to 30 mL/min). This approach can be used as a rough clinical guide in monitoring the progress of a patient's renal function and determining drug dosage adjustments.

Although Cr_s is easy to determine, requiring collection of only a single blood sample, measurement of Cl_{cr} is more difficult. The standard method consists of a continuous 24-hr urine collection for urine creatinine with a single blood sample for Cr_s at approximately the middle of the urine collection period. The most difficult problem from a practical standpoint is obtaining a complete urine collection. Almost invariably, urine collection is incomplete and consequently the Cl_{cr} is underestimated. However, the accuracy of the Cl_{cr} and urine collection can be estimated by determining the creatinine index. This is simply done by calculating the amount of creatinine (in mg/day) excreted in the urine over the 24-hr collection period. This total amount should be compared to the expected amount of creatinine to be excreted, which is approximately 20–25 mg/kg/day ideal body weight in males and 15–20 mg/kg/day in females. For example, in a 70-kg man, the expected creatinine production and excretion in the urine is approximately 1.4 g/day. If the patient's total creatinine excretion is less than this value, the possibility exists of an inadequate urine collection and correspondingly underestimated Cl_{cr}. The use of the creatinine index applies only under steady-state conditions, that is, when creatinine production and excretion are equivalent. Therefore, even if a patient's creatinine clearance were only 25% of normal (approximately 30 mL/min) at steady state, the production and excretion of creatinine are the same. At this level of renal function, the patient's Cr_s would be approximately 4 mg/dL and the excretion of creatinine would still be 1.4 g/day, matching creatinine production.

Another approach for estimating a patient's renal function is to use equations based upon the patient's age and physical data. Many of these equations exist; however, the one that is most frequently used for adults is by Cockcroft and Gault, which requires knowing the patient's age, weight, and Cr_s.[9] Equations are given for men, women, and children in Appendix 2, Anthropometrics. These equations assume steady-state serum creatinine values and are not considered valid under conditions of fluctuating renal function. Also, in patients undergoing hemodialysis, the Cr_s can vary widely during and between dialyses, thereby limiting the usefulness of these equations.

PHARMACOKINETIC/PHARMACODYNAMIC ALTERATIONS OF DRUGS IN RENAL FAILURE

The presence of decreased renal function may affect the disposition of drugs by altering the processes of absorption, distribution, protein binding, metabolism, or excretion. Furthermore, the pharmacologic effect of a drug may be different in patients with renal impairment, because of biochemical or pathophysiologic changes associated with renal disease.

The bioavailability of drugs may be altered in renal failure because of associated GI disturbances such as nausea, vomiting, and diarrhea. Furthermore, patients with decreased renal function have an increased gastric pH because of increased salivary urea levels caused by their increased BUN. Drugs best absorbed in an acidic medium, such as ferrous sulfate, may have diminished absorption. In addition, these patients routinely take aluminum or calcium antacids (for calcium-phosphorus abnormalities), which may also alter drug bioavailability. Finally, certain drugs, such as propoxyphene and possibly some β-blockers, may have an altered first-pass effect in renal failure that can lead to increased bioavailability compared with control subjects.[10-13]

The plasma protein binding of drugs in renal failure may be altered. This may be caused by hypoalbuminemia; accumulation of acidic byproducts of uremia, resulting in competitive displacement of drugs from binding sites; or changes in the structure of albumin, resulting in a decreased number of effective binding sites.[10,12-14] Most weak organic acid drugs, such as cefazolin, phenytoin, salicylate, valproic acid, and warfarin exhibit decreased plasma protein binding in uremia. Weak organic basic drugs have either decreased or unchanged binding in uremia. For example, the binding of carbamazepine, dapsone, diazepam, and morphine is decreased, whereas the binding of propranolol, quinidine, verapamil, and trimethoprim is unchanged. Some of these drugs, such as propranolol and lidocaine, are primarily bound to α_1-acid glycoprotein from which little displacement occurs in renal disease or hypoalbuminemia. The effects of altered protein binding of drugs may lead to an increased pharmacologic effect, an increased apparent volume of distribution (V_d), and either increased or unchanged total body clearance depending on whether it is a high or low extraction ratio drug.

The V_d of drugs may be increased, decreased, or unchanged in renal failure patients.[11,14] Examples of drugs with an increased V_d include cefazolin, furosemide, naproxen, and phenytoin. Digoxin exhibits a decreased V_d in renal impairment. Gentamicin, minoxidil, and procainamide are examples of drugs whose V_d does not change markedly in uremia.

Phenytoin is an example of a drug whose altered protein binding results in important differences in dosage in uremia.[15] The percentage of unbound phenytoin in plasma is normally 10%, but is 20–35% in renal failure patients. This results in an increase in the V_d from 0.65 L/kg in those with normal kidney function to 1–1.8 L/kg in renal failure patients. Furthermore, the apparent half-life decreases from 11–16 hr to 6–10 hr and the apparent plasma clearance increases from 28–41 mL/hr/kg to 64–225 mL/hr/kg in controls and renal failure patients, respectively. These pharmacokinetic changes in phenytoin result in a change in its therapeutic concentration range. In patients with normal kidney function, the usual therapeutic plasma concentration range for phenytoin is 10–20 mg/L, while in those with end-stage renal disease, it is approximately 4–8 mg/L. Both of these ranges of total drug yield the same concentration of unbound drug which is approximately 1–2 mg/L.

Drugs are eliminated from the body by two primary pathways: renal excretion and nonrenal elimination (predominantly through hepatic metabolism).[4] The degree to which renal failure impairs drug elimination depends largely on the percentage of drug excreted unchanged by the kidney. For example, the aminoglycoside antibiotics are greater than 95% excreted unchanged by the kidney; cephalosporins range from 70–100%; penicillins from 85–100%; vancomycin from 95–100%; acyclovir from 75–80%; lithium from 95–100%; and ranitidine 80%. For many of these drugs, linear correlations have been established between the half-life of the drug and serum creatinine or between plasma clearance of the drug and Cl_{cr}. These specific correlations are then used as guides to determine drug dosage in renal failure. For example, the linear correlation between gentamicin serum half-life and Cr_s demonstrates that the half-life of gentamicin can change from 2 hr in normals to as much as 60 hr in renal failure patients. This correlation has led to a simple dosage guide, which indicates that the half-life of gentamicin can be estimated by multiplying the Cr_s by 3 or 4. This can then be used to determine the dosage of gentamicin in patients with varying degrees of renal insufficiency.

Drug metabolism typically involves enzymatic conversion of drugs to more water-soluble compounds. These metabolites are formed through processes of oxidation, reduction, synthesis (eg, conjugation) or hydrolysis and are, to a large extent, excreted by the kidney.[4,14] Most metabolites are inactive or have minimal pharmacologic activity. However, some metabolites that are active may accumulate in renal impairment and lead to toxicity. Examples of drugs metabolized to active or toxic compounds that are excreted by the kidney include allopurinol to oxypurinol, which is an active inhibitor of xanthine oxidase; cefotaxime to desacetylcefotaxime, which is microbiologically active; meperidine to normeperidine, which may cause seizure activity in renal failure; and procainamide to N-acetylprocainamide, which has antiarrhythmic properties. These metabolites may accumulate to toxic levels in renal failure patients unless appropriate dosage reductions are made.

The presence of renal failure may also lead to alterations in drug metabolism because of the abnormalities associated with the uremic state. For example, both the antiviral agent acyclovir and the antihypertensive agent captopril demonstrate a 50% decrease in nonrenal clearance in patients with end-stage renal disease.[16,17] As a consequence, the elimination half-life for both these drugs is unexpectedly increased sixfold in the presence of renal failure. This shows that predictions of the disposition of drugs in renal failure based on general principles and nomograms are subject to unexpected error. The pharmacokinetics of several newer drugs and changes caused by renal failure have recently been reviewed.[18,19]

The pharmacodynamics of a drug may be altered in uremia, causing its pharmacologic effects to be different from those expected in patients with normal renal function. One well-defined example is that of nifedipine, where marked differences in E_{max} (maximal effect change in diastolic blood pressure) were observed with averages of 12% and 29% in control and severe renal failure patients, respectively.[20,21] Thus, at the same plasma concentration of unbound nifedipine, a greater effect on blood pressure lowering occurs in patients with renal insufficiency. The response of these patients to nifedipine may be different than anticipated, requiring dosage modification because of drug effect changes rather than pharmacokinetic changes.

DOSAGE APPROACHES THAT ARE USEFUL AND PRACTICAL FOR SPECIFIC DRUGS

The general approaches for dosage adjustments of drugs in renal insufficiency are to (1) decrease the dose and maintain the usual dosage interval, (2) lengthen the dosage interval and maintain the usual dose, or (3) use a combination of modifying both the dose and interval. The primary goal of these approaches is to provide similar average steady-state plasma concentrations or areas under the curve for a drug in renal failure compared with normal kidney function. The choice of approach depends upon the type of drug and the desirability, from a therapeutic or toxic standpoint, of having small or large fluctuations in peak and trough plasma drug concentrations. Other considerations are that the dosage regimen adjustment should be practical and the reduced dose or prolonged dosage interval should be relatively easy to implement.

When presented with a patient with impaired renal function for whom drug dosage regimen decisions must be made, the most practical and efficient approach is to first consult published tables or guidelines on specific drugs.[4,12,18,19] This may be accomplished by referring to tables by Bennett and colleagues,[5] which provides a quick reference source for drug dosage in renal failure. Additional sources are the appendices of *Handbook of Drug Therapy in Liver and Kidney Disease*[4] and "Use of Drugs in Renal Failure" in *Diseases of the Kidney*,[12] which describe specific pharmacokinetic alterations of drugs in kidney disease, recommended dosage, and the effects of dialysis. The reader is also advised to refer to specific drug monographs in this book, which briefly describe the effect of renal failure on drug disposition and dosage recommendations. These sources allow the user to determine whether dosage adjustments are necessary and whether there are any important toxicities or precautions in using a particular drug in the renal failure patient. These sources, however, serve only as general guidelines.

For drugs requiring dosage adjustment in renal insufficiency, the reader should consult the original publications, which provide specific data on individual drugs. Consulting the original publications will provide details regarding the relationship of renal function and drug elimination, and may provide a dosage nomogram or specific dosage recommendations and precautions for the use of a drug with varying degrees of renal insufficiency.

A final approach for dosage of drugs in renal impairment is to use general dosage equations provided by Rowland and Tozer.[22] This approach is recommended when specific guidelines for the use of a drug in renal failure have not been established. Basic pharmacokinetic information about the drug is needed—primarily the fraction of available dose that is normally excreted unchanged in the urine, f_e(normal), and the fraction of normal renal function (RF) in a given patient. The RF is the ratio of the diseased patient's creatinine clearance to that of a normal value: RF = Cl_{cr}(failure)/Cl_{cr}(normal). The patient's Cl_{cr} may be determined from Cr_s values at steady state using the method of Cockcroft and Gault.[9]

Next, the following equation, which takes into consideration the renal unbound clearance and the extrarenal unbound clearance of the drug, is used:

$$R_d = \frac{RF \times f_e(normal) + [1 - f_e(normal)] \times [(140 - age) \times \text{weight in kg}^{0.7}]}{1660}$$

where R_d is the ratio of the unbound drug clearance in the patient to that normally observed, or Cl_u(failure)/Cl_u(normal), and age and weight are that of the patient. Once the value of R_d is obtained, the dosage regimen adjustment can be made using the following equation:

$$(D_M/\tau)(\text{failure}) = R_d \times (D_M/\tau)(\text{normal})$$

where D_M/τ is the maintenance dosage rate in the renal failure patient (failure) and under normal circumstances (normal). An example will clarify the use of this approach. An 80-kg, 45-year-old man with a serum creatinine of 5.4 mg/dL requires treatment with ceftazidime for a pseudomonal infection. This drug is 70% excreted unchanged in the urine, and the usual dosage is 1 g q 8 hr intravenously. Using the equation of Cockcroft and Gault, his Cl_{cr} is calculated as

$$Cl_{cr} = \frac{(140 - 45) \times 80}{(5.4 \times 72)} = 20 \text{ mL/min}$$

Therefore

$$RF = \frac{20 \text{ mL/min}}{120 \text{mL/min}} = 0.17$$

so

$$R_d = \frac{0.17 \times 0.7 + (1 - 0.7) \times ([140 - 45] \times 80^{0.7})}{1660}$$

$$R_d = 0.12 + 0.3 \times 1.2 = 0.49$$

and

$$(D_M/\tau)(\text{failure}) = 0.49 \times (D_M/\tau)(\text{normal})$$

which means that in this patient the maintenance dosage of ceftazidime should be halved. Thus, the maintenance regimen could be 0.5 g q 8 hr or 1 g q 16 hr for this patient. The dosage could also be modified for practical reasons to 1.5 g q 24 hr.

This general equation approach provides a reasonable initial method for adjusting the dosage in patients with renal insufficiency until more specific guidelines can be consulted. This method is based on several assumptions: (1) bioavailability is unchanged in renal failure; (2) metabolites are not therapeutically active or toxic; (3) decreased renal function does not alter metabolism of the drug; (4) metabolism or renal excretion does not exhibit concentration-dependent pharmacokinetics; (5) renal function is constant with time; and (6) the renal clearance of the drug is directly proportional to the renal clearance of the compound used to measure renal function. The method above provides the best mathematical estimate of dosage in renal impairment. A simpler, but less complete, nomogram method has also been published (Fig. 3–4). All of the above limitations also apply to the nomogram.

For drugs having a much longer half-life than usual in renal failure, the time to reach steady state is much longer than in a patient with normal renal function.

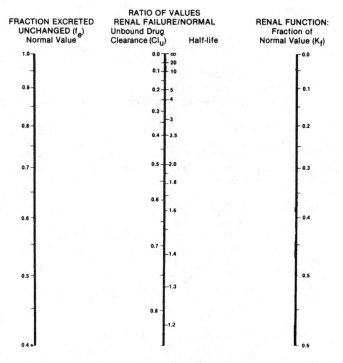

Figure 3–4. Estimation of Dosage Regimens in Patients with Renal Function Impairment. For Conditions for Use of Nomogram, How to Use Nomogram, and Modification of Dosage Regimen, see below.
From Rowland M, Tozer TN. Clinical pharmacokinetics: concepts and application. *Philadelphia: Lea & Febiger, 1980, reproduced with permission. To be used to determine how to change a normal dosage regimen. The normal dosage regimen depends upon age, weight, and condition being treated.*

Consequently, it is common to initiate therapy for many drugs with a loading dose in order to shorten the time to reach therapeutic plasma concentrations. The amount of the loading dose will obviously depend on the particular drug being used and the desired therapeutic objectives.

Finally, it should be stated that any dosage modification in renal failure may require plasma concentration determination of the drug, if available, and necessitates close clinical observation for assessment of toxicity and achievement of maximum therapeutic effect.

Conditions for Use of Nomogram (Fig. 3–4)

This nomogram should be used only if the following conditions are met:

1. Metabolites are inactive and nontoxic.
2. Individual variation in metabolism or response are not significant.
3. Altered protein binding, metabolism, or distribution do not occur.
4. Cardiac output, hepatic function, and all other physiologic factors that might affect absorption or distribution are normal.
5. Renal function is reasonably constant.
6. Pharmacokinetics of the drug are linear.
7. The renal clearance of the drug is proportional to creatinine clearance.

How to Use Nomogram

With a ruler, connect the fraction of drug normally excreted unchanged and the patient's kidney function, expressed as a fraction of normal value in a person of the same age. Read off from the center line the clearance of unbound drug (Cl_u) and the half-life relative to their normal values in a patient of the same age.

Modification of Dosage Regimen

I. Initial dose—no change (see text)
II. Adjustment of rate of administration for maintenance of drug in body.
   A. Change in dosage interval, τ, only:

$$\tau(\text{failure}) = \frac{t_{\frac{1}{2}}(\text{failure})}{t_{\frac{1}{2}}(\text{normal})} \times \tau(\text{normal})$$

   B. Change in maintenance dose, D, only:

$$D(\text{failure}) = \frac{Cl_u(\text{failure})}{Cl_u(\text{normal})} \times D(\text{normal})$$

   C. Change in rate of administration D/τ:

$$\frac{D}{\tau}(\text{failure}) = \frac{Cl_u(\text{failure})}{Cl_u(\text{normal})} \times \frac{D}{\tau}(\text{normal})$$

■ REFERENCES

1. Anderson RJ et al. Prescribing medication in long-term dialysis units. *Arch Intern Med* 1982;142:1305–8.
2. Smith JW et al. Studies on the epidemiology of adverse drug reactions: V. Clinical factors affecting susceptibility. *Ann Intern Med* 1966;65:629–40.
3. Jick H. Adverse drug effects in relation to renal function. *Am J Med* 1977;62:514–7.
4. Schrier RW, Gambertoglio JG, eds. *Handbook of drug therapy in liver and kidney disease.* Boston: Little, Brown; 1991.
5. Bennett WM et al. *Drug prescribing in renal failure: dosing guidelines for adults,* 2nd ed. Philadelphia, PA: American College of Physicians; 1991.

6. Benet LZ, Williams RL. Design and optimization of dosage regimens: pharmacokinetic data. In Gilman AG et al., eds. *Goodman and Gilman's the pharmacological basis of therapeutics,* 8th ed. New York: Pergamon Press; 1990:1650–735.

7. Kassirer JP, Harrington JT. Laboratory evaluation of renal function. In Schrier RW, Gottschalk CW, eds. *Diseases of the kidney.* Boston: Little, Brown; 1988:393–441.

8. Wesson LE. Electrolyte excretion in relation to diurnal cycles of renal function. *Medicine* 1964;43:547–92.

9. Cockcroft DW, Gault MH. Prediction of creatinine clearance from serum creatinine. *Nephron* 1976;16:31–41.

10. Matzke GR, Millikin SP. Influence of renal disease and dialysis on pharmacokinetics. In Evans WE et al., eds. *Applied pharmacokinetics,* 2nd ed. Vancouver, WA: Applied Therapeutics; 1991.

11. Gambertoglio JG. Effects of renal disease: altered pharmacokinetics. In Benet LZ et al., eds. *Pharmacokinetic basis for drug treatment.* New York: Raven Press; 1984:149–71.

12. Gambertoglio JG et al. Use of drugs in patients with renal failure. In Schrier RW, Gottschalk CW, eds. *Diseases of the kidney.* Boston: Little, Brown; 1993:3211–68.

13. Talbert RL. Drug dosing in renal insufficiency. *J Clin Pharmacol* 1994;34:99–110.

14. Aweeka F. Drug dosing in renal failure. In Young LY, Koda-Kimble MA, eds. *Applied therapeutics: the clinical use of drugs,* 5th ed. Vancouver, WA: Applied Therapeutics; 1992.

15. Flaherty JF et al. Neuropsychiatric drugs. In Schrier RW, Gambertoglio JG, eds. *Handbook of drug therapy in liver and kidney disease.* Boston: Little, Brown; 1991.

16. Laskin OL et al. Acyclovir kinetics in end-stage renal disease. *Clin Pharmacol Ther* 1982;31:594–600.

17. Duchin KL et al. Elimination kinetics of captopril in patients with renal failure. *Kidney Int* 1984;25:942–7.

18. Fillastre JP, Singlas E. Pharmacokinetics of newer drugs in patients with renal impairment (part I). *Clin Pharmacokinet* 1991;20:293–310.

19. Singlas E, Fillastre JP. Pharmacokinetics of newer drugs in patients with renal impairment (part II). *Clin Pharmacokinet* 1991;20:389–410.

20. Kleinbloesem CH et al. Nifedipine: relationship between pharmacokinetics and pharmacodynamics. *Clin Pharmacokinet* 1987;12:12–29.

21. Kleinbloesem CH. Nifedipine: influence of renal function on pharmacokinetic/hemodynamic relationship. *Clin Pharmacol Ther* 1985;37:563–74.

22. Rowland M, Tozer TN. Disease. In *Clinical pharmacokinetics, concepts and applications,* 2nd ed. Philadelphia: Lea & Febiger; 1989:238–54.

■ DIALYSIS OF DRUGS

Dialysis Removal of Drugs and Dosage Supplementation

As noted in the previous section, this is the fourth area involved in formulating a practical approach to drug therapy in patients with renal insufficiency. Dialysis is an important therapy in the treatment of patients with end-stage renal disease. These patients are primarily managed with hemodialysis, but the use of continuous ambulatory peritoneal dialysis is now common. Although the purpose of dialysis is to remove unwanted toxic waste products from the body, it also has the effect of removing drugs used therapeutically. Thus, it is important to know to what extent a drug is removed by dialysis, because this may affect the patient's therapy. Supplemental doses or a revised dosage regimen may be required under these circumstances.

Dialysis procedures, including hemoperfusion, have also been used in the drug overdose situation as a means of eliminating drugs from the body. It is therefore important to consider how effective these procedures are and whether they offer any substantial advantage over conventional means of treating overdoses.

The objectives of this section are to review various factors involved in assessing the removal of drugs by dialysis and to illustrate how the use of pharmacokinetic information can be useful for determining the dialyzability of a drug. Additionally, the accompanying table lists the effect of hemodialysis and peritoneal dialysis on the removal of specific drugs.

Methodologic Problems

Several problems are encountered in attempting to assess the literature on removal of drugs by dialysis. First, for some drugs, only anecdotal reports are available. This is primarily true in the overdose setting, in which the effect of dialysis on drug removal is determined primarily by clinical response. For example, a comatose patient awakens during or shortly after dialysis and it is assumed that dialysis removed the drug, accounting for the improved clinical status. Second, the amount of drug ingested and/or the amount of drug recovered in the dialysate are often unknown. Third, the type of dialysis system employed is frequently not specified—this is important when comparing the system being used with published data. With advances in newer dialysis technology such as high-flux hemodialysis, earlier data evaluating conventional methods are not applicable. Fourth, there is often a lack of patient data, such as weight, hematocrit, and renal and liver function. The method used to calculate drug clearance is often unspecified. For example, was clearance determined from the amount of drug recovered in the dialysate or from differences in arterial and venous plasma concentrations across the dialyzer? The proper method for clearance calculations in hemodialysis has been described.[1]

A common error is misinterpretation of plasma drug concentrations obtained before and after dialysis. A declining plasma level during dialysis is often believed to be the result of the dialysis procedure. However, a declining level could be caused by drug elimination by metabolism or renal excretion, and the contribution of dialysis to this decline may be very small. The situation in which drug concentrations are relatively unchanged during dialysis usually means that little or no drug is being removed by dialysis. However, it is also possible that the drug continues to be absorbed from the GI tract as dialysis is being carried out, as in the delayed and prolonged absorption observed in drug overdose cases.[2] Another problem is that of interpreting drug removal rate by dialysis. If 200 mg of a drug were removed in the first hour of dialysis, one might assume that 5 hr of dialysis would remove five times as much (ie, 1000 mg). This is incorrect, because drug removal by dialysis occurs by a first-order process; as the amount of drug in the body declines, so does its removal rate. Thus, the total amount removed is less than that calculated from the initial estimates.

For many drugs, there is a lack of correlation between plasma drug concentrations and clinical response. Some drugs have been found to have active or toxic metabolites that correlate well with the toxic effects of the drug.[2] In attempting to collect information on dialysis removal of drugs, attention must be given to metabolites as well. A final point relative to the overdose situation is that the pharmacokinetic disposition of a drug may be altered.[2] In making predictions of drug dialyzability, pharmacokinetic data are usually derived from healthy subjects receiving therapeutic dosages. However, during an overdose, there may be changes in drug metabolism, V_d, or protein binding. For example, large amounts of drug in the body may saturate plasma protein binding, which could in turn alter drug distribution and metabolism.

Pharmacokinetic Factors

Certain properties of a drug can be used to make some predictions about drug dialyzability.[3-12] Drugs with a small molecular weight, usually less than 500, cross conventional cuprophane dialysis membranes readily. Large molecular weight drugs, such as vancomycin (MW 3300) and amphotericin B (MW 960) cross these membranes poorly and are not effectively removed by conventional hemodialysis. The use of high-flux dialysis systems with polysulfone membranes, however, allows for removal of large molecular weight compounds such as vancomycin.

Drugs with high water solubility are more easily removed to the aqueous dialysate than more lipid-soluble compounds. In addition, the latter usually have larger volumes of distribution than more water-soluble drugs. A large V_d such as that of digoxin (approximately 500 L) impairs the ability of dialysis to remove a drug from the body. Because the majority of drug is contained in tissue compartments rather than in the blood, it is not accessible for removal. A large V_d limits the use of hemoperfusion as well.[13] Hemoperfusion may rapidly clear the blood compartment of a drug (evidenced by a dramatic decrease in plasma levels); however, once hemoperfusion has ended, plasma drug concentrations can increase as a result of reequilibration of drug from tissue stores.

Plasma protein binding of a drug also determines how effectively it can be dialyzed.[12] Drugs with a high degree of protein binding, such as propranolol (90–94%) and warfarin (99%), are poorly removed by dialysis because the drug-protein complex is too large to cross most dialysis membranes. This is not a limitation of hemoperfusion, because the drug is removed from plasma proteins as the complex passes through the high surface area adsorbent material.[9]

The clearance of a drug by dialysis can be compared to the clearance of the drug by the body. Clearance terms are additive:

$$Cl_{TD} = Cl_T + Cl_D$$

where

Cl_{TD} = total body clearance of drug during dialysis
Cl_T = total body clearance of drug
Cl_D = dialysis clearance of drug.

Thus, if dialysis clearance adds substantially to body clearance, forming a much larger total clearance, then the drug will be eliminated that much faster. For example, if the dialysis clearance of a drug is 50 mL/min and the body clearance is 50 mL/min, then the drug would be eliminated from the body twice as fast during the dialysis period. In order to relate clearance to drug half-life ($t_{1/2}$), the following equations are useful:

$$t_{\frac{1}{2}} = \frac{0.693 \times V_d}{Cl_T} \qquad \text{(off dialysis)}$$

$$t_{\frac{1}{2}} = \frac{0.693 \times V_d}{Cl_T + Cl_d} \qquad \text{(on dialysis)}$$

Thus, the more the dialysis clearance adds to the body's clearance, the shorter the drug half-life will be on dialysis (assuming V_d remains constant). A further extension of this gives the following equation:

Fraction lost during a dialysis period $= 1 - e^{-(Cl_T + Cl_D)(\tau/V_d)}$

where τ is the duration of the dialysis period.

This allows calculation of the fraction of drug in the body that is lost during a dialysis period by all routes of elimination (ie, dialysis, metabolism, and renal excretion). Thus, it is necessary to acquire from literature sources (keeping in mind the limitations discussed previously) values for V_d, Cl_T, and Cl_D. If renal or liver function are diminished, this must be taken into consideration. In addition, changes in V_d in certain disease states (eg, the decreased V_d of digoxin in renal failure) must also be taken into account.

Clearance data are not always available in the literature. Many authors report only the half-lives of the drugs, on and off dialysis. The following equation may be used to estimate the fraction of drug removed by dialysis alone using half-life data:[13]

$$f = \frac{t_{\frac{1}{2}(off)} - t_{\frac{1}{2}(on)} \times (1 - e^{-([0.693/t_{\frac{1}{2}(on)}] \times \tau)})}{t_{\frac{1}{2}(off)}}$$

where

f = fraction of drug removed by dialysis
$t_{\frac{1}{2}(on)}$ = half-life on dialysis
$t_{\frac{1}{2}(off)}$ = half-life off dialysis
τ = duration of dialysis.

The assumptions made when using this equation are that

1. all drug elimination (including dialysis removal) occurs by first-order processes, and
2. dialysis is initiated after the completion of the absorption and distribution phases.

The primary limitation of this equation is that inaccurate values of half-lives result in incorrect estimates of drug removal by dialysis. It is important to note the duration of dialysis in relation to the estimate of $t_{\frac{1}{2}(on)}$. For example, if the $t_{\frac{1}{2}(on)}$ is reported as 24 hr, but the dialysis duration is only 4 hr, the half-life value is probably not accurate. On the other hand, if the $t_{\frac{1}{2}(on)}$ is reported as 1 hr during a 4-hr dialysis period, the half-life value might be more reliable.

Two examples illustrate the use of pharmacokinetic data to calculate drug clearance during dialysis. Phenobarbital has a V_d of approximately 50 L, a total body clearance of 0.3 L/hr, and a hemodialysis clearance of 4.2 L/hr. The half-life off dialysis is 115 hr and would decrease to 8 hr with dialysis. Approximately 50% of the drug would be removed from the body during 8 hr of dialysis. As another example, digoxin has a V_d of about 300 L and Cl_T of 2.4 L/hr in an anephric patient. The hemodialysis clearance of digoxin is 1.2 L/hr. Therefore, the half-life of digoxin in this patient off dialysis is 86 hr, while on dialysis it declines to 58 hr. Although this appears to be a substantial decrease in half-life, it means that the patient would have to be dialyzed 58 hr continuously in order to remove one-half the digoxin in the body. The fraction of drug lost during a routine hemodialysis period of 4 hr would be only 5%. Thus, a supplemental dose of digoxin following hemodialysis is not warranted.

High-Flux Hemodialysis

High-flux dialyzers, which use more permeable polysulfone membranes, allow for greater removal of middle molecular weight compounds. For example, data are available comparing the dialysis clearance of vancomycin (MW 3300) using a conventional cuprophane membrane and the new polysulfone membranes. Conventional methods resulted in a dialysis clearance of 0.58 L/hr whereas high-flux dialysis produced a mean vancomycin dialysis clearance ranging from 2.7–5.1 L/hr. With conventional methods, only 7% of a dose of vancomycin was removed, compared to 26–50% using the polysulfone dialyzers. This enhanced removal of vancomycin by high-flux dialysis could be used as an effective means of drug removal in the overdose setting and suggests the need for vancomycin dosage supplementation posthemodialysis in the renal failure patient. Other antibiotics studied, such as ceftazidime and gentamicin, have also demonstrated increased removal using high-flux polysulfone dialyzers (see Dialysis of Drugs table).

Use of the Table

The table that follows should be consulted for data on specific drugs. For each drug, a qualitative statement of the range of drug removal by dialysis was derived using pharmacokinetic parameters taken from the literature. Drug removal is intentionally described in a qualitative fashion for a number of reasons. First, much of this information changes quite rapidly (eg, as new dialysis techniques are developed). Second, a given value for the amount of drug removed or the dialysis clearance determined in one study may differ from that found in another study, because of differences in dialysate or blood flow during dialysis, or the duration of the dialysis. The usual duration of dialysis has changed since earlier studies. Most conventional hemodialysis runs are 4 hr whereas high-flux dialysis procedures last 2–2.5 hr. Also, data vary on the amount of drug removed by peritoneal dialysis, because estimates of removal were determined from the literature in which both constant dialysis for long periods of time (such as in an overdose situation) and intermittent dialysis for shorter periods each day were used. Finally, the table contains comments for clarification of certain points and selected references are provided for more specific information.

Dialysis information is *not* currently available for the following drugs: alprazolam, amlodipine, betaxolol, bumetanide, carteolol, chlorpheniramine, cisplatin, clarithromycin, clofazimine, clorazepate, clozapine, codeine, cytarabine, dapsone, diltiazem, dopamine, ethacrynic acid, felbamate, fenoprofen, fluorouracil, glipizide, glyburide, griseofulvin, guanethidine, hydralazine, hydrochlorothiazide, indomethacin, levodopa, lovastatin, melphalan, metolazone, milrinone, misoprostol, morphine, muromonab-CD3, nitrofurantoin, odansetron, paromomycin, penicillamine, pentazocine, piroxicam, pravastatin, prazepam, primaquine, probenecid, ramipril, simvastatin, spironolactone, stavudine, sulfisoxazole, sulindac, tamoxifen, triamterene, and triazolam.

The following abbreviations and drug removal ranges are used in the table beginning on page 821:

- D—Dialyzed, 50–100%
- HD—Hemodialysis
- MD—Moderately Dialyzed, 20–50%
- ND—Not Dialyzed, 0–5%
- PD—Peritoneal Dialysis
- SD—Slightly Dialyzed, 5–20%

DIALYSIS OF DRUGS

DRUG	HEMODIALYSIS	PERITONEAL DIALYSIS	COMMENTS AND REFERENCES
Acebutolol	SD–MD		[Ref. 15,16]
Acetaminophen	SD–MD	ND	HD has not been shown to prevent hepatic or renal toxicity. Concentration-dependent kinetics. [Ref. 14]
Acetazolamide	MD		Data from single case study. [Ref. 14]
Acetohexamide		ND	Active metabolite also not dialyzed. [Ref.14]
Acyclovir	D	SD	Give one-half usual dose post-HD. [Ref. 14]
Alcohol	D		[Ref. 14]
Allopurinol			
Oxypurinol *(active metabolite)*	MD		Oxypurinol dialyzed as well as creatinine. [Ref.14]
Amantadine	ND–SD	SD	[Ref.14]
Amikacin	D	SD–MD	Give 50–75% of the loading dose postdialysis; use plasma levels as a guide. [Ref. 14–17]
Amiloride			No data; this drug is not recommended for patients on dialysis.
Amiodarone	ND	ND	[Ref. 14)
Amitriptyline			No data; limited removal because of high protein binding and large V_d. [Ref.18–22]
Amoxicillin	MD	SD	Give 1-g dose post-HD. [Ref. 14]
Amphotericin B	ND		[Ref.14]
Ampicillin	MD	ND–SD	Give 1-g dose post-HD. [Ref. 14,17]
Antidepressants,			
Heterocyclic	ND	ND	Multiple metabolites. [Ref. 12]
Aspirin	D	MD	Concentration-dependent kinetics. [Ref. 14]
Astemizole	ND		Limited data for HD. [Ref. 23]
Atenolol	MD	ND	[Ref.14,24–26]
Atovaquone			No data; limited HD removal due to high protein binding.
Azathioprine			
Mercaptopurine *(active metabolite)*	SD–MD		Data for azathioprine and metabolites using a nonspecific assay. [Ref. 14]
Azithromycin			No data; limited removal because of large V_d.
Aztreonam	MD	SD	Give one-half usual dose post-HD. [Ref.14]
Bacampicillin	MD	ND–SD	*See* Ampicillin.
Baclofen			No data; toxicity has been reported in patients on dialysis.

(continued)

DIALYSIS OF DRUGS (continued)

DRUG	HEMODIALYSIS	PERITONEAL DIALYSIS	COMMENTS AND REFERENCES
Bleomycin			No data; probably poorly dialyzed because of large MW.
Bretylium	MD		[Ref. 14]
Captopril	MD	SD	[Ref. 14,27]
Carbamazepine	SD		Active epoxide metabolite. [Ref. 14]
Carisoprodol			No data; multiple metabolites, one of which is meprobamate.
Cefaclor	MD		Give usual dose post-HD. [Ref. 14,28]
Cefadroxil	D		[Ref. 29]
Cefamandole	MD		Give one-half usual dose post-HD. [Ref. 14]
Cefazolin	MD	SD	Give a 0.5–1 g dose post-HD. [Ref. 14,30]
Cefixime	ND	ND	[Ref. 31]
Cefmetazole	D		[Ref. 32]
Cefonicid	ND–SD	ND–SD	No supplemental dose postdialysis. [Ref. 14]
Cefoperazone	SD	ND	[Ref.14,33]
Cefotaxime	MD	SD	Give one-half usual dose post-HD. [Ref. 14,34–37]
Desacetylcefotaxime *(active metabolite)*	MD	SD	
Cefoxitin	MD	SD	Give one-half usual dose post-HD. [Ref. 14,38]
Cefpodoxime	MD	ND–SD	[Ref. 39,40]
Cefprozil	MD		[Ref. 41]
Ceftazidime	D	SD	Give one-half usual dose post-HD. [Ref. 14,42–44]
Ceftizoxime	SD	ND	[Ref. 45–47]
Ceftriaxone	MD	ND	Give usual dose post-HD. [Ref. 17,48–52]
Cefuroxime	MD	SD	[Ref. 53–55]
Cephalexin	MD	SD	Give usual dose post-HD. [Ref. 14,56]
Cephalothin	MD	SD	Give one-half usual dose post-HD; slightly active desacetyl metabolite. [Ref. 14,57,58]
Cephapirin	MD		Give one-half usual dose post-HD; slightly active desacetyl metabolite. [Ref. 14]
Cephradine	MD	SD	[Ref. 14]
Chloral Hydrate	MD–D		[Ref. 14]
Trichloroethanol *(active metabolite)*	MD–D		[Ref. 14]
Chloramphenicol	SD	ND	No supplemental dose required; increased dialysis removal in hepatic failure. [Ref. 14]

(continued)

DIALYSIS OF DRUGS (continued)

DRUG	HEMODIALYSIS	PERITONEAL DIALYSIS	COMMENTS AND REFERENCES
Chlordiazepoxide	ND–SD		Active metabolites. [Ref. 14]
Chloroquine	ND	ND	[Ref. 14,59]
Chlorpromazine			No data; because of high protein binding and large V_d, little removal expected.
Chlorpropamide		ND	Active metabolite; single case of PD did not decrease plasma levels. [Ref. 14,60]
Cimetidine	SD	ND–SD	Supplemental postdialysis dose unnecessary; coincide doses around dialysis. [Ref. 14]
Ciprofloxacin	SD	ND–SD	Therapeutic levels achieved in the peritoneal fluid following oral doses. [Ref. 14,61]
Clindamycin	ND	ND	[Ref. 14,62]
Clonidine	ND		[Ref. 14,26]
Cloxacillin	ND		[Ref. 14]
Colchicine	ND		Insufficient data. [Ref. 63]
Cyclophosphamide	MD		[Ref. 14]
Cyclosporine	ND		Because of large MW and large V_d, little removal expected. [Ref. 14]
Desipramine			No data; because of high protein binding and large V_d, little removal expected.
Diazepam	ND		Active metabolites. [Ref. 64,65]
Dicloxacillin	ND		[Ref. 14]
Digitoxin	ND	ND	[Ref. 14]
Digoxin	ND	ND	Post-HD rebound in plasma levels. [Ref. 14]
Diltiazem		ND	[Ref. 66]
Dipyridamole			No data; because of extensive protein binding, little removal by HD expected.
Disopyramide	ND		Concentration-dependent kinetics. [Ref. 14]
Doxepin	ND		[Ref. 67]
Doxycycline	ND	ND–SD	[Ref. 14]
Enalapril	SD–MD		[Ref. 14,68–70]
Enoxacin	ND		[Ref. 71,72]
Epoetin Alfa		ND	Limited removal expected by HD because of large MW. [Ref. 73,74]
Erythromycin	SD	ND	[Ref. 14,75]
Esmolol	ND	ND	[Ref. 76]
Ethambutol	SD		No supplemental dose after HD. [Ref. 14]
Ethchlorvynol	ND–SD	ND	Concentration-dependent kinetics. [Ref.14]
Ethosuximide	MD–D		Administer dose after dialysis. [Ref. 14]

(continued)

DIALYSIS OF DRUGS (continued)

DRUG	HEMODIALYSIS	PERITONEAL DIALYSIS	COMMENTS AND REFERENCES
Ethylene Glycol	D		Toxic metabolites formed. [Ref. 14]
Etodolac	ND		Limited data. [Ref. 77]
Famotidine	SD	ND	[Ref. 14,78–80]
Felodipine	SD		[Ref. 81]
Fenoprofen			Probably not removed by HD because of high protein binding.
Filgrastim	ND		Limited removal because of large MW. [Ref. 82]
Flecainide	ND	ND	[Ref. 14,83]
Fluconazole	MD	SD	Administer daily dose post-HD. [Ref. 14,84,85]
Flucytosine	D	MD	Give 20 mg/kg post-HD. [Ref. 14]
Flurazepam			No data; probably not dialyzed.
Flurbiprofen	ND		High protein binding likely to limit HD removal. [Ref. 86]
Foscarnet	MD		[Ref. 87,88]
Furosemide	ND		[Ref. 14]
Ganciclovir	D		Administer dose post-HD. [Ref. 14,89]
Gemfibrozil	ND		Data limited to one patient on HD. [Ref. 90]
Gentamicin	D	SD–MD	*See* Amikacin; increased clearance with high-flux dialysis (unpublished). Clinically important plasma levels achieved following intraperitoneal doses. [Ref. 14,91–93]
Glutethimide	ND–SD	ND	Active metabolite formed. [Ref. 14]
Glyburide	ND		[Ref. 94]
Haloperidol			No data; probably minimal removal because of large V_d.
Heparin			No data; probably poorly dialyzed because of large MW.
Ibuprofen	ND		Two metabolites (believed inactive) well dialyzed. [Ref. 14,95]
Imipenem	MD–D	SD	Give one-half usual dose post-HD. [Ref. 14]
Cilastatin	MD	SD	
Insulin			No data; probably poorly dialyzed because of large MW.
Isoniazid	D	MD	Give usual dose post-HD. [Ref. 14]
Isopropyl Alcohol	D		Major toxic metabolite is acetone. [Ref. 14]
Isradipine	ND		Little removal by PD expected because of high plasma clearance and V_d. [Ref. 96]
Itraconazole	ND	ND	[Ref. 97]

(continued)

DIALYSIS OF DRUGS (continued)

DRUG	HEMODIALYSIS	PERITONEAL DIALYSIS	COMMENTS AND REFERENCES
Kanamycin	D	SD–MD	*See* Amikacin. [Ref. 14]
Ketoconazole	ND	ND	[Ref. 14,98]
Labetalol	ND	ND	[Ref. 14]
Lidocaine	ND		Active metabolites. [Ref. 14]
Lisinopril	MD		[Ref. 70,99]
Lithium	MD–D	MD	Rebound rise in plasma levels postdialysis; case reports suggest 300–600 mg lithium carbonate after each HD. [Ref. 14,100,101]
Lomefloxacin	ND		[Ref. 102,103]
Lorazepam	SD		[Ref. 104]
Meperidine			No data; active metabolite accumulates in renal failure.
Meprobamate	SD–MD	ND–SD	Limited information; mostly case reports. [Ref. 14]
Mercaptopurine			*See* Azathioprine.
Methadone	ND	ND	[Ref. 14]
Methanol			[Ref. 14]
Methaqualone	SD	SD	Insufficient data. [Ref. 14]
Methicillin	ND		[Ref. 14]
Methotrexate	ND–SD	ND	HD–SD as shown by single case report using combination hemodialysis-hemoperfusion procedure. [Ref. 14]
Methyldopa	SD–MD	SD	Parent drug and metabolite data. [Ref. 14]
Methylprednisolone	SD		[Ref. 14]
Metoprolol	ND		Data indicate HD removal of metabolites. [Ref. 14,26]
Metronidazole	MD	SD	Adjust dosage to administer post-HD; active hydroxy metabolite removed by HD to same extent. [Ref. 14,105–108]
Mezlocillin	MD	SD	Give dose post-HD. [Ref. 14,17,109,110]
Miconazole	ND		[Ref. 14]
Midazolam			No data; because of high protein binding, little removal by HD expected.
Minocycline	ND	ND	Insufficient data. [Ref. 14]
Minoxidil	MD		[Ref. 111]
Nadolol	MD		[Ref. 14]
Nafcillin	ND		[Ref. 14]
Naproxen	ND		[Ref. 14]

(continued)

DIALYSIS OF DRUGS (continued)

DRUG	HEMODIALYSIS	PERITONEAL DIALYSIS	COMMENTS AND REFERENCES
Neomycin	D		*See* Amikacin. [Ref. 14]
Netilmicin	D		*See* Amikacin. [Ref. 14,112]
Nifedipine	ND	ND	[Ref. 113,115]
Nitroprusside			HD useful in overdose. [Ref. 14]
Cyanide	ND		
Thiocyanate *(toxic metabolites)*	MD		
Norfloxacin	ND		Insufficient data. [Ref. 14]
Nortriptyline			No data; because of high protein binding and large V_d, little removal expected. [Ref. 116]
Ofloxacin	MD	ND	[Ref. 117–120]
Omeprazole	SD–MD		HD data limited to one patient. [Ref. 121]
Oxacillin	ND	ND	[Ref. 14,122]
Oxazepam	ND		*See* Diazepam. [Ref. 14]
Penicillin G	MD		Give 500,000 units post-HD. [Ref. 14]
Pentamidine			No data; probably not dialyzed because of very large V_d.
Pentobarbital	SD	ND–SD	[Ref. 14]
Pentoxifylline	MD		Limited data from one patient on HD. [Ref. 123]
Phenobarbital	MD–D	SD–MD	Administer dose after dialysis. [Ref. 14]
Phenothiazines	ND		Numerous metabolites; toxicity and dialyzability unknown. [Ref. 14]
Phenytoin	ND	ND	Concentration-dependent kinetics. [Ref. 14]
Piperacillin	MD	ND	[Ref. 14,124–126]
Prazosin			Insufficient data; probably not dialyzed. [Ref. 14]
Prednisone			
Prednisolone *(active metabolite)*	SD		[Ref. 14]
Primidone	MD		Partly metabolized to phenobarbital. [Ref. 14]
Procainamide	MD	ND	Post-HD dose may be necessary to maintain therapeutic levels. [Ref. 14]
N-Acetylprocainamide *(active metabolite)*	MD	ND	Has class III antiarrhythmic activity.
Propoxyphene	ND	ND	Active metabolite poorly dialyzed. [Ref. 14]
Propranolol	ND		[Ref. 14]
Pseudoephedrine		SD	Limited data. [Ref. 127]

(continued)

DIALYSIS OF DRUGS (continued)

DRUG	HEMODIALYSIS	PERITONEAL DIALYSIS	COMMENTS AND REFERENCES
Pyrazinamide	D		[Ref. 128]
Quinapril	ND	ND	[Ref. 129,130]
Quinidine	ND–SD	ND	[Ref. 14]
Ranitidine	SD	ND	[Ref. 14,131]
Reserpine			Insufficient data; probably not dialyzed. [Ref. 14]
Rifabutin	ND		No data; little removal by dialysis is expected because of large V_d.
Rifampin			Not dialyzed because of large MW and V_d.
Rimantadine	ND		[Ref. 132]
Sargramostim			No data; little removal is expected by HD because of large MW.
Secobarbital	SD	ND–SD	[Ref. 14]
Sotalol	MD		[Ref. 133–135]
Streptomycin	MD–D		See Amikacin. [Ref. 14]
Sulfadiazine	MD		Limited data. [Ref. 136,137]
Sulfamethoxazole	MD	ND	Give in 2 divided doses, 1 pre- and 1 post dialysis. [Ref. 14,138–140]
Sulindac	ND		[Ref. 141]
Tacrolimus	ND		Limited data available for HD. High degree of protein binding and large MW limit HD removal. [Ref. 142]
Teicoplanin		SD	[Ref. 143,144]
Temazepam	ND	ND	[Ref.145]
Tetracycline	SD	SD	[Ref. 14]
Theophylline	D	SD–MD	Nonlinear disposition; supplemental doses needed post-HD. [Ref. 14,146–149]
Thiabendazole	ND		Slight removal of metabolites by HD. [Ref. 150–152]
Ticarcillin	MD	ND–SD	Give a 0.75–1.5 g dose post-HD. [Ref. 14]
Timolol	ND		[Ref. 153]
Tobramycin	D	MD	See Amikacin. [Ref. 14,93]
Tocainide	SD–MD	ND	[Ref. 14,154]
Tolazamide	ND		Inactive and less active metabolites. [Ref. 14]
Tolmetin			No data; high protein binding limits removal by HD.
Torsemide	ND		Data from the manufacturer.

(continued)

DIALYSIS OF DRUGS (continued)

DRUG	HEMODIALYSIS	PERITONEAL DIALYSIS	COMMENTS AND REFERENCES
Triazolam	ND	ND	[Ref. 155]
Trimethoprim	SD–MD	ND	Give daily dose after dialysis. [Ref. 14,138–140]
Valproic Acid	SD	ND	[Ref. 14]
Vancomycin			
(conventional)	ND–SD		Removal depends upon type of dialysis. [Ref. 14,156–168]
(high-flux)	MD		
Verapamil	ND		[Ref. 14,169–171]
Vinblastine			No data; probably poorly dialyzed because of large V_d.
Vincristine			No data; probably poorly dialyzed because of large V_d.
Warfarin			Probably poorly dialyzed because of high protein binding.
Zidovudine	ND	ND	[Ref. 14,172]

■ REFERENCES

1. Lee CS et al. Clearance calculations in hemodialysis: application to blood, plasma, and dialysate measurements for ethambutol. *J Pharmacokinet Biopharm* 1980;8:69–82.
2. Rosenberg J et al. Pharmacokinetics of drug overdose. *Clin Pharmacokinet* 1981;6:161–92.
3. Takki S et al. Pharmacokinetic evaluation of hemodialysis in acute drug overdose. *J Pharmacokinet Biopharm* 1978;6:427–42.
4. Gibson TP, Nelson HA. Drug kinetics and artificial kidneys. *Clin Pharmacokinet* 1977;2:403–26.
5. Tilstone WJ et al. The use of pharmacokinetic principles in determining the effectiveness of removal of toxins from blood. *Clin Pharmacokinet* 1979;4:23–37.
6. Gwilt PR. General equation for assessing drug removal by extracorporeal devices. *J Pharm Sci* 1981; 70:345–50.
7. Lee CS. The assessment of fractional drug removal by extracorporeal dialysis. *Biopharm Drug Disp* 1982;3:165–73. Abstract.
8. Gibson TP et al. Artificial kidneys and clearance calculations. *Clin Pharmacol Ther* 1976;20:720–3.
9. Reetze-Bonorden P et al. Drug dosage in patients during continuous renal replacement therapy. Pharmacokinetic and therapeutic considerations. *Clin Pharmacokinet* 1993;24:362–79.
10. Paton T et al. Drug therapy in patients undergoing peritoneal dialysis. Clinical pharmacokinetic considerations. *Clin Pharmacokinet* 1985;10:404–25.
11. Keller E. Peritoneal kinetics of different drugs. *Clin Nephrol* 1988;30(suppl 1):S24–8.
12. Gwilt PR, Perrier D. Plasma protein binding and distribution characteristics of drugs as indices of their hemodialyzability. *Clin Pharmacol Ther* 1978;24:154–61.
13. Pond S et al. Pharmacokinetics of haemoperfusion for drug overdose. *Clin Pharmacokinet* 1979;4:329–54.
14 Aweeka FT, Gambertoglio JG. Drug overdose and pharmacologic considerations in dialysis. In Cogan MG, Schoenfeld P, eds. *Introduction to dialysis*, 2nd ed. New York: Churchill Livingstone; 1991.
15. Roux A et al. Pharmacokinetics of acebutolol after intravenous bolus administration. *Br J Clin Pharmacol* 1980;9:215–7.
16. Roux A et al. Pharmacokinetics of acebutolol in patients with all grades of renal failure. *Eur J Clin Pharmacol* 1980;17:339–48.
17. Keane WF et al. Peritoneal dialysis-related peritonitis treatment recommendations. 1993 update. *Perit Dial Int* 1993;13:14–28.

18. Oreopoulos DG, Lal S. Recovery from massive amitriptyline overdosage. *Lancet* 1968;2:221. Letter.

19. Halle MA, Collipp PJ. Amitriptyline hydrochloride poisoning. Unsuccessful treatment by peritoneal dialysis. *N Y State J Med* 1969;69:1434–6.

20. Sunshine P, Yaffe SJ. Amitriptyline poisoning: clinical and pathological findings in a fatal case. *Am J Dis Child* 1963;106:501–6.

21. Comstock TJ et al. Severe amitriptyline intoxication and the use of charcoal hemoperfusion. *Clin Pharm* 1983;2:85–8.

22. Bailey RR et al. Haemodialysis and forced diuresis for tricyclic antidepressant poisoning. *Br Med J* 1974;4:230–1. Letter.

23. Zazgornik J et al. Plasma concentrations of astemizole in patients with terminal renal insufficiency, before, during, and after hemodialysis. *Int J Clin Pharmacol Ther Toxicol* 1986;24:246–8.

24. Salahudeen AK et al. Atenolol pharmacokinetics in patients on continuous ambulatory peritoneal dialysis. *Br J Clin Pharmacol* 1984;18:457–60.

25. Campese VM et al. Pharmacokinetics of atenolol in patients with chronic hemodialysis or peritoneal dialysis. *J Clin Pharmacol* 1985;25:393–5.

26. Niedermayer W et al. Pharmacokinetics of antihypertensive drugs (atenolol, metoprolol, propranolol and cloni-dine) and their metabolites during intermittent hemodialysis in humans. *Proc Eur Dial Transplant Assoc* 1978;15:607–9.

27. Drummer OH et al. The pharmacokinetics of captopril and captopril disulfide conjugates in uraemic patients on maintenance dialysis: comparison with patients with normal renal function. *Eur J Clin Pharmacol* 1987;32:267–71.

28. Spyker DA et al. Pharmacokinetics of cefaclor in renal failure: effects of multiple doses and hemodialysis. *Antimicrob Agents Chemother* 1982;21:278–81.

29. Leroy A et al. Pharmacokinetics of cefadroxil in patients with impaired renal function. *J Antimicrob Chemother* 1982;10(suppl B):39–46.

30. Paton TW et al. The disposition of cefazolin and tobramycin following intraperitoneal administration in pa-tients on CAPD. *Perit Dial Bull* 1983;3:73–6.

31. Guay DR et al. Pharmacokinetics of cefixime (CL284,635; FK 027) in healthy subjects and patients with renal insufficiency. *Antimicrob Agents Chemother* 1986;30:485–90.

32. Halstenson CE et al. Disposition of cefmetazole in healthy volunteers and patients with impaired renal func-tion. *Antimicrob Agents Chemother* 1990;34:519–23.

33. Hodler JE et al. Pharmacokinetics of cefoperazone in patients undergoing chronic ambulatory peritoneal dialy-sis: clinical and pathophysiological implications. *Eur J Clin Pharmacol* 1984;26:609–12.

34. Heim KL et al. Disposition of cefotaxime and desacetyl cefotaxime during continuous ambulatory peritoneal dialysis. *Antimicrob Agents Chemother* 1986;30:15–9.

35. Petersen J et al. Pharmacokinetics of intraperitoneal cefotaxime treatment of peritonitis in patients on continu-ous ambulatory dialysis. *Nephron* 1985;40:79–82.

36. Overgaard S et al. Cefotaxime disposition pharmacokinetics during peritoneal dialysis. *Pharmacol Toxicol* 1987;60:321–4.

37. Hasegawa H et al. Pharmacokinetics of cefotaxime in patients undergoing haemodialysis and continuous am-bulatory peritoneal dialysis. *J Antimicrob Chemother* 1984;14(suppl B):135–42.

38. Vlasses PH et al. Disposition of intravenous and intraperitoneal cefoxitin during chronic intermittent peritoneal dialysis. *Am J Kidney Dis* 1983;3:67–70.

39. Hoffler D et al. Cefpodoxime proxetil in patients with endstage renal failure on hemodialysis. *Infection* 1990;18:157–62.

40. Johnson CA et al. Pharmacokinetics and ex vivo susceptibility of cefpodoxime proxetil in patients receiving continuous ambulatory peritoneal dialysis. *Antimicrob Agents Chemother* 1993;37:2650–5.

41. Shyu WC et al. Pharmacokinetics of cefprozil in healthy subjects and patients with renal impairment. *J Clin Pharmacol* 1991;31:362–71.

42. Ohkawa M et al. Pharmacokinetics of ceftazidime in patients with renal insufficiency and in those undergoing hemodialysis. *Chemotherapy* 1985;31:410–6.

43. Comstock TJ et al. Ceftazidime pharmacokinetics during continuous ambulatory peritoneal dialysis (CAPD) and intermittent peritoneal dialysis (IPD). *Drug Intell Clin Pharm* 1983;17:453.

44. Demotes-Mainard F et al. Pharmacokinetics of intravenous and intraperitoneal ceftazidime in chronic ambula-tory peritoneal dialysis. *J Clin Pharmacol* 1993;33:475–9.

45. Gross ML et al. Ceftizoxime elimination kinetics in continuous ambulatory peritoneal dialysis. *Clin Pharmacol Ther* 1983;34:673–4.

46. Johnson CA et al. Pharmacokinetics of intravenous ceftizoxime in patients on continuous ambulatory peri-toneal dialysis. *Clin Nephrol* 1985;23:120–4.

47. Cutler RE et al. Pharmacokinetics of ceftizoxime. *J Antimicrob Chemother* 1982;10(suppl C):91–7.

48. Albin H et al. Pharmacokinetics of intravenous and intraperitoneal ceftriaxone in chronic ambulatory peritoneal dialysis. *Eur J Clin Pharmacol* 1986;31:479–83.

49. Koup JR et al. Ceftriaxone pharmacokinetics during peritoneal dialysis. *Eur J Clin Pharmacol* 1986;30:303–7.

50. Losno Garcia R et al. Single-dose pharmacokinetics of ceftriaxone in patients with end-stage renal disease and hemodialysis. *Chemotherapy* 1988;34:261–6.

51. Ti T-Y et al. Kinetic disposition of intravenous ceftriaxone in normal subjects and patients with renal failure on hemodialysis or peritoneal dialysis. *Antimicrob Agents Chemother* 1984;25:83–7.

52. Cohen D et al. Pharmacokinetics of ceftriaxone in patients with renal failure and in those undergoing hemodialysis. *Antimicrob Agents Chemother* 1983;24:529–32.

53. Weiss LG et al. Pharmacokinetics of intravenous cefuroxime during intermittent and continuous arteriovenous hemofiltration. *Clin Nephrol* 1988;30:282–6.

54. Chan MK et al. Cefuroxime pharmacokinetics in continuous and intermittent peritoneal dialysis. *Nephron* 1985;41:161–5.

55. Local FK et al. Pharmacokinetics of intravenous and intraperitoneal cefuroxime in patients undergoing peritoneal dialysis. *Clin Nephrol* 1981;16:40–3.

56. Bunke CM et al. Pharmacokinetics of common antibiotics used in continuous ambulatory peritoneal dialysis. *Am J Kidney Dis* 1983;3:114–7.

57. Imada A et al. Comparative study of the pharmacokinetics of various beta-lactams after intravenous and intraperitoneal administration in patients undergoing continuous ambulatory peritoneal dialysis. *Drugs* 1988;35(suppl 2):82–7.

58. Aziz NS et al. Pharmacokinetics of cephalothin and its metabolite in uremic patients undergoing hemodialysis using an HPLC assay. *Perubatan UKM* (Medical Journal, National Univ. of Malaysia) 1980;2:82–9.

59. Akintonwa A et al. Hemodialysis clearance of chloroquine in uremic patients. *Ther Drug Monit* 1986;8:285–7.

60. Ludwig SM et al. Chlorpropamide overdose in renal failure: management with charcoal hemoperfusion. *Am J Kidney Dis* 1987;10:457–60.

61. Drusano GL et al. Pharmacokinetics of intravenously administered ciprofloxacin in patients with various degrees of renal function. *Antimicrob Agents Chemother* 1987;37:860–4.

62. Schwartz MT et al. Clindamycin phosphate kinetics in subjects undergoing CAPD. *Clin Nephrol* 1986;26:303–6.

63. Ellwood MG, Robb GH. Self-poisoning with colchicine. *Postgrad Med J* 1971;47:129–38.

64. Cutler RE, Blair AD. Pharmacokinetics of diazepam in normal and uremic humans. *Clin Pharmacol Ther* 1979;25:219–20. Abstract.

65. Ochs HR et al. Diazepam kinetics in patients with renal insufficiency or hyperthyroidism. *Br J Clin Pharmacol* 1981;12:829–32.

66. Grech-Belanger O et al. Pharmacokinetics of diltiazem in patients undergoing continuous ambulatory peritoneal dialysis. *J Clin Pharmacol* 1988;28:477–80.

67. Faulkner RD et al. Hemodialysis of doxepin and desmethyldoxepin in uremic patients. *Artif Organs* 1984;8:151–5.

68. Kelly J et al. Chronic dose pharmacokinetics of enalapril in renal impairment. *Proc Br Paedod Soc* 1985;Apr:264.

69. Sica DA et al. Comparison of the steady-state pharmacokinetics of fosinopril, lisinopril and enalapril in patients with chronic renal insufficiency. *Clin Pharmacokinet* 1991;20:420–7.

70. Kelly JG et al. Pharmacokinetics of lisinopril, enalapril and enalaprilat in renal failure: effects of haemodialysis. *Br J Clin Pharmacol* 1988;26:781–6.

71. van der Auwera P et al. Pharmacokinetics of enoxacin and its oxometabolite following intravenous administration in patients with different degrees of renal impairment. *Antimicrob Agents Chemother* 1989;34:1491–7.

72. Nix DE et al. The effect of renal impairment and haemodialysis on single dose pharmacokinetics or oral enoxacin. *J Antimicrob Chemother* 1988;21(suppl B):87–95.

73. Stockenhuber F et al. Pharmacokinetics and dose response after intravenous and subcutaneous administration of recombinant erythropoietin in patients on regular haemodialysis treatment or continuous ambulatory peritoneal dialysis. *Nephron* 1991;59:399–402.

74. Macdougall IC et al. Pharmacokinetics of recombinant human erythropoietin in patients on continuous ambulatory peritoneal dialysis. *Lancet* 1989;1:425–7.

75. Kroboth PD et al. Hearing loss and erythromycin pharmacokinetics in a patient receiving hemodialysis. *Arch Intern Med* 1983;143:1263–5.

76. Covinsky JO. Esmolol: a novel cardioselective, titratable, intravenous beta-blocker with ultrashort half-life. *Drug Intell Clin Pharm* 1987;21:316–21.

77. Brater DC. Evaluation of etodolac in subjects with renal impairment. *Eur J Rheumatol Inflamm* 1990;10:44–5.

78. Halstenson CE et al. Disposition of famotidine in renal insufficiency. *J Clin Pharmacol* 1987;27:782–7.

79. Gladziwa U et al. Pharmacokinetics and dynamics of famotidine in patients with renal failure. *Br J Clin Pharmacol* 1988;26:315–21.

80. Hachisu T et al. Optimal therapeutic regimen of famotidine based on plasma concentrations in patients with chronic renal failure. *Clin Ther* 1988;10:656–63.

81. Buur T et al. Pharmacokinetics of felodipine in chronic hemodialysis patients. *J Clin Pharmacol* 1991;31:709–13.

82. Shishido K et al. The effects and pharmacokinetics of rhG-CSF on the treatment of neutropenia in patients with renal failure. *Nippon Jinzo Gakkai Shi* 1991;33:973–81.

83. Bailie GR, Waldek S. Pharmacokinetics of flecainide in a patient undergoing continuous ambulatory peritoneal dialysis. *J Clin Pharm Ther* 1988;13:121–4.

84. Toon S et al. An assessment of the effects of impaired renal function and haemodialysis on the pharmacokinetics of fluconazole. *Br J Clin Pharmacol* 1990;29:221–6.

85. Debruyne D et al. Pharmacokinetics of fluconazole in patients undergoing continuous ambulatory peritoneal dialysis. *Clin Pharmacokinet* 1990;18:491–9.

86. Cefali EA et al. Pharmacokinetic comparison of flurbiprofen in end-stage renal disease subjects and subjects with normal renal function. *J Clin Pharmacol* 1991;31:808–14.

87. MacGragor RR et al. Successful foscarnet therapy for cytomegalovirus retinitis in an AIDS patient undergoing hemodialysis: rationale for empiric dosing and plasma level monitoring. *J Infect Dis* 1991;164:785–7.

88. Aweeka FT et al. Pharmacokinetics (PK) of foscarnet in patients (PTS) with varying degrees of renal function. *Int Conf AIDS* 1993:485. Abstract PO-B26-2097.

89. Swan SK et al. Pharmacokinetics of ganciclovir in a patient undergoing hemodialysis. *Am J Kidney Dis* 1991;17:69–72.

90. Knauf H et al. Gemfibrozil absorption and elimination in kidney and liver disease. *Klin Wochenschr* 1990;68:692–8.

91. Indraprasit S et al. Gentamicin removal during intermittent peritoneal dialysis. *Nephron* 1986;44:18–21.

92. Lockwood WR, Bower JD. Tobramycin and gentamicin concentrations in the serum of normal and anephric patients. *Antimicrob Agents Chemother* 1973;3:125–9.

93. Matzke GR et al. Hemodialysis elimination rates and clearance of gentamicin and tobramycin. *Antimicrob Agents Chemother* 1984;25:128–30.

94. Pearson JG et al. Pharmacokinetic disposition of ^{14}C-glyburide in patients with varying renal function. *Clin Pharmacol Ther* 1986;39:318–24.

95. Senekjian HO et al. Absorption and disposition of ibuprofen in hemodialyzed uremic patients. *Eur J Rheumatol Inflamm* 1983;6:155–62.

96. Schonholzer K, Marone C. Pharmacokinetics and dialysability of isradipine in chronic haemodialysis patients. *Eur J Clin Pharmacol* 1992;42:231–3.

97. Boelaert J et al. Itraconazole pharmacokinetics in patients with renal dysfunction. *Antimicrob Agents Chemother* 1988;32:1595–7.

98. Daneshmend TK, Warnock DW. Clinical pharmacokinetics of ketoconazole. *Clin Pharmacokinet* 1988;14:13–34.

99. Gautam PC et al. Pharmacokinetics of lisinopril (MK521) in healthy young and elderly subjects and in elderly patients with cardiac failure. *J Pharm Pharmacol* 1987;39:929–31.

100. Jaeger A et al. Toxicokinetics of lithium intoxication treated by hemodialysis. *Clin Toxicol* 1985–1986;23:501–17.

101. Jaeger A et al. When should dialysis be performed in lithium poisoning? A kinetic study in 14 cases of lithium poisoning. *J Toxicol Clin Toxicol* 1993;31:429–47.

102. Blum RA et al. Pharmacokinetics of lomefloxacin in renally compromised patients. *Antimicrob Agents Chemother* 1990;34:2364–8.

103. Leroy A et al. Lomefloxacin pharmacokinetics in subjects with normal and impaired renal function. *Antimicrob Agents Chemother* 1990;34:17–20.

104. Morrison G et al. Effect of renal impairment and hemodialysis on lorazepam kinetics. *Clin Pharmacol Ther* 1984;35:646–52.

105. Roux D et al. Metronidazole kinetics in patients with acute renal failure on dialysis: a cumulative study. *Clin Pharmacol Ther* 1984;36:363–8.

106. Kreeft JH et al. Metronidazole kinetics in dialysis patients. *Surgery* 1983;93(1 pt 2):149–53.

107. Lau AH et al. Hemodialysis clearance of metronidazole and its metabolites. *Antimicrob Agents Chemother* 1986;29:235–8.

108. Cassey JG et al. Pharmacokinetics of metronidazole in patients undergoing peritoneal dialysis. *Antimicrob Agents Chemother* 1983;24:950–1.

109. Thorsteinsson SB et al. Pharmacokinetics of mezlocillin during hemodialysis. *Scand J Infect Dis* 1981;29(suppl):59–63.

110. Brogard JM et al. Pharmacokinetics of mezlocillin in patients with kidney impairment: special reference to hemodialysis and dosage adjustments in relation to renal function. *Chemotherapy* 1982;28:318–26.

111. Lowenthal DT, Affrime MB. Pharmacology and pharmacokinetics of minoxidil. *J Cardiovasc Pharmacol* 1980;2(suppl 2):S93–106.

112. Were AJ et al. Netilmicin and vancomycin in the treatment of peritonitis in CAPD patients. *Clin Nephrol* 1992;37:209–13.

113. Spital A et al. Nifedipine in continuous ambulatory peritoneal dialysis. *Arch Intern Med* 1983;143:2025. Letter.

114. Martre H et al. Haemodialysis does not affect the pharmacokinetics of nifedipine. *Br J Clin Pharmacol* 1985;20:155–8.

115. Kleinbloesem CH et al. Influence of haemodialysis on the pharmacokinetics and haemodynamic effects of nifedipine during continuous intravenous infusion. *Clin Pharmacokinet* 1986;11:316–22.

116. Dawling S et al. Nortriptyline metabolism in chronic failure: metabolite elimination. *Clin Pharmacol Ther* 1982;32:322–9.

117. Kampf D et al. Multiple dose kinetics of ofloxacin and ofloxacin metabolites in haemodialysis patients . *Eur J Clin Pharmacol* 1992;42:95–9.

118. Dorfler A et al. Pharmacokinetics of ofloxacin in patients on haemodialysis treatment. *Drugs* 1987;34(suppl 1):62–70.

119. Chan MK et al. Ofloxacin pharmacokinetics in patients on continuous ambulatory peritoneal dialysis. *Clin Nephrol* 1987;28:277–80.

120. Bandai H et al. Pharmacokinetics of ofloxacin in severe chronic renal failure. *Clin Ther* 1989;11:210–8.

121. Roggo A et al. The effect of hemodialysis on omeprazole plasma concentrations in the anuric patient: a case report. *Int J Clin Pharmacol Ther Toxicol* 1990;28:115–7.

122. Bulger RJ et al. Effect of uremia on methicillin and oxacillin blood levels. *JAMA* 1964;187:319–22.

123. Silver MR, Kroboth PD. Pentoxifylline in end-stage renal disease. *Drug Intell Clin Pharm* 1987;21:976–8.

124. Giron JA et al. Pharmacokinetics of piperacillin in patients with moderate renal failure and in patients undergoing hemodialysis. *Antimicrob Agents Chemother* 1981;19:279–83.

125. Heim KL. The effect of hemodialysis on piperacillin pharmacokinetics. *Drug Intell Clin Pharm* 1985;19:455.

126. Johnson CA et al. Single-dose pharmacokinetics of piperacillin and tazobactam in patients with renal disease. *Clin Pharmacol Ther* 1992;51:32–41.

127. Sica DA, Comstock TJ. Pseudoephedrine accumulation in renal failure. *Am J Med Sci* 1989;298:261–3.

128. Stamatakis G et al. Pyrazinamide and pyrazinoic acid pharmacokinetics in patients with chronic renal failure. *Clin Nephrol* 1988;30:230–4.

129. Swartz RD et al. Pharmacokinetics of quinapril and its active metabolite quinaprilat during continuous ambulatory peritoneal dialysis. *J Clin Pharmacol* 1990;30:1136–41.

130. Blum RA et al. Pharmacokinetics of quinapril and its active metabolite, quinaprilat, in patients on chronic hemodialysis. *J Clin Pharmacol* 1990;30:938–42.

131. Comstock TJ et al. Ranitidine bioavailability and disposition kinetics in patients undergoing chronic hemodialysis. *Nephron* 1989;52:15–9.

132. Capparelli EV et al. Rimantadine pharmacokinetics in healthy subjects and patients with end-stage renal failure. *Clin Pharmacol Ther* 1988;43:536–41.

133. Blair AD et al. Sotalol kinetics in renal insufficiency. *Clin Pharmacol Ther* 1981;29:457–63.

134. Tjandramaga TB et al. The effect of end-stage renal failure and haemodialysis on the elimination kinetics of sotalol. *Br J Clin Pharmacol* 1976;3:259–65.

135. Singh SN et al. Sotalol-induced torsades de pointes successfully treated with hemodialysis after failure of conventional therapy. *Am Heart J* 1991;121(2 pt 1):601–2.

136. Canfield CJ et al. Acute renal failure in *Plasmodium falciparum* malaria. Treatment of peritoneal dialysis. *Arch Intern Med* 1968;122:199–203.

137. Adam W, Dawborn J. Urinary excretion and plasma levels of sulphonamides in patients with renal impairment. *Australas Ann Med* 1970;19:250–4.

138. Nissenson AR et al. Pharmacokinetics of intravenous trimethoprim-sulfamethoxazole during hemodialysis. *Am J Nephrol* 1987;7:270–4.

139. Svirbley JE et al. Co-trimoxazole (sulfamethoxazole plus trimethoprim) peritoneal barrier transfer pharmacokinetics. *Clin Pharmacokinet* 1989;16:317–25.

140. Halstenson CE et al. Trimethoprim-sulfamethoxazole pharmacokinetics during continuous ambulatory peritoneal dialysis. *Clin Nephrol* 1984;22:239–43.

141. Ravis WR et al. Pharmacokinetics and dialyzability of sulindac and metabolites in patients with end-stage renal failure. *J Clin Pharmacol* 1993;33:527–34.

142. Venkataramanan R et al. Pharmacokinetics of FK 506: preclinical and clinical studies. *Transplant Proc* 1990;22:52–6.

143. Brouard RJ et al. Teicoplanin pharmacokinetics and bioavailability during peritoneal dialysis. *Clin Pharmacol Ther* 1989;45:674–81.

144. Traina GL et al. Pharmacokinetics of teicoplanin in patients on continuous ambulatory peritoneal dialysis. *Eur J Clin Pharmacol* 1986;31:501–4.

145. Kroboth PD et al. Effects of end-stage renal disease and aluminum hydroxide of temazepam kinetics. *Clin Pharmacol Ther* 1985;37:453–9.

146. Anderson JR et al. Effects of hemodialysis on theophylline kinetics. *J Clin Pharmacol* 1983;23:428–32.

147. Lee CS et al. Comparative pharmacokinetics of theophylline in peritoneal dialysis and hemodialysis. *J Clin Pharmacol* 1983;23:274–80.

148. Slaughter RL et al. Hemodialysis clearance of theophylline. *Ther Drug Monit* 1982;4:191–3.

149. Blouin RA et al. Theophylline hemodialysis clearance. *Ther Drug Monit* 1980;2:221–3.

150. Bauer LA et al. The pharmacokinetics of thiabendazole and its metabolites in an anephric patient undergoing hemodialysis and hemoperfusion. *J Clin Pharmacol* 1982;22:276–80.

151. Schumaker JD et al. Thiabendazole treatment of severe strongyloidiasis in a hemodialyzed patient. *Ann Intern Med* 1978;89(5 pt 1):644–5.

152. Leapman SB et al. *Strongyloides stercoalis* in chronic renal failure: safe therapy with thiabendazole. *South Med J* 1980;73:1400–2.

153. Lowenthal DT et al. Timolol kinetics in chronic renal insufficiency. *Clin Pharmacol Ther* 1978;23:606–15.

154. Raehl CL et al. Tocainide pharmacokinetics during continuous ambulatory peritoneal dialysis. *Am J Cardiol* 1987;60:747–50.

155. Kroboth PD et al. Effects of end stage renal disease and aluminium hydroxide on triazolam pharmacokinetics. *Br J Clin Pharmacol* 1985;19:839–42.

156. Glew RH et al. Vancomycin pharmacokinetics in patients undergoing chronic intermittent peritoneal dialysis. *Int J Clin Pharmacol Ther Toxicol* 1982;20:559–63.

157. Blevins RD et al. Pharmacokinetics of vancomycin in patients undergoing continuous ambulatory peritoneal dialysis. *Antimicrob Agents Chemother* 1984;25:603–6.

158. Rogge MC et al. Vancomycin disposition during continuous ambulatory peritoneal dialysis: a pharmacokinetic analysis of peritoneal drug transport. *Antimicrob Agents Chemother* 1985;27:578–82.

159. Harford AM et al. Vancomycin pharmacokinetics in continuous ambulatory peritoneal dialysis patients with peritonitis. *Nephron* 1986;43:217–22.

160. Whitby M et al. Pharmacokinetics of single dose intravenous vancomycin in CAPD peritonitis. *J Antimicrob Chemother* 1987;19:351–7.

161. Quale JM et al. Removal of vancomycin by high-flux hemodialysis membranes. *Antimicrob Agents Chemother* 1992;36:1424–6.

162. Torras J et al. Pharmacokinetics of vancomycin in patients undergoing hemodialysis with polyacrylontrile. *Clin Nephrol* 1991;36:35–41.

163. Bohler J et al. Rebound of plasma vancomycin levels after haemodialysis with highly permeable membranes. *Eur J Clin Pharmacol* 1992;42:635–9.

164. Barth RH et al. Vancomycin pharmacokinetics in high-flux hemodialysis. *Clin Res* 1990;38:a339. Abstract.

165. Figg WD et al. The effect of hemodialysis using polysulfone dialyzers on vancomycin clearance and the significance of rebound post-dialysis. *Pharmacotherapy* 1991;11:34.

166. Tan CC et al. Pharmacokinetics of intravenous vancomycin in patients with end-stage renal failure. *Ther Drug Monit* 1990;12:29–34.

167. Bailie GR et al. Prediction of serum vancomycin concentrations following intraperitoneal loading doses in continuous ambulatory patients with peritonitis. *Clin Pharmacokinet* 1992;22:298–307.

168. Morse GD et al. Comparative study of intraperitoneal and intravenous vancomycin pharmacokinetics during continuous ambulatory peritoneal dialysis. *Antimicrob Agents Chemother* 1987;31:173–7.

169. Shah GM, Winer RL. Verapamil kinetics during maintenance hemodialysis. *Am J Nephrol* 1985;5:338–41.

170. Beyerlein C et al. Verapamil in antihypertensive treatment of patients on renal replacement therapy—clinical implications and pharmacokinetics. *Eur J Clin Pharmacol* 1990;39(suppl 1):S35–7.

171. Hanyok JJ et al. An evaluation of the pharmacokinetics, pharmacodynamics, and dialyzability of verapamil in chronic hemodialysis patients. *J Clin Pharmacol* 1988;28:S31–6.

172. Kremer D et al. Zidovudine pharmacokinetics in five HIV seronegative patients undergoing continuous ambulatory peritoneal dialysis. *Pharmacotherapy* 1992;12:56–60.

4 Immunization

■ GENERAL RECOMMENDATIONS ON IMMUNIZATION*

Recommendations for immunizing infants, children, and adults are based on characteristics of immunobiologics, scientific knowledge about the principles of active and passive immunization, and judgments by public health officials and specialists in clinical and preventive medicine. Benefits and risks are associated with the use of all immunobiologics: no vaccine is completely safe or completely effective. Benefits of vaccination range from partial to complete protection against the consequences of infection, which range from asymptomatic or mild infection to severe consequences, such as paralysis or death. Risks of vaccination range from common, minor, and inconvenient side effects to rare, severe, and life-threatening conditions. Thus, recommendations for immunization practices balance scientific evidence of benefits, costs, and risks to achieve optimal levels of protection against infectious disease. These recommendations describe this balance and attempt to minimize the risks by providing information regarding dose, route, and spacing of immunobiologics and delineating situations that warrant precautions or contraindicate the use of these immunobiologics. These recommendations are for use only in the United States because vaccines and epidemiologic circumstances often differ in other countries. *Individual circumstances may warrant deviations from these recommendations.* Tables 4–1 and 4–2 list the immunobiologics available in the United States.

■ IMMUNOBIOLOGICS

The specific nature and content of immunobiologics can differ. When immunobiologics against the same infectious agent are produced by different manufacturers, active and inert ingredients in the various products are not always the same. Practitioners are urged to become familiar with the constituents of the products they use.

Suspending Fluids

These may be sterile water, saline, or complex fluids containing protein or other constituents derived from the medium or biologic system in which the vaccine is produced (eg, serum proteins, egg antigens, and cell-culture-derived antigens).

---

*Excerpted from reference 1.

TABLE 4–1. LICENSED VACCINES AND TOXOIDS AVAILABLE IN THE UNITED STATES, BY TYPE AND RECOMMENDED ROUTES OF ADMINISTRATION

VACCINE	TYPE	ROUTE
Adenovirus[a]	Live virus	Oral
Anthrax[b]	Inactivated bacteria	Subcutaneous
Bacillus of Calmette and Guérin (BCG)	Live bacteria	Intradermal/percutaneous
Cholera	Inactivated bacteria	Subcutaneous or intradermal[c]
Diphtheria-tetanus-pertussis (DTP)	Toxoids and inactivated whole bacteria	Intramuscular
DTP–*Haemophilus influenzae* type b conjugate (DTP-Hib)	Toxoids, inactivated whole bacteria, and bacterial polysaccharide conjugated to protein	Intramuscular
Diphtheria-tetanus-acellular pertussis (DTaP)	Toxoids and inactivated bacterial components	Intramuscular
Hepatitis B	Inactive viral antigen	Intramuscular
H. influenza type b conjugate (Hib)[d]	Bacterial polysaccharide conjugated to protein	Intramuscular
Influenza	Inactivated virus or viral components	Intramuscular
Japanese encephalitis	Inactivated virus	Subcutaneous
Measles	Live virus	Subcutaneous
Measles-mumps-rubella (MMR)	Live virus	Subcutaneous
Meningococcal	Bacterial polysaccharides of serotypes A/C/Y/W-135	Subcutaneous
Mumps	Live virus	Subcutaneous
Pertussis[b]	Inactivated whole bacteria	Intramuscular
Plague	Inactivated bacteria	Intramuscular
Pneumococcal	Bacterial polysaccharides of 23 pneumococcal types	Intramuscular or subcutaneous
Poliovirus vaccine, inactivated (IPV)	Inactivated viruses of all 3 serotypes	Subcutaneous
Poliovirus vaccine, oral (OPV)	Live viruses of all 3 serotypes	Oral
Rabies	Inactivated virus	Intramuscular or intradermal[e]
Rubella	Live virus	Subcutaneous
Tetanus	Inactivated toxin (toxoid)	Intramuscular[f]
Tetanus-diphtheria (Td or DT)[g]	Inactivated toxins (toxoids)	Intramuscular[f]

(continued)

TABLE 4–1. LICENSED VACCINES AND TOXOIDS AVAILABLE IN THE UNITED STATES, BY TYPE AND RECOMMENDED ROUTES OF ADMINISTRATION (continued)

VACCINE	TYPE	ROUTE
Typhoid (parenteral)	Inactivated bacteria	Subcutaneous[h]
(Ty21a oral)	Live bacteria	Oral
Varicella[i]	Live virus	Subcutaneous
Yellow fever	Live virus	Subcutaneous

[a]Available only to the U.S. Armed Forces.

[b]Distributed by the Division of Biologic Products, Michigan Department of Public Health.

[c]The intradermal dose is lower than the subcutaneous dose.

[d]The recommended schedule for infants depends on the vaccine manufacturer; consult the package insert and ACIP recommendations for specific products.

[e]The intradermal dose of rabies vaccine, human diploid cell (HDCV), is lower than the intramuscular dose and is used only for preexposure vaccination. **Rabies vaccine, absorbed (RVA) should not be used intradermally.**

[f]Preparations with adjuvants should be administered intramuscularly.

[g]Td = tetanus and diphtheria toxoids for use among persons ≥7 years of age. Td contains the same amount of tetanus toxoid as DTP or DT, but contains a smaller dose of diphtheria toxoid. DT = tetanus and diphtheria toxoids for use among children <7 years of age.

[h]Booster doses may be administered intradermally unless vaccine that is acetone-killed and dried is used.

[i]A live, atttenuated varicella vaccine is currently under consideration for licensure. This vaccine may be available for use through a special study protocol to any physician requesting it for certain pediatric patients with acute lymphocytic leukemia. Additional information about eligibility criteria and vaccine administration is available from the Varivax Coordinating Center; telephone: (215) 283–0897.

TABLE 4–2. IMMUNE GLOBULINS AND ANTITOXINS* AVAILABLE IN THE UNITED STATES, BY TYPE OF ANTIBODIES AND INDICATIONS FOR USE

IMMUNOBIOLOGIC	TYPE	INDICATION(S)
Botulinum antitoxin	Specific equine antibodies	Treatment of botulism
Cytomegalovirus immune globulin, intravenous (CMV-IGIV)	Specific human antibodies	Prophylaxis for bone marrow and kidney transplant recipients
Diphtheria antitoxin	Specific equine antibodies	Treatment of respiratory diphtheria
Hepatitis B immune globulin	Specific human antibodies	Hepatitis B postexposure prophylaxis
Immune globulin (IG)	Pooled human antibodies	Hepatitis A pre- and postexposure prophylaxis; measles postexposure prophylaxis
Immune globulin, intravenous (IGIV)	Pooled human antibodies	Replacement therapy for antibody deficiency disorders; immune thrombocytopenic purpura (ITP); hypogammaglobulinemia in chronic lymphocytic leukemia; Kawasaki disease
Rabies immune globulin[†] (HRIG)	Specific human antibodies	Rabies postexposure management of persons not previously immunized with rabies vaccine
Tetanus immune globulin (TIG)	Specific human antibodies	Tetanus treatment; post-exposure prophylaxis of persons not adequately immunized with tetanus toxoid
Vaccinia immune globulin (VIG)	Specific human antibodies	Treatment of eczema vaccinatum, vaccinia necrosum, and ocular vaccinia
Varicella zoster immune globulin (VZIG)	Specific human antibodies	Postexposure prophylaxis of susceptible immunocompromised persons, certain susceptible pregnant women, and perinatally exposed newborn infants

*Immune globulin preparations and antitoxins are administered intramuscularly unless otherwise indicated.
[†]HRIG is administered around the wounds in addition to the intramuscular injection.

Preservers, Stabilizers, Antibiotics

These components of vaccines, antitoxins, and globulins are used to inhibit or prevent bacterial growth in viral cultures or the final product or to stabilize the antigens or antibodies. Allergic reactions can occur if the recipient is sensitive to one of these additives (eg, mercurials [thimerosal], phenols, albumin, glycine, and neomycin).

Adjuvants

Many antigens evoke suboptimal immunologic responses. Efforts to enhance immunogenicity include mixing antigens with a variety of substances or adjuvants (eg, aluminum adjuvants such as aluminum phosphate or aluminum hydroxide).

Storage and Handling of Immunobiologics

Failure to adhere to recommended specifications for storage and handling of immunobiologics can make these products impotent. Recommendations included in a product's package insert, including reconstitution of vaccines, should be followed closely to assure maximum potency of vaccines. In general, all vaccines should be inspected and monitored to assure that the cold chain has been maintained during shipment and storage. Vaccines should be stored at recommended temperatures immediately upon receipt. Certain vaccines, such as oral polio vaccine (OPV) and yellow fever vaccine, are very sensitive to increased temperature. Other vaccines are sensitive to freezing, including diphtheria and tetanus toxoids and pertussis vaccine, adsorbed (DTP); diphtheria and tetanus toxoids and acellular pertussis vaccine, adsorbed (DTaP); diphtheria and tetanus toxoids for pediatric use (DT); tetanus and diphtheria toxoids for adult use (Td); inactivated poliovirus vaccine (IPV); *Haemophilus influenzae* type B conjugate vaccine (Hib); hepatitis B vaccine; pneumococcal vaccine; and influenza vaccine. Mishandled vaccine may not be easily distinguished from potent vaccine. When in doubt about the appropriate handling of a vaccine, contact the manufacturer.

■ ADMINISTRATION OF VACCINES

General Instructions

Persons administering vaccines should take the necessary precautions to minimize risk for spreading disease. They should be adequately immunized against hepatitis B, measles, mumps, rubella, and influenza. Tetanus and diphtheria toxoids are recommended for all persons. Hands should be washed before each new patient is seen. Gloves are not required when administering vaccinations, unless the persons who administer the vaccine will come into contact with potentially infectious body fluids or have open lesions on their hands. Syringes and needles used for injections must be sterile and preferably disposable to minimize the risk of contamination. A separate needle and syringe should be used for each injection. Different vaccines should not be mixed in the same syringe unless specifically licensed for such use.* Disposable needles and syringes should be discarded in labeled, puncture-proof containers to prevent inadvertent needlestick injury or reuse.

---

*The only vaccines currently licensed to be mixed in the same syringe by the person administering the vaccine are PRP-T *Haemophilus influenzae* type b conjugate vaccine, lyophilized, which can be reconstituted with DTP vaccine produced by Connaught.

Routes of administration are recommended for each immunobiologic (*see* Table 4–1). To avoid unnecessary local or systemic effects and to ensure optimal efficacy, the practitioner should not deviate from the recommended routes. Injectable immunobiologics should be administered where there is little likelihood of local, neural, vascular, or tissue injury. In general, vaccines containing adjuvants should be injected into the muscle mass; when administered subcutaneously or intradermally, they can cause local irritation, induration, skin discoloration, inflammation, and granuloma formation. Before the vaccine is expelled into the body, the needle should be inserted into the injection site and the syringe plunger should be pulled back. If blood appears in the needle hub, the needle should be withdrawn and a new site selected. The process should be repeated until no blood appears.

Subcutaneous Injections

Subcutaneous injections are usually administered into the thigh of infants and into the deltoid area of older children and adults. A 5/8- to 3/4-inch, 23- to 25-gauge needle should be inserted into the tissues below the dermal layer of the skin.

Intramuscular Injections

The preferred site for intramuscular (IM) injections are the anterolateral aspect of the upper thigh and the deltoid muscle of the upper arm. *The buttock should not be used routinely for active vaccination of infants, children, or adults because of the potential for injury to the sciatic nerve.* In addition, injection into the buttock has been associated with decreased immunogenicity of hepatitis B and rabies vaccines in adults, presumably because of inadvertent subcutaneous injection or injection into deep fat tissue. If the buttock is used for passive immunization when large volumes are to be injected or multiple doses are necessary (eg, large doses of immune globulin [IG]), the central region should be avoided; only the upper, outer quadrant should be used, and the needle should be directed anteriorly (ie, not inferiorly or perpendicular to the skin) to minimize the possibility of involvement with the sciatic nerve.

For all IM injections, the needle should be long enough to reach the muscle mass and prevent vaccine from seeping into subcutaneous tissues, but not so long as to endanger the underlying neurovascular structures or bone. Vaccinators should be familiar with the structural anatomy of the area into which they are injecting vaccine. An individual decision on needle size and site of injection must be made for each person based on age, the volume of material to be administered, the size of the muscle, and the depth below the muscle surface into which the material is to be injected.

Infants (<12 months of age). Among most infants, the anterolateral aspect of the thigh provides the largest muscle mass and is therefore the recommended site. However, the deltoid can also be used with the thigh, for example, when multiple vaccines must be administered on the same visit. In most cases, a 7/8- to 1-inch, 22- to 25-gauge needle is sufficient to penetrate muscle in the thigh of a 4-month-old infant. The free hand should bunch the muscle, and the needle should be directed inferiorly along the axis of the leg at an angle appropriate to reach the muscle while avoiding nearby neurovascular structures and bone.

Toddlers and Older Children. The deltoid may be used if the muscle mass is adequate. The needle size can range from 22 to 25 gauge and from 5/8 to 1¼ inches, based on the size of the muscle. As with infants, the anterolateral thigh may be used, but the needle should be longer—generally ranging from 7/8 to 1¼ inches.

Adults. The deltoid is recommended for routine intramuscular vaccination among adults, particularly for hepatitis B vaccine. The suggested needle size is 1 to 1½ in and 20–25 gauge.

Intradermal Injection. Intradermal injections are generally administered on the volar surface of the forearm, except for human diploid cell rabies vaccine (HDCV), for which reactions are less severe when the vaccine is administered in the deltoid area. With the bevel facing upward, a 3/8- to 3/4-inch, 25- or 27-gauge needle can be inserted into the epidermis at an angle parallel to the long axis of the forearm. The needle should be inserted so that the entire bevel penetrates the skin and the injected solution raises a small bleb. Because of the small amounts of antigen used in intradermal injections, care must be taken not to inject the vaccine subcutaneously, because it can result in a suboptimal immunologic response.

Multiple Vaccinations. If more than one vaccine preparation is administered or if live vaccine and an immune globulin preparation are administered simultaneously, it is preferable to administer each at a different anatomic site. It is also preferable to avoid administering two IM injections in the same limb, especially if DTP is one of the products administered. However, if more than one injection must be administered in a single limb, the thigh is usually the preferred site because of the greater muscle mass; the injections should be sufficiently separated (ie, 1–2 in. apart) so that any local reactions are unlikely to overlap.

Regurgitated Oral Vaccines. Infants may sometimes fail to swallow oral preparations (eg, oral poliovirus vaccine [OPV]) after administration. If, in the judgment of the person administering the vaccine, a substantial amount of the vaccine is spit out, regurgitated, or vomited shortly after administration (ie, within 5–10 min), another dose can be administered at the same visit. If this repeat dose is not retained, neither dose should be counted, and the vaccine should be readministered at the next visit.

Nonstandard Vaccination Practices. The recommendations on route, site, and dosages of immunobiologics are derived from theoretical considerations, experimental trials, and clinical experience. The Advisory Committee on Immunization Practices (ACIP) strongly discourages any variation from the recommended route, site, volume, or number of doses of any vaccine.

Varying from the recommended route and site can result in (a) inadequate protection (eg, when hepatitis B vaccine is administered in the gluteal area rather than deltoid muscle or when vaccines are administered intradermally rather than intramuscularly) and (b) increased risk for reactions (eg, when DTP is administered subcutaneously rather than intramuscularly). Administration of volumes smaller than those recommended, such as split doses, can result in inadequate protection. Use of larger than the recommended dose can be hazardous because of excessive local or systemic concentrations of antigens or other constituents. The use of multiple reduced doses that together equal a full immunizing dose or the use of smaller divided doses is not endorsed or recommended. The serologic response, clinical efficacy, and frequency and severity of adverse reactions of such schedules have not been adequately studied. Any vaccination using less than the standard dose of a nonstandard route or site of administration should not be counted, and the person should be revaccinated according to age. If a medically documented concern exists that revaccination may result in increased risk of adverse effects because of repeated prior exposure from nonstandard vaccinations, immunity to most relevant antigens can be tested serologically to assess the need for revaccination.

■ AGE AT WHICH IMMUNOBIOLOGICS ARE ADMINISTERED

Recommendations for the age at which vaccines are administered are influenced by several factors: age-specific risks of disease, age-specific risks of complications, ability of persons of a given age to respond to the vaccine(s), and potential interference with the immune response by passively transferred by maternal antibody. In general, vaccines are recommended for the youngest age group at risk for developing disease whose members are known to develop an adequate antibody response to vaccination (Tables 4–3, 4–4, and 4–5).

■ SPACING OF IMMUNOBIOLOGICS

Interval Between Multiple Doses of Same Antigen

Some products require administration of more than one dose for development of an adequate antibody response. In addition, some products require periodic reinforcement or booster doses to maintain protection. In recommending the ages and intervals for multiple doses, the ACIP takes into account risks from disease and the need to induce or maintain satisfactory protection (*see* Tables 4–3, 4–4, and 4–5).

Longer-than-recommended intervals between doses do not reduce final antibody concentrations. Therefore, an interruption in the immunization schedule does not require reinstitution of the entire series of an immunobiologic or the addition of extra doses. However, administering doses of a vaccine or toxoid at less than recommended minimum intervals may decrease the antibody response and therefore should be avoided. Doses administered at less than recommended minimum intervals should not be counted as part of a primary series.

Some vaccines produce increased rates of local or systemic reactions in certain recipients when administered too frequently (eg, adult Td, pediatric DT, tetanus toxoid, and rabies vaccine). Such reactions are thought to result from the formation of antigen-antibody complexes. Good recordkeeping, maintaining careful patient histories, and adherence to recommended schedules can decrease the frequency of such reactions without sacrificing immunity.

**TABLE 4–3. RECOMMENDED CHILDHOOD VACCINATION SCHEDULE[a]—
UNITED STATES, JANUARY–JUNE 1996**

VACCINE	Birth	1 Mo	2 Mo	4 Mo	6 Mo	12 Mo	15 Mo	18 Mo	4–6 Yr	11–12 Yr	14–16 Yr
Hepatitis B[b]	Hep B-1										
		Hep B-2			Hep B-3					Hep B[c]	
Diptheria and tetanus toxoids and pertussis vaccine[d]		DTP	DTP	DTP	DTP (DTaP at ≥15 mo)			DTP or DTaP	Td	
Haemophilus influenzae type b[e]		Hib	Hib	Hib	Hib					
Poliovirus[f]		IPV[g] or OPV	OPV					OPV		
Measles-mumps-rubella[h]					MMR			MME or MMR	
Varicella zoster virus[i]					Var			Var[i]	

░░░ Range of Acceptable Ages for Vaccination

▓▓▓ "Catch-Up" Vaccination[c,i]

[a]Vaccines are listed under the routinely recommended ages.

[b]**Infants born to hepatitis B surface antigen (HBsAg)-negative mothers** should receive 2.5 µg of Recombivax HB (Merck & Co.) or 10 µg of Engerix-B (SmithKline Beecham). The second dose should be administered ≥1 month after the first dose. **Infants born to HBsAg-positive mothers** should receive 0.5 mL hepatitis B immune globulin (HBIG) within 12 hr of birth, and either 5 µg of Recombivax HB or 10 µg of Engerix-B at a separate site. The second dose is recommended at age 1–2 mo and the third dose at age 6 mo. **Infants born to mothers whose HBsAg status is unknown** should receive either 5 µg of Recombivax HB or 10 µg of Engerix-B within 12 hr of birth. The second dose of vaccine is recommended at age 1 mo and the third dose at age 6 mo.

[c]Adolescents who have not received three doses of hepatitis B vaccine should initiate or complete the series at age 11–12 yr. The second dose should be administered at least 1 mo after the first dose, and the third dose should be administered at least 4 mo after the first dose and at least 2 mo after the second dose.

[d]The fourth dose of diphtheria and tetanus toxoids and pertussis vaccine (DTP) may be administered at age 12 mo, if at least 6 mo have elapsed since the third dose of DTP. Diphtheria and tetanus toxoids and acellular pertussis vaccine (DTaP) is licensed for the fourth and/or fifth vaccine dose(s) for children aged ≥15 mo and may be preferred for these doses in this age group. Tetanus and diphtheria toxoids, absorbed, for adult use (Td) is recommended at age 11–12 yr if ≥5 yr have elapsed since the last dose of DTP, DTaP, or diphtheria and tetanus toxoids, adsorbed, for pediatric use (DT).

[e]Three Haemophilus influenzae type b (Hib) conjugate vaccines are licensed for infant use. If PedvaxHIB (Merck & Co.) Haemophilus b conjugate vaccine (Meningococcal Protein Conjugate) (PRP-OMP) is administered at ages 2 and 4 mo, a dose at 6 mo is not required. After completing the primary series, any Hib conjugate vaccine may be used as a booster.

[f]Oral poliovirus vaccine (OPV) is recommended for routine infant vaccination. Inactivated poliovirus vaccine (IPV) is recommended for persons—or household contacts of persons—with a congenital or acquired immune deficiency disease or an altered immune status resulting from disease or immunosuppressive therapy, and is an acceptable alternative for other persons. The primary three-dose series for IPV should be given with a minimum interval of 4 weeks between the first and second doses and 6 mo between the second and third doses.

[g]The Advisory Committee on Immunization Practices (ACIP) of the Centers for Disease Control and Prevention (CDC) recommends the use of enhanced inactivated poliomyelitis vaccine (IPV) injection for the first 2 doses of the series to minimize OPV-related paralysis.[5]

[h]The second dose of measles-mumps-rubella vaccine (MMR) is routinely recommended at age 4–6 yr or at age 11–12 yr but may be administered at any visit provided ≥1 month has elapsed since receipt of the first dose.

[i]Varicella zoster virus vaccine (Var) can be administered to susceptible children any time after age 12 mo.

[j]Unvaccinated children who lack a reliable history of chickenpox should be vaccinated at age 11–12 yr.

Use of trade names and commercial sources is for identification only and does not imply endorsement by the Public Health Service or the U.S. Department of Health and Human Services.

From Advisory Committee on Immunization Practices, American Academy of Pediatrics, and American Academy of Family Physicians.

TABLE 4–4. RECOMMENDED ACCELERATED IMMUNIZATION SCHEDULE FOR INFANTS AND CHILDREN <7 YEARS OF AGE WHO START THE SERIES LATE[a] OR WHO ARE >1 MONTH BEHIND IN THE IMMUNIZATION SCHEDULE[b] (ie, children for whom compliance with scheduled return visits cannot be assured)

TIMING	VACCINE(S)	COMMENTS
First visit (≥4 mo of age)	DTP,[c] IPV[d] or OPV, Hib,[c,e] Hepatitis B, MMR (should be given as soon as child is age 12–15 mo)	All vaccines should be administered simultaneously at the appropriate visit.
Second visit (1 mo after first visit)	DTP,[c] Hib,[c,e] Hepatitis B	
Third visit (1 mo after second visit)	DTP,[c] OPV,[d] Hib,[c,e]	
Fourth visit (6 weeks after third visit)	OPV	
Fifth visit (≥6 mo after third visit)	DTaP[c] or DTP, Hib,[c,e] Hepatitis B	
Additional visits (Age 4–6 yr)	DTaP[c] or DTP, OPV, MMR	Preferably at or before school entry.
(Age 14–16 yr)	Td	Repeat every 10 yr throughout life.

DTP, diphtheria-tetanus-pertussis; DTaP, diphtheria-tetanus-acellular pertussis; Hib, *Haemophilus influenzae* type b conjugate; MMR, measles-mumps-rubella; OPV, poliovirus vaccine, live oral, trivalent; Td, tetanus and diphtheria toxoids (for use among persons ≥7 years of age).

[a]If initiated in the first year of life, administer DTP doses 1, 2, and 3 and OPV doses 1, 2, and 3 according to this schedule; administer MMR when the child reaches 12–15 mo of age.

[b]See individual ACIP recommendations for detailed information on specific vaccines.

[c]Two DTP and Hib combination vaccines are available (DTP/HbOC [TETRAMUNE]; and PRP-T [ActHIB, OmniHIB] which can be reconstituted with DTP vaccine produced by Connaught). DTaP preparations are currently recommended only for use as the fourth and/or fifth doses of the DTP series among children 15 mo–6 yr of age (before the seventh birthday). DTP and DTaP should not be used on or after the seventh birthday.

[d]The Advisory Committee on Immunization Practices (ACIP) of the Centers for Disease Control and Prevention (CDC) recommends the use of enhanced inactivated poliomyelitis vaccine (IPV) injection for the first 2 doses of the series to minimize OPV-related paralysis.[5]

[e]The recommended schedule varies by vaccine manufacturer. For information specific to the vaccine being used, consult the package insert and ACIP recommendations. Children beginning the Hib vaccine series at age 2–6 mo should receive a primary series of three doses of HbOC [HibTITER] (Lederle-Praxis), PRP-T [ActHIB, OmniHIB] (Pasteur Merieux; SmithKline Beecham; Connaught), or a licensed DTP-Hib combination vaccine; or two doses of PRP-OMP [PedvaxHIB] (Merck, Sharp, and Dohme). An additional booster dose of any licensed Hib conjugate vaccine should be administered at 12–15 mo of age *and* at least 2 mo after the previous dose. Children beginning the Hib vaccine series at 7–11 mo of age should receive a primary series of two doses of a vaccine containing HbOC, PRP-T, or PRP-OMP. An additional booster dose of any licensed Hib conjugate vaccine should be administered at 12–18 mo of age *and* at least 2 mo after the previous dose. Children beginning the Hib vaccine series at ages 12–14 mo should receive a primary series of one dose of a vaccine containing HbOC, PRP-T, or PRP-OMP. An additional booster dose of any licensed Hib conjugate vaccine should be administered 2 mo after the previous dose. Children beginning the Hib vaccine series at ages 15–59 mo should receive one dose of any licensed Hib vaccine. Hib vaccine should not be administered after the fifth birthday except for special circumstances as noted in the specific ACIP recommendations for the use of Hib vaccine.

TABLE 4–5. RECOMMENDED IMMUNIZATION SCHEDULE FOR PERSONS ≥7 YR OF AGE NOT VACCINATED AT THE RECOMMENDED TIME IN EARLY INFANCY[a]

TIMING	VACCINE(S)	COMMENTS
First visit	Td,[b] OPV,[c] MMR,[d] and Hepatitis B[e]	Primary poliovirus vaccination is not routinely recommended for persons ≥18 yr of age.
Second visit (6–8 weeks after first visit)	Td, OPV, MMR,[d,f] Hepatitis B[e]	
Third visit (6 mo after second visit)	Td, OPV, Hepatitis B[e]	
Additional visits	Td	Repeat every 10 yr throughout life.

MMR, measles-mumps-rubella; OPV, poliovirus vaccine, live oral, trivalent; Td, tetanus and diphtheria toxoids (for use among persons ≥7 yr of age).

[a]See individual ACIP recommendations for details.

[b]The DTP and DTaP doses administered to children <7 yr of age who remain incompletely vaccinated at age ≥7 yr should be counted as prior exposure to tetanus and diphtheria toxoids (eg, a child who previously received two doses of DTP needs only one dose of Td to complete a primary series for tetanus and diphtheria).

[c]When polio vaccine is administered to previously unvaccinated persons ≥18 yr of age, inactivated poliovirus vaccine (IPV) is preferred. For the immunization schedule for IPV, see specific ACIP statement on the use of polio vaccine.

[d]Persons born before 1957 can generally be considered immune to measles and mumps and need not be vaccinated. Rubella (or MMR) vaccine can be administered to persons of any age, particularly to nonpregnant women of childbearing age.

[e]Hepatitis B vaccine, recombinant. Selected high-risk groups for whom vaccination is recommended include persons with occupational risk, such as health care and public safety workers who have occupational exposure to blood, clients and staff of institutions for the developmentally disabled, hemodialysis patients, recipients of certain blood products (eg, clotting factor concentrates), household contacts and sex partners of hepatitis B virus carriers, injecting drug users, sexually active homosexual and bisexual men, certain sexually active heterosexual men and women, inmates of long-term correctional facilities, certain international travelers, and families of HBsAg-positive adoptees from countries where HBV infection is endemic. Because risk factors are often not identified directly among adolescents, universal hepatitis B vaccination of teenagers should be implemented in communities where injecting drug use, pregnancy among teenagers, and/or sexually transmitted diseases are common.

[f]The ACIP recommends a second dose of measles-containing vaccine (preferably MMR to assure immunity to mumps and rubella) for certain groups. Children with no documentation of live measles vaccination after the first birthday should receive two doses of live measles-containing vaccine not less than 1 mo apart. In addition, the following persons born in 1957 or later should have documentation of measles immunity (ie, two doses of measles-containing vaccine [at least one of which being MMR], physician-diagnosed measles, or laboratory evidence of measles immunity): (a) those entering post–high school educational settings; (b) those beginning employment in health-care settings who will have direct patient contact; and (c) travelers to areas with endemic measles.

Simultaneous Administration

Experimental evidence and extensive clinical experience have strengthened the scientific basis for administering certain vaccines simultaneously. Many of the commonly used vaccines can safely and effectively be administered simultaneously (ie, on the same day, *not* at the same anatomic site). Simultaneous administration is important in certain situations, including (a) imminent exposure to several infectious diseases, (b) preparation for foreign travel, and (c) uncertainty that the person will return for further doses of vaccine.

Killed Vaccines

In general, inactivated vaccines can be administered simultaneously at separate sites. However, when vaccines commonly associated with local or systemic side effects (eg, cholera, parenteral typhoid, and plague) are administered simultaneously, the side effects might be accentuated. When feasible, it is preferable to administer these vaccines on separate occasions.

Live Vaccines

The simultaneous administration of the most widely used live and inactivated vaccines has not resulted in impaired antibody responses or increased rates of adverse reactions. Administration of combined measles, mumps, and rubella (MMR) vaccine yields results similar to administration of individual measles, mumps, and rubella vaccines at different sites. Therefore, there is no medical basis for administering these vaccines separately for routine immunization instead of the preferred MMR combined vaccine.

Concern has been raised that oral live attenuated typhoid (Ty21a) vaccine theoretically might interfere with the immune response to OPV when OPV is administered simultaneously or soon after live oral typhoid vaccine. However, no published data exist to support this theory. Therefore, if OPV and live oral typhoid vaccine are needed at the same time (eg, when international travel is undertaken on short notice), both vaccines may be administered simultaneously or at any interval before or after each other.

Routine Childhood Vaccines

The simultaneous administration of routine childhood vaccines does not interfere with the immune response to these vaccines. When administered at the same time and at separate sites, DTP, OPV, and MMR have produced seroconversion rates and rates of side effects similar to those observed when the vaccines are administered separately. Simultaneous vaccination of infants with DTP, OPV (or IPV), and either Hib vaccine or hepatitis B vaccine has resulted in acceptable response to all antgens. Routine simultaneous administration of DTP (or DTaP), OPV (or IPV), Hib vaccine, MMR, and hepatitis B vaccine is encouraged for children who are the recommended age to receive these vaccines and for whom no specific contraindications exist at the time of the visit, unless, in the judgment of the provider, complete vaccination of the child will not be compromised by administering different vaccines at different visits. Simultaneous administration is particularly important if the child might not return for subsequent vaccinations. Administration of MMR and Hib at 12–15 months of age, followed by DTP (or DTaP, if indicated) at 18 months of age remains an acceptable alternative for children with caregivers known to be compliant with other health care recommendations and who are likely to return for future visits; hepatitis B vaccine can be administered at either of these two visits. DTaP may be used instead of DTP only for the fourth and fifth doses for children 15 months of age through 6 years (ie, before the seventh birthday). Individual vaccines should not be mixed in the same syringe unless they are licensed for mixing by the U.S. Food and Drug Administration (FDA).*

Other Vaccines

The simultaneous administration of pneumococcal polysaccharide vaccine and whole-virus influenza vaccine elicits satisfactory antibody responses without increasing the frequency or severity of adverse reactions in adults. Simultaneous administration of the pneumococcal vaccine and split-virus influenza vaccine can be expected to yield satisfactory results in both children and adults.

Hepatitis B vaccine administered with yellow fever vaccine is as safe and efficacious as when these vaccines are administered separately. Measles and yellow fever vaccines have been administered together safely and with full efficacy of each of the components.

The antibody response to yellow fever and cholera vaccines is decreased if they are administered simultaneously or within a short time of each other. If possible, yellow fever and cholera vaccinations should be separated by at least 3 weeks. If time constraints exist and both vaccines are necessary, the injections can be administered simultaneously or within a 3-week period with the understanding that antibody response may not be optimal. Yellow fever vaccine is required by many countries and is highly effective in protecting against a disease with substantial mortality and for which no therapy exists. The currently used cholera vaccine provides limited protection of brief duration; few indications exist for its use.

Antimalarials and Vaccination

The antimalarial mefloquine (Lariam) could potentially affect the immune response to oral live attenuated typhoid (Ty21a) vaccine if both are taken simultaneously. To minimize this effect, it may be prudent to administer Ty21a typhoid vaccine at least 24 hr before or after a dose of mefloquine. Because chloroquine phosphate (and possibly other structurally related antimalarials, such as mefloquine) may interfere with the antibody response to human diploid cell rabies vaccine (HDCV) when HDCV is administered by the intradermal route, HDCV should not be administered by the intradermal route when chloroquine, mefloquine, or other structurally related antimalarials are used.

Nonsimultaneous Administration

Inactivated vaccines generally do not interfere with the immune response to other inactivated vaccines or to live vaccines except in certain instances (eg, yellow

*The only vaccines currently licensed to be mixed in the same syringe by the person administering the vaccine are PRP-T *Haemophilus influenzae* type b conjugate vaccine, lyophilized, which can be reconstituted with DTP vaccine produced by Connaught.

fever and cholera vaccines). In general, an inactivated vaccine can be administered either simultaneously or at any time before or after a different inactivated vaccine or a live vaccine. However, limited data indicate that prior or concurrent administration of DTP vaccine may enhance anti-PRP antibody response following vaccination with certain *Haemophilus influenzae* type b conjugate vaccines (ie, PRP-T, PRP-D, and HbOC). For infants, the immunogenicity of PRP-OMP appears to be unaffected by the absence of prior or concurrent DTP vaccination.

Theoretically, the immune response to one live-virus vaccine might be impaired if administered within 30 days of another live-virus vaccine. Whenever possible, live-virus vaccines administered on different days should be administered at least 30 days apart. However, OPV and MMR vaccines can be administered at any time before, with, or after each other, if indicated. Live-virus vaccines can interfere with the response to a tuberculin test. Tuberculin testing, if otherwise indicated, can be done either on the same day the live-virus vaccines are administered or 4–6 weeks later.

Immune Globulin

Live Vaccines. OPV and yellow fever vaccines can be administered at any time before, with, or after the administration of immune globulin or specific immune globulins (eg, hepatitis B immune globulin [HBIG], rabies immune globulin [RIG]). The concurrent administration of immune globulin should not interfere with the response to Ty21a typhoid vaccine. Recent evidence suggests that high doses of immune globulin can inhibit the immune response to measles vaccine for more than 3 months. Administration of immune globulin can also inhibit the response to rubella vaccine. The effect of immune globulin preparations on the response to mumps and varicella vaccines is unknown, but commercial immune globulin preparations contain antibodies to these viruses.

Blood (eg, whole blood, packed RBCs, and plasma) and other antibody-containing blood products (eg, immune globulin; specific immune globulins; and immune globulin, intravenous [IGIV]) can diminish the immune response to MMR or its individual component vaccines. Therefore, after an immune globulin preparation is received, these vaccines should not be administered before the recommended interval. However, postpartum vaccination of rubella-susceptible women with rubella or MMR vaccine should not be delayed because anti-Rho(D) IG (human) or any other blood product was received during the last trimester of pregnancy or at delivery. These women should be vaccinated immediately after delivery and, if possible, tested at least 3 months later to ensure immunity to rubella and, if necessary, to measles.

If administration of an immune globulin preparation becomes necessary because of imminent exposure to disease, MMR or its component vaccines can be administered simultaneously with the immunoglobulin preparation, although vaccine-induced immunity might be compromised. The vaccine should be administered at a site remote from that chosen for the immune globulin inoculation. Unless serologic testing indicates that specific antibodies have been produced, vaccination should be repeated after the recommended interval.

If administration of an immune globulin preparation becomes necessary after MMR or its individual component vaccines have been administered, interference can occur. Usually vaccine virus replication and stimulation of immunity occurs 1–2 weeks after vaccination. Thus, if the interval between administration of any of these vaccines and subsequent administration of an immune globulin preparation is less than 14 days, vaccination should be repeated after the recommended interval unless serologic testing indicates that antibodies were produced.

Killed Vaccines. Immune globulin preparations interact less with inactivated vaccines and toxoids than with live vaccines. Therefore, administration of inactivated vaccines simultaneously with or at any interval before or after receipt of immune globulins should not substantially impair the development of a protective antibody response. The vaccine or toxoid and immune globulin preparation should be administered at different sites using the standard recommended dose of the corresponding vaccine. Increasing the vaccine dose volume or number of immunizations is not indicated.

Interchangeability of Vaccines from Different Manufacturers. When at least one dose of a hepatitis B vaccine produced by one manufacturer is followed by subsequent doses from a different manufacturer, the immune response has been shown to be comparable with that resulting from a full course of vaccination with a single vaccine.

Both HDCV and rabies vaccine, adsorbed (RVA) are considered equally efficacious and safe. When used as licensed and recommended, they are considered interchangeable during the vaccine series. *RVA should not be used intradermally.* The full 1-mL dose of either product, administered by IM injection, can be used for both preexposure and postexposure prophylaxis.

When administered according to their licensed indications, different diphtheria and tetanus toxoids and pertussis vaccines as single antigens or various combinations, as well as the live and inactivated polio vaccines, also can be used interchangeably.

Currently licensed *Haemophilus influenzae* type b conjugate vaccines have been shown to induce different temporal patterns of immunologic response in infants. Limited data suggest that infants who receive sequential doses of different vaccines produce a satisfactory antibody response after a complete series. The primary vaccine series should be completed with the same Hib vaccine, if feasible. However, if different vaccines are administered, a total of three doses of Hib vaccine is considered adequate for the primary series among infants, and any combination of Hib conjugate vaccines licensed for use among infants (ie, PRP-OMP, PRP-T, HbOC, and combination DTP-Hib vaccines) may be used to complete the primary series. Any of the licensed conjugate vaccines can be used for the recommended booster dose at 12–18 months of age.

■ HYPERSENSITIVITY TO VACCINE COMPONENTS

Vaccine components can cause allergic reactions in some recipients. These reactions can be local or systemic, and can include mild to severe anaphylaxis or anaphylacticlike responses (eg, generalized urticaria or hives, wheezing, swelling of the mouth and throat, difficulty breathing, hypotension, and shock). The responsible vaccine components can derive from (a) vaccine antigen, (b) animal protein, (c) antibiotics, (d) preservatives, and (e) stabilizers.

The most common animal protein allergen is egg protein found in vaccines prepared using embryonated chicken eggs (eg, influenza and yellow fever vaccines) or chicken embryo cell cultures (eg, measles and mumps vaccines). Ordinarily, persons who are able to eat eggs or egg products safely can receive these vaccines; persons with histories of anaphylactic or anaphylacticlike allergy to eggs or egg proteins should not. Asking persons whether they can eat eggs without adverse effects is a reasonable way to determine who might be at risk for allergic reactions from receiving measles, mumps, yellow fever, and influenza vaccines. Protocols requiring caution have been developed for testing and vaccinating with measles, mumps, and MMR vaccines those persons with anaphylactic reactions to egg ingestion. A regimen for administering influenza vaccine to children with egg hypersensitivity and severe asthma has also been developed. Rubella vaccine is grown in human diploid cell cultures and can be safely administered to persons with histories of severe allergy to eggs or egg proteins.

Some vaccines contain trace amounts of antibiotics (eg, neomycin) to which patients may be hypersensitive. The information provided in the vaccine package insert should be carefully reviewed before deciding if the uncommon patient with such hypersensitivity should receive the vaccine(s). No currently recommended vaccine contains penicillin or penicillin derivatives.

MMR and its individual component vaccines contain trace amounts of neomycin. Although the amount present is less than would usually be used for the skin test to determine hypersensitivity, persons who have experienced anaphylactic reactions to neomycin should not be administered these vaccines. Most often, neomycin allergy is a contact dermatitis—a manifestation of a delayed-type (cell-mediated) immune response—rather than anaphylaxis. A history of delayed-type reactions to neomycin is not a contraindication for these vaccines.

Certain parenteral bacterial vaccines, such as cholera, DTP, plague, and typhoid, are frequently associated with local or systemic adverse effects, such as redness, soreness, and fever. These reactions are difficult to link with a specific sensitivity to vaccine components and appear to be toxic rather than hypersensitive. Urticarial or anaphylactic reactions in DTP, DT, or Td or tetanus toxoid recipients have been reported rarely. When these reactions are reported, appropriate skin tests should be performed to determine sensitivity to tetanus toxoid before its use is discontinued. Alternatively, serologic testing to determine immunity to tetanus can be performed to evaluate the need for a booster dose of tetanus toxoid.

Exposure to vaccines containing the preservative thimerosal (eg, DTP, DTaP, DT, Td, Hib, hepatitis B, influenza, and Japanese encephalitis) can lead to induction of hypersensitivity. However, most patients do not develop reactions to thimerosal given as a component of vaccines even when patch or intradermal tests for thimerosal indicate hypersensitivity. Hypersensitivity to thimerosal usually consists of local delayed-type hypersensitivity reactions.

■ VACCINATION IN SPECIAL POPULATIONS

Preterm Infants

Infants born prematurely, regardless of birth weight, should be vaccinated at the same chronologic age and according to the same schedule and precautions as full-term infants and children. Birth weight and size generally are not factors in deciding whether to postpone routine vaccination of a clinically stable premature infant. The full recommended dose of each vaccine should be used. Divided or reduced doses are not recommended. To prevent the theoretical risk of poliovirus transmission in the hospital, the administration of OPV should be deferred until discharge.

Any premature infant born to a hepatitis B surface antigen (HBsAg)-positive mother should receive immunoprophylaxis with hepatitis B vaccine and HBIG beginning at or shortly after birth. For premature infants of HBsAg-negative mothers, the optimal timing of hepatitis B vaccination has not been determined. Some studies suggest that deceased conversion rates might occur in some premature infants with low birthweights (ie, <2000 g) following administration of hepatitis B vaccine at birth. Such low-birthweight premature infants of HBsAg-negative mothers should receive the hepatitis B vaccine series, which can be initiated at discharge from the nursery if the infant weighs at least 2000 g or at 2 months of age along with DTP, OPV, and Hib vaccine.

Breastfeeding and Vaccination

Neither killed nor live vaccines affect the safety of breastfeeding for mothers of infants. Breastfeeding does not adversely affect immunization and is not a contraindication for any vaccine. Breast-fed infants should be vaccinated according to routine recommended schedules.

Inactivated or killed vaccines do not multiply within the body. Therefore they should pose no special risk for mothers who are breastfeeding or for their infants. Although live vaccines do multiply within the mother's body, most have not been demonstrated to be excreted in breastmilk. Although rubella vaccine virus may be transmitted in breastmilk, the virus usually does not infect the infant, and if it does, the infection is well tolerated. There is no contraindication for vaccinating breastfeeding mothers with yellow fever vaccine. Breastfeeding mothers can receive OPV without any interruption in feeding schedule.

Vaccination During Pregnancy

Risk from vaccination during pregnancy is largely theoretical. The benefit of vaccination among pregnant women usually outweighs the potential risk when (a) the risk for disease is high, (b) infection would pose a special risk to the mother or fetus, and (c) the vaccine is unlikely to cause harm.

Combined tetanus and diphtheria toxoids are the only immunobiologic agents routinely indicated for susceptible pregnant women. Previously vaccinated pregnant women who have not received a Td vaccination within the last 10 years should receive a booster dose. Pregnant women who are unimmunized or only partially immunized against tetanus should complete the primary series. Depending on when a woman seeks prenatal care and the required interval between doses, one or two doses of Td can be administered before delivery. Women for whom the vaccine is indicated but who have not completed the required three-dose series during pregnancy should be followed up after delivery to assure they receive the doses necessary for protection.

There is no convincing evidence of risk from immunizing the pregnant woman with other inactivated virus or bacteria vaccines or toxoids. Hepatitis B vaccine is recommended for women at risk for hepatitis B infection, and influenza and pneumococcal vaccines are recommended for women at risk for infection and for complications of influenza and pneumococcal disease.

OPV can be administered to pregnant women who are at substantial risk of exposure to natural infection. Although OPV is preferred, IPV may be considered if the complete vaccination series can be administered before the anticipated exposure. Pregnant women who must travel to areas where the risk of yellow fever is high should receive yellow fever vaccine. In these circumstances, the small theoretical risk from vaccination is far outweighed by the risk of yellow fever infection. Known pregnancy is a contraindication for rubella, measles, and mumps vaccines. Although a theoretical concern, no cases of congenital rubella syndrome or abnormalities attributable to rubella vaccine virus infection have been observed in infants born to susceptible mothers who received rubella vaccine during pregnancy.

Persons who receive measles, mumps, or rubella vaccines can shed these viruses, but generally do not transmit them. These vaccines can be administered safely to the children of pregnant women. Although live polio virus is shed by persons recently immunized with OPV (particularly after the first dose), this vaccine can also be administered to the children of pregnant women because experience has not revealed any risk of polio vaccine virus to the fetus.

All pregnant women should be evaluated for immunity to rubella and tested for the presence of HBsAg. Women susceptible to rubella should be immunized immediately after delivery. A woman infected with hepatitis B virus should be followed carefully to assure that the infant receives HBIG and begins the hepatitis B vaccine series shortly after delivery.

There is no known risk to the fetus from passive immunization of pregnant women with immune globulin. Further information regarding immunization of pregnant women is available in the American College of Obstetricians and Gynecologists Technical Bulletin Number 160, October 1991.[2]

Altered Immunocompetence

This section is a summary of the more extensive recommendations on vaccines and immune globulin preparations for immunocompromised persons found in reference 3.

Severe immunosuppression can be the result of congenital immunodeficiency, HIV infection, leukemia, lymphoma, generalized malignancy, or therapy with alkylating agents, antimetabolites, radiation, or large amounts of corticosteroids. Severe complications have followed vaccination with live, attenuated-virus vaccines and with live-bacteria vaccines among immunocompromised patients. In general, these patients should not be administered live vaccines except in certain circumstances that are noted below. In addition, OPV should not be administered to any household contact of a severely immunocompromised person. If polio immunization is indicated for immunosuppressed patients, their household members, or other close contacts, IPV should be administered. MMR is not contraindicated in close contacts of immunocompromised patients. The degree to which a person is immunocompromised should be determined by a physician.

Limited studies of MMR vaccination in HIV-infected patients have not documented serious or unusual adverse events. Because measles may cause severe illness in persons with HIV infection, MMR vaccine is recommended for all asymptomatic HIV-infected persons and should be considered for all symptomatic HIV-infected persons. HIV-infected persons on regular IGIV therapy may not respond to MMR or its individual component vaccines because of the continued presence of passively acquired antibody. However, because of the potential benefit, measles vaccination should be considered approximately 2 weeks before the next monthly dose of IGIV (if not otherwise contraindicated), although an optimal immune response is unlikely to occur. Unless serologic testing indicates that specific antibodies have been produced, vaccination should be repeated (if not otherwise contraindicated) after the recommended interval.

An additional dose of IGIV should be considered for persons on routine IGIV therapy who are exposed to measles 3 or more weeks after administration of a standard dose (100–400 mg/kg) of IGIV.

Killed or inactivated vaccines can be administered to all immunocompromised patients, although response to such vaccines may be suboptimal. All such childhood vaccines are recommended for immunocompromised persons in usual doses and schedules; in addition, certain vaccines such as pneumococcal vaccine or Hib vaccine are recommended specifically for certain groups of immunocompromised patients, including those with functional or anatomic asplenia.

Vaccination during chemotherapy or radiation therapy should be avoided because antibody response is poor. Patients vaccinated while on immunosuppressive therapy or in the 2 weeks before starting therapy should be considered unimmunized and should be revaccinated at least 3 months after therapy is discontinued. Patients with leukemia in remission whose chemotherapy has been terminated for 3 months may receive live-virus vaccines.

The exact amount of systemically absorbed corticosteroids and the duration of administration needed to suppress the immune system of an otherwise healthy child are not well defined. Most experts agree that corticosteroid therapy usually does not contraindicate administration of live virus vaccine when it is short-term (ie, <2 weeks); low to moderate dose; long-term, alternate day treatment with short-acting preparations; maintenance physiologic doses (replacement therapy); or administered topically (skin or eyes), by aerosol, or by intra-articular, bursal, or tendon injection. Although of recent theoretical concern, no evidence of increased severe reactions to live vaccines has been reported among persons receiving corticosteroid therapy by aerosol, and such therapy is not in itself a reason to delay vaccination. The immunosuppressive effects of corticosteroid treatment vary, but many clinicians consider a dose equivalent to either 2 mg/kg of body weight or a total of 20 mg/day of prednisone as sufficiently immunosuppressive to raise concern about the safety of vaccination with live virus vaccines. Corticosteroids used in greater than physiologic doses can also reduce the immune response to vaccines. Physicians should wait at least 3 months after discontinuation of therapy before administering a live-virus vaccine to patients who have received high systemically absorbed doses of corticosteroids for 2 or more weeks.

Vaccination of Persons with Hemophilia

Persons with bleeding disorders such as hemophilia have an increased risk of acquiring hepatitis B and at least the same risk as the general population of acquiring vaccine-preventable diseases. However, because of the risk of hematomas, intramuscular injections are often avoided among persons with bleeding disorders by using the subcutaneous or intradermal routes for vaccines that are normally administered by the intramuscular route. Hepatitis B vaccine administered intramuscularly to hemophiliacs using a 23-gauge needle, followed by steady pressure at the site for 1–2 min, has resulted in a 4% bruising rate with no patients requiring factor supplementation. Whether an antigen that produces more local reactions, such as pertussis, would produce an equally low rate of bruising is unknown.

When hepatitis B or any other intramuscular vaccine is indicated for a patient with a bleeding disorder, it should be administered intramuscularly if, in the opinion of a physician familiar with the patient's bleeding risk, the vaccine can be administered with reasonable safety by this route. If the patient received antihemophilic or other similar therapy, intramuscular vaccination can be scheduled for shortly after such therapy is administered. A fine needle (≤23 gauge) can be used for the vaccination and firm pressure applied to the site (without rubbing) for at least 2 min. The patient or family should be instructed concerning the risk of hematoma from the injections.

■ REFERENCES

1. General recommendations on immunization. Recommendations of the Advisory Committee on Immunization Practices (ACIP). *MMWR.* 1994;43(RR-1):1–38.
2. Immunization during pregnancy. ACOG technical bulletin number 160—October 1991. *Int J Gynaecol Obstet* 1993;40:69–79. Also available from the American College of Obstetricians and Gynecologists, Attention: Resource Center, 409 12th Street SW, Washington, DC 20024–2188.
3. Recommendations of the Advisory Committee on Immunization Practices (ACIP): use of vaccines and immune globulins for persons with altered immunocompetence. *MMWR.* 1993;42(RR-4):1–18.
4. Recommended childhood immunization schedule—United States, January–June 1996. *MMWR.* 1996;44:940–3.
5. Marwick C. Switch to inactivated polio vaccine recommended. *JAMA* 1996;276:89. News.

Medical Emergencies: Anaphylaxis, Cardiac Arrest, Poisoning, Status Epilepticus

5

Outline of Drug Therapy

The clinical management of medical emergencies is an area in which there continues to be some variability in treatment philosophy. Thus, the therapeutic approaches, drugs, and adult dosages given here are based on somewhat divergent and conflicting sources of information. In addition, some recommendations have been made based upon the authors' experience and suggestions from specialists and researchers in the field. As a result, the therapeutic concepts and dosages contained herein, although conforming to medical standards, may differ from those advocated by specific practitioners and institutions.

Anaphylaxis

Lawrence R. Borgsdorf

An anaphylactic reaction is an *urgent* medical problem that can be fatal. Although the onset of symptoms can vary from minutes to hours, most reactions occur within 5–30 minutes following ingestion or parenteral administration of an antigen. Symptoms may progress from extreme apprehension and cutaneous reactions to more severe systemic manifestations, such as severe respiratory distress and/or profound shock. Reactions include conjunctivitis, GI edema (nausea, vomiting, diarrhea), cutaneous reactions (urticaria, pruritus, angioedema), rhinitis, laryngeal edema, and bronchospasm (coughing, wheezing, dyspnea, cyanosis), vascular collapse, cardiac arrhythmias, and cardiac arrest (*see* the following section on Cardiac Arrest.)

Definitive Therapy

(*See also* Adjunctive Therapy.)
Adult dosages only are given in this section.

1a. Treatment of anaphylaxis is always initiated with *immediate* **epinephrine HCl (aqueous), SC or IM, 0.3–0.5 mg** (0.3–0.5 mL of 1:1000); may repeat q 10–15 minutes,

or, for nonresponding or severe reactions,

epinephrine HCl, IV slow push, 0.2–0.5 mg (0.2–0.5 mL of 1:1000 diluted to 10 mL with NS, or 2–5 mL of 1:10,000); may repeat q 5–20 minutes.

1b. Patient should be in a recumbent position with legs elevated, patent airway established, and oxygen given; if applicable, a tourniquet should be placed proximal to the antigen injection site (remove temporarily q 10–15 minutes), and give

epinephrine HCl, infiltrate 0.1–0.3 mg (0.1–0.3 mL of 1:1000) at antigen injection site.

2. *Bronchospasm* alone (no cutaneous or cardiovascular manifestations) may respond to **albuterol,** via nebulization (0.5 mL of 0.5% solution in 2.5 mL of NS); may repeat q 20 minutes.

3a. *Hypotension* not responding to epinephrine may be treated by the use of fluids (see 3b) and vasopressor agents; for example, **dopamine HCl, IV slow infusion,** adjust rate to response (400 mg in 500 mL NS or D5W = 800 mg/L),

or, if dopamine fails to maintain blood pressure,

norepinephrine bitartrate, IV infusion, adjust rate to maintain a systolic blood pressure of about 90–100 mm Hg (2 mL of 0.2% solution in 500 mL D5W = 4 mg base/L).

3b. *Hypovolemia* may be the underlying cause of hypotension and this requires rapid expansion of the intravascular fluid volume with **NS** or **lactated Ringer's injection,**

or, for failure to respond to above or in severe hypotension,

hetastarch or **albumin human.** Monitor cardiac filling pressures to avoid hemodynamic pulmonary edema (ie, keep pulmonary capillary wedge pressure between 15–20 mm Hg).

Adjunctive Therapy

Adult dosages only are given in this section.
There is no clear evidence that the following measures are effective in the treatment of acute, life-threatening anaphylaxis; therefore, use only after life-threatening symptoms have been controlled.

1. To prevent prolonged antigen-antibody reactions, give **hydrocortisone phosphate or succinate, IV, 100 mg;** may repeat q 6 hours.

2. To prevent further cutaneous reactions, give **diphenhydramine HCl, PO, IM, or slow IV, 25–50 mg;** may repeat q 6 hours.

3. To manage urticarial manifestations, give **cimetidine, PO, IM, or slow IV, 300 mg;** may repeat q 6 hours (unlabeled indication).

4. To manage prolonged bronchospastic manifestations, give **aminophylline, IV slow infusion, 5 mg/kg** (0.2 mL/kg of 25 mg/mL solution in 250 mL fluid) over 20 minutes, followed by continuous infusion for maintenance (*see* Theophylline monograph.)

■ REFERENCES

1. Carlson RW et al. Anaphylactic, anaphylactoid, and related forms of shock. *Crit Care Clin* 1986;2:347–72.

2. Kelly JS, Prielipp RC. Is cimetidine indicated in the treatment of acute anaphylactic shock? *Anesth Analg* 1990;71:104–5. Letter.

3. Bochner BS, Lichtenstein LM. Anaphylaxis. *N Engl J Med* 1991;324:1785–90.

4. Yunginger JW. Anaphylaxis. *Ann Allergy* 1992;69:87–96.

Cardiac Arrest

Lawrence R. Borgsdorf

A cardiac arrest is a medical emergency requiring a systematic approach. Early recognition (unconsciousness, apnea, no pulse) must be followed by prompt, effective application of Basic Cardiac Life Support (BCLS) techniques to sustain the patient until Advanced Cardiac Life Support (ACLS) capabilities are available. With ACLS capabilities, a definitive treatment plan can then be attempted.

Thus, management of cardiac arrest is a four-step approach:

- **Diagnosis**
- **Emergency Treatment (BCLS)**
- **Definitive Therapy (ACLS)**
- **Postresuscitation Care**

■ DIAGNOSIS

Verify that respiration and perfusion have ceased:

1. Loss of consciousness.
2. Loss of functional ventilation (apnea).
3. Loss of functional perfusion (no pulse).

■ EMERGENCY TREATMENT (BCLS)

The findings listed above are sufficient to justify the immediate application of BCLS techniques listed below. The goal of BCLS is to rapidly and effectively reperfuse the CNS with oxygenated blood. It is well recognized that delays in initiating BCLS or in providing ineffective BCLS can result in irreversible hypoxic brain damage in an otherwise "successful" resuscitation.

1. Summon help and resuscitation equipment.
2. If this is a witnessed arrest and a defibrillator is readily available:
    a. Defibrillate with 200 joules of direct current shock if ventricular tachycardia or ventricular fibrillation are documented.
    b. If the first shock fails to terminate the dysrhythmia, a second shock with 200–300 joules should be attempted. If the first two shocks fail, a third shock of 360 joules should be attempted.
3. If this is a witnessed arrest and a defibrillator is *not* readily available:
    Deliver a sharp precordial blow.
4. If no response to above, or if an unwitnessed arrest, start artificial ventilation:
    a. Establish an adequate airway.
    b. Ventilate by mouth-to-mask or bag-valve-mask technique.
    c. The first two ventilations should be slow and deep, then ventilate at approximately 12 per minute.

5. Begin artificial perfusion via external chest compressions:
   a. Position patient supine on firm surface.
   b. Ensure proper placement of hands on sternum.
   c. Depress sternum at rate of 80–100 cycles per minute (50% of cycle should be compression).

■ DEFINITIVE THERAPY (ACLS)

Adult dosages only are given in this section.

Initiate attempts by trained personnel to maintain a patent airway, establish an intravenous route for administration of fluids and drugs, establish an electrocardiographic diagnosis, and apply specific treatments to correct a recognized electrical and/or mechanical abnormality.

Definitive therapy can be divided into **General Therapy**—modalities to be considered in all cases of cardiac arrest before a specific electrical abnormality has been identified, and **Specific Therapy**—modalities designed for specific electrocardiographic or mechanical abnormalities.

General Therapy

Management of Acidosis. Severe acidosis can develop within 5 minutes after cardiac arrest and will continue unless BCLS is provided. Acidosis is due primarily to a respiratory component (hypoventilation) and to a lesser extent to a metabolic component (lactic acidosis), which occurs later.

1. *Respiratory acidosis:*
   a. Etiology: Accumulation of CO_2 secondary to hypoventilation.
   b. Treatment: Adequate ventilation; *no* role for sodium bicarbonate.
2. *Metabolic acidosis:*
   a. Etiology: Slow accumulation of lactic acid secondary to anaerobic metabolism within hypoperfused (hypoxic) tissues.
   b. Treatment: Adequate perfusion of oxygenated blood will delay development of clinically important lactic acidosis. Thus, early administration of sodium bicarbonate (buffer) is not indicated unless preexisting acidosis, hyperkalemia, or tricyclic antidepressant (TCA) overdose is documented. There are no proven benefits of bicarbonate, and it can produce devastating complications, including shift of the oxyhemoglobin saturation curve to the left (decreasing release of oxygen); hyperosmolarity; hypernatremia; paradoxical intracellular acidosis (because of production of carbon dioxide, which diffuses readily into cells); exacerbation of central venous acidosis; and possible inactivation of simultaneously administered catecholamines.

Therefore
   • Do *not* administer sodium bicarbonate until after specific therapy (eg., intubation; antidysrhythmics) has been employed and only at the discretion of the team leader after considering the possible complications noted above.

If the decision to use bicarbonate is made, then the following guidelines should be followed:

- *If arterial blood gases (ABGs) not available,* then empiric administration of **sodium bicarbonate, IV slow push, 1 mEq/kg initially,** then not more than **0.5 mEq/kg** q 10 minutes (50 mL of 7.5% solution = 44.6 mEq [0.9 mEq/mL]; 50 mL of 8.4% solution = 50 mEq [1 mEq/mL]).
- *If ABGs available,* then sodium bicarbonate doses can be calculated from the base deficit:

$$NaHCO_3 \text{ dose in mEq} =$$
$$\text{Base deficit in mEq/L} \times 0.2 \times \text{Body weight in kg}$$

Epinephrine—Empiric Use

Epinephrine is often given empirically at the start of definitive therapy, even before an ECG diagnosis has been made. The basis for this empiric use is epinephrine's α-adrenergic receptor agonist activity, which increases systemic vascular resistance, enhancing perfusion of the myocardium and CNS during CPR. Thus, the following is appropriate:

- **epinephrine HCl, IV push, 1 mg** (10 mL of 1:10,000 solution, or 1 mL of 1:1000 diluted to 10 mL with NS); may repeat q 3–5 minutes. (*See* Special Considerations/Precautions: high-dose epinephrine.)

If IV access has not been established or has been lost, *then:*

- **epinephrine HCl, via endotracheal tube, 2–2.5 mg** (20–25 mL of 1:10,000 solution), followed by 3 or 4 rapid ventilations to disperse drug. If neither IV nor endotracheal access is available, consider intraosseous administration (*see* Special Considerations/Precautions).

Specific Therapy

In order to simplify the pharmacologic management of cardiopulmonary arrest, disturbances of cardiac activity associated with cardiac arrest may be grouped into three major categories, each of which can be approached in a logical manner: ventricular tachydysrhythmias, bradydysrhythmias (including asystole), and pulseless electrical activity.

Ventricular Tachydysrhythmias. Considered in this category, and treated in the same way, are ventricular fibrillation, ventricular flutter, and ventricular tachycardia when associated with ineffective cardiac output.

1. *Electrical defibrillation, 200 joules delivered.* If tachydysrhythmias persist, then subsequent defibrillation should deliver more energy (eg, 200–300 joules for second shock; 360 joules for third shock).
2. Epinephrine HCl, IV push, 1 mg (10 mL of 1:10,000 solution) is commonly stated to be an effective adjunct for successful defibrillation, especially when ventricular fibrillation is monitored as "fine" fibrillatory waves. There are no scientific data to support this concept; *thus, epinephrine is not recommended as an aid to defibrillation specifically, but rather as an aid to myocardial perfusion* (*see* Epinephrine—Empiric Use).

3. In intractable ventricular tachydysrhythmias or when there is repeated re-version to tachydysrhythmias following electrical defibrillation, an irritable focus in the myocardium may be the source of persistent tachydysrhythmias and an antidysrhythmic drug is indicated (if digitalis toxicity is suspected, *see* item 7):

   - **lidocaine HCl, IV push, 50–100 mg (1–1.5 mg/kg)** (2.5–5 mL of 2% or 5–10 mL of 1% solution); may repeat q 3–5 min to a total of 3 mg/kg.

   If IV access has not been established or has been lost, *then:*

   - **lidocaine HCl via endotracheal tube, 150–300 mg (3 mg/kg)** (7.5–15 mL of 2% solution), followed by 3 or 4 rapid ventilations to disperse drug.

   If neither IV nor endotracheal access is available, consider intraosseous administration (*see* Special Considerations/Precautions).

   If response to loading dose occurs, *then maintenance:*

   - **lidocaine HCl, IV infusion, 2–4 mg/minute (20–50 µg/kg/minute)** (10 mL of 20% in 500 mL D5W = 4 mg/mL).

4. If lidocaine fails to maintain electrical stability, *then:*

   - **bretylium tosylate, IV push, 350–500 mg (5 mg/kg)** (50 mg/mL, 7–10 mL); may repeat with 10 mg/kg q 5 minutes to total of 30–35 mg/kg. Note that bretylium frequently has a slow onset of action (>10 min). While waiting for this effect, one could administer procainamide HCl (*see* item 5) in an attempt to gain control of the dysrhythmia rapidly. The important point to recognize is that once primary therapy fails, second-line agents are not predictably effective. Should procainamide fail to suppress tachydysrhythmias, the slower acting bretylium will already have been administered. Should procainamide be effective, then subsequent doses of bretylium will not be necessary.

   If response to loading dose occurs, *then maintenance:*

   - **bretylium tosylate, IV infusion, 1–2 mg/minute.**

5. If lidocaine- and bretylium-resistant dysrhythmias persist, or if one elects to administer procainamide concurrently with bretylium, *then:*

   - **procainamide HCl, IV push, 500 mg** (5 mL of 100 mg/mL vial, or 1 mL of 500 mg/mL vial); may repeat in 5 minutes to a total of 1 g. Note that this rate is greater than the commonly reported 20–50 mg/minute; however, this is a life-threatening dysrhythmia and a delay in drug administration may result in treatment failure.

   If response to loading dose occurs, *then maintenance:*

   - **procainamide HCl, IV infusion, 1–5 mg/minute** (20–80 µg/kg/minute).

6. If lidocaine-, bretylium- and procainamide-resistant dysrhythmias persist, *then:*

- **propranolol HCl, IV push, 1 mg over 1 minute** (1 mg/mL ampule); may repeat q 5 minutes to a total of 0.1 mg/kg.

7. If all of the above fail or if digitalis toxicity or hypomagnesemia is suspected, *consider:*

  - **magnesium sulfate, IV push, 1–2 g (8–16 mEq) over 1–2 minutes** (2–4 mL of 50% solution diluted in 10 mL D5W); may repeat after 5 minutes if no response.

Bradydysrhythmias. Considered in this category, and treated in the same way, are asystole, complete heart block, slow ventricular focus, sinus bradycardia, and agonal rhythm. In dealing with any of these dysrhythmias (except asystole), transvenous pacing is probably the best long-term approach, but is usually not readily available. Thus, drugs are used to enhance or initiate cardiac activity, at least until transvenous or transthoracic pacing equipment becomes available.

It is important to note that true asystole, unless it is the result of excessive vagal tone (bradysystole event), is frequently associated with irreversible cardiac damage.

1. Treatment of bradydysrhythmias should be initiated with:

  - **atropine sulfate, IV push, 0.5–1 mg** (5–10 mL of 0.1 mg/mL solution); may repeat with 0.5–1 mg q 3–5 minutes to a total of 3 mg.

    If IV access has not been established or has been lost, *then:*

  - **atropine sulfate, via endotracheal tube, 1–2.5 mg** (10–25 mL of 0.1 mg/mL solution), followed by 3 or 4 rapid ventilations to disperse drug.

    If neither IV nor endotracheal access is available, consider intraosseous administration (*see* Special Considerations/Precautions).

2. For bradydysrhythmias failing to respond to atropine, *then:*

  - **epinephrine HCl, IV push, 0.5–1 mg** (5–10 mL of 1:10,000); may repeat after 3–5 minutes (*see* Special Considerations/Precautions: high-dose epinephrine).

3. For bradydysrhythmias failing to respond to the above, some experts have recommended isoproterenol. The use of isoproterenol, although supported by AHA-ACLS guidelines, is probably inappropriate, because β-adrenergic agonist mediated vasodilation may actually lower perfusion pressures during CPR. Thus, the use of isoproterenol cannot be justified.

Pulseless Electrical Activity (PEA). PEA was previously known as electromechanical dissociation. Considered in this category are ineffective cardiac output (hypotension) in the face of ECG evidence of electrical myocardial activity, hypotension secondary to inadequate peripheral vasoconstriction, volume depletion cardiac tamponade, tension pneumothorax, or massive pulmonary embolism.

1. Rapidly assess volume status—if depleted, fluid challenge with crystalloid (**NS** or **lactated Ringer's injection**) or colloid (**hetastarch** or **albumin human**).

2. If volume is adequate and no evidence of tamponade, then consider cardiac sympathomimetics for vasoconstricting and inotropic/chronotropic effects. Begin with:

   - **dopamine HCl, IV infusion, 5 µg/kg/minute initially,** increasing prn to maximum of 20 µg/kg/minute, adjusting rate to keep systolic blood pressure between 90–100 mm Hg (400 mg in 500 mL D5W = 800 µg/mL).

3. If dopamine fails, *then:*

   - **norepinephrine bitartrate, IV infusion, 8 µg/minute initially,** adjusting, as needed, to keep systolic blood pressure between 90 and 100 mm Hg (8 mL of 0.1% solution [1 mg/mL] in 500 mL D5W = 16 µg/mL).

4. If norepinephrine fails, consider high-dose epinephrine (*see* Special Considerations/Precautions).

5. Calcium administration in the therapy of pulseless electrical activity has not been shown to be effective and, in fact, may be harmful. Therefore, its use should be confined to situations in which acceptable therapy has failed or in situations in which calcium therapy is antidotal (eg, hyperkalemia, hypocalcemia, calcium-channel blocker toxicity), in which case add:

   - **calcium chloride, IV slow push, 0.5–1 g** (5–10 mL of 10% solution = 6.8–13.6 mEq), *or*
   - **calcium gluconate, IV slow push, 1–2 g** (10–20 mL of 10% solution = 4.7–9.4 mEq), *or*
   - **calcium gluceptate, IV slow push, 1.1–2.2 g** (5–10 mL = 4.5–9 mEq).

■ POSTRESUSCITATION CARE

Patients who have been successfully resuscitated are at great risk of experiencing subsequent events. Thus, if the patient is not already in an intensive care setting with constant monitoring, readily available resuscitation equipment, and skilled nursing staff, transport the patient to such an area as soon as possible. The cause of the initial episode must be sought and corrected if possible.

■ SPECIAL CONSIDERATIONS/PRECAUTIONS

Because of concern regarding the possibility that dextrose-containing fluids administered during ACLS may worsen neurologic outcome, NS or lactated Ringer's injection should be considered the fluids of choice, with dextrose-containing solutions reserved for patients believed to be hypoglycemic.

Systemic circulation times are grossly prolonged during external chest compression. Remember to allow *at least* 2 minutes between the time of peripheral injection of pharmacologic agents and anticipated response. To enhance the onset and activity of peripherally administered medications, they should be administered by rapid bolus injection, followed by a 20-mL bolus of IV fluid and elevation of the extremity, if possible.

Initial studies of **high-dose epinephrine** (up to 0.2 mg/kg IV q 5 minutes) indicated that the higher doses may be more effective than standard ACLS doses.

However, more recent studies have found no advantage of high-dose over standard-dose epinephrine. In any event, ACLS guidelines allow options for **intermediate** (2–5 mg IV push q 3–5 minutes); **escalating** (1 mg, then 3 mg, then 5 mg separated by 3 minutes); or **high-dose** (0.1 mg/kg IV push q 3–5 minutes) epinephrine.

Endotracheal administration of epinephrine, lidocaine, or atropine can be used in situations in which IV access has not been established or has been lost. Doses 2–3 times the IV dose and diluted in 10 mL NS or distilled water are advised. Endotracheal administration may not be as effective as IV administration.

Intraosseous administration of epinephrine, atropine, sodium bicarbonate, lidocaine, vasopressors, or calcium via the distal tibia can be used in situations in which IV access and endotracheal intubation have not been established.

Intracardiac injections of drugs play *no* role in modern management of cardiopulmonary arrest. Drugs do not work within the chambers of the heart, but rather at the cellular level after delivery via the coronary circulation. Stopping BCLS to attempt intracardiac injections only serves to interrupt vital CNS perfusion.

Be aware of the possible **physical incompatibilities** of sodium bicarbonate and catecholamines. In addition, sodium bicarbonate and calcium-containing solutions may form a precipitate if infused at the same time in the same IV line.

REFERENCES

1. Otto CW et al, eds. Wolf Creek III conference on cardiopulmonary resuscitation. *Crit Care Med* 1985;13:881–951.
2. Raehl CL. Endotracheal drug therapy in cardiopulmonary resuscitation. *Clin Pharm* 1986;5:572–9.
3. Iserson KV. Intraosseous infusions in adults. *J Emerg Med* 1989;7:587–91.
4. Callaham ML. High-dose epinephrine therapy and other advances in treating cardiac arrest. *West J Med* 1990;152:697–703.
5. Anon. Adult advanced cardiac life support. *JAMA* 1992;268:2199–41.
6. Niemann JT. Cardiopulmonary resuscitation. *N Engl J Med* 1992;327:1075–80.
7. Grillo JA, Gonzalez ER. Changes in the pharmacotherapy of CPR. *Heart Lung* 1993;22:548–53.

Poisoning

William G. Troutman

Management of the poisoned patient involves procedures designed to prevent the absorption, minimize the toxicity, and hasten the elimination of the suspected contaminant. The prompt employment of appropriate emergency management procedures can often prevent unnecessary morbidity and mortality.

A regional poison center is a practitioner's best source of definitive treatment information and should be consulted in all poisonings, regardless of the apparent simplicity of the case. Contact the regional poison center in your area to learn of its staffing, resources, and capabilities before a need for its services arises. Well-qualified regional centers are certified by the American Association of Poison Control Centers.

In all cases, every attempt should be made to accurately identify the contaminant, estimate the quantity involved, and determine the time that has passed since the exposure. These data, plus patient-specific parameters such as age, weight, sex, and underlying medical conditions or drug use, will assist you and the regional poison center in designing an appropriate therapeutic plan for the patient.

The techniques described below are intended for the initial management of the poisoned patient using materials that should be readily available.

■ TOPICAL EXPOSURES

1. *Immediately* irrigate affected areas with a copious amount of water; use soap only if a stubborn, oily substance is the contaminant. Skin should be gently washed, not scrubbed, and special attention should be given to the hair, skin folds, umbilicus, and other areas where the contaminant might be trapped.
2. If the patient's clothes have been contaminated, remove them during the irrigation and either clean them before they are worn again or destroy them. Clothing can interfere with the irrigation process and can serve as a reservoir of toxic material.
3. Do not attempt to "neutralize" the contaminant with another chemical (eg, acids and alkalis). Attempts at neutralization waste valuable time, are of no benefit, and may be harmful.
4. Do not cover the affected area with emollients. These may trap unremoved contaminant against the skin. Severely damaged skin may be temporarily covered with a light, dry dressing.
5. Protect yourself from contamination. Gloves, aprons, or a change of clothes may be necessary.
6. After the irrigation is complete, contact a regional poison center for definitive treatment information.

■ EYE EXPOSURES

1. *Immediately* irrigate the eye; damage can occur within seconds. The stream of water from the tap or a pitcher should strike the patient on the forehead, temple, or bridge of the nose and then flow into the eye.
2. The eyelids should be open with frequent blinking during the irrigation.
3. The irrigation should continue for at least 15 minutes (by the clock) to ensure adequate removal of the contaminant and normalization of the conjunctival pH. Body temperature water or saline may be substituted for tap water as the irrigation proceeds, but only if they can be obtained without interrupting the irrigation.
4. After the irrigation is complete, contact a regional poison center for definitive treatment information.

■ INHALATION EXPOSURES

1. Remove the patient from the suspected contaminated area, regardless of its apparent safety. Carbon monoxide, a common inhaled toxin, cannot be detected by sight, smell, or taste.
2. Institute artificial ventilation, if necessary, and provide supplementary humidified oxygen if available and needed.
3. Protect yourself from contamination at all times.
4. Contact a regional poison center for definitive treatment information.

■ INGESTIONS

1. Remove any remaining contaminant from inside and around the mouth of the patient.
2. Give a small amount of water to clear the mouth and esophagus.
3. Contact a regional poison center for definitive treatment information.
4. In many cases, it will not be necessary to take further steps. The following information can be utilized if additional care is recommended by the regional poison center.

■ GASTROINTESTINAL DECONTAMINATION

Gastrointestinal (GI) decontamination may be accomplished by the administration of activated charcoal, gastric lavage, ipecac-induced emesis, and whole-bowel irrigation. Indications for GI decontamination are ingestion of a known toxic dose, ingestion of an unknown dose of a known toxic substance, and ingestion of a substance of unknown toxicity. For all methods of GI decontamination, the value of the procedure diminishes rapidly with time. Some authors now question the usefulness of gastric lavage or ipecac-induced emesis more than 1 hour after ingestion. None of these techniques should be presumed to provide complete removal or binding of the ingested toxin(s). Comparative experimental studies have shown only limited success with these techniques and there is considerable interpatient variability in the results. In general, activated charcoal is the most useful agent for preventing absorption of ingested toxic substances. Other methods of GI decontamination may be considered if the ingested contaminant is not adsorbed by activated charcoal or if circumstances do not permit its prompt administration.

Activated Charcoal. Activated charcoal is a nonspecific adsorbent that binds unabsorbed toxins within the GI tract. Attempts to administer it outside a health care facility have met with minimal success.

1. Activated charcoal is administered orally or by gastric tube in doses that range from 30–120 g.
2. Activated charcoal is commercially supplied as a slurry in water or a concentrated solution of sorbitol. The water-based products are preferred because the large amount of sorbitol that accompanies a typical dose of activated charcoal may result in excessive sorbitol-induced catharsis, producing fluid and electrolyte imbalance. Gentle encouragement may be needed to make children swallow the charcoal. Having the child take the liquid through a drinking straw from an opaque container is sometimes helpful.
3. Activated charcoal administration is commonly followed by the administration of a cathartic (eg, sorbitol, magnesium citrate, or magnesium sulfate) to hasten the elimination of the activated charcoal-toxin complex. There is no evidence to support cathartic use.
4. Alert the patient that charcoal will cause the stools to turn black.
5. Repeated oral doses of activated charcoal (eg, 20–30 g q 4 hours) have been used to enhance the elimination of some drugs, most notably carbamazepine, phenobarbital, salicylate, and theophylline. Multiple-dose activated charcoal is only suitable for patients with active bowel sounds.

Gastric Lavage. Lavage may be more effective in recovering toxin than ipecac-induced emesis, and it has the advantage of being useful in patients with CNS depression.

1. If the patient's gag reflex is weak or absent, the airway must be protected by the use of a cuffed endotracheal tube.
2. The largest possible orogastric tube should be used (26–28 F for children and 34–42 F for adults): the larger the tube diameter, the more efficient the lavage. The tube may be introduced through either the mouth or nose with the aid of a water-soluble lubricant.
3. Gastric lavage may be done with water, but a solution like 0.45% NaCl may be used to minimize the risk of dilutional hyponatremia, especially in children. Aliquots of fluid up to 100 mL in children and 200 mL in adults are introduced through the tube and then removed by gravity or suction-assisted drainage. The lavage should be continued for several cycles after the returning fluid is clear. Warming the lavage fluid will reduce the risk of hypothermia.

Induction of Emesis. *Do not induce emesis if the patient is experiencing or is at risk for CNS depression, seizures, or loss of gag reflex, or if the patient has ingested a caustic substance.*

1. Induce emesis only with syrup of ipecac. Salt water, mustard water, other "home remedies," or gagging have no place in the management of the poisoned patient. These techniques are ineffective and can be dangerous.

Ipecac-induced emesis is the only form of GI decontamination suitable for home use.

2. The usual initial dose of **syrup of ipecac is 30 mL in persons over 5 years of age, 15 mL in children 1–5 years old, and 10 mL in children between 6 months and 1 year of age.**

3. Give the patient additional water to drink: 125–250 mL (4–8 fl oz) in children, 250–500 mL (8–16 fl oz) in adults. Activated charcoal should not be given until after ipecac-induced emesis has occurred.

4. Emesis usually occurs within 15–20 minutes. If 30 minutes have passed without emesis, administer an additional dose of syrup of ipecac and more water.

5. Have the patient vomit into a bowl or other container so that the vomitus can be inspected for the presence of the ingested toxin.

Whole-Bowel Irrigation. Whole-bowel irrigation with an orally administered polyethylene glycol electrolyte solution (eg, GoLYTELY or CoLyte) is commonly used prior to bowel procedures. It has drawn attention as an alternative to other methods of GI decontamination in the management of acute poisoning. Results of studies are promising and the technique may have value in cases of ingestion of iron, enteric-coated, or sustained-release products, foreign bodies, and drug-smuggling packets. Instillation rates have ranged from 500 mL/hour in children to 2 L/hour in adults. Typically, 4–6 L of fluid are administered.

■ REFERENCES

1. Smilkstein MJ, Flomenbaum NE. Techniques used to prevent absorption of toxic compounds. In Goldfrank LR, Flomenbaum NE, Lewin NA, et al., eds. *Goldfrank's toxicologic emergencies,* 5th ed. Norwalk, CT: Appleton & Lange; 1994:47–59.

2. Olson KR. Comprehensive evaluation and treatment of poisoning and drug overdose, In Olson KR, ed. *Poisoning and drug overdose,* 2nd ed. Norwalk, CT: Appleton & Lange; 1994:1–58.

3. Haddad LM, Roberts JR. A general approach to the emergency management of poisoning. In Haddad LM, Winchester JF, eds. *Clinical management of poisoning and drug overdose,* 2nd ed. Philadelphia: WB Saunders; 1990:2–22.

4. Gut decontamination. In Ellenhorn MJ, Barceloux DG. *Medical toxicology. Diagnosis and treatment of human poisoning.* New York: Elsevier; 1988:53–61.

5. Herrington AM, Clifton GD. Toxicology and management of acute drug ingestions in adults. *Pharmacotherapy* 1995;15:182–200.

6. Oderda GM. Gastrointestinal decontamination. *J Pharm Pract* 1993;6:48–56.

7. Kulig K. Initial management of ingestions of toxic substances. *N Engl J Med* 1992;326:1677–81.

8. Nejman G et al. Journal club: gastric emptying in the poisoned patient. *Am J Emerg Med* 1990;8:265–9.

9. Wheeler-Usher DH et al. Gastric emptying. Risk versus benefit in the treatment of acute poisoning. *Med Toxicol* 1986;1:142–53.

10. Palatnick W, Tenenbein M. Activated charcoal in the treatment of drug overdose. An update. *Drug Saf* 1992;7:3–7.

11. Merigian KS et al. Prospective evaluation of gastric emptying in the self-poisoned patient. *Am J Emerg Med* 1990;8:479–83.

12. Shannon M et al. Cathartics and laxatives. Do they still have a place in management of the poisoned patient? *Med Toxicol* 1986;1:247–52.

13. Tenenbein M et al. Efficacy of ipecac-induced emesis, orogastric lavage, and activated charcoal for acute drug overdose. *Ann Emerg Med* 1987;16:838–41.

14. Tandberg D, Troutman WG. Gastric lavage in the poisoned patient. In Roberts JR, Hedges JR, eds. *Clinical procedures in emergency medicine,* 2nd ed. Philadelphia: WB Saunders; 1991:655–62.

15. Kirshenbaum LA et al. Whole-bowel irrigation versus activated charcoal in sorbitol for the ingestion of modified-release pharmaceuticals. *Clin Pharmacol Ther* 1989;46:264–71.

Status Epilepticus

Brian K. Alldredge

Status epilepticus is defined as more than 30 minutes of (a) continuous seizure activity, or (b) two or more sequential seizures without full recovery of consciousness between seizures. Status epilepticus is a medical emergency in which prompt recognition and effective medical intervention are required to reduce the risk of permanent sequelae and death.

Status epilepticus can be divided into two major types: convulsive and nonconvulsive. Convulsive status epilepticus is associated with the highest risk of morbidity and mortality, so this section focuses on the clinical features and management of this form of status epilepticus.

In about one-half of patients, status epilepticus is the first manifestation of seizures. The causes of status epilepticus are similar to those for new-onset seizures and include CNS infection, cerebral tumor, trauma, stroke, metabolic disorders, cardiopulmonary arrest, and drug toxicity. In the remainder of patients, status occurs in the setting of a preexisting seizure disorder. Among persons with a history of epilepsy, antiepileptic drug withdrawal (usually noncompliance with prescribed therapy) is the most common cause of status epilepticus.

The primary determinant of patient outcome after status epilepticus is the underlying cause of the episode. In general, patients with status caused by an acute or progressive neurologic insult (eg, cardiopulmonary arrest, stroke) have poorer outcomes than patients in whom status epilepticus occurs in the setting of a more chronic or stable underlying condition (eg, antiepileptic drug withdrawal or medically refractory epilepsy). Nonetheless, aggressive medical intervention and administration of effective antiepileptic drug therapy are important to reduce status-related morbidity and mortality, regardless of the etiology.

Status epilepticus should be managed in an emergency department or in an environment where continuous skilled medical and nursing support are available. The emergency management of status epilepticus should include the following:

- Ensure airway patency and adequate oxygenation.
- Obtain blood specimens for baseline laboratory measurements, including CBC, serum electrolytes (including calcium and magnesium), toxicologic screen, and anticonvulsant serum levels.
- Establish IV access.
- Administer IV glucose (100 mg thiamine followed by 50 mL of 50% glucose in adults).
- Administer IV antiepileptic drugs.
- Monitor blood pressure and temperature.
- Obtain other diagnostic studies as needed.
- Treat precipitating factors.

■ DRUG THERAPY OF STATUS EPILEPTICUS

Adult doses only are given in this section.

If a treatable cause of status epilepticus can be identified rapidly, then drug therapy to terminate seizures may be unnecessary. In these situations, treatment of the underlying cause may be sufficient to stop status. Examples include status caused by an acute metabolic derangement (where correction of the underlying abnormality often stops seizures) or status following isoniazid overdose (where IV pyridoxine is usually effective). However, when a treatable cause is not found, drug therapy should begin immediately. The goal of drug treatment is to terminate seizures as rapidly as possible. Evidence from animal and human studies indicate that 60–120 minutes of status epilepticus is associated with neurologic sequelae and that the risk increases as status continues. Thus, it is important to have a clear, stepwise plan for the administration of effective drug therapy. Figure 5–1 is an example of a status epilepticus treatment protocol. Additionally, adequate support should be available to manage cardiac and respiratory complications that may occur during drug administration.

1. For rapid termination of seizures:

   - **lorazepam, IV, 0.1 mg/kg (4–8 mg) at rate of 2 mg/minute;** may repeat in 10 minutes if seizures continue (to maximum of 0.2 mg/kg). Lorazepam has a longer duration of anticonvulsant effect than diazepam and is often preferred for this reason.

   or

   - **diazepam, IV, 0.2 mg/kg (5–10 mg) at rate of 5 mg/minute;** may repeat in 10 minutes if seizures continue (to maximum of 20 mg). Diazepam has a short duration of anticonvulsant effect (15–60 minutes) and must be immediately followed by a long-acting agent (eg, phenytoin).

2a. Following benzodiazepine administration, give

   - **phenytoin, IV infusion, 20 mg/kg at rate of 50 mg/minute** or fosphenytoin 20 mg/kg phenytoin equivalents IV at a rate of 150 mg/minute. Monitor blood pressure and ECG during administration of phenytoin loading dose. Elderly and severely ill patients are predisposed to phenytoin-related hypotension.

2b. If status persists, *then:*

   - **phenytoin** or fosphenytoin, **IV,** up to two additional doses of 5 mg/kg, to a total dosage of 30 mg/kg.

2c. If status is terminated, then begin maintenance phenytoin therapy.

3. If seizures are not terminated after administration of phenytoin 30 mg/kg, *then:*

   - **phenobarbital, IV, 20 mg/kg at rate of 100 mg/minute.** The risk of hypoventilation is increased markedly when phenobarbital is administered after benzodiazepines; respiratory support is often required.

4. For patients who continue in status epilepticus despite the above recommendations, anesthetic doses of barbiturates or benzodiazepines are often required to suppress seizure activity. Ventilatory assistance and vasopressor drug therapy are usually required; therefore, the patient should be admitted to the ICU and the following therapies considered:

4a. **pentobarbital, IV infusion, 15 mg/kg over 1 hour,** *then maintenance:*

- **pentobarbital, IV infusion, 1–2 mg/kg/hour.** Hypotension is a frequent complication of high-dose pentobarbital therapy; vasopressors (eg, dopamine) may be required.

or

4b. **midazolam, IV slow push, 200 μg/kg,** *then maintenance:*

- **midazolam, IV slow push, 0.75–10 μg/kg/minute.** High-dose midazolam is probably associated with a lower risk of hypotension than high-dose pentobarbital; however, there is less experience with its use.

The ECG should be monitored continuously during the first 1–2 hours of therapy, and infusion rates should be adjusted until suppression of electrographic seizures is evident. After seizures are terminated, the rate of the maintenance infusion can be slowed periodically to determine if status has remitted.

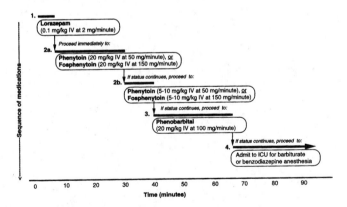

Figure 5–1. Timeline for Administration of Drug Therapy for Convulsive Status Epilepticus. Heavy bars (■■■■) indicate duration (in minutes) of intravenous drug administration.

■ REFERENCES

1. Working Group on Status Epilepticus. Treatment of convulsive status epilepticus. Recommendations of the Epilepsy Foundation of America's working group on status epilepticus. *JAMA* 1993;270:854–9.
2. Lowenstein DH, Alldredge BK. Status epilepticus at an urban public hospital in the 1980s. *Neurology* 1993;43(3 pt 1):483–8.
3. Lowenstein DH et al. Barbiturate anesthesia in the treatment of status epilepticus: clinical experience with 14 patients. *Neurology* 1988;38:395–400.
4. Parent JM, Lowenstein DH. Treatment of refractory generalized status epilepticus with continuous infusion of midazolam. *Neurology* 1994;44:1837–40.
5. Shorvon SD. *Status epilepticus: its clinical features and treatment in children and adults.* New York, NY: Cambridge University Press; 1994.

Nutrition Support

Fred Shatsky

Nutrition status is a major determinant of patients' morbidity and mortality. Morbidity increases with malnutrition as is manifested by depressed immunocompetence and impaired wound healing.[1,2] Conditions that indicate a possible need for nutrition support include inadequate oral nutrition for longer than 7 days, recent body weight loss >10%, an illness lasting more than 3 weeks, recent major surgery, a lymphocyte count <1.2 × 10³/µL, serum albumin <3 g/dL, serum transferrin <150 mg/dL, and serum prealbumin <15 mg/dL. Sepsis, trauma, and other factors that induce hypermetabolism may intensify the need.

The term "nutrition support" can be applied to any nutrition regimen that is provided for conditions that preclude the use of regular foods. There are two broad categories of nutrition support, enteral and parenteral, determined by their route of administration. Enteral nutrition applies to regimens provided via any portion of the gastrointestinal (GI) tract. Parenteral nutrition (PN), although implying all routes other than the GI tract, refers primarily to regimens that are provided directly by the intravenous route of administration. Less frequently used modes of PN such as intradialytic parenteral nutrition (IDPN) and intraperitoneal nutrition (IPN) are not discussed in this chapter.

Whenever possible, maintenance rather than repletion should be the primary objective of nutrition support. Early provision of nutrition requirements without exceeding energy balance promotes the synthesis of lean body mass rather than adipose tissue.[3]

■ NUTRITION ASSESSMENT

Nutrition assessment of the patient can aid in diagnosing malnutrition and determining its degree of severity, so that a proper nutrition support regimen can be formulated. The patient's physical and dietary history should be obtained to establish baseline data. Clinical parameters for assessing the patient's nutrition status can be evaluated through the use of an assessment form (Table 6–1). Because a patient's nutrition status is best reflected by body protein,[4] nutrition assessment should focus on the protein compartments. Protein compartments are classified into two types: somatic (muscle protein) and visceral (all other protein).

TABLE 6–1. NUTRITION ASSESSMENT*

NAME: AGE: HT (CM): DATE: SEX: WT (KG):	STANDARD	DEPLETION		
		Mild	*Moderate*	*Severe*
Triceps Skinfold (TSF), mm =	M 12.5	11.3	11.3–7.5	<7.5
Ideal Body Weight:	F 16.5	14.9	14.9–9.9	<9.9
$\dfrac{ABW}{IBW} \times 100 =$	100%	90%	90–60%	<60%
Mid–Upper Arm Circumference	M 29.3	26.4	26.4–17.6	<17.6
(MUAC), cm	F 28.5	25.7	25.7–17.1	<17.1
Mid–Upper Arm Muscle Circumference:	M 25.3	22.8	22.8–15.2	<15.2
MUAC (cm) − [0.314 × TSF (mm)] =	F 23.2	21.0	21.0–13.9	<13.9
Creatinine/Height Index:				
$\dfrac{Cr_u}{ICr_u \text{ for height}} \times 100 =$	100%	90%	90–60%	<60%
Serum Albumin, g/dL =	3.5–5.0	3.5–3.0	3.0–2.1	<2.1
Serum Prealbumin, mg/dL =	>20	20–15	15–10	<10
Serum Transferrin, mg/dL =	200–400	200–150	150–100	<100
Total Lymphocyte/μL:	1800–3000	1800–1200	1200–800	<800
$\dfrac{WBC/\mu L \times \% \text{ Lymphocytes}}{100}$				

*The standards specified represent those of healthy persons. Measurements in patients may be additionally affected by nonnutritional as well as nutritional factors.
ABW, actual body weight; Cr_u, urinary creatinine; IBW, ideal body weight; ICr_u, ideal urinary creatinine; MUAC, mid–upper arm circumference; TSF, triceps skinfold.

Somatic Protein Assessment Parameters

Percentage Ideal Body Weight. A simple initial measurement of a patient's nutrition status is body weight expressed as a percentage of ideal body weight (*see* Appendix 2, Anthropometrics).

$$\text{Percentage Ideal Body Weight} = \frac{\text{Actual Body Weight}}{\text{Ideal Body Weight}} \times 100$$

Creatinine/Height Index. Creatinine/height index (CHI), when accurately obtained, is a more sensitive indicator of somatic protein and nutrition status than is percent ideal body weight.[5] Creatinine, a product of muscle metabolism, is normally excreted in urine at a constant rate proportional to the amount of skeletal muscle and lean body mass catabolized. CHI is calculated from a 24-hr urinary creatinine measurement and the ideal urinary creatinine value found in Table 6–2, using the following formula:

$$CHI = \frac{\text{Actual Urinary Creatinine}}{\text{Ideal Urinary Creatinine for Height}} \times 100$$

It is important that the urine sample be an aliquot drawn from a 24-hour collection of urine rather than a random sample.

TABLE 6–2. IDEAL URINARY CREATININE

MALES*		FEMALES†	
Height (cm)	Ideal Creatinine (mg/24 hr)	Height (cm)	Ideal Creatinine (mg/24 hr)
157.5	1288	147.3	830
160.0	1325	149.9	851
162.6	1359	152.4	875
165.1	1386	154.9	900
167.6	1426	157.5	925
170.2	1467	160.0	949
172.7	1513	162.6	977
175.3	1555	165.1	1006
177.8	1596	167.6	1044
180.3	1642	170.2	1076
182.9	1691	172.7	1109
185.4	1739	175.3	1141
188.0	1785	177.8	1174
190.5	1831	180.3	1206
193.0	1891	182.9	1240

*Creatinine coefficient (men) = 23 mg/kg of ideal body weight.
†Creatinine coefficient (women) = 18 mg/kg of ideal body weight.
From Blackburn GL et al., Nutritional and metabolic assessment of the hospitalized patient. JPEN 1977;1:11–22, reproduced with permission.

There are limitations in using CHI as an indicator of malnutrition. Patients sometimes excrete amounts of creatinine and nitrogen that vary with different diets, medications, or degrees of renal function, conditions of illness, or stress. Certain drugs interfere with urine creatinine determinations (*see* Chapter 2, Drug–Laboratory Test Interferences).

Anthropometric Measurements. Anthropometric measurements may be of questionable value because of slow change over time and interobserver variability. If used, the triceps skinfold (TSF) and mid–upper arm circumference (MUAC) should be taken on the mid-upper portion of the nondominant arm by trained personnel. Detailed procedures and methods of measurement are available.[6,7] TSF measurement with calipers is compared to the standards in Table 6–1 to give a reasonable estimate of subcutaneous fat reserves.[4] Both TSF and MUAC, obtained with a metric tape measure, can be used to derive the mid-upper arm muscle circumference (MUAMC) by the formula:[4]

$$MUAMC = MUAC \text{ (cm)} - (0.314 \times TSF \text{ [mm]})$$

Visceral Protein Assessment Parameters

The status of visceral protein reflects the patient's ability to respond to stress by means such as immunocompetence and wound healing. Visceral protein status can be determined by measurements of serum albumin, serum thyroxine-binding prealbumin (also referred to as transthyretin or prealbumin), and serum transferrin. These visceral protein indicators usually decrease after trauma or surgical procedures; however, consistently low levels for a period of at least 1 week may indicate a degree of malnutrition.[7] Serum albumin is unreliable as an assessment parameter in certain patients. Serum albumin may be elevated as a result of dehydration, shock, hemoconcentration, or administration of anabolic hormones or IV albumin. Decreased albumin levels can result from chronic illness, malabsorption, pregnancy, nephrotic syndrome, hepatic insufficiency, protein-losing enteropathy, overhydration, or severe burns.[8,9]

Prealbumin and transferrin are visceral proteins with a more rapid turnover than albumin; they are effective assessment parameters with half-lives of approximately 2 and 8 days, respectively.

Visceral protein levels and nitrogen balance are expected to decline postoperatively. In a comparison between postoperative prealbumin and transferrin serum levels, the decline in prealbumin was much greater, and changes in transferrin were more closely correlated with changes in nitrogen balance.[10] Transferrin levels may be elevated in patients who are iron deficient, pregnant, or taking estrogens or oral contraceptives. Serum albumin, prealbumin, and transferrin values indicative of varying degrees of depletion are given in Table 6–1.

■ PERIODIC REASSESSMENT

An initial assessment can be made prior to beginning a nutrition support regimen. Periodic reassessment of the patient, using some or all of the previously mentioned parameters, can provide a means of objectively evaluating the efficacy of nutrition support. Additional parameters to consider during this stage of assessment are nitrogen balance and body weight.

Nitrogen Balance

Nitrogen balance determinations indicate the extent to which exogenous protein is being used and can serve as a method for evaluating the efficacy of nutrition support. Because nitrogen balance data are subject to errors of collection and other variables, they should be used only as a relative index of daily change and not an absolute measure of depletion or improvement. Nitrogen balance is calculated for a 24-hr period using the following formula:[7]

Nitrogen Balance = Total Nitrogen In − Total Nitrogen Out

Urinary urea nitrogen (UUN), although a less sensitive indicator of nitrogen output than total urea nitrogen, is a more simplified laboratory procedure and is therefore a more frequently used measurement to estimate nitrogen balance. Nitrogen balance is calculated as follows:

$$\text{Nitrogen Balance} = \frac{\text{Protein Intake (in g)}}{6.25} - [\text{UUN (in g)} + 4]$$

Urinary urea nitrogen is usually reported in mg/dL; therefore, to derive the amount in grams for use in the above formula, the value must be multiplied by the total 24-hr volume of urine output. The urine sample sent to the laboratory should be an aliquot drawn from an accurate 24-hr urine collection. The factor 4 is added as an empirical number to account for nonurinary nitrogen such as that excreted in feces, sweat, and other normal losses. Excessive nitrogen losses that cannot be measured, such as nitrogen lost in exudates from severe burns or other fluid losses, render nitrogen balance data less reliable.

Positive nitrogen balance can indicate a retention of nitrogen, both as newly synthesized body protein tissue and as nitrogen retained in body fluids. A positive nitrogen balance of 4–6 g/day is the maximum that should be expected;[11] greater amounts are not considered efficient. Because only synthesized protein is of therapeutic interest, increments in blood urea nitrogen (BUN) above baseline (in grams) should be subtracted from total nitrogen balance. This calculation is summarized as follows:

Corrected Nitrogen Balance = Nitrogen Balance − BUN Increment (g)

To derive the BUN increment above baseline in grams, the total body water volume of the patient must be considered. Body water can be estimated to be 55% of total body weight (0.55 L/kg).[11] A BUN of 10 mg/dL above baseline in a 70-kg patient represents a BUN increment of 3.85 g (70 kg × 0.55 L/kg × 100 mg/L = 3850 mg).

Body Weight

The weight difference between body water and tissue is indistinguishable unless water balance is measured. Body weight gain alone is therefore not a reliable maintenance assessment parameter. It is known, however, that weight gain in excess of 200 g/day is undesirable because patients cannot synthesize lean body tissue at a greater rate.[11] Despite its shortcomings as a monitoring parameter, body weight should nevertheless be measured throughout the support regimen at the same time each day, and intake and output should be considered in the interpretation of body weight changes.

■ NUTRIENT REQUIREMENTS

The nutrients required for enteral and parenteral nutrition are virtually the same. Either mode of nutrition support must consist of the basic components of a normal diet: water, carbohydrate, fat, protein, electrolytes, vitamins, and trace elements.

Caloric Requirements

Accurate estimation of caloric requirements is essential, particularly for the severely stressed or depleted patient, to avoid problems associated with overfeeding as well as underfeeding.[12] Requirements can be calculated accurately by indirect calorimetry using instruments that measure respiratory gas exchange. When this is not possible, requirements can be estimated as a multiple of the patient's basal energy expenditure (BEE). BEE is the amount of energy required to maintain basic metabolic functions in the resting state and can be derived from the Harris-Benedict equations:[12]

BEE (Men): $66 + (13.8 \times$ wt in kg$) + (5 \times$ ht in cm$) - (6.8 \times$ age in yr$)$

BEE (Women): $655 + (9.6 \times$ wt in kg$) + (1.8 \times$ ht in cm$) - (4.7 \times$ age in yr$)$

Mechanically ventilated nonsurgical patients without stress or sepsis should receive a total caloric intake no greater than the calculated BEE.[12] Trauma and sepsis increase energy and protein requirements, and the nutrition support regimen should be adjusted accordingly. One means of determining the severity of catabolism in stress conditions is by measurement of UUN excreted per 24 hr. Caloric requirements can then be estimated as a multiple of BEE as shown in Table 6–3.[13]

TABLE 6–3. CALORIC REQUIREMENTS DURING CATABOLISM

24-HR UUN	DEGREE OF NET CATABOLISM	CALORIC REQUIREMENTS
0–5 g	1° (normal)	1 × BEE
5–10 g	2° (mild)	1.5 × BEE
10–15 g	3° (moderate)	1.75 × BEE
>15 g	4° (severe)	2 × BEE

In estimating the calories to be provided by each substrate, yields may be considered as follows: dextrose, 3.4 kcal/g; fat, 9 kcal/g; and protein, 4 kcal/g. Although protein is considered a calorigenic substrate, it is not usually included in estimating caloric goals because the main role of protein is for preservation or synthesis of lean body mass.

Protein Requirements

The minimum requirement for protein is about 0.8 g/kg/day of a balanced mixture of amino acids (AAs), and can be as high as 2.5 g/kg/day in severely stressed or traumatized patients. For optimal synthesis of protein, concurrent provision of nonprotein calories must be sufficient. To calculate the nonprotein calorie to nitrogen ratio, it may be assumed that the nitrogen content is 1 g/6.25 g of AAs. The optimal ratio of nonprotein calories to nitrogen for efficient nitrogen retention and nitrogen balance is not definite, but varies with the metabolic state of the patient. Nonprotein calorie to nitrogen ratios of standard enteral and PN formulas are typically about 150:1. Lower ratios are indicated for stress or trauma, and higher ratios for nonstressed patients and those with impaired protein metabolism.

■ ENTERAL NUTRITION

For physiologic and economic reasons the enteral route should be used whenever possible, but adequacy of the GI tract must be established before enteral nutrition is provided. The IV route should be strictly reserved for patients who cannot be adequately nourished by the enteral route.

Formulas for enteral nutrition are available for supplemental oral feeding or enteral feeding through various types of tubes. When the oral route is not feasible, transnasal passage of a feeding tube into the stomach (nasogastric) or intestine (nasoduodenal or nasojejunal) are generally the feeding routes employed. Feeding ostomies, most commonly the gastrostomy, jejunostomy, or combination gastrostomy-jejunostomy, are generally indicated when insertion through the nares is not feasible or when long-term feeding is anticipated.

Formula Selection

The abundance of products and lack of an ideal system of categorization may present confusion in selecting the most appropriate enteral formula for a patient. It is not within the scope of this chapter to fully describe criteria for formula selection or to provide a complete compendium of formulas.

Some nutritionally complete, ready-to-use liquid enteral formulas that are suitable for a variety of patients are presented in Table 6–4. Carbohydrate, fat, and protein sources differ with products and may be important criteria for selecting a product. Because patients with abnormal intestinal function are usually lactose intolerant, only lactose-free products are included. Disease-specific formulas, such as those with high content of branched chain amino acids for liver disease or essential amino acids for renal disease, may be nutritionally incomplete and are not included because of inadequate evidence of their superiority.

Administration

Either of two types of feeding schedules may be employed, continuous or intermittent. Continuous drip infusion is the preferred method of administration, particularly for patients who have not eaten for a long time. Large 24-hr volumes may be given by infusion without challenging the GI tract, thereby allowing readaptation of the starved gut. Although gravity may be used, an infusion pump is recommended when initiating therapy. For most patients, it is recommended that the first day's feeding be infused at a rate of 50 mL/hr using a lactose-free, nutrient-intact, isotonic formula of 1 kcal/mL. Many protocols recommend diluting the initial formula to one-half strength; however, this practice has been questioned.[14]

TABLE 6–4. REPRESENTATIVE ENTERAL FORMULAS

PRODUCT	CALORIES (PER ML)	PROTEIN (G/L)	FAT (G/L)	CARBOHYDRATE (G/L)	NONPROTEIN CALORIES:N (CAL/G NITROGEN)	SODIUM (MEQ/L)	POTASSIUM (MEQ/L)	CALCIUM (MG/L)	PHOSPHORUS (MG/L)	OSMOLARITY (MOSM/L)
Compleat Modified	1.07	43	37	140	131	29	36	670	930	300
Criticare HN	1.06	38	5	220	149	28	34	530	530	650
Ensure Plus	1.5	55	53	200	146	50	54	705	705	690
Ensure Plus HN	1.5	63	50	200	125	51	47	1057	1057	650
Impact	1.0	56	28	132	71	48	33	800	800	375
Isocal	1.06	34	44	133	167	23	34	630	530	300
Isocal HCN	2.0	75	91	225	145	35	43	1000	1000	690
Isosource HN	1.2	53	41	157	115	31	43	670	670	390
Jevity	1.06	44	37	152	126	40	40	910	760	310
Magnacal	2.0	70	80	250	154	43	32	1000	1000	590
Nitrolan	1.24	60	40	160	104	30	30	800	800	310
Osmolite	1.06	37	38	145	153	28	26	528	528	300
Osmolite HN	1.06	44	37	141	125	41	40	758	758	300
Pulmocare	1.5	63	92	106	125	57	49	1060	1060	490
Reabilan	1.0	31	39	131	174	30	32	500	500	350
Suplena	2.0	30	96	255	342	34	29	1386	728	600
Sustacal	1.3	61	23	140	78	40	54	1010	930	620
Sustacal HC	1.5	61	58	190	134	37	38	850	850	650
TraumaCal	1.5	83	68	142	91	52	36	750	750	490
Ultracal	1.06	44	45	123	126	40	41	850	850	310

Incremental advances in rate and strength can be attempted daily until the desired rate of a full-strength formula is achieved. To minimize the risk of aspiration, proper placement of the tube must be confirmed, and the patient's head and shoulders must be kept at a 30 to 45° angle during and for 1 hr after feeding. The stomach should be checked periodically for residual volumes during gastric feedings.

Once a patient has been stabilized on maintenance therapy, intermittent infusions may be used, allowing the patient to rest from feedings at selected hours. A volume of 250–400 mL may be administered five to eight times per day. This method is preferred for ambulatory patients, because it permits more freedom of movement than does continuous feeding.

Formulas should be given at room temperature and should be kept no longer than 12 hr after the time of preparation and 6 hr from the start of administration to avoid excessive bacterial growth. The delivery system, including bag and tubing, should be changed every 24 hr.

Complications

Mechanical and GI complications known to occur with tube feedings are summarized in Table 6–5. Metabolic complications that occur with enteral nutrition are similar to those of parenteral nutrition and are included in Table 6–12.

TABLE 6–5. TUBE FEEDING COMPLICATIONS AND MANAGEMENT

COMPLICATION	PREVENTION OR MANAGEMENT
Mechanical	
Clogged Tube	Flush with water, replace tube if necessary. Avoid passing crushed tablets through small bore feeding tubes.
Nasal, Pharyngeal, Esophageal Irritation	Use small lumen flexible tube. Provide daily care of nose and mouth.
Aspiration	Ensure proper tube placement and verify location. Maintain patient's head and shoulders at 30–45° upright position during and for 1 hr after feeding. Monitor for gastric reflux and abdominal distention. Stop infusion if vomiting occurs. Check residual gastric volume prior to and q 2–4 hr during infusion. Hold if the residual exceeds the hourly volume or 150 mL.
Dislocated Tube	Verify tube location and mark tube at insertion site.
Gastrointestinal	
Diarrhea and Cramps	Reduce flow rate, dilute formula, or consider alternative formula. Rule out alternative causes. If persistent, add antidiarrheal agent.
Vomiting or Bloating	Check stool output and measure residual formula in gut q 2–4 hr. If necessary, stop or reduce flow.
Constipation	Consider different formula or a laxative.

To prevent metabolic complications, monitoring of the patient as suggested in Table 6–13 is recommended.

■ PARENTERAL NUTRITION

Parenteral Nutrition (PN) may be administered by either of two routes of access: peripheral veins or larger central veins. The peripheral route is indicated for those patients who require only short-term supplementation or supplementation in addi-

tion to enteral support, or for those in whom the risks of central venous administration are too great. Peripheral veins are susceptible to thrombophlebitis, particularly when the osmolarity of the solution exceeds 600 mOsm/L. Therefore, it is
recommended that formulas for peripheral administration not exceed final concentrations of 10% dextrose and 4.25% amino acids plus electrolyte and vitamin additives. A number of techniques to prevent or delay onset of peripheral vein thrombophlebitis have been reported.[15] Addition of small amounts of hydrocortisone (5
mg/L) and heparin (1000 units/L) to PN formulas, as well as the topical use of
agents such as transdermal nitroglycerin, have demonstrated success. Concurrent
administration of IV fat emulsion, which is a concentrated, isoosmotic calorie
source, is vital, because it increases the caloric content of a peripheral regimen
while minimizing the risk of thrombophlebitis.

The complete nutrition needs of the malnourished or hypermetabolic patient
are difficult to provide via peripheral vein for long periods of time. The concentrated, hyperosmolar solutions required by such patients for PN *must* be administered into a large central vein, such as the superior vena cava, where rapid dilution
occurs.

Administration

Initiation of PN should be gradual, particularly in the malnourished patient to
avoid glucose intolerance and the dangers of refeeding syndrome.[16] With high
concentrations of dextrose and amino acids intended for central vein administration, an initial rate of 40 mL/hr for the first 24 hr is suggested. Infusion rates may
then be increased daily in accordance with assessment goals. Less concentrated
formulas that are suited for peripheral vein administration do not warrant such
slow initial rates of infusion.

A variety of catheters exist for infusion of PN formulas by central or peripheral vein. Use of an in-line filter is recommended to minimize adverse consequences in case precipitation occurs in the PN solution.[17]

Parenteral Nutrients

Each of the following nutrient substrate groups are required in formulas for effective PN.

Water. The average healthy adult can tolerate a fluid infusion volume of about 5
L/day. The patient who is fluid restricted might be limited to an intake of 2 L/day
or less. This may be the deciding factor in selecting a hypertonic concentrated solution for infusion through a large central vein rather than a more dilute solution
for peripheral administration.

Carbohydrate. Presently, the preferred carbohydrate substrate for PN is dextrose.
The concentration of dextrose should be determined by the osmotic limitation of
the administration route and the nonprotein calorie requirement of the patient. The
concentrations of available dextrose solutions with their corresponding caloric
concentrations and osmolarities are as shown in Table 6–6.

TABLE 6–6. IV DEXTROSE SOLUTIONS

CONCENTRATION	KCAL/L	MOSM/L
5%	170	252
10%	340	505
20%	680	1010
40%	1360	2020
50%	1700	2520
60%	2040	3030
70%	2380	3530

Dextrose remains the primary source of calories for PN via central vein, and the rate of infusion should be limited to its maximum rate of oxidation, which is 5 mg/kg/min or 7.2 g/kg/day.[18] On a calorie-for-calorie basis, carbohydrate is more efficient than fat in sparing body protein during hypocaloric feedings.[19] The inclusion of both dextrose and fat is recommended in PN regimens, but the optimal proportion of each has not been established.

Fat. Fat is an important parenteral substrate for three major reasons: (1) it is a concentrated source of calories in an isotonic medium, which makes it useful for peripheral administration; (2) it is a source of essential fatty acids (EFAs) required for prevention or treatment of EFA deficiency, which may develop during prolonged fat-free PN;[20] and (3) it is a useful substitute for carbohydrate when dextrose calories must be limited because of glucose intolerance or diminished ventilatory capacity. When a patient's ventilatory effort is hampered, it is important to avoid excessive calories of any type. In comparison to dextrose, the metabolism of fat results in an increase in heat production, a decrease in respiratory quotient (RQ), and an increase in oxygen consumption. Having a lower RQ, fat produces less CO_2 for a given number of calories, thereby minimizing the ventilatory effort required to eliminate CO_2. The RQ of fat is 0.7 versus 1 for carbohydrate. An RQ in excess of 1 indicates net lipogenesis and is undesirable.[21]

Fat is available as emulsions of 10, 20, or 30% soybean oil, or 10 or 20% soybean–safflower oil mixtures. Clinical studies have not shown any major advantages of one lipid source over the other. The major differences between these products are their fatty acid contents, which are summarized in Table 6–7. The 20 and 30% emulsions are more readily cleared than the 10% because of the lower proportion of phospholipid to triglyceride.[22]

Fat emulsions that are currently marketed in the United States contain only long-chain triglycerides (LCTs); however, the use of fat emulsions that contain both LCTs and **medium-chain triglycerides** (MCTs) is being investigated. MCTs are reported to be more rapidly cleared from the blood and more ketogenic than LCTs, and emulsions containing both MCTs and LCTs have greater protein-conserving properties than pure LCT emulsions.[23] LCTs are required for their essential fatty acid content, however.

TABLE 6–7. IV FAT EMULSIONS

FATTY ACID	SOYBEAN OIL	SOYBEAN OIL/ SAFFLOWER OIL
Linoleic Acid	54%	65.8%
Linolenic Acid	8%	4.2%
Oleic Acid	26%	17.7%
Palmitic Acid	9%	8.8%
Stearic Acid	2.5%	3.4%

The caloric density of 10% fat emulsions is 1.1 kcal/mL, of which 1 kcal is supplied by lipid and 0.1 kcal by glycerol (carbohydrate); the 20 and 30% emulsions have caloric densities of 2 and 3 kcal/mL, respectively, of which 0.1 kcal/mL is glycerol. The average particle size (0.5 micron) is the same in all concentrations, and all are nearly isoosmotic.

Fat emulsion may be infused concurrently with amino acid/dextrose solution through peripheral or central veins. The 10 or 20% emulsion may be infused separately or combined with amino acids and dextrose in a single container to form a total nutrient ("3-in-1") admixture (TNA).[24] The 30% concentration is intended only for compounding TNA. Because lipid emulsion is isoosmolar, it reduces the thrombophlebitic effect of hyperosmolar amino acid/dextrose solutions on the endothelium of peripheral veins when they are infused concurrently.[25] For this reason as well as its potential adverse effect on the immune system, fat emulsion should be infused as slowly as possible.[26] Product literature suggests that fat be provided in quantities no greater than 3 g/kg or 60% of total calories. For further information on dosage, administration, and precautions of fat emulsion, the product literature should be consulted.

Protein. Various brands and concentrations of amino acid solutions are available as sources of protein for parenteral use. The AA profile differs in each, and therefore their nitrogen contents are not equivalent. A comparison of formulations is summarized in Table 6–8. Amino acid solutions >3.5% concentration should be diluted to a lower final concentration with dextrose and other additives.

TABLE 6-8. AMINO ACID SOLUTIONS COMPARISON CHART

AA SOLUTION AND OSMOLARITY CONCENTRATION	TOTAL BCAAs (G/DL)	TOTAL ESSENTIAL AAs (G/DL)	TOTAL N (G/DL)	ELECTROLYTES (MEQ/L)					PO_4 (mmol/L)	Osmolarity (mOsm/L)
				Na^+	K^+	Mg^{++}	Cl^-	Ac^-		
FOR GENERAL PURPOSE										
Aminosyn 3.5%*	0.86	1.65	0.55	7	—	—	—	46	—	357
Aminosyn 5%*	1.23	2.35	0.79	—	5.4	—	—	86	—	500
Travasol 5.5%	0.86	2.15	0.95	—	—	—	22	48	—	575
(with electrolytes)				70	60	10	70	102	30	850
Aminosyn 7%*	1.73	3.32	1.1	—	5.4	—	—	105	—	700
(with electrolytes)				70	66	10	96	124	30	1013
Aminosyn 8.5%*	2.11	4.06	1.34	—	2.7	—	11.7	90	—	856
(with electrolytes)				70	66	10	98	142	30	1160
Travasol 8.5%	1.32	3.34	1.43	—	—	—	34	73	—	890
(with electrolytes)				70	60	10	70	141	30	1160
FreAmine III 8.5%	1.92	3.94	1.43	10	—	—	<3	73	10	810
(with electrolytes)				60	60	10	60	125	20	1045
Aminosyn 10%	2.46	4.7	1.57	—	5.4	—	—	148	—	1000
Aminosyn II 10%	2.16	4.3	1.53	87	66	10	86	72	30	1130
(with electrolytes)										

(continued)

TABLE 6-8. AMINO ACID SOLUTIONS COMPARISON CHART (continued)

AA SOLUTION AND OSMOLARITY CONCENTRATION	TOTAL BCAAs (G/DL)	TOTAL ESSENTIAL AAs (G/DL)	TOTAL N (G/DL)	ELECTROLYTES (MEQ/L)					PO_4 (mmol/L)	Osmolarity (mOsm/L)
				Na^+	K^+	Mg^{++}	Cl^-	Ac^-		
FreAmine III 10%	2.26	4.63	1.53	10	—	—	<3	89	10	950
Travasol 10%	1.91	4.05	1.65	—	—	—	40	87	—	1000
Novamine	2.09	5.11	1.8	—	—	—	—	114	—	1057
Aminosyn II 15%	3.24	6.42	2.3	63	—	—	—	107	—	1300
Novamine 15%	2.75	6.72	2.37	—	—	—	—	151	—	1388
FOR PROTEIN SPARING										
ProcalAmine 3%[b]	0.68	1.4	0.46	35	24	5	41	47	3.5	735
FreAmine III 3% (with electrolytes)	0.68	1.4	0.46	35	24	5	41	44	3.5	405
Aminosyn 3.5% M[a]	0.86	1.65	0.55	47	13	3	40	58	3.5	477
3.5% Travasol (with electrolytes)	0.55	1.38	0.59	25	15	5	25	52	7.5	450
FOR RENAL FAILURE										
Aminess 5.2%	1.95	5.18	0.66	—	—	—	—	50	—	416
Aminosyn RF 5.2%	1.72	4.83	0.79	—	5.4	—	—	105	—	475
NephrAmine 5.4%	2.08	5.33	0.65	5	—	—	<3	44	—	435

(continued)

TABLE 6–8. AMINO ACID SOLUTIONS COMPARISON CHART (continued)

AA SOLUTION AND OSMOLARITY CONCENTRATION	TOTAL BCAAs (G/DL)	TOTAL ESSENTIAL AAs (G/DL)	TOTAL N (G/DL)	Na$^+$	K$^+$	Mg^{++}	Cl$^-$	Ac$^-$	PO$_4$ (mmol/L)	Osmolarity (mOsm/L)
							ELECTROLYTES (MEQ/L)			
RenAmin 6.5%	1.92	4.32	1.0	—	—	—	31	60	—	600
FOR TRAUMA										
BranchAmin 4%[c,d]	4.0	4.0[d]	0.44	—	—	—	—	—	—	316
FreAmine HBC 6.9%[c]	3.01	4.28	0.97	10	—	—	<3	57	—	620
Aminosyn HBC 7%[c]	3.15	4.21	1.12	7	40	—	—	72	—	665
FOR LIVER DISEASE										
HepatAmine 8%[c]	2.84	4.17	1.2	10	—	—	<3	62	10	785
FOR PEDIATRICS										
Aminosyn PF 7%	1.82	3.2	1.07	3.4	—	—	—	33	—	586
Aminosyn PF 10%	2.63	4.61	1.52	3.4	—	—	—	46	—	834
TrophAmine 6%	1.8	4.28	0.93	5	—	—	<3	56	—	525
TrophAmine 10%	3.0	7.2	1.55	5	—	—	<3	97	—	875

[a]BCAAs, branched-chain amino acids.

[a]Also available as Aminosyn II which contains glutamic and aspartic acids, and differs slightly in content of other amino acids, acetate, and chloride.

[b]Contains glycerol as a nonprotein calorie source.

[c]Branched-chain amino acid–enriched products. Each of these products has distinct indications for use and should not be interchanged.

[d]Contains only the branched-chain amino acids. Other essential amino acids are not included.

887

Special Amino Acid Solutions

Special amino acid solutions are available for specific metabolic or disease states. Discretion is recommended in the use of these solutions, because they are expensive and clinical benefit is not proved.

Protein Sparing. It has been demonstrated that a low concentration of amino acids infused with or without concurrent nonprotein calories conserves endogenous nitrogen more efficiently than the traditional 5% dextrose infusion alone.[27] For a limited infusion of no more than 1 week's duration in patients who are not severely catabolic, low-concentration AA formulas merit consideration. Low-concentration AA formulas are available with or without electrolytes and with or without a nonprotein calorie source (*see* Table 6–8).

Renal Failure. The objective of PN in patients with renal failure is to provide sufficient amino acids and calories for protein synthesis without exceeding the renal capacity for excretion of fluid and metabolic wastes. Four parenteral products that contain primarily essential amino acids have been developed for this purpose (*see* Table 6–8), but controversy exists regarding their use. Patients who undergo renal replacement therapy such as peritoneal or hemodialysis require both essential and nonessential amino acids and should receive standard amino acid solutions.

Hepatic Failure. Patients with hepatic failure, in whom muscle breakdown and an altered serum and CNS amino acid profile may contribute to hepatic encephalopathy, may benefit from a special AA formula. This formula has relatively greater amounts of branched-chain amino acids (BCAAs—leucine, isoleucine, and valine) and smaller amounts of the aromatic amino acids (ie, phenylalanine, tyrosine, tryptophan), and methionine.[28] One parenteral formula, HepatAmine, is currently available specifically for therapeutic and nutrition support of patients with liver disease (*see* Table 6–8).

Stress and Trauma. The hypermetabolism that occurs in response to stress and trauma presents difficulty in providing nutrition support. BCAAs, in addition to their useful effect in metabolic support of the patient with liver disease, are reported to be useful for patients with stress and trauma.[29,30] Three BCAA-enriched products are available (*see* Table 6–8). FreAmine HBC and Aminosyn HBC are solutions of nonessential and essential AAs enriched with BCAAs. BranchAmin 4% is a solution of only BCAAs intended for use as a supplement to be admixed with a complete amino acid and a nonprotein caloric source. These products are indicated only for stress and trauma, and should not be confused with the BCAA-enriched product that is indicated for hepatic encephalopathy.

Pediatrics. It is beyond the scope of this chapter to describe procedures for nutrition support of pediatric patients except in this brief mention of parenteral amino acid products. Crystalline AA solutions marketed for infants are based on the essentiality of certain AAs in these patients (*see* Table 6–8).[31] Compared to adult AA formulations, these products contain taurine and glutamic and aspartic acids. Increased amounts of tyrosine and histidine, and lower amounts of phenylalanine, methionine, and glycine are included. Although cysteine is also assumed to be essential for infants, adequate amounts cannot be included in AA formulas, because of its limited solubility. A cysteine solution (50 mg/mL) is available separately for admixture to the formula prior to administration.

Electrolytes

Formulas are also available with standard electrolyte compositions that may be suitable for most patients, after the addition of certain additives. Electrolyte provision, however, should be based on close monitoring of patients' laboratory values. Average daily requirements are summarized in Table 6–9.

TABLE 6–9. ELECTROLYTES AND REQUIREMENTS

ELECTROLYTES	AVERAGE DAILY REQUIREMENT	DOSAGE FORMS	COMMENTS
CATIONS			
Sodium	60–150 mEq	Sodium chloride concentrate (4 mEq/mL) Sodium acetate (2 mEq/mL) Sodium phosphate (4 mEq Na$^+$/mL)	Requirements during parenteral nutrition should not differ from normal fluid therapy requirements unless there is excessive sodium loss. Lactate and bicarbonate salts of sodium should not be used.
Potassium	40–240 mEq	Potassium chloride (2 mEq/mL) Potassium acetate (2 mEq/mL) Potassium phosphate (4.4 mEq K$^+$/mL)	Requirements are related to glucose metabolism and therefore increase with higher concentrations of dextrose infused.
Magnesium	10–45 mEq	Magnesium sulfate (4 mEq/mL)	Requirements increase with anabolism; however, with less variation than does potassium.
Calcium	5–30 mEq	Calcium gluconate 10% (4.5 mEq/10 mL) Calcium chloride 10% (13 mEq/10 mL)	Requirements increase only slightly during parenteral nutrition. Limited amounts of calcium and phosphate, as determined by compatibility references, may be combined in solutions that contain AAs.
ANIONS			
Phosphate	10 mmol/1000 kcal	Potassium phosphate (3 mmol P/mL, Abbott) Sodium phosphate (3 mmol P/mL, Abbott) (other concentrations may vary according to manufacturer)	Requirements increase with anabolism. Safe empirical dosage guidelines should be developed, taking into account the sodium or potassium content of the phosphate solution.
Acetate and Chloride:	The amounts of acetate and chloride contained in each amino acid solution vary (see Table 6–8). Acetate is metabolized to bicarbonate. Bicarbonate salts should not be added to PN solutions because of incompatibility.		

Vitamins

Vitamin requirements for PN have been suggested in a report by an advisory group to the American Medical Association (AMA).[32] Multiple vitamins are available in adult and pediatric formulations for once-daily IV administration (*see* Table 6–10). The usual daily dosage of the adult formulation is 10 mL to provide the amounts of vitamins specified in Table 6–10. The daily dosage of the pediatric formulation for infants who weigh <1 kg is 1.5 mL. For infants weighing 1–3 kg, the daily dosage is 3 mL. For infants and children weighing ≥3 kg up to 11 yr of age, the daily dosage is 5 mL. Vitamin K is included in the pediatric product only. Phytonadione 5 mg may be given to adults weekly in the PN formula, or by IM or SC administration.

TABLE 6–10. IV MULTIVITAMINS

	AMOUNT	
TYPICAL FORMULA	Adult (per vial)	Pediatric (per 5 mL)
Ascorbic Acid (C)	100 mg	80 mg
Vitamin A	3300 IU	2300 IU
Vitamin D	200 IU	400 IU
Vitamin E	10 IU	7 IU
Thiamine (B_1)	3 mg	1.2 mg
Riboflavin (B_2)	3.6 mg	1.4 mg
Niacinamide (B_3)	40 mg	17 mg
Pantothenic Acid (B_5)	15 mg	5 mg
Pyridoxine (B_6)	4 mg	1 mg
Biotin	60 µg	20 µg
Folic Acid	400 µg	140 µg
Cyanocobalamin (B_{12})	5 µg	1 µg
Phytonadione (K)	0	200 µg

Trace Elements

Solutions of individual trace elements are available in several concentrations from various manufacturers. Solutions of multiple trace elements are also commercially available in products containing 2, 3, 4, 5, 6, or 7 elements and in concentrations suitable for adult or pediatric use. Guidelines for the use of trace elements in PN have been reported in an AMA statement[33] and the recommended daily dosages appear in Table 6–11. Although a need for molybdenum and iodine in long-term PN has been described, there are no officially recommended requirements for these elements.[34-36]

TABLE 6–11. SUGGESTED DAILY IV DOSAGE OF TRACE ELEMENTS

TRACE ELEMENT	PEDIATRIC PATIENTS (µG/KG)[a]	STABLE ADULT	ADULT IN ACUTE CATABOLIC STATE[b]	STABLE ADULT WITH INTESTINAL LOSSES[b]
Zinc	400 (preterm)[c] 250 (<3 mo)[d] 100 (>3 mo–1 yr)[d] 50 (>1 yr)[d]	2.5–4 mg	Additional 2 mg	Add 12.2 mg per liter small-bowel fluid lost; 17.1 mg per kg of stool or ileostomy output.[e]
Copper	20	0.5–1.5 mg	—	—
Chromium	0.14–0.2	10–15 µg	—	20 µg[f]
Manganese	1	0.15–0.8 mg	—	—
Selenium	2	20–60 µg	—	—

[a]Limited data are available for infants weighing <1500 g. Their requirements may be more than the recommendations because of their low body reserves and increased requirements for growth.
[b]Frequent monitoring of plasma levels in these patients is essential to provide proper dosage.
[c]Premature infants (weight <1500 g) up to 3 kg of body weight. Thereafter, the recommendations for full-term infants apply.
[d]Full-term infants and children ≤5 years old. Thereafter, the recommendations for adults apply, up to a maximum dosage of 4 mg/day.
[e]Values derived by mathematical fitting of balance data from a 71-patient-week study in 24 patients.
[f]Mean from balance study.
Modified from references 33 and 37.

Iron

Iron deficiency can occur in patients deprived of iron during long-term PN. Although other parenteral sources of iron have been tested, the only commercially available iron product for IV use in the United States at this time is iron dextran. Iron dextran can be added to PN solutions, but the advisability of its routine use as well as its compatibility with fat emulsion is questionable. Dosage recommendations by this route range from 1–12.5 mg/day of iron.[38]

Insulin

Many patients who receive PN become hyperglycemic. When feasible, the cause should be investigated and controlled by means other than insulin before insulin is employed (*see* Table 6–12). Although the efficacy of PN is reportedly enhanced by insulin,[39] it should be used cautiously to avoid hypoglycemia, and also because it promotes deposition of fatty acids in body fat stores, making them less available for important biochemical pathways.[40] When it is required, insulin may be provided separately by SC or IV administration, or added to the PN formula. Until a patient is stabilized on a consistent dosage of insulin, it is more cost-effective to provide insulin separately to avoid wasting of PN formulations that may be discarded if the insulin dosage needs to be changed.[41] Human insulin is the least immunogenic and is therefore the insulin of choice. Guidelines for dosage are empirical; one-half to two-thirds of the previous day's sliding scale requirements may be added as regular human insulin to the daily PN formula. Standardized admixture procedures should be used to minimize variations of insulin activity caused by adsorption loss.

Albumin

Albumin is compatible when admixed with PN formulas; however, its supply is too limited and its cost is too prohibitive for casual use. Although inclusion of albumin in PN is reported to rapidly increase serum albumin levels[42] and enhance tolerance of enteral feedings,[43] the clinical benefits of such treatment are not proved. For synthesis of endogenous protein, albumin is inferior to crystalline amino acids as a parenteral source of nitrogen. If administration of albumin is necessary, it should not be included in the PN formula.

Medications

There may be advantages to the admixture of certain medications such as antibiotics, chemotherapeutic agents, and H_2-receptor antagonists to PN, if there is compatibility reported with all components of the formula. Consult other sources for information regarding the stability and compatibility of medication/PN admixtures.

■ MONITORING THE PATIENT

Metabolic complications known to occur with enteral or parenteral nutrition are summarized in Table 6–12. Most of these can be avoided by proper precautions and close monitoring of the patient. Laboratory parameters for patient monitoring are summarized in Table 6–13.

TABLE 6–12. NUTRITION SUPPORT: METABOLIC COMPLICATIONS AND MANAGEMENT

COMPLICATION	FREQUENT CAUSES	MANAGEMENT
Hyponatremia	Excessive GI or urinary sodium losses, or inadequate sodium intake.	Increase sodium provision.
	Excessive water intake.	Limit free water.
Hypokalemia	Excessive GI or urinary potassium losses; deficit of potassium; or large glucose infusion.	Increase potassium provision.
Hypocalcemia	Insufficient calcium. Magnesium deficit.	Increase calcium provision. Increase magnesium provision.
Hypomagnesemia	Insufficient magnesium; or excessive GI or urinary losses.	Increase magnesium provision.
Hypophosphatemia	Inadequate phosphate.	Increase phosphate provision.

(continued)

TABLE 6–12. NUTRITION SUPPORT:
METABOLIC COMPLICATIONS AND MANAGEMENT (continued)

COMPLICATION	FREQUENT CAUSES	MANAGEMENT
Hypoglycemia	Refeeding syndrome. Abrupt interruption of formula infusion.	Refeed gradually. Begin dextrose infusion and monitor blood glucose and potassium.
Hyperglycemia	Excessive insulin. Deficit of potassium or phosphorus. Insufficient insulin. Corticosteroid use. Sepsis.	Decrease insulin. Increase potassium or phosphate provision. Give insulin. Reduce rate of glucose infusion. Sepsis workup and treatment.
Elevated BUN	Dehydration. Renal dysfunction; or calorie:nitrogen ratio imbalance.	Correct dehydration. Increase nonprotein calorie:nitrogen ratio.
Elevated Liver Function Tests	Underlying disease; lack of GI use; or GI bacterial overgrowth. Essential fatty acid deficiency. Excessive nutrients.	Attempt enteral feeding. Provide lipid. Decrease PN.
Metabolic Acidosis	Excessive GI or urinary losses of base. Inadequate amount of base-producing substance in formula.	Increase acetate provision. Decrease chloride in formula or increase acetate provision.
Osmotic Diuresis	Failure to recognize initial hyperglycemia and increased glucose in urine.	Reduce infusion rate. Give insulin to correct hyperglycemia. Give 5% dextrose and 0.2% or 0.45% NaCl, rather than PN solution to correct dehydration. Continue to monitor blood glucose, sodium, and potassium.
Essential Fatty Acid Deficiency	Insufficient provision of fat during PN.	Provide lipid.

TABLE 6–13. ROUTINE PATIENT MONITORING PARAMETERS

PARAMETER	FREQUENCY*
Urinary glucose and specific gravity.	Every voided specimen until stable, then daily.
Finger stick glucose.	Every 6 hr until stable.
Vital signs, weight, intake and output.	Daily.
Serum glucose, electrolytes, creatinine and BUN.	Daily until stable, then twice weekly.
Magnesium, calcium, and phosphorus.	Daily until stable, then once weekly.
CBC, hemoglobin, WBC, platelets, and prothrombin time.	Baseline, then weekly.
Serum protein, albumin, prealbumin, and liver function tests.	Baseline, then weekly.
Serum cholesterol and triglycerides.	Baseline, then weekly.
Blood ammonia.	Baseline, then weekly in renal and hepatic patients.

*Frequency should be increased in critically ill patients.

■ FUTURE DEVELOPMENTS

Technological advancements in nutrition formulas and the means of preparing, providing, and monitoring their effects on patients continue to be made. These modifications enable safer and more cost-effective nutrition support of patients in the hospital or at home.

Body composition research is presenting innovative approaches to metabolic and nutrition assessment.[44] Formulas with specialized amino acid mixtures continue to be investigated. The benefits of using branched-chain amino acid–enriched formulas are reported for patients with hepatic encephalopathy[45] or hypermetabolism,[46] but remain unproved in terms of morbidity and mortality. Recombinant human growth factors,[47] arginine,[48] and glutamine[49] offer promise for their beneficial influences on protein synthesis rates, immunocompetence, and intestinal mucosal barrier protection, respectively.

In vitro and animal studies report an improvement in tissue protein synthesis and reduction in hypermetabolic response with the enteral use of structured lipids containing medium-chain triglycerides and omega-3 fish oil.[50,51] Because of difficulties reported with the IV use of currently available long-chain triglyceride emulsions, such as hepatic and pulmonary complications and immunosuppression, alternate shorter-chain lipid preparations have been investigated.[52] **MCTs** continue to be explored for IV use as an obligate fuel and as an important component of PN.[53] Animal studies with short-chain triglycerides such as **triacetin** show potential for better protein-sparing properties than MCTs, with less toxicity.[52] Short-chain fatty acids have also been shown to be beneficial in inhibiting small-bowel mucosal atrophy when infused IV or intracolonically.[54]

New insights into the relationship between nutrition and immune function are emerging through advances with recombinant monokines and new discoveries concerning the involvement of **interleukin-1** and **tumor necrosis factor** in energy metabolism.[51,55] Although all of these are promising areas of research, they are not yet considered to be standard therapy in nutrition support.

■ REFERENCES

1. Bistrian BR et al. Cellular immunity in semistarved states in hospitalized adults. *Am J Clin Nutr* 1975;28:1148–55.

2. Albina JE. Nutrition and wound healing. *JPEN* 1994;18:367–76.

3. Elwyn DH. Nutritional requirements of adult surgical patients. *Crit Care Med* 1980;8:9–19.

4. Bistrian BR et al. Protein status of general surgical patients. *JAMA* 1974;230:858–60.

5. Bistrian BR et al. Therapeutic index of nutritional depletion in hospitalized patients. *Surg Gynecol Obstet* 1975;141:512–6.

6. Grant JP et al. Current techniques of nutritional assessment. *Surg Clin North Am* 1981:61:437–63.

7. Blackburn GL et al. Nutritional and metabolic assessment of the hospitalized patient. *JPEN* 1977;1:11–22.

8. Traub SL, ed. *Basic skills in interpreting laboratory data.* Bethesda, MD: American Society of Hospital Pharmacists; 1992.

9. Vanlandingham S et al. Prealbumin: a parameter of visceral protein levels during albumin infusion. *JPEN* 1982;6:230–1.

10. Fletcher JP et al. A comparison of serum transferrin and serum prealbumin as nutritional parameters. *JPEN* 1987;11:144–7.

11. Bistrian BR. Recent advances in parenteral and enteral nutrition: a personal perspective. *JPEN* 1990;14:329–34.

12. Liggett SB, Renfro AD. Energy expenditures of mechanically ventilated nonsurgical patients. *Chest* 1990;98:682–6.

13. Rutten P et al. Determination of optimal hyperalimentation infusion rate. *J Surg Res* 1975;18:477–83.

14. Rees RGP et al. Elemental diet administered nasogastrically without starter regimens to patients with inflammatory bowel disease. *JPEN* 1986;10:258–61.

15. Payne-James JJ, Khawaja HT. First choice for total parenteral nutrition: the peripheral route. *JPEN* 1993;17:468–78.

16. Solomon SM, Kirby DF. The refeeding syndrome: a review. *JPEN* 1990;14:90–7.

17. Food and Drug Administration. Safety alert: hazards of precipitation associated with parenteral nutrition. *Am J Hosp Pharm* 1994;51:1427–8.

18. Barton RG. Nutrition support in critical illness. *Nutr Clin Pract* 1994;9:127–39.

19. Shizgal HM, Forse RA. Protein and calorie requirements with total parenteral nutrition. *Ann Surg* 1980;192:562–9.

20. Barr LH et al. Essential fatty acid deficiency during total parenteral nutrition. *Ann Surg* 1981;193:304–11.

21. Mattox TW, Teasley-Strausburg KM. Overview of biochemical markers used for nutrition support. *DICP* 1991;25:265–71.

22. Roulet M et al. Effects of intravenously infused egg phospholipids on lipid and lipoprotein metabolism in postoperative trauma. *JPEN* 1993;17:107–12.

23. Crowe PJ et al. A new intravenous emulsion containing medium-chain triglyceride: studies of its metabolic effects in the perioperative period compared with a conventional long-chain triglyceride emulsion. *JPEN* 1985;9:720–4.

24. Driscoll DF et al. Practical considerations regarding the use of total nutrient admixtures. *Am J Hosp Pharm* 1986;43:416–9.

25. Pineault M et al. Beneficial effect of coinfusing a lipid emulsion on venous patency. *JPEN* 1989;13:637–40.

26. Hardin TC. Intravenous lipids—depression of the immune function: fact or fantasy? *Hosp Pharm* 1994;29:182,185–6.

27. Humberstone DA et al. Relative importance of amino acid infusion as a means of sparing protein in surgical patients. *JPEN* 1989:13:223–7.

28. Freund H et al. Infusion of branched-chain enriched amino acid solution in patients with hepatic encephalopathy. *Ann Surg* 1982;196:209–20.

29. Freund H et al. Infusion of the branched-chain amino acids in postoperative patients: anticatabolic properties. *Ann Surg* 1979;190:18–23.

30. Cerra FB et al. Branched-chains support postoperative protein synthesis. *Surgery* 1982;92:192–9.

31. Heird WC et al. Pediatric parenteral amino acid mixture in low birth weight infants. *Pediatrics* 1988;81:41–50.

32. American Medical Association Department of Foods and Nutrition. Multivitamin preparations for parenteral use: a statement by the nutrition advisory group. *JPEN* 1979;3:258–62.

33. American Medical Association Department of Foods and Nutrition. Guidelines for essential trace element preparations for parenteral use: a statement by an expert panel. *JAMA* 1979;241:2051–4.
34. Lane HW et al. The effect of selenium supplementation on selenium status of patients receiving chronic total parenteral nutrition. *JPEN* 1987;11:177–82.
35. Abumrad NN et al. Amino acid intolerance during prolonged total parenteral nutrition reversed by molybdate therapy. *Am J Clin Nutr* 1981;34:2551–9.
36. Shils ME, Jacobs DH. Plasma iodide levels and thyroid function studies in long term home TPN patients. *Am J Clin Nutr* 1983;37:731. Abstract.
37. Greene HL et al. Guidelines for the use of vitamins, trace elements, calcium, magnesium, and phosphorus in infants and children receiving total parenteral nutrition: report of the Subcommittee on Pediatric Parenteral Nutrient Requirements from the Committee on Clinical Practice Issues of the American Society for Clinical Nutrition. *Am J Clin Nutr* 1988;48:1324–42.
38. Norton JA et al. Iron supplementation of total parenteral nutrition: a prospective study. *JPEN* 1983;7:457–61.
39. Shizgal HM, Posner B. Insulin and the efficacy of total parenteral nutrition. *Am J Clin Nutr* 1989;50:1355–63.
40. Rothkopf MM et al. Nutritional support in respiratory failure. *Nutr Clin Pract* 1989;4:166–72.
41. Sajbel TA et al. Use of separate insulin infusions with total parenteral nutrition. *JPEN* 1987;11:97–9.
42. Brown RO et al. Response of serum albumin concentrations to albumin supplementation during central total parenteral nutrition. *Clin Pharm* 1987;6:222–6.
43. Andrassy RJ, Durr ED. Albumin: use in nutrition and support. *Nutr Clin Pract* 1988;3:226–9.
44. Heymsfield SB, Matthews D. Body composition: research and clinical advances—1993 ASPEN research workshop. *JPEN* 1994;18:91–103.
45. Alexander WF et al. The usefulness of branched chain amino acids in patients with acute or chronic hepatic encephalopathy. *Am J Gastroenterol* 1989;84:91–6.
46. Teasley KM, Buss RL. Do parenteral nutrition solutions with high concentrations of branched-chain amino acids offer significant benefits to stressed patients? *DICP* 1989;23:411–6.
47. Hatton J et al. Growth factors in nutritional support. *Pharmacotherapy* 1993;13:17–27.
48. Daly JM et al. Immune and metabolic effects of arginine in the surgical patient. *Ann Surg* 1988;208:512–23.
49. Hammarqvist F et al. Addition of glutamine to total parenteral nutrition after elective abdominal surgery spares free glutamine in muscle, counteracts the fall in muscle protein synthesis, and improves nitrogen balance. *Ann Surg* 1989;209:455–61.
50. Teo TC et al. Administration of structured lipid composed of MCT and fish oil reduces net protein catabolism in enterally fed burned rats. *Ann Surg* 1989;210:100–6.
51. Endres S. The effect of dietary supplementation with n-3 polyunsaturated fatty acids on the synthesis of interleukin-1 and tumor necrosis factor by mononuclear cells. *N Engl J Med* 1989;320:265–71.
52. Bailey JW et al. Triacetin: a potential parenteral nutrient. *JPEN* 1991;15:32–6.
53. Mascioli EA et al. Thermogenesis from intravenous medium-chain triglycerides. *JPEN* 1991;15:27–31.
54. Koruda MJ et al. Parenteral nutrition supplemented with short-chain fatty acids: effect on the small-bowel mucosa in normal rats. *Am J Clin Nutr* 1990;51:685–9.
55. Pomposelli JJ et al. Role of biochemical mediators in clinical nutrition and surgical metabolism. *JPEN* 1988;12:212–8.

III
Part
III

APPENDICES

- CONVERSION FACTORS
- ANTHROPOMETRICS
- LABORATORY INDICES

Conversion Factors

■ MICROMOLECULES

SI units (*le Système International d'Unités*) are being introduced in the United States to express clinical laboratory and serum drug concentration data. Instead of employing units of mass (such as micrograms), the SI system uses moles (mol) to represent the amount of a substance. A molar solution contains one mole (the molecular weight of the substance in grams) of the solute in one liter of solution. The following formula is used to convert units of mass to moles (μg/mL to μmol/L or, by substitution of terms, mg/mL to mmol/L, or ng/mL to nmol/L).

Micromoles per Liter (μmol/L)

$$\mu mol/L = \frac{\text{Drug concentration } (\mu g/mL) \times 1000}{\text{Molecular weight of drug } (g/mol)}$$

■ MILLIEQUIVALENTS

An equivalent weight of a substance is that weight which will combine with or replace 1 g of hydrogen; a milliequivalent is 1/1000 of an equivalent weight.

Milliequivalents per Liter (mEq/L)

$$mEq/L = \frac{\text{Weight of salt } (g) \times \text{Valence of ion} \times 1000}{\text{Molecular weight of salt}}$$

$$\text{Weight of salt } (g) = \frac{mEq/L \times \text{Molecular weight of salt}}{\text{Valence of ion} \times 1000}$$

APPROXIMATE MILLIEQUIVALENTS—WEIGHTS OF SELECTED IONS

SALT	MEQ/G SALT	MG SALT/MEQ
Calcium Carbonate [$CaCO_3$]	20.0	50.0
Calcium Chloride [$CaCl_2 \bullet 2H_2O$]	13.6	73.5
Calcium Gluceptate [$Ca(C_7H_{13}O_8)_2$]	4.1	245.2
Calcium Gluconate [$Ca(C_6H_{11}O_7)_2 \bullet H_2O$]	4.5	224.1
Calcium Lactate [$Ca(C_3H_5O_3)_2 \bullet 5H_2O$]	6.5	154.1
Magnesium Gluconate [$Mg(C_6H_{11}O_7)_2 \bullet H_2O$]	4.6	216.3
Magnesium Oxide [MgO]	49.6	20.2
Magnesium Sulfate [$MgSO_4$]	16.6	60.2
Magnesium Sulfate [$MgSO_4 \bullet 7H_2O$]	8.1	123.2
Potassium Acetate [$K(C_2H_3O_2)$]	10.2	98.1
Potassium Chloride [KCl]	13.4	74.6
Potassium Citrate [$K_3(C_6H_5O_7) \bullet H_2O$]	9.2	108.1
Potassium Iodide [KI]	6.0	166.0
Sodium Acetate [$Na(C_2H_3O_2)$]	12.2	82.0
Sodium Acetate [$Na(C_2H_3O_2) \bullet 3H_2O$]	7.3	136.1
Sodium Bicarbonate [$NaHCO_3$]	11.9	84.0
Sodium Chloride [$NaCl$]	17.1	58.4
Sodium Citrate [$Na_3(C_6H_5O_7) \bullet 2H_2O$]	10.2	98.0
Sodium Iodide [NaI]	6.7	149.9
Sodium Lactate [$Na(C_3H_5O_3)$]	8.9	112.1
Zinc Sulfate [$ZnSO_4 \bullet 7H_2O$]	7.0	143.8

VALENCES AND ATOMIC WEIGHTS OF SELECTED IONS

SUBSTANCE	ELECTROLYTE	VALENCE	MOLECULAR WEIGHT
Calcium	Ca^{++}	2	40.1
Chloride	Cl^-	1	35.5
Magnesium	Mg^{++}	2	24.3
Phosphate	$HPO_4^=$ (80%)	1.8	96.0*
(pH = 7.4)	$H_2PO_4^-$ (20%)		
Potassium	K^+	1	39.1
Sodium	Na^+	1	23.0
Sulfate	$SO_4^=$	2	96.0*

*The molecular weight of phosphorus only is 31; that of sulfur only is 32.1.

■ ANION GAP

The anion gap is the concentration of plasma anions not routinely measured by laboratory screening. It is useful in the evaluation of acid-base disorders. The anion gap is greater with increased plasma concentrations of endogenous (eg, phosphate, sulfate, lactate, ketoacids) or exogenous (eg, salicylate, penicillin, ethylene glycol, ethanol, methanol) species. The formulas for calculating the anion gap follow:

$$\text{(A)} \qquad \text{Anion Gap} = (Na^+ + K^+) - (Cl^- + HCO_3^-)$$

or

$$\text{(B)} \qquad \text{Anion Gap} = Na^+ - (Cl^- + HCO_3^-)$$

where
the expected normal value for A is 11–20 mmol/L;
the expected normal value for B is 7–16 mmol/L.*

*Note that there is variation at the upper and lower limits of the normal range.

■ TEMPERATURE

Fahrenheit to Centigrade: $(°F - 32) \times 5/9 = °C$
Centigrade to Fahrenheit: $(°C \times 9/5) + 32 = °F$
Centigrade to Kelvin: $°C + 273 = °K$

■ WEIGHTS AND MEASURES

Metric Weight Equivalents

1 kilogram (kg)	=	1000 grams
1 gram (g)	=	1000 milligrams
1 milligram (mg)	=	0.001 gram
1 microgram (mcg, μg)	=	0.001 milligram
1 nanogram (ng)	=	0.001 microgram
1 picogram (pg)	=	0.001 nanogram
1 femtogram (fg)	=	0.001 picogram

Metric Volume Equivalents

1 liter (L)	=	1000 milliliters
1 deciliter (dL)	=	100 milliliters
1 milliliter (mL)	=	0.001 liter
1 microliter (μL)	=	0.001 milliliter
1 nanoliter (nL)	=	0.001 microliter
1 picoliter (pL)	=	0.001 nanoliter
1 femtoliter (fL)	=	0.001 picoliter

Apothecary Weight Equivalents

1 scruple (℈)	=	20 grains (gr)
60 grains (gr)	=	1 dram (ʒ)
8 drams (ʒ)	=	1 ounce (ℨ)
1 ounce (ℨ)	=	480 grains
12 ounces (ℨ)	=	1 pound (lb)

Apothecary Volume Equivalents

60 minims (♏︎)	=	1 fluidram (fl ʒ)
8 fluidrams (fl ʒ)	=	1 fluid ounce (fl ℨ)
1 fluid ounce (fl ℨ)	=	480 minims
16 fluid ounces (fl ℨ)	=	1 pint (pt)

Avoirdupois Equivalents

1 ounce (oz)	=	437.5 grains
16 ounces (oz)	=	1 pound (lb)

Weight/Volume Equivalents

1 mg/dL	=	10 µg/mL
1 mg/dL	=	1 mg %
1 ppm	=	1 mg/L

Conversion Equivalents

1 gram (g)	=	15.43 grains	0.1 mg	=	1/600 gr
1 grain (gr)	=	64.8 milligrams	0.12 mg	=	1/500 gr
1 ounce (ℨ)	=	31.1 grams	0.15 mg	=	1/400 gr
1 ounce (oz)	=	28.35 grams	0.2 mg	=	1/300 gr
1 pound (lb)	=	453.6 grams	0.3 mg	=	1/200 gr
1 kilogram (kg)	=	2.2 pounds	0.4 mg	=	1/150 gr
1 milliliter (mL)	=	16.23 minims	0.5 mg	=	1/120 gr
1 minim (♏︎)	=	0.06 milliliter	0.6 mg	=	1/100 gr
1 fluid ounce (fl oz)	=	29.57 mL	0.8 mg	=	1/80 gr
1 pint (pt)	=	473.2 mL	1.0 mg	=	1/65 gr

Anthropometrics 2

■ CREATININE CLEARANCE FORMULAS

Formulas for Estimating Creatinine Clearance
in Patients with Stable Renal Function

Adults [Age 18 Years and Older][1]

$$Cl_{cr} \text{ (Males)} = \frac{(140 - \text{Age}) \times \text{(Weight)}}{Cr_s \times 72}$$

$$Cl_{cr} \text{ (Females)} = 0.85 \times \text{Above value*}$$

where

Cl_{cr} = creatinine clearance in mL/min
Cl_s = serum creatinine in mg/dL
Age is in years.
Weight is in kg.

*Some studies suggest that the prediction accuracy of this formula for women is better *without* the correction factor of 0.85.

Children [Age 1–18 Years][2]

where

$$Cl_{cr} = \frac{0.48 \times \text{(Height)} \times \text{(BSA)}}{Cr_s \times 1.73}$$

BSA = body surface area in m^2
Cl_{cr} = creatinine clearance in mL/min
Cr_s = serum creatinine in mg/dL
Height is in cm.

Formula for Estimating Creatinine Clearance from a Measured Urine Collection

$$Cl_{cr} \ (mL/min) = \frac{U \times V \, ^*}{P \times t}$$

where

U = concentration of creatinine in a urine specimen (in same units as P)

V = volume of urine in mL

P = concentration of creatinine in serum at the midpoint of the urine collection period (in same units as U)

t = time of the urine collection period in minutes (eg, 6 hr = 360 min; 24 hr = 1440 min).

*The product of U × V equals the production of creatinine during the collection period and, at steady state, should equal 20–25 mg/kg/day ideal body weight (IBW) in males and 15–20 mg/kg/day IBW in females. If it is less than this, inadequate urine collection may have occurred and Cl_{cr} will be underestimated.

■ IDEAL BODY WEIGHT

Ideal body weight (IBW) is the weight expected for a nonobese person of a given height. The IBW formulas below, as well as various life insurance tables, can be used to estimate IBW. Most dosing methods described in the literature utilize IBW as a method in dosing obese patients.

Adults [Age 18 Years and Older][3]

IBW (Males) = 50 + (2.3 × Height in inches over 5 feet)

IBW (Females) = 45.5 + (2.3 × Height in inches over 5 feet)

where IBW is in kg.

Children [Age 1–18 Years][2]
Children Under 5 Feet Tall:

$$IBW = \frac{(Height^2 \times 1.65)}{1000}$$

where
IBW is in kg
Height is in cm

Children 5 Feet or Taller:

IBW (Males) = 39 + (2.27 × Height in inches over 5 feet)

IBW (Females) = 42.2 + (2.27 × Height in inches over 5 feet)

where IBW is in kg.

■ SURFACE AREA NOMOGRAMS

Nomograms representing the relationship between height, weight, and surface area in infants and adults. To use a nomogram, a ruler is aligned with the height and weight on the two lateral axes. The point at which the center line is intersected gives the corresponding value for surface area.

NOMOGRAM FOR DETERMINATION OF BODY SURFACE AREA FROM HEIGHT AND WEIGHT (INFANTS)[4]

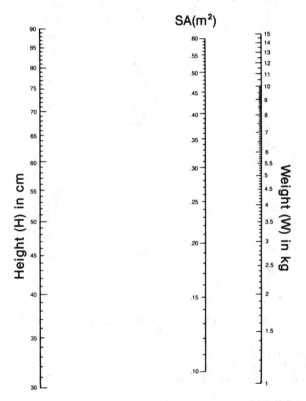

$$SA = W^{0.5378} \times H^{0.3964} \times 0.024265$$

SA(m²)
Height (H) in cm
Weight (W) in kg

Reproduced from reference 4, with permission.

NOMOGRAM FOR DETERMINATION OF BODY SURFACE AREA
FROM HEIGHT AND WEIGHT (ADULTS)[5]

Height	Body surface area	Weight

$$SA = W^{0.425} \times H^{0.725} \times 71.84$$

SA (m^2)

Height (H) in cm

Weight (W) in kg

Reproduced from reference 5, with permission.

■ REFERENCES

1. Cockcroft DW, Gault MH. Prediction of creatinine clearance from serum creatinine. *Nephron* 1976;16:31-41.
2. Traub SL, Johnson CE. Comparison of methods of estimating creatinine clearance in children. *Am J Hosp Pharm* 1980;37:195-201.
3. Devine BJ. Gentamicin therapy. *Drug Intell Clin Pharm* 1974;8:650-5.
4. From Haycock GB et al. Geometric method for measuring body surface area: a height-weight formula validated in infants, children, and adults. *J Pediatr* 1978;93:62-6.
5. DuBois and DuBois. *Arch Intern Med* 1916;17:863.

Laboratory Indices **3**

Blood, Serum, Plasma Chemistry; Urine, Renal Function Tests; Hematology

William G. Troutman

The following table includes typical reference ranges for clinical laboratory tests in common use. Reference ranges for laboratory tests may vary widely among testing facilities, often as a result of methodologic differences. It is therefore always advisable to obtain reference ranges from the laboratory preforming the analyses. Laboratory test results should never be accepted without correct identification of the units of measurement, because most tests can be reported in several systems of measurement. The table presents both conventional and international (usually the same as *Système International,* or SI) units.

The following abbreviations are used to identify the specimen:

(P)	– Plasma
(S)	– Serum
(U)	– Urine
(WB)	– Whole Blood
(WB, art)	– Whole Blood, Arterial

The table begins on page 910.

BLOOD, SERUM, PLASMA CHEMISTRY

TEST/SPECIMEN	AGE GROUP OR OTHER FACTOR	REFERENCE RANGE Conventional	REFERENCE RANGE International Units
Acid Phosphatase (S)		0.11–0.60 units/L	0.11–0.60 units/L
Alanine Aminotransferase (S)		units/L	units/L
(ALT, SGPT)	Adult	8–20	8–20
	>60 yr, M	7–24	7–24
	>60 yr, F	7–16	7–16
Alkaline Phosphatase (S)		units/L	units/L
	Child	20–150	20–150
	Adult	20–70	20–70
	>60 yr	30–75	30–75
Ammonia Nitrogen (S,P)	Adult	15–45 µg/dL	11–32 µmol/L
Amylase (S)		units/L	units/L
	Adult	25–125	25–125
	>70 yr	20–160	20–160
Anion Gap ($Na^+ - [Cl^- + HCO_3^-]$) (P)		7–16 mEq/L	7–16 mmol/L
Aspartate Aminotransferase (S)		units/L	units/L
(AST, SGOT)	Adult	8–20	8–20
	>60 yr, M	11–26	11–26
	>60 yr, F	10–20	10–20
Bicarbonate (S)		mEq/L	mmol/L
	Arterial	21–28	21–28
	Venous	22–29	22–29
(WB, art)	Adult	18–23	18–23
Bilirubin (S)		mg/dL	mmol/L
Total	Child, Adult	0.2–1.0	3.4–17.1
Conjugated (direct)	Child, Adult	0–0.2	0–3.4
Calcium (S)		mg/dL	µmol/L
Ionized	Adult	4.48–4.92	1.12–1.23
Total	Child	8.8–10.8	2.20–2.70
	Adult	8.4–10.2	2.10–2.55
Carbon Dioxide, Partial Pressure (WB, art)		mm Hg	kPa
(pCO₂)	Adult, M	35–48	4.66–6.38
	Adult, F	32–45	4.26–5.99
Chloride (S,P)		98–107 mEq/L	98–107 mmol/L
Cholesterol, Total (S,P)		mg/dL	mmol/L
	Child	120–200	3.11–5.18
	Adolescent	120–210	3.11–5.44
	Adult	140–310	3.63–8.03
	Desired, Adult	140–220	3.63–5.70

(continued)

BLOOD, SERUM, PLASMA CHEMISTRY (continued)

TEST/SPECIMEN	AGE GROUP OR OTHER FACTOR	REFERENCE RANGE	
		Conventional	*International Units*
Cortisol (S,P)		*µg/dL*	*nmol/L*
	08:00 hr	5–23	138–635
	16:00 hr	3–15	83–414
	20:00 hr	≤ 50% of 08:00 hr	≤ 50% of 08:00 hr
Creatine Kinase (CK) (S)		*units/L*	*units/L*
	Adult, M	38–174	38–174
	Adult, F	26–140	26–140
Creatinine (S,P)		*mg/dL*	*µmol/L*
	Child	0.3–0.7	27–62
	Adolescent	0.5–1.0	44–88
	Adult, M	0.7–1.3	62–115
	Adult, F	0.6–1.1	53–97
(γ)-Glutamyltransferase (S) (GGT)		*units/L*	*units/L*
	Adult, M	9–50	9–50
	Adult, F	8–40	8–40
Glucose, 2-hr Postprandial (S)		<120 mg/dL	<6.7 mmol/L

Glucose Tolerance Test (S) (Oral)		*mg/dL*		*mmol/L*	
		Normal	Diabetic	Normal	Diabetic
	Fasting	70–105	>140	3.9–5.8	>7.8
	60 min	120–170	≥200	6.7–9.4	≥11.1
	90 min	100–140	≥200	5.6–7.8	≥11.1
	120 min	70–120	≥140	3.9–6.7	≥7.8

TEST/SPECIMEN	AGE GROUP OR OTHER FACTOR	Conventional	International Units
HDL-Cholesterol (S,P)		*mg/dL*	*mmol/L*
	15–19 yr, M	30–65	0.78–1.68
	15–19 yr, F	30–70	0.78–1.81
	20–29 yr, M	30–70	0.78–1.81
	20–29 yr, F	30–75	0.78–1.94
	30–39 yr, M	30–70	0.78–1.81
	30–39 yr, F	30–80	0.78–2.07
	>40 yr, M	30–70	0.78–1.81
	>40 yr, F	30–85	0.78–2.20
	Values for Blacks 10 mg/dL higher.		
Iron (S)		*µg/dL*	*mmol/L*
	Child	50–120	8.95–21.48
	Adult, M	65–170	11.64–30.43
	Adult, F	50–170	8.95–30.43
Iron Binding Capacity, Total (S) (TIBC)		250–450 µg/dL	44.75–80.55 µmol/L
Isocitrate Dehydrogenase (S)		1.2–7.0 units/L	1.2–7.0 units/L
Lactate Dehydrogenase (S)		*units/L*	*units/L*
	Child	60–170	60–170
	Adult	100–190	100–190
	>60 yr	110–210	110–210

(*continued*)

BLOOD, SERUM, PLASMA CHEMISTRY (continued)

TEST/SPECIMEN	AGE GROUP OR OTHER FACTOR	REFERENCE RANGE Conventional	International Units
Isoenzymes (S)		% of Total	Fraction of Total
	Fraction 1	14–26	0.14–0.26
	Fraction 2	29–39	0.29–0.39
	Fraction 3	20–26	0.20–0.26
	Fraction 4	8–16	0.08–0.16
	Fraction 5	6–16	0.06–0.16
Lead (WB)		µg/dL	µmol/L
	Child	<15	<0.72
	Adult	<30	<1.45
Lipase (S)		units/L	units/L
	Adult	10–150	10–150
	>60 yr	18–180	18–180
β-Lipoprotein (LDL) (S)		28–53% of total lipoproteins.	0.28–0.53
	6–12 yr	1.38–1.74	0.69–0.87
	12–20 yr	1.35–1.77	0.67–0.89
	Adult	1.3–2.1	0.65–1.05
Magnesium (S)		mEq/L	mmol/L
Osmolality (S)		mOsmol/kg	mOsmol/kg
	Child, Adult	275–295	275–295
	>60 yr	280–301	280–301
Osmolal Gap		≤10	≤10
Measured Osmolality − Calculated Osmolality Calculated Osmolality = 2(Na$^+$) + (Glucose/18) + (BUN/2.8)			
Oxygen, Partial Pressure (WB, art) (pO$_2$) (Decreases with age and altitude)		83–108 mm Hg	11.04–14.36 kPa
pH (WB, art)		7.35–7.45	7.35–7.45
Phosphorus, Inorganic (S)		mg/dL	mmol/L
	Child	4.5–5.5	1.45–1.78
	Adult	2.7–4.5	0.87–1.45
	>60 yr, M	2.3–3.7	0.74–1.20
	>60 yr, F	2.8–4.1	0.90–1.32
Potassium (S,P)		mEq/L	mmol/L
	Child	3.4–4.7	3.4–4.7
	Adult	3.5–5.1	3.5–5.1
Protein, Total (S)		g/dL	g/L
	Adult		
	Ambulatory	6.4–8.3	64–83
	Recumbent	6.0–7.8	60–78
	>60 yr	lower by 0.2	lower by 2
Albumin	Adult	3.5–5.0	35–50
	>60 yr	3.7–4.7	37–47
Globulins	Adult	2.3–3.5	23–35

(continued)

BLOOD, SERUM, PLASMA CHEMISTRY (continued)

TEST/SPECIMEN	AGE GROUP OR OTHER FACTOR	REFERENCE RANGE	
		Conventional	International Units
Prealbumin	Adult	10–40 mg/dL	100–400 mg/L
Sodium (S,P)		mEq/L	mmol/L
	Child	138–145	138–145
	Adult	136–146	136–146
Thyroid Stimulating Hormone (S,P)		μunits/mL	munits/L
(TSH)	Child	4.5±3.6	4.5±3.6
	Adult	<10	<10
	>60 yr, M	2–7.3	2–7.3
	>60 yr, F	2–16.8	2–16.8
Thyroxine, Total (S)		μg/dL	nmol/L
(T$_4$)	5–10 yr	6.4–13.3	83–172
	Adult	5–12	65–155
	>60 yr, M	5–10	65–129
	>60 yr, F	5.5–10.5	71–135
	4–9 mo pregnant	6.1–17.6	79–227
Transferrin (S)		mg/dL	g/L
	Adult	220–400	2.20–4.00
	>60 yr	180–380	1.80–3.80

Triglycerides (S)	mg/dL		mmol/L	
	M	F	M	F
12–15 yr	36–138	41–138	0.41–1.56	0.46–1.56
16–19 yr	40–163	40–128	0.45–1.84	0.45–1.45
20–29 yr	44–185	40–128	0.50–2.09	0.45–1.45
30–39 yr	49–284	38–160	0.55–3.21	0.43–1.81
40–49 yr	56–298	44–186	0.63–3.37	0.50–2.10
50–59 yr	62–288	55–247	0.70–3.25	0.62–2.79
Desired, Adult	40–160	35–135	0.45–1.81	0.40–1.53

TEST/SPECIMEN	AGE GROUP OR OTHER FACTOR	Conventional	International Units
Triiodothyronine Resin Uptake (S)		% of Total	Fraction of Total
(T$_3$RU)	Adult	24–34	0.24–0.34
	>60 yr, M	24–32	0.24–0.32
	>60 yr, F	22–32	0.22–0.32
Triiodothyronine, Total (S)		ng/dL	nmol/L
(T$_3$)	10–15 yr	80–210	1.23–3.23
	Adult	120–195	1.85–3.00
	>60 yr, M	105–175	1.62–2.69
	>60 yr, F	108–205	1.66–3.16
Urea Nitrogen (S)		mg/dL	mmol/L urea
(BUN)	Child	5–18	0.8–3.0
	Adult	7–18	1.2–3.0
	>60 yr	8–21	1.3–3.5
Uric Acid (S)		mg/dL	mmol/L
(Uricase Method)	Child	2.0–5.5	0.12–0.32
	Adult, M	3.5–7.2	0.21–0.42

URINE, RENAL FUNCTION TESTS

TEST/SPECIMEN	AGE GROUP OR OTHER FACTOR	REFERENCE RANGE	
		Conventional	International Units
	Adult, F	2.6–6.0	0.15–0.35
Catecholamines, 24-hr (U)		<110 µg	<650 nmol
Creatinine, 24-hr (U)		mg/kg	µmol/kg
	Child	8–22	71–195
	Adolescent	8–30	71–265
	Adult, M	14–26	124–230
	Adult, F	11–20	97–177
	Decreases with age to 10 mg/kg/day at age 90.		
Creatinine Clearance (S, P, and U)		mL/min/1.73 m^2	mL/sec/m^2
	<40 yr, M	97–137	0.93–1.32
	<40 yr, F	88–128	0.85–1.23
	Decreases with age <40 yr.		
Inulin Clearance (S and U)		mL/min/1.73 m^2	mL/sec/m^2
		M　　F	M　　F
	20–29 yr	90–174　84–156	0.87–1.68　0.81–1.50
	30–39 yr	88–168　82–150	0.85–1.62　0.79–1.44
	40–49 yr	78–162　82–146	0.75–1.56　0.79–1.41
	50–59 yr	68–152　66–142	0.65–1.46　0.63–1.37
	60–69 yr	57–137　58–130	0.55–1.32　0.56–1.25
	70–79 yr	42–122　45–121	0.40–1.17　0.43–1.17
	80–89 yr	39–105　39–105	0.38–1.01　0.38–1.01
pH (U)		4.5–8	4.5–8
Protein, Total (U)		1–14 mg/dL	10–140 mg/L
	At Rest	50–80 mg/day	50–80 mg/day
Specific Gravity, Random (U)		1.002–1.030	1.002–1.030
Uric Acid, 24-hr (U)		250–750 mg	1.48–4.43 mmol

HEMATOLOGY

| TEST/SPECIMEN | AGE GROUP OR OTHER FACTOR | REFERENCE RANGE | |
		Conventional	*International Units*
Bleeding time		3–9 min	180–540 sec
Erythrocyte Count (WB)		$\times\ 10^6/\mu L$	$\times\ 10^{12}/L$
	M	4.6–6.2	4.6–6.2
	F	4.2–5.4	4.2–5.4
Erythrocyte Indices (WB)			
Mean Corpuscular Volume		80–96 μm^3	80–96 fL
Mean Corpuscular Hemoglobin		27–31 pg	27–31 pg
Erythrocyte Sedimentation Rate (WB)		*mm/hr*	*mm/hr*
	M	1–13	1–13
	F	1–20	1–20
Fibrinogen (P)		200–400 mg/dL	2.00–4.00 g/L
Hematocrit (WB)		*% Packed RBC Volume*	*Volume Fraction*
	6–12 yr	35–45	0.35–0.45
	12–18 yr, M	37–49	0.37–0.49
	12–18 yr, F	36–46	0.36–0.46
	18–49 yr, M	41–53	0.41–0.53
	18–49 yr, F	36–46	0.36–0.46
Hemoglobin (WB)		*g/dL*	*mmol/L*
	6–12 yr	11.5–15.5	1.78–2.40
	12–18 yr, M	13.0–16.0	2.02–2.48
	12–18 yr, F	12.0–16.0	1.86–2.48
	18–49 yr, M	13.5–17.5	2.09–2.71
	18–49 yr, F	12.0–16.0	1.86–2.48
Hemoglobin A$_{1c}$ (WB)		5.3–7.5% of total Hb	0.053–0.075
Leukocyte Count (WB)		4.5–$11 \times 10^3/\mu L$	4.5–$11 \times 10^9/L$
	Segs	31–71%	31–71%
	Bands	0–12%	0–12%
	Lymphocytes	15–50%	15–50%
	Monocytes	0–12%	0–12%
	Eosinophils	0–5%	0–5%
	Basophils	0–2%	0–2%
Absolute Neutrophil Count (ANC)			
ANC = (% Segst % Bands) × Leukocyte Count			
Partial Thromboplastin Time,			
Activated (WB) (aPTT)		25–37 sec	25–37 sec
Platelets (WB)		150–$440 \times 10^3/\mu L$	0.15–$0.44 \times 10^{12}/L$
Prothrombin Time (WB)		Less than 2 sec deviation from control.	
Reticulocytes (WB)		0.5–1.5% of erythrocytes	0.005–0.015

REFERENCES

1. Burtis CA, Ashwood ER, eds. *Tietz textbook of clinical chemistry,* 2nd ed. Philadelphia: WB Saunders; 1994.
2. Henry JB, ed. *Clinical diagnosis and management by laboratory methods,* 18th ed. Philadelphia: WB Saunders; 1991.
3. Preventing lead poisoning in young children: a statement by the Centers for Disease Control; 4th Rev. ed. Atlanta: Centers for Disease Control: 1991.
4. Système International (SI) units conversion table for common laboratory tests. *Ann Pharmacother* 1995;29:100–7.
5. Tietz NW, ed. *Clinical guide to laboratory tests,* 2nd ed. Philadelphia: WB Saunders; 1990.
6. Wallach J. *Interpretation of diagnostic tests: a synopsis of laboratory medicine,* 5th ed. Boston: Little, Brown; 1992.

Index

Note: Drug classes = small caps; Generic drugs = boldface; (Can) designates Canadian brand names; (BAN) = British approved names; Page numbers in boldface denote drug review monograph.

A

Abbokinase (**urokinase**), **468–469**
Abelcet (**amphotericin B lipid complex**), **54–57**
Abenol (Can), *see* **Acetaminophen**
Acarbose
drug review, **491**
interaction with lab tests, 729, 731
Accolate (**zafirlukast**), **633**
Accupril, 275, 323, *see also* **Quinapril**
Acebutolol
during breastfeeding, 782
comparison chart, 283
dialysis, 821
in lung disease, 282
ACE inhibitors, *see* ANGIOTENSIN-CONVERTING ENZYME INHIBITORS
Acenocoumarol, during breastfeeding, 777
Aceon (**perindopril**), comparison chart, 275
Acetaminophen
blood dyscrasias, 649
during breastfeeding, 776
dialysis, 821
drug review, **7–9**
hepatotoxicity, 659
interaction
drug-drug, 699
with lab tests, 729, 730, 732
with P450 enzymes, 695
nephrotoxicity, 668, 669
during pregnancy, 741

Acetazolamide
during breastfeeding, 783
dialysis, 821
with furosemide, 560
interaction
drug-drug, 699, 721, 722
with lab tests, 729, 731, 732, 733
with loop diuretics, 560
nephrotoxicity, 668
sexual dysfunction, 687
Acetohexamide
comparison chart, 500
drug review, **498–499**
interaction with lab tests, 730, 732
Acetylcysteine, 165
N-Acetylprocainamide
during breastfeeding, 782
dialysis, 826
metabolite of procainamide, 241–242
Acidosis
management of, 859–860
metabolic, 894
ACID-PEPTIC THERAPY, 406–423
Acitretin, during breastfeeding, 789
ACLS (Advanced Cardiac Life Support), 859–863
Acrivastine, comparison chart, 609
Actiprofen (Can), *see* **Ibuprofen**
Activase (**Alteplase**), **458–459**
Activated charcoal, *see* **Charcoal, activated**
Acyclovir
during breastfeeding, 780
dialysis, 821

C

Cadmium, during breastfeeding, 791

Caffeine
during breastfeeding, 790
ergotamine and, 5
interaction
with lab tests, 732
with P450 enzymes, 695
during pregnancy, 758

Calan, 288–290, see also **Verapamil**

Calcitonin, interaction with lab tests, 729

Calcitonin salmon, 526

Calcium, 574–576

Calcium carbonate, comparison chart, 410

CALCIUM-CHANNEL BLOCKERS, see also specific calcium-channel blockers
during breastfeeding, 782
comparison chart, 291–292
drug review, **286–290**
interaction, drug-drug, 706, 707, 708
during pregnancy, 749
sexual dysfunction, 686–687

Calcium chloride, for pulseless electrical activity, 863

Calcium gluceptate, for pulseless electrical activity, 863

Calcium gluconate, for pulseless electrical activity, 863

CALCIUM SALTS
interaction, drug-drug, 714
interaction with lab tests, 729, 731

Caloric requirements, 878

Camptosar (**irinotecan**), 202

Canesten (Can), see **Clotrimazole**

Capoten, **255,** see also **Captopril**

Capreomycin
comparison chart, 71
drug of choice, 42

Captopril
ACE inhibition, 262
blood dyscrasias, 650
during breastfeeding, 782–783
comparison chart, 274
for heart failure, 323

for hypertensive emergencies, 277
dialysis, 822
drug review, **255**
hepatotoxicity, 659
interaction
drug-drug, 699
with lab tests, 733
nephrotoxicity, 668
during pregnancy, 749

Carafate, **419–421,** see also **Sucral-fate**

Carbamazepine
blood dyscrasias, 650
during breastfeeding, 777
clearance, 352
comparison chart, 356
dialysis, 822
drug review, **336–338**
efficacy, 351
elimination with activated charcoal, 444
hepatotoxicity, 660
interaction
drug-drug, 702, 704, 708–709, 723
with lab tests, 729, 731, 732
with P450 enzymes, 696
oculotoxicity, 676
for partial seizures, 354
during pregnancy, 743

CARBAPENEMS, see also specific carbapenems
comparison chart, 104

Carbenicillin, drug of choice, 39, 40, 42

Carbidopa
drug review, **393–395**
interaction, drug-drug, 717, 718
with selegiline, 397

Carbimazole, during breastfeeding, 785

Carbinoxamine, comparison chart, 610

Carbohydrates, in parenteral nutrition formulas, 882–883

Carbolith (Can), see **Lithium**

CARBONIC ANHYDRASE INHIBITORS
interaction with lab tests, 729–730
sexual dysfunction, 687

RenAmin, comparison chart, 887
Renese (**polythiazide**), 565, 687, 783
Rescriptor (**delavirdine**), **79**
Reserpine
  during breastfeeding, 782
  dialysis, 827
  drug review, **273**
  interaction with lab tests, 732
  during pregnancy, 750
  sexual dysfunction, 688
Resol (**oral rehydration solutions**),
    586–588
Resorcinol, urine discoloration, 736
Respiratory acidosis, management
    of, 859–860
RESPIRATORY DEPRESSANTS, interac-
    tion with lab tests, 729
Respiratory drugs
  antiallergics, 600–616
  antihistamines, *see* ANTIHISTA-
      MINES
  bronchodilators, 617–633
  cough and cold preparations,
    638–640
  inhaled corticosteroids, 633–637
Restoril, 386, *see also* **Temazepam**
Reteplase, 466
Retinoic acid, interaction with P450
    enzymes, 695
RETINOIDS
  during breastfeeding, 789
  oculotoxicity, 680
  during pregnancy, 756
Retrovir, **89–91,** *see also* **Zidovu-
    dine**
Rhinalar (Can), *see* **Flunisolide**
Rhinocort (**budesonide**), 635
Rhythmol, **243–244,** *see also*
    Propafenone
Riboflavin, urine discoloration, 736
Rifabutin
  comparison chart, 72
  drug of choice, 43
  drug review, **68–69**
  oculotoxicity, 680
  urine discoloration, 736
Rifadin, **69–70,** *see also* **Rifampin**
Rifampicin (BAN), *see* **Rifampin**
Rifampin
  blood dyscrasias, 654
  during breastfeeding, 779

dialysis, 827
drug of choice, 38, 41, 42, 43
drug review, **69–70**
feces discoloration, 734
interaction
  drug-drug, 704, 706, 708, 712,
    713, 714, 716, 718, 720,
    721
  with lab tests, 729, 730, 731,
    732
  with P450 enzymes, 696
nephrotoxicity, 672
oculotoxicity, 680
during pregnancy, 745
urine discoloration, 736
Rimactane, **69–70,** *see also* **Ri-
    fampin**
Rimantadine
  during breastfeeding, 780
  dialysis, 827
  efficacy, 390
Ringer's solution, lactated
  for anaphylaxis, 856
  for pulseless electrical activity,
    862
Riopan (**magaldrate**), 410
Riopan Plus (**magaldrate**), 410
Riopan Plus Double Strength (**maga-
    ldrate**), 410
Risperdal, **375,** *see also* **Risperi-
    done**
Risperidone
  comparison chart, 377
  drug review, **375**
  feces discoloration, 734
  interaction with P450 enzymes,
    695
Ritodrine, during pregnancy, 757
Ritonavir
  drug review, **86–87**
  interaction with P450 enzymes,
    695, 696
Rivotril (Can), *see* **Clonazepam**
Robidex (Can), *see* **Dextromethor-
    phan**
Robidone (Can), *see* **Hydrocodone**
Robidrine (Can), *see* **Pseu-
    doephedrine**
Robitussin (**guaifenesin**), **639,** 732
Rocephin, 98, *see also* **Ceftriaxone**
Rofact (Can), *see* **Rifampin**